Advances in

Pharmaceutical Biotechnology

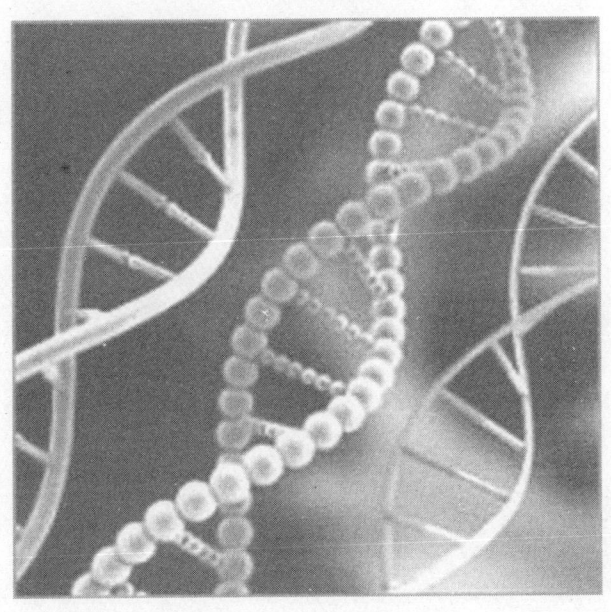

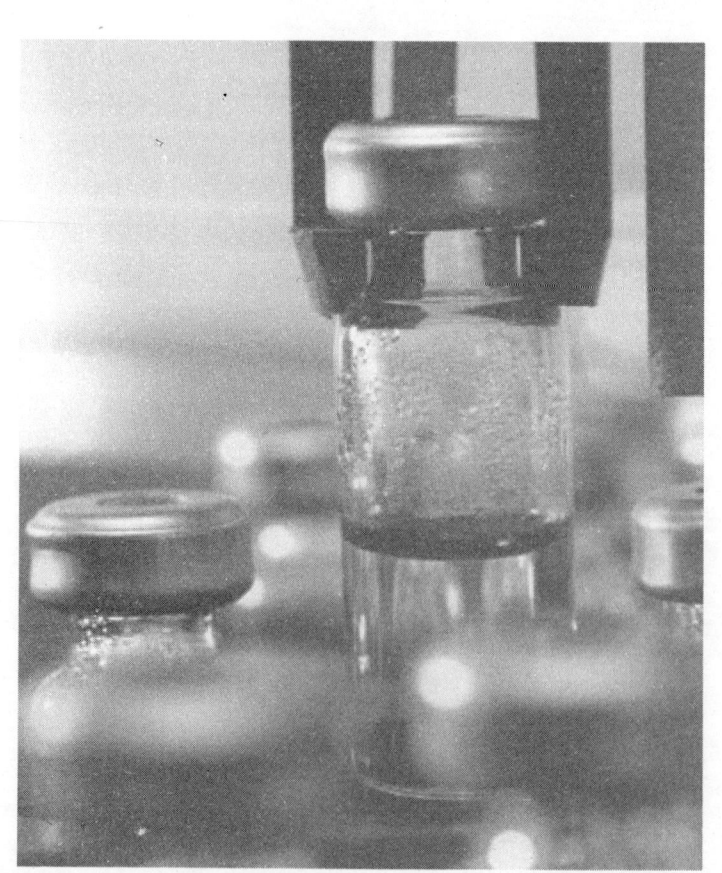

Advances in
Pharmaceutical Biotechnology

Suresh P Vyas PhD Post Doc (London)
Commonwealth Fellow, School of Pharmacy, London
Professor of Pharmaceutical Biotechnology
Department of Pharmaceutical Sciences
Dr HS Gour Vishwavidyalaya, Sagar, MP, India

HD Kumar PhD (London) FASc FNASc FNA
Professor of Biology
Ex-coordinator, Biotechnology Programme
Banaras Hindu University, Varanasi, UP, India

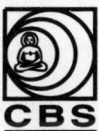

CBS

CBS Publishers & Distributors Pvt Ltd
New Delhi • Bengaluru • Pune • Kochi • Chennai

Advances in
**Pharmaceutical
Biotechnology**

ISBN: 978-81-239-1960-7

First Edition: 2011

Published by Satish Kumar Jain and produced by Vinod K. Jain for

CBS Publishers & Distributors Pvt Ltd

CBS Plaza, 4819/XI, Prahlad Street, 24 Ansari Road, Daryaganj, New Delhi 110 002, India
Website: www.cbspd.com
Ph: 23289259, 23266861/67   Fax: +91-11-23243014   e-mail: delhi@cbspd.com
cbspubs@vsnl.com
cbspubs@airtelmail.in

Branches

- Bengaluru: Seema House 2975, 17th Cross, K.R. Road,
  Banasankari 2nd Stage, Bengaluru 560 070, Karnataka
  Ph: +91-80-26771678/79   Fax: +91-80-26771680   e-mail: bangalore@cbspd.com

- Pune: Bhuruk Prestige, Sr. No. 52/12/2+1+3/2 Narhe, Haveli
  (Near Katraj-Dehu Road Bypass), Pune 411 051, Maharashtra
  Ph: 020-32404169   e-mail: pune@cbspd.com

- Kochi: 36/14 Kalluvilakam, Lissie Hospital Road,
  Kochi 682 018, Kerala
  Ph: +91-484-4059061-65   Fax: +91-484-4059065   e-mail: cochin@cbspd.com

- Chennai: 20, West Park Road, Shenoy Nagar,
  Chennai 600 030, Tamil Nadu
  Ph: +91-44-26260666, 26208620 Fax: +91-44-45530020   e-mail: chennai@cbspd.com

Printed at: India Binding House, Noida, UP

Preface

With the advances in biological sciences and also recognition of pharmaceutical biotechnology as an independent specialization it is thought to be timely and appropriate to introduce the novel concepts and basic aspects of biotechniques with their pharmaceutical applications. The biotech otherwise popularly refers to a multidisciplinary science that seeks to evolve the novel concepts and basic aspects in biosciences which relate to living organisms or their derivatives thereafter to make or modify the process or product(s) apparently beneficial to human use. The present book *Advances in Pharmaceutical Biotechnology* specifically has been a result of continual laborious quest to bring out in true sense a comprehensive introduction on a subject along with the applications and future perspectives so that it becomes a rewarding read to the students who are undertaking undergraduate or postgraduate degree programme in biochemistry, biosciences, biotechnology or related disciplines. It includes a wide spectrum of topics which are invariable components of biotechnology courses irrespective of super specialization. An attempt has been made to introduce the concepts of the subject(s), its progress and present status. It appears as a pertinent need that the applications of such concepts in context to pharmaceutical sciences should be introduced and included. Therefore, chapters are specifically designed and structured so that apart from prescribed course contents they should present additional valuable contents in very simple language to the readers.

The book comprises various chapters on topics of research, pharmaceutical industry and academic relevance. They include prerequisite biotechnology, a comprehensive detail on advents conceptually presented with possible future perspective(s) in clinical practices of therapeutics. Enzymes being of pharmaceutical relevance, their applications have been discussed in detail wherein a chapter exclusively devoted to immobilized enzymes, it elaborates upon the methodology, and applications of immobilized enzymes. Fermentation likewise discusses the fermentation technique, fermentor design and applications in novel pharmaceuticals production. Chapter on plant cell and tissue cell culture introduces the concepts, methods and applications. Similarly, animal cell, tissue and organ culture are dealt in a chapter with concepts, methods and applications. The therapeutic carbohydrates and botanical drugs and biotechnology are discussed in a separate chapter. A relatively new subject that deals with cell replacement, stem cell, cloning and regeneration is also included as a chapter. Of course, recombinant DNA technology is relevant to many allied sciences; it has been dealt in detail covering many of technological aspects with representative examples of its applications. Gene and gene therapy, the principle, vectors, disease and applications are discussed and explained with the help of schemes and diagrams. Other chapters are immunology, vaccines, traditional and new generations, proteins and proteomics, drug discovery, screening and development, immunotechniques as diagnostic tools and delivery approaches for biotechnologicals. Every chapter has a number of schemes and figure(s) to explicitly explain the concept of bioevents involved therein. Hope the contents shall be highly useful and interesting to readers being informative and near absolute in nature. It is believed that the book shall gather faith and wide acceptability by its reader.

The authors are thankful to Mr Neeraj Mishra, Miss Shailja Tiwari, Mr Abhinav Mehta, Mr Rishi Paliwal, Mrs Shivani R Paliwal, Mr Bhuvaneshwar Vaidya, Miss Devyani Dube and Miss Madhu Gupta for their valuable help in the preparation of book and designing of diagrams. We are thankful to our family members, specially Dr (Miss) Sonal Vyas, Dr (Miss) Anchal Vyas, Mr Himanshu Vyas, Mrs Vashundhara Vyas and Mrs Kavita Kumar, for their encouragement and support during the preparation of the typescript of the book. We are also thankful to Prof Pradeep Mehta for reading the proofs of the book. Our sincere thanks are due to Mr Satish Jain, CBS Publishers & Distributors, New Delhi, for his consistent involvement in the preparation and excellent production of the book.

Suresh P Vyas
HD Kumar

Contents

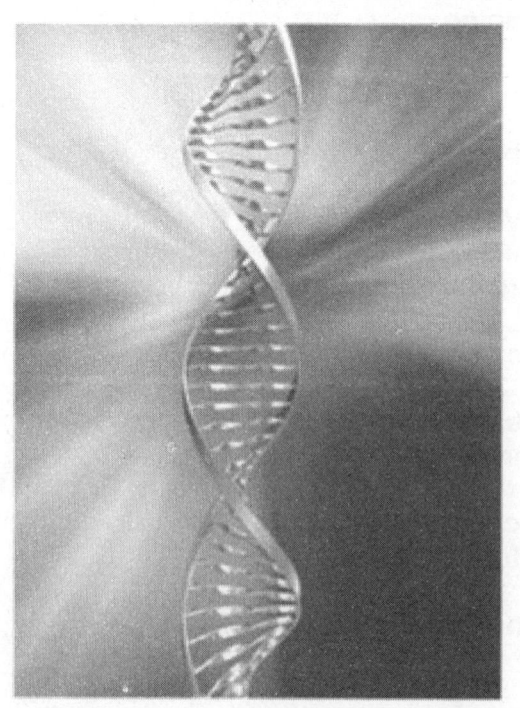

PREREQUISITE BIOTECHNOLOGY

1.1. DEFINITION AND PERSPECTIVES
1.1.1. Scope and importance
1.1.2. Medical biotechnology
1.1.3. Animal biotechnology
1.1.4. Plant biotechnology
1.1.5. Environmental biotechnology
1.1.6. Industrial biotechnology
1.2. MAJOR BREAKTHROUGHS IN MEDICINE
1.2.1. Plant cell fermentations and production of secondary metabolites
1.2.2. Plasmids and formation of secondary metabolites
1.2.3. Cell culture transformation
1.2.4. Role of yeast
1.2.5. Purification of proteins and the disruption of microbial cells
1.2.6. Fine chemicals
1.2.7. Mammalian hormones in microbial cells
1.2.8. Insulin
1.2.9. Enzyme technology
1.2.10. Proteolytic enzymes
1.2.11. Enzyme engineering
1.2.12. Redox catalysts
1.2.13. Semisynthetic antibodies
1.2.14. Cofactor engineering
1.3. GENETIC ENGINEERING
1.3.1. Recombinant DNA technology
1.3.2. Gene transfer
1.3.3. Antisense DNA and RNA
1.4. RESTRICTION FRAGMENT LENGTH POLYMORPHISM (RFLP)
1.5. RANDOM AMPLIFICATION OF POLYMORPHIC DNA (RAPD)

1.6. DNA FINGER PRINTING

1.7. *IN VITRO* AMPLIFICATION OF DNA

1.8. CATALYTIC ANTIBODIES (ABZYMES)

1.9. GENE MACHINE

1.10. DNA HYBRIDIZATION

1.11. DNA FOOTPRINTING

1.12. THE HUMAN GENOME

    1.12.1. From genomics to drugs

    1.12.2. Pharmacogenomics for healthcare

    1.12.3. Stratification

    1.12.4. The changing fortunes of pharmaceutical industry

1.13. MOLECULAR ENGINEERING

    1.13.1. Polymerase chain reaction

    1.13.2. Ominous signs

    1.13.3. The fading great promise

1.14. THE FUTURE OF BIOTECHNOLOGY

1.1. DEFINITION AND PERSPECTIVES

The term Biotechnology is derived from a fusion of biology and technology. It mainly concerns with the exploitation of biological agents or their components for generating useful products. The area covered under biotechnology is very vast and the techniques involved are highly divergent; this has often made a precise definition of subject rather difficult. Some standard definitions of biotechnology are reproduced below with a view to orient the readers to the nature and scope of the discipline.

Biotechnology consists of "the controlled use of biological agents, such as, microorganisms or cellular components, for beneficial use."

Biotechnology is "the integrated use of biochemistry, microbiology and engineering sciences in order to achieve technological application of the capabilities of microorganisms, cultured tissues/cells and parts thereof"

Biotechnology comprises the "controlled and deliberate application of simple biological agents-living or dead, cells or cell components- in technically useful operation, either of productive manufacture or as service operation."

Biotechnology may be defined as "the use of living organisms in systems or processes for the manufacture of useful products; it may involve algae, bacteria, fungi, yeast, cells of higher plants and animals or subsystems of any of these or isolated components from living matter."

It may be seen that the different definitions of biotechnology differ in their approach, content and emphasis. But, two main features, common to all of them, are (1) utilization of biological entities (microorganisms, cells of higher organisms- either living or dead), their components or constituents in such a way that (2) some products or service is generated.

Although biotechnology has ancient roots in agriculture and the brewing industry, the developments of genetic engineering and great advances in bioreactor design and computer-aided process control have given it a new dimension which greatly extends the range of technical possibilities that can revolutionize medical, agricultural, and industrial practices. Many developments in biotechnology, such as those in recombinant DNA monoclonal antibodies (MAbs), and immobilized enzymes, are aimed at producing a better product or process. Limited biological sources of hormones and growth regulators are being increasingly replaced by the use of genetically transformed microbes, thereby increasing the scale of production. Greatly increased or even complete safety of modern vaccines, resulting from the absence of ineffectively inactivated virus, is a strong merit of the genetically engineered antigen.

Following are the developments of biotechnology in chronological order-

Bread with leaven	Prehistoric period
Fermentation of juices to alcoholic beverages	Prehistoric period
Vinegar formation from fermented juices	Prehistoric period
Cultivation of vine	Before 2000 BC
Manufacture of beer in Babylonia and Egypt	3rd century BC
Wine growing promoted by Roman Emperor Marcus Aurelius Probus	3rd century AD
Production of spirits of wine (ethanol)	1150
Vinegar manufacturing industry	14th century
Discovery of the fermentation properties of yeast by Erxleben	1818
Description of lactic acid fermentation by Pasteur	1857
Detection of fermentation enzymes in yeast by Buchner	1897
Discovery of penicillin by Fleming	1928/29
Discovery of many other antibiotics	From about 1945

The essence of many biotechnological processes is the conversion of fairly cheap raw materials into highly valuable products or services (Biotransformation). It appears that the development of efficient processes is a prerequisite for the commercialization of new products or services, and requires a coordinated coupling of unit operations. The role of the process engineer to translate these discoveries into usable processes, on a large scale, is by no means insignificant. This is the area where scientists cooperate with technologists or engineers. This meaningful synthesis is diagrammatically shown in Figure 1.1. In this process, the central place is occupied by the bioreactor, whose successful operation requires adequate upstream processing. Similarly, the recovery of the final product requires a series of steps collectively called *downstream* processing.

The problems of gas liquid and solid handling prior to the use of these materials for bioconversion are important aspects of upstream processing. Over 75% of the world's total fermentation capacity is anaerobic and hence does not require gas compression, the remaining capacity being aerobic generates highly valuable products; for these aerobic processes, gas compression is critical. Other important aspects include air and media sterilization and/or filtration and removal of heat from the bioreactor.

Many of the biotechnology products produced are mainly intracellular proteins. Cells are broken up in pressure homogenizers and high-speed ball mills to release these proteins. Following fermentation, a solid-liquid separation constitutes part of the downstream processing. Centrifugation and filtration are used for separating cells from broth. Membrane filtration technology is important for concentration of protein solutions (Cooney, 1985). Humans have gainfully exploited certain microorganisms in the food and beverage industries for many centuries. Microbial activities and products have already benefited the pharmaceutical and effluent treatment industries.

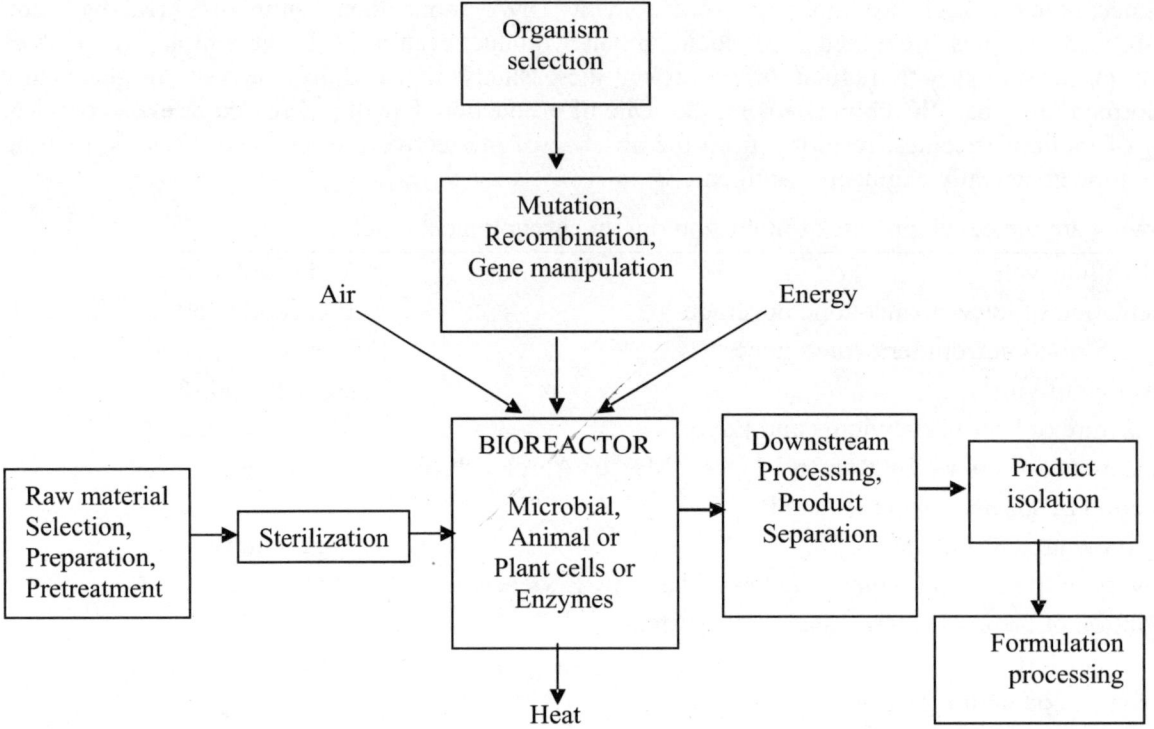

Fig. 1.1: A typical flow chart of any biotechnological process, with reference to the microbe or living cell/system employed

Another exciting possibility for exploiting microbes has been materialized following the development of recombinant DNA technology. Below is an overview of recombinant DNA based biotechnology:

1953 Double helix structure of DNA is first described by Watson and Crick.

1973 Cohen and Boyer develop genetic engineering techniques to "cut and paste" DNA and to amplify the new DNA in bacteria.

1977 The first human protein (somatostatin) is produced in a bacterium (*E. coli*).

1982 The first recombinant protein (human insulin) appears on the market.

1983 Polymerase chain reaction (PCR) technique conceived.

1990 Launch of the Human Genome Project (HGP), an international effort to sequence the human genome.

1995 The first genome sequence of an organism (*Haemophilus influenzae*) is determined.

2000 A first draft of the human genome sequence is completed.

2005 Over 40 million gene sequences are in GenBank, and genomes of hundreds of prokaryotes and dozens of eukaryotes are sequenced or in draft stage.

The potential of various microbes to produce several valuable products has been realized and, in conjunction with DNA manipulations, can enable biotechnologists to tailor microbes that might utilize some cheap substrate or waste material to synthesize a useful and costly end product. The bacterium *E. coli* acts as a suitable host for genetic material derived from other organisms, which are then expressed to produce either valuable proteins, which are excreted, or useful enzymes, which catalyze metabolic reactions to yield new products. Microbes have a valuable repertoire of primary metabolites involved in their anabolism and catabolism. Diverse aerobic microbes are known to oxidize hydrocarbons present in crude oil, using crude or heavy oil as the source of carbon and energy. These microbes produce several metabolites of utility in oil service industry; some examples include surfactants and polysaccharide biopolymers. Genetic manipulation techniques are now being pressed into service to create strains that may aid dewaxing and desulphurization in oil recovery operations, or may prove conducive to the enhanced synthesis of surfactants and biopolymers. The potential of microbial technology for gainful application in the oil service industry is high. Modern biotechnology has played a great role in the development of the health care chemical industries. It has enabled the availability of several diagnostic, prophylactic or therapeutic products. Most of the products in the pharmaceutical industry are typically high potency, low volume, (Table 1.1), and costly materials. These products are commonly made by aerobic submerged cultivation of certain microorganisms.

Table 1.1: Relationship between volume and value of some biotechnological products or activities (modified from Bull *et al.*, 1982)

Products/ Activities	Volume	Value
Methane, ethanol, biomass, animal feed	High	Low
Amino acids, organic acids, baker's yeast, acetone, butanol, polymers, foods	High	Moderate
Antibiotics, enzymes, vitamins, pharmaceuticals	Low	High

1.1.1. Scope and importance

Biotechnology has rapidly emerged as an area of activity that has been substantially realized. It has an impact on virtually all the domains of human welfare ranging from food processing, protecting the environment, to human health. As a result, it now plays a very important role in employment, production and productivity, trade, economics and economy, human health and quality of human life throughout the world. This is clearly reflected in the emergence of numerous biotechnology companies throughout the world. The total volume of trade in biotechnology products is increasing sharply every year, and it is expected to soon become the major contributor to world trade. Some of the important areas, in which biotechnology is making marked contributions, are as follows-

Human health	Agriculture
Medicines	Environment
Animal health	Renewable energy & fuels
Food processing and Beverages	Population control
Dairy	Fisheries and aquaculture

1.1.2. Medical biotechnology

a) Biotechnology has made it possible to produce monoclonal antibodies by Hybridoma Technology for diagnosis of several diseases such as venereal disease, hepatitis B, cancer and some viral diseases.

b) DNA probes, used for the diagnosis of disorders like Kala azar, sleeping sickness and malaria, are produced by Genetically Engineered microbes through Genetic Engineering (genetic manipulation). These manipulations are possible only by the advent of Molecular Biotechnology.

c) Recombinant Vaccines (Human Hepatitis B virus, *E. coli* vaccines for pigs, rabies virus) are produced only by the genetically engineered microbes.

d) Valuable recombinant drugs like human insulin, human interferon, human and bovine growth hormones are also being produced.

e) Huntington's Chorea, Cystic Fibrosis and some other diseases can be cured by **Gene Therapy.** However, cystic fibrosis is a disease whose prophylaxis and diagnosis are still to be sorted out hence it can be treated only in the advanced stages.

f) Various DNA techniques can identify the parents/criminals with the help of DNA/or autoantibody fingerprinting even from blood, semen stains and hair samples.

1.1.3. Animal biotechnology

a) Couples suffering from infertility can have babies by the Test Tube Baby technology, which involves *in vitro* fertilization and embryo transfer techniques.

b) Transgenic animals (mice, pigs, chicken rabbits, fish, and cattle) are produced for increased milk, growth rate, and resistance to diseases and for some valuable proteins in milk/ urine/ blood as well.

c) Superior genotype animals are also produced by hormone induced super ovulation and / or embryo splitting in farm animals, with the help of embryo transfer and *in vitro* fertilization techniques.

1.1.4. Plant biotechnology

a) By meristem culture (for some fruits and forest trees) rapid clonal multiplication rates are achieved as compared to the conventional techniques used.

b) Homozygous lines are isolated rapidly by chromosome doubling of haploid plants with the help of anther culture/inter specific hybridization and ovary culture techniques. Development of some new varieties of rice and wheat is an important breakthrough of Biotechnology and also has a great importance from agriculture point of view as far as food problem of the whole world is concerned.

c) For insect resistance, protection against viruses, herbicide resistance and storage protein development, Gene transfer methods such as Ti plasmid of *Agrobacterium*, Particle Gun, & Free DNA uptake are being used for Genetic Manipulations (Genetic Engineering) and some revolutionary developments in crop improvement have been achieved.

'Bt Cotton' is the best example of a Genetically Modified crop.

1.1.5. Environmental biotechnology

a) *Pseudomonas putida* strain can be used for degradation of petroleum and management of oil spills.

b) Detoxification of wastes and industrial effluents by the use of Biotechnological methodologies in which less useful products or even wastes can be transformed into useful ones.

1.1.6. Industrial biotechnology

a) Useful compounds such as Ethanol, Lactic acid, Glycerine, Citric acid, and Gluconic acid

b) Acetone is produced by microorganisms (mainly bacteria) from less useful substrates in economic and cost effective manner.

c) Antibiotics (Penicillin, Streptomycin and Erythromycin) are produced by fungi, bacteria and actinomycetes as secondary metabolites.

d) Transformation of less useful and cheaper compounds into more useful and valuable ones (steroid hormones from sterols, sorbose from sorbitol) by microorganisms or immobilized enzymes (Fermentation Biotechnology).

e) Enzymes (amylase, protease, lipase etc.) are produced from fungi/bacteria and can also be used in detergent, leather and medicines.

f) Single Cell Protein (SCP), is nothing but the total microbial biomass freed from toxic contaminants, produced from bacteria, yeast, fungi or algae for human food and animal feed.

g) Immobilization of enzymes for their repeated industrial application is more attractive and useful than the use of the whole organism.

h) Protein/enzymes engineering is used to change the primary structure of existing protein/enzymes to make them more efficient, or to change their substrate specificity e.g., T_4 Lysozyme, Trypsin subtilisin, Lactate Dehydrogenase.

This is possible only by the extensive use of computers for the generation of models of the protein molecules. It is hoped to change the RUBISCO (the most abundant protein on earth) so as to minimize its affinity for CO_2.

1) With the help of fermentation technology cheap, less useful and abundant substrate (Sugarcane, bagasse wood etc.) are transformed into more valuable fuels (Ethanol and Biogas).

2) Immunotoxins, produced by joining a natural toxin with a specific antibody, destroy a specific/targeted cell type and may prove to be a potent treatment for cancer (Immunotechnology).

The development of the technology of genetic engineering has transformed the life into a productive, vital force. Biotechnology is expected not only to exert significant effects on human and animal food, energy and chemicals, waste and pollution treatment, veterinary and medical care, and crops and minerals, but also to create entirely new industries in the not too distant future. Many more microbial synthesized mammalian proteins should become available in the next few years. Some medically important proteins that can be produced by biotechnology include interferon, hormones, vaccines, and antibodies. The bacterial cell can be used as a factory to synthesize these and other proteins. Table 1.2 lists some high value proteins in pharmaceutical applications which are being developed by Recombinant DNA Technology.

There is optimism that vaccines or other tools may soon be developed for tackling malaria, trypanosomiasis, leprosy, and cancer. The circumsporozoite gene of the malaria parasite has been cloned. We have a better understanding of the surface glycoproteins of the trypanosome parasite.

The cancer-producing virus (Rous sarcoma virus) was first detected and described over 70 years ago. Many viral oncogenes have counter parts in the genome of the host cell, often being present in the normal genetic complement of man. The *onc* gene products have been biochemically identified and found to be related to some known growth promoting substances. The product of the Rous sarcoma virus *src* gene, designated pp60, is a tyrosine specific protein phosphokinase. The product of the *v-erbB* oncogene human erythroblastosis virus resembles the receptor for epidermal growth factor, a factor already known to be a glycoprotein with an intrinsic tyrosine-specific protein kinase that is stimulated upon binding to the epidermal growth factor. This kind of relationship between growth factors and proteins can help in unraveling some of the black boxes in our understanding of cancer by precisely defining some of the components of the complex systems embracing the cell surface, the cell membrane, the cytoplast and the nucleus. The tools of biotechnology are now available to fill the gaps in our knowledge, and very soon will help find a way to prevent/cure this dreadful disease.

Table 1.2: Some high value proteins for pharmaceutical applications being developed by recombinant DNA technology

Substance(s)	Function(s)
Thymopoietins	Inhibit growth hormone secretion
Somatomedins	Mediate action of growth hormone
Growth hormone release factor	Stimulates pituitary hormone release
Calmodulin	Mediates calcium effects
Calcitonin	Inhibits bone resorption
Parathyroid hormone	Prevents excretion of calcitonin, mobilizes calcium
Luteinizing hormone	In females, induces ovulation; in males, stimulates androgen secretion
Follicle-stimulating hormone	Induces ovarian growth
Relexin	Uterine muscle relaxation
β-Endorphin	Analgesic
Encephalins	Analgesic
Interleukin-2	Promotes growth and activity of T-cells
Factor Thymic	Restores delayed-type hypersensitivity
Thrombopoietins	Inhibit B-cell differentiation

Exciting possibilities have arisen of combining genetic manipulation with fermentation technology. Progress in the culture of plant cells, tissues, and organs has boosted biotechnological applications. One example is the micropropogation of plants, and the second is concerned with the production of special chemicals. Plant micropropogation through tissue culture has made it possible to produce large number of virus-free plants. It is also possible to introduce new, desirable traits into chosen plants by the techniques of selection, protoplast and fusion and somatic cell hybridization. These traits may, *inter alia*, include disease resistance, salt tolerance, enhanced yield, and composition or yield of some natural product.

Tissue culture techniques have found commercial applications in several horticultural plants such as orchids and, in special crops, remarkable success has been achieved with oil palm, jojoba, and citrus. Biotechnology is largely concerned with a gainful exploitation of biocatalysts, which come from microbial, plant, and animal cells. Only a limited number of species have so far been developed as biocatalysts and there is a vast scope for screening many more organisms to select newer, wider range of microbial and cultured cell types for pest control, mineral processing, health care, and food production. Significant advances have occurred in introducing genetic material into plant cells. Advances in recombinant DNA research, molecular genetics, and in blastomere manipulation have likewise brought within reach the technology that can be used to insert genetic material into animal cells.

Functional proteins, or antibodies raised against such proteins, may be injected into living cells. The term microinjection means direct pressure injection of macromolecules into cells through glass micro capillaries or needles. Besides this simple needle microinjection, certain other approaches fall into two broad categories, namely, (1) membrane-vesicle methods, in which preloaded liposomes and protoplasts are fused with cultured cells and release their contents into the cytoplasm; and (2) physical diffusion of macromolecules into cells through holes transiently created in their plasma membranes through $CaCl_2$ treatment (Richardson, 1988). Lipid vesicle-mediated injection is preferred for incorporating membrane proteins into cells and protoplast fusion is advantageous for protein engineering (*vide infra*).

Antibiotics (Fig.1.2) and proteins where there is no practical alternative, where microbes can execute a number of sequential reactions, and where microbial processes give fairly high yields. The advantages of a bioprocess over conventional chemical processes are the milder reaction conditions, use of renewable resources such as biomass as raw materials for producing high-value chemicals, and less hazardous operations. Some disadvantages associated with bioprocesses relate to the frequent generation of complex product mixtures necessitating tedious separations and purifications, problems arising from the relatively dilute aqueous environments in which bioprocesses operate, prone to susceptibility of most bioprocesses to contamination by foreign organisms, and inbuilt variability of bioprocesses arising from genetic heterogeneity and raw material variability.

Biotechnology has significantly impacted clinical medicine. The cellular and molecular cloning techniques used to develop monoclonal antibodies and DNA probes have been applied in clinical medicine. Some notable developments can be broadly considered under the following four categories-

1. *Improved diagnostic tools* Monoclonal antibody kits; kits for nucleic acid hybridization (e.g., *Chlamydia trachomatis);* fluorescent and luminescent labeling of reagents.

2. *Improved laboratory techniques* Isolation and purification of antigens by monoclonal antibody methods; large-scale production of protein antigens *via* hybridomas or by cloning (e.g., herpes simplex and hepatitis B viruses); incorporation of several foreign antigens in vaccinia virus; and protein engineering for antigen design (e.g., rabies and polio).

3. *Immunological therapeutic methods* Monoclonal antibodies either for passive immunization or drug targeting.

4. *Novel vaccines* Polysaccharide-based vaccines; pneumonia infections caused by *Streptococcus* Q and *Haemophilus influenzae;* genetically attenuated or self-destructing live vaccines (typhoid, hepatitis A, and diarrhoea).

Monoclonal antibodies have greatly aided tumor diagnostics, and have also been used as probes in diagnosis of infectious diseases. DNA probes have likewise proved useful in the study and diagnosis of genetic diseases. In fact, the monoclonal antibody is a refined tool *par excellence* in the field of clinical diagnosis. The ability to study individual antigenic sites on a virus, bacterium, or parasite is sure to find application in diagnosis and in basic research. The characterization of tumor cell lines using monoclonal antibodies facilitates diagnosis. The usage of appropriate labeling methods permits easier detection and localization of tumors.

Various kinds of infectious diseases are a major cause of human mortality in several developing countries Poverty, malnutrition, starvation, and contaminated water and food all contribute to the spread of pathogens and the only economical means of preventing most infectious diseases is immunization. Biotechnology plays a major role in developing effective, cheaper, and safer vaccines that are needed for the effective immunization programmes. Rabies, dengue, encephalitis, bacterial respiratory diseases, bacterial enteric diseases, chlamydial infections, malaria, and leishmaniasis are some of the high priority human diseases against which potent vaccines are urgently needed. Research is being undertaken in several countries with the objectives of identifying and characterizing immunogenic antigens, synthesizing and producing these antigens, exploring biotechnological strategies, and formulating suitable vaccines. For animals and humans, the four diseases that deserve immediate attention are neonatal diarrhoea, bacterial respiratory diseases, African swine fever, and hemotypic diseases such as babysinosis and anaplasmosis.

Keeping above in view, research is aimed at isolation, characterization, and production of protective antigens using biotechnological techniques. In addition to the foregoing diseases of humans and animals, mycobacterial tuberculosis affects both humans and animals all over the world. It would be desirable to direct research towards (1) the development of improved diagnostic tools to distinguish in humans the BCG (Bacille Calmette Guerin) vaccine reactions from those resulting from infection; (2) improved production of TB-specific antigens; (3) proper evaluation of the potency of the BCG vaccine currently in use; and (4) production of a more effective vaccine, including bio- or organic synthesis of the immunogen, that can be used in areas of high incidence.

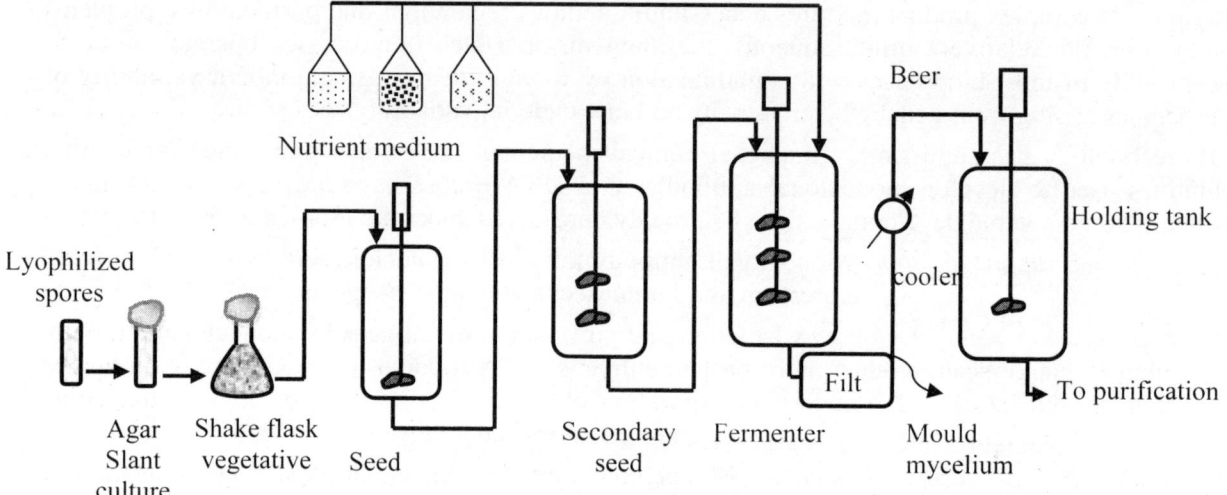

Fig. 1.2: Diagrammatic illustration of the stages in industrial antibiotic production

1.2. MAJOR BREAKTHROUGHS IN MEDICINE

Friedman and Friedland (1999) achieved the feat of whittling a long list of various discoveries in medicine to the ten greatest discoveries. These are narrated as below-

1. Dislodged anatomical errors (Andreas Vesalius)

2. The description of the proper blood circulation (William Harvey)

3. Animalcule observation in organismic and other fluids (Antony van   Leeuwenhoek)

4. Discovery of the rabies vaccine (Louis Pasteur)

5. Tubercle bacillus (Robert Koch)

6. X-Rays invention and application of Crookes tube to medicine (Roentgen)

7. *In vitro* cell based science (Ross Harrison)

8. Molecular structure (Double helical) of DNA (Watson and Crick)

9. Antibiotic production by *Penicillium* species (Fleming)

10. DNA as a genetic material in double helical form (Maurice Wilkins)

Some of the major breakthroughs in medicine in the past few decades, as listed by the Physicians Committee for Responsible Medicine, a Washington DC-based non-profit organization that promotes preventive medicine through innovative programmes and encourages higher standards for ethics and effectiveness in research, are given below:

1. Discovery of the relationship between: (i) cholesterol and heart disease; (ii) smoking and cancer; and nutrition and cancer; (iii) hypertension and smoke.

2. Discovery of the causes of trauma and the measures to prevent it.

3. Elucidation of the causes of many forms of respiratory disease.

4. Isolation of the AIDS virus and discovery of the mechanism of AIDS transmission.

5. Discovery of penicillin and its curative effect on many infectious diseases.

6. Development of X-rays.

7. Discovery of anti-depressant and anti-psychotic drugs.

8. Development of vaccine against yellow fever.

9. Discovery of the relationship between chemical exposures and birth defects.

10. Discovery of human blood groups.

11. Development of hormonal treatments of prostate and breast cancer.

12. Discovery of the chemical and physiological visual process in the eye.

13. Understanding of cholesterol bio-chemistry and familial hypercholesterolemia; and

14. Production of humulin, a synthetic copy of human insulin, which causes few allergic reactions. Humulin is widely available and is the product of choice for insulin-dependent diabetics.

1.2.1. Plant cell fermentations and production of secondary metabolites

Plants have served as valuable sources of diverse phytochemicals used in pharmacy, medicine, and industry. Recent advances in *in vitro* culture of plant cells have raised the question as to what extent the potential of plant cell culture can be used for exploitation of the plant kingdom as a source of important chemicals. The superiority of the culture system over the natural product synthesis rests on the following premises:

1. More consistent quality and yield of product;

2. Relative independence from environmental, geographical, climatic, and seasonal constraints; and

3. Controlled production systems and schedules. This results in a closer control over marketing and such other factors.

Some of the bioreactors, which have been used for the growth of plant cells, are as follows [the figures within parentheses denote volume in litres:

Nicotiana	bubble columns (65); stirred tanks (65); stainless steel (500)
Daucus	stirred tanks (75); stainless steel (15)
Catharanthus	airlift loop glass reactor (100)
Cohus	stirred tank (30)

By far the most important secondary metabolites of plants are those found in medicinal plants (secondary metabolites are usually defined as those constituents of cells which are not essential for their survival). In this context, six of the most important genera which yield frequently prescribed medicinal agents are *Dioscorea, Papaver, Atropa, Rauvolfia, Digitalis,* and *Cinchona*. Plants produce several alkaloids of pharmaceutical importance. Some of these are listed in Table 1.3.

These and some other exceptions apart, however, it is a general observation that cell suspension cultures tend to produce secondary metabolites in much lower quantities than whole plant and, furthermore, the chemicals produced are also quite often structurally different: from those of the intact plant. As a general rule, callus cultures accumulate higher levels of secondary products than cell suspension cultures. Plants form a variety of secondary compounds by biosynthetic transformations of their primary metabolites. These secondary metabolites include terpenoids, glycosides (steroids, phenolics), and alkaloids. The secondary substances usually originate in cell organelles, and are sometimes sequestered into the cytoplasm. They are either deposited in vacuoles or are excreted from gland cells. In general, dividing cells produce few, if any, secondary metabolites and hence, plant cell suspension cultures are not their good sources. However, there are some suspension cultures (Table 1.4), which do produce appreciable quantities.

Hormones exert a profound effect on the formation and release of secondary metabolites. The effect, however, depends on the relative proportions of various growth regulators, as is well known for differentiation of shoots/roots. Thus, relatively higher concentrations of 2,4-D inhibit polyphenol accumulation in rose and *Cassia* cultures, and of nicotine in tobacco. Cultured cell lines (callus cultures) of *Catharanthus roseus* produce and accumulate indole alkaloids such as corynanthe, strychnos, aspidosperma and, rarely, also catharanthine. Until recently, many valuable compounds have been either chemically synthesized or extracted from entire plants. It is now known that the potency of most plant cells to produce these compounds (secondary metabolites) remains intact when the cells are cultured in suspension. Recent research has shown the feasibility of using an airlift loop reactor as a suitable reactor for the biotechnological production of secondary metabolites from immobilized plant cells. Two advantages of this kind of reactor are (1) absence of mechanical agitation (as most cells are sensitive to shearing forces, agitation inhibits the production yields); and (2) efficient oxygen mass transfer (as oxygen is toxic at high concentrations, a suitable level is to be maintained). Immobilization of plant cells protects the cells against the damage caused by shearing and also induces a stress state, which is desirable for optimum production of secondary metabolites. The method of choice for immobilization of plant cells is their entrapment in a gel matrix. Calcium alginate, carrageenan, agarose, and chitosan are some good matrices for this purpose.

Plant cell cultures are being increasingly used for producing valuable products by biotransformation from low-cost precursors. Biotransformation of cardenolides is pharmaceutically significant because their glycosides are widely prescribed for heart diseases (*Digitalis* produces digitoxin arid digoxin). Undifferentiated cell cultures of *D. lanata* do not synthesize perceptible amounts of the medically important glycosides, but the addition of the derivative methyldigitoxin to the culture suspensions induces them to convert this derivative into the medically important methyldigoxin. Roots *of Lithospermurn erythrorhizon* yield shikonin derivatives, which are widely used as dyestuffs and medicine for wounds. The shikonin content of different cell lines of this plant varies from 17% to 23%. Table 1.5 lists some of these cases. Alkaloids, steroids, terpenoids, and other secondary metabolites are usually obtained from plants grown under tropical conditions. The advent of plant tissue culture technology in recent years has kindled the hope that commercially important colourings, flavours, fragrances and pharmaceutical products may now be obtained from plant tissue cultures, which are raised under controlled conditions.

Apart from the composition of the basal culture medium, the concentrations of auxins and cytokinins, which are added to the basal media, affect the growth and differentiation of the culture and also trigger the biosynthesis of secondary compounds. In tobacco tissue cultures, exogenous provision of 2,4-D, IAA or NAA increases the production of scopoletin, and in callus of *Panax ginseng*, 2, 4-D increases saponin production. Whereas high levels of auxins stimulate increased production of indole alkaloids in tissue cultures of *Cinchona ledgeriana*, low level of 2, 4-D tends to increase total phenols in cultures of *Digitalis purpurea* and tobacco. Reduced Levels of NAA or 2, 4-D markedly increases nicotine production in tobacco cultures.

Table 1.3: Some pharmaceutically important alkaloids obtained from plants

Alkaloid	Activity
Atropine	Blocking of cholinergic
Berberine	Antibacterial
Cocaine	Anaesthetic
Codeine	Sedative
Colchicine	Anti-inflammatory
Quinine	Antimalarial
Camptothecin	Anticancer
Theophylline	Bronchodilator
Reserpine	Hypotensive
Morphine	Analgesic
Noscapine	Antitussive
Tubucuranine	Muscle relaxant
Nicotine	Ganglion blocker
Emetine	Antiamoebic
Ajmaline (serpentine)	Antiarrythmic
Digoxine	Cardiac stimulant
Diosgenin	Steroidal
Vinblastine	Antileukaemic

Table 1.4: Some natural substances produced by plant cell suspension cultures

Plant	Product(s)
Nicotiana tabacum	Alkaloids, anthocyanins, phosphodiesterase, quinines
Datura stramonium	Alkaloids
*Vinca minor**	Alkaloids
*Catharanthus roseus**	Alkaloids, coccidiostatic compounds
Ruta graveolens	Alkaloids, furanocoumarins
Phytolacca americana	Betalains, antibiotics, antiviral agents, phosphodiesterase
Panax ginseng	Saponins
Digitalis purpurea	Cardiac glycosides
Daucus carota	Carotenoids, phosphodiesterase
Saccharum officinarum	Amylases
Triticum aestivum	Glucanases

Table 1.5: Some cell cultures, which accumulate alkaloids at levels higher than the mother plant

Plant	Alkaloid(s)	Yield	(% Dry weight)
		Cell culture	Whole plant
Ephedra	Pseudoephedrine	02.25	00.60
Nicotiana	Nicotine	03.40	02.50
Macleaya	Protopine	09.40	00.32
Stephania	Biscoclaurines	02.29	00.92
Catharanthus	Ajmalicine, serpentine	01.30	00.26
Ailanthus	Canthin-6-ones	01.27	00.01
Berberis	Jatrorrhizine	10.00	02.00

1.2.2. Plasmids and formation of secondary metabolites

Plasmids confer drug resistance, fertility, and toxin production in several bacteria. They also determine many other lesser-known properties both in prokaryotes and eukaryotes. In *Streptomyces,* genes located on plasmids determine the traits of aerial hyphae, fertility, enzymes, and antibiotics. In *S. glaucescens*, plasmid genes control melanin formation. In some species of *Streptomyces,* plasmid-borne genes determine antibiotic resistance. Some plasmids are economically valuable, e.g., those related to biodegradation of organic compounds in *Pseudomonas.* Sometimes several hydrocarbon-degrading plasmids can be maintained together in a single bacterial strain. Some eukaryotes, e.g., *Saccharomyces cerevisiae,* also harbour plasmids.

1.2.3. Cell culture transformation

Mammalian cell culture transformation systems make it possible to conduct short-term-tests for potential carcinogens, because such systems could conceivably mimic the process of neoplastic transformation *in vivo.* In. these systems, morphological transformation is the endpoint usually scored; with fibroblast cultures, this means piling up of cells in a crisscross pattern, representing some loss of growth inhibition and cell-cell orientation at confluency. Subsequent passages of the transformed cells can lead to the acquisition of other traits associated with the malignant condition; this includes the ability to grow in a semisolid medium, and also to produce tumours in immune-suppressed animals. Several workers have observed a high correlation between the known carcinogenicity *in vivo* of a given agent and its capacity to produce transformation in mammalian systems. Several assays have been developed for the screening of suspected carcinogens. Some non-epithelial cell cultures that have proved useful in studying chemical transformation are primary and secondary embryo cultures (for example, of Syrian hamster, guinea pig, and rat or mouse infected with adenovirus or murine leukaemia virus) and Fibroblast-like cell lines (including mouse prostate and hamster kidney). It should, however, be noted that no single *in vitro* transformation system is really adequate to test different types of agents suspected to be carcinogenic. It is possible now to induce the fusion of different types of animal cells to form hybrids, which have diverse applications in biotechnology. Studies on the control of gene expression and differentiation, gene mapping, malignancy, viral replication, and antibody production have greatly benefited from experimental cell fusions. Myoblasts fuse spontaneously, forming multinucleate muscle fibers. Macrophages furnish another example, as they are phagocytic, fusing around foreign bodies or bacterial cells in the tissues that are too big to be engulfed by single cells. Bone cells are also known to fuse. Viruses can induce cells growing in culture to fuse. Nucleated cells of different types sometimes fuse into a single cell, called heterokaryon. If the nuclei of a heterokaryon undergo synchronous mitotic divisions, uninucleate hybrid cells are formed. Hybrid cells from mixed cultures of two different mouse cell lines were successfully produced in the 1960s in France. By now, cells from widely different taxa can sometimes be fused. Sendai virus is the agent of choice to induce such fusions. The essence of cell fusion is that it imposes a kind of artificial sexuality on otherwise somatic cells, thereby facilitating genetic analysis of somatic cells. The fact that cells coming from taxonomically remote animals can be fused, suggests that there may not be any basic incompatibility between the membranes, nuclei, or other organelles of these different cells, Thus, there appears to be no rejection mechanism operating at the intracellular level analogous to the immunological rejection mechanism working at the tissue level in whole animals. Figure 1.3 illustrates the process of cell fusion induced by Sendai virus. A heterokaryon is produced first and may then divide synchronously to give uninucleate hybrid cells.

Polyethylene glycol and certain other chemicals can also induce fusions of cells. Quite often, removal of surface carbohydrates is a necessary prerequisite for fusion. Successful fusions have been achieved between cells in different phases of the cell cycle (e.g., in HeLa cells) mid also between mitotic and interphase cells.

1.2.4. Role of yeast

Nutritional supplements, enzymes, nucleotides, proteins, and carbohydrates are some of the derived products obtained from a variety of yeasts. The most popular and best-known yeast is the baker's yeast, *Saccharomyces cerevisiae.* This yeast is used for brewing beer, making bread, making wine, ethanol, cider, and distilled beverages. *S. carlsbergensis* is mostly used for brewing beer. Sparkling wines are made through *S. bayenus. S. lactis* yields lactase whereas nucleic acids are obtained from *Candida utilis.* Some important feed yeasts are *S cerevisiae, Kluyveromyces fragilis, Candida utilis, C. tropicalis,* and *C. pseudotropicalis.*

One opening of the hollow fibre is attached to the fresh medium reservoir and the other is used for harvesting of spent medium. Both pumps are switched alternately from a minimum-maximum level controller. A 3-way valve is used to recycle the initial small volume of fresh medium remaining in the hollow fibre, back to the reactor vessel. Yeast has been increasingly used in genetic studies and much information of great value in biotechnology has accumulated that is of great value in biotechnology. *Saccharomyces cerevisiae* grows rapidly in simple defined media, is well amenable to genetic analysis, and can serve as a recipient of genes from several sources. However, it does not have any natural viral vectors that could be used in introducing foreign DNA into its cells.

Recent work on genetic transformation in yeast has ushered in the era of molecular cloning of DNA either from yeast itself or from other sources, and has permitted incorporation of this DNA into yeast cells for studies on gene expression. Now we have a wide choice of gene vectors for yeast. Mutant lines of yeast are incubated with purified DNA from a suitable vector carrying the wild-type gene whereupon some of the DNA enters the yeast cells and often expresses itself, thereby transforming the yeast. The transformed clones are selected for further use. In the foregoing process, usually the *E. coli*-derived plasmid pBR322 is employed as a vector. This or its derivatives can be grown in *E. coli* to several thousand copies. The isolated DNA from the plasmid is returned to the yeast cell and this can be followed because the vector also has a marker gene for some selectable trait such as requirement for leucine or uracil. The vectors used in this method serve as shuttle cloning vectors as they can grow both in *E. coli* and yeast. Restriction fragments of yeast DNA are inserted into the vector by ligation. Transforming *E. coli* for antibiotic resistance amplifies the ligation mixture. Yeast cell-DNA mixture is treated with polyethylene glycol (PEG) and calcium chloride, followed by plating the suspension under selective conditions where only the transformed cells form clones. Several genes have been cloned in this manner.

1.2.5. Purification of proteins and the disruption of microbial cells

Intracellular proteins with catalytic or biological activity are of growing importance for developments in enzyme technology, as well as for the production of mammalian proteins by recombinant DNA technology. The release of these proteins from microorganisms is an important unit operation, as it is the first step in their isolation. Microorganisms can be performed by a variety of established methods based on chemical, enzymatic, physical, or mechanical principles.

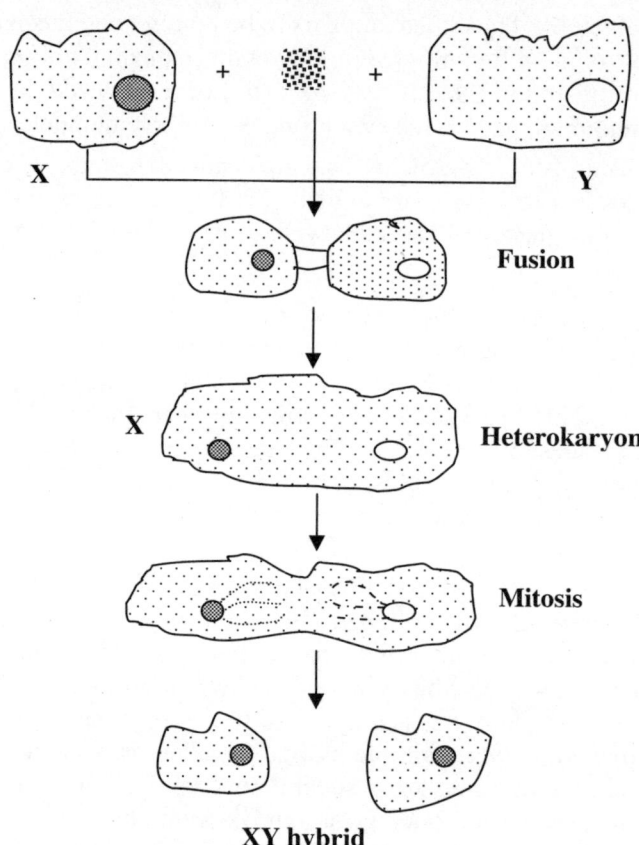

Fig. 1.3: Diagrammatic sketch of cell fusion induced by *Sendai virus*, resulting in the production of hybrid cells

Different methods can be employed to solubilize intracellular proteins, depending on the localization within the cell and the intended use of the compound of interest.

In biotechnological processes, cells are relatively expensive raw materials. Therefore, complete disintegration of the biomass is desired with high product and activity yields. Biologically active proteins usually withstand only moderate temperatures and pH values and are the target of proteolytic enzymes liberated from the same cell, which limits process conditions and process time. A selective liberation of enzymes from the periplasmic space may be achieved by treatment with water miscible solvents such as alcohol or acetone. Mechanical methods of cell disintegration are currently preferred for large scale. Two general approaches are used: high-pressure homogenization or wet milling in high-speed agitator bead mills.

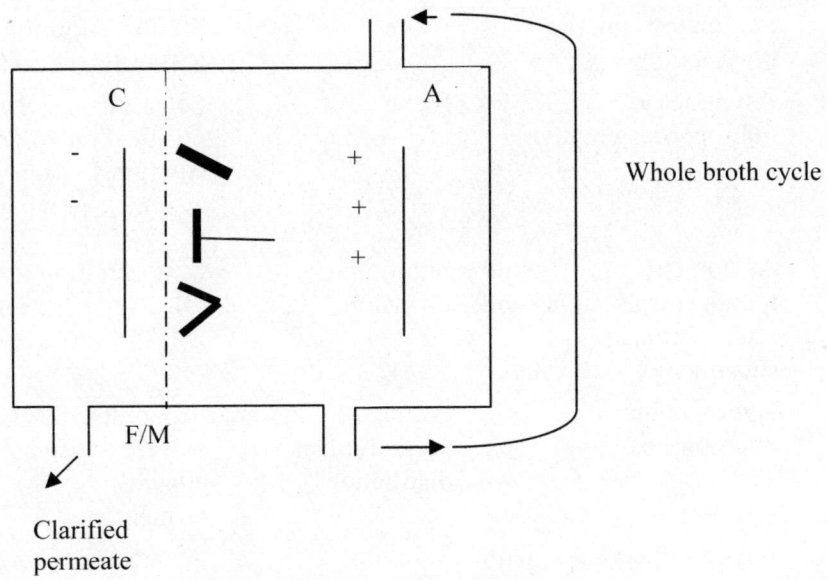

Fig. 1.4: Electrophoretically assisted cross-flow filtration (F/M, filter membrane; A, anode; C, cathode; F, electrophoretic force)

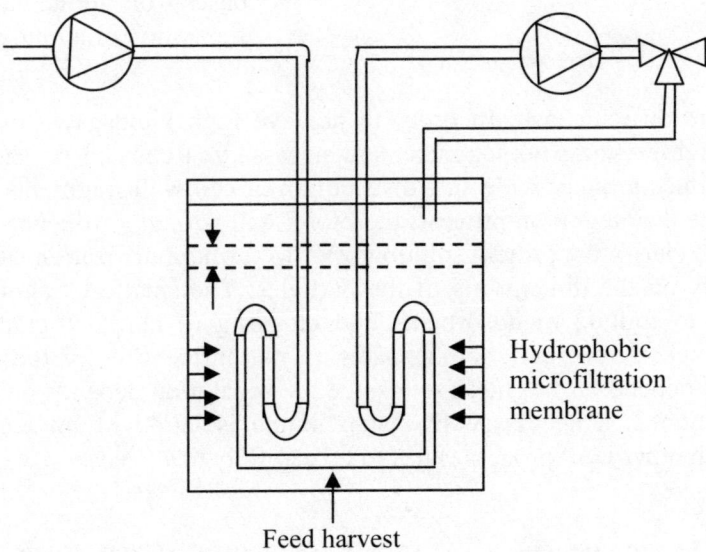

Fig. 1.5: Microfiltration membrane in stirred tank reactor

Table 1.6: Some membrane processes used in modern biotechnology

Process	Membrane type	Mass separation mechanism	Application
Microfiltration	Symmetric microporous polymeric	Sieve	Sterile filtration, clarification, harvesting of bacterial cells
Ultrafiltration	Asymmetric microporous polymeric	Sieve	Separation, concentration, and purification of macromolecular solutions such as proteins, enzymes, polypeptides
Reverse osmosis	Asymmetric, with homogeneous skin and microporous substructure	Solution diffusion	Concentration of solutes, e.g., salts, sugars, amino acids
Distillation	Hydrophobic, microporous	Partial vapour pressure, as in distillation	Separation of volatile organic solvents e.g., acetone, and ethanol from aqueous fermentation
Pervaporation	Asymmetric, with homogeneous skin and microporous substructure	Solution diffusion	Separation of organic solutions such as ethanol, butanol, and acetic acid from aqueous solution
Electrodialysis	Cation- and anion-exchange	Electric charge	Removing salts, acids, and bases from fermentation broths; separation of amino acids

Disintegration is a quite difficult task. In order to achieve high yields, two or three passages through the mill or the high-pressure homogenizer are necessary. Repeated passages through the disintegration machine produce a rather wide size distribution of cell wall fragments, extending well into the colloidal range. The disintegration process, therefore, will strongly influence any solid/liquid separation step necessary to clarify the protein solution prior to further purification steps. Solid/liquid separation depends strongly on the dimensions of the particles. The smallest fragments have to be removed, since they lead to fouling of adsorbents and clogging of chromatographic column. In contrast, extraction of proteins from cell homogenates is not influenced by the method of cell disintegration and does not depend on fragment size since the separation depends on thermodynamic properties. Cell disintegration is a necessary first step in the isolation of intracellular products; therefore its interaction with other DSP processes has to be carefully analyzed.

1.2.6. Fine chemicals

Several microbial cultures can synthesize a variety of bio-surfactants such as glycolipids, lipopeptides, and lipopolysaccharides. Hydrocarbons are commonly used as substrates for bio-surfactant production but in some cases, carbohydrates can be used as the substrate. Nitrogen deficiency often induces microbes to shift metabolism, leading to an overproduction of certain metabolites, including bio-surfactants. When *Ustilago maydis* is grown on glucose, it produces a mixture of extra-cellular cellobiose lipids called ustilagic acids. Certain lipophilic substrates such as vegetable oils are suitable substrates for the growth and glycolipid formation by this fungus. Another organism that has been frequently used for bio-surfactant production is *Pseudomonas aeruginosa.* Species of the soft rot Gram-negative bacterial genus *Erwinia,* e.g., *Erwinia carotovora* subspecies (E.ca.) and *Erwinia chrysanthemi* (E.chr.) cause economically important damage in plants in the field or after harvest, during storage. These diseases are called soft rot, blackleg or stem rot of potato, and soft rot of pumpkins, carrots and cucumber as well as of certain oranamental plants. Pathogenicity appears to depend primarily on the production of extra-cellular cell-wall degrading pectinases, cellulases, and proteases. These enzymes are actively secreted by the bacteria and depolymerize the main constituents of the plant cell wall.

These pectinolytic and cellulolytic activities may be used for plant biomass conversion: for example, in pectin/cellulose sugar beet waste, pectin and cellulose can yield simple sugars–high added value products–which can be used as animal feed or fermented to give ethanol. Applications are as diverse as protecting crops against the *Erwinia* diseases, production of enzymes such as *Erwinia* pectinases and pectin antileukaemics. These all require a fundamental knowledge of regulation systems. *Erwinia* is now attracting interest as an industrial microbe; the *Erwinia* secretory apparatus, when cloned in *E. coli,* enabled this organism to secrete heterologous *Erwinia* pectinases.

L-Asparaginase, produced since 1972 by Worthington Biochemical Corporation (see Table 1.7), is effective against acute lymphoblastic leukaemia. In early studies, using high dosages of *E. coli,* presence of glutaminase in asparaginase preparations is reported. Glutaminase free asparaginase is not hepatotoxic. The Porton Company (UK) has focused on asparaginase production using recombinant vectors enabling high expression of the *Erwinia* asparaginase gene. At Genentech, a recombinant vector has been constructed to express 2, 5-diketogluconic acid reductase gene in *Erwinia*, enabling the large-scale conversion of glucose to 2-keto-L-gulonic acid (2-KLG): 2-KLG is an intermediate in the production of ascorbic acid (vitamin C). Recombinant DNA technology has also been used for engineering the secretion of heterologous proteins by fusing the coding sequence of such protein to the leader peptide segment of the bacterial pe/B gene (pectate lyase). In this manner, a gene fusion between the leader peptide segment of pe/B gene and the mature coding sequence of chimeric mouse-human Fab antibody protein has been obtained. This particular antibody binds specifically to a human carcinoma cell line, and could be expressed and secreted. Deverse chiral substances are produced in nature by the reduction of unsaturated compounds and the production of such chiral substances has attacted the interest of biotechnologists in recent years since chemical methods for obtaining chiral

Table 1.7: Some industrial applications of *Erwinia*

Products/Derivatives	Company	Area of interest
L-Asparaginase	Worthington	Antileukaemics; glutaminase-free L-asparaginase
Pectin methylesterase	Dalgety	Depectinization of fruit juice and wine
2,5-Diketogluconic acid reductase gene	Genetech	Intermediate for vitamin C production
Polysaccharides	Rhone-Poulenc	Foodstuffs, pharmaceuticals; enhanced oil recovery; catalysts and ceramics

compounds are quite costly. A method of choice is the co-reduction of substituted unsaturated molecules with microbes metabolizing carbohydrates. Of course, co-reduction entails a few disadvantages well, viz, (1) the intended reduction is not the major step but only a side reaction, (2) the optical purity of the product can vary depending on the developmental state of the microbial cells, and (3) the product has to be separated from larger number of cells and the essential reaction without competition from the main stream of the cellular metabolism.

1.2.7. Mammalian hormones in microbial cells

Contrary to the widely held belief that hormones are exclusively the products of vertebrate endocrine organs, several hormone-like peptides occur in insects and other invertebrates. Indeed, some of these hormones exert biological actions similar to those in vertebrates. Some attention has also been given to the possible existence and role of vertebrate hormones in microbial cells (Tables 1.8 and 1.9). The evidence for the existence and activity of polypeptide and steroid hormones and catecholamines in microorganisms is extensive and falls into five general categories.

(1) Materials that cross-react with antibodies to mammalian hormones have been detected by radioimmunoassy (RIA) in cell extracts or media.

(2) Similarities in chromatographic elution behaviour, in one or more separation procedures, between the microbial substance being characterized and the corresponding mammalian hormone.

(3) The microbial substance shows biological activity similar to that of the corresponding mammalian hormone when tested on mammalian cells.

(4) Mammalian hormones induce biological responses in microbial cells.

(5) Specific, high-affinity binding proteins for the mammalian hormone in the appropriate location in microbial cells, *i.e.* in the plasma membrane for peptide hormones, has been demonstrated (in the cytosol for steroids). This points to the existence of fully developed, functional signal transduction pathways in microbial cells–paths that can recognize and respond to the corresponding mammalian hormones.

Table 1.8: Biological activity of insulin in microorganisms

Species	Chromatographic behaviour	Microbial insulin in mammalian cells	Mammalian insulin in microbial cells	Binding sites**
Tetrahymena pyriformis	+	+		
Neurospora crassa	+	+	+	+
Aspergillus fumigatus	+			
Saccharomyces cerevisiae				+
Escherichia coli	+	+		

1.2.8. Insulin

This is a ubiquitous hormone, having been found in every microorganism for which it was examined, from archaea and bacteria to microbial eukaryotes. The insulin-like material from certain bacteria shows extensive immunological similarities to mammalian insulin. The fungus *Neurospora crassa* contains an insulin responsive signal transduction system. From this organism, a plasma membrane protein that binds insulin with high affinity has been identified by cross-linking and purified. This protein binds several mammalian insulins with the same affinity.

Several metabolic responses of *N. crassa* cells to mammalian insulin have been reported. The production of CO_2 ethanol, alanine, glycogen, and other metabolites of glucose are all increased by insulin.

1.2.9. Enzyme technology

Enzyme technology involves the synthesis, purification and immobilization of enzymes and their application in industry, health care, cosmetics, diagnostics, and therapeutics. Enzymes are useful as industrial biocatalysts in view of their non-polluting biodegradable nature and in view of efficacy at physiologically mild condition such as pH, temperature, and pressure. Several factors influence the commercial production of enzymes. Animals, plants and microbes are three important biological sources of enzymes. These organisms are themselves influenced by climatic edaphical, hydrological, and other factors. Some of these influences are lessened in the case of microbes, which are usually grown in sterile cultures under controlled conditions. Figure 1.6 shows some methods of choice for the immobilization of enzymes. Until a few years ago it was only practical to use immobilized systems containing whole cells or specific enzymes. More complex systems that regenerate cofactors outside living cells have been developed; co-immobilization of enzymes cells and sub-cellular organelles from different organisms has brought within our reach notable improvements in the industrial utility of immobilized biocatalysts. Already, genetic engineers are attempting to design organisms with improved enzyme profiles and specifically tailored individual enzymes.

1.2.10. Proteolytic enzymes

Proteolytic enzymes account for over one-half of the industrial enzyme market. Commercially significant proteases are produced from microbial, animal and plant sources. The oldest known examples of proteolytic enzymes are milk-clotting enzymes used for transforming milk into cheese.

More modern examples are detergent protease, animal and microbial rennets, and protease of *Aspergillus oryzae* used in baking. Proteinases hydrolyze large polypeptides into smaller molecules that can be assimilated by the organisms. Proteolytic enzymes also regulate various metabolic processes such as blood coagulation, fibrinolysis and complement activation, Phagocytosis and blood pressure control. Proteolytic activity is quite essential during cellular differentiation. Papain, bromelain, and microbial proteases are often incorporated into animal feeds to improve their nutritional value. Urokinase is produced from kidney cells in tissue culture and is used for treatment of clotting disorders. Proteases are believed to be involved in the modulation of gene expression, and in the modification or secretion of enzymes. High yielding microbial strains are used in surface or submerged fermentation systems for the production of proteases. The enzymes are formed extra-cellularly. Their recovery involves separation of the spent medium by filtration centrifugation.

1.2.11. Enzyme engineering

One of the more exciting programmes of modern biotechnology relates to the designing and construction of enzymes to catalyze any desired reaction. Enzymes are highly specific acting in dilute aqueous solutions at ambient temperature. Substrates attach in precise orientations in the active site of an enzyme and the amino acid side chains of the enzyme assist catalysis by attacking or destabilizing the substrate molecules. In some cases, the affinity of an enzyme towards its substrate may be changed artificially, as has been possible in the case of the *Bacillus stearothermophilus* tyrosyl RNA synthetase for ATP, resulting in the change in specificity of the enzyme for tyrosine.

Table 1.9: Biological activity of other polypeptide hormones in microorganisms

Hormone	Species	Radioimmuno assays	Microbial hormone in mammalian cells	Mammalian hormone in microbial cells
Calcitonin	*Tetrahymena pyrifomis*	+		
Corticotropin	*T- pyriformis*	+		
β-Endorphin	*Amoeba proteus*			+
Glucagon	*Neurospora crassa*			+
Gonadotropin releasing hormone	*Saccharomyces cerevisiae*			
α-factor				
Relaxin	*Tetrahmena pyriformis*			
Somatostatin	*T. pyriformis Plasmodium falcipaparum E.coli, Bacillus subitlis*	+	+	
Thymosin α 1	*Tetrahymena pyrifomis*	+		
Thyrotropin	*Clostridium perfringens*	+		

Some other suitable candidates for enzyme engineering may be glucose isomerase, alpha-amylase, and para-hydroxybenzoate hydroxylase. Protein engineering may usher in the next major boom in biotechnology, offering the promise of tailor made industrial enzymes and therapeutic proteins. Already some improved proteins for specific industrial and therapeutic uses have been produced. It has been shown that tailoring enzymatic properties for the non-physiological substrate conditions, altering pH optima, changing substrate specificity and improving stability are feasible. Selecting chemical modification is now being used to design novel proteins, particularly enzymes and antibodies, with altered specificities and catalytic activities *in vitro*. Modification strategies now being developed are expected to yield a wide spectrum of novel bio-molecules with optimum activities for specific industrial processes or therapeutic application. Posttranslational modification confers a number of advantageous properties to proteins *in vivo*. Chemical cross-linking of amino acid side chains enhances the stability and overall structural integrity of these molecules. Selective chemical reactions, more generally, chemical modification of proteins represents a powerful tool for altering signal transduction mechanisms and controlling biological function and chemical reactivity within the cell.

Chemical modification may be resorted to improve the activities of proteins *in vitro* (Hilvert, 1991). The properties of enzymes are not always optimal. Covalent chemical modification of specific functional groups can often increase their stability, solubility and antigenicity; alter patterns of inhibition and activation, and change pH optima or substrate specificity. Enzymes are potentially valuable as drugs. These methods allow entirely new enzymatic activities to be engineered into naturally occurring proteins via post-translation modifications. Selective chemical reactions may be exploited for incorporation of non-natural amino acids or catalytic co-factors directly into pre-existing protein binding pockets. Metal-chemical agents, such as phenanthroline derivatives, can be attached to DNA- binding proteins by alkylation of free thiols to produce site-specific nucleases. On addition of a reducing agent, copper phenanthroline generates HO⁻ radical or metal-oxo derivatives, which cleave phosphodiester bonds. Additonal thiols can be introduced if necessary, by pretreating the protein with 2-iminothiolane. The enzymatically susceptible residues in serine and cysteine protease are highly reactive functional groups. Both being active-site nucleophile (ser or Cys), and general base (His), they undergo selective modification in the presence of bacterial protease. The subtilisin can thus be chemically converted into a Cys residue, yielding large amount of pure thiolsubtilisin. Also non-natural amino acids may be chemically introduced into the protein-binding site.

Restriction endonucleases and DNA ligases have enhanced this propensity of manageable-sized fragments of genetic material to manipulation and study. Design of new agents that bind to or cleave large DNAs site-specifically will further facilitate cloning and mapping of genomic DNA. Rationally designed catalysts able to cleave large RNAs site-specifically, should also be aided in studies of RNA structure and function.

M=Water-insoluble matrix E=Enzyme

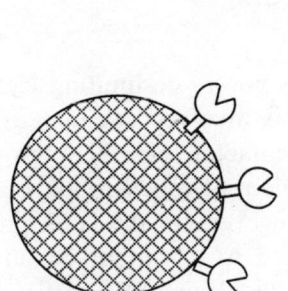

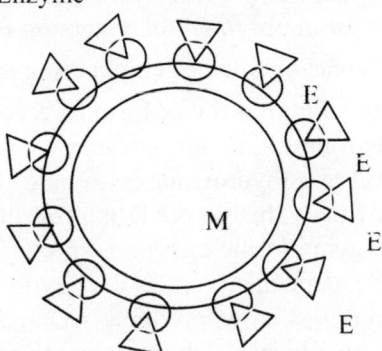

Enzyme attachment to matrix by covalent bonds

Enzyme cross-linking by multifunctional reagent

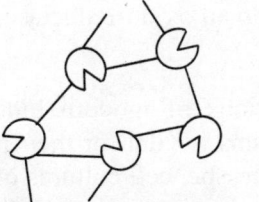

Cross-linked enzyme matrix

Fig. 1.6: Various methods of enzyme immobilization

1.2.12. Redox catalysts

Enzymes can use metal ions, vitamins, and various cofactors to catalyze certain reactions that cannot be catalyzed by protein side chains alone. This is especially true for oxidative functional group transformations. Likewise, artificial oxido-reductases can be prepared by covalently attaching redox-active prosthetic groups to existing active sites. Alkylation of protein binding sites with a reactive 10-methylisoalloxazine derivative yields semi-synthetic flavoenzymes that combine the reactivity of the catalytic cofactor (electron transfer, thiol, and dihydronicotinamide oxidation) with the specificity of the template protein. Affinity labeling is a powerful strategy for incorporating catalytic groups into antibody combining sites. Use of a cleavable affinity reagent places a free thiol proximal to the binding pocket after treatment with dithiothreitol (DTT). The thiol is a convenient handle for attaching chemical functionality (e.g., imidazoles) (Hilvert, 1991).

1.2.13. Semisynthetic antibodies

Catalytic groups can be incorporated selectively into antibody combining sites via chemical modification. Catalytic antibody technology allows the creation of catalysts for virtually any chemical transformation, even reactions that have no physiological counterpart.

1.2.14. Cofactor engineering

All enzyme-catalyzed reactions involve the interaction of the enzyme, its substrate and the immediate environment (e.g., solvent). Changing the properties of the enzymic reaction involves manipulating one or more of these three components. Some examples of engineering enzyme reactions include site-directed mutagenesis or selective chemical modification of the enzyme; derivatization of the substrate to better suit the enzyme or environment or use of organic solvents or additives to modify catalytic activity. For more than 50% of known enzymes, either a cofactor or coenzyme is also required in the reactions they catalyze: this provides yet another way of manipulating reactions. Cofactor engineering is a good approach for improving bioconversion for specific applications.

Some potential areas of cofactor engineering are listed below:

(1) Regenerating the required redox form of a coenzyme such that it is not a rate-limiting factor has long been a problem in optimizing enzyme catalysis. One approach has involved attempts to attach the coenzyme NAD to dehydrogenases so as to let NAD function as cofactor (prosthetic group). In this way, escape of the valuable NAD is prevented, although the problem of regeneration is shifted now from the coenzyme to the enzyme. An elegant solution exists, however, for the latter problem; for example, NAD dependent glucose dehydrogenase was engineered to a variant containing a cysteine residue in a postion where the NAD analogue covalently couples. It not only participates in catalysis initiated by glucose dehydrogenase, but also assists in the catalysis by NAD-dependent lactate dehydrogenase that is contained in the same solution.

(2) Enzymes may be modified by incorporating a cofactor which is normally associated with a quite different type of enzymes. An example is the alkylation of a cysteine residue in the active site of papain with a flavin derivative transforming the hydrolase into an oxido-reductase.

1.3. GENETIC ENGINEERING

Genetic engineering constitutes one of the basic foundations of modern biotechnology because genetic modification or manipulation of useful microorganisms is vital for their profitable utilization in the production of useful, high-value products. Besides microsbe, cell cultures of plants and animals can be genetically manipulated to advantage; this is possible in view of our ability in many cases to raise protoplast cultures (and fuse them), which can be handled like microbes in genetic experiments. Techniques of genetic engineering have made it possible in some cases to transfer genes from one organism to another by overcoming the species barrier. Gene manipulation experiments require the use of certain enzymes concerned with nucleic acid metabolism. These enzymes make it possible to manipulate DNA *in vitro*. The most important of these enzymes are those called restriction endonucleases, which are part of the armory that bacteria have plasmids. The nucleases hydrolyze nucleic acids into nucleotides. An exonuclease chews the DNA strand bacteria which produce these restriction endonucleases protect the specific sequences in their own DNA at specific sequences. The bacteria which produce this restriction endonuclease protect the specific sequences in their own DNA by masking them with certain chemical group with the consequence that a restriction endonuclease cannot cut the specific sequence in the bacterium's own DNA but can attack only the foreign DNA. When the DNA is cut specifically by an endonuclease, this cleavage often gives rise to DNA fragments with single-stranded sticky ends. These sticky ends may be rejoined by means of another kind of enzyme called ligase. Still other enzymes are available for cutting out and processing the required gene fragments from a donor genome. Usually, the substrates that restriction endonucleases attack are palindromic DNA sequences that read the same both backwards and forward (e.g., the word MADAM). Over 100 different endonucleases have so far been isolated and characterized. Perhaps the most popular example is EcoR1, produced by Escherichia coli. This EcoR1 attacks the sequence

5…GAATTC…3

3…CTTAAG…5

It may be noted that this sequence has symmetry around its centre. The enzyme produces single-strand cuts or nicks" between A and G:

3…CTTAA/G…5

1.3.1. Recombinant DNA technology

Molecular genetics involves direct manipulation of genetic material and the transfer of genetic information between species which cannot interbreed. One of the most widely known aspects of molecular genetics is called recombinant DNA. Certain techniques allow fragments of DNA from an animal, plant, or microbe to be transferred to a host bacterium (or some other microbe), which in turn incorporates the fragments into its own genome, thereby gaining new capabilities for synthesis or biochemical reactions. The host of choice in most experiments has been the bacterium *E. coli*, but other microorganisms or even cultured cells of higher plants and animals can now be used as hosts.

How exactly is the genetic information moved form the donor to the host? This is done by means of certain vectors such as bacteriophages and restriction enzymes. The former are viruses which infect bacteria; the latter are synthesized naturally by bacterial cells and are capable of nicking DNA molecules at specific sites where there is a complementary or specific sequence of nucleotide bases. Two characteristic properties of most vectors are the ability to move from organism to organism, and reproducing themselves as the cells divide. One can cut out a fragment from the donor DNA molecule by means of a suitable restriction enzyme and insert the fragment into a vector, which carries the donor DNA into the host cell. The host cells that have received the alien DNA through vectors by the foregoing technique can sometimes be coaxed to synthesize fairly large quantities of a novel protein, which the unmodified host does not synthesize naturally. The first noteworthy example of a tangible achievement of this technology was the production of human insulin by *E. coli*. Recombinant DNA technology and genetic engineering techniques find several useful applications in the areas of vaccines, foods, antibiotics, alcohols, hormones, and monoclonal antibodies. It has become possible in some cases to diagnose genetic defects by use of the restriction mapping technique. This is based on the fact that the base sequence in defective genes differs from that in normal genes, leading to the production of different-sized DNA fragments when a gene is cut up with a restriction endonuclease. One interesting application is the creation of gene libraries or gene banks, which store genes of rare organisms inside bacterial hosts until needed. Genetic engineering techniques have perhaps found one of the most important uses for the production of insulin and somatostatin.

It has now become possible to insert foreign genes into cells, not just anywhere in the host genome but exactly where desired. This new technique of targeting a transferred gene to some specific site on a chromosome is bound to improve the chances of achieving effective gene therapy for such hereditary diseases as sickle cell anaemia. Targeted gene transfer can also be used to introduce specific mutations into mice as well as to repair gene defects The technique has the potential to generate mice of any desired genotype; such mice could serve as models for human genetic diseases. Human beta-globin gene sequences have already been successfully inserted into the beta-globin gene of the recipient cells by homologous recombination, which is the basis for all targeted gene transfer. The vector used to introduce the new gene into cells carries nucleotide sequences identical to those of the DNA at the chromosomal site where one wants the gene to integrate.

1.3.2. Gene transfer

Gene transfer in animals involves four steps; (1) a method of cutting and joining DNA, (2) a vector (gene carrier) that can replicate itself and a foreign DNA segment that has been inserted in it, (3) a method of producing enough DNA for insertion into the germline of animals (cloning), and (4) a method of introducing the cloned DNA into germ cells. The first three of these steps became possible in the early 1970s; the fourth step could be achieved several years later in 1977. Rapid and accurate methods of identifying the precise nucleotide sequences of genes were designed by Sanger, Nicklen, and Coulson at Cambridge, and Maxam and Gilbert at Harvard. This opened the way for the molecular dissection of genes, and elucidation of the way in which they function. In the mid-1970s, it had been shown that viral DNA could be introduced into mouse embryos, for example Simian virus 40 DNA can be placed into the blastocyst cavity. The first time strategy was developed to insert a gene into a living animal albeit into bone marrow cells, rather than germ cells. At the same time, the insertion of cloned DNA into the mouse genome by microinjection of the male pronucleus of the one-celled embryo was disclosed. The way was now clear for germ line transfer of DNA to produce transgenic animals. In the procedure, embryos which survive microinjection are implanted into recipient females, and some offspring developing from injected eggs carry the foreign gene in all cells, integrated into a chromosome.

The integrated DNA usually occurs in multiple copies. In livestock, microinjection is technically more demanding than in mice, because their eggs are almost opaque, making the pronucleus difficult to see. Retroviruses can be used as gene vectors both with cell systems and also with multicellular embryos. Retroviruses have a gene coding for the enzyme reverse transcriptase, which catalyzes the production of double-stranded DNA complementary to the RNA core of the retrovirus This DNA can integrate into the DNA of host cells, as a single copy called provirus. The virus multiplies in host cells by transcribing retroviral RNA from the proviral DNA, using the host cells own RNA polymerase. Some of this RNA is used to produce the proteins required for the retrovirus envelope using the cells system for translating RNA to protein. Provirus genes coding for protein may be deleted by standard genetic engineering techniques, and replaced by foreign DNA. The provirus can no longer replicate on its own, and is then known as "defective virus". However, a non-defective helper virus can be used to infect the cells, and supplies the missing gene functions to the defective virus. Retroviruses have some limitations as vectors. The size of the foreign DNA sequence that can be inserted in provirus is limited and the nucleotide sequences at each end of the provirus, the so-called long terminal repeats, which are necessary for viral transcription, can interfere with or over ride signals determining expression of foreign DNA.

For successful commercial use, transgenes must function in the right place (the chosen target tissue) at the right time in the animal's life history, and deliver the right amount of product. When the DNA of a gene transcribes messenger RNA it does so under the action of RNA polymerase. The site on the DNA where the enzyme attaches is known as the promoter. In higher animals, the promoter alone allows only very inefficient transcription of structural genes. Other elements in the promoter alone allow only very inefficient transcription of structural genes. Other elements in the genome must regulate or open the transcription initiation site(s). Specific regulatory elements called enhancers appear to affect genes even though they are not located next to them.

1.3.3. Antisense DNA and RNA

Only one of the two strands of DNA of a gene codes for the gene's product. The other is known as antisense. It is thus possible to block gene action by creation of antisense RNA. The antisense RNA so formed is not translated into the protein product of the gene. There are two potential applications of antisense RNA. The first is in the study of gene function, by observing cells or animals with functioning and inactivated genes. The second is to use antisense inhibition for therapy in genetic diseases. Any antisense genes must be active in the same tissues as the corresponding normal gene in order for the expression of the latter to be inhibited. Also, antisense genes must produce a large excess of RNA relative to the amounts produced by the normal, or sense, gene. For such an excess to be obtained *in vivo*, the promoter and enhancer(s) attached to the antisense gene must be more active than those of the sense gene, and should have the same tissue specificity.

1.4. RESTRICTION FRAGMENT LENGTH POLYMORPHISM (RFLP)

RFLP markers are co-dominant (heterozygotes can be distinguished from either homyzygote) and provide complete genetic information at a single locus. The amount of DNA required for RFLP analysis is relatively large (5-10 µg). Multiple southern blots corresponding to hundreds of individuals can be probed simultaneously. New genetic markers or genes can easily be located within the context of an existing RFLP map, but very little is known about the distribution of markers in the germplasm. Figure 1.7 illustrates the principles of RFLP. An alternative to one of the disadvantages of RFLP markers, the need for radioactive probes, has become available with the availability of sensitive non-radioactive detection systems. Automation of RFLP mapping is difficult, and it may be more practical to turn to one of the DNA-amplification based marker·systems to provide an automated genotype assay. Sequence information is not required in either of the two systems. Types of polymorphism for both systems are single-base changes, insertions and deletions.

1.5. RANDOM AMPLIFICATION OF POLYMORPHIC DNA (RAPD)

Technology for the amplification of discrete loci with single, random-sequence, and oligonucleotide primers is simple and easy to use. The RAPD amplification reaction is performed on a genomic DNA template and primed by an arbitrary oligonucleotide primer, resulting in the amplification of several discrete DNA products. These are usually separated on agarose gels and visualized by ethidium bromide staining. Each amplification product is derived from a region of the genome that contains two short DNA segments with some sequence homology to the primer; these segments must be present on opposite DNA strands, and be sufficiently close to each other to allow DNA amplification to occur. The polymorphism between individuals results from sequence differences in one or both of the primer binding sites, and manifests as the presence or absence of a particular RAPD band. Such polymorphisms behave as dominant genetic markers. Analysis of RAPD is suitable for automated breeding applications because it requires only small amounts of DNA (15–25 ng) a non-radioactive assay that can be performed in several hours, and a simple experimental set-up.

RAPD technology enables researchers to screen for DNA sequence based polymorphisms at a large number of loci. Sets of short primers (usually 10 mers) suitable for RAPD amplification are available commercially or may be readily synthesized. RAPD markers are dominant (profiles are scored for the presence or absence of a single allele). When a marker linked to a trait of interest is available, it becomes easy to turn the RAPD assay into a more reproducible PCR-type assay based on secondary DNA sequence, by use of allele-specific PCR (AS-PCR), allele-specific ligation, or sequence characterized amplified region (SCAR) assay.

Table 1.10: Comparisons of two systems for the generation of genetic markers

	RFLP	RAPD
Principle	Endonuclease restriction, southern blotting, hybridization	DNA amplification with random primers
Genomic abundance	High	Very high
Dominance	Codominant	Dominant
Amount of DNA required	2–10 µg	10–25 ng
Development	Medium	Low
Start-up costs	Medium/High	Low

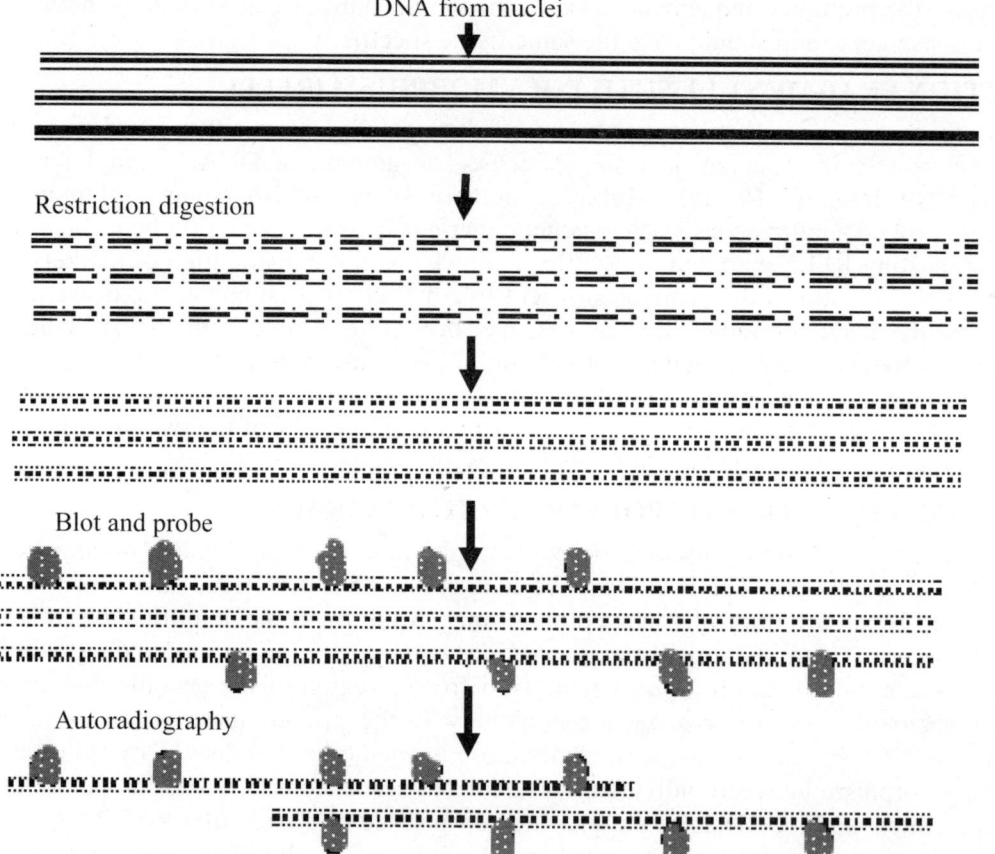

Fig.1.7: Diagram illustrating various steps involved in restriction fragment length polymorphism

1.6. DNA FINGER PRINTING

In the early 1980s, DNA regions (hypervariable minisatellite DNA) were discovered which varied in nucleotide sequences between individuals, so that two individuals, except identical twins, had identical hypervariable regions. Ten to 15 kb long core sequences were found to be common in hypervariable regions in all individuals, and therefore could be used as genetic markers of such regions, by means of DNA hybridization probes.

The hypervariable regions consist of short nucleotide sequences that are repeated many times, and it is the number of repeats that is the key to DNA fingerprinting. Use is made of restriction endoucleases to cut the DNA into pieces. These enzymes recognize specific sequences of 4–6 nucleotides, and create breaks in the double-stranded DNA. In case of variation in the number of short-sequence repeats between two sites, DNA pieces of different length will be produced. When the cut DNA is electrophoresed, DNA fragments of different length will move through the gel to different distances from the start point and occur as transverse bands in the gel. The gel is then transferred by blotting to a nitrocellulose filter, hybridized to radioactive DNA probe for a core region, and the hybridizing bands may be identified by autoradiography. The technique is used in forensic science to identify the offending male in rape cases by examination of DNA extracted from semen, and also in parenthood testing. Use of the technique in animals has followed in the wake of the human applications.

DNA fingerprinting of cattle, horses, dogs, fowls, and a fish was carried out using four probes, namely, wild type M13 bacteriophage DNA a plasmid containing a human alpha globulin hypervariable region sequence, a plasmid containing a mouse DNA fragment related to a Drosophila gene, and a plasmid containing 25 tandem copies of a core sequence. Individual specific fingerprints could be detected in all the species for one or more probes. In farm livestock, inaccuracy, particularly in artificially inseminated cattle, is often higher than is generally realized. Currently, most checking involves typing for blood groups and sometimes for polymorphic biochemical markers. In the future, DNA fingerprinting is likely to be the method of choice.

1.7. *IN VITRO* AMPLIFICATION OF DNA

A new gene amplification method has greatly facilitated DNA analysis and has found several applications. The technique is called polymerase chain reaction (PCR). It works with intact or broken DNA pieces, even as small as about 50 base pairs. It is an *in vitro* method for copying simultaneously the two complementary DNA strands which make up a gene sequence. By this technique it is possible to synthesize millions of copies of a single sequence in only a few hours. The specific DNA segment to be amplified is selected by using primers (short segments of DNA that have been synthesized to have sequences complementary to the DNA flanking the target region). These primers help define the ends of the DNA to be duplicated. Upon heating of the DNA sample, the two strands separate, allowing the primers to bind to the flanking sequences, one on each strand. Thereafter, the primers initiate the synthesis of two daughter strands, complementary to the parental strands, in the presence of DNA polymerase. This kind of cycle involving heating and DNA synthesis can be repeated several times. The enzyme DNA polymerase used in the PCR technology is that isolated from the thermophilic bacterium *Thermus aquaticus* and is quite heat-stable. Twenty cycles can amplify the DNA by a factor of about a million. The PCR technology is stimulating efforts to track down the cellular changes involved in cancer. It makes it easier to detect even a single base pair mismatch in the human genome, by amplifying it. The DNA sequences of the human Papilloma virus can be detected in samples of cervical cancer tissue by means of the PCR technique, even in old samples in which DNA may have degraded. The PCR has made it possible to perform immediate tests on hypothesis linking the presence or absence of specific DNA sequences with a disease or its prognosis.

1.8. CATALYTIC ANTIBODIES (ABZYMES)

Many industrial chemical transformations require either a promoter or catalyst. The promoter, unlike the catalyst, is usually either consumed in the reaction, or tends to show relatively low turnover efficiency. Therefore the promoter, unlike the catalyst, is used in stoichiometric (or even greater) proportions. In contrast, catalysts are usually used in subequivalent quantities. The majority of enzymatic functions are performed by proteins, which show diversity in their primary, secondary, and tertiary structure that confers specific reactivity. Little opportunity for gross improvements in efficiency, as judged by rate, seems to be available in the redesigning of enzymes though enzymes carry out specific, life enabling reactions, their applications to non-natural situations are complicated. We might distinguish between two kinds of non-natural settings. One is that of natural type of reaction (such as oxidation, reduction, or aldol condensation) with non-natural substrates. Considerable scope exists for achieving enzymatic modulation of artificial substrates undergoing natural reactions. It has been less easy to adapt protein-based enzymes to catalyze reaction types not included in their original "capability". Consequently the protein structure of enzyme has shown little adaptability in acquiring wholly unanticipated reactions. Two main complications hinder '*de novo*' protein based catalyses (that is, artificial enzymes) to accommodate unnatural reactions. It is difficult to interrelate the active site structure of the proposed protein with its ability for catalysis. For the moment the capacity to obtain peptides and proteins of defined amino acid sequence by fully synthetic or recombinant means has not helped much in obtaining novel artificial enzymes *de novo*. It is for this reason that catalytic antibodies have attracted interest. The massive power of the immune system is directed towards producing antibodies. The active sites are complementary to the antigen which on exposure to reaction substrates bind the substrate and accelerate the reaction. Virtually the full binding force of the antibody is, in principle, exploitable for purposes of catalysis. Catalytic antibodies can catalyze known but non-natural chemical reactions quite well. Till hitherto, they have been used to catalyze "typical" organic reactions, but recently catalysis by an antibody has also been achieved in an otherwise disfavoured reaction. Ribozymes destroy RNAs involved in disease. They are now are on the verge of leaving the lab for the clinic. The ability to target ribozymes to cleave viral RNA *in vitro* has generated much speculation about their potential therapeutic value as antiviral agents *in vitro*.

A specially designed ribozyme–an RNA molecule engineered to seek out and destroy the RNA genome of HIV by cutting it in two–is being tried with the expectation that lymphocytes containing the ribozyme gene will have a better chance of surviving HIV infection. RNA enzymes have potential as therapies for diseases such as AIDS, cancer, and chronic hepatitis. Many ribozymes were dubbed with terms such as hammerhead, hairpin, and exehead, inspired by their three-dimensional shapes. The key to their unique activity lies in their structure: they contain stretches of nucleotides that base-pair with a complementary RNA region, and they have a catalytic section, like the active site of a protein enzyme, that chops the bound RNA while the base pairing holds it in place. These features make catalytic RNAs ideal material for bioengineering: a ribozyme can be custom-designed to recognize and base pair with a specific cellular RNA that a researcher would like to eliminate. Once designed, the ribozyme can be turned loose in the cell to kill its target. In several clinical situations, physicians like to target and destroy" bad RNA" e.g., in chronic viral diseases. Cancers can be initiated by a mutated oncogene. HIV is another tempting target. Attempts are underway to develop a way to target a ribozyme to the site in the cell where the HIV RNA accumulates thereby improving the ribozyme's chances of hitting home. Delivering the goods to the right site in the cell and to the right cell is an important challenge for ribozyme therapy. For example, ribozymes are a potential therapy for chronic hepatitis B. But unlike white blood cells, which can be removed form the body and reintroduced for treating HIV, the liver obviously cannot be temporarily removed, and therefore ribozymes need to be delivered to the organ while it is still in the body.

1.9. GENE MACHINE

A computerized gene machine performs the function of building DNA sequences to order by combining nucleotides, one at a time into some predetermined sequence. For instance if a G (guanine) is needed, the growing sequence is placed in a solution containing modified G nucleotides. The purpose of the modification is to allow only one G to be added, in order to prevent several G s from attaching to the sequence. Following the incorporation of one G, the chemical block (modification) has to be removed before a different nucleotide (or even another G) can be added. Figure 1.8 gives an outline of a gene machine.

One such machine has a column reactor in which oligonucleotides are grown on solid support beads packed into cassettes. These prepacked cassettes can be colour-coded according to the first 3' terminal in the required gene sequence. The appropriate cassette is inserted into one of the column reactors before the start of the synthesis. At the end of the process, the cassette is removed off the solid support.

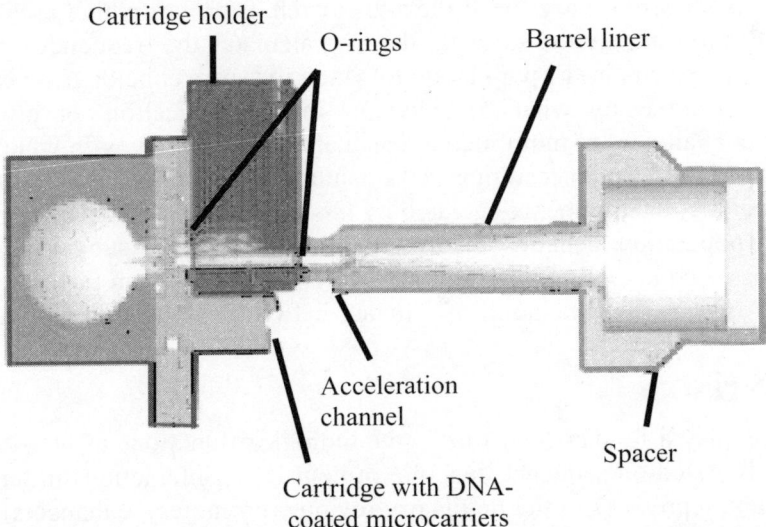

Fig. 1.8: Schematic representation of gene machine for elucidating its structure

The solid support beads are made from an inert polymer. The machine has a peristaltic pump and nine glass bottles used for washing solutions, oxidation, capping, and adenylation operations. Some bottles serve to contain waste solutions whereas others can store modified nucleotides or additional reagents. The gene assembly process involves adenylation, activation, coupling, oxidation, and capping operations, which are controlled by microprocessor. Several intervening washes are also involved. Although gene machines presently offer the quickest way of synthesizing predetermined nucleotide sequences, their limitation is that only short DNA sequences can be built.

1.10. DNA HYBRIDIZATION

An inherent part of several genetic manipulation programmes is DNA hybridization. The rate at which two-polynucleotide strands join together *in vitro* depends on the extent to which their nucleotide sequences complement each other. The relative ease with which single-stranded cDNA can be produced has catalyzed new possibilities. Often, it can be made radioactive to facilitate its proper identification, and it can then be employed as a DNA probe for locating complementary sequences elsewhere. For instance, in chromosome mapping, cDNA binds to the precise position on a chromosome where a gene is located. Again, the genes of different organisms can often be inter compared by their ability to bind to a specific sequence of cDNA, so that the relationships between them may be elucidated. One of the most useful applications of recombinant DNA technology has been the synthesis of insulin genes.

The 15-bp synthetic oligonucleotide 5-GCTGTGAGGAAATAC-3 as a probe to screen a human DNA library and detect recombinant phages containing genes of the interferon alpha family was developed. One of the clones was found to carry the interferon alpha 2 genes, which was processed to substitute the sequence encoding the leader peptide by an ATG initiating codon. They then placed this construction under the direction of suitable promoters of an expression vector generating a plasmid (pIN89) that expressed substantial amounts of the mature form of interferon alpha 2 genes in *E. coli*. Forensic DNA fingerprinting is a powerful and reliable technology to link the blood, semen, or hair left at the scene of a crime to a suspect's DNA. This new technology allows us to match two DNA samples. Successful application of the technology depends on several factors, e.g., reliable statistical analysis and very precise, high quality DNA analysis. This is done by examining the DNA at several sites where its sequence is known to vary. If all the sites match, it proves which both samples came from the same person. But to estimate the strength, the lab calculates the frequency with which each sequence variation, or allele, occurs in the population to which the suspect belongs by examining, say, the Caucasian database. Then using what is known as the multiplication, or product rule, the frequencies of the individual alleles are multiplied to calculate the frequency with which the complete pattern occurs in that population, often resulting in vanishingly small numbers. But several leading population geneticists feel that the numbers generated by this procedure are misleading and are based on misapprehension of population genetics theory. Populations contain subgroups in which the frequencies of the markers used in DNA fingerprinting vary dramatically from their frequencies in the population at large. That means the likelihood of a match between samples may be grossly over or underestimated.

1.11. DNA FOOT PRINTING

Ligand-DNA interactions play a fundamental role in the biological functions of DNA. Regulation of gene expression is largely based on sequence specific, protein-DNA interactions in terms of binding of transcription factors and repressors to the regulatory regions (promoters, enhancers) of genes. The binding of such proteins to their recognition sequences of the DNA, promotes the gene expression at the transcription level, and protects the DNA sequence from degradation by an enzyme such as DNase1. The DNA molecule is labeled on one strand at one end and cleaved (1) at a density of one cleavage per DNA molecule. Each cleavage point thus corresponds to a specific length of labeled.

DNA fragment as analyzed by gel electrophoresis in polyacrylamide (PAGE). (A, control; B, in the presence of protein (ligand) (In the case of transcription factors) or restricts (in the case of repressors) binding of RNA polymerase to the gene promoter region. Similarly, many drugs bind to DNA by sequence selective manner and thus interfere with DNA function. The structural analysis of ligand-DNA complexes can often be obtained by rather simple foot printing experiments. Fig. 1.9 illustrates the concept of a typical foot printing experiment. A DNA fragment containing the base sequence to interest is radioisotope-labelled on one strand at one end. The DNA is then treated with the footprinting probe under condition that results in one modification per DNA fragmentation average. The modificaiotn usually directly, or or can be converted to, a scission of the DNA backbone, and the positon of this modification can be determined by subsequent analysis of the DNA by high-resolution gel electrophoretic anaylsis, since each cleavage position will correspond to a band in the gel, By comparing the cleave pattern in the absence and presence of DNA binding ligand, regions and single base positions which are protected from modification by the ligand can be identified as a "footprint" in the cleavage pattern. By choce of the probe, various aspects, such as overall ligand-DNA contact region, contacts with the DNA bases, or contacts with deoxyribose or the phosphates of the DNA backbone can be analyzed. Thus the choce of footprinting probe is an essential part of a foot printing experiment. Fe (II) EDTA, UV-B radiation and psoratlens/UV-A radiation; for *in vivo* footprinting anaylysis, dimethyl sulphate is a very useful probe but enzymatic probes are unsuitable.

1.12. THE HUMAN GENOME

The publication of the human genome sequence has given us a view of the internal genetic scaffold around which every human life is moulded. This scaffold has been inherited from our ancestors; through it we are connected to all other life on earth. Actually, the human genome sequence is not complete—it is only a working draft. Much more work remains to be done to obtain a complete view of the human genome as the sequences of only two human chromosomes 21 and 22 are effective in the same state as the other genome that have been sequenced so far. But alongside the sequencing work, structural genomics, described as determining the three dimensional structure of proteins in parallel, rather than one at a time, has been boosted by such technical advances as access to genome sequence from a growing list of species. The availability of a reference human DNA sequence constitutes a milestone towards understanding how humans have evolved and it makes large-scale comparative studies possible. The major impact of such studies will be to reveal just how similar humans are to each other and to other species. The first comparisons will be between the human genome and distantly related genomes such as those of yeast, flies, worms and mice. About 26,000-38,000 genes are found in the draft version of our own genome, a number that is only 2-3 times larger than the 13,600 genes in the fruit fly genome. Some 10% of human genes are clearly related to particular genes in the fly and the worm. Obviously we share much of our genetic scaffold even with very distant relatives. The similarity between humans and other animals will become even more apparent when genome sequences from organisms such as the mouse, with which we share a more recent common ancestor, become available. For these species, both the number of genes and the general structure of the genome are likely to be very similar to ours. The close similarity of human genome to that of other organisms will reinforce unity of life, and point to the genomic view of our place in nature, as both are source of humanity and a blow to the idea of human uniqueness.

Protein structures being very illuminating from a biochemical perspective, as and when more protein structures are determined, their utility will increase. One of the most recent highlights in structural biology is the high-resolution analysis of the ribosome. Solving the structure of proteins is crucial for drug discovery. Several drugs, such as inhibitors of the influenza virus and HIV (human immunodeficiency virus), have been discovered by systematic analysis of the molecular interactions between the potential drug and target protein.   Even though the two draft human sequences are similar, their interpretation in the papers from the two groups (i.e., the public domain and the private or commercial domain) has been rather different. In the public paper, there is an ascent on repeats and genome evolution while in the commercial paper; there is more of a concentration on coding DNA.

There are, for instance, some tables listing the number of genes that code for proteins in different families. There are over 600 G protein-coupled receptors (GPCRs). For those interested in drug discovery, this kind of information is valuable. It is now essential to know how many proteins there are in those families that are already known to contain drug targets. GPCRs constitute the target for about 50% of all small molecule drugs. Other important families include nuclear hormone receptors, ion channels, phosphodiesterases, and protein kinases. The surprising conclusion is that there are only 35,000 genes in the human genome as compared to the less complex organisms—19,000 in worm,

14,000 in fly, and 7000 in yeast. But even now, new genes are being found in these genomes; so the real number of genes is still conjectural. Some help in this work may come from the comprehensive collections of full-length human complementary DNAs (cDNAs) such as those being assembled for the mouse in Japan. Some of these genes, via alternative splicing will encode multiple protein products: the precise relationship between number of genes and number of encoded proteins will require more work. We are also some time away from being able to do a simple database search to find genes in chromosomal regions involved with susceptibility to disease, or any other complex trait, and it is still quite difficult to find these regions.

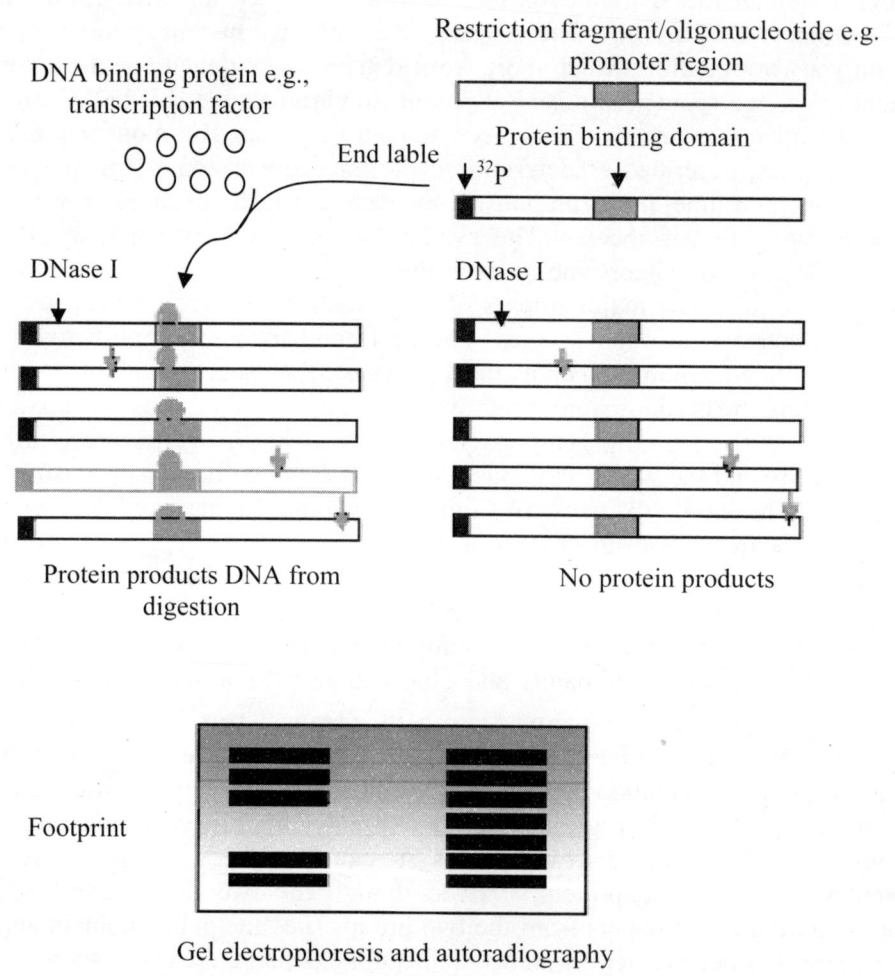

Fig. 1.9: Production of human insulin by recombinant DNA technology

If one considers the number of genes in all these organisms form a protein structure perspective, however, it is still quite high. There are around 15,000 protein structures in the Protein Data Bank but only some 3000 of these are unique. For example, there are hundreds of versions of lysozyme in the database and there are thousands of proteins for which there are no structural data at all. Only about 30% of the protein sequences in Swiss Prot Database can be assigned to a structural class on the basis of sequence homology to one of these structural templates. One aim of the structural genomics effort is to provide templates for the majority of protein sequences. One question for the structural biologist would be: How many protein folds are there? One of the primary objectives in structural genomics is to develop the ability to relate, more directly, specific amino acid sequences with protein folds. As and when many more real structures become available one could predict structure more easily from primary amino acid sequence. The strongest challenge to the notion of human uniqueness may come from comparisons of genomes of closely related species. The overall DNA sequence similarity between humans and chimpanzees is about 99%. When the genome sequence of chimpanzee becomes available, we will find that its gene content and organization are very similar (if not identical) to our own. It will be quite easy to determine the chimpanzee sequence by using the human sequence as a guide to assembly. The few difference between our genome and that of the great apes, will attract much interest because they will reveal the genetic prerequisites that make us different from all other animals, and may reveal the genetic foundation for our rapid cultural evolution, geographic isolation and our current overaccing domination of earth.

About a decade ago, structure determination used to be a slow and laborious process. The advent of simple gene cloning techniques and access to many gene sequences have now made it possible to choose the same gene from several species as the starting point to increase the chances of obtaining a soluble protein for X-ray analysis. Proteins can be labeled with histidine tags and rapid affinity-based methods used for protein purification. Automation technology is used for rapid crystallization set up and viewing: this allows the production of numerous protein crystals. From a drug discovery perspective, it is vital to obtain the structure of many members of a closely-related family of proteins because in this way one can obtain a three-dimensional view of many compounds bound to both the target protein in the family and all the relatives, some of which may mediate undesirable rather than therapeutic effects. Another possible application may be to obtain systematically the structure of proteins encoded by open reading frames (ORFs) of unknown function. As the structure database expands in size and the correlating between structure and function becomes clear, it may become possible to assign functions to unknown proteins by virtue of their structure and cross referencing to databases of gene expression protein-protein interaction, and gene deletion information. The emergence of high-throughput techniques for DNA sequence determination has made possible large-scale comparisons of human genomes from many individuals. The general picture that has emerged so far is that the gene pool in Africa contains more variation than elsewhere, and that the genetic variation found outside of Africa represents only a sub set of that found within the African continent. From a genetic perspective, all humans are therefore Africans.

1.12.1. From Genomics to Drugs

As genomics can potentially transform medicine, several programs are focusing on collecting or exploiting genomic information. One such project, for example, aims to determine gene expression profiles for normal, precancer, and cancer cells with a view to better detection, diagnosis, and treatment for cancer patients. A first step in realizing this goal of drug development is to develop the capability to modulate the functions of genes that are over expressed with temporal and spatial control in tissue culture cells or animals. Available genetic tools for eliminating function, such as knockout mice, are very slow. Some newer tools, such as RNA interference (RNAi) require additional development. As cancer results after several changes occur in the cell, testing the effects of perturbing many gene functions in different ways and in different combinations should give valuable clues, but are not possible with currently available tools. Therefore, the development of small-molecule probes to be used to study the results of activating or inactivating protein functions cells and organisms are being encouraged. As small molecular probes can activate or inactivate protein functions, they are valuable resources to identify the functions of gene products in normal and disease cells, as well as in tissues.

By using such valuable techniques as pool synthesis and combinatorial chemistry, modern synthetic organic chemistry could be exploited to increase the availability of small molecules as probes of biological systems. The monastrol, a small molecule inhibitor of the kinesin motor protein Eg5 targets a member of the kinesin family. Eg5 inhibitors have shown promising results in animal models of cancer. The process of diversity-oriented synthesis (DOS) in which small molecules are directed to large expanses of chemical descriptor space by means of a planning algorithm for efficient synthesis of stereochemically complex and skeletally diverse small molecules. Indeed, ready access to the tools of high-throughput screening, and to collections of diverse small molecules, can effectively speed up the discovery of potential drug targets.

Informative tools and valuable databases are being developed to facilitate the identification of the proteins to which small molecules discovered in cellular and organismal assays bind, and to explore the underlying principles of biological networks.

1.12.2 Pharmacogenomics for healthcare

The discipline of pharmacogenomics deals with the effect of genotype on individual drug responses with a view to improving the safety and efficacy of drug therapy. Its objective is to make drug discovery, development and delivery to patients more rational and efficient. It is still not very clear about its lofty goal of getting the right medicine, at the right dosage, to the patient will affect, and be affected by the regulatory and healthcare environment. The impact of pharmacogenomics on drug design, development and clinical trials has attracted considerable analysis, but very little effort has been directed at post-clinical trials. Pharmacogenomics interfaces with the regulatory and healthcare aspects in regard to liability and litigation. As the first products based on pharmacogenomics emerge, economic and regulatory considerations will affect and be affected by drug approval, licensing and delivery long before medicines are prescribed by physicians. The first treatments based on pharmacogenomics have now started appearing: Herceptin (Genentech, San Fransisco), is a monoclonal antibody that targets the protein product of the HER2 oncogene (also known as ERBB2) expressed in a subpopulation of breast cancer patients; Gleevec (Novartis, Basel) is designed to treat patients with chronic myeloid leukemia (CML) resulting form the so-called 'Philadelphia chromosome' translocation; and a test linking hypersensitivity reactions to the HIV/AIDS drug Abavacir (Glaxo SmithKline, Brenstfored) to the HLA B* 5701 haplotype.

1.12.3. Stratificaition

Pharmacogenomics poses a dilemma between directions towards a broad spectrum of effective, highly stratified personalized medicines and the fall in revenue resulting from market segmentation. One option is to consider an individual's response to medicines in terms of safety and/or efficacy. This 'patient' stratification can generate increased market size and revenue, while not requiring high research and development investment as a need for an entirely new drug; this makes it attractive from the perspective of regulators and industry. The other alternative involves subdividing illnesses, where patients with similar symptoms are prescribed different medicines depending on their molecular profile. Adoption of the second stratification scenario will raise the need to revamp the concept of the 'blockbuster' drug and to replace it with a number of 'minibusters'. It is also conceivable that pharmacogenomics may be channeled into the industry's tendency to develop "me-too" products, which offer incremental innovation over existing first-in-class medicines. Such products offset the high cost and probability of failure inherent in developing novel drugs, and have often generated price competition in a therapeutic category. But when genetic information can be connected with drug response data, me-toos would also be marketed as being particularly beneficial for a genetically defined subpopulation as departure from current norms.

1.12.4. The changing fortunes of pharmaceutical industry

In the pharmaceutical industry, high-throughput screening can assay many thousands of entities per day. Miniaturization and speed have increased but the numbers of high-quality leads anticipate has not materialized; even the rate of increasing such leads has not increased. If anything greater emphasis on numbers has virtually eliminated the most unique source of chemical diversity, natural products, from the playing field in favor of combinatorial chemistry. Nature does provide millions of new compounds, but it is quite difficult to harness and analyze this great resource of undiscovered chemistry by high-throughput screening. Combinatorial chemistry yields mainly minor modifications of present-day drugs, and in the absence of new scaffolds on which to build, it has not measured up to the task at hand.

No doubt, comparative genomics can reveal new targets for antimicrobials and other types of drugs, but the number of such potential targets is very large and it requires tremendous financial investments to set up all the screens necessary to exploit this resource. This can only be handled by a high- throughput screening methodology, which demands libraries of millions of chemical entities. Such targets are no doubt highly desirable for screening natural products but the industry has not exploited this opportunity and has rather opted to save funds by eliminating natural product departments or decreasing their relevance in the search for new drugs.

In the USA an increasing number of synthetic drugs have been recalled by the Food and Drug Administration because of toxicities and deaths occurring in patients after initial approval. In nature bacteria and other microbes produce thousands of novel and useful secondary metabolites whose structures are more spatially complex than those of synthetic chemicals. Microbial and plant secondary metabolites doubled our life span during the 20th century, reduced pain and suffering, and revolutionized medicine. Many of our approved drugs are either natural products or related to them even excluding biologicals, such as vaccines and monoclonal antibodies. Unfortunately the pharmaceutical industry has downgraded natural products just at the time when new assays and techniques are available for detection, characterization and purification of small molecules. With the advent of combinatorial biosynthesis, many of new derivatives can be made by a biological technique complementary to combinatorial chemistry. Also no more than about 10% of bacteria and fungi have been studied for secondary metabolites. New methods are being evolved to cultivate the so called "unculturable" microbes from the soil and sea. The selective action exerted on pathogenic bacteria and fungi by microbial secondary metabolites heralded the antibiotic era, and for several decades we have benefited from using antibiotics. But antimicrobial technology alone cannot permanently win the war against infectious microorganisms because of the development of resistance in pathogenic microbes. The search for new antibiotics must go on. New entities are continually needed as a result of the development of resistant pathogens, the existence of naturally resistant bacteria (e.g., *Pseudomonas aeruginosa,* many *enterococci, Burkholderia cepacia* and *Actinotobacter baumannii*), and the toxicity of some of the current compounds. There is increased incidence of infection by organisms that are not normally virulent but do infect immunocompromised patients. Fungal infections doubled from the 1980s to the 1990s. *Candidiasis, Cryptococcosis,* exceeds 60%. Fungal infections, usually by *Candida* and *Aspergillius* species, occur frequently after lung, kidney, heart, and liver transplant operations. Pulmonary aspergillosis can prove fatal for recipients of bone marrow transplants, and *Pneumocystis carnii* kills patients with AIDS form Europe and North America.

Current treatments include the synthetic azoles (such as fluconazole and flucytosine) or the natural polyene amphotericin B. But resistance can develop to the azoles and amphotericin B is quite toxic.

In recent years a major change has occurred in the discovery and application of secondary metabolites, broadening the scope of the search. Molecular biology has been applied to detect activities of compounds from microbes and plants for non-antibiotic applications. These include the cholesterol lowering statins (e.g., atrovastatin, preavastatin), anticancer agents (e.g., the microtubule) stabilizer (paclitaxel), immunosuppressants agents (e.g., avermectins and the polyethers) and bioherbicides (e.g., bialaphose). According to Demain, the future success of the drug industry will depend on the combination of complementary technologies, such as natural product discovery, high throughput screening, genomics, proteomics, and combinatorial chemistry. Between 1996 and 2000 several important shifts in public perception of risks and benefits of biotechnology occurred in Europe, USA and other regions.

Today, Europeans are much more negative about biotechnology than North Americans; and people respond more positively to medical biotechnology than to agricultural biotechnology. Mainstream media coverage of biotechnology has increased greatly in recent years. In 1991, 50% of Europeans surveyed believed that biotechnology would improve their lives and only 11% thought that it would make them worse. By 1999, the figures changed to 40% and 25% respectively. Over the past decade, press coverage of the fields was much higher in the United Kingdom than in other countries. Yet, during 1996, 52% of UK respondents admitted that they had never previously discussed biotechnology. By 1999, even after all the public concerns over cloning and GM foods, this figure actually rose to only 59%.

1.13. MOLECULAR ENGINEERING

Molecular engineering makes it possible to remove, insert, or substitute nucleotide sequences in target genes. The target gene is cloned. This if followed by site-specific deletion substitution or insertion of DNA obtained from other genes or synthesized *in vitro*. It is possible to construct promoters that ensure constitutive expression in specific hosts or tissues. Genetic engineering technology also has the potential to design a gene that is expressed to some predetermined level in specific subset of animal or even human cells. Molecular engineering also permits the tailoring of gene products required for specified needs. The engineered genes can be made to express by introducing the genes into cells either by themselves or in a vector. Some vectors allow the engineered gene to be inserted into a specific site in the target genome. Other vectors carry a gene that imparts to the recipient cell a selective advantage for growth in special media; these vectors furthermore may have DNA sequences that ensure that the gene is replicated along with the cellular genome. A third category of vectors (most viruses) are designed to introduce the engineered genetic engineering also involves specific deletion, replacement or insertion of DNA but by homologous recombination in cells rather than by construction *in vitro*. For instance insertional substitution or deletion proceeds by a double recombination event through the homologous flanking regions. From this it follows that viable recombinant genomes can arise only if the genome segments deleted or interrupted are dispensable with respect to replication and function.

1.13.1 Polymerase chain reaction

Polymerase Chain Reaction (PCR) is an extremely useful tool with many applications in molecular biology. Because of the potential to select and amplify sequences of DNA, starting with extremely small amount of DNA, the technique can revolutionize the manner in which molecular biology experiments are carried out. The PCR can be used in clinical genetics (including phenylketonuria screening, cystic fibrosis, Duchenne muscular dystrophy and Von Willebrand's disease). It also finds application in the study of highly polymorphic regions of the genome and for the detection of rare sequences (Fig. 1.10).

The PCR is based on the enzymatic amplification of a DNA fragment that is flanked by two oligonucleotide primers that hybridize to opposite strands of the target sequence. The primers are oriented with their 3' ends pointing towards each other. Repeated cycles of heat denaturation are given to the template. This is followed by annealing of the primers to their complementary sequences and given to the template. Annealing of the primers to their complementary sequences follows this and extension of the annealed primers with a DNA polymerase, resulting in the amplification of the segment defined by the 5'-ends of the PCR primers. The extension product of each primer serves as a template for the other primer consequently each cycle doubles the amount of the DNA fragment produced in the previous cycle. The result is an exponential accumulation of the specific target fragment up to several million folds within just a few hours. A modern version of PCR is "Ligation-mediated" PCR illustrated in Figure 1.11.

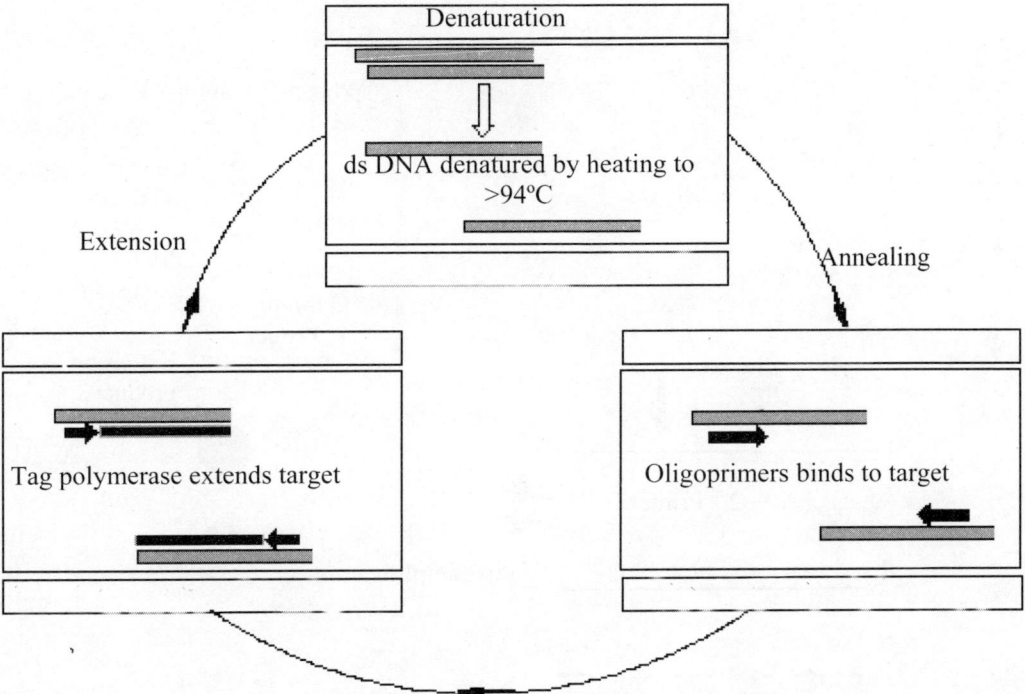

Fig. 1.10: A simplified scheme of one PCR cycle that involves denaturaion, annealing and extension

1.13.2. Ominous signs

The above account should not lead to the conclusion that the future must be bright for U.S. biotechnology. Some ominous signs have already emerged serious reservations about the commercialization of recombinant DNA research have been expresses. One of the reservations concerns the sharing of knowledge. Many see commercialization as breeding secrecy rather than scientific openness, and industrial sponsorship of academic research lead to reduce sharing of research results. Secondly many scientists believe that commercialist shifts the focus away from science and toward financial gain. This can erode the quality and status of basic research.

Collaboration with industry makes scientists gravitate towards research topics that promise patentable or practical results rather than basic scientific insight. There is genuine concern about the perceived trend toward secrecy and neglect of basic research in genetic engineering.

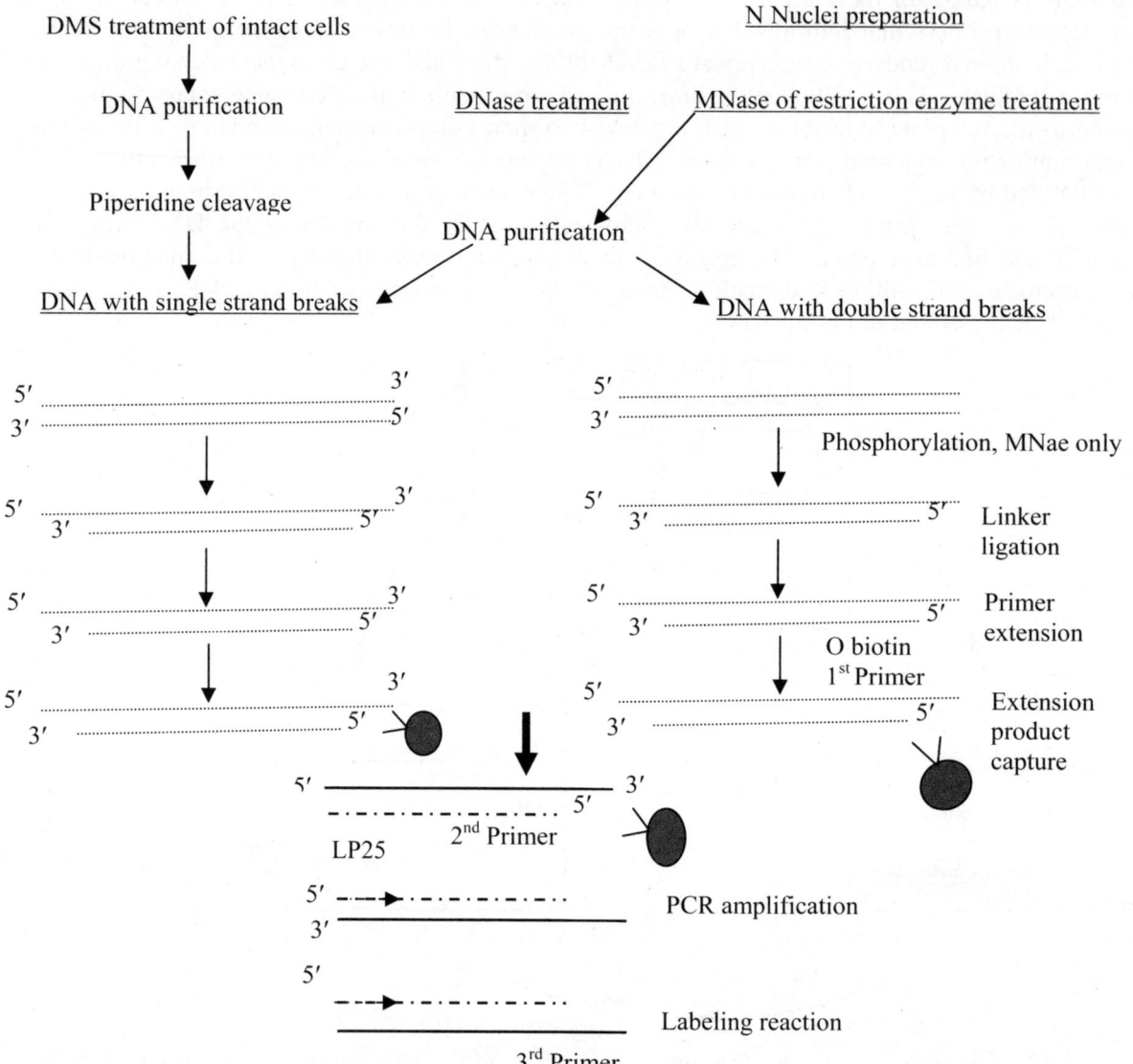

Fig. 1.11: Basic flow chart of ligation mediated-PCR describing various steps involved in the reaction

1.13.3. The fading great promise

Conceivably the greatest promise of medical biotechnology is its ability to reduce human suffering by eliminating genetic diseases such as Huntigton's disease, cystic fibrosis or sickle-cell anemia, not just for a given individual but for successive generations. Genetic repair that would have such an effect is called germ-line therapy. Such therapy is controversial but a best long-term goal of biotechnology. The majority of American scientists have voted in its favour, in various surveys. But there are obstacles to achieving this goal. One is purely financial lack of funding of basic biomedical research.

Successful germ-line therapy would go against the interests of the therapies for chronic diseases. Similar issues already have arisen in agricultural biotechnology where for instance, techniques to reduce pests by using genetically engineered seed lines have been seen to threaten future demand for pesticides. The outlook becomes dimmer in view of the shift to managed health care, which is likely to reduce funding for care and neglect the costs of medical education, vaccines or drug could possible stand up to such a short-term cost focus, but something as remote as germ-line therapy must fade into the dim future. Another obstacle to germ-line therapy is the science itself. Much effort will have to go into understanding possible long-term side effects on individuals and the species, as well as any selective benefits of inherited diseases. The greatest barriers are public resistance and the lack of rational public debate.

1.14. THE FUTURE OF BIOTECHNOLOGY

In recent years, the popular press has been filled with excitement, anxiety, and confusion about mammalian cloning. Many applications soon may be made possible by recombinant DNA technology, popularly called genetic engineering. It is no wonder; given the rapid advances in this field of research that genetic engineering is widely viewed as the science of the 21st century. But the risks involved in gene-splicing, let alone gene therapy or cloning, have led to controversy, activist pressures and litigation. A complex social climate is rapidly developing around genetic technology. The public perception about modern biotechnology differs significantly from one side of the Atlantic to the other; while there is growing optimism about public acceptance of biotechnology in the U.S.A., there is pessimism in Europe. Public attention is undoubtedly the ultimate driving force behind science and winning court battles.

SUGGESTED READING

- Arnold FH, Georgiou G, (Eds.). *Directed Enzyme Evolution: Screening and Selection Methods (Methods in Molecular Biology),* Humana Press (2003).
- Aird ELH, Hamill JD, Rhodes MJC. *Plant cell tissue organ cult* 15, 47 (1988).
- Arcamone MG. Una nuova iscrizione runica de Monte Sant "Angelo" In:(1992) *Vetena Christianorum.*, 29, 405 (1992).
- Matsiota-Bernard P, Roullet E, Ragimbeau J, *et al., Autoimmunity* 16, 237 (1993).
- Andersen B. *Sygeplejersken* 86, 4 (1986).
- Barinaga M. *Science* 262, 512 (1993).
- Berns K, Hijmans EM, Mullenders J, *et al., Nature* 428, 431 (2004).
- Birmingham K. *Nature Med* 7, 262 (2001).
- Broader S, Venter JC. *Annn Rev Pharmacol Toxicol* 40, 97 (2000).
- Bayley H. *Curr Opin Biotechnol* 10, 94 (1999).
- Bryan JA. *Arch Pathol Lab Med* 111, 1015 (1987).
- Caskey CT. *Hosp Pract* (Off Ed)., 22, 181- (1987).
- Couzin J. *Science* 299, 995 (2003).
- Cameotra SS, Makkar RS. *Appl Microbiol Biotechnol* 50, 520 (1998).
- Cooney JP. *Med Care* 23, 986 (1985).

- Chang YT. *J Natl Cancer Inst* 59, 1479 (1977).
- Cline TW. *Genetics* 96, 903 (1980).
- Clark M, King P, Buckley L., *et al.*, *Newsweek* 110, 62 (1987).
- Demain AL. *Nature Biotech* 20: 331 (2002).
- Farnsworth NR. Screening plants for new medicines. In *Biodiversity* (Wilson, E.O., ed.), National Academy Press, Washington, D.C. pp. 83 (1988).
- Fraser A. *Nature* 428, 375 (2004).
- Friedman M and Friedland G. W. Medicine's 10 Greatest Discoveries, Universities Press (1999).
- Gasker G, Bauer MW. (eds.) *Biotechnology: The Years of Controversy.* National Mus. Sci. and Industry, pp. 1996 (2001).
- Hodgson J. *Nature Biotech* 20, 1199 (2002).
- Haffner ME, Whitley J, Moses M. *Nat Rev Drug Discov* 1, 821 (2002).
- Hallman W. *Nature Biotech* 14, 35 (1996).
- Issa AM. *Nat Rev Drug Discov* 1, 300 (2002).
- Jacobsen EN, Pfaltz A, Yamamoto H. (Ed.s). *Comprehensive Asymmetric Catalysis.* Springer, New York (1999).
- Konarzycka-Bessler M, Bornscheuer UT. *Angew Chem Int Ed Engl* 42, 1418 (2003).
- Lasser *KE, et. al. JAMA* 287, 2215 (2002).
- Lindpaintner K. *Pharmacogenomics J* 1, 23 (2001).
- Lindpaintner K. *Nat Rev Drug Discov* 1, 463 (2002).
- Milen CP. *Nature Biotech* 20, 780 (2002).
- Movassaghi M, Jacobsen EN. *Science* 298, 1904 (2002).
- Norton RM. *Drug Discov Today* 6, 180 (2001).
- Northrup AB, MacMillan DWC. *J Am Chem Soc* 124, 6798 (2002).
- Paddison E. *et al., Nature* 428 (2004).
- Panke S, Wubbolts MG. *Curr Opin Biotechnol* 13, 111 (2002).
- Reetz MT. *Angew Chem Int Ed Engl* 40, 284 (2001).
- Reetz MT. *Angew Chem Int Ed Engl* 41, 1335 (2002).
- Reid H, Riggins GJ, Strausberg RL. *Hum Mol Genet* 10, 663 (2001).
- Robertson JA, Brody B, Buchanan A, Kahn J, McPherson E. *Health Aff* 21, 155 (2002).
- Rabino I. *Biotech Forum Europe* 9, 636 (1992).
- Rabino I. *American Scientist* 86, 110 (1998).
- Robert-Baudouy J, Condemine G. *Mol Microbiol* 5, 2191 (1991).
- Ron EZ, Rosenberg E. *Curr Opin Biotech* 13, 249 (2002).
- Ron EZ, Rosenberg E. *Environ Microbiol* 3, 229 (2001).
- Sato Y, Rifkin DB. *J Cell Biol* 109, 309 (1982)
- Strausberg RL, Schreiber SL. *Science* 300, 294 (2003).

- Sullenger BA, Cech TR. *Science* 262, 1566 (1993).
- Shoemaker HE *et al., Science* 299, 1694 (2003).
- Strathof AJJ *et al., Curr Opin Biotechnol* 13, 548 (2002).
- Sivakumaran TA, Kucheria K, Oefner PJ. *Current Science* 84, 291 (2003).
- Strausberg RL, Schreiber SL. *Science* 300, 294 (2003).
- Shah J. *Nature Biotechnol* 21, 747 (2003).
- Turner NJ. *Trends in Biotech* 21, 474 (2003).
- Tao H, Cornish VW. *Curr Opin Chem Biol* 6, 858 (2002).
- Tollman P, Guy P, Altshuler J, Flangan A, Steiner M. *A Revolution in R&D: How Genomics and Genetics are Transforming the Biopharmaceutical Industry.* The Boston Consulting Group, Boston (2001).
- Venter J. *el al. Science* 291, 1304 (2001).
- Veenstra DL, Higashi MK, Phillips KA. *AAPS Pharm Sci* 2, E29 (2000).
- Wolf CR, Smith G. *Br Mad Bull* 55, 366 (1999).
- Walters MJ. *Six Modern Plagues: And How We are Causing Them.* Island Press (2003).
- Yang NS. *CRC Crit Rev Biotechnol* 12, 335 (1992).
- Zhao H, Chockalingam K, Chenet Z. *Curr Opin Biotechnol* 13, 104 (2002).
- Lindpaintner K. *Pharmacogenomics J* 1, 23 (2001).
- Lindpaintner K. *Nat Rev Drug Discov* 1, 463 (2002).
- Lindpaintner K. *Br J Clin Pharmacol* 54, 221 (2002).
- Tollman P, Guy P, Altshuler J. *et al., Pharmacogenomics J* 1, 23 (2001).
- Norton RM. *Drug Discov Today* 6, 180 (2001).
- Snedden R. *Soc Sci Med* 48, 711 (1999).
- Shah J. *Nature Biotechnol* 21, 747 (2003).
- Issa AM. *Nat Rev Drug Discov* 1, 300 (2002).
- Wolf CR, Smith G. *Br Med Bull* 55, 366 (1999).
- Broder S, Venter JC. *Curr Opin Biotechnol* 11, 581 (2000).
- Spallone P, Wilkie T. *New Genetics & Society* 19, 193 (2000).
- Ward SJ. *Biotechniques* 31, 64 (2001).

ENZYMES

2.11. ENZYME INHIBITION

2.11.1. Irreversible inhibition

2.11.2. Reversible inhibition

2.11.3. Kinetic of competitive and non-competitive inhibition

2.12. REGULATION OF ENZYME ACTIVITY

2.12.1. Regulation of enzyme quantity

2.12.2. Availability of reactants

2.12.3. Regulation of catalytic efficiency

2.13. ALLOSTERIC ENZYMES

2.13.1. Effect of modulators

2.13.2. Model for allosteric enzymes

2.13.3. Kinetics of allosteric enzymes

2.14. ENZYME STABILITY

2.14.1. Stabilizing enzymes during storage

2.14.2. Enzyme inactivation during activity assays

2.15. ENGINEERING ENZYMES FOR STABILITY

2.15.1. Entropic stabilization factors

2.15.2. Enthalpic stabilization factors

2.16. ENZYME TECHNOLOGY AND BIOPROCESS ENGINEERING

2.16.1. Enzyme-catalyzed racemization

2.16.2. Enzymes in organic solvents

2.16.3. Control of water activity in process design

2.17. NANOSCALE BIOCATALYST SYSTEM

2.17.1. The perspectives of materials and methods

2.18. COMPUTATIONAL ENZYMOLOGY

2.19. FOOD PROCESSING ENZYMES FROM RECOMBINANT MICROORGANISMS

2.20. PHARMACEUTICAL APPLICATIONS

2.20.1. Diagnostic applications

2.20.2. Enzymes in therapeutics

2.21. ENZYMES IN BIOANALYTICAL CHEMISTRY

2.22. ENZYMES FOR THE TREATMENT OF EFFLUENTS

2.1. INTRODUCTION AND EARLY ENZYMOLOGY

While the ancients made much practical use of enzymatic activity, these early applications were based purely on empirical observations and folklore, rather than any systematic studies or appreciation for the chemical basis of the processes being utilized. In the eighteenth and nineteenth centuries scientists began to study the actions of enzymes in a more systematic fashion. The process of digestion seems to have been a popular subject of investigation during the years of the enlightenment. Wondering how predatory birds manage to digest meat without a gizzard, the famous French scientist Reaumur (1683—1757) performed some of the earliest studies on the digestion of buzzards. Reaumur designed a metal tube with a wire mesh at one end that would hold a small piece of meat immobilized to protect it from the physical action of the stomach tissue. He found that when a tube containing meat was inserted into the stomach of a buzzard, the meat was digested within 24 hours.

Thus he concluded that digestion must be a chemical rather than a merely physical process, since the meat in the tube had been digested by contact with the gastric juices (or, as he referred to them, ''a solvent''). He tried the same experiment with a piece of bone and with a piece of a plant. He found that while meat was digested, and the bone was greatly softened by the action of the gastric juices, the plant material was impervious to the ''solvent''; this was probably the first experimental demonstration of enzyme specificity. Reaumur's work was expanded by Spallanzani (1729—1799), who showed that the digestion of meat encased in a metal tube took place in the stomachs of a wide variety of animals, including humans. Using his own gastric juices, Spallanzani was able to perform digestion experiments on pieces of meat in vitro (in the laboratory). These experiments illustrated some critical features of the active ingredient of gastric juices: by means of a control experiment in which meat treated with an equal volume of water did not undergo digestion.

Spallanzani demonstrated the presence of a specific active ingredient in gastric juices. He also showed that the process of digestion is temperature dependent, and that the time required for digestion is related to the amount of gastric juices applied to the meat. Finally, he demonstrated that the active ingredient in gastric juices is unstable outside the body; that is, its ability to digest meat wanes with storage time. Today we recognize all the foregoing properties as common features of enzymatic reactions, but in Spallanzani's day these were novel and exciting findings. The same time period saw the discovery of enzyme activities in a large number of other biological systems. For example, a peroxidase from the horseradish was described, and the action of α-amylase in grain was observed. These early observations all pertained to materials—crude extracts from plants or animals—that contained enzymatic activity.

During the latter part of the nineteenth century scientists began to attempt fractionations of these extracts to obtain the active ingredients in pure form. For example, in 1897 Bertrand partially purified the enzyme laccase from tree sap, and Buchner, using the ''pressed juice'' from rehydrated dried yeast, demonstrated that alcoholic fermentation could be performed in the absence of living yeast cells. Buchner's report contained the interesting observation that the activity of the pressed juice diminished within 5 days of storage at ice temperatures. However, if the juice was supplemented with cane sugar, the activity remained intact for up to 2 weeks in the icebox. This is probably the first report of a now well-known phenomenon—the stabilization of enzymes by substrate. It was also during this period that Kuhne, studying catalysis in yeast extracts, first coined the term ''enzyme'' (the word derives from the Medieval Greek word enzymos, which relates to the process of leavening bread). Cell, the basic building block of living systems, effectively functions, utilizing enzymes, the biocatalysts, which are remarkable in their catalytic efficiency, and substrate as well as reaction specificity. Enzymes have extraordinary catalytic power and high degree of specificity for their substrate. They are functional units of cell metabolism. All the chemical reactions occurring in plants, micro-organisms and animals proceed at a measurable rate as a direct consequence of enzymatic catalysis.

Much of the history of biochemistry in a way is the history of enzyme research. Biological catalysis has been known for nearly 150 years. In 1837 Berzelius recognized that there were naturally occurring 'ferments' which promoted chemical reactions. Catalysis in biological systems was first recognized in the early 1800's from the studies of the digestion of meat by secretion of the stomach and the conversion of starch into sugar by saliva and various plant extracts. In 1850's Louis Pasteur concluded that fermentation of sugar into alcohol by yeast is catalyzed by '*ferments*'. He also postulated that these ferments are inseparable from the structure of yeast. These ferments were later named as *enzymes* (in yeast). The major landmark in the history of enzymes came in 1897 when Edward Buchner extracted the soluble active form from yeast cells and set of enzymes that catalysis the fermentation of sugar to alcohol. Emil Fischer carried out the first systematic studies on enzyme specificity in the early twentieth century. In 1926 James Sumner isolated *urease* in pure crystalline form from Jack beans. He also established the protein nature of urease. In 1930, John Northrop and his colleagues crystallized pepsin and trypsin and found them to be proteins.

Table 2.1: Chronology of enzyme studies

Name	Year	Work
Payen and Persoz	1833	Alcohol precipitation of thermolabile 'diastase' from malt
Berzelius	1835	Concept of catalysis
Berzelius	1837	Recognition of biological catalysis
Pasteur	1850	Fermentation of sugar into alcohol by yeast
Wilhelmy	1850	Quantitative evaluation of the rates of sucrose inversion
Kuhne	1878	Investigations of trypsin catalyzed reactions and introduction of word 'enzyme'
Fischer	1894-5	'Lock and Key' hypothesis of enzyme specificity
Bertrand	1896-7	Coenzyme or coferment (now known as cofactors)
Buchner	1897	Extraction of soluble active form of enzyme from yeast cells
Duclaux	1898	Nomenclature- substrate plus suffix 'ase'
Henri	1901-3	General procedures for the derivation of kinetic rate laws, principle of enzyme-substrate complex
Harden and Young	1906	Coezymase (NAD)
Michaelis and Menten	1913	Extension of the kinetic theory of enzyme catalysis
Briggs and Haldane	1925	Derivation of enzyme rate equations using the steady-state approximation
Sumner	1926	Crystallization of urease
Northrop and Kunitz	1930-3	Crystallization of proteolytic enzymes
Cori and Cori	1937-9	Muscle phosphorylase
Beadle and Tatum	1940	'One gene one enzyme' hypothesis
Chance	1943	Spectroscopic techniques
Koshland	1953	'Induced fit' hypothesis
Umbarger Yates, Pardee	1956	Control of enzyme activity through feedback inhibition
Sutherland	1956	Cyclic AMP adenyl cyclase
Anfinsen	1956-8	Amino acid sequence determines folding pattern and activity of ribonuclease
Jacob, Monod, and Changeux	1961	Allosterism
Phillips, Johnson, and North	1965	Three-dimensional structure of lysozyme obtained at 1.5A resolution

During the succeeding half century enzymology developed rapidly (Table 2.1). Some significant developments during this fruitful period are: elucidation of major metabolic pathways, for example glycolysis and tricarboxylic acid cycle; discovery of various biochemical events of digestion; muscular contraction; endocrine function; coagulation; and their roles in the maintenance, control and integration of complex metabolic processes; kinetic frameworks to rationalize the observations of enzyme action and inhibition; and development of procedures to analyze the structures of functionally sensitive proteins.

After this, intensive research started on the enzymes, enzyme catalyzed reactions, and enzymes involved in cell metabolism. Some 2000 different enzymes have been identified, each of which catalyzing a different chemical reaction. More recently, attention has increasingly been directed to the application of the enzymes. The high efficiency of enzymes makes them potentially valuable catalyst in industry and their specificity of action is providing benefits in clinical medicine.

2.2. THE DEVELOPMENT OF MECHANISTIC ENZYMOLOGY

As enzymes became available in pure or partially pure forms, scientists' attention turned to obtaining a better understanding of the details of the reaction mechanisms catalyzed by enzymes. The concept that enzymes form complexes with their substrate molecules was first articulated in the late nineteenth century. It is during this time period that Emil Fischer proposed the ''lock and key'' model for the stereo-chemical relationship between enzymes and their substrates; this model emerged as a result of a large body of experimental data on the stereo-specificity of enzyme reactions. In the early twentieth century, experimental evidence for the formation of an enzyme-substrate complex as a reaction intermediate was reported. One early study, reported by Brown in 1902, focused on the velocity of enzyme-catalyzed reactions. Brown made the insightful observation that unlike simple diffusion-limited chemical reactions, in enzyme-catalyzed reactions ''it is quite conceivable . . . that the time elapsing during molecular union and transformation may be sufficiently prolonged to influence the general course of the action.'' Brown then went on to summarize the available data that supported the concept of formation of an enzyme-substrate complex:

There is reason to believe that during inversion of cane sugar by invertase the sugar combines with the enzyme previous to inversion. C. O'Sullivan and Tompson have shown that the activity of invertase in the presence of cane sugar survives a temperature which completely destroys it if cane sugar is not present, and regard this as indicating the existence of a combination of the enzyme and sugar molecules. Wurtz (1880) showed that papain forms an insoluble compound with fibrin previous to hydrolysis. Moreover, the more recent conception of E. Fischer with regard to enzyme configuration and action also implies some form of combination of enzyme and reacting substrate.

Observations like these set the stage for the derivation of enzyme rate equations, by mathematically modeling enzyme kinetics with the explicit involvement of an intermediate enzyme-substrate complex. In 1903 Victor Henri published the first successful mathematical model for describing enzyme kinetics. In 1913, in a much more widely read paper, Michaelis and Menten expanded on the earlier work of Henri and redefined the enzyme rate equation that today bears their names. The Michaelis-Menten equation, or more correctly the Henri-Michaelis-Menten equation, is a cornerstone of much of the modern analysis of enzyme reaction mechanisms. The question of how enzymes accelerate the rates of chemical reactions puzzled scientists until the development of transition state theory in the first half of the twentieth century. In 1948 the famous physical chemist Linus Pauling suggested that enzymatic rate enhancement was achieved by stabilization of the transition state of the chemical reaction by interaction with the enzyme active site. This hypothesis, which was widely accepted, is supported by the experimental observation that enzymes bind very tightly to molecules designed to mimic the structure of the transition state of the catalyzed reaction.

In the 1950s and 1960s scientists reexamined the question of how enzymes achieve substrate specificity in light of the need for transition state stabilization by the enzyme active site. New hypotheses, such as the ''induced fit'' model of Koshland emerged at this time to help rationalize the competing needs of substrate binding affinity and reaction rate enhancement by enzymes. During this time period, scientists struggled to understand the observation that metabolic enzyme activities can be regulated by small molecules other than the substrates or direct products of an enzyme. Studies showed that indirect interactions between distinct binding sites within an enzyme molecule could occur, even though these binding sites were quite distant from one another. In 1965 Monod, Wyman, and Changeux developed the theory of allosteric transitions to explain these observations. Thanks in large part to this landmark paper; we now know that many enzymes, and non-enzymatic ligand binding proteins, display allosteric regulation.

2.3. NATURE OF ENZYMES

Enzymes are defined as soluble, colloidal, organic catalysts, which are produced by living cells, but are capable of acting independently of the cells. Enzymes behave as catalyst in small quantities relative to the concentration of their substrates. The total amount of substrate transformed per mass of enzyme is often very large. All enzymes are proteinaceous in nature without any exception and exhibit all properties of the protein. Disruption of characteristic folding of polypeptide chains of a native enzyme protein by extreme temperature and pH or by treatment with other denaturing agents results in total loss of catalytic activity. Thus primary, secondary, tertiary and quaternary structures of enzyme proteins are necessary for their catalytic activity. Their catalytic activity depends mainly upon the integrity of their structure as proteins. Enzymes have molecular weights ranging from about 12,000 to over 1 million. Furthermore, some enzymes consist only of polypeptides and contain two chemical groups other than amino acid residues, e.g. pancreatic ribonuclease.

Many enzymes require a specific, heat stable, low molecular weight organic molecule, a coenzyme. Furthermore, some enzymes require both a coenzyme and one or more metal ions for activity. A complete catalytically active enzyme consisting of the protein part together with the bound coenzyme or metal is known as holoenzyme. The protein part of an enzyme is referred to as apoenzyme. A coenzyme may bind covalently or non-covalently to the apoenzyme. In some enzymes the coenzyme or metal ion is only loosely and transiently bound to the protein but in others it is tightly and permanently bound, in which it is called a prosthetic group. Prosthetic group denotes a covalently bound coenzyme. Coenzymes and metal ions are stable on heating, whereas the protein part of an enzyme (apoenzyme) is denatured by heat.

Holoenzyme   =   Apoenzyme + Prosthetic group
(Total enzyme)   (Protein)   (Non-protein)

Prosthetic groups may be categorized functionally into two major classes, coenzymes and cofactors. The first may be considered biosynthetically related to the vitamins. For example, the coenzyme nicotinamide adenine dinucleotide (NAD) important for cellular energy metabolism incorporates the vitamin niacin into its chemical make up. In addition coenzyme may be regarded as co-substrate, undergoing a chemical trans-formation during the enzyme reaction (NAD is reduced to NADH) reversal of which requires a separate enzyme, possibly from different cellular location. They may therefore travel intracellularly between apoenzymes and by transferring chemical groupings integrate several metabolic processes. Table 2.2 lists the more common coenzymes and their functions.

Table 2.2: Coenzymes used in transfer of specific atoms or functional groups

Coenzyme	Entity transferred
Biotin	CO_2
Coenzyme A	Acyl groups
Flavin adenine dinucleotide	Hydrogen atoms (electrons)
5'-deoxyadenosylcobalamine (coenzyme B_{12})	H atoms and alkyl groups
Nicotinamide adenine dinucleotide	Hydrogen atoms (electrons)
Pyridoxal phosphate	Amino groups
Tetrahydrofolate	Other one carbon groups
Thiamine pyrophosphate	Aldehydes

Other enzymes, for example carboxypeptidase require metal ions as cofactors, the divalent cations Mg^{2+}, Zn^{2+}, Mn^{2+} being most common; these are often termed as enzyme *activators*. Table 2.3 lists various enzymes and their respective co-factors.

Table 2.3: Some enzymes and their cofactors

Enzyme	Cofactors	Enzyme	Cofactors
Arginase	Mn^{++}	Alcohol dehydrogenase	Zn^{++}
Carbonic anhydrase	Zn^{++}	Catalase	Fe^{++} or Fe^{+++}
Cytochrome oxidase	Cu^{++}	Cytochrome oxidase	Fe^{++} or Fe^{+++}
DNA polymerase	Zn^{++}	Glutathione peroxidase	Se
Glucose 6-phosphatase	Mg^{++}	Hexokinase	Mg^{++}
Nitrate reductase	Mo	Peroxidase	Fe^{++} or Fe^{+++}
Pyruvate kinase	K^+ and Mg^{++}	Urease	Ni^{++}

2.4. STRUCTURE OF ENZYMES

All enzymes act as catalysts and only small quantities relative to the concentrations of their substrate are needed to significantly increase the rate of chemical reactions, while they themselves undergo no net change. Like all true catalysts, an enzyme does not change the final equilibrium position of a reaction, which is thermodynamically determined, and only the *rate* of attainment of equilibrium of a feasible reaction is increased. In addition to their catalytic properties, enzymes exhibit the chemical and physical behavior of proteins, their electrolytic behaviors, solubility, electrophoretic properties and chemical reactivities. The catalytic activity of enzymes depends on the L-α-amino acid sequence and peptide bonds constituting the protein molecule (Fig. 2.1). Enzymes differ considerably from traditional chemical catalysts such as hydrogen ions, heavy metals or metal oxides. These are most effective in organic solvents, at very high temperatures or at extreme pH values; enzymes operate most efficiently under very mild conditions. Departure in terms of deviation from homogeneous aqueous solutions, physiological pH and temperature rapidly destroys their activities, but under normal conditions the increase in rate is rarely matched by their non-protein counterparts.

The linear chain of amino acid residues joined by peptide bonds which constitute a protein molecule is called the *primary structure*. Localized folding of the primary structure is referred to as *secondary structure* and the overall folding of the molecule is entitled *tertiary structure*. The agglomeration of the several folded chains is known as *quaternary structure*.

2.4.1. Primary and secondary structures

Three dimensional analysis of the amino acid sequence of hen's egg white lysozyme have illustrated several features inherent to primary structure. These are:

1. Molecules derived from the same source have similar order of amino acid residues and appear to be random with no obvious predictability.

2. Even though many enzymes are intramolecularly crosslinked through disulfide bridges of cysteine, no branching occurs.

There are indications that few of the amino acids are superfluous and most are 'functional', i.e., most co-operatively determine the higher orders of structural organization and hence the catalytic activity. On comparing the primary structures of enzymes performing similar functions, extensive structural homologies were observed in their sequence, particularly in the patterns of their non-polar residues. For example, pancreatic juice contains five inactive precursors (zymogens) viz. chymotrypsinogen A, B and C, trypsinogen and pro-elastase, all of which are activated to the respective proteases by proteolytic cleavage.

The overall folding of the amino acid sequence to give the functional enzyme appears to be unorganized, but on minute observation, it is seen that regions are organized into structures of definable symmetry (Fig. 2.2). For instance, residues 24–34 and 41–54 are folded into elements of secondary structure, α-helix and β-sheet respectively. These are named after the corresponding structures of the α- and β-keratins that were obtained by X-ray diffraction data of crystalline short polypeptides. The peptide bond was found to be shorter than the 0.14nm of a single carbon-nitrogen bond by approximately 0.001nm, and also had more double bond character. Rotation around this bond is restricted at normal temperatures, causing the peptide bond and the two adjacent α-carbon atoms to lie in one plane, with the carbonyl oxygen and amino hydrogen in the energy minimum of a *trans* configuration, as illustrated in Figure 2.1. Rotation can then only occur around those bonds close to the α-carbon atoms, and the possible types of stable structure, which maximize the number of hydrogen bonds, are restricted to the α-helix and β-plated sheet.

The sequence of the covalently linked amino acids is referred to as the primary level of structure for the protein. In writing the sequence of amino acids in a chain, it is conventional to orient the chain so that the amino acid on the left is the one with a free amino group on its carbon, while the last amino acid on the right is the one whose α-carbon carboxylate is free. In other words, the amino- or N-terminus of the peptide chain is written on the left, and the carboxylic C-terminus is written on the right. One more convention: the term "backbone" for a protein refers to the series of covalent bonds joining one α-carbon in a chain to the next α-carbon.

Secondary structure refers to regularities or repeating features in the conformation of the protein chain's backbone. Four major types of secondary structure in proteins are: (1) the Alpha (α) helix, formed from a single strand of amino acids; (2) the *beta* (β) sheet, formed from two or more amino acid strands (from either the same chain or from different chains); (3) the *beta* (β) bend or reverse turn, in a single strand; and (4) the collagen helix, composed of three strands of amino acids.

The overall folding of the polypeptide chain, which includes the organized secondary structure as well as random stretches, is attributed to the tertiary structure (Fig. 2.2). At present one of the most reliable and powerful methods to determine the three-dimensional structure of a protein, and in combination with the primary sequence, for portraying the relative stereochemical positions of the atoms is X-ray crystallography. X-rays are utilized because their wavelength and molecular dimensions in the protein crystal are of the same order of size.

The enzymes listed in Table 2.4 that catalyze dissimilar reactions possess unique tertiary structures, but several generalizations can be afforded due to the accumulated atomic details. In spite of the regional flexibility, all the compactly folded molecules have very little space inside to accommodate even small water molecules. This interior mainly consists of hydrophobic side chains (of leucine, phenylalanine, tryptophan, valine, etc.) and is surrounded by the polar amino acids (arginine, aspartic acid, etc.). The enzyme involved in catalyzing similar reaction types and possessing homology in their primary structures, especially in the sequence of their non-polar residues (the aggregation of which provides the driving force for protein folding) also possess three-dimensional homology. For instance, all the members of the serine proteases family have tertiary conformations with a common hydrophobic core.

2.4.2. Tertiary structure

A second type of localized three-dimensional homology that is not evident from amino acid sequence data has been observed with enzymes binding similar cofactors. For example, tertiary structures of dogfish-muscle lactate DH (dehydrogenase), horse-liver alcohol DH and lobster and *B. stearothermophilus* glyceraldehyde-3-phosphate DH, all of which require NADH as coenzymes, can be divided into separate domains, i.e., polypeptide regions associated with particular functions. The two domains being: a catalytic domain which is structurally unique to each individual enzyme and a coenzyme binding domain whose construction is remarkably similar to all. The coenzyme binding domain is comprised of six parallel strands of β-pleated sheet and four α-helices, and these are found arranged in the sequence β-α-β along the primary structure. The continuous amino acid sequences constituting the domain are however not located identically in the overall primary structures.

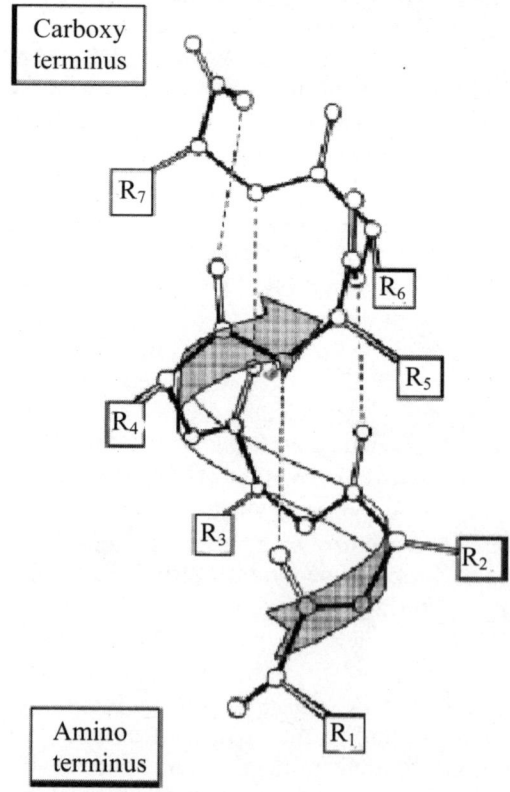

Fig 2.1: The alpha (α) helix, showing the pattern of intra-chain hydrogen bonds that stabilize the structure, and the radial extension of amino acid side chains from the helix axis

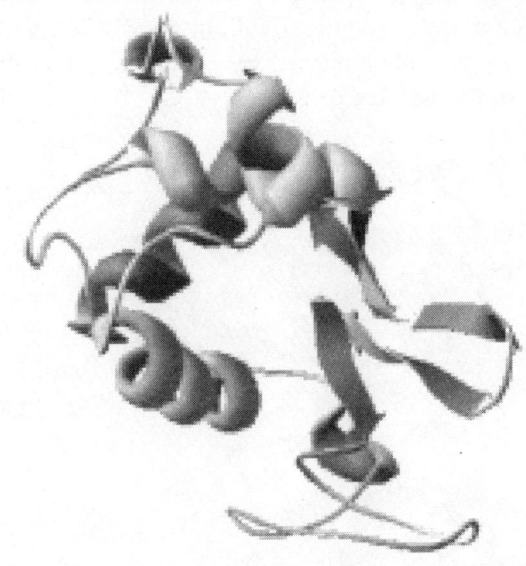

Fig. 2.2: The tertiary structure of hen egg white lysozyme, showing the packing of α helices and β sheet structures

Table 2.4: X-ray crystallography of enzymes

Enzyme	Source	Molecular weight	Resolution (A°)
Adenyl kinase	Porcine muscle	22,000	3
Alcohol dehydrogenase	Horse liver	80,000	2.9
Aspartate transcarbamoylase	*E.coli*	3,10,000	5.5
Cationic anhydrase B	Human erythrocytes	30,000	2.2
Cationic anhydrase C	Human erythrocytes	30,000	2
A- Chymotrypsin	Bovine pancreas	3,600	2, 2.8
Elastase	Porcine	25,900	3.5
Hexokinase	Yeast	51,000	2.3
Lysozyme	Bacteriophage T	18,800	2.5
	Hen's egg white	14,600	2
	Human	14,500	2.5
Papain	Papaya latex	23,000	2.8
Protease	*Rhizopus chinensis*	35,000	5.5
Pyruvate kinase	Cat muscle	2,40,000	6
Ribonuclease A	Bovine	13,600	2
Ribonuclease S	Bovine	13,600	2
Superoxide dismutase	Bovine	16,000	3, 5.5
B-Trypsin	Bovine pancreas	24,000	1.8, 2.7

2.4.3. Quaternary structure

Enzymes from intracellular origin generally also possess quaternary structure, which is an agglomeration of several units of tertiary structure. In these enzymes each of the contributing tertiary structure is termed a *subunit* or *monomer* and the complete complex as an oligomer, and a dimer, trimer, tetramer, etc. depending on the number of subunits it contains (Fig. 2.3). Oligomeric proteins are classified as *homologous* (containing identical subunits) and *heterologous* (containing different subunits). Quaternary structure cannot be stabilized by covalent bonds; on the contrary the subunits associate through combinations of the weaker forces.

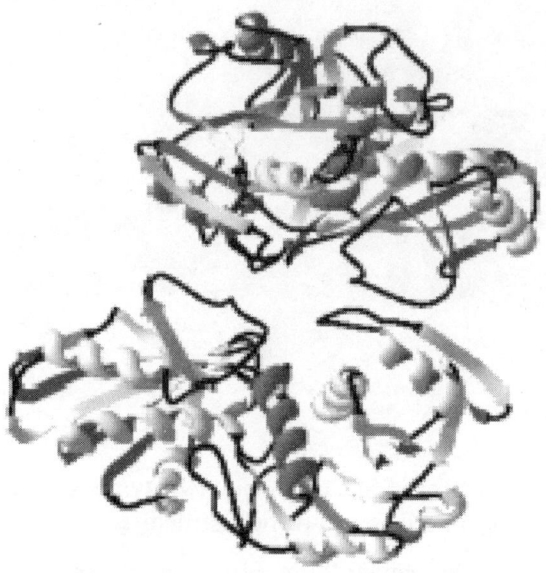

Fig.2.3: An example of quaternary structure: the dimer of
glycerol phosphate dehydrogenase from *E. coli*

2.5. ENZYMOLOGY TODAY

Fundamental questions still remain regarding the detailed mechanisms of enzyme activity and its relationship to enzyme structure. The two most powerful tools that have been brought to bear on these questions in modern times are the continued development and use of biophysical probes of protein structure, and the application of molecular biological methods to enzymology. X-ray crystallography continues to be used routinely to solve the structures of enzymes and of enzyme—ligand complexes. In addition, new NMR methods and magnetization transfer methods make possible the assessment of the three-dimensional structures of small enzymes in solution, and the structure of ligands bound to enzymes, respectively.

The application of Laue diffraction with synchrotron radiation sources holds the promise of allowing scientists to determine the structures of reaction intermediates during enzyme turnover, hence to develop detailed pictures of the individual steps in enzyme catalysis. Other biophysical methods, such as optical (e.g., circular dichroism, UV-visible fluorescence) and vibrational (e.g., infrared, Raman) spectroscopy, have likewise been applied to questions of enzyme structure and reactivity in solution. Technical advances in many of these spectroscopic methods have made them extremely powerful and accessible tools for the enzymologist. Furthermore, the tools of molecular biology have allowed scientists to clone and express enzymes in foreign host organisms with great efficiency. Enzymes that had never before been isolated have been identified and characterized by molecular cloning. Over-expression of enzymes in prokaryotic hosts has allowed the purification and characterization of enzymes that are available only in minute amounts from their natural sources. This has been a tremendous advance for protein science in general.

The tools of molecular biology also allow investigators to manipulate the amino acid sequence of an enzyme at will. The use of site-directed mutagenesis (in which one amino acid residue is substituted for another) and deletional mutagenesis (in which sections of the polypeptide chain of a protein are eliminated) have allowed enzymologists to pinpoint the chemical groups that participate in ligand binding and in specific chemical steps during enzyme catalysis. The study of enzymes remains of great importance to the scientific community and to society in general. We continue to utilize enzymes in many industrial applications. Moreover enzymes are still in use in their traditional roles in food and beverage manufacturing. In modern times, the role of enzymes in consumer products and in chemical manufacturing has expanded greatly. Enzymes are used today in such varied applications as stereospecific chemical synthesis, laundry detergents, and cleaning kits for contact lenses.

Perhaps one of the most exciting fields of modern enzymology is the application of enzyme inhibitors as drugs in human and veterinary medicine. Many of the drugs that are commonly used today function by inhibiting specific enzymes that are associated with the disease process. Aspirin, for example, one of the most widely used drugs in the world, elicits its anti-inflammatory efficacy by acting as an inhibitor of the enzyme prostaglandin synthase. Enzymes take part in a wide range of human pathophysiologies, and many specific enzyme inhibitors have been developed to combat their activities, thus acting as therapeutic agents. Several of the inhibitors are the result of the combined use of biophysical methods for assessing enzyme structure and classical pharmacology in what is commonly referred to as rational or structure-based drug design.

This approach uses the structural information obtained from x-ray crystallography or NMR spectroscopy to determine the topology of the enzyme active site. Next, model building is performed to design molecules that would fit well into this active site pocket. These molecules are then synthesized and tested as inhibitors. Several iterations of this procedure often lead to extremely potent inhibitors of the target enzyme. The list in Table 2.5 will continue to grow as our understanding of disease state physiology increases. There remain thousands of enzymes involved in human physiology that have yet to be isolated or characterized. As more and more disease-related enzymes are discovered and characterized, new inhibitors will need to be designed to arrest the actions of these catalysts, in the continuing effort to fulfill unmet human medical needs.

2.6. CLASSIFICATION AND NOMENCLATURE

A system of enzyme nomenclature that is comprehensive, consistent and at the same time easy to use has proved elusive. The common names for most enzymes derive from their most distinctive characteristic: their ability to catalyze a specific chemical reaction. In general, an enzyme's name consists of a term that identifies the type of reaction catalyzed followed by the suffix -*ase*. For example, dehydrogenases remove hydrogen atoms, prote*ases* hydrolyze proteins, and isomerases catalyze rearrangements in configuration. One or more modifiers usually precede this name. Unfortunately, while many modifiers name the specific substrate involved (xanthine oxidase), others identify the source of the enzyme (pancreatic ribonuclease), specify its mode of regulation (hormone-sensitive lipase), or name a distinguishing characteristic of its mechanism (a cysteine protease). When it was discovered that multiple forms of some enzymes existed, alphanumeric designators were added to distinguish between them (e.g., RNA polymerase III; protein kinase Cβ). To address the ambiguity and confusion arising from these inconsistencies in nomenclature and the continuing discovery of new enzymes, the International Union of Biochemists (IUB) developed a complex but unambiguous system of enzyme nomenclature. In the IUB system, each enzyme has a unique name and code number that reflect the type of reaction catalyzed and the substrates involved.

Table 2.5: Examples of enzyme inhibitors as potential drugs

Inhibitor/Drug	Disease/Condition	Enzyme Target
Acetazolamide	Glaucoma	Carbonic anhydrase
Acyclovir	Herpes	Viral DNA polymerase
Allopurinol	Gout	Xanthine oxidase
Argatroban	Coagulation	Thrombin
Aspirin, ibuprofen,	Inflammation, pain, fever	Prostaglandin synthase
β- Lactam antibiotics	Bacterial infections	D-Ala-D-Ala transpeptidase
Brequinar	Organ transplantation	Dihydroorotate dehydrogenase
Candoxatril	Hypertension, congestive heart failure	Atriopeptidase
Captopril	Hypertension	Angiotensin-converting enzyme
Clavulanate	Bacterial resistance	β- Lactamase
Cyclosporin	Organ transplantation	Cyclophilin/calcineurin
DuP450	AIDS	HIV protease
Enoximone	Congestive heart failure ischemia	cAMP phosphodiesterase
Nitecapone	Parkinson's disease	Catechol-O-methyltransferase
Norfloxacin	Urinary tract infections	DNA gyrase
Omeprazole	Peptic ulcers	$H^+ K^+$-ATPase

2.6.1. Enzyme commission numbers

The ultimate identification of a particular enzyme is possible through its Enzyme Commission (E.C.) number.2 The assignment of E.C. numbers is described in guidelines set out by the International Union of Biochemistry, and follows the format E.C. w.x.y.z, where numerical values are substituted for w, x, y and z. The value of w is always between 1 and 6, and indicates one of six main divisions; values of x indicate the sub-classification, and are often related to either the prosthetic group or the cofactor required for the reaction; values of y indicate a sub classification, related to a substrate or product family; and the value of z indicates the serial number of the enzyme.

Enzymes are grouped into six classes, each with several subclasses. For example, the enzyme commonly called "hexokinase" is designated "ATP:D-hexose-6-phosphotransferase E.C. 2.7.1.1." This identifies hexokinase as a member of class 2 (transferases), subclass 7 (transfer of a phosphoryl group), sub-subclass 1 (alcohol is the phosphoryl acceptor). Finally, the term "hexose-6" indicates that the alcohol phosphorylated is that of carbon six of a hexose. Listed below are the six IUB classes of enzymes and the reactions they catalyze.

1. Oxidoreductases catalyze oxidations and reductions.

2. Transferases catalyze transfer of groups such as methyl or glycosyl groups from a donor molecule to an acceptor molecule.

3. Hydrolases catalyze the hydrolytic cleavage of C.C, C.O, C.N, P.O, and certain other bonds, including acid anhydride bonds.

4. Lyases catalyze cleavage of C.C, C.O, C.N, and other bonds by elimination, leaving double bonds, and also add groups to double bonds.

5. Isomerases catalyze geometric or structural changes within a single molecule.

6. Ligases catalyze the joining together of two molecules, coupled to the hydrolysis of a pyrophosphoryl group in ATP or a similar nucleoside triphosphate.

2.7. COFACTORS IN ENZYMES

The structures of the 20 amino acid side chains can confer on enzymes a vast array of chemical reactivities. Often, however, the reactions catalyzed by enzymes require the incorporation of additional chemical groups to facilitate rapid reaction. Thus to fulfill reactivity needs that cannot be achieved with the amino acids alone, many enzymes incorporate non-protein chemical groups into the structures of their active sites. These non-protein chemical groups are collectively referred to as enzyme cofactors or coenzymes. In most cases, the cofactor and the enzyme associate through non-covalent interactions (e.g., H-bonding, hydrophobic interactions). In some cases, however, the cofactors are covalently bonded to the polypeptide of the enzyme. For example, the haeme group of the electron transfer protein cytochrome C, is bound to the protein through thioester bonds with two modified cysteine residues. Another example of covalent cofactor incorporation is the pyridoxal phosphate cofactor of the enzyme aspartate aminotransferase. Here the cofactor is covalently linked to the protein through formation of a Schiff base with a lysine residue in the active site.

In enzymes requiring a cofactor for activity, the protein portion of the active species is referred to as the apoenzyme, and the active complex between the protein and cofactor is called the holoenzyme. In some cases the cofactors can be removed to form the apoenzyme and be added back later to reconstitute the active holoenzyme. In some of these cases, chemically or isotopically modified versions of the cofactor can be incorporated into the apoenzyme to facilitate structural and mechanistic studies of the enzyme. Cofactors fulfill a broad range of reactions in enzymes. One of the more common roles of enzyme cofactors is to provide a locus for oxidation/reduction (redox) chemistry at the active site. An illustrative example of this is the chemistry of flavin cofactors. Flavins (from the Latin word *flavius*, meaning yellow) are bright yellow cofactors common to oxidoreductases, dehydrogenases, and electron transfer proteins. The main structural feature of the flavin cofactor is the highly conjugated isoalloxazine ring system. Oxidized flavins readily undergo reversible two-electron reduction to 1,5-dihydroavin, and thus can act as electron sinks during redox reactions within the enzyme active site. For example, a number of dehydrogenases use flavin cofactors to accept two electrons during catalytic oxidation of NADH. Alternatively, flavins can undergo discrete one-electron reduction to form a semiquinone radical; this can be further reduced by a second one-electron reduction reaction to yield the fully reduced cofactor. Through this chemistry, flavin cofactors can participate in one-electron oxidations, such as those carried out during respiratory electron transfer in mitochondria. There are actually two stable forms of the flavin semiquinone that interconvert, depending on pH. The blue neutral semiquinone occurs at neutral and acidic pH, while the red anionic semiquinone occurs above pH 8.4. Both forms can be stabilized and observed in certain enzymatic reactions. Additional chemical versatility is demonstrated by flavin cofactors in their ability to form covalent adducts with substrate during redox reactions. The oxidation of dithiols to disulfides by the active site flavin of glutathione reductase is an example of this. Here the thiolate anion adds to the C4a carbon of the isoalloxazine ring system. Likewise, in a number of flavoenzyme oxidases, catalytic reoxidation of reduced flavin by molecular oxygen proceeds with formation of a transient C4a peroxide intermediate. A variety of other cofactors participate in the catalytic chemistry of the enzyme active site. Some additional examples of these are listed in Table 2.6.

Table 2.6: Some examples of cofactors found in enzymes

Cofactor	Enzymatic use	Examples of enzyme
Copper ion	Redox center-ligand binding	Cytochrome oxidase, Superoxide dismutase hosphodiesterases.
Magnesium ion	Active site electrophile Phosphate binding	ATP synthases, Matrix metalloproteases
Zinc ion	Active site electrophile Redox center-proton transfer, Redox center-ligand binding	Carboxypeptidase A, Glucose oxidase Succinate dehydrogenase
Hemes	Amino group transfer, stabilizer of intermediate	Cytochrome oxidase, cytochrome P450s, alcohol dehydrogenase, ornithine cyclase
NAD and NADP	Carbanions	Aspartate transaminase, arginine
Pyridoxal phosphate	Acyl group transfer	Racemase, pyruvate dehydrogenase

2.8. FACTORS AFFECTING ENZYME ACTION

An enzyme is a catalyst and it greatly enhances the rate of a specific chemical reaction. Enzymes cannot change the equilibrium of a reaction, i.e., an enzyme accelerates the forward and backward reaction by precisely the same factor. Enzymes accelerate the attainment of equilibrium but do not shift their position. A chemical reaction of substrate S to form product P goes through a transition state S* that has a higher free energy than either S or P.

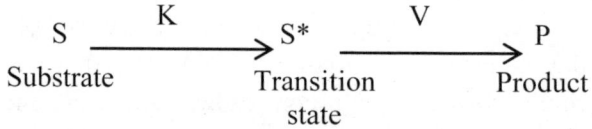

$$S \xrightarrow{\ \ K\ \ } S^* \xrightarrow{\ \ V\ \ } P$$

Substrate   Transition   Product
                   state

The transition state is the most seldom occupied species along the reaction pathway because it has the highest free energy. The activation energy of a reaction is the amount of energy in calories required to bring all the molecules in 1 M of a substance at a given temperature to the transition state at the top of the energy barrier, i.e., the Gibb's free energy of activation [G*] which is equal to the difference in free energy between the transition state and the substrate (Fig. 2.4). The rate of any chemical reaction is therefore proportional to the concentration of the transition state of species, which depends on G* because it is in equilibrium units.

There are two general ways in which the rate of a chemical reaction can be increased:

1. By increasing the temperature which increases the concentration of transition state species

2. By adding catalyst: Catalysts accelerate chemical reactions by finding a lower 'pass' over the energy barrier. The catalyst [C], combines transiently with the reactant [A] to produce a new complex [CA] whose transition state has a much lower energy of activation than the transition state

of [A] reactant molecule in uncatalyzed state (Fig. 2.4). The [CA] complex then reacts to form the product [P], releasing the free catalyst, which can then combine with another molecule of [A] to repeat the cycle.

2.8.1. Effect of substrate concentration

The effect of varying the substrate concentration on the initial rate of an enzyme-catalyzed reaction when enzyme concentration is held constant could be followed in the figure 2.5. At very low concentration of substrate the rate of reaction is very slow, but increases with an increase in substrate concentration. The rate of enzyme-catalyzed reaction however does not increase beyond a certain concentration of the substrate. No matter how high the substrate concentration is raised beyond this point, the reaction rate will tend to approach but never reach a plateau. At this plateau, called the maximum rate (V_{max}), the enzyme is 'saturated' with its substrate and can function no faster.

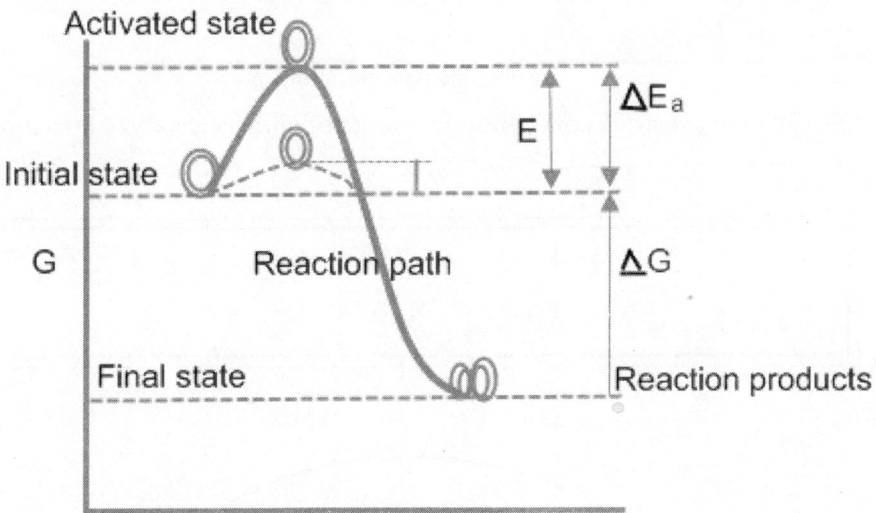

Fig. 2.4: Energy curve for catalyzed and uncatalyzed reactions

This saturation effect is exhibited by nearly all enzymes. It led Victor Henri to the conclusion (in 1903) that an enzyme combines with its substrate molecule to form an enzyme substrate complex.

$$E + S \rightarrow ES$$

The ES complex then breaks down through a second reversible reaction, which is slower to yield the reaction product P and the free enzyme E.

$$ES \rightarrow E + P$$

Since the second reaction is the rate limiting step, the overall rate of the enzyme catalyzed reaction must be proportional to the concentration of the enzyme-substrate complex. At any given point of time in an enzyme catalyzed reaction the enzyme exists in two forms, the free or uncombined form [E] and the combined or complexed form [ES]. The rate of the catalyzed reaction is maximum when virtually the entire enzyme is present as the [ES] complex and the concentration of free enzyme [E] vanishes to lowest. This condition may possibly exist at a very high concentration of the substrate (Fig. 2.6).

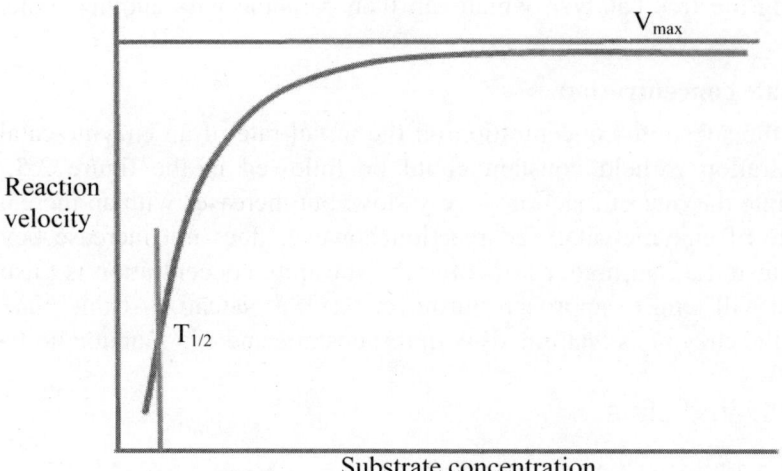

Fig. 2.5: Effect of substrate concentration on rate of enzyme catalyzed reaction

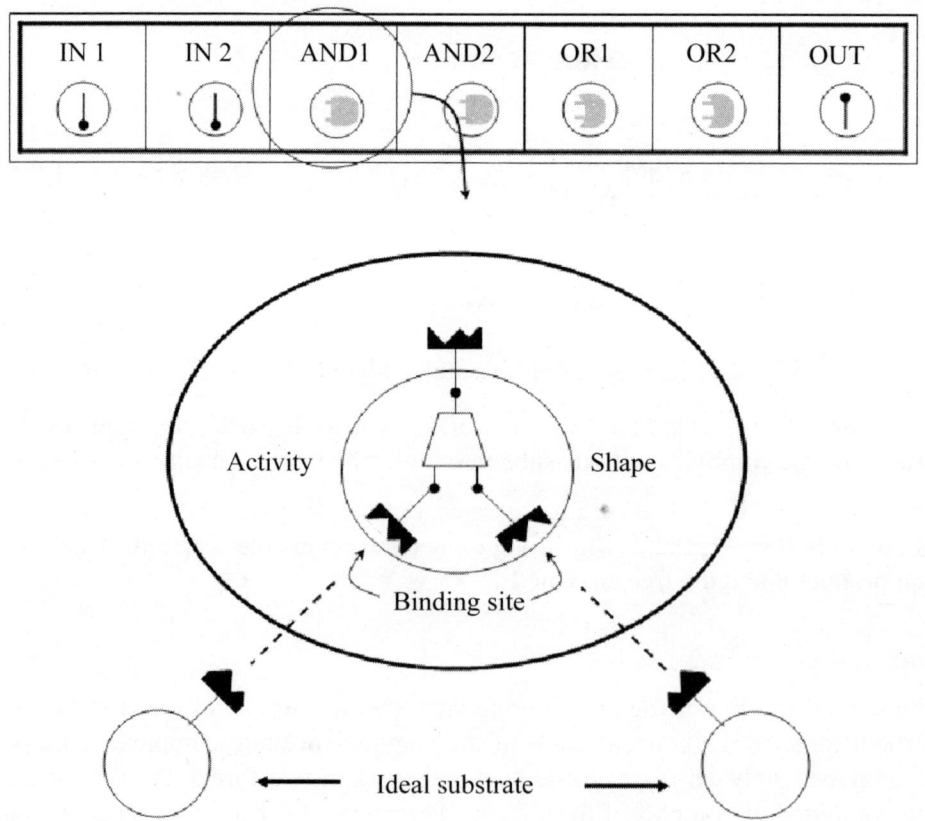

Fig. 2.6 Ideal substrate is the requisite for optimum enzyme activity

Derivation of Michaelis-Menten Enzyme Kinetics

The derivation of equation occurs at a time when the rate of formation of ES complex is equal to rate of destruction (break down), i.e., at equilibrium, when [S] >>>> [E] so that total E is bound in ES complex and reaction works like a 1st order reaction enzyme catalyzed reaction.

The rate limiting equation thus becomes $v = (dP/dt) = k_3 [ES]$

It would be easy if we could measure the concentration of [ES], say in a spectrophotometer but, its presence is fleeting. So then the real purpose of the derivation of M&M kinetics is to be able to express [ES] in terms of E & S alone, which are measurable, but measuring [ES] is very difficult.

Derivation of Michaelis-Menten Equation

$$E + S \underset{k_2}{\overset{k_1}{\rightleftarrows}} ES \underset{k_4}{\overset{k_3}{\rightleftarrows}} E + P$$

Rate limiting step is $\Delta P/\Delta t = k_3 [ES]$ (& $\Delta P/\Delta t = v$)

1. Rate of formation of ES complex $\Delta ES /\Delta t = k_1 [E_T - ES] [S]$

2. Rate of destruction ES complex $\Delta ES /\Delta t = (k_2 + k_3) [ES]$

3. Steady State Equilibrium $k_1 [E_T - ES] [S] = (k_2 + k_3) [ES]$

4. Michaelis Constant (K_m) $\dfrac{(k_2 + k_3)}{(k_1)} = \dfrac{[E_T - ES] [S]}{[ES]}$

$$K_m = \frac{(k_2 + k_3)}{(k_1)} = \frac{[E_T - ES] [S]}{[ES]}$$

5. Solve for [ES] $[ES] = \dfrac{[E_T] [S]}{(K_m) + [S]}$

6. Substitute in above $\Delta P/\Delta t = k_3 [ES]$ $v = \dfrac{k_3 [E_T] [S]}{(K_m) + [S]}$

7. Substitute V_{max} for $k_3 [E_T]$ $v = \dfrac{V_{max} [S]}{K_m + [S]}$

K_m - the Michaelis Constant

- Is a constant that is independent of [S] or [E]
- Is a mathematical interpretation of an enzyme action
- Is the substrate concentration when enzyme velocity is equal to ½ V_{max}
- Km is a characteristic physical property for each and every different enzyme
- It measures "*relative afffinity*" of an enzyme for its substrate
- Suppose there's more than 1 substrate for an enzyme [phosphatases], then each has its own K_m e.g. one enzyme with 2 substrates each with following Km's - 0.3 M & 2.0 M thus, one takes more substrate to reach same rate (½ V_{max} rate)
- Many enzymes have individual steps in a complex reaction sequence; each step has its own Km's i.e., K_m is a complex function of many individual rate constants
- Not all enzymes are treatable by M & M kinetics.
- Most regulatory enzymes (multi-subunits) are not treatable by M&M kinetics

Table 2.7: pH optima and Michaelis constants for some enzymes

Enzyme	Source	Substrate	pH optimum	K_m
Amylase	Saliva and pancreas	Starch	6.0-7.0	0.8-0.25%
Carboxylase	Yeast	α-Keto acids	4.8	0.01M for pyruvic acid
Catalase	Liver	H_2O_2	6.3-9.5	0.025M
Dipeptidase	Intestine	Dipeptides	7.3-8.1	0.02-0.07 M for glycyl-leucine
Lipase	Pancreas	Ethyl butyrate	7.0	>0.03 M in phosphate buffer
Phosphatase	Bone	Glycero-phosphate	5.5	0.09 M
Pepsin	Stomach	Various proteins	1.5-2.5	4.5 % for ovalbumin
Saccharase	Mammalian intestine	Sucrose	6.2	0.02 M
Urease	Soybean	Urea	7.2-7.9 ca.	0.025 M

2.8.2. Concentration of enzyme

The rate of an enzyme catalyzed reaction measured during initiation is directly proportional to the concentration of enzyme. The initial rate of a reaction is the rate measured when almost no substrate has been reacted to form the product and permits the reverse reaction to occur. The enzyme [E] combines with substrate [S] forming an **enzyme-substrate complex [ES]**, which decomposes to form a product, [P], and free enzyme.

$$E + S \rightleftharpoons ES \rightleftharpoons E + P$$

or

$$E + S \rightleftharpoons E + P$$

Rate of forward reaction: $Rate_1 = k_1 [E] [S]$

Rate of backward reaction: $Rate_2 = k_2 [E] [P]$

where k_1 and k_2 are the rate constants for the forward and backward reaction respectively.

The overall equilibrium constant $K_{eq} = \dfrac{k_1}{k_2} = \dfrac{[E][P]}{[E][S]} = \dfrac{[P]}{[S]}$

The enzyme concentration thus has no effect on the equilibrium constant. Impure pepsin and trypsin show reaction velocities more nearly proportional to the square root of the enzyme concentration. Northrop demon-stated that highly purified pepsin does digest protein (within limits) at a rate that is almost proportional to its concentration. In the presence of increased concentration of reaction products this linear relationship may not hold.

2.8.3. Concentration of reaction products

The addition of products of enzyme reaction to a system containing purified enzyme destroys the linear relationship between enzyme concentration and reaction rate. Thus if peptic digestion products are added to a system in which purified pepsin is hydrolyzing protein, the rate of reaction is similar to the rate obtained with a crude pepsin preparation. Addition of either glucose or fructose inhibits the hydrolysis of 2% sucrose by yeast invertase. This could be due to formation of a more stable complex of enzyme and reaction products than of enzyme and substrate, which obstructs the active centers of a certain proportion of the enzyme molecules. It is also assumed that, in the presence of high concentrations of reaction products some re-synthesis by enzyme may occur; that would result in an apparent decrease in the rate of decomposition.

2.8.4. pH

The activity of an enzyme is determined usually by the pH of the system in which it operates. Each enzyme has an optimum pH i.e., a $[H^+]$ concentration at which the enzyme reacts at maximum level. The optimum pH changes with varying conditions of time, temperature, concentration of substrate, or other factors (Table 2.7). Moderate pH changes affect the ionic state of the enzyme and frequently that of substrate also. When enzyme activity is measured at several pH values, optimal activity is generally observed between pH 5.0 and 9.0. However, a few enzymes, e.g., pepsin, are active well outside this range.

The pH-activity curve is bell-shaped (Fig. 2.7) and is governed by the following factors:

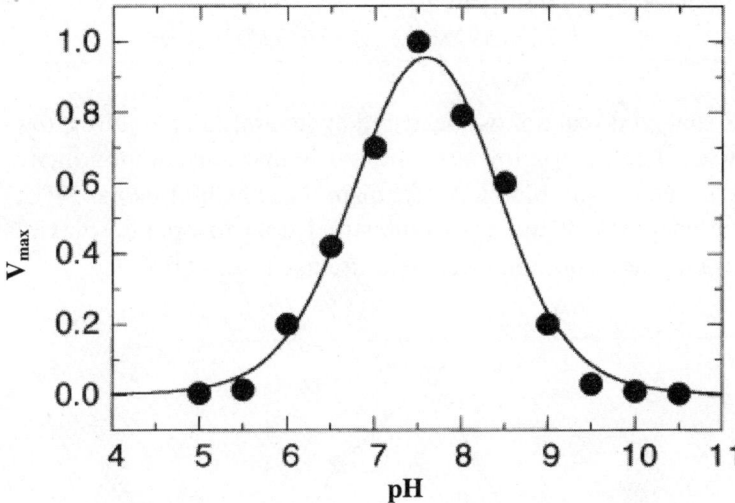

Fig. 2.7: The effects of pH on the velocity of a typical enzymatic reaction

1. Denaturation of enzyme at extremely high or low pH values.

2. Effect on the charged state of substrate or enzyme.

In the case of an enzyme, the charge changes may affect activity either by changing structure or by changing the charge on an amino acid residue that is functional in substrate-binding or catalysis. If a negatively charged enzyme $[E^-]$ reacts with a positively charged substrate $[S^+]$ then at low pH values $[E^-]$, will get protonated and would lose its negative charge. Similarly, at very high pH values, $[S^+]$ will ionize to lose its positive charge. Since the only forms that will interact are $[S^+]$ and $[E^-]$, extreme pH values will lower the reaction velocity as shown in Figure 2.7 (bell shaped curve of pH-enzyme activity). Only the area under the curve for both [E] and [S] in the appropriate ionic state, and the maximal concentration of [E] and [S] are correctly charged at X. The result is the bell-shaped pH-activity curve.

2.8.5. Temperature

Chemical reactions, both catalyzed and noncatalyzed proceed at a faster rate as the reaction temperature is increased. This is true of enzymatically catalyzed reactions. In general only up to

50°C. Above this temperature heat denaturation of enzymes starts. In a few exceptional cases, the speed of reaction slows and ceases at or around temperature 70°C to 80°C. The exact ratio by which the velocity changes for a 10°C rise is the Q_{10}, or temperature coefficient. The velocity (V_o) of many biologic reactions roughly doubles with a 10°C rise in temperature ($Q_{10} = 2$), and is halved if the temperature is decreased by 10°C. The Q_{10} values for few enzymes are listed in Table 2.8.

Table 2.8: Q_{10} values for some enzymes

Enzyme	Q_{10} value
Catalase	2.3 (0–10°), 2.19 (10–20°)
Urease	1.81 (20–30°), 1.90 (30–40°)
Maltase (Yeast)	1.90 (10–20°), 1.44 (20–30°), 1.28 (30–40°)
Succinic oxidase	2.0 (30–40°), 2.1 (40–50°)
Invertase	1.76 (15–25°), 1.62 (25–35°)

When the rate of enzyme-catalyzed reaction is measured at several temperatures, the results shown in Fig. 2.8 come to be typical. For most enzymes, optimal temperature approximates those of the environment of the cell. For the warm blooded organism i.e., man, this is 37°C. The optimal temperature for the digestive enzymes of the gastro-intestinal tract to operate maximally is around 40°C. Certain plant enzymes may have optimum temperature as high as 60°C.

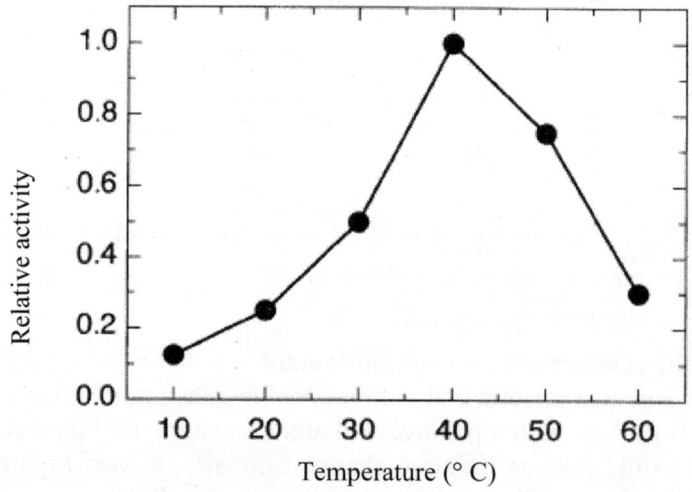

Fig. 2.8: Effect of temperature on the rate of the enzyme catalyzed reaction

The increase in the rate below optimal temperature results from the increased kinetic energy of the reacting molecules. As the temperature is raised still further, the kinetic energy of the enzyme molecule becomes so high that it exceeds the energy barrier in order to break the secondary bonds that hold the enzyme in its native or catalytically active form. However, simultaneously there is a loss of secondary and tertiary structures and a parallel loss of biological activity.

2.8.6. Time

For an enzyme catalyzed reaction, an optimum pH or an optimum temperature can not be independent of time. For example the optimum temperature of many enzymes from warm blooded animals is approximately 37°C only if the time is measured in hours; if time is measured in days, the optimum temperature may be much lower; further, if the time is measured in minutes, perhaps the optimum temperature could be as high as 70°C or above.

2.8.7. State of oxidation of enzyme

Enzymes containing sulfhydryl groups are activated by certain reducing agents and inactivated by aeration or other mild oxidizing treatments. Representative examples of this class are papain, urease and succinic dehydrogenase. Glutathione, cysteine, hydrogen sulfide, and HCN activate these enzymes. Such activation might be accounted for the removal of inactivating heavy metal ions. Recent studies suggested that actual reduction of disulfide linkage (-S-S-) in the enzyme molecules to sulfhydryl (-SH) groups may be responsible for the activation.

2.8.8. Activators

Many ions and molecules have the capacity to activate some enzymes. Metals ions are activators of a number of enzymes (Table 2.3). Pepsin (as proenzyme pepsinogen) is activated by H^+ to form the active enzyme. Many reducing agents (cysteine, glutathione) act as enzyme activators of enzyme containing sulfhydryl groups. Enzyme themselves activate other enzymes or proenzymes; e.g., enterokinase activates trypsinogen to form active trypsin. Trypsinogen, pepsinogen and chymotrypsinogen, are such enzymes known as *zymogens*.

2.8.8.1. Zymogen activation

Zymogen activation involves the hydrolysis of uniquely located peptide bond in the zymogen molecule. In bovine and porcine trypsinogen the primary activation involves the hydrolysis (by trypsin) of a lysyl-isoleucine bond which liberates an amino terminal hexapeptide in the bovine (Val-Asp_4-Lys) and an amino terminal octapeptide (Phe-Pro-Thr-Asp_4-Lys) in the porcine variety, with the subsequent liberation of active enzyme in either of case. Zymogen activation involves the procarboxypeptidase A which occurs in the pancreas in two forms which can be easily separated into larger form (S6) of molecular weight 87,000 and the smaller (S3) form of molecular weight 64,000. Activation of the S6 form with trypsin led to fractions with different catalytic activities; one fraction was an endopeptidase and the other a carboxypeptidase.

2.9. HOW ENZYMES WORK

The enzymatic catalysis of reactions is essential to living systems. Under biologically relevant conditions, uncatalyzed reactions tend to be slow—most biological molecules are quite stable in the neutral-pH, mild temperature, aqueous environment inside cells. Furthermore, many common reactions in biochemistry entail chemical events that are unfavorable or unlikely in the cellular environment, such as the transient formation of unstable charged intermediates or the collision of two or more molecules in the precise orientation required for reaction. Reactions required to digest food, send nerve signals, or contract a muscle simply do not occur at a useful rate without catalysis.

An enzyme circumvents these problems by providing a specific environment within which a given reaction can occur more rapidly. The distinguishing feature of an enzyme-catalyzed reaction is that it takes place within the confines of a pocket on the enzyme called the **active site.** The molecule that is bound in the active site and acted upon by the enzyme is called the **substrate.** The surface of the active site is lined with amino acid residues with substitute groups that bind the substrate and catalyze its chemical transformation. Often, the active site encloses a substrate, sequestering it completely from solution. The enzyme substrate complex, whose existence was first proposed by Charles-Adolphe Wurtz in 1880, is central to the action of enzymes. It is also the starting point for mathematical treatments that define the kinetic behavior of enzyme-catalyzed reactions and for theoretical descriptions of enzyme mechanisms.

2.9.1. Enzymes affect reaction rates, not equilibria

A simple enzymatic reaction might be written

$$E + S \leftrightarrow ES \leftrightarrow EP \quad E + P$$

Where, E, S, and P represent the enzyme, substrate, and product; ES and EP are transient complexes of the enzyme with the substrate and with the product. To understand catalysis, we must first appreciate the important distinction between reaction equilibria and reaction rates. The function of a catalyst is to increase the *rate* of a reaction. Catalysts do not affect reaction equilibria. Any reaction, such as S P, can be described by a reaction coordinate diagram a picture of the energy changes duhj6ring the reaction. Energy in biological systems is described in terms of free energy, *G*. In the coordinate diagram, the free energy of the system is plotted against the progress of the reaction (the reaction coordinate). The starting point for either the forward or the reverse reaction is called the **ground state,** the contribution to the free energy of the system by an average molecule (S or P) under a given set of conditions. To describe the free-energy changes for reactions, chemists define a standard set of conditions (temperature 298 K; partial pressure of each gas 1 atm, or 101.3 kPa; concentration of each solute 1 M) and express the free-energy change for this reacting system as $\Delta G°$, the **standard free energy change.** Because biochemical systems commonly involve H^+ concentrations far below 1 M, biochemists define a **biochemical standard free-energy change,** $\Delta G'°$ the standard free-energy change at pH 7.0.

The equilibrium between S and P reflects the difference in the free energies of their ground states. The free energy of the ground state of P is lower than that of S, so $\Delta G'°$ for the reaction is negative and the equilibrium favors P. The position and direction of equilibrium are *not* affected by any catalyst. A favorable equilibrium does not mean that the S → P conversion will occur at a detectable rate. The rate of a reaction is dependent on an entirely different parameter. There is an energy barrier between S and P: the energy required for alignment of reacting groups, formation of transient unstable charges, bond rearrangements, and other transformations required for the reaction to proceed in either direction. This is illustrated by the energy "hill" in Fig. 2.9. To undergo reaction, the molecules must overcome this barrier and therefore must be raised to a higher energy level. At the top of the energy hill is a point at which decay to the S or P state is equally probable (it is downhill either way). This is called the transition state. The transition state is not a chemical species with any significant stability and should not be confused with a reaction intermediate (such as ES or EP). It is simply a fleeting molecular moment in which events such as bond breakage, bond formation, and charge development have proceeded to the precise point at which decay to either substrate or product is equally likely. The difference between the energy levels of the ground state and the transition state is the activation energy, ΔG^t. The rate of a reaction reflects this activation energy: higher activation energy corresponds to a slower reaction. Reaction rates can be increased by raising the temperature, thereby increasing the number of molecules with sufficient energy to overcome the energy barrier.

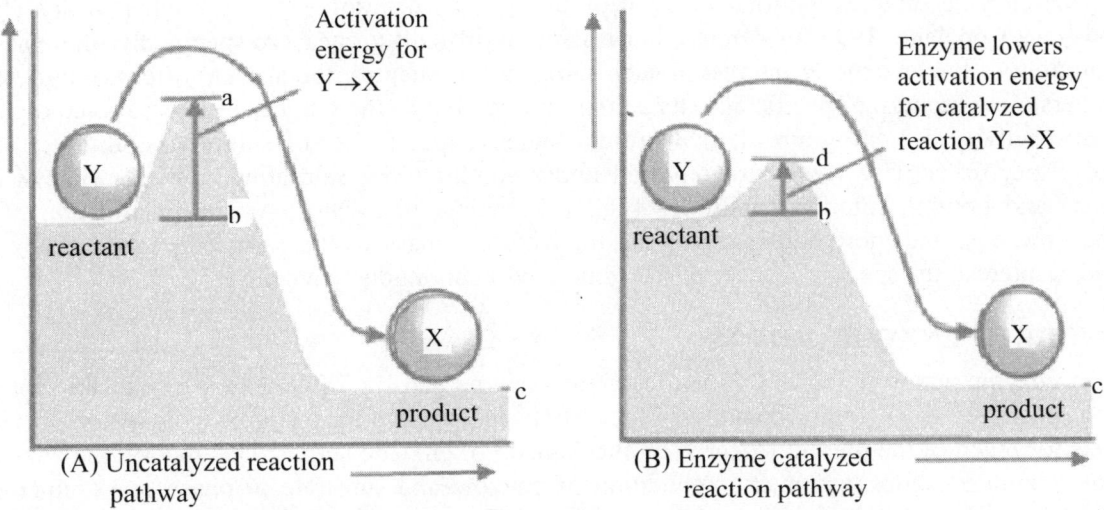

Fig 2.9: Enzyme catalyzed and uncatalyzed reaction

Alternatively, the activation energy can be lowered by adding a catalyst. Catalysts enhance reaction rates by lowering activation energies (Fig 2.9).

2.9.2. Reporting enzyme activity data

As we have seen in the preceding section, many solution conditions can affect the overall activity of an enzyme-catalyzed reaction. Thus, for investigators in different laboratories to reproduce one another's results it is critical that the data be reported in meaningful units, and be accompanied by sufficient information on the details of the assay used. In reporting activity measurements, one should always specify the buffer system used in the reaction mixture, the pH and temperature at which the assay was recorded, the time interval over which initial velocity measurements were made, and the detection method used.

Initial velocities and V_{max} values should always be reported in units of molarity (of substrate or product) change per unit time, while K_m and k_{cat} values should be reported in molarity units and reciprocal time (min^{-1}, or s^{-1}), respectively. Turnover numbers are typically reported in terms of molarity change per unit time per molarity of enzyme, moles of substrate lost or product produced per unit time per mole of enzyme, or, equivalently, molecules of substrate lost or product produced per unit time per molecule of enzyme. Many times it will be necessary to measure the enzymatic activity of samples that contain proteins other than the enzyme of interest. During the initial purification of an enzyme, for example, it is often helpful to follow the activity of the enzyme at various stages of the purification process, where multiple contaminating proteins will be present in the sample also. To standardize the reporting of activities in such cases, the International Union of Biochemistry has adapted the *international unit* (IU) as the standard measure of enzyme activity: one international unit is the amount of enzyme (or crude enzyme sample) required to catalyze the transformation of one micromole of substrate per minute or, where more than one bond of each substrate molecule is attacked, one micro equivalent of the group concerned, under a specific set of defined solution conditions. The definition allows the individual researcher to specify the solution conditions, but the IUB recommended that units be reported for measurements made at 25°C. The specific solution conditions have no intrinsic significance, but they must to be reported to ensure reproducibility.

In crude enzyme samples the total mass of protein can be determined by a number of analytical methods (see Copeland, 1994 for details), but it is often difficult to measure specifically the mass or concentration of the enzyme of interest in such samples. To quantify the amount of enzyme present, researchers often report the specific activity of the sample: that is, the number of international units of enzymatic activity per milligram of total protein under a specific set of solution conditions. Most typically, specific activity values are reported under conditions of saturating substrate (i.e., where v~Vmax) and optimal solution conditions (i.e., pH, temperature, etc.). As the purification of an enzyme proceeds, and more and more of the total protein mass of the sample is made up by the enzyme of interest, the specific activity of the sample will continuously increase.

2.10. MODE OF ENZYME ACTION

Mode of enzyme action involves the nature of the enzyme substrate interaction responsible for the reaction specificity of the biologic catalysts. The Michaelis-Menten theory of enzyme action provides the basis for much of the present research on mechanism of enzyme action. This theory, the enzyme-substrate complex theory, assumes combination of enzyme and substrate in phase one (sometimes known as transition phase) of the enzyme activity and liberation of enzyme and the products of the catalysis in phase two of the reaction:

Enzyme + Substrate $\rightleftharpoons$ Enzyme-Substrate complex $\rightleftharpoons$ Enzyme+ Product

One key factor of enzyme to act as catalyst is their ability to bind effectively one or (more frequently) both reactants in a bimolecular reaction with an accompanying increase in local reactants concentration and hence in local reaction rate. Enzymes are both extremely efficient and highly selective catalysts. To understand these distinctive properties of enzymes, the concept of 'active' or 'catalytic site' must be introduced. Fig. 2.10a illustrates the mode of enzyme action.

2.10.1. The catalytic site

The region of an enzyme concerned with substrate binding and catalysis is termed as **active site**. The large size of proteins relative to substrates led to the concept that a restricted region of the enzyme is concerned with the catalysis. This region, 'the catalytic site', has been recognized from three dimensional models of enzymes that suggest that a far greater portion of the protein interacts with the substrate than was formerly supposed. Different models of the catalytic sites have been proposed so far, the most relevant models are discussed here.

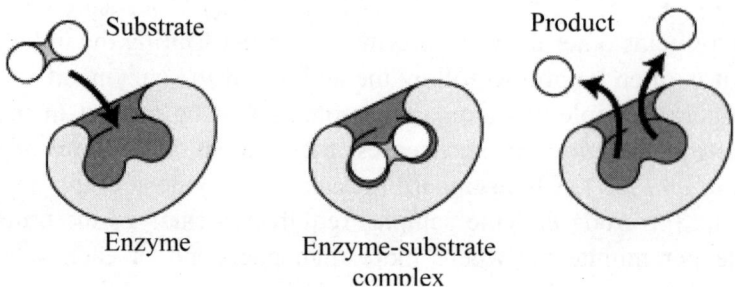

Fig 2.10a: Mode of enzyme action

2.10.1.1. The lock and key or template model

Many properties of enzymes can be explained in terms of the rigid 'lock and key' model of an active site. The model of a catalytic site proposed by Emil Fischer visualized interaction between substrate and enzyme in terms "**lock and key**" analogy. This lock and key, or rigid template, model (Fig. 2.10b), is still useful for understanding certain properties of enzymes. The ordered binding of two or more substrates can be explained by this model. It states that the enzymatic specificity lies in a strict conformity of the substrate with the active center of enzyme.

According to Fischer, the enzyme is a rigid structure whose active center is a replica of the substrate. The enzymatic reaction is feasible if the substrate matches the active center as the key fits into the lock. If the substrate ('key') becomes slightly modified, it no longer fits the active center ('lock'), and no reaction takes place. The Fischer's hypothesis is rather attractive since it provides a simple explanation of the specificity of enzymatic action.

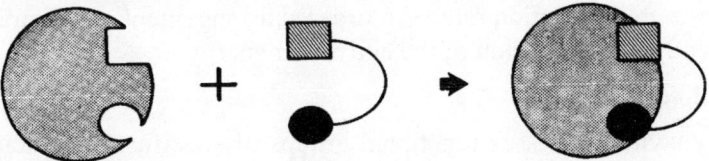

Fig. 2.10b: Formation of enzyme substrate complex according to lock and key mode

2.10.1.2. The 'Induced fit' model

In the induced fit model of a catalytic site, the substrate induces a conformational change in the enzyme that creates the catalytic site. Koshland found an unfortunate feature of Fischer's model in the form of rigidity of the catalytic site and gave a more general model, i.e., 'induced fit' model. This model has considerable experimental support. In the Fischer model, the catalytic site is presumed to be oriented and pre-shaped to fit the substrate but in the Koshland model, the substrate induces a conformational change in the enzyme (Fig. 2.11). Changes in tertiary or quaternary structure of the relatively large enzyme molecule thus can exert mechanical leverage on the substrate.

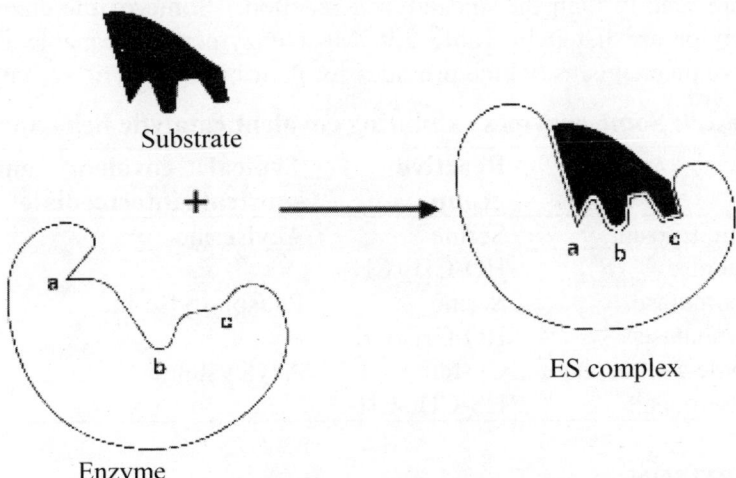

Fig. 2.11: Enzyme substrate interaction according to 'Induced fit model'

This concept may explain why enzymes are proteins and thus much larger than most substrate molecules. The conformational changes align amino acid residues or other groups on the enzyme in the correct spatial orientation for substrate binding, catalysis, or both.

2.10.2. Proximity and orientation

Mutual orientation of reactants is a very specific property of enzymes enabling them to accelerate the conversion (to increase the reactivity of substrates) by a few orders of magnitude. The contact site of the enzyme active center binds the substrate specifically, thereby providing for their mutual orientation and approach so as to facilitate the intervention of catalytic groups. The formation of enzyme substrate complex may take place in such a way that the susceptible bond is in a close proximity to the catalytic group and also is precisely oriented, greatly increasing the probability that the ES complex will enter the transition state. Orientation of two or more molecules, incapable of realization via chaotic collisions in an aqueous medium or on the surface of an inorganic catalyst, favors a drastic increase in the reaction rate. An ordered arrangement of substrates leads to a drop in entropy and, consequently, to diminution of the activation energy.

2.10.3. General acid-base catalysis

The active site of an enzyme possesses functional groups of specific amino acid residues capable of acting both as an acid (good proton donors) and as a base (good proton acceptors). When the substrate is anchored at the active site, its molecule becomes liable to the influence of electrophilic and nucleophilic groups of the catalytic site, which results in an electron density redistribution in the substrate molecule regions accessible to attack by acid base groups. Such general-acid or general-base groups are powerful catalysts for many organic reactions in aqueous systems. Histidine exhibits clearly defined acid-base properties. Blocking of the histidine residue entails the enzyme inactivation. The acid-base catalysis is typical of hydrolases, lyases and isomerases.

2.10.4. Covalent catalysis

Covalent catalysis is observed in the enzymes capable of forming covalent bonds between the substance and the catalytic group of the active site. Some enzymes react with their substrates to form very unstable, covalently joined enzyme-substrate complexes, which undergo further reaction to form the products much more readily than the uncatalyzed reaction. Some of the enzymes exhibiting a covalent catalytic behavior are listed in Table 2.9. Most enzymes are capable of a simultaneous involvement in the above mechanisms, which provides for their high catalytic activity.

Table 2.9: Some enzymes exhibiting covalent catalytic behavior

Enzyme	Reactive group	Typical covalent enzyme-substrate intermediate
Chymotrypsin, trypsin, thrombin, esterase	Serine $HO-CH_2-CH-$	Acylserine
Phosphoglucomutase, alkaline phosphatase	Serine $HO-CH_2-CH-$	Phosphorylserine
Glyceraldehyde-3-phosphate dehydrogenase papain	Cysteine $HS-CH_2-CH-$	Acylcysteine

2.11. ENZYME INHIBITION

The normal state of living matter is a delicately balanced, spatially and temporally coordinated organization. If a substance causes an adverse effect on this balance it is usually termed a poison;

alternatively if it redresses a pathologic imbalance it is regarded as a drug. Both may be enzyme inhibitors. An enzyme inhibition decreases the activity of an enzyme without significantly disrupting its three-dimensional macromolecular structure. Inhibition is therefore distinct from denaturation and is the result of a specific action by a reagent directed or transmitted to the active site region. Studies of enzymes can yield much information about:

1. The substrate specificity of enzymes

2. The nature of functional group at the active site

3. Mechanism of the catalytic activity.

4. Usefulness in elucidating metabolic pathways in cells

5. Some drugs, useful in medicine appear to function because they can inhibit certain enzymes in malfunctioning cells.

The pharmacological action of drugs is based largely on enzyme inhibition. Common examples are found in the action of the sulfonamides and other antibiotics. In the great majority of cases, the enzyme (or coenzyme) inhibited is not known. The development of nerve gases, insecticides and herbicides (weed killer) is based on enzyme inhibition studies.

There are two major types of enzyme inhibition;

1. Irreversible

2. Reversible

2.11.1. Irreversible inhibition

Irreversible inhibitors are those which combine with or destroy a functional group on the enzyme molecule that is necessary for its catalytic activity. An irreversible inhibitor dissociates very slowly from its target enzyme because it becomes very tightly bound to the enzyme, either covalently or non-covalently. Chemical modification is particularly valuable for probing the physico-chemical character of an enzyme and for determining the nature and reactivity of its constituent amino acids. It is therefore an important part of the investigation of proteins that have yet to be crystallized and of membrane bound proteins.

Modification of the enzyme can indicate the position of the active site and which of several possible amino acids are essential to its function. In addition the preparation of derivatives for peptide sequencing, the production of isomorphous heavy atom derivatives for X-ray analysis and crosslinking stabilization of the enzyme depends on the application of modifying reagents. These reagents can be divided into groups and site selective types.

2.11.1.1. Group specific reagents

There are several methods of determination for the groups essential to enzymatic activity. One most widely used method is differential labeling. Group selective modification of the enzyme is generally performed in the presence of a substrate analog, to protect the active site. The protector is then removed and the enzyme again exposed to the modifier. If the activity is retained by the substrate protected enzyme but lost when deprotected, then the group tested for activity is presumed to be present at or near the active site. If prior to the second treatment, both inhibitor and excess reagent are removed and the latter replaced by radioisotope labeled modificant, the active site will be specifically tagged. Table 2.10 gives a representative list of the more selective reagents.

Table 2.10: Chemical modification of amino acid side chains

Amino Acid	Reagent
Arginine	Nitromalondialdehyde, phenylglyoxal
Aspartic acid/ Glutamic acid	Triethyloxonium fluoroborate, water soluble carbodiimide plus glycine methyl ester
Cysteine/ Cystine	Phosphorothioate, performic acid; 5,5'-dithio*bis*(2-nitrobenzoic acid); *p*-chloromercurybenzoate
Histidine	Iodoacetamide, diazonium-1 H-tetrazole
Lysine	Methyl acetimidate maleic anhydride
Methionine	Hydrogen peroxide, β-propiolactone
Tryptophan	Iodine, *N*-bromosuccinimide

These methods have several drawbacks. First is the lack of absolute specificity shown by a modifier for a given functional group. Alkyl halide preferentially reactive with lysine and α-amino groups will also modify cysteine and threonine. This leads to considerable complication in the isolation procedures and in the interpretation of labeling patterns. Another drawback is that a lack of reactivity cannot be taken as an evidence for the absence of a functional group. Neighboring residues may either sterically hinder reagent approach to a 'buried' group or restrict formation of the transition state for reaction even though the residue may be initially accessible.

2.11.1.2. Site specific modification

Four types of compounds specifically modify active sites: (a) substrate, (b) pseudosubstrate, (c) affinity labels, and (d) 'suicide' or 'k_{cat}' inhibitor.

2.11.1.2.1. Substrate

The substrate is the almost perfect site-specific reagent but the bonds formed in the Michaelis complex are often labile and transitory making isolation of an enzyme bound species almost impossible. In certain cases however it has proven possible to trap an intermediate in the enzyme reaction. Reasonable mechanisms proposed for acetoacetate decarboxylase catalyzed decarboxylation and class I aldolase catalyzed reactions envisage initial schiff base formation between the incoming substrate and an amino group in the enzyme.

In the presence of their substrates both enzymes were inhibited by sodium borohydride which reduced the imines to the stable secondary amines E--NH--CHR_1R_2. The carbon-nitrogen single bonds, being resistant to the catalytic action of the enzymes and the protein degradative and sequencing procedures, permitted the isolation and identification of active site sequences.

Another example is iodoacetamide, which can react with sulfhydryl (-SH) groups of essential cysteine residues or with the imidazole group of essential histidine residues. With the help of such inhibitors the hydroxyl group of serine, the thiol group of cysteine and the imidazole group of histidine have been identified as participating in the catalytic activity of different classes of enzymes

2.11.1.2.2. Pseudosubstrates

Pseudosubstrates possess certain characteristics which are common with the actual enzyme substrate. The designation pseudosubstrate has been particularly applied to di-isopropyl fluorophosphate (DFP) and its analogues. DFP is also known as Di-isopropyl phosphofluoridate (DIPF). These agents react with hydroxyl group of an essential serine residue at the active site of enzyme acetylcholine-esterase to form a catalytically inactive derivative. These organohalophosphates react rapidly and irreversibly with enzymes trypsin, chymotrypsin, thrombin and acetylcholinesterase. In each case the reaction is stoichiometric, resulting in the loss of a single active site serine residue.

Acetylcholine catalyses the hydrolysis of acetylcholine which is a neurotransmitter functioning in certain portions of the nervous system. Acetylcholine is released by a stimulated nerve cell into the synapse, with another nerve cell. Once the acetylcholine has been secreted into the synapse, it binds to receptor sites on the next nerve cell, causing the latter to propagate the nerve impulse. Before a second impulse can be transmitted through a synapse, the Ach secreted after the first impulse must be hydrolyzed by the acetylcholinesterase to acetate and choline which have no transmitter activity.

Animals treated with DFP, become paralyzed in certain functions because of failure of nerve impulses to be transmitted properly. This has led to the development of **Malathion** and other insecticides that are relatively nontoxic for human and animals. Malathion is inactivated and is degraded by higher animals into products that are believed to be harmless to them, but it is converted by enzymes of insects into an active inhibitor of their Acetylcholine esterase. DFP has been found to inhibit a whole class of enzymes, many of them capable of catalyzing hydrolysis of peptide or ester linkages. They include not only acetylcholine hydrase but also trypsin, chymotrypsin, elastase, phosphoglycomutase and cocconase. All the DFP inhibited enzymes have an essential serine residue in their active site, which participates in their catalytic activity.

2.11.1.2.3. Affinity labels

Reversible binding does not provide good information concerning the active site. A more fruitful approach reported by Schoellman and Shaw suggested the synthesis of substrate analog possessing molecular requisites complementary to the active site and in addition incorporated chemically reactive groupings. By mimicking the substrate, they argued, such molecules would be held at high concentrations in the sites and once in position the reactive group(s) would then form irreversible covalent attachment to amino acid side chains in their vicinities. Hence, such compounds are designated as *affinity labels*. Various enzymes and their affinity labels are listed in Table 2.11.

Table 2.11: Various affinity labels

Enzyme	Reagent	Residue modified
Carboxypeptidase B	α-*N*-Bromoacetyl-D-arginine	Glutamate
	Bromoacetyl-*p*-aminobenzylsuccinate	Methionine
α-Chymotrypsin	Tosyl-L-phenylalanine chloromethyl ketone (TPCK)	Histidine 57 Methionine 192
	Glycidol phenyl ether	Serine 195
	Phenylmethanesulphonyl fluoride	
Fumarase	Bromomesaconate	Methionine, histidine
β-Galactosidase	*N*-Bromoacetyl-β-D-galactosylamine	Methionine
Lactate dehydrogenase	3-Bromoacetylpyridine	Cysteine, histidine
Lysozyme	2',3'-Epoxypropyl-β-D-(*N*-actylglucosamine)$_2$	Aspartate 52
RNA polymerase	5-Formyl-uridine-5'-triphosphate	Lysine
Triose phosphate isomerase	Glycidol phosphate	Glutamate

An example of affinity label is the chloromethyl ketone of tosylphenylalanine (TPCK) as a possible affinity label for chymotrypsin.

$$CH_3- C_6H_4 - SO_2 - HN - CH - CO - CH_2 - Cl$$
$$CH_2C_6H_5$$

Tosyl-L-phenylalanine chloromethyl ketone(TPCK)

The specificity requirement is fulfilled by incorporation of large aromatic benzyl group because chymotrypsin preferentially cleaves peptide bonds adjacent to phenylalanine, tryptophan and tyrosine. The enzyme-inhibitor complex is probably stabilized by hydrogen bond formation between the ketone and the active site serine. The proteases irreversibly and rapidly inactivated by TPCK, amino acid analysis indicated that one histidine molecule had been modified.

2.11.1.2.4. 'Suicide' or 'k-cat' inhibitors

This term was coined first by Abeles and Maycock and then by Rando. The two main characteristics of this type of irreversible inhibitor are (i) non-reactivity of the precursor before it interacts with the enzyme active site and (ii) activation and subsequent inhibition catalyzed by the same active site residues as those responsible for substrate transformation. This second characteristic thus adds an extra dimension to the specificity of inhibition, in that the catalytic reactivity of the enzyme is employed to effect its modification. Such compounds can therefore be regarded as catalytic inhibitors as opposed to affinity labels or transition-state analogs whose selectivity reside in their binding powers. Suicide inhibitors can then provide additional evidence on the mechanism of an enzymatic reaction.

The postulated intermediary catalytic formation of activated double bonds causing the observed inhibition is a common feature of suicide inhibitors, and the selectivity opens up a fascinating approach to the design of pharmacologically active agents. For example, pargyline, currently employed clinically in anti hypertension therapy inhibits monoamine oxidase stoichiometrically via enzymatic formation of a relatively stable flavin-allene adduct (Fig. 2.12). Once formed the electrophilic allene is in a favorable position to attack any adjacent nucleophile and thus inactivates the enzyme.

The natural antibiotic, rhizobitoxine NH_2-$CH(CH_2OH)$-CH_2-O-CH:CH-$CH(NH_2)CO_2H$ which resembles the substrate cystathionine NH_2-$CH(CO_2H)$-CH_2-S-CH_2-$CH(NH_2)CO_2H$ of bacterial β-cystathionine, irreversibly prevents its cleavage into homocysteine and pyruvate probably also by acting as a suicide inhibitor.

$$C_6H_5\text{-}CH_2\text{-}N(CH_3)CH_2\text{-}C\text{:}CH$$

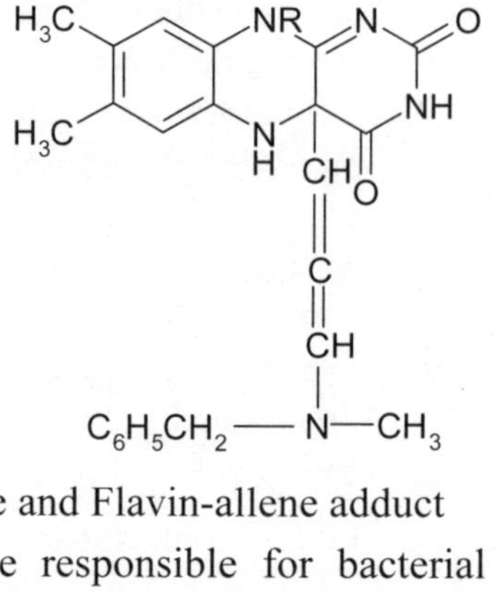

Fig. 2.12: Structure of pargyline and Flavin-allene adduct

Penicillin irreversibly inactivates a key enzyme responsible for bacterial cell-wall synthesis. Penicillin consists of a thiazolidine ring fused to a β-lactam ring, to which a variable R group is attached by a peptide bond. In benzyl penicillin, R is a benzyl group. The β-lactam ring is very labile and this property is closely tied to the antibiotic action of penicillin.

Penicillin interferes with the synthesis of the bacterial cell wall. The cell wall macromolecule called peptidoglycan consists of linear polysaccharide chains that are cross linked by short peptides. The enormous bag shaped peptidoglycan confers the mechanical support and prevents bacteria from bursting due to high internal osmotic pressure.

In 1965, James Park and Jack Storming deduced that penicillin blocks the last step in cell wall synthesis namely the cross-linking of different peptidoglycan strands. This cross-linking reaction is catalyzed by glycopeptide transpeptidase. Penicillin inhibits the cross-linking transpeptidase (Fig. 2.13).

2.11.2. Reversible inhibition

Reversible inhibition is characterized by a rapid dissociation of the enzyme inhibitor complex. In this type of inhibition, the enzyme can bind with the substrate, forming an [ES] complex. Reversible inhibitors of enzymes have also provided much important information on enzyme structure in regard to the active site present on different enzymes.

There are two types of reversible inhibition

1. Competitive and

2. Non-competitive

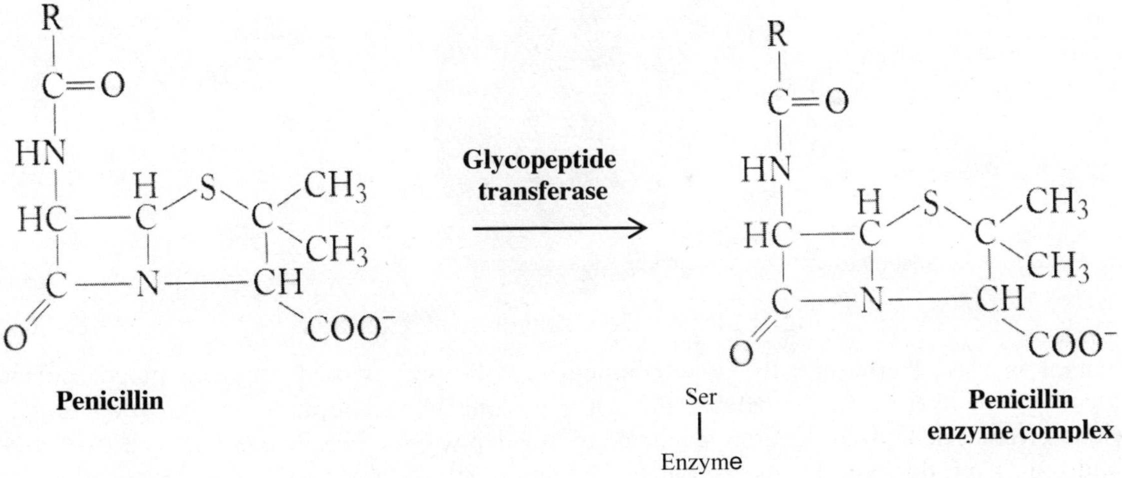

Fig. 2.13: Inhibition of glycopeptide transpeptidase by penicillin

2.11.2.1. Competitive inhibition

A competitive inhibitor competes with the substrate for binding to the active site but, once bound, cannot be transformed by the enzyme. In competitive inhibition, the enzyme can bind substrate (forming an [ES] complex) or inhibitor (EI complex) but not both at a time (ESI). Competitive inhibitors resemble the substrate and bind to the active site of the enzyme preventing the substrate from binding to the same active site. A competitive inhibitor diminishes the rate of catalysis by reducing the proportion of enzyme molecules bound to a substrate. Competitive inhibition can be reversed or relieved by increasing the substrate concentration. For example if an enzyme is 50% inhibited at a given concentration of the substrate and competitive inhibitor, we can diminish the percent inhibition by raising the substrate concentration.

Competitive inhibitors usually resemble the normal substrate in three-dimensional structure. Because of this resemblance the competitive inhibitor 'tricks' the enzyme in binding to it. Competitive inhibition can be quantitatively analyzed by the Michaelis-Menten theory. The competitive inhibitor [I] simply combines reversibly with the enzyme to form [EI] complex. However, the inhibitor [I] cannot be attacked by the enzyme to form new reaction products.

$$E + I \rightleftharpoons EI$$

The classic example of competitive inhibition is the action of malonate on succinate dehydrogenase, a member of the group of enzymes catalyzing the citric acid cycle. These enzyme catalyses the removal of two hydrogen atoms from each of the methylene (-CH₂-) groups of succinate.

Succinate dehydrogenase is inhibited by malonate, which resembles succinate in having two ionized carboxyl groups at pH 7.0, but differs in having only three carbon atoms. Malonate occupies the active site, keeping the enzyme away from acting on its normal substrate. The reversibility of the inhibition by malonic acid is shown by the fact that increasing the succinate concentration will reduce the extent of inhibition by a given concentration of malonate (Fig. 2.14).

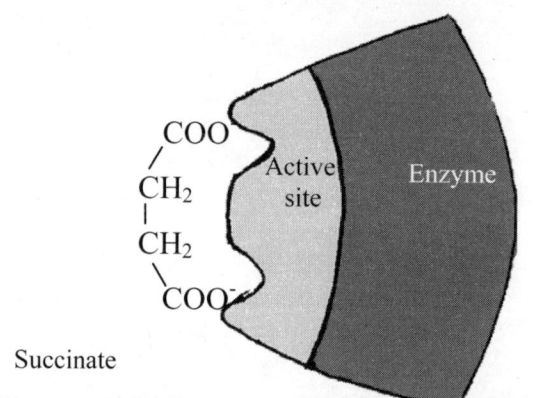

Fig. 2.14: Succinate dehydrogenase reaction

Ethanol is used therapeutically as a competitive inhibitor to treat ethylene glycol poisoning. Ethylene glycol itself is not lethal but the harm is done by oxalic acid, an oxidation product of ethylene glycol. Kidneys are severely damaged by the deposition of oxalate crystals. Ethylene glycol is oxidized to an aldehyde by the action of enzyme alcohol dehydrogenase. This reaction can be effectively inhibited by administering an intoxicating dose of ethanol (Fig 2.15). Ethanol is a competing substrate for alcohol dehydrogenase and therefore it blocks the oxidation of ethylene glycol to aldehyde products. The ethylene glycol is then excreted harmlessly. Ethanol is also used as a competing substrate for treating methanol poisoning.

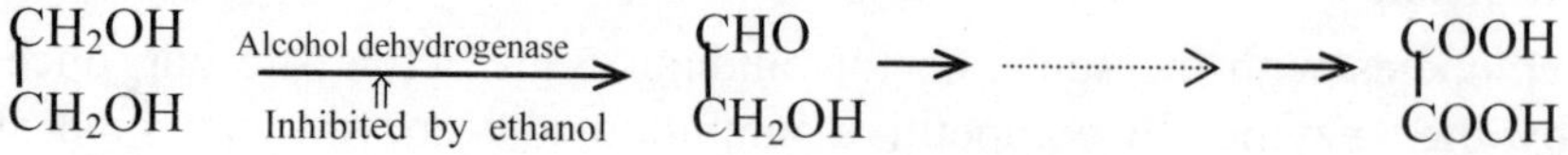

Fig. 2.15: Enzymatic conversion of ethylene glycol to oxalic acid is competitively inhibited by ethanol

In gout, uric acid accumulates in tissues and causes symptoms of gout. Uric acid is formed by oxidation of hypoxanthine by xanthine oxidase. Allopurinol, which has a structural resemblance to hypoxanthine, decreases the formation of uric acid by competitive inhibition (Fig. 2.16). Allopurinol also inhibits the enzymatic oxidation of mercaptopurine, which is used as an antineoplastic antimetabolite.

Monoamine oxidase (MAO) oxidizes pressor amines like adrenaline and noradrenaline. Ephedrine and amphetamine which have similar structure as adrenaline and noradrenaline inhibit monoamine oxidase and thus prolong the action of the pressor amines.

The sulfonamides and sulfones act as antibacterials by competitively inhibiting the incorporation of PABA to form dihydropteroic acid. Similarly trimethoprim is an inhibitor of folate reductase needed to convert dihydrofolic acid (FAH_2) into tetrahydrofolic acid (FAH_4) in bacteria.

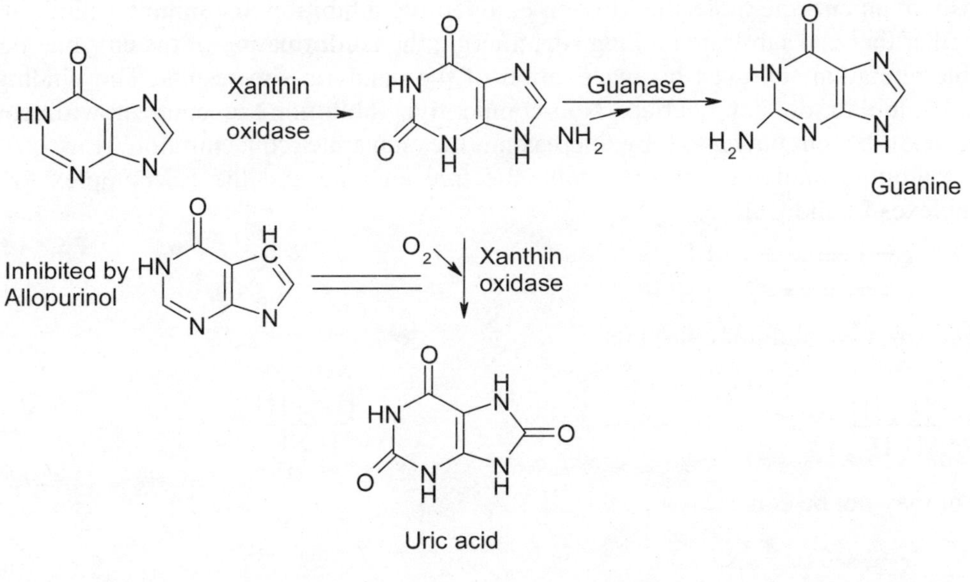

Fig. 2.16: Inhibition of conversion of xanthin to uric acid by allopurinol

In the chemotherapy of malaria tetrahydrofolate synthesis inhibitors are widely used e.g., pyrimethamine, chloroguanide, cycloguanil, trimethoprim, sulfadoxine, sulfadiazine, 4,4'-diaminodiphenylsulfone (DDS) etc. Malarial dihydrofolate reductase is structurally different from mammalian dihydrofolate reductase and is 2,000 times more sensitive to the antimalarial drugs. The malarial protozoa are unable to use pyrimidine nucleoside of host and therefore must synthesize its own, which requires the folinic acid and other tetrahydrofolic acid cofactors. Thus any drug that inhibits the synthesis of dihydrofolic acid in malarial protozoa or selectively inhibits the dihydrofolate reductase of malarial protozoa in turn will inhibit the growth and kill the protozoa. The biguanides (chloroguanide), diamino-pyrimidines (pyrimethamine) and dihydrotriazines (cyloguanil) are selective inhibitors of malarial protozoa.

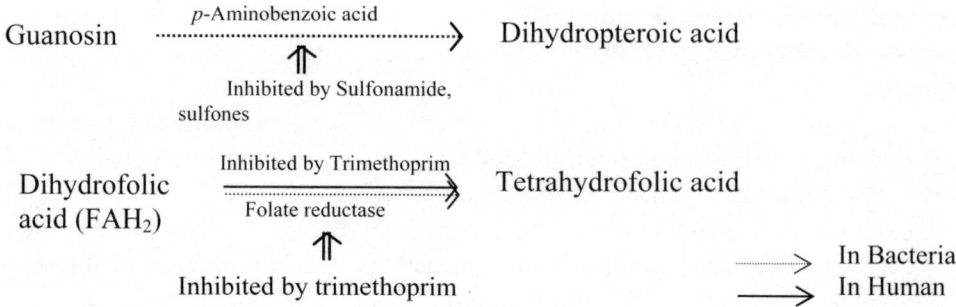

2.11.2.2. Noncompetitive inhibition

In non-competitive inhibition, which is a reversible process, the inhibitor substrate can bind simultaneously to an enzyme molecule. In non-competitive inhibition, the inhibitor binds at a site on the enzyme other than the substrate binding site, altering the conformation of the enzyme molecule so that reversible alteration followed by inactivation of the catalytic site results. The binding sites of substrate and inhibitor do not overlap. Non-competitive inhibition, in contrast with competitive inhibition, cannot be circumvented by increasing the substrate concentration (Fig. 2.17). Non-competitive inhibitors bind reversibly to both, the free enzyme and the ES complex to form the inactive complexes EI and ESI:

$$E + I \rightleftharpoons EI$$
$$ES + I \rightleftharpoons ESI$$

for which there are two inhibitor constants:

$$K_I^{ES} = \frac{[E]\,[I]}{[EI]}$$

$$K_I^{ES} = \frac{[ES]\,[I]}{[ESI]}$$

Which may or may not be equal.

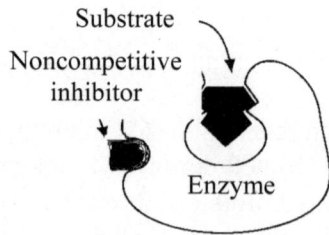

Fig. 2.17: Noncompetitive inhibition

The most important non-competitive inhibition is given by reagents that can combine reversibly with some functional group of the enzyme (outside the active site) that is essential for maintaining the catalytically active three dimensional conformation of the enzyme molecule. Some enzymes possessing -SH groups are non-competitively inhibited by heavy metal ions. Some enzymes that require metal ions for activity are inhibited noncompetitively by agents capable of binding the essential metal. For example, the chelating agent EDTA reversibly binds Mg^{++} and other bivalent cations and thus non-competitively inhibits some enzymes requiring such ions for activity.

Noncompetitive inhibitors are exemplified by cyanides which are capable of strongly binding with the trivalent iron forming part of the catalytic moiety of hemin enzyme, cytochrome oxidase. Blocking of this enzyme switches the respiratory chain off, and the cell can no longer exist. Heavy metal ions and their organic compounds belong to noncompetitive inhibitors of enzymes and due to this reason they are very toxic in nature (mercury, lead, arsenic, etc.). For example, they can block the S-H groups that make part of the catalytic site of an enzyme (Fig. 2.18). The complex enzyme-inhibitor can add a substrate, but subsequently no conversion of the substrate occurs, since the catalytic site of enzyme remains blocked.

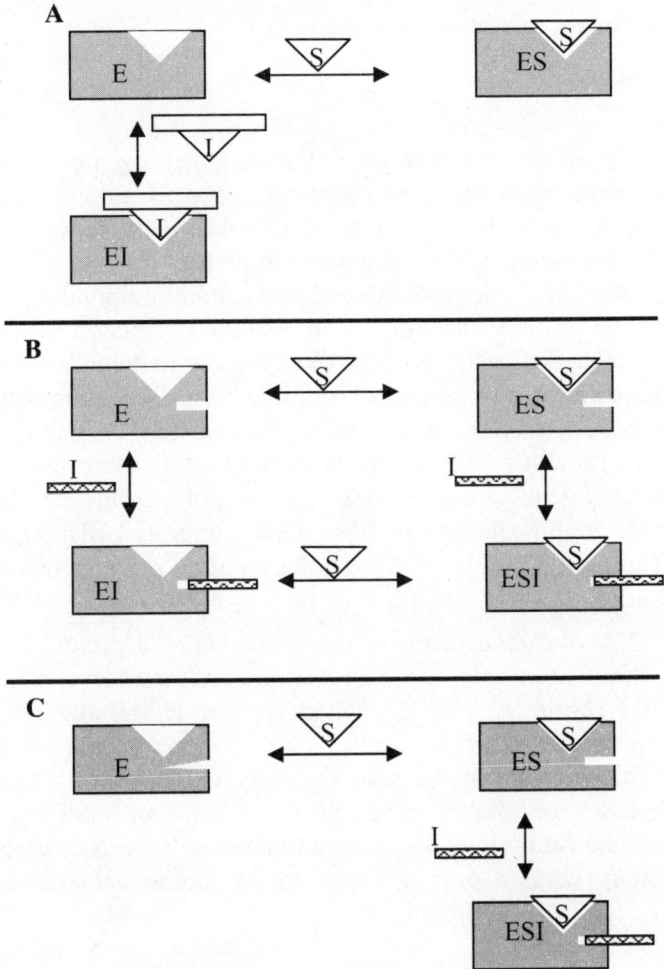

Fig. 2.18: Representations of the three major forms of inhibitor interactions with enzymes: (A) competitive inhibition, (B) noncompetitive inhibition, and (C) uncompetitive inhibition

2.12. REGULATION OF ENZYME ACTIVITY

The net flow of carbon through any enzyme-catalyzed reaction might be influenced by

1. Changing the absolute quantity of enzyme present

2. Altering the pool size of reactants other than enzyme, and

3. Altering the catalytic efficiency of enzyme.

2.12.1. Regulation of enzyme quantity

Regulation of enzyme quantity is determined by the net balance between enzyme synthesis and enzyme degradation. The enzyme level in a cell can be changed by either increasing its rate of synthesis or by decreasing its rate of degradation, or a combination of both. The net result will be an increased enzyme level. The enzyme quantity at a particular time in a particular cell can be affected by various factors outlined below:

1. Genetic basis - Increased rate of enzyme synthesis

2. Induction - Increased rate of enzyme synthesis

3. Repression and depression - Decreased rate of enzyme degradation

2.12.1.1. Control of enzyme synthesis

2.12.1.1.1. Genetic basis

An enzyme that is protein in nature is essentially expressed by its respective gene contained in master genome. The expression typically remains to be the same as discussed for protein synthesis later in this book. The structure of enzyme is determined by the trinucleotide code contained in RNA that is attached to polyribosomes. The ribosomal RNA contains anticodon for the tRNA-amino acid complex. Thus serves as adapter molecule. The mRNA contains codon component of gene whereas tRNA bears anticodon to mRNA. The primary structure of an enzyme is dictated by the trinucleotide (triplet) code of necessary RNA attached to polyribosomes and by the matching bases of a transfer RNA-amino acid complex. The sequence of purine and pyrimidine bases of the messenger RNA is in turn dictated by a complementary base sequence that is part of a master DNA template or gene in the nucleus of the cell. Information for protein synthesis stored in DNA, thus determines a cell's ability to synthesize a particular enzyme. One gene generally codes for one polypeptide, and two genes for a protein containing two dissimilar polypeptides. It has been suggested that proteins of the bacteriophage ϕX 174 are coded not for a single protein; however they are coded for two different polypeptides. For example, the sequence GAAUAGA is read both as GAA-UAG and AAU-AGA.

Mutational changes alter the DNA code and result in the synthesis of a protein molecule with a modified primary structure. In some cases, this may result in altered structures at higher levels of organization also. If the mutation results in change, which is not lethal, the modified genetic information is transmitted to the progeny of the cell. As a result, there frequently arises a transmissible metabolic defect, which occurs at the step formerly catalyzed by the new defective enzyme. Many human genetic diseases are known in which one enzyme or another is either totally inactive or is otherwise defective in the catalytic or regulatory functions. In such diseases (Table 2.12) the defective enzyme molecule may contain one or more wrong amino acids in its polypeptide chain(s) as a result of a mutation of the DNA coding for it.

2.12.1.1.2. Induction

The rate of enzyme synthesis can be induced by various molecules which act as inducers. For a molecule to be metabolized or for an inducer to act, it must first enter the cell. In some cases, a specific transport system or **permease** is needed. The permease itself may be inducible. Permeases share many properties in common with enzymes and appear to perform functions analogous to the cytochromes in electron transport insofar as they appear to transport substrates without causing a net change in substrate structure.

Table 2.12: Some human genetic disease with specific defective enzyme

Disease	Defective enzyme
Albinism	Tyrosine 3-monooxygenase
Alkaptonuria	Homgentisate 12-dioxygenase
Galactosemia	Galactose 1-phosphate uridylyl transferase
Homocysteinuria	Cystathionine β-synthase
Phenylketonuria	Phenylalanine 4-monooxygenase
Tay-Sachs disease	Hexosaminidase A

The phenomenon of enzyme induction is explained with the help of the example of *Escherichia coli* (*E. coli*). *E. coli* grown on glucose does not ferment lactose, due to the absence both of a specific permease for a *β*-galactoside (lactose) and of the enzyme β-galactosidase, which hydrolyses lactose to glucose and galactose. If lactose or certain other β-galactosidase are induced, the culture can ferment lactose. Although, in general inducers serve as substrates for the enzymes or permeases, they induce compounds structurally similar to the substrate which may be inducers but not substrates. They are termed as **gratuitous inducers**.

Variations in induction patterns in bacteria also occur at the genetic level where the structured genes which specify a group of catabolic enzymes comprise of an operon, all the enzymes expressed by operon are induced by a single inducer. This phenomenon is termed as co-ordinate induction.

2.12.1.1.3. Repression and depression

Presence of specific amino acids in the culture media curtails the synthesis of amino acid by bacteria via **repression**. A small molecule such as histidine or leucine, acting as a co-repressor, can ultimately block the synthesis of the enzymes involved in its own biosynthesis. In *Salmonella* species, addition of histidine, and addition of leucine represses synthesis of the first three enzymes unique to leucine biosynthesis. In both cases, these biosynthetic enzymes comprised of operons; co-ordinate repression occurs following addition of the end products histidine or leucine. However, this mode is not general for all biosynthetic pathways since the genetic information specifying the structure of biosynthetic enzymes may be organized into more than one operon. Following removal or exhaustion of an essential biosynthetic intermediate from the medium, the genetic information coding for the biosynthesis of enzymes is again expressed. This constitutes, what is termed **depression**, which may be co-ordinate or non-coordinate.

2.12.1.2. Enzyme turnover

The combined processes of enzyme synthesis and degradation constitute enzyme turnover. While turnover occurs both in bacteria and mammals, the enzyme levels are regulated on this basis. **Schoenheimer's classical work** suggests that body proteins are in a state of 'dynamic equilibrium', a concept extended to other body constituents, including lipids and nucleic acids. In man and other animals, the regulation of intracellular levels of enzymes thus involves regulation of both enzyme synthesis and of enzyme degradation.

There is now considerable evidence that enzyme levels in mammalian tissues may be altered by a wide range of physiologic, hormonal or dietary manipulations. Glucocorticoids increase the concentration of tyrosine transaminase by stimulating its rate of synthesis. Insulin and glucagon despite their mutually antagonistic physiologic effects, both independently increase the rate of synthesis by 4 to 5 folds. Similarly, the activity of 8-aminolevulinate synthase, is increased as much as 50 fold by drugs which produce experimental prophyria, and this effect is blocked by glucose.

2.12.2. Availability of reactants

Kinetic and regulatory properties of enzymes have value with respect to insights into physiological processes in intact cells, tissues and organisms. The localization of specific metabolic processes in the cytosol or within specific cellular organelles permits regulation of these processes. The extensive compartmentation of metabolic processes has potential for a sophisticated and finely tuned regulation of metabolism. The translocation of essential metabolites across compartmental barriers may be achieved via **shuttle mechanisms**. In general, these shuttle mechanisms involve conversion of the material to be translocated in a form permeable to the compartmental barrier. This is followed by transport and conversion back to the original form on the other side of the barrier. Consequently, these inter conversions require, for example, cytosolic and mitochondrial forms of the same catalytic activity.

2.12.2.1. Effective concentrations of substrates and coenzymes

The mean cellular concentrations of a substrate, coenzyme or metal ion do not have any significant relationship with respect to the *in vivo* enzyme activity. However, the concentration of essential metabolites in the neighborhood of the enzyme in question is crucial. Measuring this metabolite concentration within the cellular compartments is however of little importance. The total concentration of 2,3-diphosphoglycerate in erythrocytes is extremely high, although the concentration of free diphosphoglycerate is probably comparable to that of other tissues. This is due to the binding of diphosphoglycerate with hemoglobin.

A more sophisticated kinetic approach for *in vivo* situation employs an equation of the Michaelis-Menten form, but assumes steady state kinetics: where S_f, is the concentration of free substrate but it does not hold for macromolecular complexes.

$$V = \frac{K\,E_t\,S_f}{K_m + S_f}$$

2.12.2.2. Compartmentation of enzyme and enzyme system

In eukaryotic cells, different enzymes and enzyme systems are segregated into various organelles and intracellular structures. This facilitates regulation of various processes independently. Table 2.13 lists the intracellular distribution of some important enzymes and metabolic sequences in a model mammalian cell.

Some processes such as urea biosynthesis and gluconeogenesis, depend on the interplay of reactions occurring in more than one compartment. A further extension of spatial organization occurs in multicellular organisms in which different tissues have their distinctive metabolic characteristics that are subjected to control in response to special needs of the organism.

2.12.2.3. Role of metal ions

Bacterial glutamine synthetase offers a well documented example of metal ion regulated enzyme activity. In the absence of metal ions *E. coli* glutamine synthetase assumes a relaxed configuration that is catalytically inactive. Addition of Mg^{2+} or Mn^{2+} converts the synthetase to the active 'tightened' form. In addition to metal ion regulated conformational changes, adenylation of the synthetase completely changes divalent cation specificity. Another example is carbonic anhydrase which requires zinc ion for its activity. Removal of zinc from carbonic anhydrase leads to the loss of activity. Furthermore, no other ion has been found to replace zinc from the enzyme. Some other similar enzymes are listed in table 2.2 which require metal ions for their activity.

Table 2.13: Compartmentation of some major enzymes and metabolic processes

Cell structure	Enzyme
Plasma membrane	Amino acid transport systems, Na^+-K^+ATPase
Cytosol	Glycolysis, gluconeogenesis and glycogenesis, HMP pathway fatty acid synthesis, purine and pyrimidine catabolism, amino acyl-tRNA synthetase
Mitochondria	Tricarboxylic acid cycle, electron transport and oxidative phosphorylation, fatty acid oxidation, urea synthesis
Nucleus	DNA and RNA synthesis
Endoplasmic reticulum (Rough and Smooth)	Protein synthesis, steroid synthesis, glycosylation, detoxification
Lysosomes	Hydrolases
Golgi apparatus	Glycosyl transferases, glucose-5-phosphatase, formation of plasma membrane and secretory vesicles
Peroxisomes	Catalase, D-amino oxidase, urate oxidase

2.12.2.4. Macromolecular complexes

Organization of enzymes catalyzing a protected sequence of metabolic reactions in a macromolecular complex series that co-ordinates the activities of the enzymes concerns and channelizes intermediates along a chosen metabolic pathway. Appropriate alignment of the enzymes can facilitate transfer of product from one enzyme to another without prior equilibration and without the formation of a metabolic pool of the intermediates. This permits a finer level of metabolic control than is possible without the isolated components of the complex.

Conformational changes in one component of the complex may be transmitted by protein-protein interaction to other enzyme of the complex. Amplification of regulatory effects is thus readily achieved. Consider the case of the combined dehydrogenation and decarboxylation of pyruvate to acetyl-CoA isomer: there is a segmental action of three different enzymes of pyruvate dehydrogenase complex viz. pyruvate dehydrogenase E1, dehydrolipoyl transacetylase E2, dihydrolipoyl dehydrogenase together working with five different coenzymes thiamine pyrophosphate (TPP), flavin adenine dinucleotide (FAD), coenzyme-A (CoA), nicotinamide adenine dinucleotide (NAD) and lipoic acid. These enzymes and coenzymes are organized into a multi-enzyme cluster.

2.12.3. Regulation of catalytic efficiency

Changes in the enzyme activity that occur independently of the quantity of enzyme present can be designated as effects on catalytic efficiency. In cell metabolism, groups of enzymes work together in sequential chain or systems to carry out a given metabolic process, such as the conversion of glucose into lactic acid in skeletal muscles or the synthesis of an amino acid from simpler precursors. In such enzyme systems the reaction product of the first enzyme becomes the substrate of the next and so on.

In each enzyme system there is at least one enzyme, the **pacemaker** that sets the rate of the overall reaction because it catalyses the slowest or rate-limiting step. Such pacemaker enzymes not only have a catalytic function but also have capabilities of increasing or decreasing their catalytic activity in response to certain signals. These pacemaker enzymes, whose activity is modulated through various types of molecular signals, are called **regulatory enzymes**. There are two major classes of regulatory enzymes: allosteric or noncovalently regulated enzymes (described elsewhere) and covalently regulated enzymes.

2.12.3.1. Cascade system or covalent modification

The catalytic properties of some enzymes are markedly altered by the covalent attachment of some small groups. Enzyme activity is regulated by cyclic interconversion of the enzyme into two forms-modified and unmodified. The interconversions brought about by a "converting enzyme" which together with the two forms of the enzyme (modified and unmodified), constitutes a cascade system.

In many of these enzymes, the modification involves phosphorylation of the enzyme at a -OH group of serine, threonine or tyrosine. Such cascade systems include liver phosphorylase, glycogen synthetase, etc. The converter enzymes are usually protein kinases and they exist in an inactive form and require to be activated by substances such as cyclic AMP. The production of cyclic AMP is in turn regulated by an enzyme adenyl cyclase under hormonal control.

Regulatory enzyme glycogen phosphorylase of muscle and liver catalyses the reaction:

(Glucose)$_n$ + Phosphate $\longrightarrow$ Glucose)$_{n-1}$ + glucose-1-phosphate

Glycogen   Shortened glycogen chain

The glucose-1-phosphate so formed is then broken down into lactic acid in the muscles or into free glucose in the liver.

The enzyme glycogen phosphorylase occurs in two forms:

1. The active form phosphorylase *a*, and

2. The relatively inactive form phosphorylase *b*.

Phosphorylase *a* has two polypetide chain subunits, each with one specific serine residue in its sequence that is phosphorylated at its hydroxyl group. These serine phosphate residues are required for maximum activity of the enzyme. The phosphate group can be hydrolytically removed from phosphorylase-*a* by an enzyme called phosphorylase phosphatase.

Phosphorylase *a* + 2H$_2$O $\longrightarrow$ Phosphorylase *b* + 2Pi

  (More active)   (Less active)

Thus the active form of glucagon phosphorylase is converted into the relatively inactive form due to the cleavage of the two covalent bonds between the phosphoric acid and the two specific serine residues in the enzyme. Phosphorylase *b* can intern be reactivated i.e., covalently transformed back into active phosphorylase *a* by another enzyme phosphorylase kinase. The enzyme catalyses the transfer of phosphate groups from ATP to the hydroalkyl groups of the specific serine residue in phosphorylase *b* (Fig. 2.21).

2ATP + Phosphorylase *b* $\longrightarrow$ 2ADP + Phosphorylase *a*

    (less active)   (more active)

The breakdown of glycogen in skeletal muscles and in the liver is regulated by alteration in the ratio of the active and inactive forms of enzyme.

2.12.3.2. Isoenzymes (multiple form)

Many enzymes occur in more than one molecular form in the same species, at the same time or even in the same cell. In such cases the different forms of the enzymes may catalyze the same reaction; however, they have different kinetic properties and different sequences of amino acids. These can be distinguished and separated by the application of appropriate procedures. These multiple forms of enzymes are termed **isoenzymes** or **isozymes**.

Isoenzymes are physically distinct forms having the same catalytic activity, thus they catalyze the same reaction. Medical interest in isoenzyme was stimulated by the discovery in 1957 that human serum contained several lactate dehydrogenase isoenzymes and that their relative proportions change significantly in certain pathologic conditions. Lactate dehydrogenase catalyses the reversible oxidation of lactate to pyruvate.

$$\text{Lactate} + \text{NAD}^+ \rightleftharpoons \text{Pyruvate} + \text{NADH} + \text{H}^+$$

Lactate dehydrogenase occurs in animal tissue as five different isoenzymes separable by electrophoresis at pH 8.6, using a starch agar or a polyacrylamide gel supporting medium. The isoenzymes have different charges at this pH and migrate to 5 regions of the electrophoretogram. Isoenzymes are then identified by enzyme catalyzed reduction of a colorless dye to a specific colored form. All the lactate dehydrogenase isoenzymes contain four polypeptide chains, each of molecular weight 33,500, but the five isoenzymes contain varying ratios of two kinds of polypeptides which differ in composition and sequence. The active lactate dehydrogenase molecule consists of 4 subunits of 2 types, A chains (also designated as M) and B chains (also designated as H). Only the tetrameric molecule possesses catalytic activity. In skeletal muscle the lactate dehydrogenase isoenzyme that predominates contains four A chains, and in heart the predominately isoenzyme contains four B chains. In other tissues it exists as a mixture of five possible forms, which may be designated as AAAA, AAAB, AABB, ABBB and BBBB.

2.12.3.3. Proenzymes

Regulation of the activity of the enzymes could be achieved by the synthesis of the enzyme in a catalytically inactive or proenzyme form. Conversion of the proenzyme to the active enzyme is catalyzed either by proteolytic enzymes or by hydrogen ions. Various proenzymes and their respective enzymes are listed in Table 2.14.

Table 2.14 : Various proenzymes and their enzymes

Proenzyme		Enzyme
Pepsinogen	$\xrightarrow{\text{H+ or pepsin}}$	Pepsin
Trypsinogen	$\xrightarrow{\text{Trypsin or enterokinase}}$	Trypsin
Chymotrypsinogen	$\xrightarrow{\text{Trypsin}}$	Chymotrypsin
Procarboxypeptidase	$\xrightarrow{\text{Trypsin}}$	Carboxypeptidase

Similarly, conversion of fibrinogen to fibrin involves limited proteolysis catalyzed by thrombin. Under normal physiologic conditions, thrombin exists as the inactive precursor of prothrombin. These involve a cascade of activation reactions, many of which are based on proteolysis. Limited proteolysis is thus one of the key regulatory factors in the complex process of blood coagulation.

2.13. ALLOSTERIC ENZYMES

The term 'Allosteric' is derived from Greek 'allo' which means other and 'stereos' which means space or site. Allosteric enzymes are those having other sites. The properties of allosteric enzymes are significantly different from those of simple non-regulatory enzymes and they include:

1. Like all enzymes allosteric enzymes have catalytic sites which bind the substrate and transform it but they also have one or more regulatory or allosteric sites for binding the regulating metabolites which are called the **effectors** or **modulators**. The allosteric enzymes are specific in regard to their modulators just as the catalytic sites are specific for the substrate (Fig. 2.19). Many allosteric

enzymes have the substrate binding site and the modulator binding site on different subunits, which are referred as the catalytic [C] and regulation [R] subunits respectively. Binding of the positive modulator M to its specific site on the regulatory subunit is communicated to the catalytic subunit through a conformational change rendering the catalytic subunit active and capable of binding the substrate S with high affinity. On dissociation of the modulator M from the regulatory subunit the enzyme reverts to its inactive or less active form. The enzyme is specific for its substrate, whereas the allosteric site is specific for its modulator.

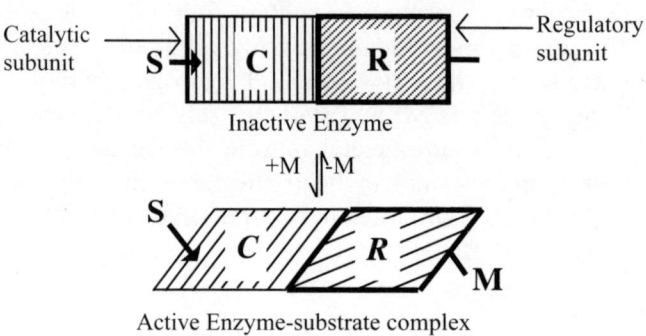

Fig. 2.19: Activation of allosteric enzyme by conformational change

2. Allosteric enzyme molecules are generally larger and more complex than those of simple enzymes. Most have two or more polypeptide chains or subunits.

3. Allosteric enzymes usually show significant deviation from classical Michaelis-Menten theory.

4. They are inhibited by the end product of multienzyme system.

5. Treatment with mercurials, urea, proteolytic enzymes, high or low pH, etc. may produce loss of feedback control with retention of catalytic activity.

6. Many allosteric effectors confer enhanced resistance to heat denaturation of the allosteric enzyme.

7. Unlike most enzymes, regulatory enzymes undergo reversible inactivation at 0°C.

8. All known allosteric enzymes possess tertiary and, in some cases, also quaternary structure.

In some multienzyme systems the first or regulatory enzyme is inhibited by the end product of the multienzyme reaction process. When the concentration of the end product of such a metabolic sequence increases above its normal steady state concentration, indicating that it is being produced in an excess of the cell's needs. The end product of the sequence acts as a specific inhibitor of the first, (i.e. regulatory enzyme) of the sequence. The whole enzyme system thus slows down to reduce the rate of end product formation. This is known as *feedback inhibition* mechanism.

A classical example of this type of inhibition is the conversion of L-threonine to L-isoleucine using bacterial enzyme system. In this sequence of five enzymes, the first, threonine dehydrogenase, is inhibited by isoleucine, the end product of enzyme reaction. No other enzyme of this sequence gets inhibited by isoleucine, nor the intermediates in this sequence of reaction, are inhibitory to the threonine dehydrogenase. This inhibition is reversible, when the isoleucine concentration decreases, the activity of threonine dehydrogenase increases. As the binding of isoleucine to the regulatory site of threonine dehydrogenase is non-covalent, it is readily reversible.

2.13.1. Effect of modulators

Allosteric enzymes may be inhibited or stimulated by their modulators. When the allosteric site is occupied by a specific inhibitory or negative modulator (which happens when the modulator concentration in the cell rises) the enzyme undergoes a change to a less active or inactive form; in other words, it is 'turned off'. When the inhibitory modulator leaves the allosteric site with decreasing modulator concentration in the cell, the enzyme is switched back to its active or 'on' form. The negative modulator is generally the end product of the enzyme reaction. These types of allosteric enzymes are known as **heterotropic enzymes**.

There are also allosteric enzymes which are stimulated by their modulator molecules. In this case the stimulatory or positive modulator is not the end product of the enzymes, reaction sequence but some other metabolite that serves as the molecular signal to the enzyme to speed up the catalytic activity. The stimulatory modulation of this type is often brought about by the substrate molecule itself. Allosteric enzymes belonging to **homotropic class** (because the substrate and modulator are identical), involve two or more steps for substrate binding, particularly when modulator is not the substrate (heterotropic).

Some allosteric enzymes may have two or more modulators and may be opposite in effect, so that one or more modulators of the enzyme are stimulatory. Likewise one or more may be inhibitory. In these more complex enzyme reactions, each modulator has its own specific allosteric site, which when occupied, signals the enzyme either to speed up its catalytic action or slow it down.

Hemoglobin is an allosteric protein. Once the first haem-polypeptide subunit of a hemoglobin molecule binds an oxygen molecule, it communicates this information to the remaining subunits, which respond by greatly increasing their oxygen affinity. Such communication amongst the four haem-polypeptide subunits of hemoglobin is the result of co-operative interaction between the subunits. Because binding of one molecule of oxygen increases the probability that further molecules of oxygen will be bound to the remaining subunits, so this is known as **positive co-operativity**.

Aspartate transcarbamoylase is feedback inhibited by cytidine-s-triphosphate (CTP), the final product of the pyrimidine pathway. Pryimidine biosynthesis begins with the formation of N-carbamoyl-aspartate from aspartate and carbamoyl phosphate. The reaction is catalyzed by aspartate transcarbamoylase (ATCase). The enzyme ATCase is feed back inhibited by the final product of the synthesis cytidine-s-triphosphate (CTP) (Fig. 2.20).

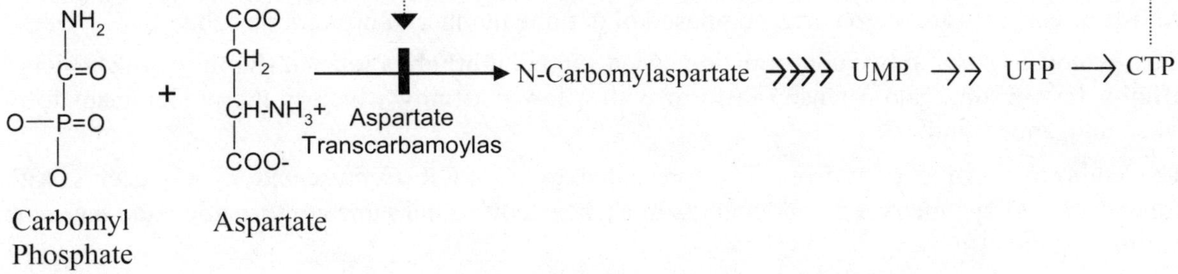

Fig. 2.20: Feedback inhibition of aspartate transcarbamoylase by CTP

The binding of carbamoyl phosphate and aspartate is co-operative as reflected in sigmoidal dependence of reaction velocity on substrate concentration. Co-operative binding seems to switch on the synthesis of N-carbamoylaspartate, over a narrow range of concentration of substrates. The regulation of the rate of pyrimidine nucleotide synthesis operates through the enzyme aspartate trancarbamoylase which catalyses the first reaction of the sequence. This enzyme is inhibited by cytidine-s-triphosphate (CTP) the end product of this sequence of reactions.

The ATCase molecule consists of six catalytic subunits and six regulatory subunits. The catalytic subunits bind the substrate molecules and the allosteric subunits bind the allosteric inhibitor CTP. The entire ATCase molecule, as well as its subunits, exists in two conformations, active and inactive. When the regulatory subunits are unoccupied, the enzyme is maximally active. However, when CTP accumulates it is bound to the regulatory subunits to cause a change in their conformation. This change is transmitted to the catalytic subunits which then transform to an inactive conformation. The presence of ATP prevents the changes induced by CTP (Fig. 2.21).

2.13.2. Model for allosteric enzymes

Two models have been proposed to explain the mechanism of regulation of allosteric enzymes:

1. Concerted model proposed by Monod-Wyman-Changeux and

2. Sequential model proposed by Koshland, Nemethy and Filmer.

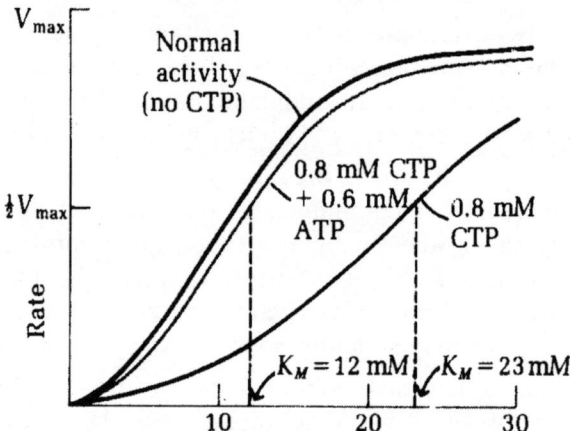

Fig. 2.21: Effect of various modulators on the catalytic activity of aspartate transcarbamoylase

2.13.2.1. The Monod-Wyman-Changeux (MWC) concerted model

The simple model explains the sigmoid binding curve by assuming:

1. Allosteric enzymes are oligomeric, composed of definite number of protomeric subunits.

2. Each protomer exists in two conformational states in equilibrium, a relaxed (R) form with a higher affinity for substrate and a tense (T) form with a lower affinity which is the predominant form when unliganded, and

3. The conformational change from T (represented by □) to R (represented by O) occurs with conservation of symmetry, i.e., all subunits in each state have the same conformation and the same intrinsic ligand affinity.

According to this model, the binding of one molecule enhances the rate of binding of other substrate molecules as a result of binding site interaction in which conversion from one state to another is concerned with all subunits underlying a simultaneous transition. For an allosteric dimer the substrate binding can be represented as shown in Figure 2.27.

It is also proposed that substrate molecules have higher binding affinity for the relaxed state than with the tense state. Formation of RS will reduce the R-state concentration of enzyme, but since this state is in equilibrium with the T-form some of this will be relaxed. If initially very little of the R-state is present i.e., if the ratio T/R of the unliganded species is large, the relative amount of the T-state converted to the R-state on substrate binding will also be large, however if the enzyme already exists predominately in the relaxed state the relative amount of conformational change will be small. The ratio T/R is called the *allosteric constant* (L). Greater is the numerical value of L, the greater is the degree of the co-operativity between subunits and if the L is small so that essentially the entire enzyme is in the R-state then there will be no co-operative subunit interaction.

This model explains the theoretical curves based on the allosteric constant (L), the dissociation constant (K_R) for substrate binding to the tense state, which is suitable for the hemoglobin oxygen binding. The limitation of this model is that only positive and negative co-operativity is predicted. This model can be applied to symmetrical enzymes only.

2.13.2.2. The Koshland-Nemethy-Filmer (KNF) sequential model

This model makes four assumptions:

1. Only two conformational states (R and T) are accessible to any subunit.

2. Only one unliganded conformational state exists for an enzyme.

3. The association of a ligand molecule with one subunit induces a conformational change in that subunit which is transmitted to adjacent unfilled subunits so altering their ligand association.

4. The conformational change elicited by the binding of substrate in one subunit can decrease the substrate-binding affinity of other subunits in the same enzyme molecule.

The binding process in an allosteric enzyme according to this model is shown in Figure 2.22 where K_1 and K_2 are association constants.

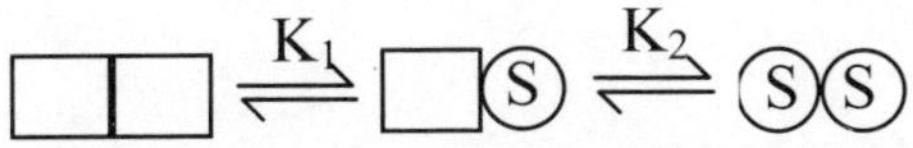

Fig. 2.22: Binding of substrate to an allosteric dimer according to the sequential model

Each subunit can exist in two conformational states, □ and O; binding of the substrate to a subunit changes its conformation, in this case from □ to O. The result of this conformational change is an alteration in the specificity and strength of the inter subunits contacts. They could facilitate subsequent substrate binding, to elicit positive co-operativity.

The differences between this and concerted model are:

1. It does not assume an equilibrium between R and T forms in the absence of substrate;

2. The involvement of mixed intermediate formed as a consequence of the subunits undergoing conformational changes in sequence; and

3. Negative co-operativity can be accounted for, since the model assumes that symmetry is not conserved on ligand binding, the conformational transition each subunit undergoes depends on the energy of activation.

2.13.3: Kinetics of allosteric enzymes

Allosteric enzymes usually differ from classical Michaelis-Menten relationship between substrate concentration and reaction rate, because their rate is dependent on enzyme modulator whether it is inhibitory or stimulatory in nature. Many allosteric enzymes (especially homologous) exhibit a sigmoid curve (Fig. 2.23 A) relating initial velocity to substrate concentration, as compared to the rectangular hyperbola yielded by the Michaelis-Menten relationship. The sigmoid curve implies the binding of the first substrate molecule to the enzyme, supports the binding of the subsequent substrate molecules to the other substrate molecules or the enzyme as well as other molecule to the other substrate sites e.g., binding of oxygen to hemoglobin enhances the binding of subsequent oxygen molecules. Such sigmoid curves are examples of positive co-operativity. This accounts for the sigmoid rather than hyperbolic increase in the rate of enzyme activity on increasing the substrate concentration (Fig. 2.23 A). In some types of allosteric enzymes, binding one substrate molecule decreases the binding of subsequent substrate molecules. This exemplifies negative co-operativity and results in a flattened plot of initial reaction velocity versus substrate concentration. A small change in substrate concentration is ineffective and saturation is achieved more slowly as compared to non regulatory or positively co-operative enzymes (Fig. 2.23 B).

A homotropic allosteric enzyme has multiple binding sites for its substrate and acts co-operatively, so that the binding of one molecule of the substrate greatly enhances the binding of subsequent substrate molecules. In case of heterotropic enzymes, where the modulator is some metabolite other than the substrate itself, the shape of the curve is related to whether the modulator is positive (stimulatory) or negative (inhibitory). If the modulator is positive, it may cause the substrate saturation the curve to become more hyperbolic, with a decrease in $K_{0.5}$ but no change in V_{max}, thus resulting in an increased rate at a fixed substrate concentration (Fig. 2.23 B). Other allosteric enzymes respond to a stimulatory modulator by an increase in V_{max}, with little change in $K_{0.5}$ (Fig. 2.23 C). If the modulator is negative or inhibitory, the substrate saturation curve may become more sigmoid, with an increase in $K_{0.5}$ (Fig. 2.23B). Allosteric enzymes therefore show different types of responses in their substrate activity curves because some have inhibitory modulators, some have stimulatory modulators, and some have both.

2.14. ENZYME STABILITY

One of the most common practical problems facing the experimental biochemist is the loss of enzymatic activity in a sample due to enzyme instability. Enzymes, like most proteins, are prone to denaturation under many laboratory conditions, and specific steps must be taken to stabilize these macromolecules as much as possible. The following general recommendations for the storage and handling of enzymes can help to maintain the catalytic activities of these proteins.

2.14.1 Stabilizing enzymes during storage

Like all proteins, enzymes in their native states are optimally stabilized by specific solution conditions of pH, ionic strength, anion/cation composition, and so on. No generalities can be stated with respect to these conditions, and the best conditions for each enzyme individually must be determined empirically. Note, however, that the solution conditions that are optimal for protein stability may not necessarily be the same as those for optimal enzymatic activity. When this caveat applies, enzyme stocks should be stored under the conditions that maximally promote stability, while the enzyme assays should be conducted under conditions of optimal activity.

For long-term storage, enzymes should be kept at cryogenic temperatures i.e. a 70°C freezer or under liquid nitrogen. Conventional freezers operate at nominal temperature of -20°C, but most of these cycle through higher temperatures to keep them ''frost free.'' This can lead to unintentional freeze-thaw cycling of the enzyme sample, which can be extremely denaturing. If enzymes are stored in such a freezer, protein stability can be greatly enhanced by adding an equal volume of glycerol to the sample and mixing it well. This 50% glycerol solution will maintain the enzyme sample in the liquid phase at 20°C, and thus will prevent repeated freezing and thawing. In fact, many enzymes display optimal stability when stored at -20°C as 50% glycerol solutions. Before the samples are frozen, they should be sterile-filtered through a 0.22 μm filter composed of a low protein-binding material, and then placed in sterilized cryogenic tubes to avoid bacterial contamination. To avoid protein denaturation during the freeze-thaw process, it is critical that the samples be frozen quickly and thawed quickly. Rapid freezing is best accomplished by immersing the sample container in slurry of dry ice and ethanol. Rapid thawing is best done by placing the sample in a 37°C water bath until most, but not all, of the sample is in the liquid state. When there is just a small bit of frozen material remaining, the sample should be removed from the bath and allowed to continue thawing on ice (i.e., 4°C).

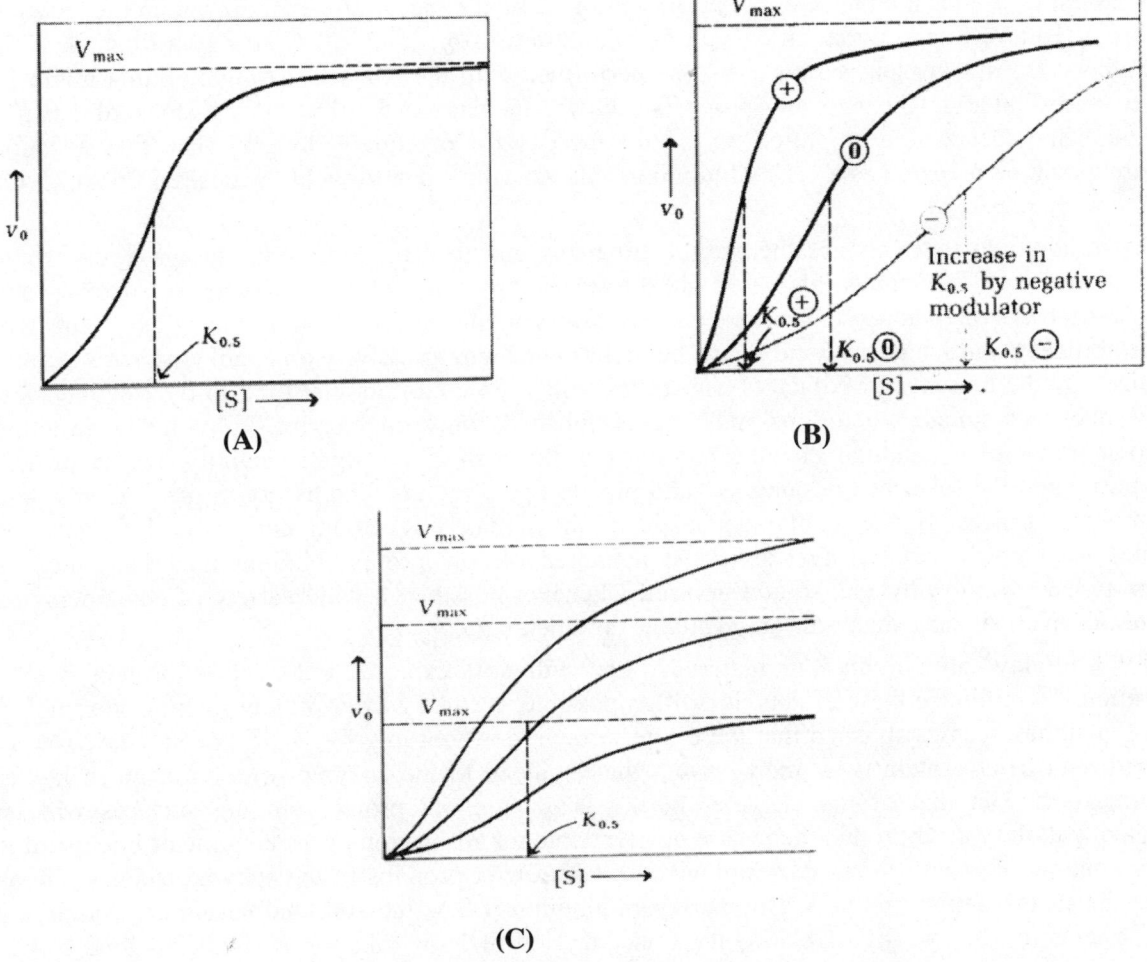

Fig. 2.23: Double reciprocal plot for allosteric enzymes

A. Sigmoid curve given by homotropic enzymes

B. Effect of positive (+), negative (-) and no modulator (O) on an allosteric enzyme

C. A rare type of modulation in which V_{max} is modulated but $K_{0.5}$ is not changed

Repeated freeze-thaw cycles are extremely denaturing to proteins and must be avoided. Thus, a frozen enzyme sample should be thawed once and used promptly. Sample remaining at the end of the experiment should not be refrozen. An enzyme that can be maintained in stable conditions for several days at 4°C, however, may be used in an experiment run soon after the first. If a particular enzyme is not stable under these conditions, any sample remaining at the end of an experiment must be discarded. To avoid wasting enzyme sample material, samples should be stored in small volume, high concentration aliquots. This way the volume of sample that is needed for each day's experiments can be thawed, while the bulk of the sample aliquots remain frozen. Once thawed, the enzyme should be kept at ice temperature (4°C) for as long as possible before equilibration to the assay temperature. Again, if the enzyme is stored at high concentration, only a small volume of the enzyme stock will be needed for dilution into the final reaction mixture.

For example, a typical enzyme assay might require a final concentration of enzyme in the reaction mixture of 10 nM. Suppose that an enzyme is in long-term storage at -70°C as a 100µM stock in 50 µL aliquots. On the day that assays are to be performed with the enzyme, a single aliquot might be thawed and diluted 1:100 with an appropriate buffer to make a 5 mL working stock of 1.0 µM enzyme. This stock would be stored on ice for the day (or potentially longer). The final reaction mixture would be prepared as a 1:100 dilution of this working stock to yield the desired final enzyme concentration of 10 nM.

Certain additives will enhance the stability of many enzymes for long-term storage at cryogenic temperatures and sometimes also for short-term storage in solution. Glycerol, sucrose, and cyclodextrans are often added to stabilize enzyme samples; the exact concentrations of excipients that best stabilize a particular enzyme must be determined empirically. Some enzymes are greatly stabilized by the presence of cofactors, substrates, and even inhibitors that bind to their active sites. Again, the best storage conditions must be established for each enzyme individually. Another common problem in handling enzyme solutions is the loss of enzymatic activity due to protein adsorption onto the surfaces of containers and pipette tips. Proteins bind avidly to glass, quartz, and polystyrene surfaces. Hence, containers made of these materials should not be used for enzyme samples. Containers and transfer devices constructed of low protein binding materials, such as polypropylene or polyethylene, should be used whenever possible; a wide variety of containers and pipette tips made of these materials are available commercially.

Even with low protein binding materials, one will still experience losses of protein due to adsorption. To minimize these effects, it is often possible to add a carrier protein to enzyme samples, as long as it has been established that the carrier protein does not interfere with the enzyme assay in any way. A carrier protein is an inert protein that is added to the enzyme solution at much higher concentrations than that of the enzyme. In this way potential protein binding surfaces will be saturated with the carrier protein, hence are not available for adsorption of the enzyme of interest. It is a very common practice among enzymologists to add carrier proteins to the enzyme stock solutions and to the final reaction mixtures. Bovine serum albumin (BSA), gelatin, and casein are commonly used proteins for this purpose. Gelatin, at a concentration of 1 mg/mL, is a particularly good carrier protein for many enzymes. The lack of aromatic amino acids in the gelatin makes this a useful carrier protein for enzyme studies utilizing ultraviolet absorption or fluorescence spectroscopy. Gelatin, casein, and BSA are available commercially in highly purified forms from a number of suppliers.

Some workers have found polyethylene glycol, molecular weight 8000 Da (PEG-8000), to be a useful alternative to carrier proteins for minimizing enzyme adsorption to container surfaces. Addition of 0.1 % PEG-8000 has been for several enzymes. If PEG-8000 is to be used for this application, a high grade (i.e., molecular biology grade or the equivalent) should be used, since lower grades may contain impurities that can have deleterious effects on enzyme activity. Our own experience with the use of PEG-8000 suggests that this additive works well to stabilize some, but not all, enzyme activities. Hence, again, the reader is left to explore the utility of this approach on a case-by-case basis.

2.14.2. Enzyme inactivation during activity assays

Certain enzymes that are stable under optimized conditions of long-term storage will inactivate during the course of an activity assay. This behavior is characterized by progress curves that plateau early, before significant substrate loss has occurred. There are two common reasons for this type of enzyme inactivation. First, the active conformation of the enzyme may not be stable under the specific conditions (i.e., temperature, pH, ionic strength, and dilution of enzyme concentration) used in the assay. For example, if the active form of the enzyme is a dimer, dilution to low concentration at the initiation of an activity assay may cause simultaneous dissociation of the dimeric enzyme to monomers. If the time course of dimer dissociation is slow, hence similar to that of the enzymatic assay, a diminution of activity may be seen over the time course of the activity measurements. Sometimes minor adjustments in final enzyme concentration can help to ameliorate this situation. Likewise, minor adjustments in other solution conditions can help to extend the lifetime of the active enzyme species during activity assays. For multisubstrate enzymes, the stability of the enzyme can sometimes also be greatly augmented by preforming a binary enzyme-substrate complex and initiating the reaction by addition of a second substrate.

The second cause of activity loss during assay is spontaneous enzyme inactivation that results directly from catalytic turnover. For some enzymes, the chemistry associated with turnover can lead to inactivation of the enzyme by covalent adduct formation, or by destruction of a key active site amino acid residue or cofactor. For example, some oxidoreductases form highly damaging free radical species as a by-product of their catalytic activity. When this occurs, the radicals that build up during turnover can attack the enzyme active site, rendering it inactive. In these cases, the radical-based inactivation can sometimes be minimized by the addition of free radical scavengers, such as phenol, to the reaction mixture. Addition of a small amount of a peroxidase enzyme, such as catalase, can also sometimes help to stabilize the enzyme of interest from radical-based inactivation. Of course, it is critical to determine that addition of such species does not affect the measurement of enzyme activity in other ways.

Regardless of the cause, enzyme inactivation during activity assays can be diagnosed by two simple tests. The first test is to allow the progress curve to go to its premature plateau and then add a small volume of additional enzyme stock that would double the final enzyme concentration in the reaction mixture (i.e., addition of a mass of enzyme equal to the initial enzyme mass in the reaction mixture). If enzyme inactivation during the assay is the cause of the premature plateau, a second phase of reaction should be realized after the addition of the second volume of fresh enzyme. The second test, known as Selwyn's test, consists of measuring the reaction progress curve at several different concentrations of enzyme. The test makes use of the fact that regardless of its complexity for individual enzymatic reactions, the integrated rate equation has the general form:

$$[E]t = f([P])$$

when all other conditions are held constant. Hence the concentration of product, [P] is some constant function of the multiplicative product of enzyme concentration and assay time. The term [E] in Equation refers to the concentration of active enzyme molecules in solution. If the enzyme is stable over the course of the assay, a plot of [P] as a function of [E]*t* should give superimposable curves at all concentrations of enzyme. If, however, the enzyme is undergoing unimolecular inactivation during the course of the activity assay, the concentration of active enzyme will itself show first-order time dependence. Thus, the dependence of [P] on [E] will have the more complex form of Equation that is given below

$$[P] = k[E](1-e^{\lambda t}) / \lambda$$

where *k* is a constant of proportionality and is the first-order decay constant for enzyme inactivation. Now plots of [P] as a function [E]*t* will vary with changing enzyme concentration. The lack of superposition of the data plots is a clear indication that enzyme inactivation has occurred during the assay time period.

2.15. ENGINEERING ENZYMES FOR STABILITY

There have been many recent developments in elaborating the approaches for stabilizing enzymes by stabilizing the folding state, destabilizing the unfolded state and altering the kinetics of unfolding. However, these represent a series of rules of thumb rather than the reliable principles that would be expected of 'engineering'. Stability is taken to include thermodynamic stability as measured by reversible denaturation, and kinetic stability as measured by the unfolding rate for enzymes that are subject to irreversible denaturation. As such, the factors that affect stability of the folded state versus the unfolded state, as well as factors affecting rates of folding and unfolding, all play a role in maintaining stability. Recent studies on the role of kinetics and the effect that site-specific substitutions have on transition-state free energies add to our understanding of the factors that determine whether or not a particular substitution will result in the measurable stabilization of a protein.

Enzymes are catalysts that can enhance reaction rates by many orders of magnitude, usually display exquisite specificity and have, therefore, many potential biomedical, chemical and industrial applications. For these applications, enzymes are frequently required to catalyze reactions in distinctly different environments to those in which they have evolved to function in nature. Thus, there is an important need to engineer enzymes that can function in non-natural environments, so that their full potential can be realized. A major limitation to enzyme function in non-natural environments is stability. The enhancement of enzyme stability is therefore an important goal of protein engineering.

In many industrial applications, stability is defined as having a sufficiently long lifetime under specified conditions to complete a reaction. As such, the factors affecting kinetic stability are as important as those that affect the thermodynamic equilibrium. Simple model systems, such as phospholipase A2, chymotrypsin inhibitor 2, GCN4, and P22 *arc* repressor have a reversible two-state folding mechanism that is amenable to rigorous thermodynamic analysis, and have been used to understand how the folded state of a protein can be stabilized. There are now several recent examples that illustrate the role kinetics can play in stabilizing proteins. From such information, engineering guidelines for stabilizing the folded state can be separated into thermodynamic factors (both entropic and enthalpic factors), for systems in rapid equilibrium, and kinetic factors that alter the stability of transition states in the folding/unfolding pathway for systems that slowly equilibrate or irreversibly denature.

2.15.1. Entropic stabilization factors

Entropy is a driving force in protein folding. When unfolded, the polypeptide has more degrees of freedom, but is extensively hydrated, particularly at hydrophobic residues around which water clathrate structures form, so that the entropy of the solvent is lowered. When folded, the protein has much fewer degrees of freedom, but sequestration of hydrophobic group releases bound water molecules, so that the entropy of the solvent is increased. The result is a net increase in the entropy of the system in the folded state. Makhatadze and Privalov (1990) have presented evidence that the hydration of polar groups also makes major contributions to entropy changes. Mutations that decrease the entropy of the system of the unfolded protein, or increase the entropy of the system of the folded protein, will result in a larger ΔS for folding, which, in the absence of complementary enthalpic contributions, will stabilize the structure.

A strategy for lowering the entropy of the unfolded protein is to reduce the degrees of freedom in the main chain. One can replace glycines with residues that have side chains, such as alanine which reduce the conformational degrees of freedom. This approach has been successful in T4 lysozyme and *Bacillus cereus* oligo-1,6-glucosidase. Corroboration for the rationale of this approach can be seen from protease substrate interaction studies. We assume that the thermodynamic factors that affect the stability of a polypeptide substrate binding to a protease are the same as those that hold different segments of a protein together. In a recent study on the binding of various peptide-like inhibitors with thrombin, it was shown that inhibitors that have side chains with more degrees of freedom in solution bind less tightly than those that have more restricted side chains. The lower affinity has been attributed to the higher entropy of inhibitors with side chains with more degrees of freedom when unbound relative to those having more restricted side chains in a manner analogous to the factors affecting the free energy of the unfolded state in proteins.

Thermostable enzymes, such as the thermostable triosephosphate isomerase from *Bacillus stearothermophilus*, have fewer internal cavities than their mesophilic counterparts, so that the removal of water trapped in internal cavities increases the entropy of the folded structure. Also, filling in cavities with larger residues will result in an unfolded polypeptide with a larger side chain to hydrate, lowering its entropy. Strategies devised to fill in internal cavities have been successful for subtilisin. In addition, thermostable enzymes often have shorter loops, leading to folded molecules that are more compact than their mesophilic counterparts and often have larger, more hydrophobic interfaces. This results in a smaller overall surface to be hydrated, leading to an increase in the entropy of the folded protein. Disulfide bonds are believed to play an important role in protein stabilization by increasing the entropy of folding by decreasing the entropy of the unfolded state.

2.15.2. Enthalpic stabilization factors

The free energy of a folded protein is lowered by favorable enthalpic interactions within the structure. These include extensive hydrogen bonding, complementary van der Waals interactions and electrostatic charge interactions, such as ion pairs. Homology modeling predicted that d-glyceraldehyde-3-phosphate from *Thermotoga mahtima* has 12 more surface ion pairs than the equivalent enzyme from *B. stearothermophilus*. The interaction of barnase with the inhibitor barstar forms a very tight complex (KD=10-14M) that may also serve as a paradigm for internal protein stabilization. It was found from extensive mutagenesis studies that the interaction between barnase and barstar is stabilized predominantly by a series of coupled ion-pair interactions.

Helices figure prominently in the folding intermediates of the prosubtilisin-subtilisin complex, chymotrypsin inhibitor 2 (CI$_2$) and alpha-lactalbumin are factors in thermodynamic stabilization and folding kinetics. Certain amino acids appear with higher frequency in different elements of secondary structures such as the N caps and C caps of alpha-helices. The introduction of a negatively charged side chain at the N cap, which can neutralize the partial dipole created by the unpaired amide protons, has been shown to increase stability in T4 lysozyme. Similar results have been reported for the complementary removal of negatively charges side chains near the C cap of alpha helices in ribonuclease T1. Comparisons of tire amino acid preferences of helices from thermophiles with those from mesophiles have been made. Tyrosine, glycine and glutamine have increased frequency in the alpha-helices of thermophilic proteins whereas valine, glutamic acid, histidine, cyteine and aspartic acid have decreased frequency. The increased frequency of glycine residues at the C termini of seven helices in thermophilic citrate synthetases was attributed to the capacity of glycine to adopt the alpha conformation at the C cap without strain. A related analysis of the N- and C-capping preferences for all 20 amino acids in alpha-helical peptides found that the N cap preferences of peptides and protein are retained, but that glycine was not preferred in the C cap of peptide helices. This may reflect a greater need for correct helix termination in proteins and its role in structure stabilization.

2.16. ENZYME TECHNOLOGY AND BIOPROCESS ENGINEERING

The impact of directed evolution and site-specific mutagenesis on the industrial utility of enzymatic catalysis through the modification of enzyme structure and function is clearly an important area of research in bioprocess engineering. High throughput screening for novel or improved enzyme activities, both by more efficiently exploring nature's diversity and by creating new diversity in the test tube, allow new bioprocesses to be developed. Similarly, innovations in enzyme technology that address novel ways to apply enzymes in bioprocesses also have an impact on bioprocess engineering. Several recent developments have been made in this latter aspect of bioprocess engineering.

2.16.1. Enzyme-catalyzed racemization

The combined use of *Pseudomonas* sp. lipase and mandelate racemase for deracemization of *rac*-mandelic acid to (*S*)-*O*-acetylmandelic acid (80% yield, enantiomeric excess) has previously been described by Strauss and Faber (1999). The utility of mandelate racemase from *Pseudomonas putida* ATCC 12336 for DKR has been increased by binding the enzyme to anion-exchange resins, thus activating and stabilizing the enzyme. In addition, the scope of this particular mandelate racemase has been studied and substrates were shown to include 2-heteroaryl analogs of mandelic acid as well as mandelic amide and *p*-bromomandelic amide enabling its application in novel DKRs.

N-Acylamino acid racemases, which racemize *N*-acylamino acids but not the free amino acids, are used in combination with D- or L-aminoacylases for the production of enantiomerically pure D- and L-amino acids. The *N*-acylamino acid racemase from *Amycolatopsis* sp. TS-1-60, which is particularly useful because it is thermostable, has been immobilized on DEAE anion exchanger resin in combination with either D-aminoacylase from *Amycolatopsis* sp. TS-1-60 or L-aminoacylase from *Streptomyces atratus* Y-53. These two combinations of enzymes can be used for the production of D-methionine (90% yield) and L-methionine (99% yield), respectively. The nucleotide sequence of the *N*-acylamino acid racemase from *Amycolatopsis* sp. TS-1-60 was used to isolate related enzymes with improved properties with respect to substrate and product inhibition and dependency on divalent cations.

2.16.2. Enzymes in organic solvents

2.16.2.1. Improving the activity

Enzymes in neat organic liquids are generally orders of magnitude less active than in the aqueous phase; however, this observation is now challenged by recent findings. In a series of papers, Clark and coworkers (Ru et al., 1999, 2000, 2001) investigated the effects of lyophilization conditions on the catalytic efficiency of subtilisin Carlsberg. They investigated the addition of inorganic salts such as KCl to an enzyme solution before freeze-drying, which can lead to a dramatic increase of activity in organic solvents. The salts were added in amounts up to 98% (wt/wt) of the preparation at the end of lyophilization. In their systematic study, the authors found that the extent of the activating effect correlates with the kosmotropicity of the salts. Kosmotropic salts possess a positive Jones–Dole viscosity B coefficient and interact strongly with water, leading, for example, to an increase in viscosity.

The addition of the salts had several effects: the number of catalytically active sites increased, as also the catalytic constants and the catalytic efficiency. Part of the effect was explained by the preferential hydration of the protein as a result of the addition of kosmotropes. This would help to maintain the native conformation of the protein during the lyophilization process. The effects of different kosmotropic salts could be combined such that the effect is larger than the effect of two salts separately. Furthermore, optimization of cooling rate, water content of the lyophilized material, and buffering capacity of the additive contributed to an increase in specific activity of the lyophilized material. In total, the experiments led to a catalytic efficiency of lyophilized subtilisin Carlsberg that was within one order of magnitude of the enzyme's activity in aqueous media.

2.16.3. Control of water activity in process design

Obviously, the control of water activity is one of the main issues for enzymatic reactions in organic solvents, as it has a strong effect on the specific activity and the inactivation rate of the biocatalyst. Control is particularly important if water is produced during the reaction as, for example, in esterification reactions. Lipase biocatalysts are frequently immobilized on a matrix that itself can act as an adsorbent for water. This can be very practical, but complicates the analysis. An ideal reaction system would rapidly remove the water produced from the reaction mixture. One recent approach to achieve this is the development of the chromatographic reactor, in which water is removed by adsorption to, for example, an ion exchanger. Models have been developed to evaluate this option for lipase esterification in a fixed-bed reactor: lipozyme, a *Mucor mihei* lipase immobilized on a phenolic macroporous weak anion exchanger, and a gel-type polystyrene-divinylbenzene cation-exchange resin was combined in a column. The ion exchanger adsorbed the water produced and so maintained the water activity below a critical activity (above which the enzyme would become deactivated).

This concept was successfully applied for the quasi-irreversible esterification of propionic acid with isoamyl alcohol to form isoamyl propionate in hexane. A detailed model of the system was used to construct a continuous three-fixed-bed reactor system that was superior in productivity per unit mass enzyme. Two sequential reactors were used for the simultaneous reaction/adsorption. The third reactor was regenerated by removing the adsorbed water with isoamyl alcohol. Periodically, the status of one reactor was changed from reaction to regeneration. Although in this case the critical issue was to prevent enzyme inactivation, the same principle can also be used for reactions where the esterification is equilibrium-limited because the solubility of water remains high during the reaction. Thus, the conversion of propionic acid and 2-ethyl-1,3-hexanediol in hexane could be increased by water adsorption, relative to the situation without water adsorption, especially when the reactors were operated in transient fashion.

2.17. NANOSCALE BIOCATALYST SYSTEMS

Since the large-scale application of immobilized enzymes in the1960s, substantial research efforts have aimed to optimize the structure of carrier materials for better catalytic efficiency. In this regard, nanoscale materials provide the upper limits in balancing the key factors that determine the efficiency of biocatalysts, including surface area, mass transfer resistance, and effective enzyme loading. Various nanomaterials such as nanoparticles, nanofibers, nanotubes and nanoporous matrices have shown potential for revolutionizing the preparation and use of biocatalysts. Beyond their high surface area : volume ratios, nanoscale biocatalyst systems exhibit unique behaviors that distinguish them from traditional immobilized systems. The Brownian motion of nanoparticles, confining effect of nanopores and self-assembling behaviors of discrete nanostructures are providing exciting opportunities in this field. The development of catalyst systems that are highly stable, efficient, and self-targeting, or that function as molecular machines to catalyze multiple reactions, is rapidly reshaping our vision of biocatalysts.

2.17.1. The perspective of materials and methods

Materials of various compositions, shapes and structures and with modified surfaces have been used to support biocatalysts (Fig. 2.24). Nanoparticles made of silica, magnetite and gold, comprise the first group of nanomaterials employed for biocatalysis. Nanoparticles provide an ideal remedy to the usually contradictory issues encountered in the optimization of immobilized enzymes, as high surface area and enzyme loading are usually accompanied with high mass transfer resistance within the supports. There are drawbacks, however; often the dispersion of nanoparticles in the reaction media and their recovery after the reaction are daunting tasks. The handling of dry powders of nanoparticles also presents certain health and environmental concerns. Carbon nanotubes, which exist in powder form when in a pure state, share similar concerns when used as enzyme supports. Some of these problems can be overcome by using one-dimensional nanomaterials, such as polymeric nano-fibers. The surface area volume ratio of nanofibers is also high, representing two-thirds of that of nanoparticles of the same diameter when considering equivalent amounts of material. Nanofibers, however, have the benefit of being much easier to produce and handle. They can be applied in the form of coils, sheets or dispersed fibers and can also be attached to the surface of other materials or blended with them, thus offering very flexible design of reactors.

Many methods have been developed to incorporate enzymes into nanostructures. Surface attachment was employed in many of the earlier studies and is often the method of choice. Another way to develop nanoscale biocatalysts is to entrap enzymes within nanopores. Mesoporous silica gels have been used to host enzymes through physical adsorption or chemical binding. Using carefully designed synthetic routes, enzymes were also entrapped within the cores of discrete polymeric and silica particles. More sophisticated structures, such as porous materials hosting enzyme-carrying nanoparticles and cross-linked enzyme aggregates, have been developed by applying enzyme modification and fabrication procedures. The functionalization and modification of nanomaterials have been pursued with great interest to improve the performance of nanoscale biocatalysts in their application environments. The use of magnetic nanoparticles to facilitate handling of materials and reaction control, surface modification for better dispersion or assembly properties, and the fabrication of multienzyme systems have all been reported.

Overall, many earlier studies followed the concepts and mechanisms underlying traditional enzyme immobilization and modification. The type and format of materials and methods for enzyme attachment have been applied on a random trial basis. At the same time, several unique properties that distinguish nanoscale biocatalyst systems from traditional immobilized systems can be gleaned from recent studies. Examining these unique properties and behaviors might eventually help us to identify key factors that control the performance of nanoscale biocatalyst systems, and could provide the basis for the rational design of biocatalyst systems that better realize the power of nanoscale science and engineering.

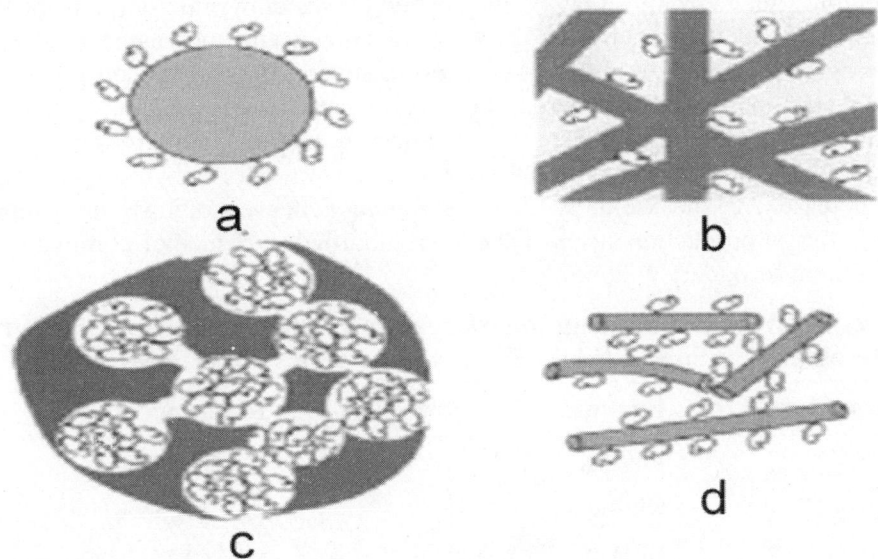

Fig. 2.24: Basic structures of nanoscale biocatalysts. (a) Nanoparticles with surface-attached enzymes. (b) Nanofibers carrying enzymes. (c) Nanoporous matrix with entrapped enzymes. (d) Carbon nanotube–enzyme hybrid materials

2.18. COMPUTATIONAL ENZYMOLOGY

Numerical simulations of enzyme reaction mechanisms are beginning to provide quantitative as well as qualitative insights. Methods based on a hybrid quantum mechanical/molecular mechanical technique permit the natural inclusion of protein solvation effects. Coupled with modern experimental techniques, the numerical simulations are providing details at the atomic level about how enzyme structure influences its function.

Various approaches have been developed to study the key chemical steps in enzyme-catalyzed reactions, as one might imagine, as computational resources have improved, so have the complexity and sophistication of numerical simulation methods. One method involves incorporating both a quantum-mechanical (QM) description of atoms in the active site of the enzyme and a molecular-mechanical (MM) description of the remaining atoms. The principal assumption of the method is that changes in the electronic structure during the reaction are localized to the vicinity of the active site. In this scheme, the bulk of the protein/solvent system is represented by a molecular mechanics potential; only a small number of atoms in the active site are treated quantum mechanically. While this hybrid QM/MM technique is not as complete a model as one might wish, it has proven quite capable of providing the sort of detailed information about reaction mechanisms previously unavailable from experimental measurement.

2.19. FOOD-PROCESSING ENZYMES FROM RECOMBINANT MICROORGANISMS

Enzymes are commonly used in food processing and in the production of food ingredients. Enzymes traditionally isolated from culturable microorganisms, plants, and mammalian tissues are often not well adapted to the conditions used in modern food production methods. The use of recombinant DNA technology has made it possible to manufacture novel enzymes suitable for specific food-processing conditions. Such enzymes may be discovered by screening microorganisms sampled from diverse environments or developed by modification of known enzymes using modern methods of protein engineering or molecular evolution. As a result, several important food-processing enzymes such as amylases and lipases with properties tailored to particular food applications have become available (Table 2.15). Another important achievement is improvement of microbial production strains. For example, several microbial strains recently developed for enzyme production have been engineered to increase enzyme yield by deleting native genes encoding extracellular proteases. Moreover, certain fungal production strains have been modified to reduce or eliminate their potential for production of toxic secondary metabolites.

Table 2.15: Enzymes from recombinant microorganisms (based on FDA regulations, Generally Recognized as Safe (GRAS) affirmation petitions, and GRAS notices)

Source microorganism	Enzyme	Reference
Aspergillus niger	Phytase	GRASP 2G0381
	Chymosin	21 CFR 184.1685
	Lipase	GRN 158
Aspergillus oryzae	Esterase-lipase	GRASP 7G0323
	Aspartic proteinase	GRN 34
	Glucose oxidase	GRN 106
	Laccase	GRN 122
	Lipase	GRN 43; GRN 75; GRN 103
Bacillus licheniformis	Amylase	GRASP 0G0363;
	Pullulanase	GRN 22; GRN 24;
Escherichia coli K-12	Chymosin	21 CFR 184.1685
Fusarium venenatum	Xylanase	GRN 54
Trichoderma reesei	Pectin lyase	GRN 32

2.20. PHARMACEUTICAL APPLICATIONS

2.20.1. Diagnostic applications

The assay of enzyme levels in the extracellular body fluids (blood plasma and serum, urine, digestive juices, amniotic fluid and cerebrospinal fluid) are important aids to the clinical diagnosis and management of diseases. Although the majority of enzyme catalyzed reactions take place within living cells, whenever an energy imbalance occurs in the cells as a result of exposure to infective agents, bacterial toxins, etc., enzymes 'leak' out through the membranes into the circulation. This causes their fluid level to be raised above the normal cellular level. Measurement of the type, extent and duration of these raised enzyme activities can then provide information about the identity of the damaged cell and indicate the degree of injury. Enzyme assay can make significant contribution to the diagnosis of diseases because a minute change in enzyme concentration can be easily measured. Measurement of the changes in enzyme level therefore, offers a greater degree of organ and disease differentiation as compared to other possible clinico-chemical parameters such as albumin or gamma globulin.

Now a days, the diagnostic specificity of enzyme tests is such that they are restricted mainly to confirming diagnosis providing data to be weighed with other clinical evidences due to lack of disease specific enzymes. Table 2.16 lists some diagnostically important enzymes which are most frequently assayed in clinical laboratories.

Table 2.16: Diagnostically important enzymes

Enzyme and abbreviation	Tissue source*	Reaction
Acetylcholinesterase ACHE	BE	Acetylcholine to acetate and choline
Acid phosphatase SP	Pr E	Phosphate monoester to alcohol and Pi (pH 8-10)
Alanine aminotransferase GPT (AAT)	L	Alanine to gultamate
Alkaline phosphatase AP	BILPIK	Phosphate monoester to alcohol and Pi (pH 8-10)
α-Amylase	Pa S	Starch to maltose
Aspartate aminotransferase GOT (AST)	HLMKB	Aspartate to glutamate
Cholinesterase CHE	L	Acylcholine to fatty acid and choline
Chymotrypsin CT	PA	Proteins to polypeptides
Creatine lipase CPK	MHB	Creatine to creatine phosphate
Fructose-biphosphate aldolase ALD	MH	Fructose-1,6-biphosphate to triose phosphate
γ-Glutamyl transferase GGT	KL	γ-Glutamyl peptide to γ-glutamylamino acid
Hydroxybutyrate dehydrogenase HBD (LD1)	H	2-Hydroxybutyrate to 2-oxybutyrate
Isocitrate dehydrogenase ICD	L	Isocitrate to oxoglutarate
Lactate dehydrogenase LD	HLMK	Lactate to pyruvate
5'-Nucleosidase 5.N	Ht Pa	5'-Ribonucleotide to ribonucleoside
Ornithine carbamoyltransferase OCT	L	Carbamoyl-P to citrulline
Triacylglycerol lipase	Pa	Triacylglycerol to diacylglycerol and fatty acid

* *B, brain; E, erythrocytes; H, heart muscle; Ht, hepatobiliary tract; I, intestinal mucosa; K, kidney; L, liver; M, skeletal muscle; Pa, pancreas; Pl, placenta; Pr, prostate gland; S, saliva.*

2.20.1.1. Enzymes in the diagnosis of liver and biliary system disorders

Liver diseases were among the first to which serum enzyme tests were applied. They have proved to be most successful due to the large size of the organ and wide variety and abundance of enzymes. The liver-function enzymes GOT, GPT and AP are assayed to determine the site and nature of liver disease. LD, GGT, OCT and CHE are also monitored. Various enzymes used in the diagnosis of liver diseases along with their respective levels are listed in Table 2.17.

2.20.1.2. Enzymes in heart disease

No single entirely specific enzyme has yet been found for myocardial damage and a combination of results from assays of CPK, GOT and HBD, each of which are elevated in more than 90% of cases, is used for diagnostic purposes. The elevated enzyme activities in serum after acute myocardial infarction are shown in Figure 2.25.

Table 2.17: Liver diseases and enzymes used for diagnosis

Disease	Enzyme used	Enzyme level
Acute hepatitis	GOT and GPT	20 to 50 times of normal level
Chronic hepatitis and cirrhosis	All liver transaminases	3 to 12 fold than normal level and inflammation of the liver
Fatty liver	GPT	2 fold than normal
Solvent poisoning of liver	GOT GPT LD	GOT:GPT:LD 6500:3000:10000 (U/ml)
Hepatobiliary disease (obstructive jaundice)	GOT and GPT	5 to 10 fold

The level of CPK starts rising after three to four hours of the initial onset of pain, followed in order by GOT and AST (HBD) which appear after a lapse of approximately eight hours. The maximum level reached in same sequence, CPK after 24 hours, LD 1 after 36 hours and AST after about two days. The rise in enzyme levels is fairly moderate AST and CPK rise four to ten fold above their respective normal levels and LD 1 approximately five fold higher than normal.

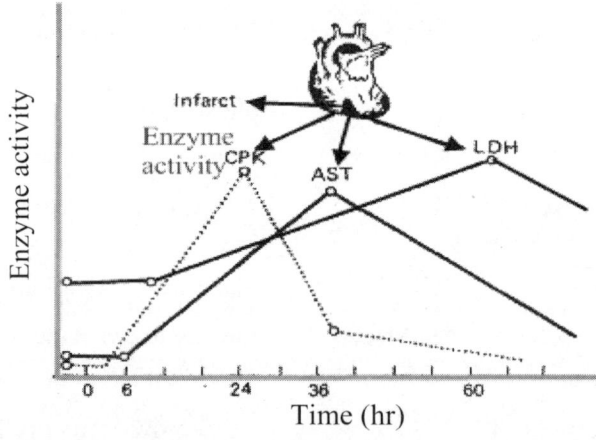

Fig. 2.25: Serum enzyme activities after myocardial infarction

2.20.1.3. Diagnosis of muscle disease

Skeletal muscle disorders include the diseases of the muscle fibers (myopathies) or of the muscle nerves (neurogenic disorders). In myopathies CPJ, LD, ALD, GOT and GPT levels are raised. In the case of neurogenic diseases and hereditary diseases, CPK is occasionally raised (2 to 3 fold). Damage to the muscle may be due to extensive muscular exercise, drugs, physical trauma, inflammatory diseases, microbial infection or metabolic dysfunction or it may be genetically predisposed. In muscular disorders the level of CPK is elevated in serum with the highest frequency and is assayed in the diagnosis of these disorders.

2.20.2. Enzymes in therapeutics

Many enzymes are used as therapeutic agents due to some of their following specific characteristics:

1. they are specific to their substrates;
2. they can produce the desired effect without eliciting any side reaction;
3. they are water soluble; and
4. they are highly efficient in biological environment.

Enzymes as therapeutic agents also have some drawbacks which limit their utility. The large molecular structure and high molecular weight excludes them from the intracellular domains. They are highly antigenic because of their proteinaceous nature. They are rapidly cleared from blood plasma. Extensive purification from pyrogens and toxins is necessary for parenteral enzymes which increases the cost. Table 2.18 lists some therapeutically important enzymes.

2.20.2.1. Enzyme therapy of neoplastic disease

The enzyme therapy of cancer is based on the principle of depriving the abnormal cells of their essential metabolic precursors (amino acids, nucleic acid and folates). Several enzymes have been tested for and proved suitable as antitumor agents. L-asparaginase, L-arginase, carboxypeptidase G (folate depletion), L-glutaminase, L-methioninase, L-phenylalanine ammonia lyase, L-serine dehydratase, L-tyrosinase and xanthine oxidase have been tested for their anticancer activity.

Table 2.18: Therapeutically important enzymes

Enzyme preparation	Source	Therapeutic application
Asparaginase (amidase)	*E. coli*, guinea pig serum	Cytotoxic agents
Chymotrypsin (protease)	Bovine pancreas	Inflammation, oedema, ophthalmology, and upper respiratory tract diseases
Deoxyribonuclease (DNA hydrolysis)	Bovine pancreas	Reduces viscosity of pulmonary secretions
Dextranase (Dextran hydrolysis)	*Penicillum funiculosum*	Dental plaque restriction
Diastase (Starch hydrolysis)	Malt	Amylaceous dyspepsia
Galactosidase (Lactose hydrolysis)	*Aspergillus niger*	Inherited β-galactosidase deficiency
Hyaluronidase (Mucopolysaccharide hydrolysis)	Animal testes	Increase absorption rate, increase effectiveness of local anesthetics
Pancreatin	Animal pancreas	Pancreatitis
Papain (Protease)	*Carica papaya*	Dyspepsia and gastritis
Penicillinase	*Bacillus cereus*	Penicillin allergy
Plasmin(Protease)	Plasminogen	Thrombotic disorders anticoagulation
Streptodornase (DNA-ase)	*Streptococci*	Depolymerization of DNA in purulent exudates
Streptokinase (Protease)	*Streptococci*	Thromboemolic diseases
Trypsin (Protease)	Animal pancreas	Cleaning necrotic tissue
Tissue plasminogen activator (Protease)	Recombinant DNA tech.	Thromboemolic diseases
Urokinase (Protease)	Human urine	Thromboemolic diseases

L-Asparaginase is the most extensively studied enzyme. It is used in the treatment of three neoplastic diseases, acute lymphoblastic leukemia, leukemic lymphosarcoma and myeloblastic leukemia. It deprives the tumor cells of their nutritional asparagine supply. Asparagine is required by the cell for protein synthesis and impaired protein synthesis is probably responsible for the immunosuppression and toxic effects of asparaginase therapy.

$$\text{L-Asparagine} + \text{PPi} + \text{AMP} \underset{}{\overset{\text{Asparaginase}}{\rightleftharpoons}} \text{L- Aspartate} + NH_3 + \text{ATP}$$

The future of enzyme therapy in cancer is very bright but the problems of antigenicity and short circulation time remain to be overcome.

2.20.2.2. Enzymes as thrombolytic agents

The fibrinolytic system dissolves intravascular clots as a result of the action of plasmin, a nonspecific protease that digests fibrin. Plasminogen is an inactive precursor of plasmin and is converted to plasmin by cleavage of a single peptide bond. Plasmin digests fibrin clots and other plasmin proteins including several coagulation factors. Therapy with thrombolytic enzymes tends to digest fibrin clots of vascular injury.

The general clinical use of enzymes is the promotion of thrombolysis. The rationale of enzymatic fibrinolysis relies on the supposition that increasing the levels of circulating proteases should more rapidly dissolve the blood clot or preformed thrombus.

Currently, two types of enzyme are used, one with direct and general proteolytic activity such as plasmin or trypsin and another which increases the level of native plasmin such as plasminogen activator. Clinical evidence supports the second alternative. Promotion of natural lysis utilizes the avalanche effect of the cascade, and does not require a prior infusion to neutralize circulating anti-proteases and lastly it is more specific. Two lysokinase plasminogen activators streptokinase and urokinase have been used as thrombolytic agents.

2.20.2.3. Indigestion disorders and inflammation

Enzymes have been used for long to supplement enzyme deficiencies of the pancreas and small intestine. Pancreatin (obtained from alcoholic extract of animal pancreas) is administered buccally to enhance the enzymatic digestion of starch and proteins in patients with pancreatic cyst and pancreatitis. Pancreatin along with lipase is used to treat patients with fatty stools.

Hydrolytic enzymes e.g., papain and extracts from fungi *Aspergillus niger* and *A.oryzae* are used to increase absorption from the small intestine. These extracts containing amylases and proteases along with cellulases assist the degradation of the indigestible fibers of cabbages etc., and so reduce dyspepsia and flatulence.

Micro-organisms are used as large scale sources of therapeutic enzymes. *Saccharomyces cerevisiae, S. fragilis, Bacillus subtilis* and two *Aspergillus* species are recommended safe by FDA (USA) for oral administration. *β*-Galactosidase (from *A. oryzae*) is used by patients suffering from the inherited intestinal disease lactose deficiency. Children with this genetic disorder are unable to digest milk lactose. *β*-Galactosidase catalyses the conversion of lactose to glucose and galactose which are readily absorbed by the intestine. Penicillinase (from *Bacillus subtilis*) is used to treat hypersensitivity reaction caused by penicillin. The enzyme catalyzes the hydrolysis of penicillin to penicillanic acid, which is non-immunogenic.

Microbial and plant hydrolases are also used to reduce inflammation and oedema. Thrombin, trypsin, chymotrypsin, papain, streptokinase, streptodornase, and serrapeptidase have been subjected to clinical trials. They are administered orally and have significant proteolytic activity in the serum. Streptodornase has shown pain relieving action on systemic infection. The preparations have also been used to clean dirty wounds and necrotic tissue and to remove debris from second and third degree burns.

2.21. ENZYMES IN BIOANALYTICAL CHEMISTRY

Enzymes can be employed to measure substrate concentrations as well as the concentrations of species that affect the catalytic activity of the enzyme toward its substrate, such as activators and inhibitors. Enzymatic methods are popular because they are relatively simple, require little or no sample pretreatment, and do not require expensive instrumentation. The single critical advantage, however, is the lack of interferences due to the selectivity of enzymes for their natural substrates. The selectivity of glucose oxidase from *Aspergillus niger* has been studied through a comparison of the maximum rates of product formation from a variety of structurally related sugars, shown in table 2.19. Glucose oxidase is most reactive toward its natural substrate, beta-D-glucose, so that this substrate has been assigned a relative oxidation rate of 100%.

Table 2.19: Substrate Selectivity of Glucose Oxidase

Substrate	Relative rate of oxidation (%)
β-D-Glucose	100
2-Deoxy-D-glucose	25
6-Deoxy-6-fluoro-D-glucose	3
6-Methyl-D-glucose	1.85
4,6-Dimethyl-D-glucose	1.22
D-Mannose	0.98
D-Xylose	0.98
α-D-Glucose	0.22

The data in Table 2.19 show that the only substrate that would represent a significant interference in an enzymatic assay for glucose using glucose oxidase is 2-deoxy-D-glucose. It is of particular interest that the anomeric form of the enzyme's natural substrate, a-D-glucose, cannot be oxidized at a significant rate, even though the two compounds differ only in the position of the hydroxyl group at the C1 position of the sugar. It is this exquisite selectivity that is exploited in enzymatic assays, enabling their use for substrate quantitation in matrices that may be as complex as blood or fermentation broths.

2.22. ENZYMES FOR THE TREATMENT OF EFFLUENTS

There are research reports and patents that have described the use of microorganisms and/or enzymes pools developed in the laboratory for the biological treatment of effluents with high fat and oil concentrations. For example, the Japanese company Meito Sangyo Co. (41 Sasazuka- Cho 2-ChomeNishi-Ku Nagoya, Aichi, Japan) produces a lipase from Candida rugosa (Lipase-MY) for fat removal in equipment of effluent treatment plants in the United States . In addition, Neozyme International Inc. (33 Journey, Aliso Viejo, CA, USA) manufactures and sells patented bioorganic catalytic formulations that rapidly break down organic contaminants including fats, oils, and greases (FOG) due to the difficulty of successfully treating these substances with conventional products and equipment.

Enzymes and pure cultures have also been used to increase hydrolysis during or prior to biological treatment processes. Such pre- or co-treatments methods generally consist of the cultivation of lipase-producing microbial strains in the effluents. Cail *et al.* (1986) tested an enzymatic mixture containing protease, amylase, cellulase and lipase and Bacillus subtilis spores on wool scouring wastewater with high lipid content; this mixture increased the COD reduction from 59% in the control to 78%, increased grease removal from 47% to over 70%, and improved solids reduction from 34% to over 70%. Lipases have also been used for the degradation of wastewater contaminants from olive oil processing. De Felice et al. (2004) cultivated the yeast Yarrowia lipolytica ATCC 20255 on wastewater from an olive oil mill under batch culture conditions. They found that the yeast was capable of reducing the COD value (100–200 g/L) by 80% in 24 h and producing a useful biomass of 22.45 g/L as single cell protein and enzyme lipases.

SUGGESTED READING

- Axen R, Carlsson J, Janson JC, Porath J. *Enzymologia* 41, 359 (1971).
- Barman TE. *Enzyme Handbook*, Spring-Verlag, Berlin, (1969).
- Bender ML, Kezdy FJ, Wedler FC. *J Chem Educ* 44, 84 (1967).
- Blacklow SC, Raines RT, Lim WA, et al. *Biochemistry*, 27, 1158 (1988).
- Boyer PD. (Ed.) *The Enzymes*, Vol. 3, Acdemic Press, New York (1971).
- Carraway KL, Koshland DE. *Methods Enzymol* 25, 616 (1972).
- Cleland WW. *Anal Biochem* 99, 142 (1979).
- Cleland WW, O'Leary MH, Northrop DB. *Isotope Effects on Enzyme-Catalyzed Reactions*, University Park Press, Baltimore (1977).
- Cho YK, Bailey JE. *Biotechnol Bioeng* 21, 461 (1979).
- Colowick SP, Kaplan NO. (Eds.), *Methods in Enzymology*, Academic Press, New York, Vol.I. (1955).
- Copeland RA. *Methods for Protein Analysis: A Practical Guide to Laboratory Protocols*, Chapman & Hall, New York (1994).
- Copeland RA, Lombardo D, Giannaras J, Decicco CP. *Bioorg. Med Chem Lett* 5, (1947).
- Copeland RA, Williams JM, Giannaras J, et al., *Proc. Natl. Acad. Sci.* USA 91, 11202 (1994).
- Coulet PR, Sternberg R, Thevenot DR. *Biochim Biophys Acta* 612, 317 (1980).
- Caravajal SG, Leyden DE, Quinting GR, et al., *Anal. Chem.* 60, 1766 (1988).
- Cornish-Bowden A. *Biochem J* 130, 637 (1972).
- Dixon M, Webb EC. *Enzymes*, 3rd ed., Academic Press, New York (1979).
- Duggleby RG. *Biochem J* 228, 55 (1985).
- Duggleby RG. *Biochim Biophys Acta* 1205, 268 (1994).
- Duggleby RG, Morrison JF. *Biochim Biophys Acta* 481, 297 (1977).
- Degani Y, Miron T, *Biochim Biophys Acta* 212, 362 (1970).
- Easterby JS. *Biochim Biophys Acta* 293, 552 (1973).
- Enzyme Nomenclature : Recommendations of the Nomenclature of the International Union of Biochemistry on the Nomenclature and Classification of Enzymes, Academic Press, New York, (1978).
- Fersht A. *Enzyme Structure and Mechanism*, Freeman, San Francisco (1977).
- Foster RL. *The Nature of Enzymology*, Croom Helm, London (1980).
- Fernandez-Lafuente R, Guisan JM, Ali S, Cowan D, *Enz Microb Technol* 26, 568 (2000).
- Giuseppi-Elie A, Sheppard NF, Brahim S, Narinesingh D, *Biotechnol Bioeng* 75, 475 (2001).
- Guilbault GG, Das J. *Anal Biochem* 33, 341 (1970).

- Goldstein L, Katchalski E, Fresenius Z. *Anal Chem* 243, 375 (1968).
- Guilbault GG. *Handbook of Enzymatic Methods of Analysis*, Marcel Dekker, New York, pp. 510–517 (1976).
- Godfrey T, Reichelt J. (eds), *Industrial Enzymology*, Macmillan London (1983).
- Greenberg DM, Harper HT. (Eds.), *Enzymes in Health and Disease*, Charles C. Thomas, Springfield (1960).
- Habeeb AFSA, Hiramoto R. *Arch Biochem Biophys* 126, 16 (1968).
- Hatchikian EC, Monsan P. *Biochem Biophys Res Commun* 92, 1091 (1980).
- Hugo WB. (Ed.), *Inhibition and Destruction of Microbial Cells*, Academic Press, London, p 39-70 (1971).
- Inman JK, Dintzis HM. *Biochemistry* 8, 4074 (1969).
- Innerfield I. *Enzymes in Clinical Medicine*, McGraw Hill, Blakiston Division, New York (1960).
- Ishikawa E, Hashida S, Kohno T, Tanaka ., *Methods for enzyme-labeling of antigens, antibodies and their fragments*, in *Nonisotopic Immunoassay*, T. T. Ngo, (Ed), Plenum Press, New York, pp. 27–55 (1988).
- Joseph MD, Kasprzak D, Crouch SR. *Clin Chem* 23, 1033 (1977).
- Johansson G. *Appl Biochem Biotechnol* 7, 99 (1982).
- Kohn J, Wilchek M. *Appl Biochem Biotechnol* 9, 285 (1984).
- Kula MR. *Enzymes,* In *Fundamentals of Biotechnology* P. Prave, U. Faust, W. Sittings, D.A. Sukatsch (Eds.), VCH Verlagsgesellschaft mbH, Weinheim Germany, p 473 (1987).
- Lomant AJ, Fairbanks G. *J Mol Biol* 104, 243 (1976).
- Lehninger AL. *Principles of Biochemistry*, CBS, New Delhi, p 207-241 (1990).
- Lilly MD, Hornby WE, Crook EM. *Biochem J* 100, 718 (1966).
- Line WF, Kwong A, Weetall HH. *Biochim Biophys Acta* 242, 194 (1971).
- Melling J, Phillips BW. *Practical aspect of large-scale enzyme purification* In *Handbook of Enzyme Biotechnology*, A. Wiseman (Ed.), Ellis Harwood. Chichester, p 181-202 (1975).
- Moran LA, Scringeous KG. *Biochemistry Resource Book*, Neil Patterson Publishers, Prentice Hall, NJ, USA, p 27-57 (1994).
- Murary PK, Mayes PA, Granner DK, Rodwell VM. (Eds.), *Harper's Biochemistry*, 22nd edition, Prentice-Hall International, p 58-89 (1990).
- Neilands JB, Stumpf PK. *Outline of Enzyme Chemistry*, 2nd edition, John Wiley & Sons, New York, p 132-169 (1958).
- Ngo T. *Int J Biochem* 11, 459 (1980).
- Ozawa H. *J Biochem* 62, 531 (1967).
- Ottaway and Apps DK. *Biochemistry*, Fourth edition, The English Language Book Society and Bailler Tindall, p 24-44 (1984).
- Patel PR. *Enzyme Isolation and purification*, In *Biotechnology: Application and Research*, P.N. Cheremisinoff and R.P. Ouellette (Eds.), Technomic Publising, Lancaster, Basel, p 534-564 (1985).
- Patel RP, Lopiedes DV, Brown SP, et al., *Biopolymers* 5, 577 (1967).
- Royer GP, Ikeda S, Aso K. *FEBS Lett.* 80, 89 (1977).
- Rosevear A, Kennedy JF, Cabral JMS. *Immobilized Enzymes and Cells*, IOP Publishing, Philadelphia, pp. 83–97 (1987).
- Ru MT, Dordick JS, Reimer JA, et al. *Biotechnol Bioeng* 63, 233 (1999).
- Ru MT, Hirokane SY, Lo AS, et al., *J Am Chem Soc* 122, 1565 (2000).

- Ru MT, Wu KC, Lindsay JP, et al., *Biotechnol Bioeng* 75,187 (2001).
- Shimizu SY, Lenhoff HM. *J Solid Phase Biochem* 4, 75 (1979).
- Strauss UT, Faber K. *Tetrahedron: Asymmetry* 10, 4079 (1999).
- Strove EA. *Biochemistry,* Mir Publications, Moscow, p 125-163 (1989).
- Stryer L. *Biochemistry*, Third edition, W.H. Freeman and Company, New York, p 177-257 (1988).
- Silman IH, Albu-Weissenberg M. Katchalski E. *Biopolymers* 4, 441 (1966).
- Sundaram PV, Hornby WE. *FEBS Lett* 10, 325 (1970).
- Trehan MD, Grover S. *Trans Biochem Soc* 7, 28 (1979).
- Weber G. (Ed.), *Advances in Enzyme Regulation*, Vol. 1-4, Pergamon Press (1963-1977).
- West ES, Todd WR, Mason HS, VanBruygen JT. *Textbook of Biochemistry*, fourth edition, The Macmillan Company, Collier-Macmillan Ltd., London, p 419-490 (1966).
- Weetall HH. *Nature* (London) 223, 959–960 (1969).
- Zaborski OR. *Immobilized Enzymes*, CRC Press, Cleveland, Ohio, pp. 49–60 (1973).
- Zingaro RA, Uziel M. *Biochim Biophys Acta* 213, 371 (1970).

ENZYME AND CELL IMMOBILIZATION

3.1. IMMOBILIZATION OF ENZYMES

3.2. IMMOBILIZATION METHODS

  3.2.1. Adsorption and ionic binding

  3.2.2. Entrapment and occlusion

  3.2.3. Microencapsulation

  3.2.4. Covalent bonding

    3.2.4.1. Azo linkage

    3.2.4.2. Isocyanates and isothiocyanates

    3.2.4.3. Carboxy methylazides

    3.2.4.4. Carbodiimides

    3.2.4.5. Covalent immobilization through glutaraldehyde

    3.2.4.6. Covalent coupling employing N-succinimide activation

    3.2.4.7. Covalent coupling through diacyl fatty anhydrides

    3.2.4.8. Covalent coupling through sulfhydryl group

    3.2.4.9. Covalent immobilization of glycoenzyme through carbohydrate chains

    3.2.4.10. Covalent immobilization by plasma deposition methods

    3.2.4.11. Photochemical immobilization

3.3. CELL IMMOBILIZATION

  3.3.1. Cell immobilization in polymeric beads

  3.3.2. Coacervation

  3.3.3. Emulsion/interfacial polymerization

  3.3.4. Pre gel dissolving: two-step method

  3.3.5. Covalent bonding

  3.3.6. Adsorption

  3.3.7. Entrapment

  3.3.8. Photo cross-linking

3.4. APPLICATIONS OF IMMOBILIZATION

  3.4.1. Immobilized enzymes and industrial processes

    3.4.1.1. Changes in enzyme kinetics after immobilization

    3.4.1.2. Enzyme reactors

3.1. IMMOBILIZATION OF ENZYMES

Soluble enzymes are employed in a wide variety of substrate and enzyme activity assays. In addition to the unquestionable advantages, there exist a number of practical problems in the use of enzymes. To these belong: the high cost of isolation and purification of enzymes, the instability of their structures once they are isolated from their natural environments, and their sensitivity both to process conditions other than the optimal ones, normally narrow-ranged, and to trace levels of substances that can act as inhibitors. Also, unlike conventional heterogeneous chemical catalysts, most enzymes operate dissolved in water in homogeneous catalysis systems, which is why they contaminate the product and as a rule cannot be recovered in the active form from reaction mixtures for reuse. Several methods have been proposed to overcome these limitations, one of the most successful being enzyme immobilization. The term "immobilized enzymes" refers to "enzymes physically confined or localized in a certain defined region of space with retention of their catalytic activities, and which can be used repeatedly and continuously." Immobilization is achieved by fixing enzymes to or within solid supports, as a result of which heterogeneous immobilized enzyme systems are obtained. By mimicking the natural mode of occurrence in living cells, where enzymes for the most cases are attached to cellular membranes, the systems stabilize the structure of enzymes, hence their activities. Thus, as compared to free enzymes in solution immobilized enzymes are more robust and more resistant to environmental changes. More importantly, the heterogeneity of the immobilized enzyme systems allows easy recovery of enzyme and product, multiple reuses of enzymes, continuous operation of enzymatic processes, rapid termination of reactions and greater variety of bioreactor designs. There are number of factors which influence performance of immobilized enzymes (Table 3.1). Besides the application in industrial processes, the immobilization techniques are the basis for making a number of biotechnological products with applications in diagnostics, bioaffinity chromatography, and biosensors. There are a number of immobilization techniques by which the properties of enzymes can be improved (Fig. 3.1).

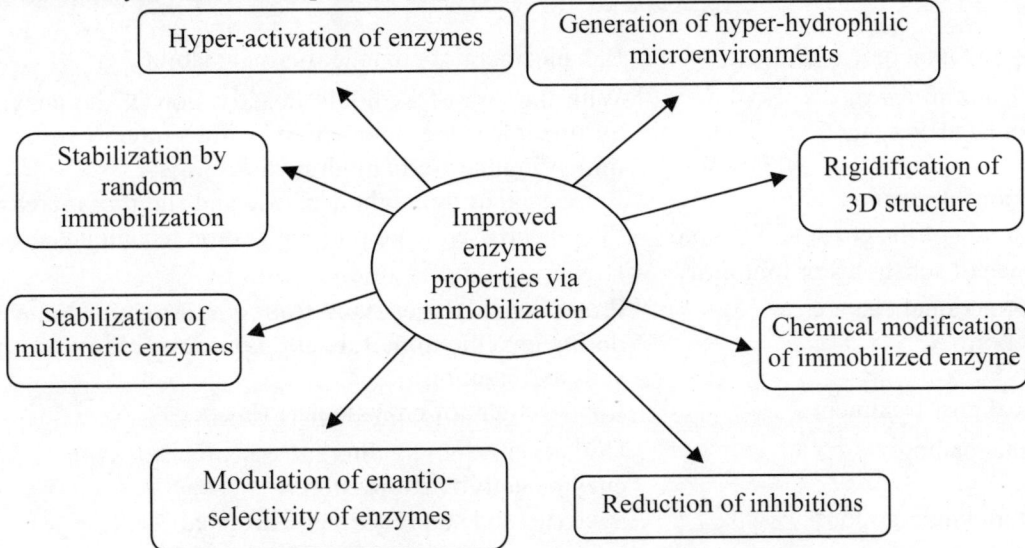

Fig. 3.1: Possible use of immobilization techniques to improve enzyme properties

Although the basic methods of enzyme immobilization can be categorized into a few different methods only, for example adsorption, covalent bonding, entrapment, encapsulation, and cross-linking, hundreds of variations based on combinations of these original methods have been developed. Correspondingly, many carriers of different physical and chemical nature or different occurrence have been designed for a variety of bio-immobilizations and bio-separations. The main goal of enzyme immobilization is the industrial re-use of enzymes for many reaction cycles. Several hundred enzymes have been immobilized in different forms, for example amino acylase, penicillin G acylase, many lipases, protease, nitrilase, amylase, invertase, etc. have been increasingly used as indispensable catalysts in several industrial processes. In this way, simplicity and improvement of enzyme properties have to be strongly associated with the design of protocols for enzyme immobilization. In spite of their excellent catalytic properties, enzymes have many other characteristics that are not very suitable for their use in chemical industries: low stability, inhibition by high concentrations of substrates and products, low activity and selectivity toward non-natural substrates under nonconventional conditions, and so on. The possibility of improving these unsuitable characteristics via the design of simple immobilization protocols is a very exciting goal. There are many protocols for immobilization of enzymes but very few are also very simple and/or very capable of improving enzyme properties. Novel immobilization protocols are still needed in order to achieve a massive implementation of enzymes as catalysts of the most complex chemical processes under the most benign experimental and environmental conditions. Table 3.1 lists the criteria for robust immobilized enzymes. A critical review of enzyme immobilization under this point of view is still necessary.

Table 3.1: Important factors influencing performance of immobilized enzymes

Factors	Implication or application
Hydrophobic partition effect	Enhancement of reaction rate of hydrophobic substrate
Microenvironment effect of the carrier	Hydrophilic nature often stabilizes the enzyme, whereas hydrophobic nature often destabilizes the protein
Multipoint attachment effect	Enhancement of enzyme thermal stability
Spacer or arm various types of immobilized enzyme	With the aim of avoiding deactivation of the enzyme by incompatible interaction with protein-carrier or mitigating the steric hindrance
Diffusion constraints	Enzyme activity might decrease and stability increases
Orientation of the enzyme featured	Site-specific enzyme immobilization techniques
Presence of substrates or inhibitor	Higher activity retention
Conformational changes or protection	Protection of the enzyme from conformational change during enzyme immobilization process leading to high activity retention
Physical post-treatments	Improvement of enzyme performance
Enzyme loading	Higher enzyme loading is essential to avoid lower enzyme activity expression
Different binding mode	Activity and stability can be affected
Enzyme modification	Suitable chemical modification often leads to the improvement of enzyme stability
Enzyme modification/ immobilization	Formation of active enzyme, which can be covalently bound to the inert carrier, can control the binding mode, thus improving the activity retention
Physical structure of the carrier	Activity retention was often pore-size-dependent
Stabilization-immobilization	Enzyme can, moreover, be stabilized before binding of enzyme to carrier
Physical nature of the carrier	Carriers with large pore size mitigates diffusion limitation, leading to higher activity retention
Hydrophilic-hydrophobic balance of the carrier	A delicate balance of hydrophilic and hydrophobic character of the selected carrier is essential for the activity and stability

It has recently been demonstrated that rational combination of methods can often solve a problem that cannot be solved by an individual method. Despite better understanding of enzyme-immobilization techniques and the numerous possible means of obtaining robust immobilized enzymes, development of a robust immobilized biocatalyst which can meet the requirements of modern biocatalytic processes – mild reaction conditions, high activity, high selectivity, high operational stability, high productivity, and low cost still relies on laborious trial-and-error experimental approaches. Consequently, a crucial question is whether it is possible to develop a generic method or to establish generic guidelines for enzyme immobilization. Obviously, the answer to this question lies both in the reality of different immobilization techniques and the peculiarity of each individual application.

On the other hand, the peculiarities of applications, for example the types of reaction (hydrolytic reaction or reverse reaction), reaction medium (aqueous or organic solvents), reaction system (solid-to-solid, liquid-to-solid, and liquid-to-liquid), reactor configuration (stir-tank, plug-flow), economic viability (cost contribution of the immobilized enzyme, space-time yield and productivity) and the intrinsic characteristics of the enzymes selected might differ from case to case. Thus differences between the peculiarities of each application also require specific solution of each individual application.

Table 3.2: Criteria for robust immobilized enzymes

Parameter	Requirement	Benefits
Non-catalytic function	Suitable particle size and shape, Suitable mechanical properties, Low water regain capability, High stability in a variety of organic solvents	Aid separation, easy control of the reaction, Flexibility of reactor design, Easy removal of water, No change of pore radius and thus fewer diffusion constraints
Catalytic function	High volume activity, High selectivity, Broad substrate specificity, Stability in organic solvents, Thermostability, Operational stability, Conformational stability	High productivity and space–time yield, Fewer side reactions, easier downstream processing and separation of products, and less pollution, Shift of reaction equilibrium with the use of organic solvents, Short reaction time by increasing temperature, Cost-effective and lower cost-contribution for the product, Modulation of enzyme properties
Immobilized enzyme	Recyclability, Broad applicability, Reproducibility, Easy and quick design	Low cost-contribution of catalyst, Tolerance of process variation, Guaranteed product quality, Early insight into process development and avoidance of learning process
Economical and Ecological consideration	Lower volume, Easy disposal, Rational design, Safety for use	Lower cost for solid handling, Less environmental concern, Easy biodegradability, Avoidance of laborious screening Meeting safety regulations

It must, therefore, be expected that choice of the method of immobilization is mainly dictated by the specific conditions and requirements of each application, which should selectively employ the positive attributes of the method selected. In this sense, the diversity of enzyme-immobilization techniques could be a powerful asset in the design of robust immobilized enzymes, because changes in the peculiarities of the applications often require design of new immobilized enzymes, which fit the new applications.

3.2. IMMOBILIZATION METHODS

Several methods are available for the immobilization of enzymes on a variety of natural and synthetic supports. Enzyme immobilization methods are classified as chemical or physical. Chemical methods involve the formation of covalent bonds between functional groups on the support material (also called as the matrix or the carrier) and functional groups on the enzyme. Chemical methods are sub-classified as either non-polymerizing or cross-linking methods. Non-polymerizing methods involve the formation of covalent bonds only between enzyme and support, but not between individual enzyme molecules, while cross-linking methods allow the formation of both enzyme-support bonds as well as enzyme–enzyme cross-links. Immobilization methods may be represented by the illustrations shown in Figure 3.2.

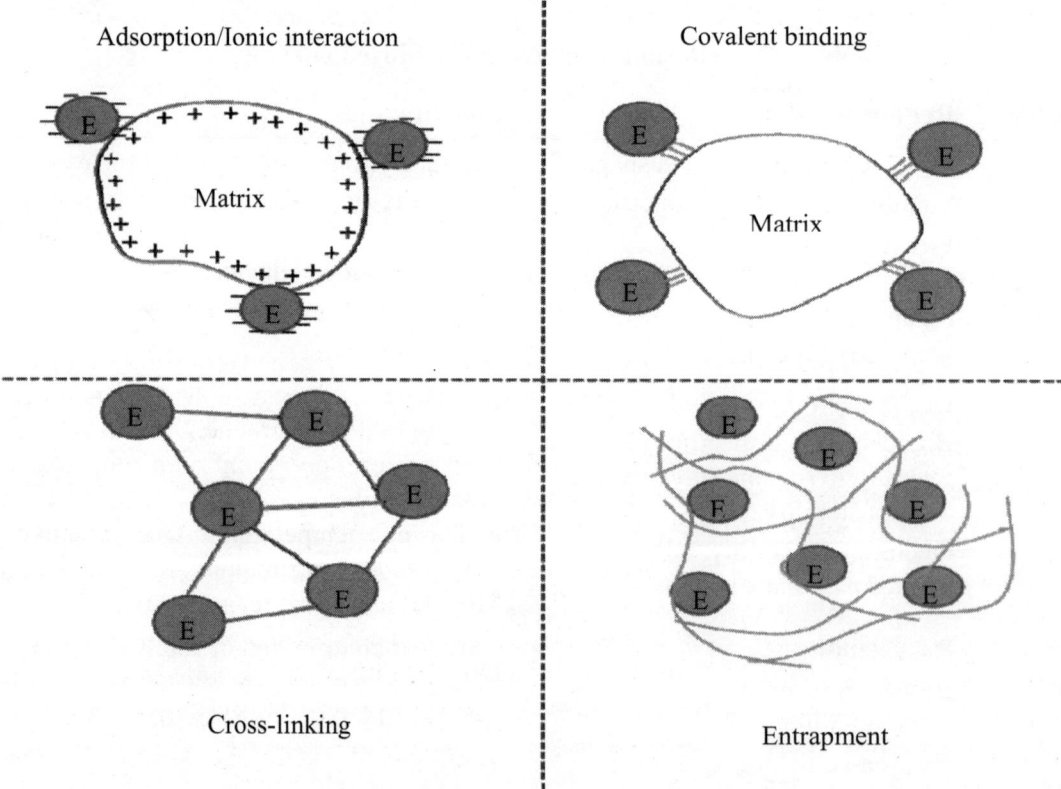

Fig. 3.2: Methods of enzyme immobilization

Physical immobilization methods do not involve covalent bond formation with the enzyme, so that the native composition of the enzyme remains unaltered. Physical immobilization methods are sub-classified as adsorption, entrapment, and encapsulation methods. Adsorption of proteins to the surface of a carrier is, in principle, reversible but careful selection of the carrier material and the immobilization conditions can render desorption negligible. Entrapment of enzymes in a cross-linked polymer is accomplished by carrying out the polymerization reaction in the presence of enzyme; the enzyme becomes trapped in the network polymer matrix. Encapsulation of enzymes results in regions of high enzyme concentration being separated from the bulk solvent system by a semi-permeable membrane, through which substrate, but not enzyme, may diffuse. The following sections consider each immobilization method in detail.

Numerous other methods which are combinations of the ones listed or are original and specific for a given support or enzyme has been devised. No single method and support is best for all enzymes and their applications because of the widely different chemical characteristics and composition of enzymes, the different properties of substrates and products, and the different uses to which the product can be applied. Table 3.3 gives a comparison of different immobilization techniques. Besides, all of the methods present advantages and drawbacks of their own. Adsorption is simple, cheap and effective but frequently reversible, covalent attachment and cross-linking are effective and durable but are expensive and may easily worsen the enzyme performance, and in membrane reactor-confinement, entrapment and micro-encapsulations diffusional problems are inherent. Consequently, as a rule the optimal immobilization conditions for a chosen enzyme and its application are found empirically by a process of trial and error in a way to ensure the highest possible retention of activity of the enzyme, its operational stability and durability.

Table 3.3: Comparison of the attributes of different immobilization techniques

Characteristic	Cross-linking	Physical adsorption	Ionic binding	Chelation or metal binding	Covalent binding
Preparation	Intermediate	Simple	Simple	Simple	Difficult
Binding force	Strong	Weak	Intermediate	Intermediate	Strong
Enzyme activity	Low	Intermediate	High	High	High
Regeneration of carrier	Impossible	Possible	Possible	Possible	Rare
Cost of immobilization	Intermediate	Low	Low	Intermediate	High
Stability	High	Low	Intermediate	Intermediate	High
General applicability	No	Yes	Yes	Yes	No
Protection of enzyme from microbial attack	Possible	No	No	No	No

The surface of the supports, on which the enzyme is immobilized, has an important role in retaining the tertiary structure of the enzyme which influences the thermal stability and catalytic activity of the immobilized enzyme. Indeed an immobilized enzyme is known to acquire novel kinetic properties, which can modify the Michaelis–Menten constant (Km) and maximum velocity (V_{max}) and cause a shift of the pH and temperature-activity profile. Likewise, the groups involved in the attachment of proteins to the support must be different from the active sites of enzymes. The types of bonds formed between carriers and enzymes are dependent on the support materials selected for immobilization. Mainly three forces are involved in internal surface immobilization- attractive, diffusive and multiple hydrogen bonds (Fig. 3.3). Therefore, the choice of the support as well as the technique depends on the nature of enzyme, support and on its ultimate application. For this reason it is not possible to recommend any universal immobilization method. Although it is recognized that there is no universal support for all enzymes and their applications, a number of desirable characteristics should be common to any material considered for immobilizing enzymes. These include: high affinity to proteins, availability of reactive functional groups for direct reactions with enzymes and for chemical modifications, hydrophilicity, mechanical stability and rigidity, ability to regenerate, and ease of preparation in different geometrical configurations that provide the system with permeability and surface area suitable for a chosen biotransformation. Understandably, for food, pharmaceutical, medical and agricultural applications, non-toxicity and biocompatibility of the materials are also required. Furthermore, to respond to the growing public health and environmental awareness, the materials should be biodegradable, and should be economical and inexpensive.

3.2.1. Adsorption and ionic binding

This is perhaps the simplest of all the techniques and one which does not grossly alter the activity of the bound enzyme. An enzyme solution is incubated with an adsorbent for several hours; the adsorbent is then removed and rinsed with a buffer. The yields are however low and the enzyme is often partially or totally inactivated. Adsorptive interactions may be ionic, polar or hydrogen bonding or they may involve hydrophobic or aromatic stacking interactions. These interactions are all non covalent, and are, in principle, reversible. In case of enzymes immobilized through ionic interactions, adsorption and desorption of the enzyme depends on the basicity of the ion exchanger. Moreover, a dynamic equilibrium is normally observed between the adsorbed enzyme and the support, which is often affected by pH as well as the ionic strength of the surrounding medium. This property of reversibility of binding has often been used for the economic recovery of the support. With adsorptive immobilizations, the activity yield of the immobilized enzyme is not directly related to the amount of protein adsorbed, since drastic conformational changes can occur upon adsorption that causes significant loss in activity.

The adsorption of a protein onto a given surface depends on ionic strength, pH, temperature, and type of solvent system and enzyme concentration. The most commonly used adsorbents are carbon, alumina, cellulose, clay, polystyrene, hydroxyapatite and glass. The binding forces may be ionic, hydrophobic, hydrogen bonds or van der Wall's interactions (Table 3.4).

Table 3.4: Interactions and carriers used for enzyme immobilization by adsorption

Interaction	Adsorbents
Physical adsorption	Activated carbon, silica gel, alumina, starch clay and glass
	Modified materials: tannins, aminohexyl cellulose, concanavalin-A, sepharose
Ionic binding	Cation exchange: carboxymethyl cellulose, cellulose citrate, P-cellulose, Amberlite, CG-50, Dowex-50
	Anion exchange: DEAE cellulose, TEAE cellulose, DEAE-sephadex, polyaminopolystryene, Amberlite IR-45

Tables 3.5 and 3.6 list some therapeutically important enzymes immobilized by adsorption and ionic bonding method. Cellulose based ion exchange resins e.g., carboxy methyl cellulose, diethyl amino ethyl (DEAE)-cellulose; have been extensively used for immobilization of enzymes with

higher adsorption capacity (up to 15% w/w protein: cellulose). Catalase was immobilized by binding it to the DEAE-cellulose. Ionic binding is influenced by many of the same factors that influence physical adsorption. Most commonly used carriers for ionic binding include polysaccharides and a variety of synthetic polymers having ion exchange group attached. The ionic binding is usually carried out under relatively mild conditions as compared to covalent coupling and it causes very little or no effect on conformational structure of the protein and yield of immobilized enzyme systems (Table 3.6).

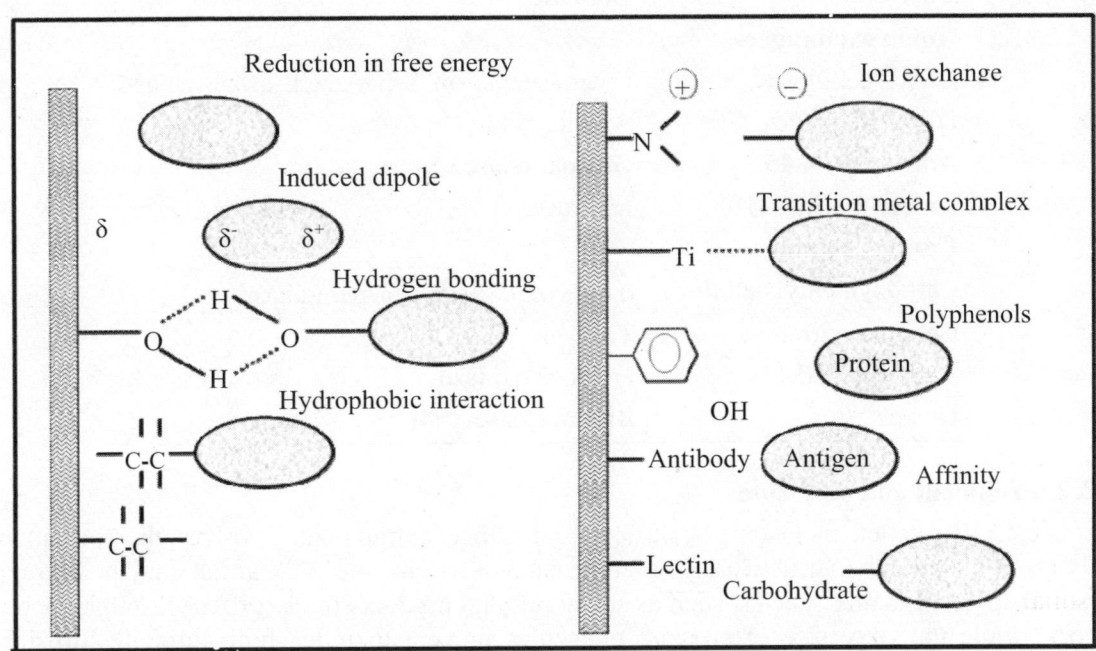

Fig.3.3: Forces involved in the adsorption of biocatalyst

Table 3.5: Some therapeutic enzymes immobilized by physical adsorption

Carrier	Enzyme
Organic supports	
Concanavalin-A	Arylsulfatase
Gluten	β-amylase
Concanavalin A-sepharose	Phosphodiesterase
Butyl sepharose	Lipoamide dehydrogenase
Starch	α-amylase
Activated carbon	Glucose oxidase, α-amylase, β-amylase
Inorganic supports	
Alumina	Glucose oxidase
Kaolin	Lysozyme
Porous glass	Glucose oxidase
Silica gel	Aspartase
Bentonite	Invertase

Another development in immobilization technologies by adsorption has been the use of an effector or activator of an enzyme, attached to a water insoluble polymer; to bind that enzyme. Tyrosinase and tryptophanase were immobilized by adsorption to an insoluble derivative of pyridoxal-5'-phosphate, an activator of these enzymes. This method has an added advantage that the enzyme is not only specifically adsorbed on to the polymer, but it is activated by the same process.

Table 3.6: Some therapeutic enzymes immobilized by ionic binding

Carrier	Enzyme
Anion exchangers	
DEAE cellulose	Invertase, pepsin, aspartase L-asparaginase,
DEAE-sephadex	Aminoacylase
Amberlite IR-45	Glucoamylase
Amberlite IRA-410	Invertase
Cation exchangers	
Carboxymethyl cellulose	α- chymotrypsin, L-asparaginase
Cellulose citrate	Trypsin
Amberlite CG-50	Glucose oxidase
Dowex 50	Ribonuclease

3.2.2. Entrapment and occlusion

Entrapment, also called inclusion, occlusion, and lattice entrapment, involves the formation of a highly cross-linked polymer network in the presence of an enzyme, so that the enzyme is trapped in interstitial spaces. Smaller species, such as substrates and products freely diffuse through the polymer network, while the large size of enzyme molecules prevent their leaching through diffusion. The entrapment of enzyme molecules can be achieved using one of the following six ways: 1) Inclusion within the matrix of a highly cross-linked polymer, 2) Separation from the bulk phase by a semi-permeable membrane, 3) Dissolution in a distinct non-aqueous phase, 4) Liposomes, 5) Reverse micelles and 6) Resealed erythrocytes.

Enzyme immobilization by physical entrapment has the benefit of applicability to many enzymes and may provide relatively small perturbation of their native structure and function, per se.

3.2.2.1. Entrapment within the matrix of highly cross linked polymer

The most widely used system for enzyme entrapment in a polymer lattice is polyacrylamide gel produced by cross-linking acrylamide in the presence of enzyme. Potassium persulfate is used as a polymerization initiator and β-dimethylamino propionitrile (DMAPN) as an accelerator. The pore size in immobilized enzyme gels remains sufficiently small to retain many enzymes, which have molecular diameter in the range of 200-300 nm.

3.2.2.2. Separation from the bulk phase by a semi-permeable membrane

In this method, the enzyme stays in solution, while a semi-permeable membrane physically confines solution so that the enzyme cannot escape. There is a biological analog of these techniques. The lysosome within the cell confines hydrolytic enzymes, which would otherwise kill the cell immediately if they were released. In an immobilization method known as microencapsulation, the enzymes are entrapped in small capsules with diameters ranging up to 30–50 μm. The capsules are surrounded by spherical membranes, which have pores permitting small substrates and product molecules to enter and leave the capsule. The pores are too small, however, for enzymes and other large molecules, to permeate. There are different methods for the preparation of microcapsules.

A) Emulsion polymerization method

In this method, a semi-permeable membrane is formed by condensation co-polymerization reaction at the interface between an organic phase and a dispersed aqueous phase containing enzyme. By choosing a water-insoluble monomer as one of the reactants and a monomer slightly soluble in both phases for the other, the co-polymerization occurs only at the interface. Alternatively, an aqueous solution of enzyme dispersed in a solution of PVC or cellulose triacetate may be extruded to form fibers containing droplets of enzymes.

B) Coacervation phase separation method

The term coacervate is derived from Latin word *Acervus*, meaning a heap or an aggregation. In coacervation a colloidal dispersion is caused to collapse and separate into colloidal rich and colloidal poor regions by careful control of temperature, pH, electrolytes addition, or other factors. The coacervate or colloidal rich region forms as droplets making the system opaque and sediment to form a separate lower layer. The phase boundary formed is unlike that between immiscible liquids; the solvent is continuous on both sides of the interface, facilitating free migration of solute between layers.

C) Interfacial poly-condensation

Interfacial poly-condensation involves the reaction of various monomers at the interface between two immiscible liquid phases to form a film of polymer that encapsulates the dispersed phase. Usually two reactive monomers are employed, one dissolved in the aqueous disperse phase containing a solution or dispersion of core material, and the other dissolved after the emulsification step in the non-aqueous continuous phase. The water-in-oil (w/o) emulsion formed requires the addition of a suitable emulsifying agent as dispersion stabilizer.

D) Emulsion solvent evaporation

In this method, the polymer is dissolved in a volatile organic solvent and emulsified with the aqueous phase (W_1) containing enzyme to be immobilized. The resulting W_1/O emulsion is again emulsified with another aqueous phase (W_2) containing suitable stabilizer to form a $W_1/O/W_2$ multiple emulsion. The emulsion is magnetically stirred to evaporate the organic solvent leaving a thin film of polymer around the phase W_1.

E) Dissolution in a distinct non-aqueous phase

Non-permanent microcapsules can be prepared by emulsifying the aqueous enzyme solution with a surfactant. These liquid-surfactant membranes based capsules can then be added to an aqueous substrate solution. Microcapsules have the potential advantage of a very large surface area (e.g., 2500 cm^2 per milliliter of enzyme solution) and the possibility of added specificity: the membrane can be made in some cases to admit some substrate selectively while exclude other. Moreover, these methods are applicable to a large variety of enzymes. Various therapeutic enzymes immobilized in microcapsules are given in Table 3.7.

3.2.3. Microencapsulation

Enzymes may be immobilized by encapsulation in nonpermeant (e.g., liposomes) or permeant (e.g., nylon) microcapsules. The enzyme is trapped inside by a semi-permeable membrane, where substrates and products are small enough to freely diffuse across the boundary. Microcapsules developed for use in medicine consist of a solid or fluid core material containing one or more drugs enclosed in coating. They usually have a particle size range between 1-2000 nm. In enzymology the microencapsulated enzymes are known as "artificial cells". This term, introduced by Chang (1964) initially included impermeable and semi-permeable microcapsules, into the inner space of which an enzyme is encapsulated. Recently the term normal cells, cell ghosts and liposomes are implicated. An active enzyme intended for ingestion should be protected against inactivation by the multiple actions of the digestive proteases, including chemical attack (pH), bacterial action and proteolytic enzymes. The microencapsulated enzymes possess a number of advantages for therapeutic dimension.

Table 3.7: Therapeutic enzymes immobilized in microcapsules

Polymer	Enzyme
Agarose	Urokinase
Albumin	L-Asparaginase, Urokinase
Collagen	L-Asparaginase
Polydextran	L-Asparaginase
Nylon 6-10	Urease
Nylon 6-10	L-Asparaginase
Poly DL lactide-co-glycolide	L-Asparaginase, Superoxide dismutase
Poly vinyl pyrrolidone	Lysozyme
Poly acrylamide	L-Asparaginase
Polyhydroxyethyl-methacrylate	Urokinase

The microcapsule membrane on one hand protects an enzyme from contact with an aggressive physiological medium and on the other hand, protects tissues and organs from undesirable effects of the immobilized enzymes. Considerable amounts of the enzyme may be encapsulated or microencapsulated into microcapsules, which increase the enzyme/carrier ratio up to 10,00,000:1. The surface area/volume ratio of microcapsules is maximal at a given volumes as a result there is a fast penetration of substrates and exiting products of enzymatic reaction *via* the membrane. An enzyme may be encapsulated into microcapsules as an additionally stabilized form, moreover, multienzyme complexes, enzyme mixtures or even intact cells may be encapsulated inside 'artificial cells'. The disadvantages associated with the microparticles are: the use of synthetic material (polyamides, polyurethanes, etc.) in the body and the risk of vessel embolism upon accumulation of microcapsules in the circulation as a result of prolonged and repeated application. Figure 3.4, represents some peculiarities of enzyme encapsulation in synthetic semi-permeable microcapsules.

Because of these problems, a great deal of work is progressing in the field of biodegradable microcapsules (made from polylactic acid, polylactide-co-glycolide alginates, etc.). Microencapsulated enzymes can be administered intravenously, intramuscularly, intraperitoneally, perorally or applied locally as a fine suspension. This immobilization method requires a high-protein concentration in an aqueous phase (10 mg/mL), resulting in a high osmotic pressure that prevents the collapse of the microcapsules, and also acts as an emulsifier. Particles are spherical, with diameters ranging from 2 mm to several millimeters (mm), while pore sizes are of the order of nanometers (nm).

3.2.4. Covalent bonding

The most intensely studied of the immobilization techniques is the formation of covalent bonds between the enzyme and the support matrix. Enzymes are covalently linked to the support through the functional groups in the enzymes, which are not essential for catalytic activity. The conditions for immobilization by covalent binding are much more complicated and less mild than in the cases of physical adsorption and ionic binding. Covalent immobilization methods rely on functional groups on both the enzyme and the support material for the formation of stable covalent bonds (Table 3.8). When trying to select the type of reaction by which enzymes should be immobilized, the choice is limited by two characteristics: (1) the binding reaction must be performed under conditions that do not cause loss of enzymatic activity, and (2) the active site of the enzyme must be unaffected by the reagents used. For this reason, the choice of a support is crucial in that it determines the immobilization chemistry and the stability of the enzyme-support bonds (Fig. 3.5).

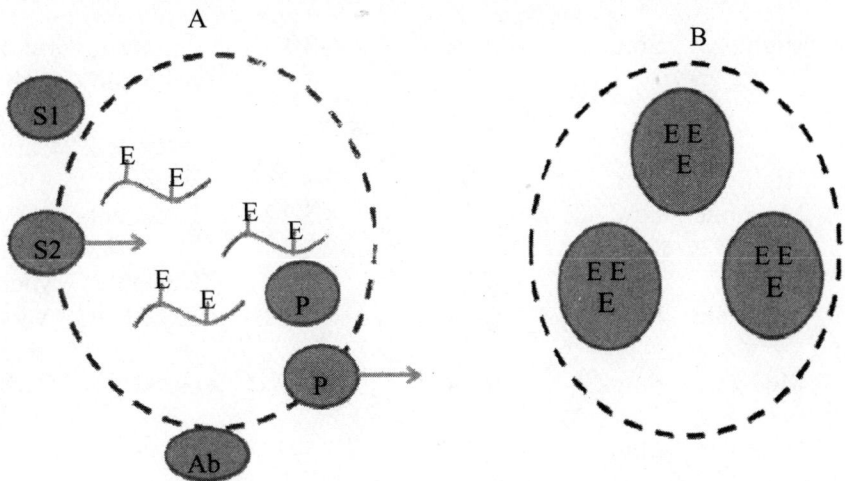

Fig. 3.4: Schematic representation of enzyme (E) entrapment in to microcapsules. A: semi-permeable microcapsules. The enzyme can be immobilized in the native form (1), as intermolecularly cross-linked derivative (2), being immobilized on a soluble carrier (3), or as a component of an immobilized multienzyme complex (4), low molecular substrates (S_1) and product can easily penetrate the membrane; at the same time the high-molecular substrates (S_2) and antibodies (Ab) cannot enter the microcapsule; B: Double entrapment of enzymes into polymeric microcapsules

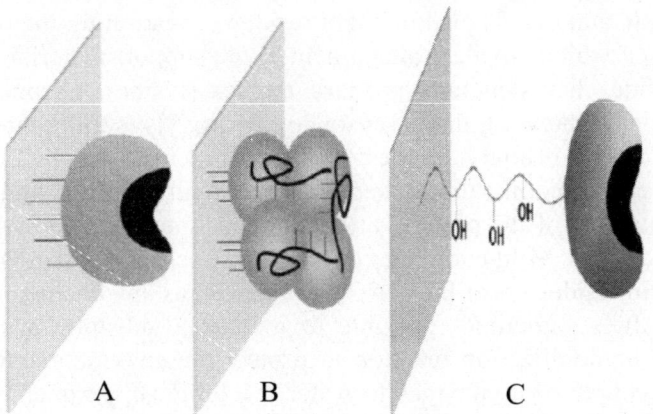

Fig. 3.5: Covalent Coupling; A: Multipoint covalent attachment, B: multisubunit covalent immobilization plus additional cross-linking, C: Coupling without altering properties

Table 3.8: Details of various covalent immobilization techniques

Activation method	Reagent toxicity	Technical difficulties	Activation times (Hrs)	pH of coupling	Stability of complex	Types of ligand bond
Glutaraldehyde	Moderate	Few	5-18	6.5-8.5	Excellent	Michael Adduct alkylamine
Cyanogen bromide	High	Some	0.2-0.4	8-10	Unstable pH 5 and >10	Imido-carbonate, Isourea, Carbamate
Hydrazine	High	Many	1-3	7-9	Excellent	Amide
Bisoxiranes	Moderate	Few	5-18	8.5-12	Excellent	Alkylamide ether Thioether
Divinylsulfone	High	Few	0.5-2	8-10	Unstable	Micheal adduct
Epichlorohydrin Epibromohydrin	Moderate	Few	2-24	8.5-12	Excellent	Alkylamide ether Thioether
Carbonyl Diimidazole	Moderate	Some	0.2-0.4	8-9.5	Good	Carbamate
Trichloro s triazine	High	Many	0.5-2	7.5-9	Good	Triazinyl
Diazonium	Moderate	Some	0.5-0.8	6-8	Moderate	Azo
Tosylchloride	Moderate	Some	0.5-0.8	7.5-10.5	Good	Alkylamine Alkyl mercaptane
Periodate	Non toxic	Few	14-20	7.5-8.5	Good	Schiff base alkylamine

Carriers may be activated under harsh conditions, to convert relatively unreactive functional groups into activated species that will then readily react with proteins under mild conditions of temperature, ionic strength, and pH. The amino acid residues constituting the polypeptide component of enzymes provide sites at which covalent attachment to the support material may occur. Functional groups present on the side chains include primary amines (lysine), phenol hydroxyls (tyrosine), carboxylic acids (aspartate, glutamate), thiols (cysteine), hydroxyls (serine, threonine), and imidazole nitrogen (histidine). Of these, primary amines, carboxylic acids, and hydroxyl groups are most commonly used for protein immobilizations, because their hydrophilic character suggests that they will occur in an accessible area of the protein, at the aqueous interface, and will therefore be readily available for chemical reactions. Mild coupling conditions are essential in order to avoid the chemical modification of amino acid residues near the active site, as well as any change in tertiary structure that may affect the activity. It is sometimes possible to include a substrate analogue, or competitive inhibitor, in the enzyme immobilization reaction to protect the enzyme's active site from coupling reagents. The chemical coupling of enzymes to water insoluble supports and even to water-soluble polymers is the most commonly employed method of enzyme immobilization. Higher activities result from prevention of inactivation reactions with amino acid residues of the active sites. It is possible in some cases to increase the number of reactive residues of an enzyme in order to increase the yield of the immobilized enzyme. By the careful selection of supports with appropriate physical and chemical characteristics, bioreactors with variety of therapeutic applications can generated. This is true even if very little is known about the protein structure or active site of the enzyme to be coupled. Table 3.9 lists several materials, which have been employed for covalent enzyme immobilization, and some of their surface functional groups. Other materials, which have been used as support for immobilization of enzymes, include ceramics, glass and other metal oxides.

Table 3.9: Insoluble materials and some of their surface functional groups useful for covalent enzyme attachment

Natural supports	Synthetic supports
Cellulose (-OH)	Polyacrylamide derivatives ($-CONH_2$)
CM-Cellulose (-COOH)	Polystyrene ($-NH_2$)
Agarose (-OH)	Maleic anhydride copolymer (R-COO-CO-RO)
Dextran (-OH)	Polyethylene glycol
Dextrans	Polyaspartic acid, Polyglutamic acid,
	Carboxymethylcellulose (-COOH)

The most important and conventional methods of covalent attachment include azo linkage, isocyanates and isothiocynates, carboxymethylazides and carbodiimides coupling.

3.2.4.1. Azo linkage

Any arylamine can be treated with nitrous acid to form a diazonium salt. Diazonium salt will react with, and couple with many aromatic compounds, particularly phenols such as L-tyrosine, and other abundant constituent of proteins. The most widely used supports include: polyamino polystyrene, aryl aminocellulose, arylamine glass and ceramics. Several therapeutic enzymes immobilized by this method are shown in Figure 3.6 and Table 3.10.

3.2.4.2. Isocyanates and isothiocyanates

Both alkyl and arylamines can be converted in to isocyanates and isothiocyanates. These active compounds covalently bind with available amine groups. Such groups are common on proteins and are usually provided by the ε-amino group of L-lysine residues of the protein backbone, or by N-terminal α-amino nitrogen atoms. Therapeutically important enzymes, which are immobilized by this method, are given in Table 3.11.

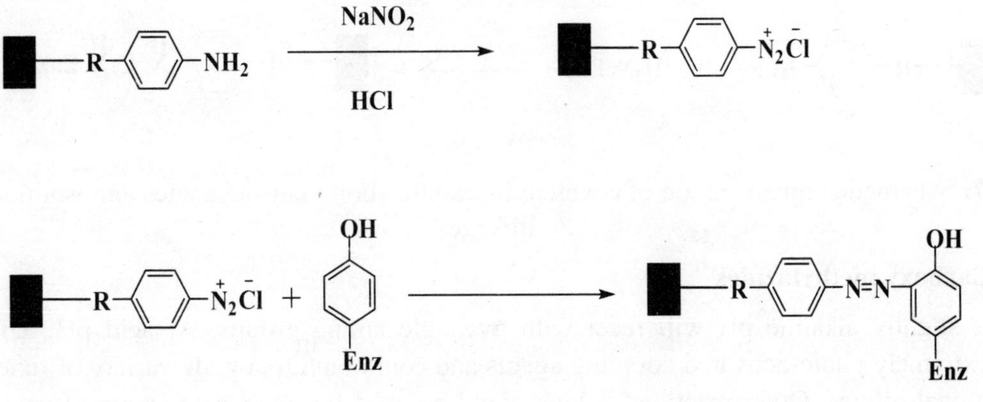

Fig. 3.6: Schematic representation of covalent immobilization via azo linkage

Table 3.10: List of therapeutic enzymes immobilized via Azo linkage

Carrier	Enzyme
Polysaccharide derivative	
M- Aminoanisole cellulose	α-Chymotrypsin, Trypsin
P-Amino benzyl cellulose	α-Amylase, Lysozyme, Trypsin, Chymotrypsin
Amino acid co-polymer	
p-amino-DL-phenylalanine L-Leucine	Trypsin, α-Chymotrypsin, Prothrombin, Streptokinase, Urease
Polyacrylamide derivatives	Lysozyme, α-Amylase

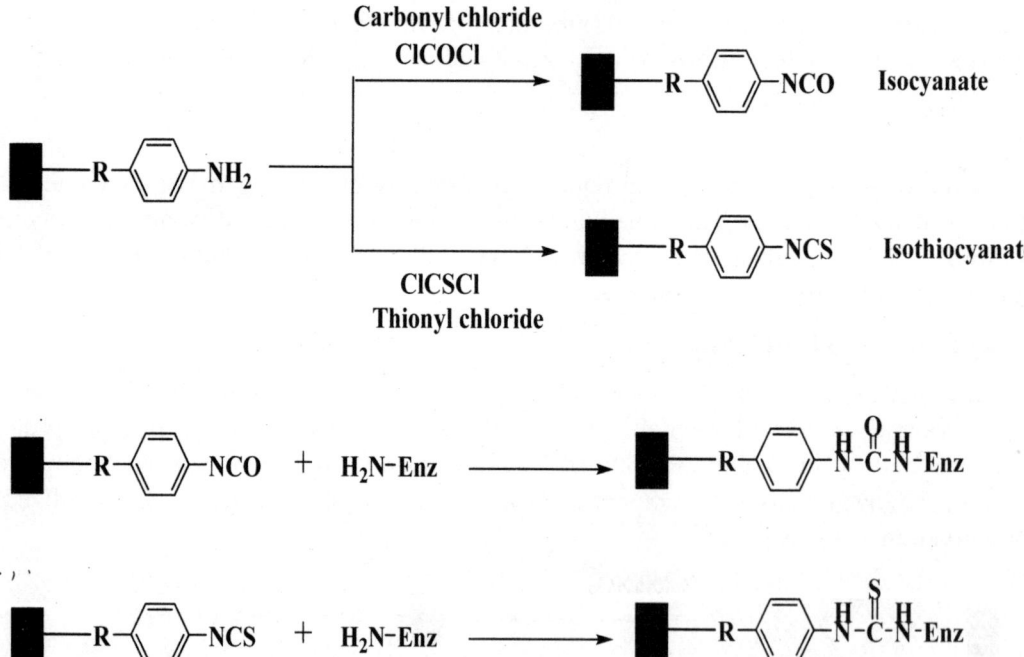

Fig. 3.7: Schematic representation of covalent immobilization via isocyanates and isothiocyanates linkages

3.2.4.3. Carboxy methylazides

Azides at slightly alkaline pH will react with available amine groups. At acid pH, azide groups become extremely photo-activated coupling agents and could bind to a wide variety of functional and non-functional groups. Other reactions, which could be used for anchoring enzymes, include CNBr and dihydroquinoline (Fig. 3.8). Table 3.12 lists some enzymes immobilized by amide linkages.

Table 3.11: Therapeutic enzymes immobilized by amide linkage

Carrier	Enzyme
Co-polymer of methacrylic acid and m-isocyanate styrene	Trypsin
Isothiocyanate derivatrive of Enzacryl amino acid	α-Amylase
Isothiocyanate derivartive of amino silanized hydroxylapalite	Glucose oxidase
Isothiocyanate derivative of amino silanized porous glass	Glucose oxidase, Trypsin, Papain
Isothiocyanate derivative of amino silanized silica	Papain
CM-Cellulose isocyanate derivative	ATPase
Sephadex-isocyanate derivative	Trypsin
Polyaminopolystyrene isocyanate derivative	Catalase

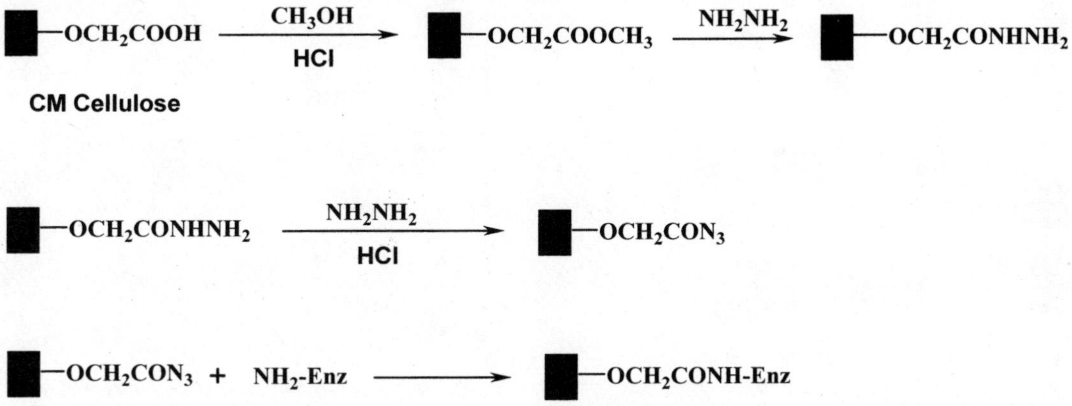

$$\blacksquare-OCH_2COOH \xrightarrow[HCl]{CH_3OH} \blacksquare-OCH_2COOCH_3 \xrightarrow{NH_2NH_2} \blacksquare-OCH_2CONHNH_2$$

CM Cellulose

$$\blacksquare-OCH_2CONHNH_2 \xrightarrow[HCl]{NH_2NH_2} \blacksquare-OCH_2CON_3$$

$$\blacksquare-OCH_2CON_3 + NH_2-Enz \longrightarrow \blacksquare-OCH_2CONH-Enz$$

Fig. 3.8: Schematic representation of covalent immobilization via carboxy methylazides

Table 3.12: Some enzymes immobilized by amide linkage

Carrier	Enzyme
Aceto Azide derivative	
CM-Cellulose	Glucose oxidase, α-amylase, Trypsin, Bromelain, Streptokinase, Urokinase
CN-Br-Activated Polysaccharides	
CN-Br Activated Cellulose	Xanthine oxidase, β-D-Glucosidase, α-Chymotrypsine, Glucoamylase
CN-Br Activated Sephadex	Lactate dehydrogenase, Carboxy peptidase A, α-Chymotrypsine, Glucose 6-Phosphate dehydrogenase
CN-Br Activated Sepharose	Lactate dehydrogenase, Glucose oxidase, Maleate dehydrogenase,

3.2.4.4. Carbodiimides

Carbodiimide reagent has been extensively used in covalent coupling and thus in immobilization. Carbodiimides soluble in both aqueous and organic solvents are commonly available. These compounds react with free carboxyl groups forming a pseudourea intermediate adduct, which can be coupled with available amines via an amide linkage (Fig. 3.9). Table 3.13 lists some enzymes immobilized by carbodiimide coupling.

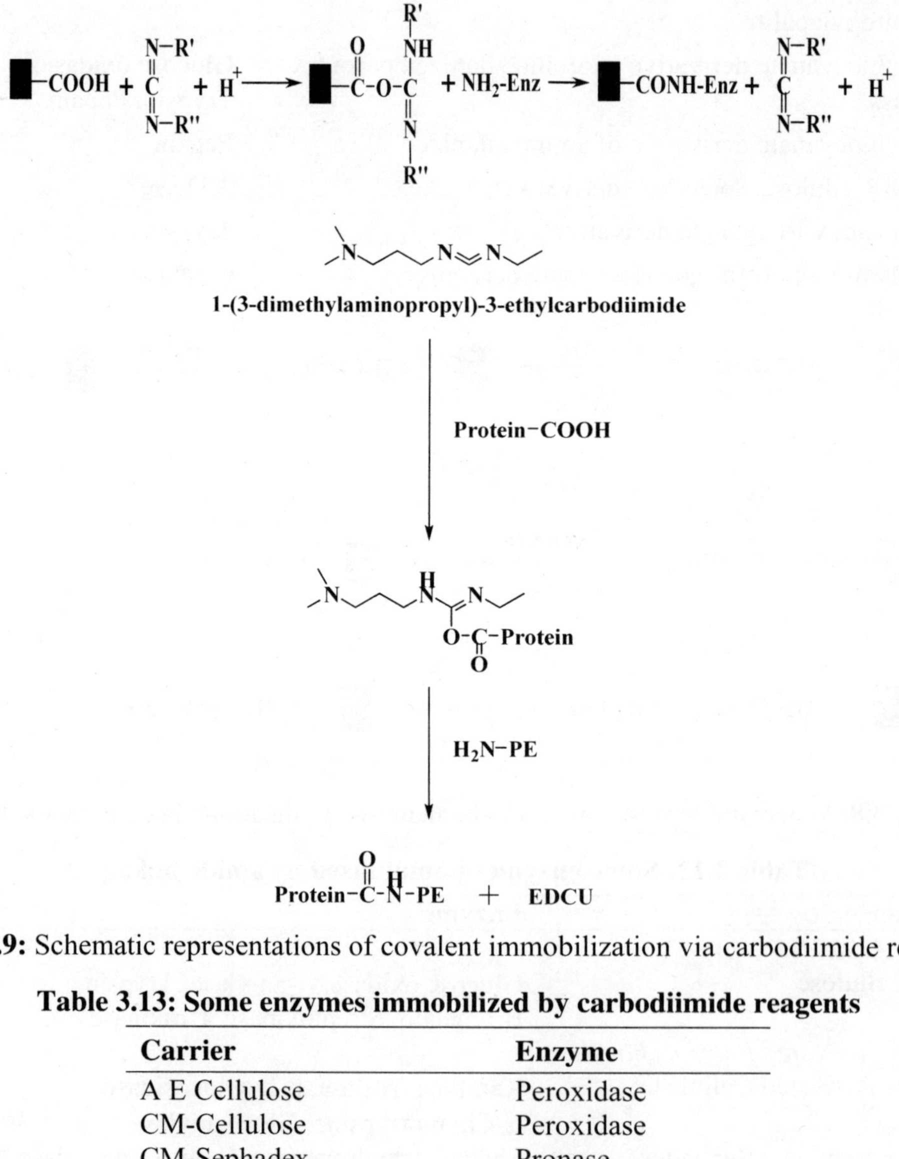

1-(3-dimethylaminopropyl)-3-ethylcarbodiimide

Fig. 3.9: Schematic representations of covalent immobilization via carbodiimide reagent

Table 3.13: Some enzymes immobilized by carbodiimide reagents

Carrier	Enzyme
A E Cellulose	Peroxidase
CM-Cellulose	Peroxidase
CM-Sephadex	Pronase
Bio-GelCM-100	β-Amylase, Trypsin
Copolymer of acrylamide and acrylic acid	β-D-Glucosidase, Trypsin, Urease

3.2.4.5. Covalent immobilization through glutaraldehyde

Agents with bifunctionality like glutaraldehyde can be used as an anchoring agent for immobilizing proteins possessing free amino/amine groups. It could effectively hook-up the amino group of two adjacent molecules; one is protein and the other one will be the support. One of the problems associated with the use of such agent is that it could lead to cross-linking as well as cross-bridging amongst other adjacent protein molecules. The functional character of glutaraldehyde initiated covalent anchoring is schematically presented in Figure 3.10.

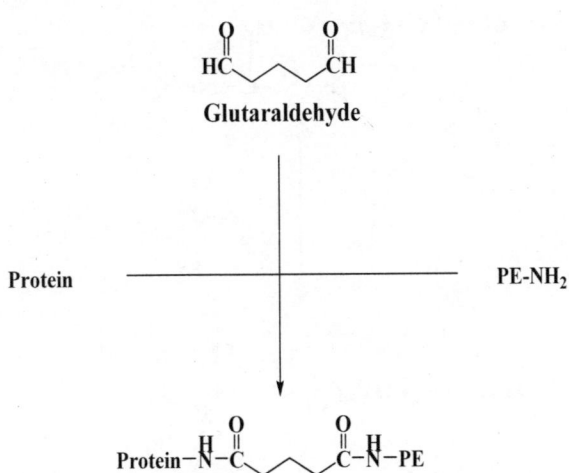

Fig. 3.10: Schematic representation of covalent immobilization via glutaraldehyde

3.2.4.6. Covalent coupling employing N-succinimide activation

Where surface fatty acylation is adapted as a strategy for protein or enzyme immobilization, the amino group of the protein could be covalently linked to the activated carboxyl group of a fatty acid. However, the latter needs preactivation which could be brought about by reacting fatty acids with N-hydroxy succinimide. The most widely used reaction is schematically presented in figure 3.11.

3.2.4.7. Covalent coupling through diacyl fatty anhydrides

The free amino groups of the enzymes and the protein could directly be reacted and conjugated with diacyl fatty anhydride(s). The covalent conjugation employing this method is shown in figure 3.12. Dodecanoic acid anhydride reacts with free amino group imparting fatty acylation to the protein molecule(s).

3.2.4.8. Covalent coupling through sulfhydryl group

Disulfide linkage offers useful strategies where sulfide reactive agents could be used for covalent conjugation without disrupting the reactivity (Figs 3.13 to 3.15). For this, the general prerequisite is thiol modification prior to treatment of proteins with disulfide reducing agent such as; dithiothreitol. However, the pretreatment step could be avoided by adapting the procedure which introduces new preactivated sulfhydryl group into the protein molecule. Ellman's reagent, 5,5'-dithio bis-2-nitrobenzoic acid can be coupled to the carrier which has been activated at amine residue using 2-iminothiolane. The method is presented schematically in Figure 3.13. Disulfide coupling with available sulfhydryl group of proteins occurs together with the production of thionitrobenzoate, which is water soluble, hence could be removed through washings.

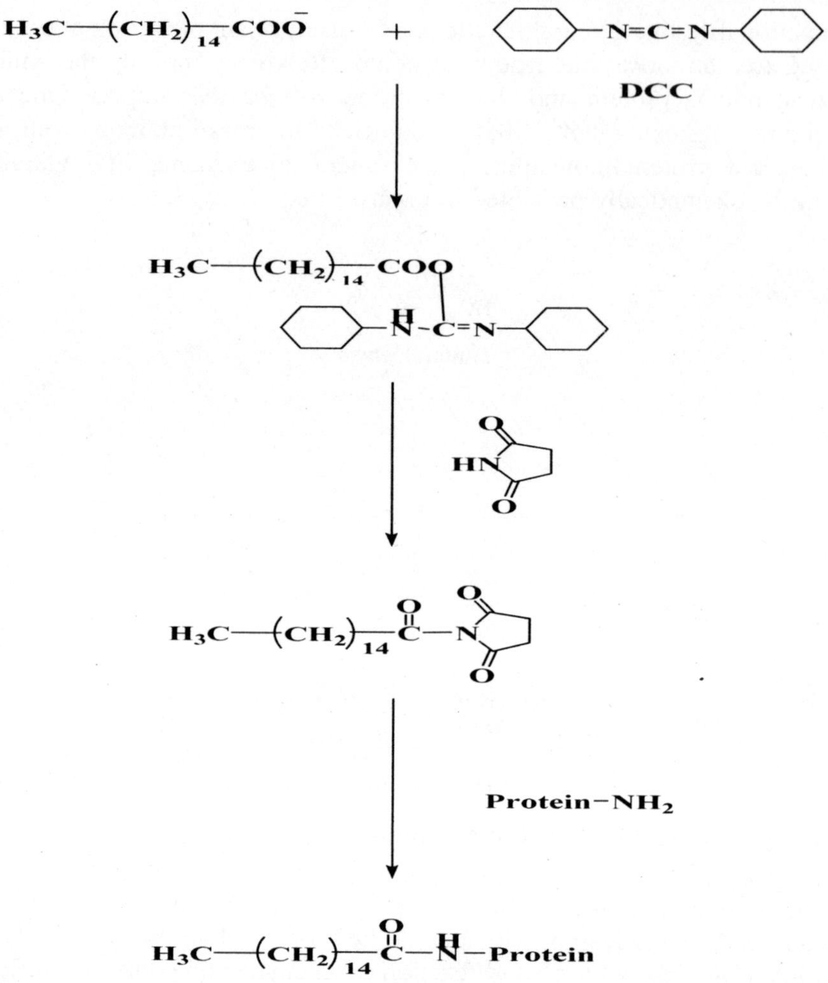

$$H_3C-(CH_2)_{14}-COO^- \quad + \quad \bigcirc-N=C=N-\bigcirc$$

DCC

$$H_3C-(CH_2)_{14}-COO$$

$$\bigcirc-\overset{H}{N}-C=N-\bigcirc$$

$$HN\overset{O}{\underset{O}{\diagdown}}$$

$$H_3C-(CH_2)_{14}-\overset{O}{\overset{\|}{C}}-N\overset{O}{\underset{O}{\diagdown}}$$

Protein−NH₂

$$H_3C-(CH_2)_{14}-\overset{O}{\overset{\|}{C}}-\overset{H}{N}-\text{Protein}$$

Fig. 3.11: Covalent coupling of the amine residue of protein to fatty acids via N-succinimide

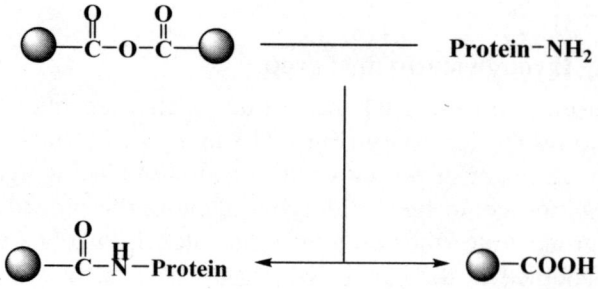

Fig. 3.12: Reaction of diacyl acid anhydrides with the free amino group of protein

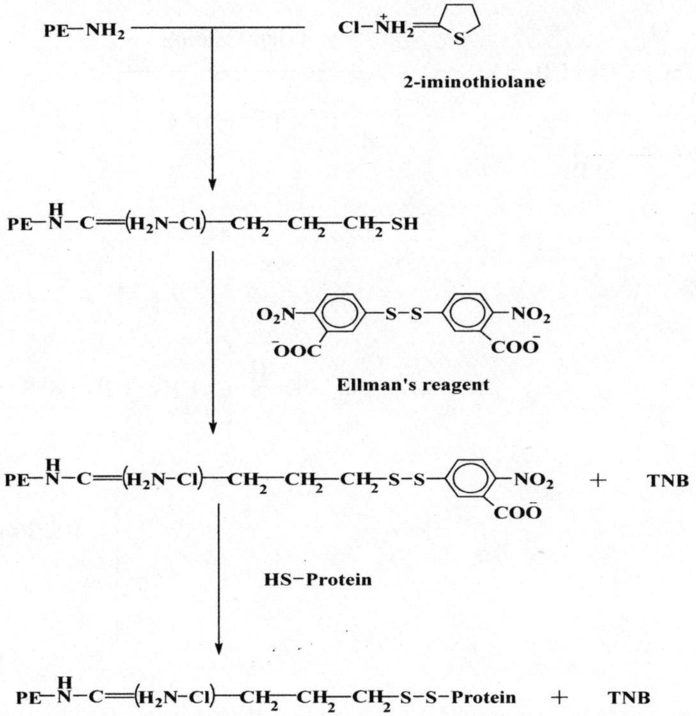

Fig. 3.13: Thiolation of phospholipids and subsequent activation for reaction with the sulfhydryl functions of the protein

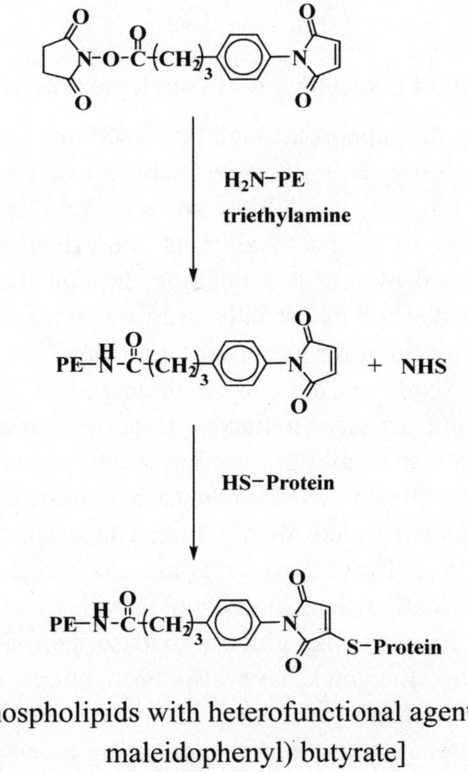

Fig. 3.14: Activation of phospholipids with heterofunctional agent SMPB [N-succinimidyl 4-(p-maleidophenyl) butyrate]

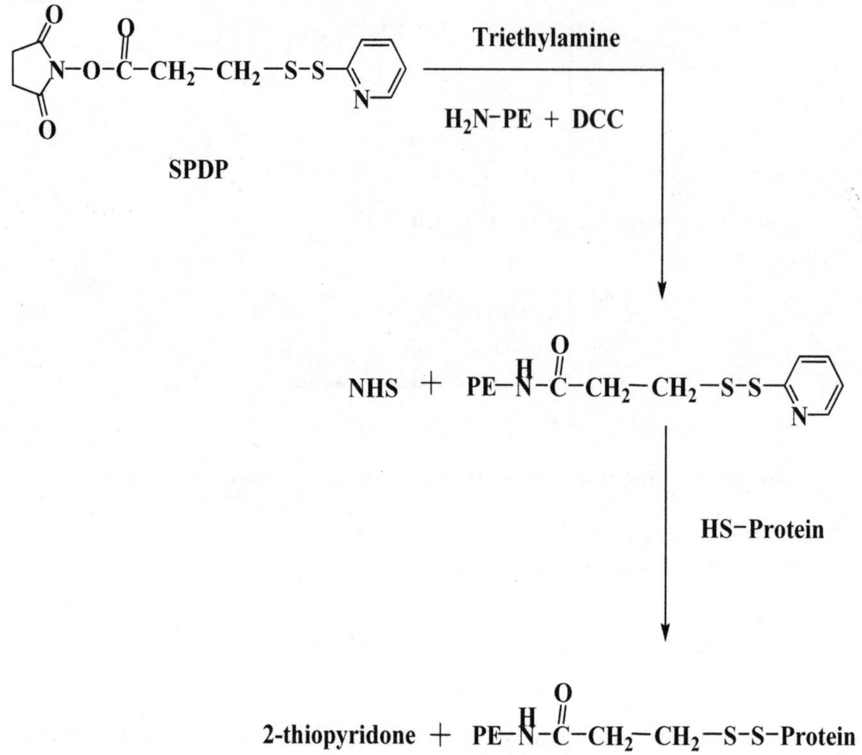

Fig. 3.15: Activation of phospholipids with heterofunctional agent SPDP (N-succinimidyl proprionyl dithiopyridine)

3.2.4.9. Covalent immobilization of glycoenzyme through carbohydrate chains

Enzymes are covalently linked to the support through the functional groups in the enzymes which are not essential for the catalytic activity. It is often advisable to carry out the immobilization in the presence of its substrate or a competitive inhibitor so as to protect the active site. The covalent binding should also be optimized so as not to alter its conformational flexibility. Some of these problems however, can be obviated by covalent bonding through the carbohydrate moiety when a glycoprotein is concerned. A number of industrially useful enzymes are glycoproteins wherein the carbohydrate moiety may not be essential for its activity. In general, functional aldehyde group can be introduced in a glycoprotein by oxidizing the carbohydrate moiety by periodate oxidation without significantly affecting the enzyme activity. It makes glycol-enzymes reactive. Generally Sodium metaperoxidate or other periodates or iodates are used as oxidizing agent. The stable derivatives are formed by attachment of EDTA or glycyltyrosine to the carbohydrate chain in the presence of Sodium borohydrate. The enzyme could then be covalently linked to a support containing an alky amine group through Schiffs base reaction. These derivatives are enzymatically active and react well with solid subject. EDTA adducts are finally reacted and coupled with an active ester derivative of agarose by covalent binding (Fig. 3.16). Enzymes like glucose oxidase, peroxidase, invertase, etc. have been immobilized using this technique. Enzymes have also been bound to synthetic membranes, thus integrating biconversion and downstream processing. Large-scale processes using such an approach have been demonstrated for the preparation of invert sugar using invertase.

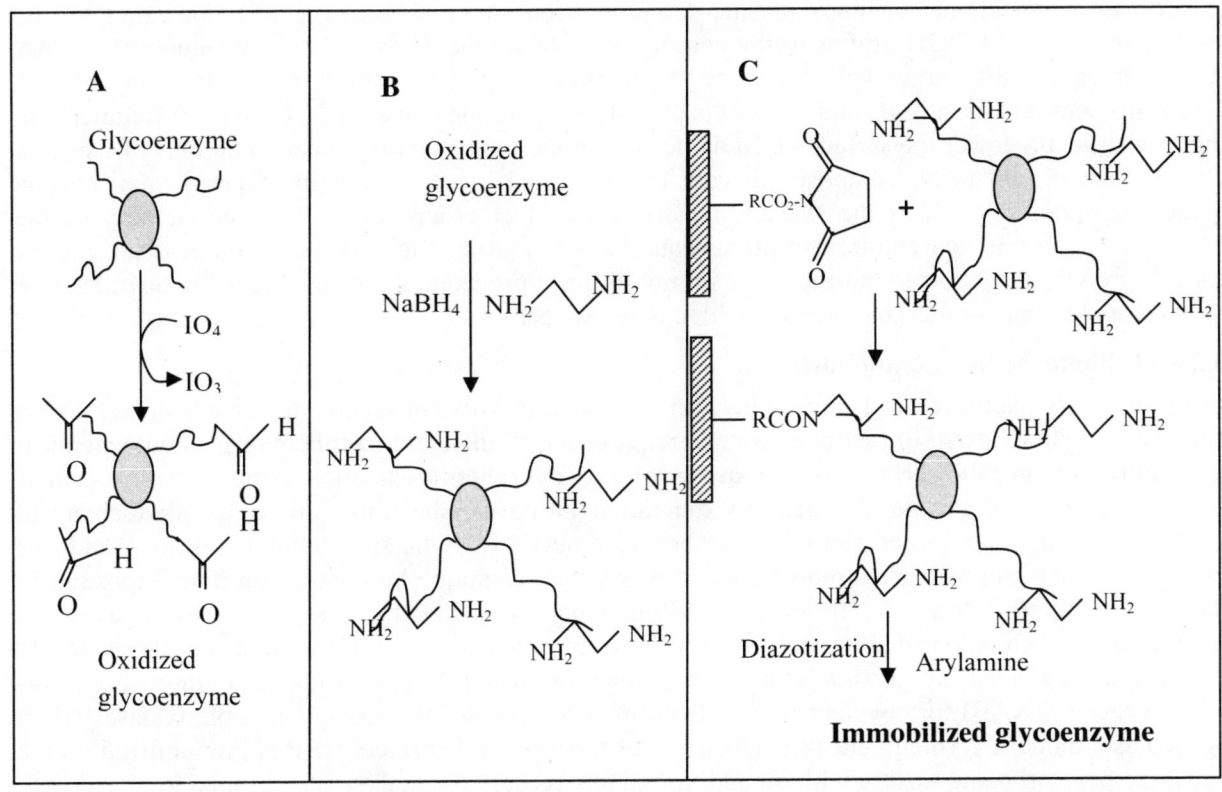

Fig. 3.16: Immobilization of glycoenzyme through carbohydrate chains (a) oxidation of glycoenzyme (b) formation of EDTA/ glycyltyrosine adduct (c) enzyme immobilization

3.2.4.10. Covalent immobilization by plasma deposition methods

Low temperature plasma deposition and treatment processes can be successfully employed in order to modify surfaces of enzymes as well as to improve cells. Low temperature plasma processes such as the deposition of thin films (PE-CVD, Plasma Enhanced Chemical Vapor Deposition) from volatile organic compounds, and the grafting of polar functional groups (i.e., –NH₂, –OH, etc.) onto hydrophobic polymers (Plasma Treatments) are very popular modification techniques in the field of biomedical materials, as well as in the field of membranes, for many different applications, due to their ability to functionalize in specific and controlled way the surface of materials and devices with a negligible influence on their bulk properties, to their easy scalability to industrial production plants, and to their negligible impact on the environment. Plasma deposition and treatment processes can be duly optimized to improve the adhesion, spreading and proliferation of cells at the surface of materials of biomedical interest, as well as to improve membrane properties such as hydrophilic/ hydrophobic character, non fouling properties, transport and capability of immobilizing molecules (catalysts, peptides, etc.). In certain research areas, such as that of bioreactors, membranes themselves are the substrates of interest for cell substrate biological interactions to be adapted to the best performances.

By varying properly external plasma parameters such as power input, pressure, gas feed flow rate and composition, etc., it is possible to tune internal process parameters such as the distribution and density of atoms, radicals and ions produced in the discharge, to the requested surface modification. In the case of functional coatings plasma-deposited from Acrylic Acid (pdAA), for example, the surface density of –COOH groups in the coating depends on the degree of fragmentation of the AA monomer in the discharge, which can be monitored by Optical Emission Spectroscopy of AA fragments such as CH radicals and CO molecules. The higher the density of CO and CH fragments in the discharge, the lower the surface –COOH density in the pdAA coating. pdAA coatings of tuneable CH_xO_y overall chemical composition can be deposited under different experimental plasma conditions; features such as the surface density of –COOH groups as well as the stability of the coating in water and cell-culture conditions can also be optimized to surfaces of biomedical interest for cell growth, as well as to bio-molecule immobilization procedures for membranes to be utilized in bioreactors to improve their interactions with eukaryotic cells.

3.2.4.11. Photochemical immobilization

In recent years photochemical immobilization has become a useful technique for covalently fixing enzymes, cells, DNA or carbohydrates required for different applications. Photochemical immobilization on solid surface offer unique advantage over thermo-chemical immobilization such as (i) any biomolecule irrespective of their functional group can be immobilized by photochemical method, (ii) it is non-invasive method and there is no need of any harsh reaction conditions, and (iii) micro patterning can be carried out easily for microarray technique by controlling light exposure. In the last couple of years, 1- fluoro-2-nitro-4-azidobenzene (FNAB) has been widely used for photochemical activation of solid supports for different applications. Polycarbonate—a thermostable polymer is activated by a simple and rapid method using a photo-linker, 1-fluoro-2-nitro-4-azidobenzene (FNAB) for covalent immobilization of a biomolecule. Horseradish peroxidase (HRP) is used as a model enzyme to check the efficacy of the activated surface. HRP is immobilized on the activated polycarbonate surface without addition of any reagent or catalyst and is found to give 2–2.5-fold increase in absorbance with the substrate as compared to the directly adsorbed enzyme.

Optimized concentration of the photolinker is found, as 6 µmol of FNAB per well and time of photo irradiation is 8 min for activation of a PCR polycarbonate plate. PC bound HRP has shown enhanced thermal and storage stability. Kinetic studies of the immobilized HRP show improved catalytic activity. The potential application of activated polycarbonate surface includes immobilization of biomolecules for biosensors, immunoassays, and protein and DNA micro-arrays. Due to the stability of the polycarbonate at high temperature, the activated polycarbonate has an advantage for immobilization of thermostable biomolecule such as thermostable enzyme for reaction at elevated temperature.

3.3. CELL IMMOBILIZATION

Immobilization of microbial/plant/animal cells in biological processes can occur either as a natural phenomenon or through artificial process. While the attached cells in natural habitat exhibit significant growth, the artificially immobilized cells are allowed restricted growth. Various immobilization protocols and numerous carrier materials have been developed. Immobilization of cells is the attachment of cells or their inclusion in distinct solid phase that permits exchange of substrates, products, inhibitors, etc., but at the same time separates the catalytic cell biomass from the bulk phase containing substrates and products. Therefore it is expected that the microenvironment surrounding the immobilized cells do not necessarily their free-cell counterparts experience the same. Immobilizing microbial/plant cells in high density not only improve the productivity of a bioreactor but also provide many benefits over free cells. A large number of techniques are now available for the immobilization of cells on a variety of natural and synthetic supports. Entrapment/encapsulation method has been commonly used for the preparation of immobilized microbial cells. A matrix for immobilization can alter microbial physiology. The immobilization of cells can be obtained by encapsulation or entrapment into polymeric supports such as alginate, carrageenan, agarose, etc. The microbial cells immobilized in a polymer matrix/ supports can be protected from harsh environmental conditions such as pH, temperature, organic solvent and poison. Immobilized microbial cells can be handled more easily; recovered from the solution without difficulty and operated in a high cell density without loss of microbial cells even at high dilution rates, which results in a higher bioreactor volumetric productivity.

3.3.1. Cell immobilization in polymeric beads

Cells have been commonly entrapped in the gel matrix through which substrates and products diffuse in and out easily. The gel matrix is usually composed of agar, agarose, k-carrageenan, collagen, alginate, chitosan and cellulose (Table 3.14). Some of them are expensive but have weak mechanical strength. The components of gel matrix, polyacrylamide and polyurethane are toxic to the immobilized cells. Calcium alginate is very mild and used for the entrapment of animal cells, microbial cells, mitochondria, chloroplasts, protoplasts and red blood cells. Calcium alginate gelled by ionic bond swells in the solution and dissolves in a solution containing a chelating agent such as phosphate. Cells grow usually on the surface and in the pore of the matrix where the space available for the cell growth is limited. The cells immobilized in a large bead proliferate only in the periphery of the bead because of the substrate and oxygen limitation. The maximum cell loading in the entrapped beads is limited to 25% by volume because of weak mechanical strength. Post-treatment of the calcium alginate bead with triethylene tetramine and glutaric dialdehyde increases mechanical strength and prevents the bead from swelling and dissolving.

Table 3.14: Encapsulation techniques

Method/Material	Cell
Pre gel dissolving, two-step method	
Alginate/poly-L-lysine/alginate	*E. coli,* Rat hepatocytes, *Erwinia herbicola*
Alginate/poly-L-lysine/polyethylenimine	Rat pancreatic tissue; Mouse erythroleukemia
Alginate/poly-L-lysine	Hybridoma cell
Liquid droplet forming, one-step method	
Chitosan/carboxymethyl cellulose	Hybridoma cell
Calcium alginate	Monkey kidney cell, *Saccharomyces cerevisiae, Corynebacterium glutamicum, E. coli, Aspergillus niger, Zoogloea ramigera*
Barium alginate	*Lactobacillus casei*
Interfacial polymerization	
1,6-Hexanediamine/poly(allylamine hydrochloride)/dodecanedioyl dichloride	Erythrocyte hemolysate, *Saccharomyces cerevisae*
Chitosan/hexamethylene diisocyanate	*Lactococcus lactis*
Gelatin/toluene2,4diisocyanate	*Lactococcus lactis*
Coacervation	
Collodion	Erythrocyte haemolysate

Polyvinyl alcohol, which is cheap and nontoxic to cells, is not mechanically strong. Cross-linking the beads of polyvinyl alcohol with boric acid solution makes the beads strong and durable but damages cells in a lengthy cross-linking process. Addition of some alginate or phosphate to the boric solution during the cross-linking procedure prevents the polyvinyl alcohol beads from aggregation. The monoclonal antibodies produced by hybridoma cells entrapped in the alginate beads leaked from the hydrogel, but those from the encapsulated cells stayed inside the capsule without leaking. The encapsulated cells grew and the dry cell weight reached a limiting value, but the cells entrapped in the gel matrix burst the beads in the end.

3.3.3. Emulsion/interfacial polymerization

Interfacial polymerization occurs between monomers dissolved in the respective immiscible phases. Aqueous drops containing the water-soluble monomer are dispersed in the organic phase by stirring. The capsule membrane is then formed by addition of the other organic solvent-soluble monomer to the continuous organic phase (Fig. 3.17). Polymer membrane, such as polyamide, nylon, poly-terephthaloyl chloride, polyester, poly-phenylester is produced by the reaction between water-soluble monomer, such as polyamine, 1,6-hexamethylenediamine, piperidine, L-lidine, polyphenol, 2,2-bis (4-hydroxyphenyl)-propane, and organic solvent-soluble monomer, such as sebacoyl chloride, terephthaloylchloride, bischloropormate, 2,2-dichloroether. Erythrocyte cells has been encapsulated in aqueous droplets containing monomer, 1, 6-hexanediamine and erythrocyte haemolysate in the mixture of chloroform and cyclohexane and added sebacoyl chloride to the organic phase by interfacial polymerization and not detected the leakage of proteins from the capsule. The replacement of the monomer with nontoxic chitosan also enables the encapsulated microbial cell to maintain the initial activity.

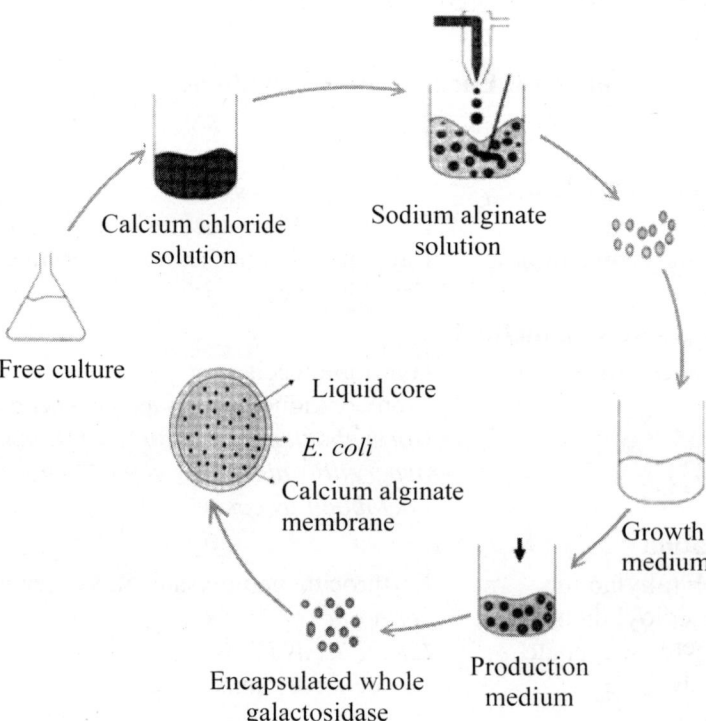

Fig. 3.17: Schematic capsule preparation method by emulsion/interfacial polymerization

3.3.4. Pre gel dissolving: two-step method

Recently, Some improvemnt has been made in the cell immobilization techniques by modifying encapsulation techniques like pre gel dissolving two-step method, liquid droplet forming one-step method (Fig. 3.18). In pre gel dissolving two-step method, the calcium alginate beads containing cells are made by the same procedure employed for the preparation of conventional calcium alginate beads. The carboxyl group of the calcium alginate bead reacts with acid-reactive amine or imine group in the poly-L-lysine or polyethylenimine and as a result, polyelectrolyte complex membrane is formed on the surface of the calcium alginate bead. The cross-linked beads are retreated with sodium alginate to crosslink the residual poly-L-lysine on the surface of the bead. The liquid core capsule is accomplished when the calcium alginate core is dissolved in a sodium citrate solution. The capsules prepared by pre gel dissolving two-step method have been widely used for immobilizing animal cells. Microbial cells have also been encapsulated using the pre gel dissolving two-step method.

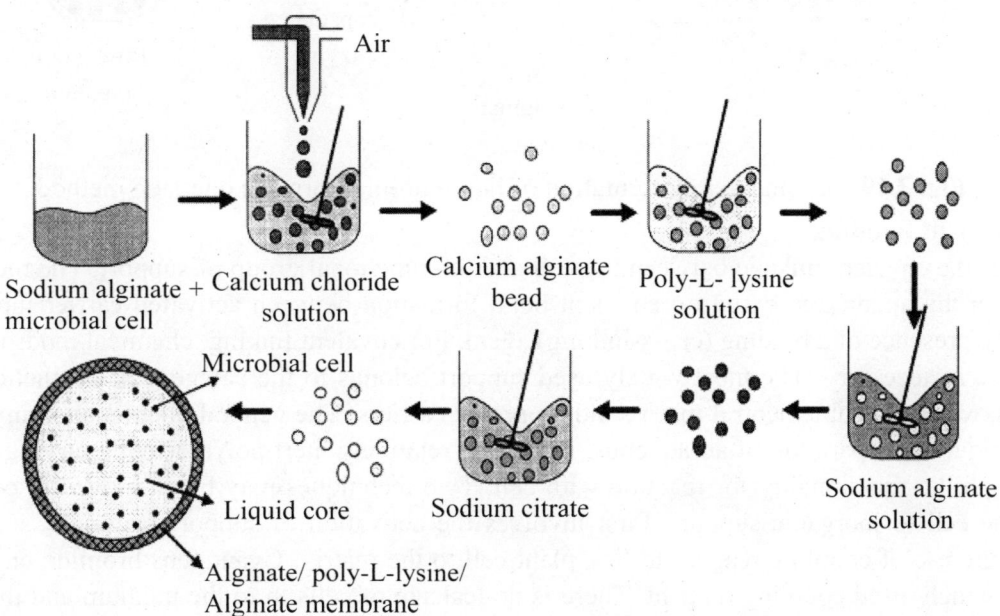

Fig. 3.18: Schematic capsule preparation method by pregel dissolving two-step method

In Liquid droplet forming: one-step method, encapsulation of cells prepared by the reverse procedure of the formation of conventional calcium alginate beads (Fig. 3.19). In this method, cells mixed in a solution of calcium chloride were dropped into a swirling sodium alginate solution. A calcium alginate membrane is formed immediately on the surface of the micro aqueous droplet by ionic interaction. Biomaterials such as living tissue, cell, hormone, enzyme and antibody can be immobilized inside the capsule and do not come into contact with the ionic prepolymer which is converted to the capsule membrane. Wall thickness, pore size, surface charge and mechanical strength of the capsules can easily be controlled by alteration of the concentrations of alginate, calcium and gel-forming polymer. These methods have been utilized for encapsulation of animal cells microbial cells such as yeasts, bacteria, and fungi (Table 3.14).

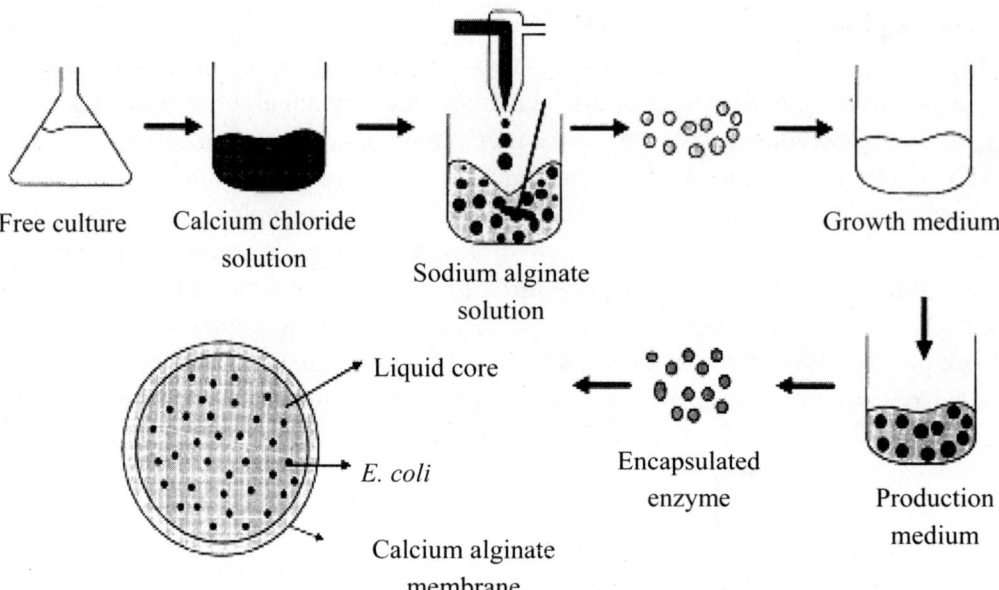

Free culture   Calcium chloride   Growth medium
solution

Sodium alginate
solution

Liquid core

E. coli

Encapsulated
enzyme

Production
medium

Calcium alginate
membrane

Fig. 3.19: Schematic representation of liquid droplet forming one-step method

3.3.5. Covalent bonding

It involves the covalent linkage between the cell and the functional group of support. The mechanism involved in this method is based on covalent bond formation between activated carrier/support and cells in the presence of a binding (cross-linking) agent. For covalent linking, chemical modification of the surface is necessary. The most widely used support belongs to the category of synthetic organic polymers, water insoluble neutral matrix and inorganic carriers. The general phenomenon involved in this technique is preparation of an aqueous, insoluble, relatively inert polymer with varying amounts of electrophillic functionality for reaction with cell. Two techniques may be employed to covalently couple the cell to inorganic support. First involves the activation of support materials, and second involves the use of coupling reagent to link plant cell to the matrix. Cyanogens bromide or isonitrile are most widely used coupling reagent. There is no leakage of cells in to the medium and the system provides greater stability during continuous use.

Cells of *S. cerevisiae* have been immobilized by coupling with silica beads. The reaction requires introduction of reactive organic group on inorganic silica surface for the reaction between the activated support material and yeast cells. α-aminopropyltriethoxy silane is generally used as the coupling agent. This inorganic functional group condenses with hydroxyl group on silica surface. As a result, the organic group is available for covalent bond formation on the surface of silica (Fig. 3.20). Covalent bonding can also be achieved by treating the silica surface with glutaraldehyde and isocyanate. A system of more general interest has been developed using inorganic carrier system. The addition of Ti^{4+} or Zr^{4+} chloride salts to water results in pH-dependent formation of gelatinous polymeric metal hydroxide precipitates wherein the metals are bridged by hydroxyl or oxide groups. By conducting such a precipitation in a suspension of microbial cells, the cells have been entrapped in the gel-like precipitate formed. In continuous operation, titanium hydroxide-immobilized cells of *Acetobacter* were employed to convert alcohol to acetic acid.

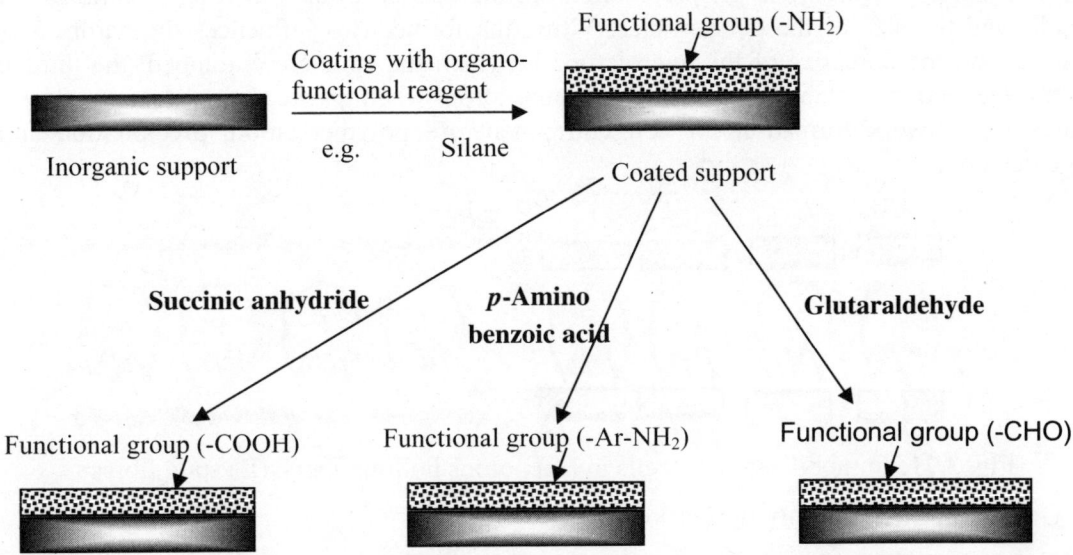

Fig. 3.20: Processing of inorganic supports for cell immobilization

3.3.6. Adsorption

This was apparently the first example of cell immobilization with the binding of *Escherichia coli* cells onto an ion exchange resin. Subsequently, a variety of microbial cells were immobilized by adsorption on different supports like kieselguhr, wood, glass, ceramic, plastic materials, etc.

Since the adsorption phenomenon is based on electrostatic interactions (van der Walls forces) between the charged support and microbial cells, the actual zeta potential of both plays a significant role in cell-support interactions. Unfortunately, the actual charge on support surfaces is still unknown and this limits the proper choice for microbial attachment. Along with charge on the cell surface, the composition of cell wall carrier will also play a predominant role. Cells of *Saccharomyces cerevisiae* and *Candida utilis* contain mannans in the cell wall. The cells of latter have a strong affinity to Concanavalin-A-activated carrier. Carrier properties, other than zeta potential, will also greatly influence cell-support interaction. All glass or ceramic supports are comprised of varying proportions of oxides of alumina, silica, magnesium, zirconium, etc. which result in bond formation between the cell and the support. Several procedures of cell adsorption based on pH dependence are reported in literature.

3.3.7. Entrapment

The most extensively studied method in cell immobilization is the entrapment of microbial cells in polymer matrices. The matrices used are agar, alginate, carrageenan, cellulose and its derivatives, collagen, gelatin, epoxy resin, photo cross-linkable resins, polyacrylamide, polyester, polystyrene and polyurethane. Among the above matrices, polyacrylamide has been widely used by several workers. Cells are entrapped within the interstitial spaces of a network of cross-linked water insoluble polymers (Fig. 3.21).

As a rule, the entrapment methods are based on the inclusion of cells within a rigid network to prevent the cells from diffusing into surrounding medium while still allowing penetration of substrate. The precise mode of entrapment of cells in polyacrylamide is critical for satisfactory retention of activity. The factors affecting the gel preparation are the content of acrylamide, the ratio of cells to acrylamide, and the size of the gel particles. While the former two influences the hardness of the resulting gel and the pore size of the microlattice in which the cells are entrapped, the third factor determines the activity, stability, and the pressure drop when packed in a reactor. The other procedures for network formation for cell entrapment are polymerization, precipitation and ion exchange gelation.

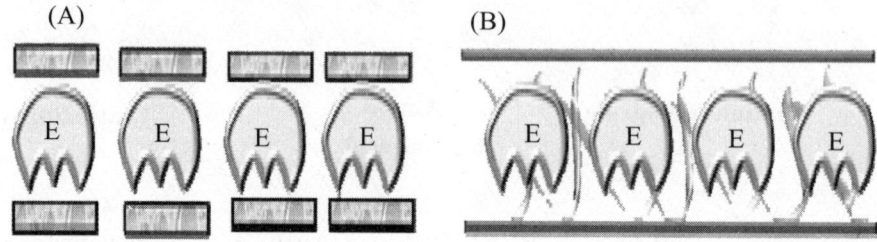

Fig. 3.21: Immobilization of cells in (A) porous hollow fibers, (B) spun fibres

3.3.7.1. Gel entrapment by polymerization

A monomer or a mixture of monomer is polymerized in the presence of a cell suspension, which is entrapped inside the lattice of a polymer. The preparation involves the cross linking of the polymer in the presence of cell, thus physically entrapping it. In all the protocols, enzymes are well mixed with monomers/polymers and cross-linking agents in a solution. Inclusion of cells in a gel such as cross-linked polyacrylamide or starch has the advantage of requiring very mild conditions to impose minimal constraints on the immobilized plant cells. To entrap plant cells either a cross-liked polymeric network around the cell molecule must be formed, or a cell should be placed inside a polymer chain and then cross-linked in the polymer chain.

The most common example is polyacrylamide. The method is based on the free radical polymerization of acrylamide in an aqueous solution. As this linear polymer is soluble in water, they have to be insolubilized with bi-functional compounds such as N, N'-ethylene bisacrylamide. The free radical polymerization of acrylamide is conducted in an aqueous solution containing the cells and the cross-linking agent. Polymerization is commonly carried out in the absence of oxygen and at lower temperature (10°C) to avoid damage to the cell during the operation. An initiator N,N,N'N' - tetramethylethylene diamine (TEMED) is used. Both the initiation and the cross-linking agents are toxic to the cells and therefore, their viability can be lost e.g. *C. roseus* and *Silybum marianum*.

The process also has some disadvantages, such as:
1. It is difficult to avoid the continuous leakage of cells from the immobilizes system,
2. Difficult to make the reproducible results,
3. Activity is limited to only those cells, which are entrapped at near the periphery.

3.3.7.2. Gel entrapment by ionic network formation

In this method, polymerization of polyelectrolytes is achieved by addition of multivalent ions. The most common method is the entrapment in calcium alginate. This is a non-toxic process in which sodium alginate solution containing the cell suspension is dropped into a mixture of counter ion solution such as calcium chloride. A uniform, spherical and highly micro porous structure is formed, which retains the cells. The method may be inconvenient over long run in media containing calcium-chelating agents, such as phosphates and certain cations such as Mg^{2+} that may accelerate disruption of gel by solubilizing bound Ca^{2+}. Carrageenan is also a suitable matrix for the immobilization of cells. k-carrageenan is one of the polymeric gel materials used for cell immobilization for continuous production of l-lactic acid by *Escherichia coli*. The gels of calcium and potassium carrageenates are very stable at room temperature and at a pH above 4.5.

The immobilization procedure is similar to alginate, and several other groups have used this polysaccharide as a preferred gel matrix either alone or in combination with other gums because of the mild conditions required and good gel stability. Immobilized *Brevibacterium flavum* using k-carrageenan attained high stability against several denaturing chemicals. The rate of cell leakage could be lowered by hardening the gel with potassium cations. Similarly several other natural polymers such as agar, agarose, pectin and gelatin were also employed for cell immobilization. Gel as a carrier material is employed for the immobilization of *Kluyveromyces fragilis* for β-galactosidase activity and *E. coli* for penicillin acylase.

3.3.7.3. Gel entrapment by precipitation

Gels may be formed by precipitation of some natural and synthetic polymers by changing one or more parameters in the solution, such as temperature, salinity or pH of solvent. The precipitation techniques are exemplified by collagen, cellulose and carrageenan. Polymer precipitate can be prepared from a homogeneous solution of linear chain polymers. The networks are primarily formed by precipitation with salt solutions, ones that are constituted by secondary valence forces ranging from dispersion to hydrogen bonding. Network formation procedures where the cross-linking is established by ionic bonds between linear polyelectrolytes and multivalent cations have been extensively tried.

3.3.7.4. Entrapment in preformed structures

Hollow fiber reactors can be used to immobilize cells by entrapment. The cells are placed on the shell side of the reactor and nutrient medium is rapidly re-circulated through the fibers. This may have important applications in large-scale operation. In other examples, the cells are added to preformed polymerized structures such as polyurethane foam. When cells in suspension are mixed with these materials, they are rapidly incorporated into the network and subsequently grown into the cavities of the mesh and are entrapped by physical restriction and attachment to the matrix material.

The mechanism of this involvement is at first a mechanical entrapment and later, the fixation of the cells due to mechanisms of adsorption and adhesion or even due to their natural tendency for aggregation. These methods of immobilization have several advantages over other methods in that they are simple, cheap, gentle and rapid and maintain cellular functions.

3.3.7.5. Intermolecular cross-linking

Cells can be immobilized by cross-linking with bi-functional groups, producing covalent bonds with intermolecular cross-linking between the cells and the reagents. The reagents may possess two different functional groups or groups of different reactivities. The agent used for this method is glutaraldehyde, this process is of little applicability as large quantities of cells are used and the insoluble form is too fine to make mechanical separation. The toxicity of the chemicals used for cross-linking obviously imposes limitations for the general applicability of these procedures. Apart from chemical cross-linking, procedures employing physical processes, such as flocculation and pelletization, also benefit the immobilization techniques because of strong mutual adherence forces of some microbial cell cultures.

3.3.8. Photo cross-linking

Some research groups in Japan have developed a novel immobilization procedure involving photo cross linkage resins. A prominent feature of glycolic cross linked with polyethylene resins is that not only cells but also enzymes can readily be immobilized in their three-dimensional matrix, the size of which can be changed freely by adjusting the degree of polymerization of the polyethylene glycol molecules located between the two isophorone isocyanate molecules. Immobilized cells are produced by irradiating a mixture of such cells and the resin, using 300–400 nm wave length from a low pressure mercury lamp. By this method immobilized cell sheets of 50 cm width are prepared under aseptic conditions.

3.4. APPLICATIONS OF IMMOBILIZATION

The potential applications of immobilization techniques are well recognized. Practical use of immobilization techniques for enzymes, cells and other biomolecules has been realized in various industrial, therapeutic, analytical processes and is being expanded in new fields: chemical synthesis, pharmaceuticals, biosensors, bioremediation, biobleaching, polymerase chain reaction, protein digestion in proteomic analysis, and biofuel cells. Enzyme and cell immobilization have been a popular strategy for most large-scale applications due to the ease in catalyst recycling, continuous operation, and product purification. The specificities of immobilization techniques promise their practical application in improvements of enzyme and cell stability. It can reduce the required amount of enzymes, prolong the lifetime of enzyme reactors, increase the potential for enzyme reuse, or maintain the good signal of biosensors.

3.4.1. Immobilized enzymes and industrial processes

The use of immobilization technology has gained a wide range of applications in industrial, medical and analytical fields (Table 3.15). A brief discussion on the use of immobilized enzymes in the field of industrial processes is presented below.

3.4.1.1. Changes in enzyme kinetics after immobilization

The study on enzymes artificially bound onto or within solid supports has attracted considerable attention owing to the potential of these water-insoluble preparations as highly specific reusable and removable reagents. For the rational design of processes using immobilized enzymes a mechanistic kinetic model is required, which accounts for all kinetic and thermodynamic phenomena, including the enzyme reaction, the mass transfer of the reactants between both the phases, and their diffusion inside the immobilizate.

Enzymes are usually attached covalently to a porous particle support to increase their thermodynamic stability and for easy separation from the reaction system so that they can be reused. Since the catalytic reaction occurs inside the particles, the reaction rate is a function of the local substrate and product concentrations, and the process is commonly influenced by external and internal diffusional limitations. Most theoretical models developed for estimating the effectiveness factor for heterogeneous enzymatic systems are based on the following assumptions:

- The catalytic particle is a porous sphere.
- The enzyme is uniformly distributed throughout the whole catalytic particle.
- Diffusion reaction takes place at a constant temperature and under steady-state conditions.
- The substrate and product diffusion inside the catalytic particle can be modelled by Fick's first law assuming that effective diffusivity remains the same throughout the particle.
- The enzymatic reaction is mono-substrate and hence yields only one product.

Table 3.15: Applications of immobilized enzymes

Industry	Application
Pharmaceuticals	Selective hydrolysis of penicillin G
	Steroid modification
	Production of monoclonal antibodies
	Animal vaccines
Food	Isomerization of glucose to fructose
	Hydrolysis of sucrose
	Inversion of sucrose
	Amino acid synthesis
	Ethanol production
Fine chemicals	Optical isomer resolution by hydrolysis of esters and amide
	Redox reaction using dehydrogenase
	Cyanide detoxification
	Iodination of proteins
	Radioactive chemicals
Analytical	Enzyme electrode based on changes in pH, redox potential, oxygen tension
	Enzyme thermistor based on heat of reaction
	Bioprobes based on cellular metabolism
Medical	*In vivo* devices to treat failure of kindney, or pancreas
	Detoxification following drug overdose
	Body monitor for key electrolytes and glucose
Fundamental biochemistry	Study of enzyme interaction with other tissue

The effects of immobilization on the kinetic behaviour of an enzyme can be classified as follows:

1. Conformational and steric effects: The enzyme may be conformationally different when fixed on a support; alternatively it may be attached to the solid carrier in a way that would render certain parts of the enzyme molecule less accessible to substrate or effector. These effects are however the least well understood.

2. Partitioning effects: The equilibrium substrate, or effector concentrations within the support, may be different from those in the bulk solution. Such effects, related to the chemical nature of the support material, may arise from electrostatic or hydrophobic interactions between the matrix and low-molecular-weight species present in the medium, leading to a modified microenvironment, i.e., to different concentrations of substrate, product or effector, hydrogen and hydroxyl ions, etc., in the domain of the immobilized enzyme particle.

3. Microenvironmental effects on the intrinsic catalytic parameters of the enzyme: Such effects due to the perturbation of the catalytic pathway of the enzymic reaction would reflect events arising from the fact that enzyme-substrate interactions occur in a different microenvironment when an enzyme is immobilized on a solid support.

4. Diffusional or mass-transfer effects: Such effects would arise from diffusional resistances to the translocation of substrate, product, or effector to or from the site of the enzymatic reaction and would be particularly pronounced in the case of fast enzymatic reactions and configurations, where the particle size or membrane thickness is relatively large. An immobilized enzyme functioning under conditions of diffusional restrictions would hence be exposed, even in the steady state, to local concentrations of substrate product or effector different from those in the bulk solution. This would be reflected in the values of the kinetic parameters which are usually employed to characterize enzymatic reactions.

These effects depend on the properties of the support, the properties of the substrate and its concentration, and the immobilization procedure, however the mass transfer limitation effects on the observed reaction rates are due to external mass transfer resistance of the substrate from the bulk fluid phase to the external surface of support pellets and internal mass transfer resistance arising from pore diffusion. The extent of mass transfer limitations depends on the physical properties of the substrate and its concentration, the shape and size of the support pellets, and the velocity of the fluid phase over the pellets.   With respect to the above effects, in the case of immobilized enzymes, where the apparent kinetic behaviour can be controlled by both microenvironmental and mass-transfer effects, it is useful to distinguish between (1) *intrinsic* rate parameters of the enzyme reaction, i.e., the kinetic parameters characteristic of the native enzyme in solution; (2) *inherent* rate parameters, those pertaining to the immobilized enzyme in the absence of any diffusional limitations; and (3) *effective* rate and kinetic parameters, observed in an immobilized enzyme when diffusional limitations are significant.

A) Conformational and steric effects

The decrease in specific activity often encountered when enzymes are covalently bound to solid supports is usually attributed to changes in the tertiary structure of the protein and to steric effects resulting from limitations on the accessibility of substrate. When the activity is measured with low-molecular-weight substrate, these effects are difficult to separate except in the cases when the number of catalytically active bound molecules can be determined by an independent method, e.g., active-site titration. Conformational changes arising from strains on the tertiary structure of the immobilized protein have been invoked by several authors to explain the low specific activities observed with bound enzymes. Such approaches, however, did not always take into account the denaturation effects, induced by contact with the support, which in the case of hydrophobic carriers may be of considerable importance.

The reduced enzyme activity observed with high-molecular-weight substrates can in most cases be related to steric limitations on the penetration of substrate. Thus a water-insoluble derivative of trypsin hydrolyzed casein at 15% of the rate that would have been expected on the basis of the amount of the enzymically active bound protein, determined by rate assay using low-molecular-weight substrate. Similar results have been reported for immobilized derivatives of ficin, bromelain, papain, and subtilopeptidase A.

Additional effects might become prominent in the case of enzymes immobilized on charged supports, e.g., electrostatic interactions between charged carrier and charged high-molecular-weight substrate; in the digestion of casein by polyanionic derivatives of trypsin, the rate of hydrolysis was found to depend on the carrier-to-enzyme ratio. Preparations of high enzyme content (60-70% protein by weight) showed caseinolytic activities close to those of native trypsin, while preparations of low enzyme content (5-10% protein by weight) had only about 20% of the expected proteolytic activity. Raising the pH, and thus increasing the charge density on the support, led to a marked decrease in the caseinolytic activity of both polyanionic-trypsin preparations. The data suggested that the number of peptide bonds split could be monitored by controlling the magnitude of charge-charge interactions between charged substrate and charged immobilized enzymes by varying the charge density on the support.

B) Partitioning effects

The observed kinetic behaviour of an enzyme embedded in a charged support may differ from that of the same enzyme in solution even in the absence of diffusional effects. This modified behaviour can be attributed to the fact that the concentration of charged species, substrates, products and effectors, hydrogen and hydroxyl ions, etc., in the domain of the immobilized enzyme is different from that in the outer solution, owing to electrostatic interactions with the fixed charges on the support. Such differences in the equilibrium concentrations of charged solutes may be conveniently described by the partition coefficient, P, given by

$$P = C_i / C_o \tag{1}$$

where, C_i and C_o are the local and bulk concentrations, respectively.

Assuming the Boltzmann distribution, the partitioning of hydrogen ions between a charged immobilized-enzyme particle and the outer solution can be described by

$$a_i^{H+} = a_o^{H+} exp(-e\varphi / kT) \tag{2}$$

Where, a_i^{H+} and a_o^{H+} are the hydrogen ion activities in the charged solid phase and the outer solution, respectively; φ is the electrostatic potential; e, the electronic charge; k, the Boltzmann constant; and T, the absolute temperature. Introducing the partition coefficient for hydrogen ions, P_{H+}, Eq. (2) can be rewritten as

$$P_H = a_i^{H+} / a_o^{H+} = exp(-e\varphi / kT) \tag{2a}$$

Equations (2) and (2a) show that the local hydrogen ion concentration in the domain of a polyanionic enzyme derivative would be higher than that measured in the bulk solution. The local pH would hence be lower. The reverse would be true for a polycationic enzyme derivative. Consequently, the pH-activity profile of an enzyme immobilized within a charged carrier would be displaced toward more alkaline or toward more acidic pH values for a negatively or positively charged carrier, respectively. Quantitatively this may be expressed in the form

$$\Delta pH = pH_i - pH_o = 0.43 e\varphi / kT \tag{3}$$

Where, pH_i and pH_o are the local and outer (bulk) pH values.

The displaced pH-activity profiles of a polyelectrolyte enzyme derivative can be alternatively represented in terms of changes in the values of the apparent acidic dissociation constant of an active-site ionizing group BH^+, given by $K = [B][H^+]/[BH^+]$. In analogy to Eq. (3) it can therefore be written as

$$\Delta pK = pK - pK' = 0.43 e\varphi / kT \tag{3a}$$

Where, pK' is the dissociation constant of the ionizing group on the bound enzyme. It can be easily seen that for a positively charged support $(\varphi > 0)$, $pK' < pK$; conversely for a negatively charged support $(\varphi < 0)$, $pK' > pK$. Active-site ionizing group $pK's$ can be estimated from the midpoints of the appropriate pH-rate curves and by a number of other procedures.

By a similar argument, the partitioning of charged substrate between a charged enzyme particle and the outer solution can be represented in the form

$$S_i = S_o \, exp(-ze\varphi / kT) \tag{4}$$

Where, S_i and S_o are the substrate concentrations in the domain of the polyelectrolyte enzyme particle and the outer solution and ze is the substrate charge. In terms of the partition coefficient for substrate, P_s, Eq. (4) becomes

$$P_s = S_i / S_o = exp(-ze\varphi / kT) \tag{4a}$$

Comparison of (4) and (4a) shows that when $S_i > S_o$; the immobilized enzyme and substrate are of opposite charge, conversely when $S_i < S_o$; enzyme and substrate are of the same charge. Assuming that the Michaelis-Menten scheme is obeyed by the charged enzyme derivative and that diffusional limitations can be neglected, the observed rate of the reaction, V', will depend on the local equilibrium concentration of substrate, S_i, hence

$$V' = V_{max} S_i / (K_m + S_i) \tag{5}$$

Insertion of Eq. (4) into Eq. (5) leads to

$$V' = \frac{V_{max} S_o \, exp(-ze\varphi/kT)}{K_m + S_o \, exp(-ze\varphi/kT)} \tag{6}$$

Where, the observed rate, V', is expressed in terms of the bulk concentration of substrate. From Eq. (6) it follows that

$$V' = \tfrac{1}{2} V_{max} \text{ when } S_o = K_m exp(ze\varphi/kT)$$

Thus the bulk concentration of substrate, S_o, at which the half-maximal rate is attained, leads to an apparent Michaelis constant, K_m', related to the intrinsic Michaelis constant of the native enzyme, K_m, by the expression

$$K'_m = K_m exp(ze\varphi/kT) \tag{7}$$

Equation (7) shows explicitly that in the case of similar charge on substrate and supported enzyme; $K'_m > K_m$, conversely for dissimilar charges; $K'_m < K_m$. In analogy to Eqs (3) and (3a), Eq (7) can be written in the form

$$\Delta pK_m = pK_m - pK'_m = log(K'_m / K_m) = 0.43 exp(ze\varphi / kT) \tag{7a}$$

The pH-activity profiles of polyanionic derivatives of several enzymes acting on their specific low-molecular-weight substrates at low ionic strength were displaced toward more alkaline pH values by 1-2.5 pH units, as compared to the native enzymes. Polycationic derivatives of the same enzymes exhibited the reverse effect, i.e., displacement of the pH-activity profiles towards more acidic pH values. As expected, the anomalies were abolished at high ionic strength.

C) Microenvironmental effects

When an enzyme is embedded in a solid support, the protein is in effect removed from its native aqueous milieu, being now exposed to a different local *microenvironment,* whose characteristics are determined by the chemical nature of the support material. This may have rather far-reaching kinetic consequences, since microenvironmental effects may lead to unequal distribution, viz. partitioning, of substrate, product, and low-molecular-weight effectors between the two phases--the immobilized enzyme particles and the bulk solution. Such a phenomenon related, for example, to electrostatic or hydrophobic interactions between the matrix and low-molecular-weight species in solution--would be reflected in the concentration-dependence of the rate parameters. Furthermore, the intrinsic kinetic parameters of an enzyme, as well as its apparent specificity, might be changed as a result of perturbations of the catalytic pathway of an enzyme reaction induced by a modified microenvironment.

Microenvironmental effects on the intrinsic kinetic parameters of immobilized enzymes

In the simple electrostatic models employed to explain the perturbed kinetics of charged immobilized enzyme derivatives, it was assumed that the intrinsic catalytic properties of the bound protein were independent of the charge characteristics of the microenvironment and identical with those of the native enzyme. The generality of such assumptions is, however, questionable. In some cases the intrinsic catalytic properties of an enzyme might be affected by the chemical characteristics of the microenvironment.

The kinetic behaviour of charged enzyme derivatives was reinvestigated, using a series of water-soluble polyanionic and polycationic derivatives of chymotrypsin. The amount of active enzyme in these preparations could be determined by the conventional spectrophotometric "active- site" titration methods; thus the intrinsic kinetic parameters of the polyelectrolyte derivatives of chymotrypsin and those of the native enzyme could be compared on an absolute basis. The kinetic data indicated that the overall rate constants (k_{cat}) of the polyanionic derivatives of chymotrypsin were higher than the k_{cat} value of the native enzyme; conversely the k_{cat} values of the polycationic derivatives were lower. The perturbation of k_{cat} was greater with amide than with ester substrates, suggesting that the acylation step was more strongly and effectively affected by electrostatic perturbations. Moreover, an increase in the ionic strength of the medium caused an increase in the values of k_{cat} of both native chymotrypsin and the positively charged polyornithyl chymotrypsin derivatives; the k_{cat} values of the negatively charged EMA-chymotrypsin and polyglutamyl chymotrypsin, on the other hand, were not affected by ionic strength. The simplest kinetic model that accommodated these findings was based on the assumption that a kinetically significant step in chymotrypsin catalysis involves the interaction of two positively charged residues. By this model, the high k_{cat} values of the polyanionic derivatives of chymotrypsin could be related to the screening of the above interactions by the negative charges on the support, this being analogous to the effect of high salt concentration on the native enzyme. In the case of a polycationic derivative, however, the charge-charge interaction between two positive residues would be enhanced and k_{cat} would be lower.

The model thus assumed, in effect, that catalytically significant steps in an enzyme reaction could in principle be modified by perturbations arising from the chemical nature of the matrix. This view found indirect support in experiments originally intended to establish the magnitude of product inhibition effects in systems where both product and support are charged. In these studies the hydrolysis of acetyl-L-tyrosine ethyl ester by a-chymotypsin, by the polyanionic polyglutamyl- and EMA-chymotrypsin derivatives, and by a polycationic polyornithylchymotypsin derivative was investigated in the presence of increasing amounts of acetyl- L-tyrosine anion (AcTyr), the product of the enzymic reaction. As expected, the kinetic parameters of native chymotrypsin and of the polyanionic chymotrypsin derivatives were not significantly affected even at fairly high concentrations of acetyltyrosine. In the case of polyornithylchymotrypsin, however, both K_m' and k_{cat} increased hyperbolically with increasing AcTyr concentration, suggesting a saturation phenomenon. Several aliphatic and aromatic anions, e.g., acetate, propionate, benzoate, and 1-anilino-8-naphthalene sulfonate (ANS), caused a similar increase in the k_{cat} values of polyornithylchymotrypsin. The common feature of all anionic modifiers tested was that they all contained an apolar hydrocarbon core attached to the ionizing carboxyl or sulfonate group. The data could be explained by assuming that the strong binding of AcTyr (and the other anions) was the result of a combination of electrostatic and hydrophobic interactions between relatively hydrophobic acetyltyrosine anion and the positively charged polyornithyl side chains on the enzyme. This could also explain the hyperbolic increase of k_{cat} with increasing AcTyr concentration; strong and essentially stoichiometric binding of AcTyr anions onto the cationic ornithyl residues of the side chains would result in, at least partial, cancellation of the positive charge on the matrix, hence abolishing its deleterious effects on the catalytic activity of the bound enzyme.

D) Mass-transfer effects

When an enzyme is immobilized on or within a solid support, the substrate has to diffuse from the bulk solution to the site of the enzyme reaction. Hence when the rate of diffusion of substrate is slower than the rate of its transformation by the enzyme, the observed rate of the reaction would be lower than that expected for a given amount of enzyme in solution, since not all enzyme molecules would be in contact with substrate at a concentration level identical with that of the bulk solution. This phenomenon can be expressed quantitatively by the effectiveness factor, η, defined as the ratio of the actual reaction rate, V' to the rate, V_{kin}, which would obtain if no mass-transfer limitations were present and hence all enzyme molecules were exposed to the same substrate concentration as that in the bulk solution. This relationship is expressed by

$$V' = \eta V_{kin} \tag{8}$$

For a reaction obeying Michaelis-Menten kinetics, V_{kin} is given by

$$V_{kin} = V_{max} S /(K_m + S) \tag{9}$$

Where, V_{max}, K_m, and S have their usual meaning.

Since, in the presence of diffusional limitations, the observed rate, V', is not the true rate of the reaction, the conventional methods of treating enzyme kinetic data, whereby the characteristic rate parameters V_{max} and K_m are deduced from the slopes and intercepts of the appropriate linear plots, would be misleading. This can be easily seen by introducing the effectiveness factor, η, from Eq (8) into the Michaelis-Menten expression:

$$V_{kin} = \eta[V_{max} S /(K_m + S)] \tag{10}$$

The kinetics of an enzyme embedded in a porous medium are governed by two types of diffusional resistances to transport of substrate: (1) *external* diffusional resistances arising from the fact that substrate must be transported from the bulk solution to the surface of catalyst across a boundary layer of liquid; (2) *internal* diffusional resistances, i.e., diffusional limitations pertaining to the transport of substrate inside the porous catalytic medium.

In the case of external diffusional limitations, the chemical reaction occurs *after* the substrate has reached the catalyst's surface. The depletion of substrate across the boundary layer can in many cases be approximated by a linear gradient. Moreover, partial cancellation of external diffusional limitations can be effected by increasing the rate of stirring of a suspension of immobilized enzyme particles or increasing the rate of flow of substrate solution through an enzyme column. With internal transport limitations the diffusion process occurs *simultaneously* with the chemical reaction, so that the two events are coupled in the mathematical sense and would normally give rise to nonlinear substrate concentration gradients within the porous catalyst. Hence the theoretical approaches to the analysis of the interplay of enzyme catalyzed reaction with external or internal transport of substrate are different.

3.4.1.2. Enzyme reactors

A) Batch reactors

These are enzyme reactors (Fig. 3.22) in which the immobilized enzymes and substrates are placed and the reaction is allowed to take place under constant stirring. Once the reaction is completed, the reactor is drained and the product is separated from the enzyme. Separation of enzymes is usually done by denaturing the enzymes. Again this is possible only with soluble enzymes. This type of separation when required at large scale can be carried not only when the enzyme used is less. In an enzyme reactor, the highest specific enzyme activity is desirable. It is considered an added bonus if the support that is used also aides in separation. If the availability of enzyme used is low, then such process would lead to a severe loss in production. To overcome such problems the use of immobilization technique is highly appreciated. Using this technique the enzyme can be recovered intact without any significant loss in activity. For an industrial reactor, it is preferable to use supports that are non-biodegradable such as glass, silica, Celite, Bentonite, alumina, or titanium oxide, if possible. Even the linkages between enzyme and support can be non-biodegradable, as they are in the case of titanium. In some of these supports the physical nature of the surface becomes a major problem. Thus, some supports that form excellent packed beds fail to do so when coated with enzyme. Particles, which ideally self-suspend in a fluid bed may form aggregates during use and thus require more power to pump through substrate. Many problems were encountered using porous glass supports until someone realized that the glass itself could dissolve. This problem has been eliminated by treatment of the glass surface with zirconium.

B) Continuous flow reactors

In a continuous flow enzyme reactor, the substrate is added continuously to reactor while simultaneous removal of product is taking place. Among the various types of continuous flow reactors, a few are discussed here:

i) *Continuous flow stirred tank*

These are reactors consisting of a continuously stirred tank with separate inlets for substrate entry and product exit. The yield obtained can be increased by varying the input substrate quantity to minimum while the enzyme available to convert the same into a product will ultimately lead to higher yield. Immobilized enzyme can be retained in the reactor while the product is recovered by either filtering the product outlet or by using magnetically active particles for immobilization, which can later be retained actively within a magnetic field whilst the product is still recovered.

ii) *Cell- free system and bioreactors*

A typical cell free bioreactor for gene cloning works on the principle of immobilization of the required component(s) in chambers traditionally built by using semi-permeable membrane. The immobilization technique has effectively made it possible to synthesize and clone up the gene or other peptides which are amenable to the factoring and modifications.

C) Other reactors

A *recycle reactor* is a reactor that is not seen very often, but is very important to consider when studying immobilized enzymes. It is especially important in chemical engineering because it allows certain substrates to be processed, which could not be processed in other reactor types. In a recycle reactor, a portion of the product stream is recycled and mixed with the inlet flow to the reactor. If the entire product stream is recycled back to the inlet stream, then it is called a total recycle reactor. This can obviously only be used in a batch process, because if the entire product stream is recycled back into the reactor in a continuous reactor, the volume of the reactor would increase to infinity. Therefore, only partial recycle streams are recycled in a continuous reactor. This type of rector is used when one has a substrate that cannot be completely processed on a single pass, such as with an insoluble substrate. These reactors continue to move the same substrate through the reactor so that the effective contact time is long enough to allow the substrate to be processed. Recycle reactors also allow the reactor to operate at high fluid velocities. This is important because it minimizes the bulk mass transfer resistance to the transport of the substrate.

The *packed bed reactor* is an enzyme reactor in which the immobilized enzyme particles and immobilized microbial cells are packed inside the column while the substrate is allowed to pass through the column. In these systems, it is necessary to consider the pressure drop across the packed bed or column, and the effect of the column dimensions on the reaction rate. The recycling method is advantageous when the linear velocity of the substrate solution affects the reaction flow rate. This is because the recycling method allows the substrate solution to be passed through the column at a desired velocity. For industrial applications, upward flow is generally preferred over downward flow because it does not compress the beds in enzyme columns as downward flow does. When gas is produced during an enzyme reaction, upward flow is preferred.

A *stirred tank reactor* is the simplest type of reactor. It is composed of a reactor and a mixer such as a stirrer, a turbine wing or a propeller. This reactor is useful for substrate solutions of high viscosity and for immobilized enzymes with relatively low activity. However, a problem that arises is that an immobilized enzyme tends to decompose upon physical stirring. The batch system is generally suitable for the production of rather small amounts of chemicals. The continuous stirred tank reactor is more efficient than a batch stirred tank reactor but the equipment is slightly more complicated.

A *fluidized-bed reactor* is a combination of the two most common, packed-beds and stirred tank, continuous flow reactors. The fluidized bed reactor is most suitable when a high viscosity substrate solution and a gaseous substrate or products are used in a continuous reaction system. In a fluidized-bed reactor, the substrate is passed upward through the immobilized enzyme bed at a high enough velocity to lift the particles. However, the velocity must not be so high that the enzymes are swept away from the reactor entirely. In this system, care must be taken to avoid the destruction and decomposition of immobilized enzymes. The particle size of immobilized enzymes is an important factor for the formation of a smooth fluidized bed. This type of reactor is ideal for highly exothermic reactions because it eliminates local hot spots; due to its mass and heat transfer characteristics mentioned before. It is most often applied in immobilized-enzyme catalysis where viscous, particulate substrates are to be handled.

The *hollow fiber reactor* is a variant of the packed bed reactor, which uses walls made up of fibers permeable to the substrate and product while being impermeable to enzyme molecule. The substrate passes over the enzyme to react with it producing the required product. Further, the substrate diffuses out through the fibrous wall, reacts with the enzymes and the product diffuses through the fibrous wall.

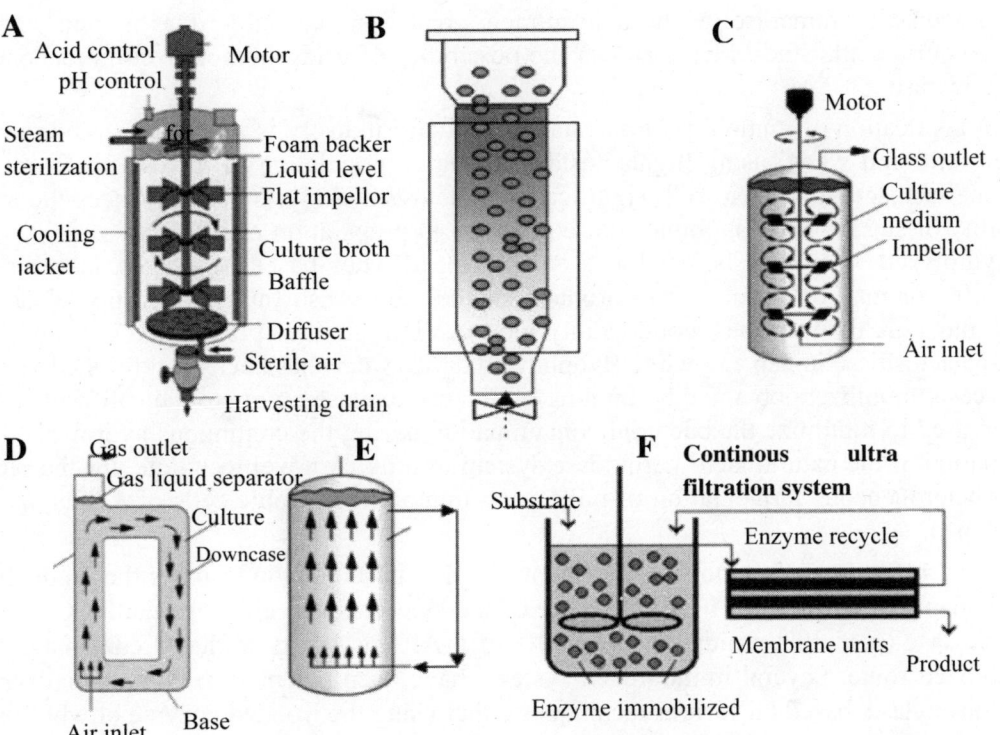

Fig. 3.22: Various types of bioreactors (A) Basic assembly of bioreactor(Batch flow reactor), (B) Packed bed reactor, (C) Air left reactor, (D) Fluidized bed reactor, (E) Recycler bioreactor, (F) Continuous flow hollow fiber reactor

3.4.1.3. Industrial processes

Several large-scale industrial processes that employ immobilized-enzyme catalysts at some point are already in operation. Cells of *Saccharomyces cerevisiae* and *Kluyveromyces marxianus*, inulase, glucose oxidase, chloroplasts, and mitochondria have been immobilized in calcium alginate gels. By far the most important application of immobilized enzymes in industry is the conversion of glucose syrups to high fructose syrups by the enzyme glucose isomerase. Application of glucose isomerase technology is particularly important in non tropical countries that have abundant starchy raw materials. Unlike these countries, in tropical countries like India, where sugarcane cultivation is abundant, high fructose syrups can be obtained by a simpler process of invertase mediated hydrolysis of sucrose. Compared to sucrose, invert sugar has higher solubility and osmotic pressure. A large number of immobilized invertase systems have been patented. The possible use of whole cells of yeast as a source of invertase was demonstrated as early as 1978.

L-aspartic acid is widely used in medicine and as a food additive. A one-step stereospecific addition of ammonia to the double bond of fumaric acid is catalysed by the enzyme aspartase. The whole cells of *E. coli* can be immobilized for this and considered to be the first industrial application of immobilized microbial cells. The initial process made use of polyacrylamide entrapment which was later substituted by treating carrageenan with glutaraldehyde and hexamethylenediamine.

Immobilized fumarase has been used for the production of malic acid for pharmaceutical use. These processes make use of immobilized nonviable cells of *Brevibacterium ammoniagenes* or *B. flavus* as a source of fumarase. Malic acid attracts greater market interest as a food acidulant as compared to citric acid. Studies have shown the possibility of using immobilized mitochondria as a source of fumarase.

A major application of immobilized biocatalysts in dairy industry is in the preparation of lactose-hydrolyzed milk and whey, using β-galactosidase. A large population of lactose intolerant humans can consume lactose-hydrolyzed milk significantly. Lactose hydrolysis also enhances the sweetness and solubility of sugars, and has found future potential in preparation of a variety of dairy products. Lactose-hydrolyzed whey may be used as a component of whey-based beverages, leavening agents and feedstuffs, or may be fermented to produce ethanol and yeast, thus converting an inexpensive byproduct into a highly nutritious, good quality food. An immobilized preparation obtained by cross-linking β -galactosidase in hen egg white (lyophilized dry powder) has been used for the hydrolysis of lactose. A co-immobilizate obtained by binding of glucose oxidase on microbial cell walls using Con A has been used to minimize the bacterial contamination during the continuous hydrolysis of lactose by the initiation of the natural lacto-peroxidase system in milk. A novel technique for the removal of lactose by heterogeneous fermentation of milk using immobilized viable cells of *K. fragilis* has also been developed.

One major application of immobilized enzymes in pharmaceutical industry is the production of 6-aminopenicillanic acid (6-APA) by deacylation of the side chain in either penicillin G or V, using penicillin acylase (penicillin amidase). Over 50% of 6-APA is being produced enzymatically using the immobilized route. Several immobilized systems have been patented or commercially produced for penicillin acylase, based on various techniques either using the isolated enzyme or whole cells.

Lipases have industrial potential including use in detergents; leather treatment; controlled hydrolysis of milk fat for acceleration of cheese ripening; hydrolysis, glycerolysis and alcoholysis of bulk fats and oils; production of optically pure compounds and flavors, etc. Lipases are spontaneously soluble in aqueous phase but their natural substrates (lipids) are not. Although use of proper immobilization techniques helps in overcoming the problem of intimate contact between the substrate and enzyme, the practical use of lipases in such pseudo-homogeneous reactions poses technological difficulties.

Immobilized oxidoreductases are gaining importance in biotechnology for synthetic transformations. Of particular significance are oxidoreductase-mediated asymmetric synthesis of amino acids, steroids and other pharmaceuticals and a host of specialty chemicals. Enzymes entrapped either in radiation-polymerized acrylamide, Ca-alginate or gelatin has shown promise in clinical diagnosis and other analytical applications including biosensors. They play a major role in immobilized glucose oxidase and can find application in the production of gluconic acid, removal of oxygen from beverages and the removal of glucose from eggs prior to dehydration in order to prevent Maillard reaction.

3.4.2. Analytical applications

3.4.2.1. Enzyme electrode

Enzyme electrodes are probes that generate an electrical potential as a result of a reaction catalyzed by an immobilized enzyme that is fixed onto or around the probe. The use of immobilized enzymes in automated analysis implies that the immobilized enzyme is used to replace the soluble enzyme in an existing automatic analyzer system (Fig. 3.23). Two important challenges in enzyme electrodes are: (1) the durable immobilization of the enzyme on the transducer while maintaining its biological activity and ensuring good diffusional properties for substrates and (2) the establishment of satisfactory communication between the active sites of the enzyme and the electrode surface.

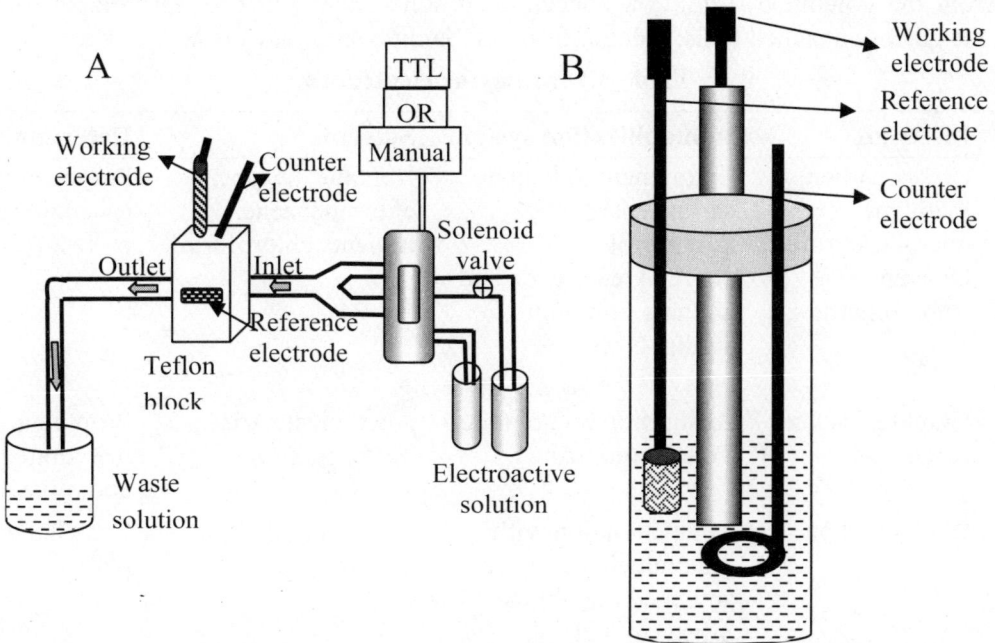

Fig. 3.23: (A) Principle and mechanism of enzyme electrode, (B) Basic structure of enzyme electrode

Many of these have used conventional immobilization techniques to localize the enzyme at the electrode surface; examples include the physical entrapment of the enzyme behind a dialysis membrane, the covalent attachment of the enzyme to the electrode surface or to a polymeric support, or the cross-linking of the enzyme in a protein matrix using glutaraldehyde (Tables 3.16 and 3.17). Frequently, these approaches have been combined with the use of a discrete macroscopic membrane to reduce electrode fouling and to alleviate problems of interference caused by electro-active species present in the sample. The first enzyme electrode to be reported was the glucose sensitive electrode. In this electrode, the enzyme glucose oxidase was immobilized in a polyacrylamide gel and held in around electrode by a piece of cellulose acetate. The principle involved is the removal of oxygen from solution at a rate dependent upon the concentration of glucose present. Where a redox enzyme confined close to the tip reduces the flux of oxygen reaching the detector by catalyzing a specific oxidation. This "enzyme electrode" was then combined with the selective the enzyme for its substrate such as D-glucose and the sensitivity of potentiometric measurements. Another example is the urea electrode, in which immobilized urease decomposes urea into ions which can be detected using standard electrochemical techniques. Also, using immobilized enzyme electrodes, standard biochemical tests can be automated. Examples of determining glucose or lactate levels by employing immobilized glucose oxidase or lactate dehydrogenase respectively substantiate practical application potentials of immobilized enzyme systems in the estimation of bioeluates.

3.5.2.2. Affinity chromatography and purification

Immobilized enzymes are also used in affinity chromatography. This technique is extremely efficient at removal of the material from solution which permits purification or analysis of enzyme inhibitors, cofactors; antigens, antibodies and other substances. For example, Con A, a plant protein can be purified by passing the crude extract of the plant containing the protein through a column of beads containing covalently attached glucose residues. Con A has affinity to glucose and gets bound to the beads while the other proteins pass through the column (Fig. 3.24). The bound Con A can then be released from the column by adding a concentrated solution of glucose. The glucose in solution displaces the glucose attached to the column from the binding sites on Con A.

Table 3.16: Enzyme electrodes

Enzyme	Electrode	Immobilization system	Solvents	Determination
PPO	Glassy carbon, Platinum microdisk array, Oxygen amperometric	Entrapment in kappa-carrageenan, Polypyrrol, polyethylene oxide and alginate film with avidin–biotin interactions	Heptane, hexane, chlorobenzene, toluene, chloroform	Polyphenols (phenol, catechol, p-cresol)
PPO	Graphite–Teflon composite	Adsorption on graphite–Teflon composite	Acetonitrile–tris buffer mixtures	Propyl gallate in dehydrated broth and olive oil
PPO	Glassy carbon	Covalent union with glutaraldehyde to pre-activated membrane, Silica sol–gel	n-Hexane, Chloroform	Catechol and phenol
Catalase	Oxygen amperometric, Platinum	Entrapment in kappa-carrageenan gel, polyacrylamide gel	Acetonitrile or dioxane	Hydrogen peroxide in cosmetic, food and pharmaceutical formulations
HRP	Glassy carbon, Platinum, Graphite	Entrapment in ferrocene-phenylenediamine film and N-methyl-pyrrole, Adsorption on graphite	Acetonitrile–buffer mixture; Reversed micelles, Acetonitrile	Hydrogen peroxide and other organic peroxides, Lauryl peroxide
GOx	Screen-printed electrode: rhodinised-carbon	Adsorption	Methanol, ethanol and isopropanol aqueous buffer mixtures	Glucose
SOD	Oxygen amperometric, GDE	Entrapment in kappa-carrageenan gel	Dimethylsulfoxide	Antioxidant or radical scavenging capacity of phytotherapeutic products
AChE	Screen-printed electrode	Entrapment in polyvinyl alcohol styryl-pyridinium polymer	Acetonitrile and ethanol	p-Aminophenol

Table 3.17: Some examples of immobilized enzymes used in electrode constructs

Substance assayed	Enzyme immobilized	Electrode base
Adenosine monophosphate	AMP deaminase	NH_4^+
Alcohols	Alcohol oxidase	Pt/O_2
D-amino acid	D-amino acid oxidase	NH_4^+
L-amino acid	L-amino acid oxidase	NH_4^+
D-Glucose	Glucose oxidase	Pt/quinine
Glucose-6-phosphate	Alkaline phosphatase/glucose oxidase	Pt/O_2
Lactate	LDH	Pt/ferricyanide
Penicillin	Penicillinase	pH
Urea	Urease	pH or CO_2
Uric acid	Urease	Pt/O_2

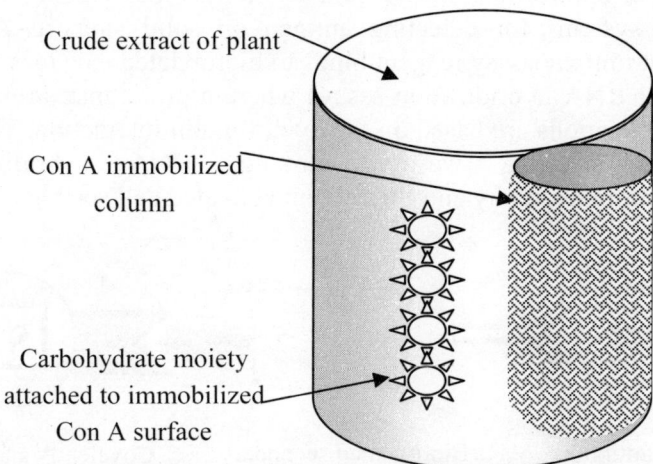

Fig. 3.24: Con A immobilized column for carbohydrate purification

3.4.2.3. Immobilized receptor ligands for affinity cell sorting

The cell isolation affinity chromatography media are principally based on immobilization of affinity ligands corresponding to the receptors that are specifically expressed by a particular cell line. The cells containing receptor or positive with regard to receptor are actively retained in the column and these without specific receptors are eluted out of column. Thus with the combination of cell affinity media, cells can be isolated free of identified cellular contaminants. Some commercially available affinity media are Isocell™ for human T cell isolation, Isocell ™ for CD8, Isocell™ for CD4, etc.

3.4.2.4. Immobilization in affinity purification

Based on avidin-biotin binding, immobilized systems have been developed where affinity binding is exploited for separation/purification. Avidin is covalently attached to a solid support, a biotinylated product or conjugate passing through is held strongly which can later be detected to let immobilized affinity support freely eluting 6M guanidine HCl. The biotinylated ligands include antigen, antibody, carbohydrates, cells, DNA, enzymes, haptens, lectins, peptides, proteins and receptors.

3.4.2.5. Immobilized avidin-biotin based systems

Immobilized avidin can be used in various applications for the affinity purification of biotinylated macromolecules. Principally, an antibody that has an affinity for a particular antigen is labeled with biotin. Cells containing the antigen are lysed, and then incubated with the biotinylated antibody to form a typical antigen/antibody complex. To isolate the antigen the crude mixture is passed through an immobilize avidin or streptavidin column, which will bind the complex. After appropriate washing, the antigen can be eluted from the column with a pH 2.8-elution buffer. The biotinylated antibody is retained by the column. Immobilized avidin is used for various purposes. They are:

- Purification of double-strand DNA
- Binding biotinyl peptides and elution with a SDS/urea solution
- Binding biotinylated antitransferrin for purifying transferrin from serum
- Hybridization of biotinylated RNA to its complementary DNA and binding to immobilized avidin, with subsequent elution of the single-stranded DNA

The interaction between biotin (a vitamin) and avidin (hen-egg white protein) has been extensively exploited to produce a variety of applications in the field of immunology. Figure 3.25 exemplifies avidin-biotin complex (ABC) systems for detecting antigen on solid support. A similar assay procedure can develop where an immunoassay reagent binds to biotinylated enzymes or conjugates to enzymes. For example, DNA or RNA hybridization assays where a probe instead of an antibody is biotinylated and a few other applications are based on the avidin-biotin interaction. These are ELISA assays, immunohistochemical staining, western blotting, DNA hybridization assays, immunoprecipitation, affinity chromatography and fluorescent activated cell sorting (FACS).

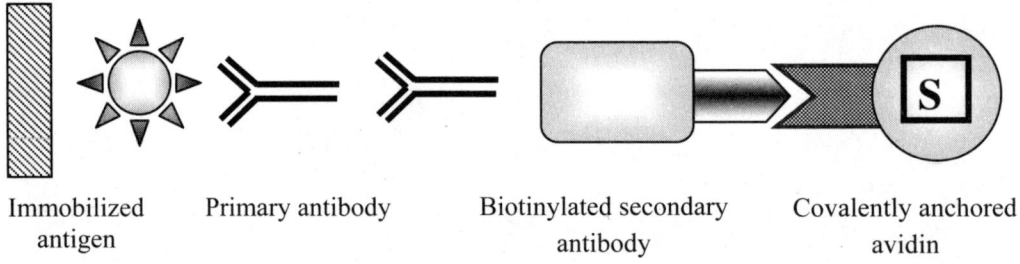

| Immobilized antigen | Primary antibody | Biotinylated secondary antibody | Covalently anchored avidin |

Fig. 3.25: ABC system (Avidin biotin based system)

Similarly, purified streptavidin and lectin can be used in place of avidin in the above system (ABC system). This modified system is broadly used in:

- Enzyme immuno staining,
- Cell and tissue staining (for light microscope),
- Blot immuno staining,
- Tissue staining, and
- Cell staining for fluorescent activated cell sorting

3.4.2.6. Autoanalysis

The conventional method has the disadvantage that an aliquot of enzyme is added to each sample, which is subsequently lost. The alternative is to immobilize the enzyme and fix it in the sample stream. The enzyme may also be conveniently attached to the inner wall of a narrow bore nylon tube, through which the sample stream is made to pass. Immobilized hexokinase and glucose-6-phosphate dehydrogenase have been used for the autoanalysis of glucose concentration. When large volumes are analyzed continuously the principle involved is the measurement of heat generated by an enzyme reaction. If a thermistor is held in the middle of a column of an immobilized enzyme as a substrate solution is passed through column, the reaction catalyzed around the thermistor raises the temperature. The rise in temperature created by the reaction could be a measure of the substrate concentration. The disadvantage of using such a system is in checking contaminants in the production stream where the solvent stream is not required to be optically cleared (used to monitor substances in blood). Immobilized enzymes arc mainly useful in two areas:

- Repeated autoanalysis of small samples (e.g., blood samples)
- Continuous stream monitoring of large volume

3.4.2.7. Biosensors

A biosensor is a device, probe or electrode having immobilized biocatalyst which, upon making contact with an appropriate simple, converts the presence of the desired analyte into physical, chemical or electrical signals, which can be measured. The concentration in the sample is measured as the electrical signal or could be measured with the help a suitable combination of a biological recognition system and an electrochemical transducer. Biosensors essentially respond in reversible and specific manner to the concentration variation of biochemical event of great practical utility. There are two types of biosensors, depending on the nature of the recognition event. Bioaffinity devices rely on the selective binding of the target analyte to a surface-confined ligand partner (e.g. antibody, oligonucleotide). In contrast, in biocatalytic devices, an immobilized enzyme is used for recognizing the target substrate. For example, sensor strips with immobilized glucose oxidase are widely used for personal monitoring of diabetes. The research drive has been propelled vigorously towards designing and development of precise biosensors as there is a continuous need of them. One common use of biosensor is quantitation of a drug substance in the finished drug product. Accurate measurements of drugs have become possible by applying biosensors for all traditional dosage forms such as liquids, tablets, powders and ointments.

Biological recognition systems are typically some enzymes, organelles, microbial, plant or animal cells, tissue, slice, section or immune binding or receptor protein. The system is responsible for the specific recognition of the analyte and subsequent response with a change in some measurable parameters. Some detection systems that can be used in biosensing are electrochemical detection system, thermal and mass detection, photometric detection, infra-red, fluorescence, surface plasmon systems and those based on signal processing and instrumentation (Fig. 3. 26).

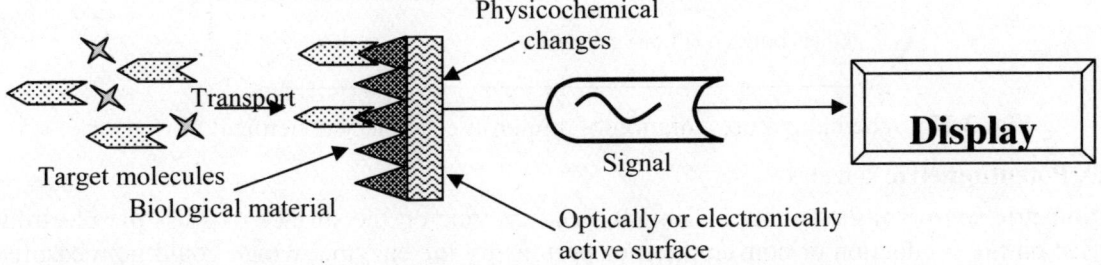

Fig. 3.26: Schematic representation of genetic biosensor showing major components and the processes that contributes to signal generation

A combination of immobilized antibody (or antigen) with an electronic device yields an immunosensor. In this system, the antigen acts as an analyte. Immunosensors are of two main types, namely labeled and non-labeled. The frequently used labels are radioisotopes, enzyme, particles, and precipitins. Non-labeled immunosensors include potentiometric immunosensors with antigen (or antibody) coated membrane or potentiometric immunosensor with antibody-coated electrode. An interesting immunosensor has been developed for the diagnosis of syphilis. Principally, the antigen analyte due to affinity selectively immobilized antibody and generates signals via labeled immunsorbent(s), which could be monitored electronically. This enables estimation to be rapid, precise, reproducible and continuous in nature.

3.4.2.8. Electrochemical sensors

Electrochemical sensors are subdivided into amperometric, potentiometric, and conductometric types. In the amperometric category, an enzyme is typically coupled to an amperometric electrode and as the enzyme reacts with the substrate, a current is produced that is correlated to analyte concentration (Fig. 3.27). There are four common ways for making an amperometric device:

a) Immobilizing an oxygen-consuming enzyme on a platinum electrode where the reduction of oxygen produces a current that is inversely proportional to the analyte concentration,

b) Directing or mediating electron transfer from electrode to enzyme, thus eliminating the oxygen consumption at the electrode,

c) Utilizing an enzyme directly immobilized on to a polarized anode to produce hydrogen peroxide based sensors. This is generally better than oxygen sensing systems, but the selectivity is usually poorer,

d) Using the analyte along with a dehydrogenase enzyme to produce a concomitant reduction of NAD to NADH.

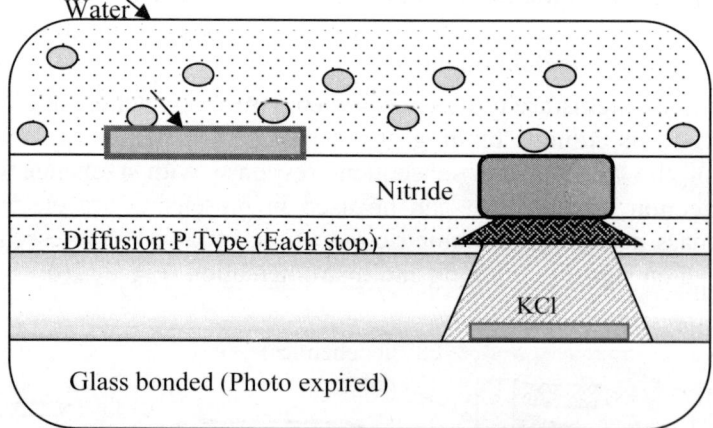

Fig. 3.27: Schematic representation of amperometric electrochemical biosensor

3.4.2.9. Potentiometric sensors

Potentiometric sensors utilize either an immobilized enzyme on the surface of glass pH electrode or are based on tile production or consumption of protons by the enzyme, which could be measured by the electrode. Measurements are usually done in the 'zero current' mode for both liquid and gaseous configurations. One of the major limitations of the potentiometric approach is that enzyme activity is sensitive to pH, ammonia, carbon dioxide and some other endogenous analyte present in the sample (Fig. 3.28). Potentiometric biosensors can be miniaturized with ion-selective field effect transistors

(ISFETs). Hundreds of sensors configurations have been proposed and developed for a wide variety of applications such as chiral amine salt detection, enzyme inhibitors of acetyl choline esterases, anionic surfactants like sodium dodecyl sulfate and dodecyltrimethyl ammonium bromide, concentrations in pharmaceutical preparations for cationic anesthetics such as procaine, tetracaine and lidocaine sensors for cardiovascular applications have also been developed. The intramyocardial pH is monitored by an ISFET biosensor during human open-heart surgery.

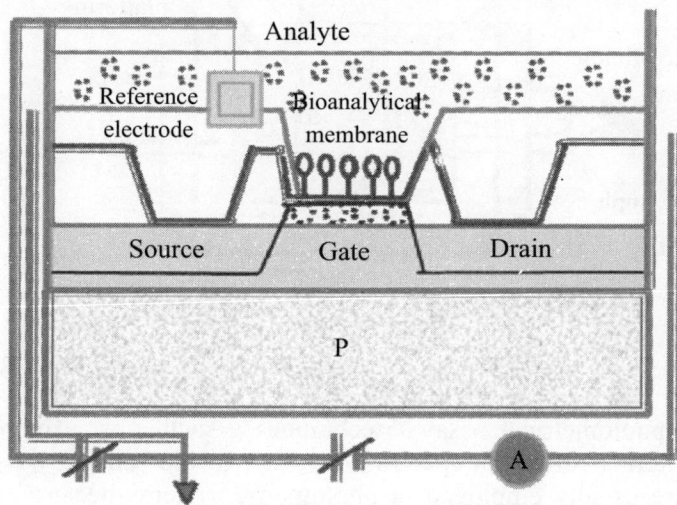

Fig. 3.28: Schematic representation of potentiometric biosensor

3.4.2.10. Thermal and mass calorimetric biosensor

In these biosensors the heat generated during enzyme/substrate reactions is used. Changes in solution temperature caused by the enzyme/substrate reactions are measured using thermistor or transistor and compared to a sensor with no enzyme to determine the analyte concentration. Calorimetric microsensors have been manufactured for detection of cholesterol in blood serum based on enzymatically-produced heat of oxidation and decomposition (Fig. 3.29). Industrial applications are possible for monitoring sugars and amino acids in biotechnology based processes and for determination of water content in foods like jelly, chicken and fish. Femtogram levels of drug vapors have been detected with SAW resonators for forensic use and sub-nanogram amounts of particulates are detectable as a function of temperature and pressure. In liquid based systems, piezoelectric mass sensors based on AT shear quartz crystals are used as miniature viscometers. The system has been successfully used for the study of interfacial processes.

The concept of generating physical changes in close vicinity of a detector by a biocatalytic process has been well appreciated. Thermistors that register the heat of an enzyme-catalyzed exothermic reaction have proved effective detectors and it is conceivable that other physical factors might also be useful. Bioprobes consisting of living cells held close to oxygen or pH probes have also been suggested. Although they detect interesting metabolites directly they are far more susceptible to deactivation interference and contaminative infections.

3.4.2.11. Optical biosensor

It is a small device along with its measuring instrument that uses optical principles quantitatively to convert chemical or biochemical concentrations or activities into electrical signals. This type of sensor often incorporates biological molecules such as antibodies and enzymes as transducing elements (Fig. 3.30).

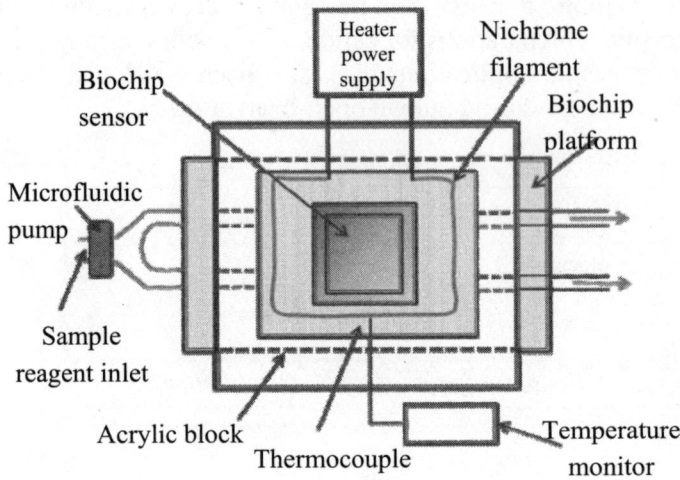

Fig. 3.29: Assembly and process of thermal biosensor

Application of photometric assay techniques such as fluorescence, absorbance, chemiluminescence, internal reflection spectroscopy, etc. to bio-sensing has been adopted. Optical fibers or light pipes are usually employed in photometric systems because of the added flexibility since the transducer element can be separated from the actual measuring instrument by relatively large distances with virtually no losses in sensitivity or selectivity. Optical based biosensors have many advantages over electrical based sensor. The biocatalyst or bio-receptor does not have to be in intimate contact with the optical fiber, which allows for a wider range of non-invasive sensor configurations. Optical fibers permit the scientist to bring the spectrometer to the sample and apply many of the spectroscopic techniques on a sample volume of a few micro liters. No interference from electrical noise occurs in optical based biosensors.

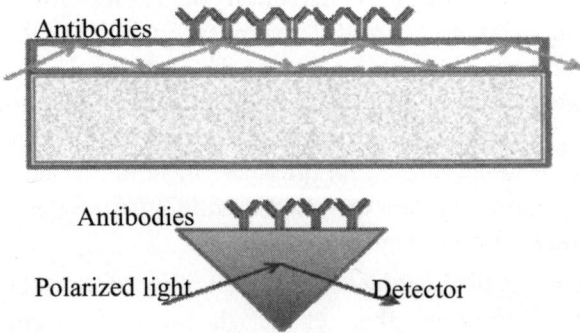

Fig. 3.30: Schematic representation of optical biosensor

NIR (near infrared) spectroscopy is a valuable tool for real-time process control when combined with fiber optic probes or on-line flow-through cells. Diffuse reflected and transmissive IR absorption measurements have been simultaneously applied to blood samples to measure blood analyte concentrations such as glucose. *In vivo* oxyhaemoglobin measurements were first made using NIR reflection spectroscopy in conjunction with balloon catheters. ATR spectroscopy and IR spectroscopy were used in developing a biosensor based on the immobilization of enzymes on a chalcogenide optical fiber. NIR Raman spectroscopy is an effective medical diagnostic tool for identifying silicone gel materials in biopsy specimen taken from women who possess leaking breast implants. A personnel vapor detector badge has been developed for detecting the accumulated exposure to benzene vapor using small sections of optical fibers coated with a membrane that adsorbs ambient benzene vapor. After exposure, the badge is passed into a FT-IR spectrometer for quantitation, enabling estimation of degree of exposure.

An application of optical fiber sensing that has already become a commercial reality is in the area of blood gas monitoring. Combining three optical fibers and a thermocouple with an appropriate gas sensing dye has produced systems that accurately measure *in vivo* concentration of pH, pCO_2 and pO_2 for use in critical care and surgical monitoring. Respiratory gas measurements for the volatile anesthetic halothene have become possible by using the absorbance of UV radiation at 230 nm as measured by change in fluorescence of a polymer film. Optical fibers have also been applied to immunoassay systems.

One most interesting application of optical biosensors is to combine bacterial magnetite with a chromophoric system to measure a patient's blood glucose level through a colour development. Briefly, glucose oxidase is immobilized on to bacterial magnetites, which act as a reaction phase. The levels of glucose (in the range of 0.56–22 mM) are linearly proportional to the quantity of H_2O_2 produced, which moves through the inner membranes and alters the color of the chromphore, o-dianisidine. The intensity of color is proportional to the quantity of glucose and can be calculated.

3.4.2.12. Acoustic biosensors

Piezoelectric devices have been made that show sensitivity to frequency of interactions relating to surface mass. Principally, piezoelectric phenomena based on acoustic principles that essentially rely on establishing vibrational wave in material, i.e., under the influence of alternative current voltage is applied through a surface coated electrode depending on the characteristics of acoustic waves and on the structure of the device. They are known as quartz micro valence Saw (surface acoustic wave) lamb wave or acoustic plate based devices (Fig. 3.31). When antibodies are coated on to the surfaces resulting constructs it could selectively pickup the load of complementary antigens. The resultant increment in the surface mass loading decreases the vibrational wave, which could be quantified and has been found to be proportional to the mass.

3.4.2.13. Surface plasmon

Surface plasmon is a quasi-free electron cloud prepared by coating the core with a thin layer of silver approximately 600 A° thick. Surface plasmon resonance is used to measure concentration of sulfamethazine in bovine milk with standard digestion as low as 2.2%. It is also used for kinetic analysis of low molecular weight compounds by immobilizing receptors to the sensor surface. Kinetic measurements with an optical fiber sensor for the IgG anti-tetanus antibody gave approximately a 10-fold difference in the dissociation rate constant when compared with affinity constants determined by conventional solid phase enzyme immunoassays.

Biosensors are applied successfully in various fields. They replaced the existing inconvenient bioassays; they are used for monitoring of pollutants in water, monitoring of fermentation products and cell cultures and estimation of the concentration of various ions. Near infrared is used as an in-process quality control tool for pharmaceuticals to measure particle size, moisture content, identity and quantitation of blends of poly-alcohols, celluloses and thickening agents. The polymer films and monolayers of metals can be analyzed by applying polarization modulation FTIR to the reflection spectra from the films.

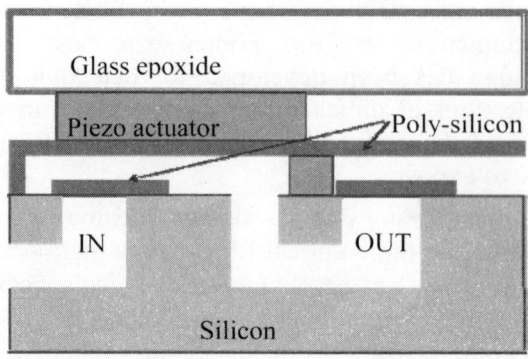

Fig. 3.31: Assembly of acoustic biosensor

3.4.2.14. Genosensor

Wide-scale DNA testing requires the development of small, fast and easy-to-use devices. Genosensors (Fig. 3.32) based on nucleic acid recognition processes are being developed for rapid, simple and inexpensive testing of genetic and infectious diseases and for the detection of DNA damage and interactions. Various methods for the attachment of oligonucleotide probe DNAs to the surface of the electrode, such as adsorption, direct covalent binding, entrapment in a polymer matrix or indirect binding by the use of intermediate systems of polypyrrole films, have been developed. In this kind of biosensor, a DNA probe is immobilized on a transducer and its hybridization with target DNA can be monitored by optical, electrochemical, piezoelectric, impedimetric and surface plasmon resonance techniques. However, the immobilization of the nucleic acid probe onto the transducer surface plays an important role in the overall performance of DNA biosensors (genosensor) and gene chips. The immobilization step should lead to a well-defined probe orientation, readily accessible to the target. The environment of the immobilized probes at the solid surface depends upon the mode of immobilization and can differ from that experienced in the bulk solution. Depending upon the nature of the physical transducer, various schemes can be used for attaching the DNA probe to the surface. These include the use of thiolated DNA for self assembly onto gold transducers (gold electrodes or gold-coated piezoelectric crystals), covalent linkage to the gold surface via functional alkanethiol-based monolayers, the use of biotylated DNA for complex formation with a surface-confined avidin or strepavidin, covalent (carbodiimide) coupling to functional groups on carbon electrodes, or a simple adsorption onto carbon surfaces. As in solution-based hybridization assays, conditions for interfacial hybridization events (e.g. ionic strength, temperature, presence of accelerators) have to be optimized. Chemical and thermally induced dehybridization of the resulting duplex is often used for regenerating the interface. Recent advances in nucleic acid recognition can enhance the power of genosensor. For example, the introduction of peptide nucleic acid (PNA) has opened up exciting opportunities for genosensor. PNA is a DNA mimic in which the sugar–phosphate backbone is replaced with a pseudopeptide one. DNA dendrimers can be used for imparting higher sensitivity to the genosensor. These tree-like superstructures possess numerous single-stranded arms that can hybridize to their complementary DNA sequence. A greatly increased hybridization capacity and hence a substantially amplified response is achieved by immobilizing these dendritic nucleic acids onto the physical transducer.

Commercial tests available for the qualitative detection of genes are based on detection of the amplified gene product through the use of genosensor. Commercially available kits for detection of HCV RNA are based on qualitative (PCR: Amplicor HCV v2.0 Roche Molecular Systems or

Transcription-mediated amplification: Versant HCV RNA Bayer Diagnostics) and quantitative (PCR: LCx HCV RNA Abbott Diagnostics, SuperQuant National Genetics Institute, Amplicor HCV Monitor v2.0 Roche Molecular Systems) and Cobas Amplicor HCV Monitor Roche Molecular Systems, or Branched DNA: Versant HCV RNA 3.0 Bayer Diagnostics).

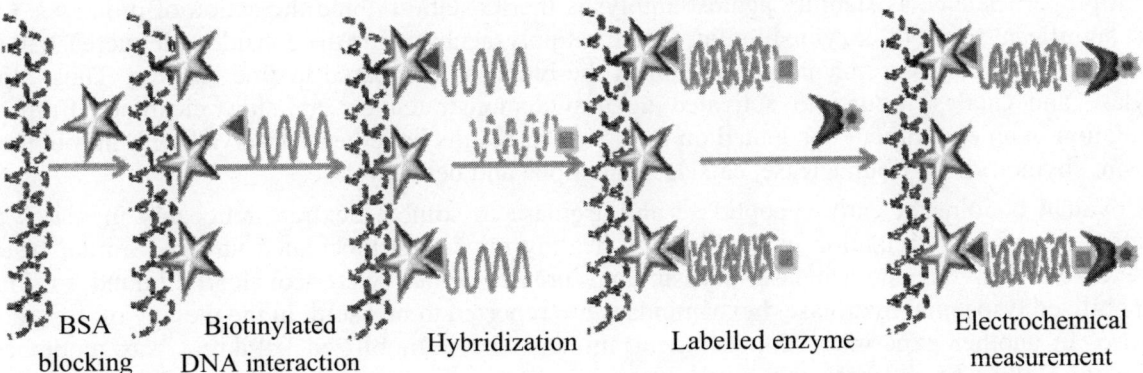

BSA blocking   Biotinylated DNA interaction   Hybridization   Labelled enzyme   Electrochemical measurement

Fig. 3.32: Schematic presentation of DNA biosensor for HCV detection

3.4.2.15. Glucose sensor

The determination of glucose is important for the process control pertaining to the metabolism of many nutrients. An oxygen electrode can determine assimilation of glucose by microorganisms because respiration activity increases after assimilation of organic compounds. Therefore, it is possible to construct a microbial electrode sensor for glucose using immobilized whole cells which utilize mainly glucose and an oxygen electrode. A microbial electrode consisting of immobilized whole cells of *Pseudomonas fluorescens* was developed for the determination of glucose. Furthermore, the microbial sensor was applied for continuous determination of glucose in molasses.

A typical membrane electrode consists of bacterial membranes and an oxygen electrode. The bacterial membrane remains in direct contact with the oxygen electrode and is tightly secured with the help of rubber rings. The microbial sensor is inserted into a sample solution which is saturated with dissolved oxygen and stirred magnetically. The temperature of the system is maintained at 30.0 ± 0.5 °C. The current is measured with the help of a milliammeter; the signal is magnified and recorded.

3.4.3. Therapeutic applications

The clinical uses of enzymes are still limited by certain of factors, such as:

a) Availability of the enzymes at the site of interest is generally very poor unless a high therapeutic dose is administered; which is often undesirable;

b) The sensitivity of enzymes to the action of various natural inhibitors;

c) The immunogenicity of many enzymes;

d) The destruction of the enzymes under the action of endogenous proteases;

e) *in-vivo* inactivation and fast clearance considerably increase the consumption of the enzyme in the course of treatment, and

f) The high cost and low availability of pure enzymes.

In order to address the above problems, the immobilization of enzymes can be used to a great extent as this makes it possible to decrease the total dose of enzyme used, prolong enzymatic activity at the site of interest, and reduce undesirable side effects. Preparation of immobilized enzymes, for example streptokinase and urokinase in microgranules of sephadex can be effectively used for treatment of thromboses and thromboemboli of any vessels (for example atherosclerosis of coronary arteries, which is often the cause of myocardial infarction) that is accessible with the help of modern methods of catherization.

An *ex-vivo* experimental result demonstrated that enzymes bound to polysaccharides acquire many useful properties such as stability against autolysis, thermostability, and the action of proteases. One most significant result of enzyme binding to natural polysaccharide is the considerable increase in the duration of immobilized enzyme circulation in the blood as compared to free enzyme. Thus, alpha amylase and catalase bound to activated dextran demonstrated a very slow clearance from the circulation in an experiment conducted on rats. Similar results have been observed with immobilized trypsin, chymotrypsin, ribonuclease, catalase, and alpha and beta amylase.

Covalent bonding of carboxypeptidase and arginase to soluble dextran noticeably increases the duration of enzyme circulation in the blood in healthy mice with inoculated tumors. Similar results were noted with enzyme catalase, trypsin and urease, which were covalently bound to PEG. Immobilized lysosomal hydrolase, hexoamindase are reported to be useful in the therapy of Tay-sache disease. In another experiment conducted in animals, the immobilized kallikrein was reported to retain the ability to decrease the blood pressure. A most impressive study involved the use of glucocerebrosidase accumulated in the cells of the RES as a result of a deficiency of the corresponding lysosomal enzymes.

3.4.3.1. Immobilization based novel drug delivery systems

A) Urea-urease modulated system

Urea-urease modulated system suggests the interesting possibility of using immobilized enzymes to alter local pH and consequently to change the pH-sensitive polymer erosion rates. Urease converts urea to NH_4HCO_3 and NH_4OH, causing an increase in pH. To utilize this reaction a polymer whose erosion rate increases with pH is selected. A partially esterified copolymer of methylvinyl ether and maleic anhydride undergoes surface erosion at an erosion rate that is extraordinarily sensitive to small increase in external pH. The polymer dissolves by ionization of the carboxylic acid group as shown below and results in release of incorporated therapeutic agent.

B) Glucose oxidase-glucose modulated system

The search for a delivery system to replace parenteral administration of insulin by periodic injections has led to the development of an erodible polymeric system containing insulin, which is modulated by glucose-glucose oxidase reaction (Fig. 3.33). In this system a polymer is selected which shows increased erosion rates with decreasing pH. The pH is lowered by production of gluconic acid from glucose. The conversion is catalyzed by the enzyme glucose oxidase. Poly (ortho esters) prepared by the reaction between polyols and the diketene acetal. 3,9-bis (ethyldiene 2,4,8,10-tetraoxaspiro undecane) are ideal polymers for this system because of the pH sensitive linkage in the polymer backbone. Cross-linked poly (ortho esters) are produced by first preparing a ketene acetal-terminated prepolymer that is a viscous liquid at room temperature, followed by its cross linking with a triol. A therapeutic agent can be mixed into the prepolymer at room temperature and the mixture can be cross linked at temperatures as low as 40°C; mild conditions are important for proteinaceous therapeutic agents like insulin.

Acid sensitivity of these polymers can be studied by incorporating a marker molecule such as 1'-nitroacetanilide in the polymer and observing its release at different pH values. Magnitudes of change and response times in the process are not adequate. A self-regulated insulin delivery system should respond in less than 15 minutes. In order to increase the pH sensitivity of the system, polymers prepared by using n-alkyl diethanolamines and triethanolamines were prepared. The acid sensitivities of polymers prepared from N-N-butyldiethanolamines and from N-methyldiethylanolamines can be observed. Changing the size of alkyl group on the amino portion of the diol has a significant effect on both degree of acid sensitivity and the pH range where maximum sensitivity occurs. The pH sensitivity of the polymer can be explained by swelling of the polymers induced by protonation of the tertiary amines in the polymer backbone. The observed effect of N-alkyl group size is consistent with decreased hydrophilicity as the size of N-alkyl group increases, and to a lesser extent by changes in the pKa values. Polymers of varying degrees of cross-linking and consequently varying degrees of swelling have been prepared by varying the ratio of triol cross-linker and the bifunctional ketene acetal terminated pre-polymer.

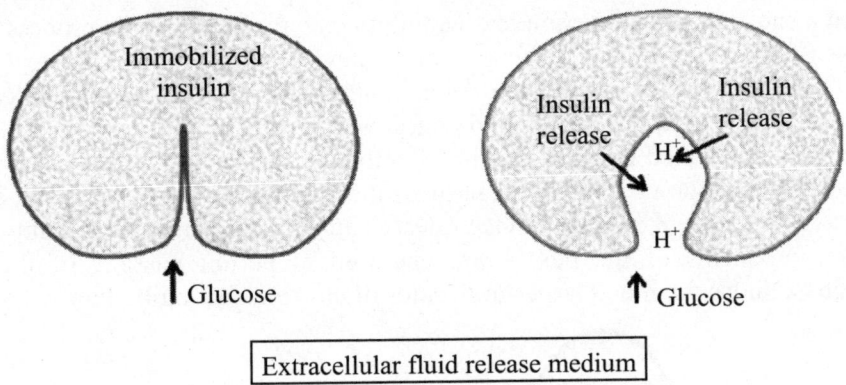

Fig. 3.33: Schematic representation of one dimensional model for the release of insulin from polymeric systems

C) Triggered drug delivery system

Triggered drug delivery systems are based on a device containing the active agent placed in other appropriate body site where it remains passive until a specific molecule appears in tissues surrounding the device. This molecule triggers the programmed release of therapeutic agent from the device. The device utilizes highly selective sensing mechanisms to recognize the specific trigger molecule in a complex mixture of physiologic fluids. Antibodies to the trigger molecule provide high selectivity (Fig. 3.34). Such triggered devices may have many potential applications.

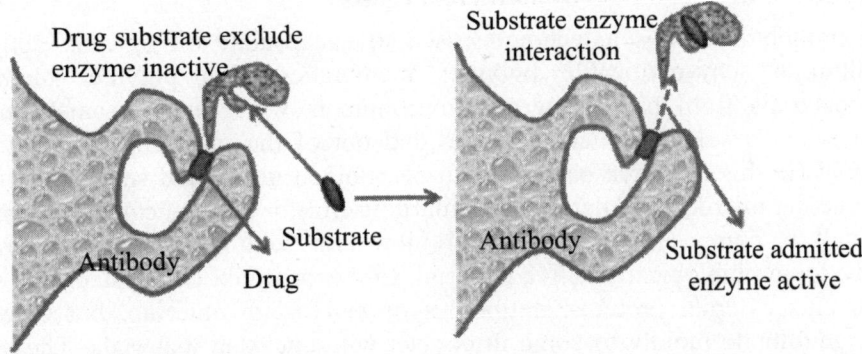

Fig. 3.34: Reversible enzyme inactivation by hapten-antibody interaction

A device containing the narcotic antagonist naltrexone can be implanted in opiate addicts undergoing rehabilitation after the withdrawal therapy. The device is so designed that the release is triggered by morphine. Such device remains passive as long as the individual refrains from heroin; and naltrexone is released upon heroin intake when morphine is produced metabolically and triggers the release of naltrexone in amounts sufficient to replace morphine from its receptors and thus neutralizes the heroin induced pleasurable effect.

In designing such a device, a hapten (morphine in this case) is covalently attached to the enzyme close to its active sites and the hapten is complexed with its antibody. Being a very large molecule, the antibody sterically hinders access of enzyme substrate to the enzyme active site, thereby rendering the enzyme inactive. In the presence of free hapten the complex dissociates to form separate antibody hapten complex and a substrate enzyme complex leading to enzyme action. This process is illustrated in figure 3.35 shows the design of a bioerodible polymeric device. This device contains a pH sensitive polymer capable of releasing naltrexone by an erosion controlled process at the physiological pH 7.4 but is stable at a lower pH; so that no erosion and consequently drug release takes place. This device also contains reversibly inactivated enzyme that in its activated state can degrade the hydrogel. This enzyme is activated when morphine appears in tissues surrounding the device and the enzyme then removes the protective hydrogel. Activated device releases an antigenic enzyme and antibody, so it is necessary that the components of the device are enclosed to permit passage of the opiate and naltrexone but which excludes the much larger molecules of enzyme and antibody.

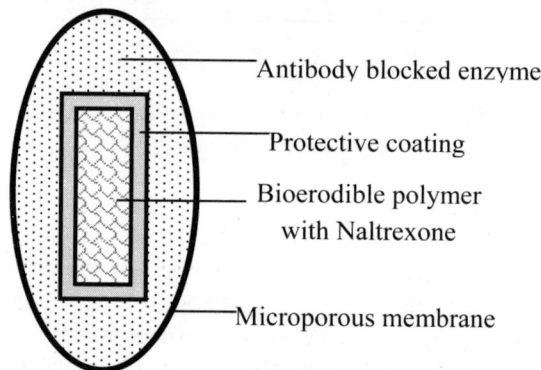

Fig. 3.35: Schematic representation of triggered drug delivery device

D) Immobilization of artificial cells as artificial organs

Artificial cell immobilization is a technique used to encapsulate biologically active materials in specialized ultrathin semi-permeable polymer membranes. The polymer membrane protects encapsulated materials from harsh external environments while at the same time allowing the metabolism of selected solutes which pass into and out of the microcapsule. In this manner, the enclosed material (in this case live bacteria) can be retained inside and separated from the external environment, making microencapsulation particularly useful for biomedical and clinical applications. An artificial cell is composed of a spherical ultra thin semi-permeable membrane of cellular dimensions enveloping biologically active material. In this artificial cell system, the semi-permeable membrane prevents external proteins, antibodies or cells from entering, but external permanent molecules can equilibrate rapidly to come in contact with enclosed materials. The artificial cellular units could be developed using various permselective membranes preferably based on biodegradable polymers. Some polymers of synthetic and biological origins have been identified for such use.

Artificial cell microcapsules can be used for live cells (plant, animal, human, and microbial) or other bioactives useful for therapeutic functions. Artificial cells are being used as detoxifiers, artificial kidney, artificial liver, immunosorbents, and blood substitutes and in other areas.

Almost any biologically active material such as enzymes or proteins can be enclosed within artificial cells. Magnetic materials have also been incorporated within artificial cells to allow external magnetic fields to direct the movements of the artificial cells. Other materials which can be incorporated include radioisotope labeled enzymes, proteins, antigens, vaccines and hormones. The artificial cells can be used to immobilize enzymes and proteins. The enzymes so immobilized remain in enzyme systems in red blood cells especially as complex multienzyme systems. The advantage is that there is no limit to the number of different enzyme systems that can be enclosed and immobilized together in a single artificial cell.

Enzyme adsorbents or other material can be incorporated together with target enzyme into artificial cells. Using artificial cells combining activated charcoal or ion exchange resin, toxic materials can be removed. Using the principle of artificial cells extremely compact, efficient and simple artificial organs can be designed and constructed as for example blood detoxifier, artificial liver, artificial kidney and immunosorbents. Artificial cells containing multienzyme systems are used for the sequential conversion of substrates into products and also to recycle the required cofactors.

Immobilized enzymes are generally recommended in replacement therapy needed in hereditary enzyme deficiency conditions in the form of microencapsulated enzyme as cell immobilized catalase is used to effectively replace a hereditary catalase deficiency. Artificial cells containing tyrosinase have been used in extracorporeal haemoperfusion to lower tyrosine levels in rats. The therapeutic applications of artificial cells for tumor suppression are well appreciated being distinctive and of therapeutic value. Artificial cells containing tyrosinase immobilized in a carrier system have been used for haemoperfusion in galactosamine-induced fulminate hepatic failure (FHF) in rats.

3.4.3.2. Immobilized enzymes and multienzymes in artificial cells

In the body, enzymes and proteins are mostly located in the intracellular spaces. These proteins act sequentially on substrates, oozing out through the cell wall by passive transportation or by special transport mechanism. In their absence one cannot inject solution of enzyme(s) into the body. Since, exogenously administered enzyme(s) are considered as foreign proteins in free form, they induce hypersensitivity reactions. Production of antibodies is followed by rapid removal and inactivation. Free enzymes in solution cannot be kept at the sites where the action is desired. Enzymes in free solution are not stable, especially at body temperature of 37°C. Furthermore, multienzyme systems require the enzymes and substrates to be in close proximity and also for cofactor recycling preferably in an intracellular environment. In order to device maximum benefits of treatment, possible use of artificial cells as a system to immobilize enzymes and proteins deserves consideration. Unlike those immobilized by a conventional method, enzymes immobilized in artificial cells may remain in free solution as suspended cellular units. Therefore, the systems function more like enzyme systems similar to the one which operates in RBC, especially similar to a complex multienzyme system. There is no limit to the class of different enzyme systems that can be enclosed in one artificial cell. Artificial cells containing simple enzyme systems may be obtained by selecting one of the many methods available. All single enzymes tested so far can be successfully encapsulated within artificial cells.

A 10 gdl^{-1} haemoglobin solution is usually present in standard artificial cells. This simulates an intracellular environment, comparable to that in red blood cells. Thus, the enzymes enclosed in the artificial cells are stabilized by the high concentration of protein(s). Similarly, multienzyme systems can also be generated. Most metabolic functions are carried out in cells by complex multienzyme systems in coordination with cofactor; for example, artificial cells containing hexokinase and pyruvate kinase recycle ATP for the continuous conversion of glucose into G-6-P and phosphoenol pyruvate into pyruvate; and artificial cells containing alcohol dehydrogenase and maleic dehydrogenase recycle NADH making use of NAD^+ multienzyme system consisting of urease, glutamate dehydrogenase, and glucose-6-phosphate dehydrogenase all within each artificial cell can convert urea into ammonia which then serves as substrate to alpha-keto glutarate which in the presence of NADPH forms an amino acid, glutamate with glucose-6-phosphate dehydrogenase to recycle the cofactor.

The above system suggests that it is feasible to prepare artificial cells containing multienzyme systems for the sequential conversion of substrate into products and at the same time to recycle the required cofactors. This principle is also applicable in the conversion of waste metabolites in liver failure and renal failure or other metabolic disorders. The concept opens up possibilities of management of disease related to organ failure via application of immobilized cellular unit(s).

3.4.3.3. Artificial pancreas

Endocrine cells from heterogeneous sources could be enclosed within artificial cells and implanted. In this form the cells inside the artificial cells can respond to external substance concentrations (e.g. blood glucose) and the required hormone (e.g. insulin) can be secreted into the systemic circulation. The microencapsulated rat-islet cells when implanted intraperitoneally into diabetic rats avoid rejection and maintain normal glucose levels in the diabetic animals.

3.4.3.4. Blood detoxifier

Artificial cells containing activated charcoal have formed the basis for the construction of a novel detoxifier. A simple and inexpensive system uses 0.005m thick collodion membrane coating on activated charcoal granules. An albumin coating can be applied to the collodion membrane to make the surface more blood compatible. In coating activated charcoal with polymer membranes, the thickness and permeability are extremely important factors. One of the most effective blood detoxifiers consists of 80g of spherical petroleum-based charcoal (1 mm diameter) coated by an ultra-thin collodion membrane. The principle of microencapsulation of ion exchange resin inside artificial cells can also be used, so that it prevents the ion exchange resin from adversely affecting blood cellular components. Circulating the blood from patients through these detoxifying devices in artificial cells purifies it. This has prompted use of detoxification based on artificial cellular detoxifier units in patients needing treatment for acute drug intoxication.

3.4.3.5. Artificial liver

The first partial success with an artificial liver support system was attained when a patient with grade IV hepatic coma was treated by haemoperfusion with an artificial cell detoxification device. Artificial cells containing multienzyme systems with cofactor recycling characteristics are being studied *in-vivo* for the sequential conversion of ammonia into different amino acids.

3.4.3.6. Artificial kidney

The blood detoxifier consisting of artificial cells containing activated charcoal can reduce terminal renal failure as it eliminates uremic symptoms related to nausea, vomiting, fatigue, bleeding and others. But these artificial cells containing activated charcoal fail to remove coated electrolytes and urea. In patients who develop uremic symptoms despite standard haemodialysis treatment, the artificial cells approach can eliminate the complications of pericarditis, nausea, vomiting, peripheral neuropathy and others.

However, the best device may be an artificial cell blood detoxifier combined in series with a small ultrafiltrator. In this, the artificial cell removes uremic water metabolites and toxins while the ultrafiltrator would effectively remove sodium chloride and water (Fig. 3.36). The problems of removal of potassium, phosphate and urea will however remain. Potassium could be removed by the oral administration of potassium adsorbent, and the urea is removed by the use of artificial cells containing urease.

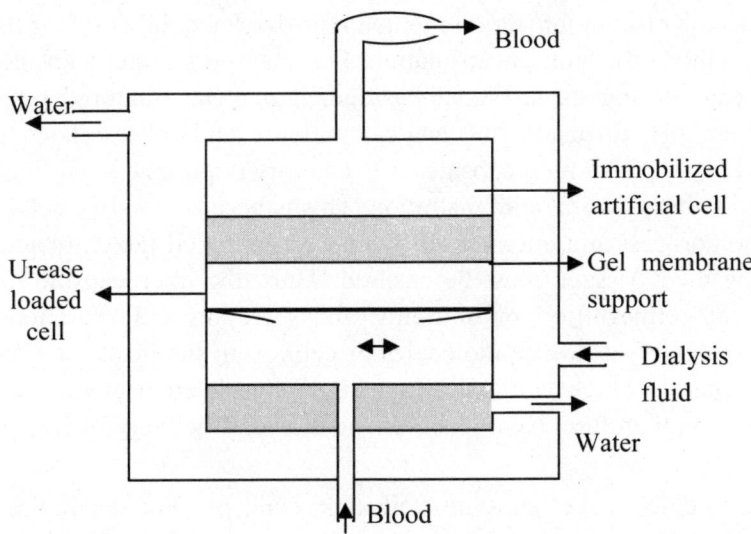

Fig. 3.36: Schematic representation of artificial kidney

3.3.3.7. Artificial cells used as blood substitutes (surrogates)

Artificial cells with haemoglobin and those with organic material are two systems being investigated as possible red blood cell substitutes. In the preparation of haemoglobin artificial cells, microdroplets of haemolysate solution with spherical ultrathin membrane of cellular dimensions can be developed or cross-linking may be used for the same objective. There was no agglutination when these two types of haemoglobin artificial cells were placed in contact with plasma even when the artificial cells were prepared by using haemoglobin obtained from the blood of heterogeneous sources with varied blood groups.

The cross-linked haemoglobin artificial cells, each consisting of soluble poly-haemoglobin, survive significantly longer in the circulation when compared to free haemoglobin. A fine emulsion of fluorocarbon was used for the development of artificial cells based on organic material. These fine fluorocarbon emulsions were evaluated to be effective oxygen carriers. Fluorocarbon artificial cells represent the first artificial cells ready for clinical trial as a blood cell substitute. One of the advantages of haemoglobin artificial cell is the biodegradability of the haemoglobin content. Artificial cells have been prepared to perform many functions but only comparatively simple artificial cells have been developed to a stage of actual application. Some classical examples of such systems are liposomes, nylon capsule, lipid nanocapsules, cross-linked microspheres and aquasomes.

3.4.3.8. Artificial cells: Immobilized bacterial cells

Live bacterial cells have been increasingly used for therapeutic purposes. The fact that these cells can be genetically engineered to synthesize products with therapeutic potential has aroused much interest and excitement among clinicians and health professionals. Hopefully, a wide range of disease-modifying substrates such as enzymes, hormones, antibodies, vaccines, and other genetic products will be used successfully and will impact health care substantially. However, a major limitation in the use of these bacterial cells is the difficulty of delivering them to the correct target tissues. Considerable research interest has been dedicated to the immobilization of bacterial cells for therapeutic applications such as in kidney failure, uremia, cancer therapy, diarrhea, cholesteremia, and other diseases. Success of immobilization methods for live bacterial cells for therapy depends on the suitability of the methods for their encapsulation. For example, a microcapsule can be disrupted by many different means during its intestinal passage; it may be fractured by enzymatic action, chemical reactions, heat, pH, diffusion, mechanical pressure and other related physiological and biochemical stresses. The safety of microcapsules is even more important when live cells are intended for use in the intestinal system by oral administration. This is because the live cells must be protected during the encapsulation process and microcapsules must reach the GI intact. In addition, the survival of the live cells during their passage must be ensured. Thus, the microcapsule membrane must be provided with sufficient permeability for nutrients, and secretion and excretion products to pass through, yet prevent, the entry of hostile molecules or cells from the host, for example, products of the host's immune response, which could destroy the encapsulated bacterial cells. The problems inherent with oral delivery, therefore, have made the goal of oral delivery of live bacterial cells very challenging.

Several promising studies have substantiated this concept. For example, oral feeding of *Lactobacillus* bacteria has been used for prevention and treatment of diarrhea in children. Similarly, feeding on *Lactobacillus casei* strain Shirota enhances innate immunity. Bacteria such as *Bifidobacteria* have been successfully used to treat intestinal disorders and to prevent rotaviral diarrhea in children. In premature infants feeding on lyophilized strains of *B. breve* or *B. longum* can restore the imbalance in the gut microflora. These latter strains can also suppress azomethane-induced colon carcinogenesis in rats. Cultures of *B. longum* reduced carcinogenesis by a food mutagen, 2-amino-3-methylimidazoquinoline. Certain strains of *Lactobacilli* also significantly suppress intestinal tumors induced by chemical mutagens. Some human feeding studies with *Lactobacilli* suggest a possible effect in lowering cholesterol. Oral feeding of freeze-dried live *Lactobacillus acidophilus* (LB) cells in subjects with advanced chronic kidney failure has lowered elevated levels of uremic toxins. In another study, the level of a carcinogen, nitrosodimethylamine (NDMA) and the level of the toxin dimethylamine (DMA) were lowered significantly by oral feeding of LB cells, and there were no side effects of the therapy. *Lactococcus lactis* bacteria have been genetically engineered to produce cytokine interleukin-10 (IL-10) so that it can be orally delivered for the therapy of inflammatory bowel disease (IBD).

Several delivery systems for oral delivery of live bacterial cells have been proposed. For example, microcapsule immobilization of *Bifidobacteria* to protect them against adverse effects of acid during oral administration has been proposed. Encapsulated freeze-dried *B. pseudolongum* using cellulose acetate phthalate (CAP) coated with beeswax has shown that survival of the encapsulated *B. pseudolongum* in the simulated gastric environment was greater than of non-encapsulated cells.

Calcium alginate and k-carrageenan gel beads are the two most commonly used polymers for immobilizing viable cells. However, alginate beads are not acid resistant, and it has been reported that the beads undergo shrinkage and have decreased mechanical strength. In order to overcome this, coating bacteria by cross-linking with a carboxyvinyl polymer carrier has been suggested. The carboxyvinyl polymer has, however, proved effective only for intestinal delivery and release. k-carrageenan gel beads are less sensitive to acid than alginate and hence are used for làctic fermentation. However, two major limitations preclude their use. Firstly, in the formation of k-carrageenan, Locust bean gum beads require high potassium ions. The latter could potentially damage the cells of *B. longum* during lactic fermentation. Second, as potassium ions are important in maintaining electrolyte equilibrium, their inclusion in the diet in large amounts is not advisable. Gelatin and xanthan gum beads are not only acid resistant but are also stabilized by calcium ions, suggesting that they could be a good candidate for immobilizing microbial cells and protecting them against acid injury. But, they do not protect against immunorejection which is a primary requirement for probiotic oral delivery of live cells for therapy. Similarly agarose capsules prepared by emulsification/internal gelatinization for oral delivery of Bacillus Calmette-Guerin (BCG) cells, although stable for up to 12 months *in vitro*, are not suitable for oral delivery as agarose membranes do not provide immunoprotection. A host of other formulations using poly(lactide-co-glycolides), carrageenan, alginate-poly-L-lysine, starch polyanhydrides, polymethacrylates, polyamino acids, enteric coating polymers, etc. have been developed for the immobilization of microbial cells.

3.4.4. G*ene probes*

Gene probes are used to find genes of particular interest by applying the molecular hybridization technique which allows two strands of DNA to be dissociated and reassociated *in vitro*. The gene of interest can be identified by constructing a DNA with identical sequence which will anneal only to that particular gene but not to the rest of the DNA. Similarly, using the enzyme RNA-dependent-DNA-polymerase, cDNA has been synthesized from mRNA isolated from mammalian cells. Furthermore, if radioactive bases are added to the reaction, the synthesized cDNA could be used as a probe to look for complementary sequences. The technique is quite versatile and useful for gene identification. At first, when the technology was introduced it was based on solution. Utilizing the latest technology in which DNAs are immobilized over nitrocellulose fibers, which can support for DNA for a longer period of time. Human responses to foreign chemicals vary depending on their genetic make-up, predisposition and environmental exposures. Such individual variations reflect differing degrees of expression. The kind and amount of expression of these enzymes determines whether a chemical is detoxified or activated to toxic metabolites. Using this, one can determine the gene or other biologically active system responsible for the metabolism or inactivation of the drug. One such example is the identification of specific cytochromes p-450 responsible for xenobiotic and endobiotic metabolism.

MAbs and cDNA have been used as bioprobes to identify the specific cytochrome p-450 responsible for xenobiotic and endobiotic metabolism. MAbs are specific to each phenotype and epitope of p-450 can quantify levels of expression of individual p-450. MAbs inhibitory to enzyme activity can determine the contribution of the MAbs specific p-450 to the total reaction of an individual substrate in a tissue preparation such as microsomes. Inhibitory MAbs can also be added to the tissue preparation at saturating levels and inhibition can be observed. In addition to examining intertissue differences, interspecies comparisons can be made with activity inhibition experiments for different animal species. While MAbs can be used as probes for the detection of p-450 proteins, p-

450 cDNAs isolated from cDNA libraries and immobilized on a proper support can also be used as probes for the detection of mRNA transcripts of p-450 genes in different human organs and tissues and DNA fragments present in cells can be amplified by specific polymerase chain reactions (PCR).

3.4.5. Microarrays

In the late 1990s the genomic century hit its peak with several large sequencing projects and the development of global gene expression profiling techniques. While classical genetics focused on the examination of single genes, novel technologies such as the DNA microarray enabled the analysis of several thousand genes simultaneously. Differential expression profiling, in which the mRNA profiles of diseased cells is compared with those from healthy donors, has led to the identification of numerous disease specific genes and biomarkers.

3.4.5.1. DNA microarray

DNA microarray has become a well-established technique not only in fundamental and applied medical science, such as cancer research, but also in other biological disciplines such as microbiology and plant research. These arrays can for example be used to compare expressed genes in a genome of a healthy tissue with those in the genome of a diseased tissue in a miniaturized way. Thus, important insights into the character of the disease can be gained and help significantly in the development of therapeutic strategies and potential drugs. Two different methodologies have been established. In cDNA microarray PCR-generated cDNA-probes are robotically spotted onto solid supports such as glass slides or nylon membranes. The samples to compare are labeled with two different fluorescent dyes, co-hybridized to the same array and the relative abundance of sample vs. control is measured. In 1996, Affymetrix Inc. launched the so-called oligonucleotide or Gene Chip R array, in which several short oligonucleotide probes representing one gene are synthesized *in-situ* by photolithography. The samples under comparison are labeled with the same dye and hybridized to different arrays. Thereby the absolute mRNA-content is measured, which requires careful data processing and normalization.

3.4.5.2. Protein microarray

Following the continuous growth and demand of new technologies in the field of proteomics, the next logical step on the way to global proteome analysis was the establishment of protein microarrays in analogy to DNA microarrays. The major advantages of protein microarray technologies include a highly parallel and miniaturized solid-phase assay, high-throughput approaches, and low consumption of reagents and samples. In 1999, Ciphergen Biosystems (Fremont, CA) launched the SELDI Protein Chip R System. The protein chip R is available with different chromatographical properties (hydrophobic, hydrophilic, anion exchange, cation exchange and metal affinity) to purify crude samples directly on the chip. A special TOF-mass spectrometer, the surface enhanced laser desorption ionization (SELDI) mass spectrometer, is used as read-out. With Ciphergen being one of the first protein chip companies, there are 140 companies meanwhile involved in protein arrays and related technologies. To avoid certain inherent problems with the immobilization of thousands to millions of different proteins, antibodies are utilized as structurally uniform catcher molecules for the protein analytes. Antibodies are important components of the immune system as they bind to and disarm a great variety of potentially harmful pathogens. In antibody microarrays these highly specific molecules are spotted to the chip in an array-format with each spot representing one antigen-specificity, i.e., one protein-analyte. In analogy to DNA microarrays the resulting pictures of present and absent proteins in the individual proteome (of e.g. healthy and diseased tissue) can easily be compared and used as a foundation for further in depth studies.

Protein microarrays are prepared by immobilizing hundreds or thousands of different proteins to a common substrate that allow highly parallel experiments with small amounts of proteins and reagents. A series of proteins has been immobilized on aldehyde-terminated glass slides and showed that these proteins were able to interact with other molecules in solution. More recently, a library of oligohistidine fusion proteins from *Saccharomyces cerevisiae* has been immobilized onto Nitrilotriacetic acid (NTA) surfaces and used the array to identify several calmodulin and phospholipid-binding motifs. These examples demonstrate the potential of protein arrays, but have also highlighted the need for methods that present proteins in a well-defined environment and simultaneously prevent unwanted nonspecific protein interactions.

The important key-component for the production of high-density DNA, protein and antibody microarrays is the carrier or solid support. Immobilized on a surface, interacting biomolecules differ in their reaction kinetics and affinities, mainly due to lower reaction volumes and changes in the molecular configuration of the reactants. As immobilized biomolecules (DNA/enzyme/protein/ antibodies) are exposed to enormous local forces, they are often distorted on the surface and the concentration of functional reactant is reduced. Thus, a careful evaluation of solid supports suitable for the immobilization of biomolecules and biocompatible with the probe of choice is a prerequisite for successful microarray analysis. Several methods for immobilization of biomolecules have already been developed.

Six new surfaces for the attachment of nucleic acids, proteins, and small molecules have been developed and these surfaces were divided into two groups: 1) "dendrimer-like" linkers so-called for their high functional group capacity and 2) triamino based linker systems. To evaluate the performance of these slides in a microarray application, benzamidine and biotin were printed amongst a library of small molecules and screened with their respective receptor fluorophore conjugates, streptavidin and trypsin and specific ligand-receptor recognition has been observed. New immobilization strategies are required as the diversity of small molecule libraries increases and where only a limited number of functional groups are compatible with previously described microarray surfaces. It was reported that a new small-molecule immobilization strategy involve using a Staudinger ligation that couples azide derivative molecules with a phosphane-modified glass surface through the formation of a stable amide bond. This method clearly demonstrated selective immobilization and the ability of the molecules to retain their functionality. It has opened up yet another functional group to small molecule array assembly. In typical microarray applications, the surface must be so derivatized as to accommodate the relevant functional group of the desired probe. For example, a hydroxy functionalized probe and a chlorinated microarray surface would allow covalent attachment, but an acid functionalized ligand with the same surface would fail to form a covalent bond. In order for most microarray surface/probe systems to operate, every member of the printed library must possess the operable functional group. Exciting advances in probe immobilization have been accomplished by immobilization of probes by using photoactive substances through the use of photoaffinity reactions. Using such a photoaffinity reaction, the small molecules are immobilized "non-selectively" and provide many facet of the molecule toward the target protein. Practical immobilization has been achieved by using a suite of natural products and their known protein complements. These include: digoxigenin, digoxin and digitoxin, binders of the mouse monoclonal antibody DI-22 (Sigma), FK506 and rapamycin, binders of protein FKBP12, and the cyclic peptide cyclosporin A recognized by the monoclonal antibody. All compounds showed specific recognition with their respective proteins and demonstrated for the first time the immobilization of complex natural products in a uniform manner. The technique offers great promise in the immobilization of diverse libraries without the need for specific functional groups. It was described *the work done at Graffinity Pharmaceutical AG on the use of small molecules immobilized on reactive self-assembled monolayers on gold-coated glass.*

3.4.5.3. Immunoassays

Immunoassays are currently the predominant analytical technique for the quantitative determination of a broad variety of analytes of clinical, medical, biotechnological, and environmental fields. A very large proportion of modern immunoassays involve the use of solid materials to immobilize one of the reactants. For many applications, the adsorption of the first reagent to the solid materials is the essential step and depends on chemical functionality, charge, energy and morphology of the solid surface. A basic requirement of a successful assay is a strong bonding of this reagent to the surface in its active state. Additionally, sensitivity, specificity, good reproducibility and low cost are necessary important parameters to be considered for the future application of the solid materials. A wide variety of matrices, including inorganic surfaces, organic polymers and other commercially available solid supports have been used for the design of immunoassays. Of the various solid-phase immunoassay formats, the enzyme-linked immunosorbent assays (ELISA) typically carried out in microliter plates have been widely used in immunoassay with respect to specificity and sensitivity. The most commonly utilized solid support is polystyrene because of its optical clarity and range of surface properties. As a long chain hydrocarbon, non-modified polystyrene tends to repel water and hydrophilic molecules and attract hydrophobic molecules. Large bimolecular considered hydrophilic will inevitably have stretches of hydrophobic regions that allow the molecule to adsorb to the polystyrene surface. But to enable stable binding of hydrophilic molecules, assay conditions such as high molecule concentration, long incubation time and critical temperature conditions might be required to prevent the molecule from washing off the polystyrene surface. Therefore, the use of alternative methods of immobilization is attractive. Despite the growing interest in this area, relatively few studies have been published covering the optimization of support materials for ELISA assay. In recent years, metal nanoparticles, especially gold nanoparticles; have been extensively studied in analytical chemistry as they have size dependent unique chemical, electrical and optical properties. Gold nanoparticles have been intensively studied for immobilization of bio-reagents via the large specific interface area, desirable biocompatibility and high surface free energy of nano sized particles. They have been widely used in immunoassay.

3.4.5.4. Carrier systems

Various novel delivery systems, generally providing a large surface area for the immobilization of enzyme and cell biomolecules, have been actively developed for biomolecules stabilization. This strategy is particularly applicable in the case of poorly absorbed enzymes/cells which are unstable in the GI lumen and their targeting to a specific tissue or organ is to be affected. The proper designing of the biomolecules through immobilization not only protects the biomolecules from harsh environments prior to absorption but also localizes the cells/ enzymes at or near the cellular membrane to maximize the driving force for passive permeation. Some delivery systems that have been explored include lipid vesicles, resealed erythrocytes, emulsions, nanoparticles, and other particulate carriers systems.

A) Nanoparticles

Nanoparticles with different compositions and characteristics have been explored for immobilization of biomolecules for various therapeutic applications. Several different types of biodegradable polymers including bio-polymers (e.g. gelatin, albumin, casein, polysaccharide, lectin, etc.) and synthetic polymers (polycaprolactone, polyesters, polyanhydrides, polycynoacrylates) with drug release characteristics ranging from several hours to several months have been used to immobilize the cells and enzymes. It is the sub-micron size of this delivery system which makes it so efficient in certain drug therapy applications such as in intracellular localization of therapeutic agents. These systems in addition to sustained drug delivery have been investigated for various other therapeutic applications. Enzymes are increasingly seen as therapeutic drugs. Being susceptible to proteolytic degradation they can create problems of physicochemical and bio-stability coupled with their short biological half-life and inability to pass through most biological barriers (Fig. 3.37). For enzyme delivery, nanoparticles offer an attractive possibility. Most studies however deal with the stability of the nanoparticle associated enzymes against challenges from the luminal proteases in the GIT. Polyalkylcyanoacrylate nanoparticles and nanocapsules have been developed with L-asparaginase, trypsin and other enzymes. Most studies with nanoparticles have been concerned with the improvement of enzyme activity and loading, rather than enzyme stabilization. The final immobilization exhibited high stability for a month, and can be easily separated from the reaction medium. Further, nanoparticles can cross the gut lumen by paracellular pathway and enter the blood circulation thus, demonstrating a systemic drug effect. This strategy is under investigation for an oral administration of other proteins and peptides, and receptor mediated transport through gut wall by using glycoprotein and glycopeptide conjugated nanoparticles. Nanoparticle-bound peptides can in fact be used for sustained oral delivery and to improve bioavailability.

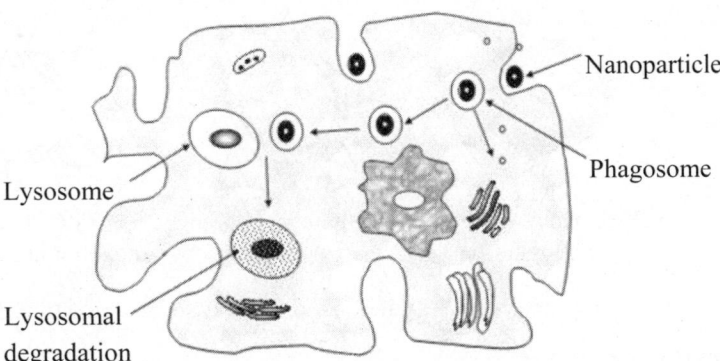

Fig. 3.37: Schematic representation of cellular uptake and fate of nanoparticle immobilized biomolecules

Superoxide dismutase (SOD) protects against cytotoxic effects of superoxide anions. SOD encapsulated into nanoparticles demonstrated improved pharmacokinetics including longer plasma half-life and slower release of SOD with no side effects. Nanoparticles-entrapped SOD reduces ischemia reperfusion oxidative stress in gerbil brain upon intraperitoneal bolus injection by increasing enzyme activity and decreasing membrane peroxidation in various regions of the brain. Nanoparticles are also used for transmembrane intracellular delivery of superoxide dismutase and catalase, so important for elimination of oxygen-derived free radicals inside cells; their increased generation causes ischemia of endothelial and many other cells. A variety of protein antigens have been incorporated into nanoparticles (such as diphtheria toxoid, hepatitis B antigens, influenza virus antigens, tumor-associated antigens, and many others) have been used as a delivery vehicle for the transfection of plasmid DNA and to improve its stability in the bio-environment. A novel system has been developed for gene delivery based on the use of DNA-gelatin nanoparticles (nanospheres) formed by salt-induced complex coacervation of gelatin and plasmid DNA. Nanosphere-DNA incubated in bovine serum was more resistant to nuclease digestion compared to naked DNA. Various bioactive agents could be encapsulated in the nanospheres through ionic interaction with the matrix components, physical entrapment or covalent conjugation. Oral administration of DNA nanoparticles synthesized by complexing plasmid DNA with chitosan, a natural biocompatible polysaccharide, resulted in transduced gene expression in the intestinal epithelium. Mice receiving nanoparticles containing a dominant peanut allergen gene (pCMVArah2) produced secretory IgA and serum IgG2a. Compared with non-immunized mice or mice treated with 'naked' DNA, mice immunized with nanoparticles showed a substantial reduction in allergen-induced anaphylaxis associated with reduced levels of IgE, plasma histamine and vascular leakage.

After synthesis of silica nanoparticles (SiNP) with covalently linked cationic surface modifications and demonstration of its ability to electro statically bind, condense and protect plasmid DNA it was postulated that these particles can be utilized as DNA carriers for gene delivery (Fig. 3.38). The ability of colloidal silica particles with covalently attached cationic surface modifications to transfect plasmid DNA *in vitro* has been investigated and the complex is termed nanoplex. DNA-based gold nanoparticle assembly approach has also been used for the detection of specific DNA sequences and to analyze combinatorial DNA arrays (or "gene chips"). DNA-functionalized gold nanoparticles assemble onto a sensor surface only in the presence of a complementary ligand. By using a patterned sensor surface of multiple DNA strands, it is possible to detect different DNA sequences simultaneously. Figure 3.38 illustrates different mechanisms for DNA delivery using nanoparticles.

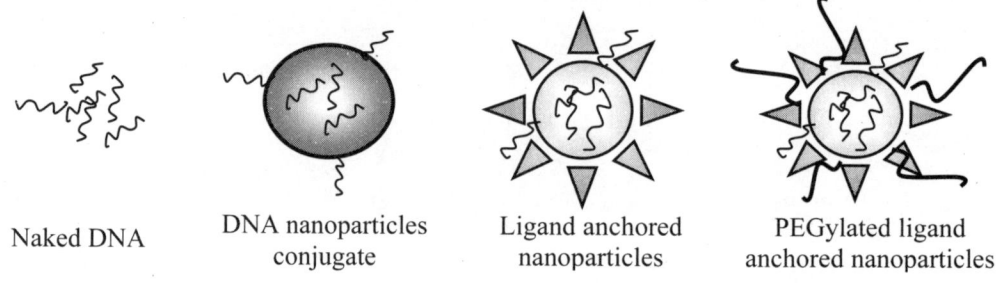

| Naked DNA | DNA nanoparticles conjugate | Ligand anchored nanoparticles | PEGylated ligand anchored nanoparticles |

Fig. 3.38: DNA nanoparticle conjugates used for transfection of plasmid DNA

B) Resealed erythrocytes

Erythrocytes have been utilized as carriers for a wide range of bioactive components including drugs, enzymes, pesticides, DNA molecules and others. Their ability for prevention of premature degradation or inactivation, slow release of loaded drug(s), targeting potential to reticulo-endothelial system (RES) and serving as circulatory bio-vectors for enzymes make them highly versatile delivery systems in modern pharmaceutical research and development. Erythrocytes could be used as circulating carriers to disseminate bioactive agents over a prolonged period of time in circulation or selectively to liver, spleen and lymph nodes. They are difficult to engineer for a non-RES target but innovations based on biophysically modulated devices may render them suitable for targeting to organs other than RES. Resealed erythrocytes may soon find many possible applications in various fields of human and veterinary medicine.

Resealed erythrocytes serve as an ideal carrier for enzymes in the treatment of inherited metabolic diseases. Enzymes can be injected into the blood stream to replace the missing or deficient enzyme in a metabolic disorder. Lysosomal storage disorders (such as Gaucher's disease), hyperargininaemia, hyperuricaemia, hyperphenylalaninaemia, and kidney failure are some examples of metabolic disorders that can be treated by enzyme(s) based therapy. The entrapment of catalase, urease, uricase, invertase, arginase, asparaginase, β-glucuronidase, β-fructouronidase, and β-galactosidase in erythrocytes using hypotonic lysis method has proved that erythrocytes could operate as enzyme carriers. Alcohol dehydrogenase and acetaldehyde dehydrogenase encapsulated into human erythrocytes can be used *in vivo* for complete metabolization of ethanol. Glutamate dehydrogenase (GDH) encapsulated in erythrocytes can be used as a potential carrier systems for the *in vivo* removal of high levels of ammonia from blood. Lightly damaged or modified erythrocytes are sequestered by spleen similar to normal senescent erythrocytes, whereas liver sequesters/recognizes heavily modified erythrocytes. Circulatory half-life is shortened by coating resealed erythrocytes with antibodies. Lightly coated (modified) resealed erythrocytes cause a reduction of the half-life from 27 days to several minutes and the majority of the erythrocytes are sequestered by the spleen macrophages. On the other hand, heavily modified cells cause a similar reduction in circulating half-life while in this case; the majority of the erythrocytes are sequestered by the liver macrophages, and as a result accommodated in these organs. Enzymatically modified cell surface carbohydrates of erythrocytes exhibit a different biodistribution as compared against their plain version. Sialidase, an enzyme that removes sialic acid from external glycoproteins and glycolipids, causes a significant reduction in the circulatory half-life of the erythrocytes, and make them prone to macrophage uptake especially in liver and spleen. The external sulfhydryls of erythrocytes can be oxidized to differing degree and the circulatory half-life of the cells thus can be manipulated from a normal value of 27 days to several minutes (8 min).

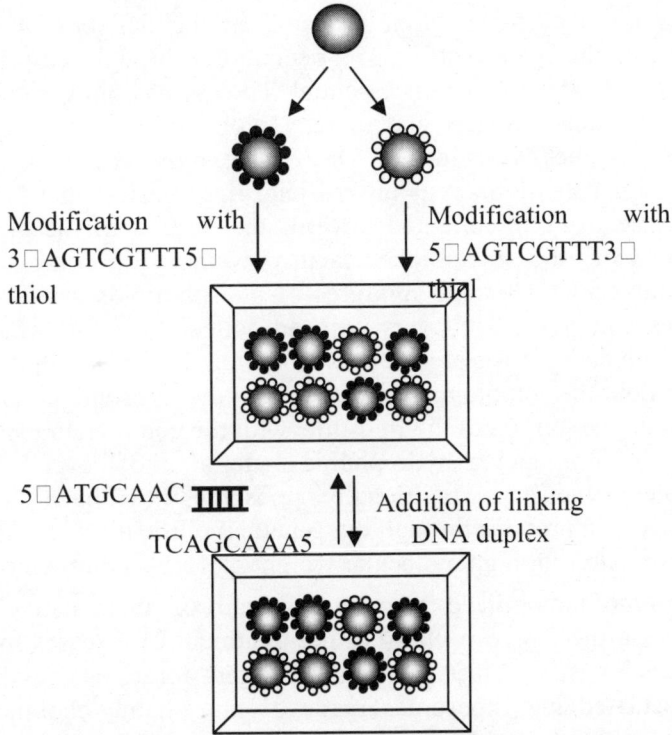

Fig. 3.39: DNA based nanoparticle assembly strategy

Delivery of encapsulated substances to macrophages can easily be obtained by cross-linking of loaded erythrocytes. The delivery of ^{125}I-labelled carbonic anhydrase (Iodine[125]I-CA) carried by mouse erythrocytes, either loaded, or loaded and cross-linked with bis (sulphosuccinimidyl) suberate (BS3) and 3,3'-dithiobis-(sulphosuccinimidyl propionate), into homologous peritoneal macrophages has been done. Hypotonically loaded mouse erythrocytes showed a weak recognition by macrophages, similar to native erythrocytes. CA loaded in erythrocytes is thus delivered to a limited extent into macrophages. In contrast, cross-linking of these loaded erythrocytes stimulates phagocytosis by macrophages as assessed by microscopic observations, producing a markedly increased amount of targeted enzyme. Thus these cross-linking treatments improve the capacity of loaded mouse erythrocytes to deliver significant amounts of targeted enzyme to macrophage cells, and so increase the therapeutic potential of carrier erythrocytes. The disease caused due to accumulation of glucocerebroside in liver and spleen can be combated by the use of glucocerebrosidase encapsulated in erythrocytes. The resealed erythrocytes have been used for replacement of enzyme in lysosomes. α-glucuronidase, α-galactosidase and α-glucosidase were encapsulated in erythrocytes for lysosomal disorders.

Erythrocytes have been demonstrated as circulating carriers for enzymes to serve as circulating bioreactors. Sometimes it is desirable to decrease the level of circulating metabolites that can enter erythrocytes. The immobilization of enzymes which catalyze these reactions can be used in a bioreactor. It is the perm-selectivity of the erythrocyte membrane, which allows it to act as a portal for enzyme allowing selective action on excessive pool of substrate and thus lowering down their blood levels. Arginase-loaded erythrocytes have been proved to be efficacious in reducing plasma arginine levels by 40% within 2 hrs of infusion into a patient with hyperargininaemia.

C) Lipidic carriers

These delivery systems have shown great potential in the delivery of enzymes/cells. Before a biomolecule can exert its therapeutic effects, its penetration through the plasma membrane (a lipoid bilayer) or uptake through carrier system is essential. The use of lipid vesicular carriers has paved the way to circumvent membrane barriers and thereby promote the uptake of this 'difficult' class of therapeutics such as enzymes, proteins, or DNA. The most common type of lipid vesicles is liposomes. A liposome can be defined as an artificial lipid vesicle that has a bilayer phospholipid arrangement with the head groups oriented towards the interior of the bilayer and the acyl group towards the exterior of the membrane facing water. Liposomes are usually made of phosphatidylcholine molecules although mixtures of phospholipids can also be employed to make liposomes. Liposomes comprise of bilayers with an aqueous core in which enzymes or cells are encapsulated. Fusion and endocytosis are the most common methods of liposome interaction with cell membrane. During fusion, the soluble material carried in the liposome is released into the cytoplasm of the target cell through the joining of the liposome with the cell membrane lipids (Fig. 3.40). Such a mechanism is useful for introducing hydrophobic material into the cell, and it has been already adapted by the petroleum industry. Traditionally, liposomes have been used in the bioengineering field to over-produce certain proteins through the genetic modification of cells. They have thus solved the inconvenience of transferring high molecular weight molecules through cell membranes.

The use of liposome-immobilized enzymes instead of their native precursors opens new opportunities for enzyme therapy, especially in the treatment of diseases localized in some specific area like tumor, liver, lungs, etc. that are natural targets for liposomes. Lysozyme was the first enzyme to be encapsulated into liposomes made of phosphatidylcholine, dicetyl phosphate and cholesterol, in 1970. Since then, liposomal forms of various enzymes have been prepared and investigated: glucose oxidase, glucose-6-phosphate dehydrogenase, hexokinase and β-galactosidase, glucuronidase, glucocerebrosidase, α-mannosidase, amyloglucosidase; hexoseaminidase A, peroxidase, α-d-fructofuranosidase, neuraminidase, superoxide dismutase and catalase, asparaginase, cytochrome oxidase, ATPase, dextranase as well as many other enzymes from different sources.

The following parameters are usually considered as a proof of enzyme incorporation into the inner aqueous phase of liposomes or its firm and irreversible association with the liposomal membrane: the possibility of chromatographic separation of liposome-encapsulated and free enzyme; the latency of liposome-encapsulated enzymes; the correlation between protein incorporation and a change in net surface charge of the lipid bilayer. From the clinical point of view, the potential ability of liposome-encapsulated enzymes to enter the cytoplasm or lysosomes of live cells is of primary importance for the treatment of inherited diseases caused by the abnormal functioning of some intracellular enzymes. Despite relative rarity of these diseases, together they pose a serious medical problem.

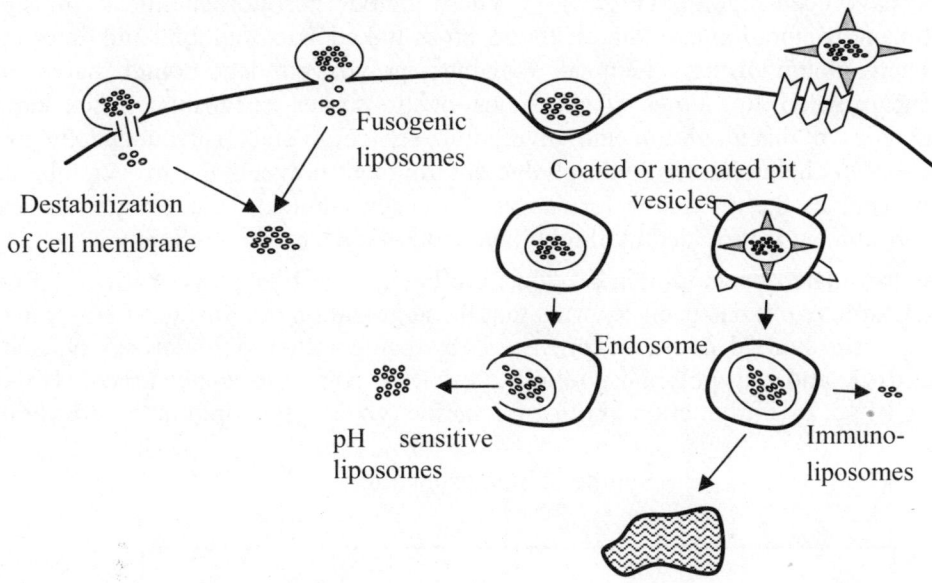

Fig. 3.40: Endocytosis of liposomal immobilized biomolecules

Animal experiments have also clearly demonstrated the suitability of liposomes for immobilization of enzymes used for the therapy of tumor diseases. L-asparaginase used for the treatment of asparagine dependent tumors is a good example. Thus, an increase in the circulation half-life of the liposomal L-asparaginase (in lecithin-dicetylphosphate liposomes, a negative charge of the liposomes was used to inhibit the liposome interaction with cells and to keep them in the blood longer), and decrease in its antigenicity and susceptibility towards proteolytic degradation together with the increase in the efficacy of experimental tumor therapy in mice have been shown.

The use of unilamellar vesicles made of cationic lipids have improved the transfection efficiencies and prevented interactions with DNA molecules. Therefore, the possibility of introducing genes to cure diseases (genetic therapy) is not far from becoming a reality if the patient being treated were found not to suffer from severe side effects. Vaccine formulations based on liposomes have been successfully tested in animal immunization, and such studies are currently undergoing clinical testing. The benefits and limitiations of liposomes as drug carriers in a system as complex as the human body depend basically on their interactions with the cells, their immuno-compatibility, and their ability to escape detection by the human immune system.

Scientists have been using liposomes for nucleic acid and gene delivery. Recent advances in terms of genosomes (complex formulations of DNA with various cationic liposomes, lipoplex) have revolutionized DNA and gene delivery strategies. These colloidal soluble (suspended) DNA-liposome/lipid complexes (genosomes) significantly improve transfection (delivery of plasmid into cell nuclei) and gene expression (the synthesis of protein encoded in the DNA plasmid by the cell machinery). Cationic lipids used for DNA complex formation are N-(2,3-dioleyloxy)propyl)-N,N,N-trimethylammonium chloride (DOTMA) and N-(2,3-dioleyloxy)propyl)-N,N,N-trimethylammonium propane (DOTAP).

Various semi-synthetic and synthetic blood-substitutes which immobilize oxygen, i.e., red blood cell substitutes, have been reported (Fig. 3.41). These include perfluorochemical emulsion (Flusol, USA), recombinant haemoglobin, glutaraldehyde cross-linked haemoglobin and inter-molecularly cross-linked haemoglobin using chemical reagents, polyoxyethylene-bound haemoglobin and haemoglobin-encapsulated liposomes (Hb-vesicles or liposomes encapsulated liposomes, LEH). Protohaeme moieties of haemoglobin and myoglobin are completely surrounded by hydrophobic residues of the globin chain and this hydrophobic environment prevents the irreversible oxidation to ferric states and enables the reversible formation of oxygen adducts. In haemoglobin vesicles, this hydrophobic environment is provided by lipid bilayer and that's why they mimic the red cells.

Liposome encapsulated haemoglobin products are being investigated as artificial RBCs (oxygen carrying RBC substitutes). It has been reported that the aggregation and fusion of Hb-vesicles and the leakage on long-term storage could be prevented by using either polymerized phospholipids or polyphospholipids (stabilized polyphospholipid vesicles containing concentrated Hb are called "artificial red cells") or by introduction of oligosaccharide type of glycolipid in the bilayer membrane.

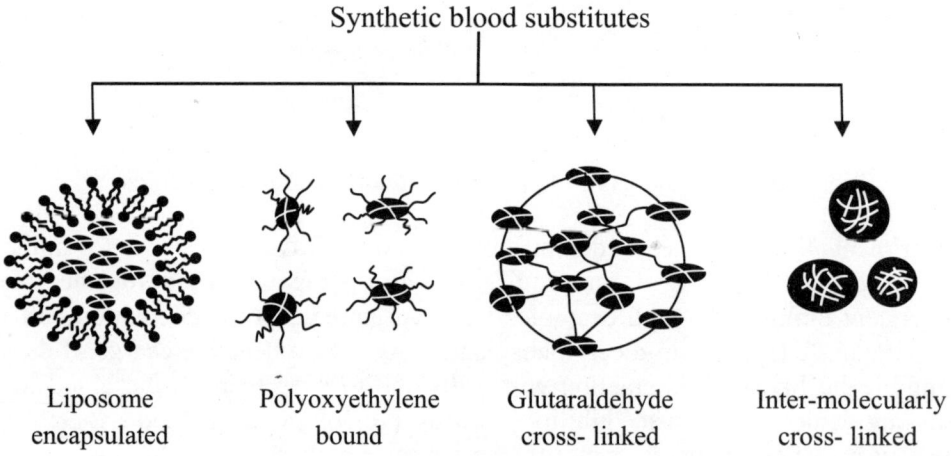

Fig. 3.41: Various synthetic blood substitutes

Sterically stabilized liposome bearing Hb (PEG-PE LEH) are even better than LEH as artificial blood substitutes as they manifest less toxicity, less platelet activating and aggregating effects and generate less haemostatic. Previously, it was reported that completely synthetic amphiphilic haeme derivatives (lipid haeme) and incorporated them into the hydrophobic centre of the bilayer membrane of the phospholipid vesicles. These vesicles have excellent oxygen transporting abilities.

Liposomes with biotin-modified lipids can be easily prepared and used to immobilize a variety of avidin/ streptividin linked targeting enzymes/ proteins. Non-specific protein based binding ligands (for example, avidin, streptividin, protein A or protein G) can be attached to liposomes using covalent conjugation methods (Fig. 3.42). In a further development, anti- transferrin antibody has been anchored to the liposomal systems (immunoliposomes) for the delivery of anti-neoplastic drug daunomycin to rat brain. Optimal brain targeting was mediated through the OX-26 monoclonal antibody to the rat transferrin receptor. The latter is selectively expressed in excess at the brain microvascular endothelium that mainly comprises the blood-brain barrier in vivo. Several attempts have been made to simplify the coupling of therapeutics to anti-transferrin receptor antibody (OX-26) by using avidin/streptividin-biotin systems.

3.4.5.6. PEG conjugates with biological macromolecules

There are three main area of application of PEG-polypeptide conjugates: (1) therapeutics, (2) enzymatic catalysis in organic solvents and (3) two-aqueous phase partitioning systems for purification and analysis of various biologically derived mixtures. Covalent coupling reactions between amino groups (or other nucleophiles) of proteins and mPEG equipped with an electrophilic functional group (also termed "activated PEGs') have been used in most cases of PEG-protein conjugates.

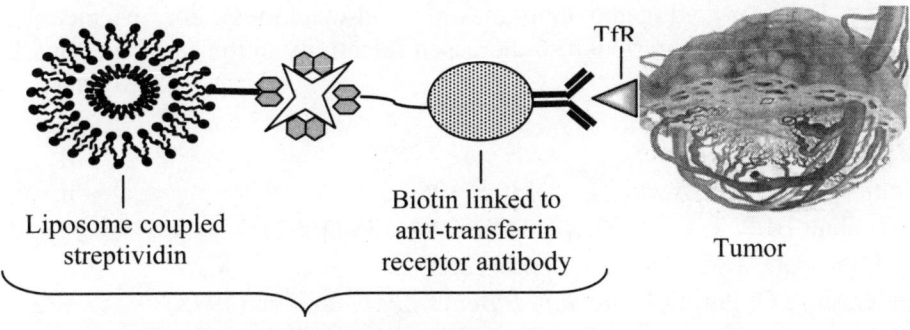

Liposome coupled streptividin

Biotin linked to anti-transferrin receptor antibody

Tumor

Sandwich Targeting Carrier

Fig. 3.42: Biotin-avidin/streptavidin conjugated carriers, where avidin/streptavidin links the delivery systems and biotinylated targeting ligand. This sandwich-targeting carrier then target receptor (or antigen) mediated through a targeting ligand (antibody)

The single largest classes of proteins, which have been subjected to covalent modifications with PEG, are enzymes. Some enzymes, e.g., peroxidase, L-asparaginase, alkaline phosphatase, gluconolactone oxidase and superoxide dismutase (SOD), in conjugation with PEG show remarkable preservation of activity with very little dependence on the method used (Table 3.18).

Table 3.18: Macromolecular derivatives of peptide/protein drug molecules

Drug	Results
Arginase	Prolonged the plasma half-life to 12 h (native enzyme-1 h)
Asparaginase	In humans the plasma half-life increased to 357 h (native -20 h); Better protease stability and a 7–10 fold prolongation in plasma clearing properties
Adenosine deaminase	Conjugate has a half-life of 48–72 h in children
Uricase	Enzymatic activity half-life increased 10 times to 7 h
Superoxide dismutase	Plasma half-life increased significantly
Streptokinase	Prolongs plasma circulation and reduces antigenicity of the enzyme
Trypsin	Resistant to anti-trypsin antibody precipitation.

However, preservation of enzyme activity of PEG-enzyme conjugates depends not only on the chemistry of PEG activation and subsequent conjugation to enzymes but also on the extent of modification. Similar results have been reported in case of PEG-tissue plasminogen activator conjugates; fibrinolytic activity was found to be independent of the type of activating reagent employed but decreased with increase in the extent of modification. PEG-conjugated acyl-plasmin-streptokinase, elastase, trypsin and chymotrypsin show a similar decrease in fibrinolytic, hydrolytic and proteolytic activities.

Site-specific PEG grafting (PEGylation) of proteins is a recent innovation to avoid random protein modification that leads to steric hindrance into essential binding sites of proteins. For example, in the case of glycoproteins (ovalbumin, glucose oxidase) it is possible to utilize the reactivity of oligosaccharide residues for the attachment of mPEG chains without affecting the polypeptide portion of the molecule. Several biological macromolecules like interleukins, interferons, oligonucleotides, polysaccharides and their analogs are conjugated with PEG and their *in vitro* and *in vivo* behaviors are well documented. Polymer-conjugated cytokines (hybrid-cytokines), for instance PEG-modified interleukin-2 and PEG-modified interleukin-6 increased selectivity in their function but did not curtail unfavorable functions.

SUGGESTED READING

- Axen R, Porath J, Ernback S. *Nature* 214, 1302 (1967).
- Bartlett PN, Tebbutt BLP, Tyrrell CH. *Anal Chem* 64, 138 (1992).
- Bengali Z and Shea LD. *MRS Bulletin* 30, 659 (2005).
- Brandt J, Andersson LO, Porath J. *Biochim Biophys Acta* 386, 196 (1975).
- Campbell DH, Luescher FL, Lerman LS. *Proc Natl Acad Sci USA* 37, 575 (1951).
- Cao L, van Rantwijk F, Sheldon RA. *Org Lett* 2, 1361 (2000).
- Chang TMS and Prakash S. *Molecular Biotechnology* 17(3), 249 (2001).
- Clark LC Jr, Lyons C. *Ann NY Acad Sci* 102, 29 (1962).
- D'Souza SE, Altekar W, D'Souza SF. *J Biochem Biophys Methods* 24, 239 (1992).
- D'Souza SF, Nadkarni GB. *Enzyme Microb Technol* 2, 217 (1978).
- Drobnik J, Saudek V, Svec F, Kalal J, Vojtisek V, Barta M. *Biotechnol Bioeng* 21, 1317 (1979).
- Dunlap BR. *Immobilised Chemicals and Affinity Chromatography*, Plenum Press, New York (1974).
- Gemeiner P. In: *Enzyme Engineering: Immobilized Biosystems*; Gemeiner P.(Ed) Ellis Horwood 167 (1992).
- Grubhofer N, Schleith L. *Hoppe-Seylers Z Physiol Chem* 297, 108 (1954).
- Hultschig C, Kreutzberger J, Seitz H, Konthur Z, Bussow K, Lehrach H. *Current Opinion in Chemical Biology* 10, 4 (2006).
- Johansson AC, Mosbach K. *Biochim Biophys Acta* 370, 339 (1974).
- Jungbae K, Hongfei J, Ping W. *Biotechnology Advances* 24, 296 (2006).
- Katchalski-Katzir E, Kraemer DM. *J Mol Catal B Enzym* 10, 157 (2000).
- Kay G, Crook EM. *Nature* 216, 514 (1967).
- Kierstan M, Bucke C. *Biotechnology and Bioengineering* 19 (3), 387 (1977).
- Kierstan MPJ, Coughlan MP: In *Protein Immobilization Fundamentals and Applications*; Taylor R F, Ed. Marcel Dekker Inc 32 (1991).
- Kipper H, Egorov Kh-R, Kivisilla K. *Tr Tallin Politekh Inst* 465, 33 (1979).

- Kircka LJ, Thorpe GHG. *Trends Biotechnol* 4, 253 (1986).
- Klein MD, Langer R. *Trends Biotechnol* 4, 179 (1986).
- Martinek K, Mozhaev VV. *Adv Enzymol* 57, 179 (1985).
- Mclaren AD. *Science* 125, 697 (1957).
- Modler HW, Vila-Gracia L. *Cult Dairy Prod* 28, 4 (1993).
- Niiolova P, Ward OP. *J Ind Microbiol* 12, 76 (1993).
- Osada Y, Lino Y, Numajiri Y. *Chem Lett* 4, 559 (1982).
- Ouyang W, Chen H, Jones ML, Metz T, Haque T, Martoni C, Prakash S. *J Pharm Pharmaceut Sci* 7(3), 315 (2004).
- Quiocho FA, Richards FM. *Biochemistry* 5, 4062 (1966).
- Rosell CM, Fernandez-Lafuente R, Guisan JM. *Biocatal Biotransform* 12, 67 (1995).
- Scardi V, Cantarella M, Gianfreda L, Palescandolo R, Alfani F, Greco G Jr. *Biochimie* 62, 635 (1980).
- Schulze B, Wubbolts MG. *Curr Opin Biotechnol* 10, 609 (1999).
- Silman IH, Katchalski E. *Ann Rev Biochem* 35, 837 (1966).
- Straathof AJJ, Panke S, Schmid A. *Curr Opin Biotechnol* 13, 548 (2002).
- Sun AM, O'Shea GM, Goosen M F. *Appl Biochem Biotechnol* 10, 87 (1984).
- Turkova J. *J Chromatogr B: Biomed Sci Appl* 722, 11 (1999).
- Vassilev N, Vassileva M, Fenice M, Federici F. *Bioresource Technology* 79, 263 (2001).
- Weetall HH. *Nature* 223, 959 (1969).
- Weliky N, Brown FS, Dale EC. *Arch Biochem Biophys* 131, 1 (1969).
- Wykes JR, Dunnill P, Lilly MD. *Biochim Biophys Acta* 250, 522 (1971).

FERMENTATION

4.8.3. Vitamins

4.8.3.1. Riboflavin

4.8.3.2. Ascorbic acid (vitamin C)

4.9. ALCOHOL FERMENTATION

4.1. INTRODUCTION

Microorganisms are capable of growing on a wide range of substrates and can produce a remarkable spectrum of products. The relatively recent advent of in vitro genetic manipulation has extended the range of products that may be produced by microorganisms and has provided new methods for increasing the yields of existing ones. The commercial exploitation of the biochemical diversity of microorganisms has resulted in the development of the fermentation industry and the techniques of genetic manipulation have given this well-established industry the opportunity to develop new processes and to improve existing ones.

The term fermentation is derived from the Latin verb fervere, to boil, which describes the appearance of the action of yeast on extracts of fruit or malted grain during the production of alcoholic beverages. Fermentation may be defined as the process of growing a culture of microorganisms in a nutrient media and thereby converting feed into a desired end product. It is sometimes described as a biochemical reaction in which microorganisms (bacteria or fungi) serve as biocatalyst. The fermentation segment forms a major part of biotechnology industry. It has been so for a long time, starting with the herbs, doctor, brewer, bakers, and cheese and wine makers of ancient civilization who used empirical fermentation methods to achieve the desired products.

The pharmaceutical industry uses fermentation for the manufacture of hormones, biologicals and biodrugs. Furthermore, microorganisms are used to convert waste products and raw material into energy or industrial chemicals. Certain microbes have special affinity for certain metals and are used to mine low-grade ores of uranium, copper, etc. and also to remove or recover metals from industrial effluents and to enhance oil recovery

Microbes are now designed to produce bioactive proteins such as human type insulin, enzymes, vitamins, amino acids or specific antibiotics on a large industrial scale. A list of major industrial products prepared from fermentation is given in Table 4.1.

Table 4.1: A list of major industrial products

Fermentation product	Name of product
Foods, beverages	Dairy product (cheese, yogurt), vitamins (B_1, B_{12}), amino acid (glutamic acid, Lysine), glucose, baker's yeast, beverages (beer, wine, whiskey)
Chemicals	Ethanol, butanol, acetone, citric acid, gluconic acid, lactic acid, enzyme, polymers (xanthan, dextran)
Pharmaceuticals	Antibiotics, vaccine, steroids, diagnostic enzymes, monoclonal antibody, enzyme inhibitors
Agriculture	Single cell protein, microbial pesticide, composing processes plant cells and tissue culture

4.2. THE FERMENTATION PROCESS AND OPTIMIZATION

Process of fermentation is based upon utilization of metabolic and catalytic activities of various micro-organisms for desirable chemical transformations. Biosynthetic techniques have revolutionized the industrial process of fermentation. The study of kinetics of cell growth has put forth possibilities of high yield production of fermentation end product(s). Similarly with the technique of genetic engineering scientists are able to improve the strains of micro-organisms responsible for protein expression to produce desired biological products. Fermentation generally encompasses processes and products. The basic principles of fermentation thus remain nearly central to all.

4.2.1. Kinetics of cell growth in fermentation optimization process

In order to design a maximal capacity fermenter, it is desired that there should be a proper understanding of the kinetics of microbial, animal or plant cell growth kinetics. Cell production kinetics revolves around the cell growth rate and it is affected by various physicochemical conditions. It is appropriate to state that cell kinetics is the consequential interaction of numerous complicated biochemical reactions and transport phenomena, involving multiple stages of multicomponent systems. The complete mathematical modeling of growth kinetics is not possible as a heterogeneous mixture of young and old cells continuously transforms and adapts to a changing environment during growth phase. Hence, in order to derive simpler models of fermenter operation and performance that can accommodate mathematical modeling, assumptions must be made regarding the involvement of various cellular components and cell population dynamics (Table 4.2).

Table 4.2: Kinetics, growth and production

Population	Cell components unstructured	Cell components structured
Distributed	Cell represented by single component, which is uniformly distributed throughout the culture	Multiple cell components uniformly distributed throughout the culture, interact with each other.
Segregated	Cells are represented by single component, but form a heterogeneous mixture.	Cells of multiple components form a heterogeneous mixture.

Among the models suggested, the simplest possible model is the unstructured distributed model. The model is classically based upon two basic assumptions.

A. All the cells can be represented by single component such as cell mass, cell number etc.

B. Cellular mass is distributed throughout the culture. In addition to the cells, the medium should be formulated such that 'one component may limit the reaction rate'. All other components should be present at sufficiently high concentrations so that minor changes do not affect the growth significantly.

Growth rates based on the number of cells and on cell weight or mass are not necessarily the same, as the average cell size may vary considerably from one stage to another. For example, when the mass of an individual cell increases without division, the growth rate based on cell weight increases while the growth rate based upon number of cells remains constant. However, during exponential growth phase, cell number based growth rate and growth rate based on cell weight are proportional. Furthermore, sometimes growth rate may be confused with division rate (rate of cell division per unit time). Take the case of a vessel in which all the cells at time t = 0 ($Cn = Cn_o$) have divided once, after a certain period of time, the cell population will have increased to Cn_0 x 2. All the cells have divided X times after time t, so the total number of cells will be:

$$Cn = Cn_0 \times 2\,M$$

Concentration versus time curve presents a relationship between growth and time where the growth rate is expressed as the slope of the curve (Fig. 4.1). If fresh sterile medium is inoculated and the cell density is measured deriving subsequent growth as against time, the results could be distinguished as representing six stages in batch growth cycle.

- **Latent period**: The phase in which the cell number does not vary.
- **Accelerated growth**: The cell number starts increasing and cell division rate accelerates.
- **Exponential growth**: It is the phase of exponential increase in cell number
- **Decelerated growth**: The phase where growth rate is higher and during this period growth and division rates start decreasing.
- **Stationary period**: Any further proliferation of cells is stopped and cell number reaches a maximum point.
- **Death period**: The period where limiting growth substances have depleted and cells begin to die.

The major applications of kinetic growth data and models are to predict the time period of fermentation stage in order to estimate the necessary fermenter size before considering other more complex factors. Furthermore, the same models could be utilized in designing batch fermentation processes as well as to predict the fermenter size necessary for continuous culture fermentations.

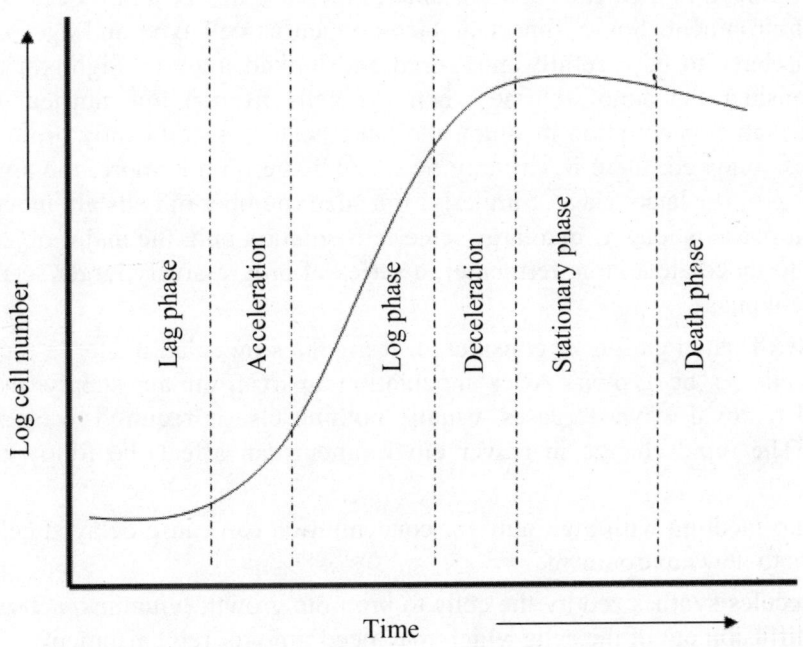

Fig. 4.1: Batch fermentation stages

The foremost objective of fermentation is to support the growth of specific culture and to promote high end point yield. In certain conditions excess of essential nutrients concentration could extensively inhibit growth (or even kill off the culture); hence essential nutrients should not always be supplied in excess. For main application of the optimization process established on the requirements of nutrients by certain microorganism and the kinetics of growth are studied by limiting the concentration of one ingredient while keeping the others in excess. Hence, growth increases exponentially until the essential (limiting) substance is depleted. The prediction of kinetics for single cell growth is quite simple

$$\mu = \frac{dX}{d\theta}$$

Where θ is time factor, μ is specific growth rate and X is the concentration of cells

However, for complex cell growth a Monod equation is utilized. It projects an empirical and simplified model for complex cell-growth.

$$\mu = \mu_m \frac{[C_1]}{[C_1 + K_1]} \frac{[C_2]}{[C_2 + K_2]}$$

The two limiting component C_1 and C_2 are the concentration.

$$\mu = \mu_m \frac{[C_i]}{[C_i + K_i]} \frac{[C_p]}{[C_p + K_p]}$$

Where, K_p is the saturation constant for the products K_i and C_p is the product concentration.

The latent state as has been pointed out earlier is the stage where cell population growth rate is either nil or negligible, although cells are still able to increase in size and it occurs while cells adjust to their newer environment. Some important factors such as cell type and age, inoculum size and culture conditions have to be carefully monitored and looked into. To highlight the importance of these factors, consider the simplest case when the cells from a low nutrient concentration are inoculated into a high concentration medium, the latent state is significantly prolonged. However, if the opposite set is followed, there is virtually no latent stage. Furthermore, the amount of inoculum affects the duration of the latent stage. Similarly, if a small number of cells are inoculated into a large volume, the latent phase is longer. In a large scale fermentation unit, the major objective is to shorten the latent phase; to inoculate a large fermenter, a series of progressively larger seed inocula are used to shorten the latent phase.

When the case of batch culture is considered, it involves inoculating sterile medium with a seed culture of the cells to be grown. After inoculation apart from air supply in case of aerobic fermentation and removal of waste gases, usually nothing else is required to be added or removed from the batch. The rapid change in newer environment can affect the following four important variables

1. Inoculation into medium with high nutrient concentration can cause delayed cell growth until the culture adapts to new environment.

2. Essential molecules synthesized by the cells to promote growth (vitamins, activators) may be lost due to their diffusion out of the cells which may need time for replenishment;

3. The inoculum size and viable cell percentage greatly affect the duration of latent stage;

4. The maturity of the inocula is highly important because newer cells are already in exponential growth.

For an optimum fermenter design, one requirement is that the latent phase should be shortened. Hence, the following three points are to be considered:

1. Inocula should be as active as possible;

2. Inoculum's medium should correspond as closely as possible to the fermenter;

3. Reasonably large volumes of inocula should be used to minimize the loss of key metabolic intermediates by diffusion.

A proper consideration of all kinetics related factors and appropriate modeling of the fermentation unit should be considered for development and design of a fermenter.

4.3. IMPROVEMENT OF MICROBIAL STRAINS

Owing to their inherent control systems, microorganisms usually produce commercially important metabolites in very low concentrations and, although the yield may be increased by optimizing the cultural conditions, productivity is controlled ultimately by the organism's genome. In order to obtain the highest possible yield of the fermented product, the major requirement is that the concerned microorganism should possess the highest production capabilities. Thus, to improve the potential productivity, the organism's genome must be modified and this may be achieved by:

(i) Classical strain improvement by mutation and selection

(ii) The use of recombination

(iii) Protoplast fusion

4.3.1. Mutations

When a microbe divides naturally, the probability of occurrence of inherited changes is low. However, due to some environmental factors, some strains suffer stable change in some characteristics. These strains are termed as mutants and the factor which caused the change is termed the mutagen; the whole process is termed mutation. The mutagenic agents could be UV radiation, ionizing radiation, chemicals like nitrous acid, nitrosoguanidine, etc. The exposure to these agents usually kills most of the cells in a culture; however, a few surviving cells may contain some of the mutants that manifest changed characteristics. A small population of these cells is sometimes the source of large amount of bioactive components of interest.

The separation of desired mutant from other survivors of mutation is similar to isolation of desired organism from the nature. Whereas possible, the mutant isolation procedure should use the improved characteristics of the desired mutant as a selective factor. Presumably, superior productivity is a result of diversion of precursor into the product or a modification of the control mechanism limiting the level of the production. Thus, knowledge of the biosynthetic route and the mechanism of control of the biosynthesis product should enable the design off isolation technique which would give desired mutant a selective advantage over the other types present. Knowledge of biosynthetic routes and control mechanisms are more detailed for primary metabolites and therefore, the use of selective pressure in mutant isolation is more common in the fields of amino acid, nucleotide and enzyme production than in secondary metabolite production. However, considerable progress has also been made in the design of such procedures for the isolation of secondary metabolite over-producers.

The selection of induced mutant synthesizing improved level of primary metabolites. Before considering the method used for the selection of mutants producing improved levels of primary metabolites it is necessary to study the mechanism of control of their biosynthesis such that the blueprints referred to above, may be drawn accurately. The levels of primary metabolites in the microorganisms are regulated by feedback inhibition and feedback repression. Feedback inhibition is situation where the end product of a biochemical pathway inhibits the activity of an enzyme catalyzing one of an enzyme catalyzing one of the reactions (normally the first reaction) of the pathway. Inhibition acts by the end product binding to the enzyme at an allosteric site which results in interference with the attachment of the enzyme to its substrate. Feedback repression is the situation where the end product (or a derivative of end products) of a biochemical pathway prevents the synthesis of an enzyme catalyzing a reaction of the pathway. Repression occur at the gene level by a derivative of the end product combining with the genome in such a way as to prevent the transcription of gene into messenger RNA, thus resulting in the prevention of enzyme synthesis.

Feedback inhibition and repression act in concert in the control of biosynthetic pathways, where inhibition may be visualized as a rapid control which switches off the biosynthesis of an end product and repression as a mechanism to then switch off the synthesis of temporarily redundant enzymes. The control of the pathways giving rise to only one product (i.e., unbranched pathways) is normally achieved by the first enzyme in the sequence being susceptible to inhibition by the end product, as shown in Figure 4.2.

The control of biosynthetic pathway giving rise to a number of end products (branched pathway) is more complex then the control of simple, unbranched sequences. The end product of the same, branched biosynthetic pathway are rarely required by the microorganism to the same extent, so that if an end product exert control over a part of the pathway common to two or more end product then the organism may suffer deprivation of the product not participating in the control. Thus, mechanisms have evolved which enables the level of end products of branched pathways to be controlled without depriving of the cell of essential intermediates. The following description of these mechanisms is based on the effect of the control, which may be arrived at by inhibition, repression or a combination of both systems.

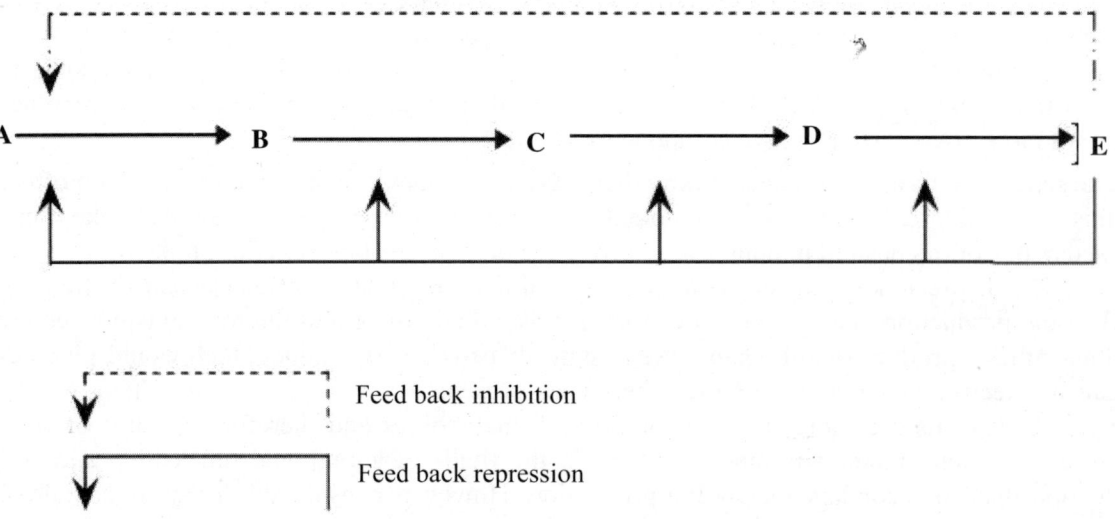

Fig. 4.2: The control of a biosynthetic pathway converting precursor A to end product E via the intermediates B, C and D. Concerted or multivalent feedback control

This control system involves the control of the pathway by more than one end product- the first enzyme of the pathway is inhibited or repressed only when all end products are in excess, as shown in Figure 4.3.

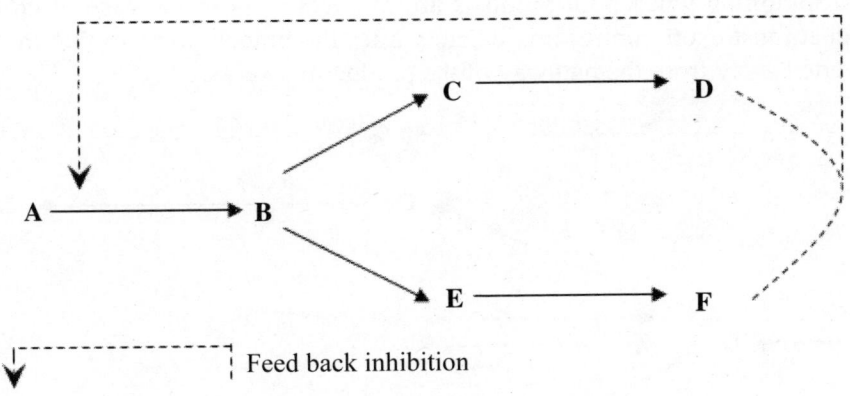

Fig. 4.3: The control of a biosynthetic pathway by concerted effects of products D and F on the first enzyme of the pathway

Co-operative feedback control

The system is similar to concerted control except that weak control may be affected by each end product independently. Thus, the presence of all end products in excess results in a synergistic repression or inhibition. The system is illustrated in Figure 4.4 and it may be seen that for efficient control to occur when one product is in excess there should be a further control operational immediately after the branch point to the excess product. Thus, the reduced flow of intermediates will be diverted to the product which is still required.

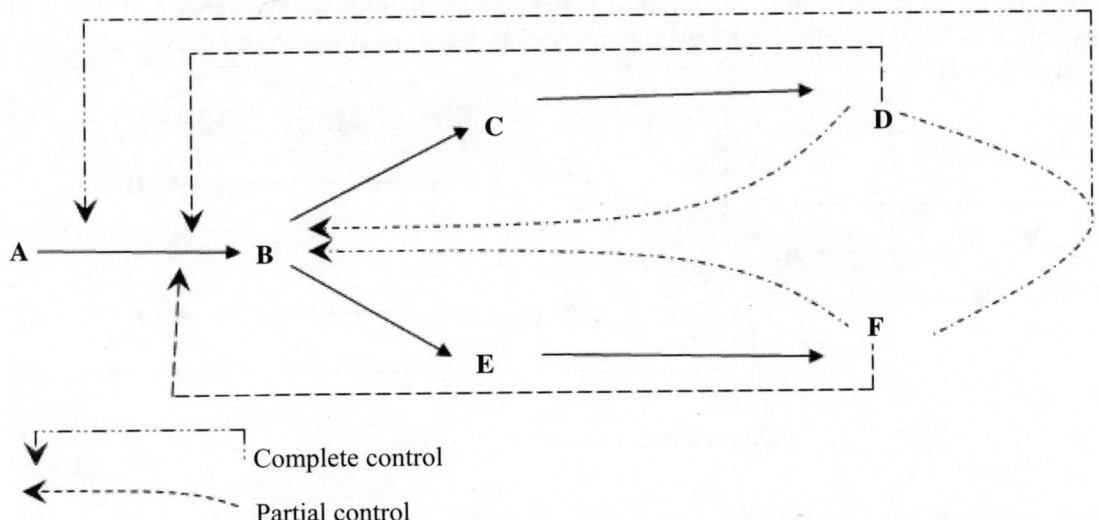

Fig. 4.4: The control of a biosynthetic pathway by co-operative control by end product D and F

Cumulative feedback control

Each of the end products inhibits the first enzyme by a certain percentage independently of the other end products. In Figure 4.5 both D and F independently reduces the activity of the first enzyme by 50%, resulting in total inhibition when both products are in excess. As in the case of co-operative control, each end product must exert control immediately after the branch point so that the common intermediate, B, is diverted away from the pathway of the product in excess.

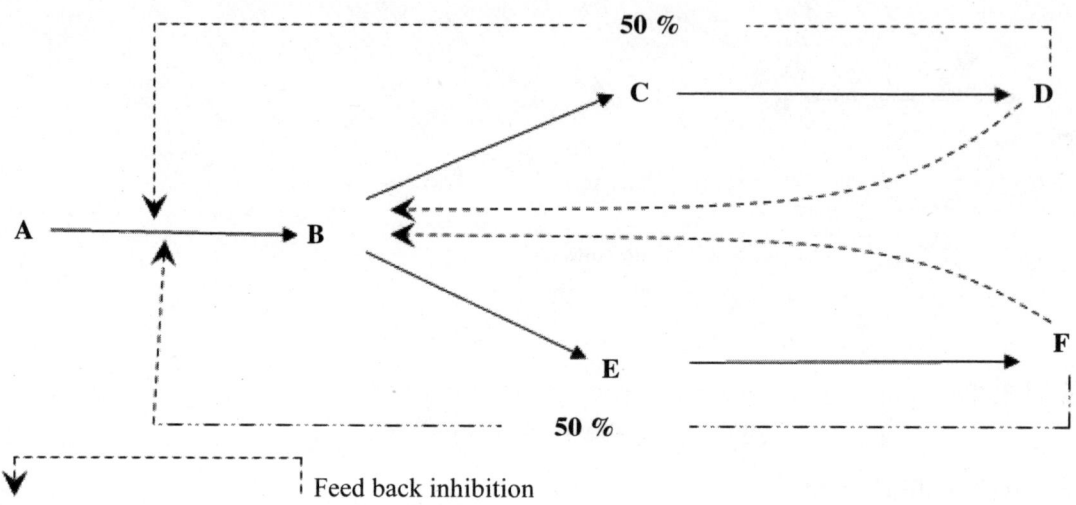

Fig. 4.5: The control of a biosynthetic pathway by cumulative control of product D and F

Sequential feedback control

Each end product of the pathway controls the enzyme immediately after the branch point to the product. The intermediates, those build up as a result of these control earlier enzymes in the pathway. Thus, in Figure 4.6, D inhibits the conversion of B to C, and F inhibits the conversion of B to E. The inhibitory action of D, F, or both would result in an accumulation of B which in turn would inhibit the conversion of A to B.

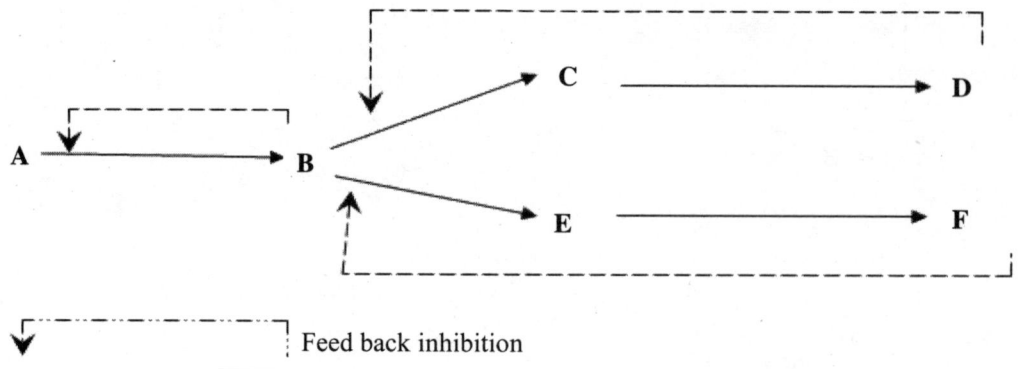

Fig. 4.6: The control of two iso-enzymes (catalyzing the conversion of A to B) by end product D and F

Isoenzyme control

Isoenzymes are enzymes which catalyze the same reaction but differ in their control characteristics. Thus, if a critical control reaction of a pathway is catalyzed by more than one isoenzyme may be controlled by the different end product (Fig. 4.7). Such a control system should be very efficient, provided that control exist immediately after the branch point so that reduced flow of intermediates is diverted away from the production excess.

Thus, the levels of microbial metabolites may be controlled by a variety of mechanisms, such that end products are synthesized in amounts not greater than those required for growth. However, the ideal industrial micro-organism should produce amount far greater than those required for growth and, as suggested earlier, an understanding of the control of production of a metabolites may enable the construction of a blueprint of the most useful industrial mutant, i.e. one where the production of the metabolite is not restricted by the organism's control systems. Such postulated mutants may be modified in three ways:

1. The organism may be modified such that the end products which control the key enzymes of the pathway are lost from the cell due to some abnormality in the permeability of the cell membrane.

2. The organism may be modified such that it does not produce the end products which control the key enzymes of the pathway.

3. The organism may be modified such that it does not recognize the presence of inhibiting of repressing level of the normal control metabolites.

One major drawback of mutation-based improvisation of cell strains is that some specific or desired mutation is not always possible by using standard mutation techniques. Mutagenesis is a random process and we cannot predict which gene will suffer. Hence, it is the task of an industrial geneticist to differentiate a few superior producers found among the survivors as mutant's target.

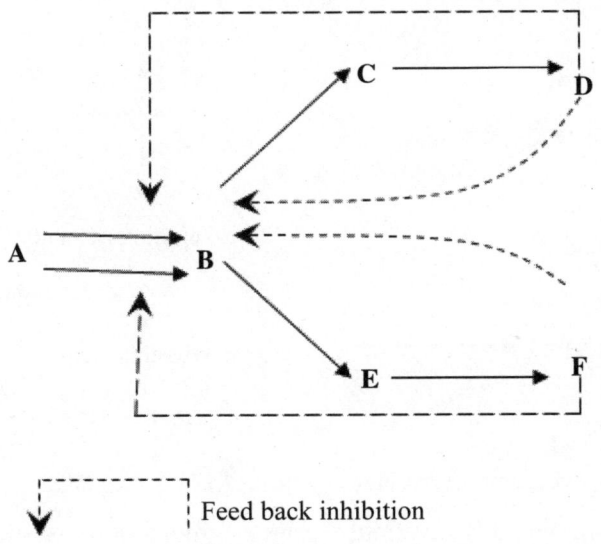

Feed back inhibition

Fig. 4.7: The control of two iso-enzymes (catalyzing the conversion of A to B) by end product D and F

4.3.1.1. Selection of mutant producing improved level of primary metabolite

The separation of desired mutant from the other survivors of the mutation is similar to the isolation of desired organism from the nature. Whereas possible, the mutant isolation procedure should use the improved characteristics of the desired mutant as a selective factor. Presumably, superior productivity is a result of diversion of precursor into the product or a modification of the control mechanism limiting the level of the production. Thus, knowledge of the biosynthetic route and the mechanism of control of the biosynthesis product should enable the design off isolation technique which would give desired mutant a selective advantage over the other types present. Knowledge of biosynthetic routes and control mechanisms are more detailed for primary metabolites and therefore, the use of selective pressure in mutant isolation is more common in the fields of amino acid, nucleotide and enzyme production than in secondary metabolite production. However, considerable progress has also been in the design of such procedures for the isolation of secondary metabolite over-producers.

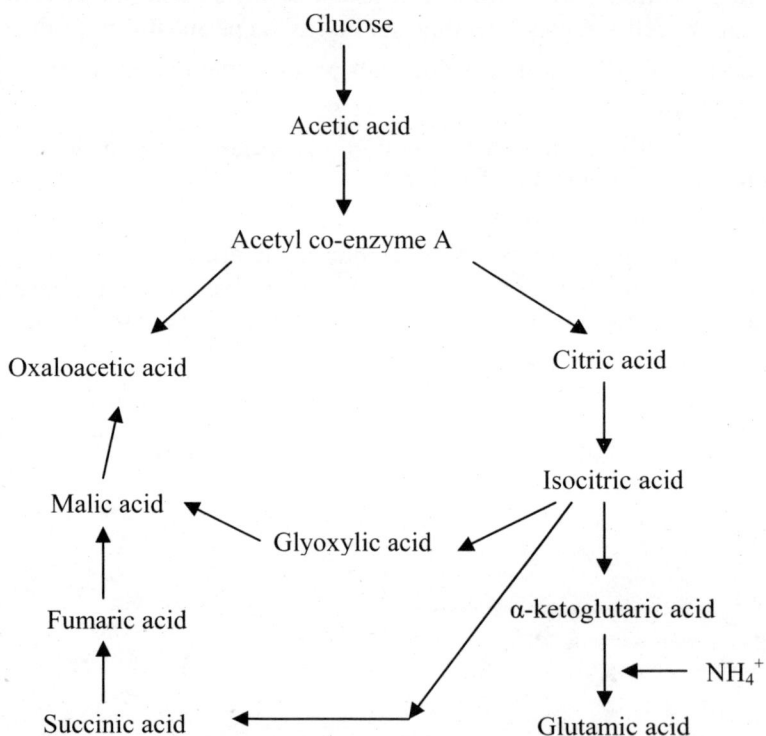

Fig. 4.8: TCA cycle and glyoxylate cycle in *Corynebacterium glutamicum*

One most important commercially available primary metabolite is glutamic acid. The most common organism that produces it is *Corynebacterium glutamicum.* Originally *C. glutamicum* was isolated by Kinoshita and associates, as a biotin auxotroph, i.e., it required biotin for production of glutamic acid. Looking into the TCA cycle, it could be inferred that glutamic acid is produced when the microbe lacks the enzyme responsible for conversion of α-ketoglutaric acid into succinic acid (Fig. 4.8). When *C. glutamicum* is grown in grown in culture medium containing high concentration of biotin (25–35 µg/mg/dry weight of cells), the conversion rate and hence the yield of glutamic acid is appreciably high. Therefore, biotin concentration is a limiting factor in the production of glutamic acid. In the absence of biotin the low yield of glutamic acid could be accounted for by the negative feedback inhibition resulting from high concentration of glutamic acid. The excretion of glutamic acid in the biotin limiting condition seems to be due to disturbance of the selective permeability of the cells.

Thus, the combination of a metabolic modification that blocks the in conversion of glutamic acid to succinic acid in the TCA cycle may result in a higher yield of glutamic acid. A major disadvantage of using biotin limitation as a controlling factor is that it precludes the use of biotin rich crude carbohydrate carbon source. As an alternative some other growth factors such as penicillin and surfactant like fatty acid derivatives have been utilized to vary the permeability of the cell membrane. Mutants of *C. glutamicum* have been extensively utilized for commercial production of a large number of amino acids. However, the wild types of strains produce the primary end product according to the requirement of the organism. The control over the production is typically a negative feedback control. Since the feedback control for *C. glutamicum* is quite easy for production of glutamic acid, the microbe shows considerable application potential for industrial usage. Furthermore, the use of mutant strains of *C. glutamicum* has been effectively and exclusively utilized for the production of lysine.

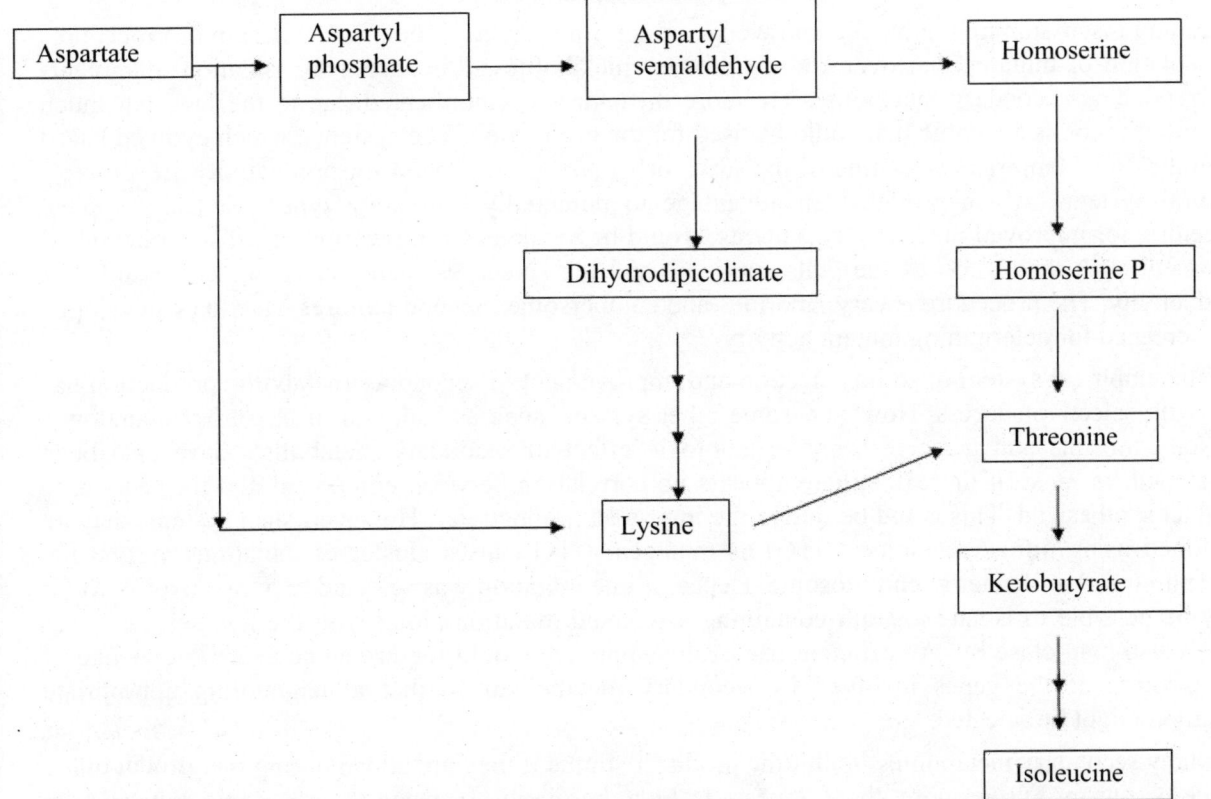

Fig. 4.9: The control of lysine production in *Corynebacterium glutamicum* (feed back inhibition)

Figure 4.9 showed the control of lysine production in *Corynebacterium glutamicum*. It could be inferred that aspartokinase, the first enzyme involved in the biosynthetic route, is inhibited only when lysine and threonine are present above their threshold control level; this is termed as an absolute feedback inhibition. An important feature of the pathway is that lysine does not exert any control over the biosynthesis of lysine from aspartyl semialdehyde. A mutant that could not catalyze the conversion of aspartic semialdehyde to homoserine would be able to grow only in homoserine supplemented medium and the organism would be referred as a homoserine auxotroph. If such an organism were grown in the presence of very low concentration of homoserine the endogenous level of threonine would not reach the inhibitory concentration of aspartokinase control, hence aspartate will be converted to lysine.

The knowledge of biosynthetic route allows the geneticist to develop a mutant with route specific desirable traits. The isolated homoserine auxotroph of *C. glutamicum* using penicillin enrichment technique developed (Davis, 1949). Under normal culture conditions an auxotroph suffers a disadvantage compared to the parental (wild type) cells. However, penicillin selectively kills growing bacterial cells and therefore, if the survivors of a mutation treatment are cultured in a medium containing penicillin that lacks essential growth elements/components needed for growth of the mutant then only the cells that do not grow would survive; these cells can be isolated as desired auxotrophs in a medium containing the specific elements. The resulting subculture would be rich in the mutant strain.

4.3.1.2. Selection of secondary metabolite producing strains

Preceding discussion highlights the knowledge of control systems of help in the design of procedures for isolation of mutants that overproduce primary metabolites. Procedures for isolation of mutants overproducing secondary metabolites are more difficult and complicated due to the fact that much less information is available that could be used for the production. The systems, which evolved based upon the direct empirical screening of the survivor's mutation treatment for productivity are valuable cultural systems, which provided an advantage to potentially producing types. Hence, a typical screening for improved productivity mutants, would be to subject a population of cells to mutational treatment such that 1–5% of the cells survived, and the screen as many survivors as possible for productivity. The procedure is very laborious and cumbersome. Several cultures have to be developed and screened for determining mutant activity.

The empirical system of strain selection and improvement of secondary metabolite production has met with selective success. However, some other systems such as isolation of auxotrophs, analogue resistant mutants and those resistant to autotoxic effect of secondary metabolites have also been developed. In most of the cases there appears no correlation between compound and the secondary product synthesized. This could be due to the improved productivity. However, such systems may be exploited using nitrosoguanidine (NTG) as mutagen. NTG causes cluster of mutations around the replicating fork of bacterial chromosome. Hence, if one mutation was selected (e.g. by auxotrophy) it may be possible to isolate a strain containing a selected mutation along with the non selected ones which also map close by. An efficient use of this approach would require an accurate knowledge of the position of the genes involved in secondary metabolism so that a neighboring appropriate mutation might be selected.

Many secondary metabolites inhibit the producer strains if they are added during the growth phase of the organism. Furthermore, there appears to be a correlation between the auxotoxic resistance in growth phase and productivity in idophase. This ability of a survivor of a mutation treatment to grow in the presence of high concentration of its secondary metabolites may be used as a selective parameter for improved productivity. The technique has successfully been combined with genetic manipulation techniques to clone the gene coding for 6'N-acetyl transferase into *Streptomyces kanamyceticus*, (a kanamycin producer). The enzyme is involved in aminoglycoside resistance and the recombinants containing the cloned gene were more resistant to, and produced more of kanamycin. Thus, the application of the technique used in improvement of primary metabolite formation has catalyzed considerable progress in secondary metabolite production.

4.3.2. Recombination

The idea of utilizing the genes in effective recombination in order to generate a new recombinant was proposed and investigated by Hopwood (1979). The practical applicability of this technique for strain improvement of industrial strains is rather low in view of the complexity of the process and paucity of genetic literature on industrial strains. Relatively little industrially important organism exhibit sexual reproduction as such, production and isolation of their recombinants is generally restricted to commercial mushrooms and yeast strains used in baking, brewing and distilling industries. Recombination systems not associated with sexual reproduction are more common in industrially important strains. Recently developed experimental methodologies make these systems easier to exploit. Some of these techniques applied for various fermentation products are described in the following paragraphs.

4.3.2.1. Recombination systems utilized in earlier days

The development of recombination systems was based upon the concept of parasexual cycle. In this cycle the nuclear fusion and gene segregation take place outside the sexual organs, for instance in the fungi *A.nidulans and P. chrysogenum*. The nuclear fusion occurs in genetically different nuclei present in the same organism. Such an organism is termed heterokaryon and is formed by fusion and migration of genetic material of two different cells when they come in contact with each other. The establishment of heterokaryon is a rare event and to assist its recognition, auxotrophic markers are used.

Nuclear fusion may occur between unlike nuclei in the heterokaryon and gives rise to a diploid clone. In rare cases the nucleus may undergo an abnormal mitosis resulting in production of a recombinant. The abnormal mitosis may involve mitotic crossing over, haploidization or a combination of both. The recombinants so formed may have the characteristics of both the nuclei.

Some agents like camphor vapor and UV light increase the frequency of nuclear fusion. Furthermore, utilization of X-rays, UV light and nitrogen mustards facilitates crossing over or haploidization. The technique has been utilized to study the genetics of *P. chrysogenum* and *A. niger*. However, the technique could not be successfully utilized due to one major difficulty in the establishment of a heterokaryon that is fusion of cells from different strains. Protoplast fusion techniques can overcome the problem effectively and successfully.

Another similar process of interest is conjugation. In bacteria, genetic information is transferred from one cell to another through cell-to-cell contact. The chromosomes of the 'donor' cell are mobilized by integration of a normal extra chromosomal DNA segment into chromosome. The transfer of genetic material is governed by the time (duration) of contact. Furthermore, the DNA is transferred in a linear fashion. Single strand of DNA is cut adjacent to the site of integration of the mobilizing factor and this strand passes into the recipient cell; the mobilizing factor is the last element to be transferred. The transferred segment is incorporated into chromosomes of the recipient cells by crossing-over. Similar to the case of parasexual cycle, different isolating procedures have to be applied to identify the most appropriate strains since the activity of the conjugate is dependent upon the linkage of gene in the chromosome fragment. However, availability of genetic maps may help the process, as the utilization of genetic markers could be used to screen certain recombinants. Moreover, genetic complexity of the strain further adds to the complexity of the process.

4.3.3. Protoplast fusion

A protoplast is a cell devoid of the cell wall that may be prepared by subjecting the cells to the action of wall-degrading digesting enzymes in an isotonic solution. Cell fusion, followed by nuclear fusion, may occur between protoplasts of cells that otherwise do not fuse. Further, following fusion the protoplasts regenerate the cell wall and can grow as normal cells. Protoplast fusion has been successfully achieved in filamentous fungi, yeasts, *Bacillus* species, *Brevibacterium flavum* and *Streptomyces*.

The process is better than parasexual cycle in facilitating heterokaryon formation. Literature presents several citations regarding strain improvement for industrially applicable strains.

4.4. FERMENTERS

The heart of a fermentation process is a fermenter. A working definition of a fermenter is a container in which an environment favorable to the operation of a desired biological process is maintained. Fermentation is typically either batch operated or continuous in operation mode. In the case of batch operated, fermentation proceeds for a defined period and is terminated when the product concentration reaches a preselected level. The fermenter contents are then harvested, separated, recovered and purified. In the case of continuous culture fermentation, there is a requirement for sterile medium for continuous feeding and medium containing desired end product should continuously be taken out through a vessel at the same rate. The major advantage with continuous culture fermentation is a steady productivity rate. However, factors like maintenance of aseptic medium and steady state environment are to be carefully considered and monitored.

A fermenter is frequently confused with a bioreactor. However, the major difference between the two is the type of cells being grown. A fermenter grows cells such as bacteria or fungi etc, while a bioreactor grows eukaryotic cells such as insects or mammalian cells. In practice, many manufacturers and bioprocess scientists still refer them as fermenters. Furthermore, the bioreactors differ from fermenters in their parts such as agitators and mixers.

The word 'fermenter' tends to conjure up the vision of large, shiny, stainless steel vessels bristling with sophisticated instrumentation. While most of the industrial fermenters are indeed like that, several large-scale biological processes are carried only in equipments which are less sophisticated and considerably cheaper. For fermentation engineering, the system should not be more complicated than really necessary.

The physico-chemical status of a fermenter is subject to manipulations. Some selected variables which can usually be measured directly in a fermenter are completed active fermentation time, temperature, pressure, and flow rate of cooling water, rate of agitation, power input, inlet air flow rate, exhaust gas composition, dissolved oxygen; pH, liquid level, mass, or volume of vessel contents, turbidity; fluorescence, various ions, product, and byproduct concentrations. Some selected variables which can be measured off-line are concentrations of sugars or other substrates, protein concentration, nitrogen level, enzyme activities, product concentrations, biomass, dry weight of unfiltered broth, and viscosity of broth.

An optimum design of a fermenter is necessary to maintain an environment suitable for the controlled growth of microorganisms, hence regulating the environment and maintaining aseptic conditions are the prime requirements regardless of size. Growth medium must be regulated with respect to agitation, temperature, aeration, pH, concentration, dissolved oxygen, foam control and other parameters. To overcome the difficulty of purifying the product, the fermenter must be made up of non-corrosive and non-toxic material that could be readily sterilized. Small fermenters are usually made from borosilicate glass while the pilot size systems are made up of stainless steel. Furthermore, each fermenter should be so assembled that most of the parts could be separated for cleaning purpose.

4.4.1. Structure of a fermenter (with appropriate configuration)

A typical fermenter consists of three major parts:

1. The culture vessel

2. Associated supply and environmental systems, its measurement and control systems.

Various important factors responsible for optimized fermenter design are listed in Table 4.3.

Table 4.3: Various important fermenter design considerations

Factor	Importance
Maintenance of sterility	To allow only desirable micro-organism to grow
Oxygen transfer rate	For optimum growth of the micro-organism in aerobic conditions
Heat transfer	For maintaining optimum temperature which changes due to growth of cells
Instrumentation and control protocols	For continuous fermentation process monitoring
Biological kinetics	To shorten latent phase
Mass transfer of the substrate to micro-organism	For attaining higher yield
Mass transfer of product out of micro-organism	For attaining higher yield
Safety (fail-safe control; pressure build up; micro-organism escape)	Production hazard

After a careful consideration of all these factors in the designing of a typical fermenter, some more operational characteristics have to be looked into. They are listed in Table 4.4. Basically, from a bench type fermenter to a production scale fermenter, they are essentially similar and are simply closed, temperature controlled culture vessels. Further, the maximum instrumentation, controls and accessory equipments differ from requirement to requirement. Figure 4.10 shows a typical fermenter design.

4.4.2. Size and scale of process

As the complexity of a fermenter increases there arises the need for increasing peripheral equipment and instrumentation, particularly measurement and control systems. Essential features that need to be considered in selecting fermenters the product reliability, multipurpose flexibility, interchange ability, level of sophistication, compatibility and range of monitoring instrumentation available for the system. Most frequent classification of fermenters is based upon their size and accordingly they are grouped as given below:

(A) Laboratory and research (bench scale) fermenters, which are generally ranging from 1-50 liter.

(B) Pilot plant fermenters that typically ranging from 50-1000 liter.

(C) Production scale fermenters, usually larger than 1000 liter.

Table 4.4: Characteristics of typical fermenter

S.No.	Characteristics	S.No.	Characteristics
1.	Alarm and fail safe system	9.	Integrated piping system
2.	Batch or continuous operation	10.	Interchangeable peripherals
3.	Computer controlled operation	11.	Multiple entry and exit ports
4.	Convenient aeration	12.	Physical integrity
5.	Ease of installation	13.	Programmable inputs
6.	Foam control	14.	Reliability
7.	Heating and cooling	15.	Sterilizable peripherals
8.	In situ sterilization	16.	Suitable contact surface

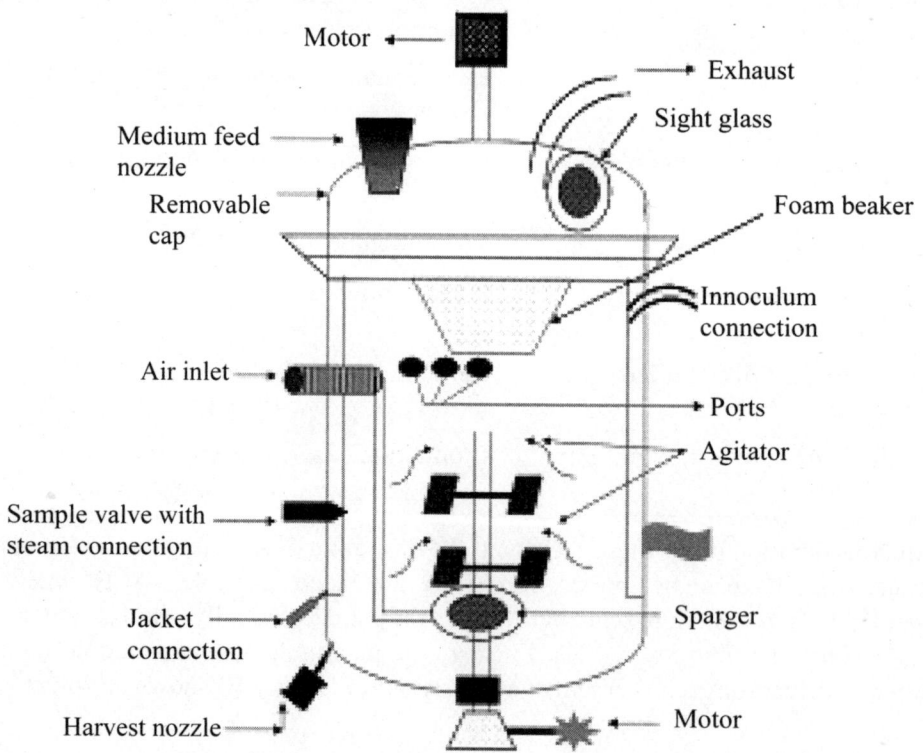

Fig. 4.10: Diagrammatic representation of a typical fermenter

While the division appears to be arbitrary, it has been generally adopted at industrial level. The large number of fermenters currently available covers a wide spectrum that blurs distinction between one class and another, especially when dealing with smaller production quantities of high value added substances such as cytokines or interferons.

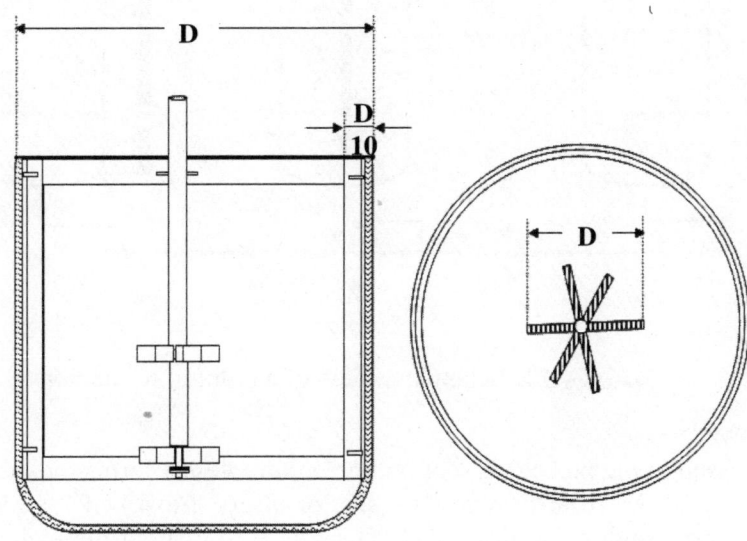

Fig. 4.11: Bench top stirred tank fermenter

A comparative account of all the three classes of fermenters is presented in Table 4.5. and Fig. 4.12.

- A. Non-agitated fermenter
- B. Mechanically agitated fermenter
- C. Fluidized air fermenter

Table 4.5: Stirred tank fermenters (STF): A comparison

Feature	Small bench	Large bench
Size	1-1- L	10–100 L
Sterilization	Autoclave	in situ
Mixing	Air lift	Bladed turbine
Drive		Direct drive or magnetically coupled
Fittings	Autoclavable	Sterilized in situ
Seals		Autoclavable O-ring seals
Jacketing		Yes, with internal baffles
Ports	4–10	4–10
Surface		Electro polished stainless steels, Pyrex
Parts		Interchangeable impellers and fittings
Others	Bottom aeration by sparging, maximized oxygen transfer, remote valve process control, view window, sterile compressed air between agitator seals, distinctive safety features.	

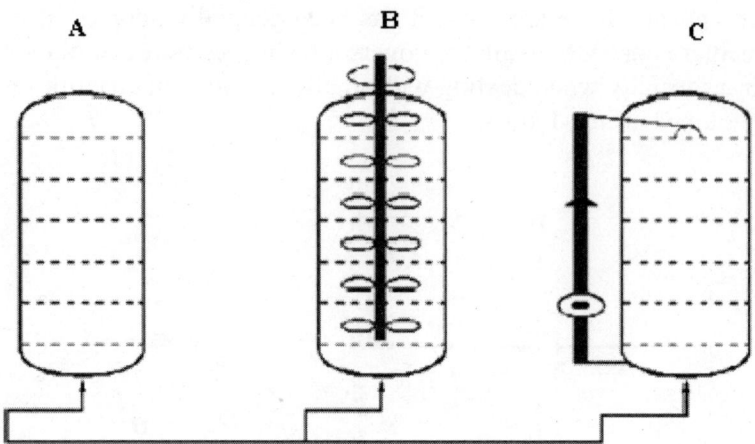

Fig. 4.12: Schematic view of a column fermenter

4.4.3. Culture vessels

As has been discussed in the preceding section, the culture vessel forms the major part of a fermenter and is common to all types regardless of their size or utility. Most bench-scale fermenters are made up of borosilicate glass and/or stainless steel. The selection of both the materials is based upon the conceptual understanding of the process as both of them are nontoxic, non-corrosive, and easily cleanable and could be steam sterilized. As an example a cheap and simple to maintain fermenter culture vessel could be made up of glass cylinder with stainless steel head and bottom plates, ending an opportunity for viewing of fermentation. The head plates provide ports for nutrient media and gas input as well as waste product removal. For linking vessel and head plate, silicon rubber O-rings are utilized, and autoclaving is used for sterilization.

Stainless steel vessels on the other hand provide strength, and make possible the use of double-jacketed steam sterilization equipments. However, the visual observation is a major drawback. To overcome the problem, many sealed glass windows could be built and utilized. Interestingly, contamination problems have been attributed to glass vessels rather than to stainless steel vessels: self-sterilizable stainless steel vessels typically offer greater protection against contamination as compared to glass vessels or silicon rubber seals.

4.4.4. Agitation systems

Agitation systems represent the major requirement for all the fermenters. On small scale units, agitation is generally accomplished by direct-drive mechanical stirring through a seal in the head plate. Some models offer either magnetically coupled agitators or air-lift systems to eliminate mechanical seals. For large-scale fermenters, baffles and paddles are used as mechanical agitators. At the lower end, LSL BioLafitte for example offers a fermenter with an overlay of pressurized sterile air between the two impeller shaft seals and an automatic monitor of seal wear.

4.4.5. Size and capacity

Regardless of size, the basic fermenter design remains invariably the same. However, as fermenter size increases, special and more complex features tend to multiply. Large fermenters usually vary in the additional devices incorporated into the large units such as additional entry and exit ports frequently used to accommodate more in process monitoring probes that are required by the large vessels, although sometimes extra ports are utilized so as to separate various components before adding them to culture vessel.

Although a large-scale fermenter adds to the complexity of operation, it also allows greater control; for example, increased thermal mass of a larger vessel permits better temperature control and its large volume facilitates closer pH regulation and buffering of the medium. A Chemp's Chemical system enables efficient bubble free medium aeration and cell separation and thereby avoids growth limitation for build up of metabolic waste products. The major consideration in large-scale equipment is proper agitation and *in situ* control monitoring.

4.4.6. Process monitoring and control

Process monitoring and control are some issues at the leading edge of fermenter development. The advent of recent bioanalytical techniques has inspired development of a vast array of probes. The controls applicable in the fermentation process are listed in table 4.6. The process monitoring parameters are listed in Table 4.7.

Table 4.6: Typical fermenter control ranges

Control	Range
Temperature	4°C above coolant to 60°±1°C
Agitator speed	0-1000 rpm
Stability	>94%
pH range	2 -12±0.1
Pressure	2000 mbar
DO_2 range	0-100%
Air flow	0-6 liters/minute

4.4.7. Cleaning and sterilization

A bioprocess facility relating to the cleaning of a fermenter is a crucial element in designing and construction. Piping, inlet and outlet ports, valves, sensors, regulators, and other components must be so designed as to eliminate dead spaces, ridges and crevices where material can accumulate and must be constructed to resist the wear and corrosion that could produce areas of surface deterioration (preferential sites for micro-organism growth and substance contamination).

Cleaning process begins when a fermenter is empty following completion of a culture run. Both systems such as clean-in-place (CIP) and sterilize-in-place (SIP) minimize disassembly and down time. CIP and SIP systems, sanitary design verification and sterile operation are critical components of fermenter system validation maintained from the start. Most industrial fermentations are carried out in pure culture. If foreign organisms proliferate in the medium then producing organisms are forced to compete with the contaminating organisms for the nutrients.

Foreign organisms also produce metabolic byproducts that limit the producing cultures growth. Therefore, before starting fermentation, the medium, additives, and all equipments must be completely sterile and aseptic conditions should be maintained. Steam sterilization is desirable because it destroys contaminants as well as affects cleaning of the system as the steam reaches all contact sites, process liquids and gases. Continuous steam flow during processing provides a sterile barrier with process liquid on one side and steam on the other. Media and equipment are generally so treated that all contaminating organisms are destroyed or killed. This is done by:

1. Dry or moist heat
2. Ultra violet radiation
3. Chemical agents
4. Ultrafiltration
5. Ultrasound (Mechanically disrupting contaminating organisms).

Table 4.7: Fermentation process control monitoring parameters and methodology

Process control	Monitoring device
Air flow	Flow meter
Coolant water flow	Flow meter
Power input	V.O.M.; torque
Temperature	Resistance thermocouples, thermistors, diodes
Rheology	Tube viscometer cone and plate viscometer, concentric cylinder viscometer, foam control.
Redox potential	pH, dissolved oxygen (DO_2), polarographic probes, Galvanic probes, Permeable tube/oxygen analyzer, Dissolved carbon dioxide (DCO_2).
Cell concentration	Gravimetric dry weight turbidity
Immunocytometry	Cell number, impedance, carbon dioxide production, oxygen production, DNA content, cell particle size distribution
Gas analysis	Oxygen analyzers, carbon dioxide analyzers, Mass spectrometry, Gas chromatography

Heat is most widely used as a means of sterilization and is employed for both medium and heatable fermenter parts. It can be applied either dry or moist (steam). Moist heat is more effective for sterilization because vegetative bacterial heat resistance is greater in dry state resulting in death kinetics that are much lower for dry cells than for moist ones. Laboratory autoclaves are usually operated at pressure of about 30 psi, corresponding to 121°C where bacterial spores are destroyed.

Cells exposed to UV radiations can suffer DNA damage leading to cell death. The best bactericidal efficiency is at wavelength around 265nm. Its use has been limited to microbial population in areas such as clean rooms and sterile chambers due to its limited ability to penetrate non-biotic matter.

Oxidizing and alkylating chemicals kill micro-organisms but they are not used for medium or fermenter sterilization because residual traces of antiseptics inhibit fermentation. Some major antimicrobial chemical agents are phenol and phenolic compounds, ethanol, halogens, detergents, dyes, quaternary ammonium compounds, acids, alkalis and gaseous sterilizing chemicals (ethylene oxide, propiolactone, formaldehyde, etc.).

Ultrafiltration is effective for removing micro-organisms from the air or from other gases and liquids. It is used for sterilization of thermolabile products such as sera and enzymes. Ultrasound of appropriate intensity can disrupt microorganisms. This technique is usually employed for extracting cellular components rather than for sterilization (Fig. 4.13).

4.5. DOWNSTREAM PROCESSING

After the fermentation is completed, the product is harvested and recovered. This is called downstream processing (DSP). The efficiency of the fermenter is mainly determined by the DSP operations, viz., how well the fermented product, and byproducts, are separated from the broth. DSP is concerned with the isolation of products either from cells (microbial, plant or animal) or from the fluid in which such cells have been grown. The latter category includes blood but most products of interest arise from the activity of cells or of cell constituents under controlled condition as reactors. Isolation of the desired product usually involves the following three stages:

1. The separation of cells from ambient fluid,
2. Isolation of an impure product from the fluid, and
3. The purification of the impure product

If the desired substance is within the cells, a procedure to release the cell contents either by mechanical disruption or lysis precedes second step. In the case of pharmaceutical products however, there will usually be a final (polishing) step involving the removal of trace impurities including heavy metal ions and pyrogens and, in many cases, a sterilization process also.

Free cell suspension cultures require rigorous DSP (down stream processing) because they usually attain rather low cell and product concentrations. In contrast, immobilized or entrapped cells give low product yields per cell but large productivity per reactor volume. This gives high product concentrations associated with lower costs of DSP.

In general, greater emphasis has been placed on genetic engineering and fermentation technology as compared to downstream processing aspects. The consequential operational limitations and high costs of DSP have therefore become grave obstacles in the process of developing commercially viable biotechnological products. In this context, the recovery of microorganisms from fermented broth presents a fairly difficult solid-liquid separation process. Roughly one-half of the total production costs of various products of medium-scale manufacturing process are accounted for by DSP. Some of these medium-scale biotechnological processes are listed in Table 4.8 along with a few large-scale and small-scale processes for comparison.

Table 4.8: A few representative large-scale, medium-scale, and small-scale biotechnological processes

Process	Approximate concentration of product in whole broth (% w/w)
Large-scale ($>200 \, m^3$ /batch, $1500 \, m^3$ /day)	
Single cell protein	3-5
Citric acid	10
Ethanol	10
Medium-scale (50-$200 \, m^3$ /batch)	
Penicillin	4
Cephalosporin	3
Extracellular enzymes	1
Small-scale (up to $50 \, m^3$ /batch)	
Riboflavin	0.1
Vitamin B_{12}	0.005

The primary stages of separation are greatly influenced by broth conditioning, whose major objective is to aggregate the cells to form larger clumps or flocs and hence reduce the separation costs. Broth conditioning techniques are based on physical, chemical or biological principles.

Examples of physical techniques include heating, freezing, mechanical (e.g., homogenizers), ultrasonics, and electrical treatments. Chemical techniques are exemplified by coagulation (by multivalent metal ions), flocculation (by organic polymers or polyelectrolytes), pH change, and lysis (by surfactants). The biological techniques of broth conditioning include the use of enzymes such as proteases, lipases and amylases, ageing, lysis (by antibiotics, e.g., penicillin), and antigen-antibody interactions between cells.

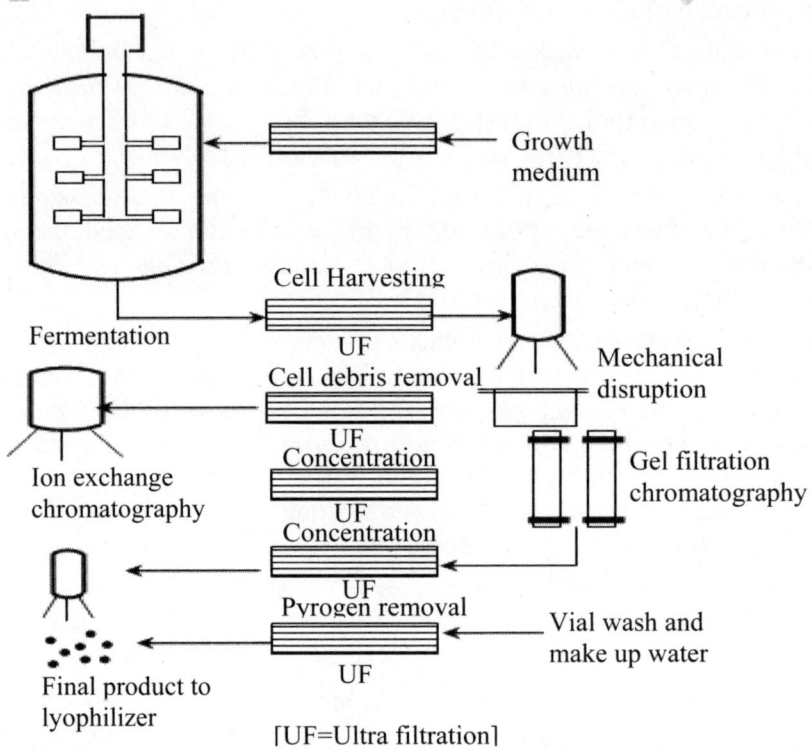

Fig. 4.13: A typical recovery process for intracellular product of fermentation

Membranes and membrane processes are a potent tool in modern biotechnology for downstream processing of bioreactor product constituents, sterilization of feed streams, or immobilization of enzymes. The advantage of membrane processes is that mass-scale separation can be achieved physically at ambient temperature without any chemical change. This makes membrane processes especially suitable for the treatment of thermally or chemically sensitive biologicals. In any typical microbial production system, there are four main areas where membranes may be used to advantage; these are (1) sterilization of bioreactor feed streams (e.g., nutrients, enzyme, oxygen, air, and water); (2) DSP of spent medium; (3) enzyme immobilization; and (4) on-line monitoring of bioreactor constituents.

4.6. TYPES OF FERMENTERS

Some commonly used fermenters are:

1. Continuous stirred tank bioreactor
2. Bubble column bioreactors
3. Airlift bioreactors

4. Tower fermenters
5. Fluidized bed bioreactor
6. Packed bed bioreactor

1. Continuous stirred tank bioreactor

Fig.4.14 showed the tank used in this system is essentially similar to that of the batch fermenter. It differs only in so far as there is provision for the inlet of medium and the outlet of broth. The airlift vessel may be baffled to improve mixing. These vessels provide very gentle mixing, and so are particularly suited to cells that are too shear sensitive to be mixed by an impeller. The number of impellers is variable and depends on the size of bioreactor i.e., height to diameter ratio. This ratio is referred to as aspect ratio. This ratio is usually 3-5 for a typical fermenter.

2. Bubble column bioreactors

In the bubble column bioreactor, the air or gas is introduced at the base of the column through perforated pipes or plates, or metal microporous spargers. The flow rate of the air/gas influences the performance factors-O_2 transfer, mixing. The bubble column bioreactor may be fitting with perforated plate to improve the performance (Fig. 4.14). The vessel used for the bubble column bioreactor is usually cylindrical with an aspect ratio of 4-6 (i.e., height to diameter ratio).

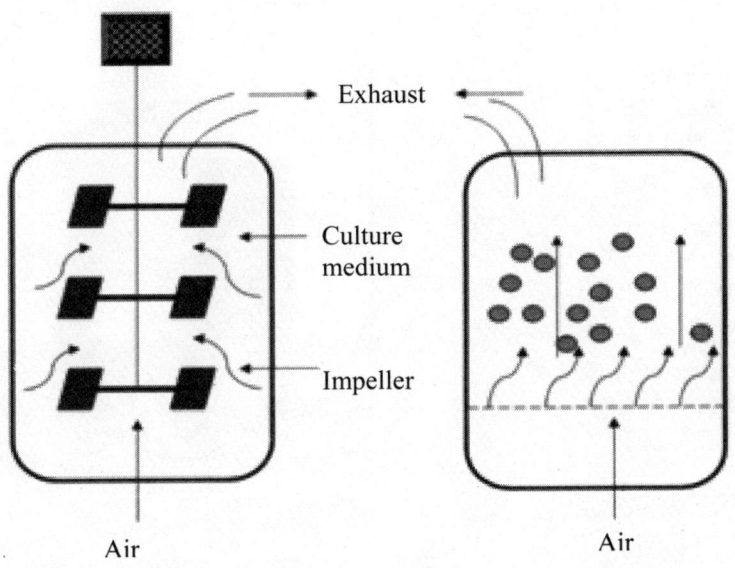

Fig. 4.14: Schematic representation of continuous stirred tank (left) and bubble column bioreactor (right)

3. Airlift bioreactors

In the airlift bioreactor, the medium of the vessel is divided into two interconnected zones by the means of a baffle or draft tube. In one of the two zones referred to a riser, the air/gas is pumped. The other zone that receives no gas is the down comer. The dispersion flows up the riser zone while the down flow occurs in the down comer. The airlift vessel may be baffled to improve mixing. These vessels provide very gentle mixing; therefore, they are particularly suited to cells that are too shear sensitive to be mixed by an impeller. The airlift bioreactors are mainly employed for aerobic bioprocess technology. They ensure a controlled liquid in a recycle system by pumping. Due to high efficiency, airlift fermenters are sometimes used preferred for the fermentation of methanol, waste water treatment and single cell protein.

There are two types of airlift bioreactor as shown in Figure 4.15.

Internal-loop airlift bioreactor has a single container with a central draft tube that creates interior liquid circulation channels. These bioreactors are simple in design, with volume and circulation at a fixed rate of fermentation.

External loop airlift bioreactors processes an external loop so that the liquid circulates through separate independent channels. These reactors can be suitably modified to suit the requirement of different fermentations. In general, the airlift bioreactors are more efficient than bubble columns, particularly for denser suspension of microorganisms. This is mainly because in these bioreactors, the mixing of the content is better compared to bubble column.

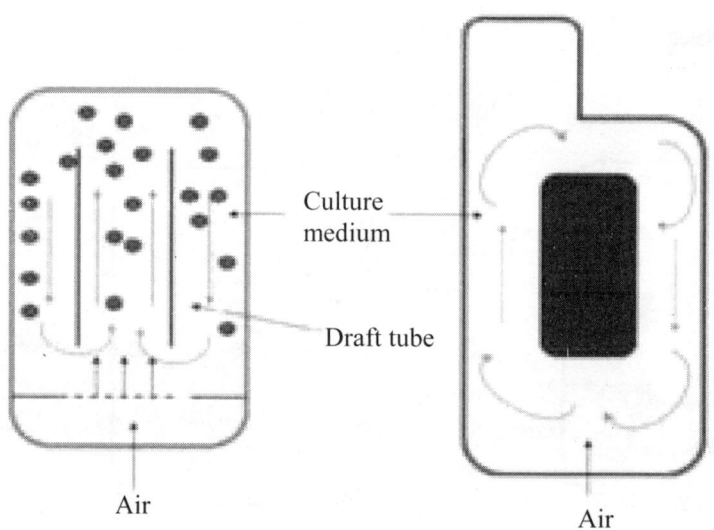

Fig. 4.15: Diagrammatic representation of internal loop airlift bioreactor (left) and external loop airlift bioreactor (right)

Two-stage airlift bioreactors

Two-stage air lift bioreactors are used for the temperature dependent formation of the products. Growing cells of one bioreactor are pumped into another bioreactor. Each one of the bioreactors is fitted with valves and they are connected by a transfer tube and pump. The cells are grown in first bioreactor and the bioprocess proper takes place in the second reactor (Fig. 4.16).

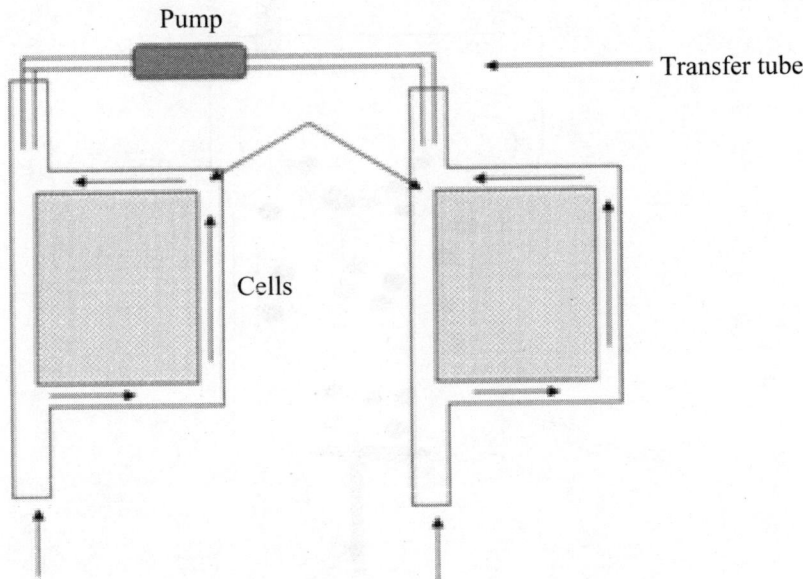

Fig. 4.16: Diagrammatic representation of two stage airlift bioreactor

4. Tower fermenter

Typically tower fermenters are vessels characterized by a high height-to diameter ratio, anywhere from 6:1 to 15:1. They are aerated by gas sparging via a simple sparger usually located near the fermenter base. These systems can be operated continuously by the creation of settling zones by using baffles, which allow the product to be taken off and the cells returned to the main body of the vessel. In *airlift fermenters* the mixing system (Motor, driveshaft and impellors) is replaced by a constant flow of gas introduced into a riser tube. Within the vessel flows develop that, as the air rises and then the medium containing cells falls ensure thorough mixing (Fig. 4.17).

5. The fluidized bed bioreactors

This is essentially similar to the tubular fermenter. In both the continuous stirred fermenter and the tubular fermenter there is a real danger of the organisms being washed out (Fig. 4.18). The fluidized bed reactor is an answer to this problem because it is intermediate in nature between the stirred tank and the tubular fermenter. The microorganisms which are in a fluidized bed fermenter are kept in suspension by a medium flow rate whose force just balances the gravitational force. If the flow were lower, the bed would remain 'fixed' and if the flow rate was at a force higher than the weight of the cells then 'elutriation' would occur with the particles being washed away from the tube. The tower fermenter for the brewing of beer and production of vinegar is an example of a fluidized bed fermenter.

6. Packed bed bioreactors

A bed of solid particles, with biocatalyst on or within the matrix of solids, packed in a column constitutes a packed bed bioreactor. The solid may be porous or non-porous gels, and they may be compressible or rigid in nature. A nutrient broth flows continuously over the immobilized biocatalyst.

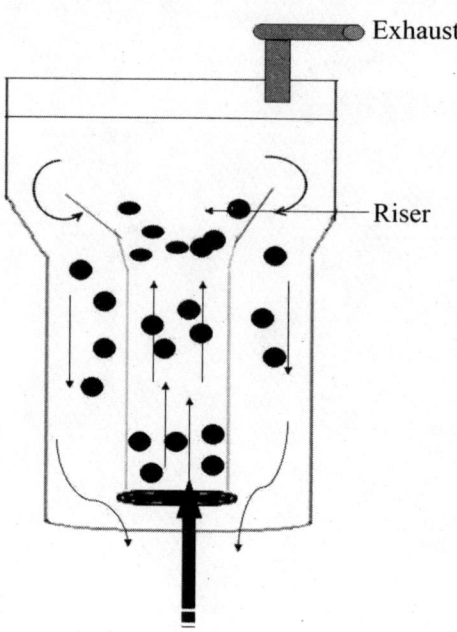

Fig. 4.17: Diagrammatic representation of tower fermenter

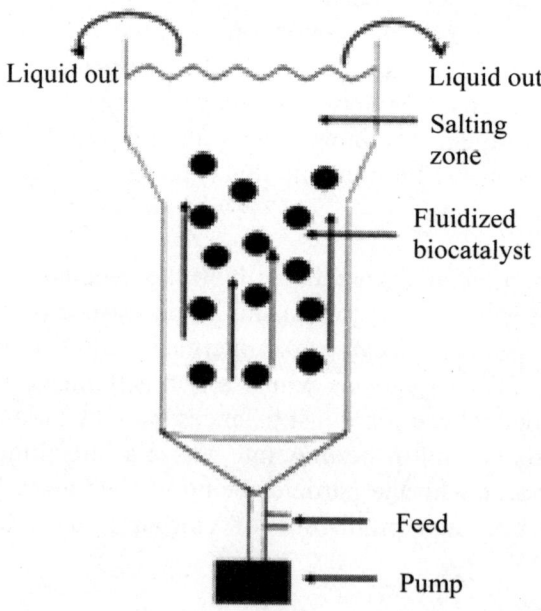

Fig. 4.18: Diagrammatic representation of fluidized bed bioreactors

The product obtained in the packed bed bioreactor are released into the fluid and removed. While the flow of the liquid can be upward or downward, down flow under gravity is preferred (Fig. 4.19).

The concentration of the nutrients (and therefore the product formed) can be increased by increasing the flow rate of nutrient broth. Because of poor mixing, it is rather difficult to control pH of the packed bed bioreactors by the addition of acid or alkali. However, these bioreactors are preferred for bioprocess technology involving product inhibited reactions. The packed bed bioreactors do not allow the significant accumulation of the product in the bioreactor.

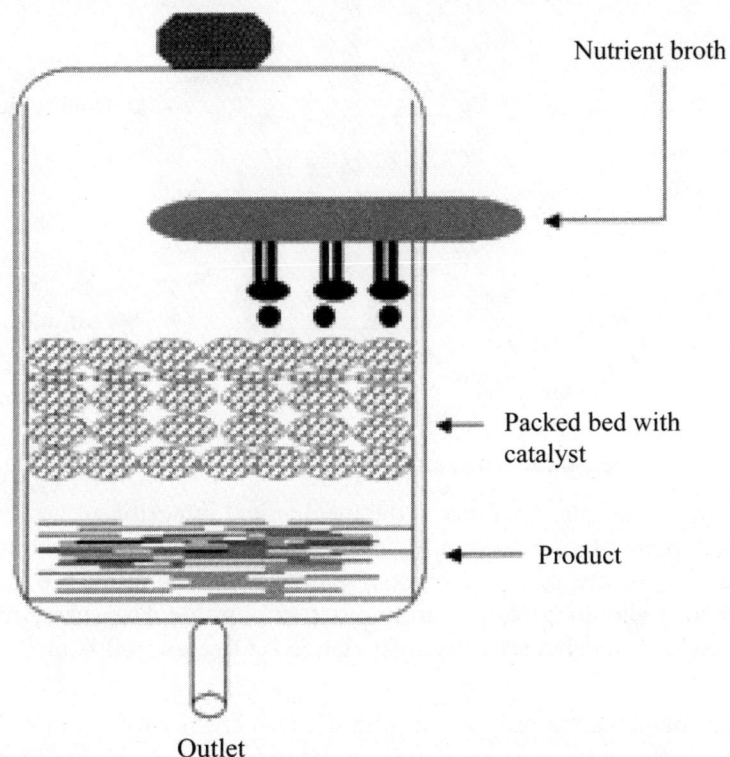

Fig. 4.19: Diagrammatic representation of packed bed bioreactors

4.7. FERMENTER DESIGNS

Environment sensitive processes require a closed and controlled environment to be maintained within the fermenter, but maintenance of an aseptic entry and outlet for the nutrient media, air, and provision for heating, cooling and agitation are required for the success of a fermentation process. Moreover, these fermenters are better maintainable as compared to chemical reactors which suffer from corrosion and contamination. The fermenter design is quite simple and much effort has been devoted to an efficient fermenter design so as to increase the versatility of the process and to evolve a generalized design for a fermenter that is applicable to all the biological processes (Fig. 4.20).

4.7.1. Fundamental rules in designing of a fermenter

The fundamental basis for the design and construction of any aseptically operated plant are based on the principle that micro-organisms are extremely small dimensions much less than normal engineering tolerance which are permitted in case of tight closed container in a non-biological process. Strictly aseptic conditions have to be maintained. Yet, the maintenance of such conditions entails high expenditure and inconvenience in building, operation and maintenance of the plant.

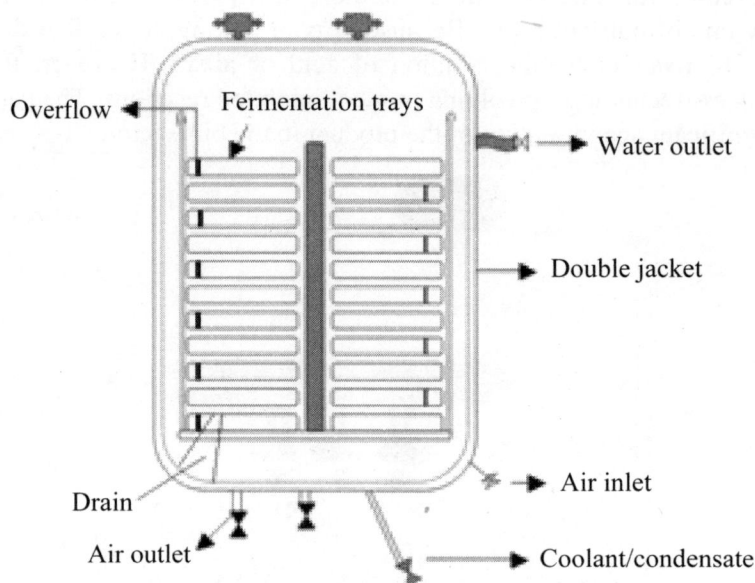

Fig. 4.20: Diagrammatic representation of tray fermenter

In order to conduct aseptic operations, the mechanical integrity of the fermentation plant should be maintained. Entry points to the aseptic region of the plant such as mechanical seals for agitators and pump shafts, valve closures, probe insertions, sample ports and joints are loci prone for contamination risks and hence they should be as few in number as possible The structure as far as possible should not be all welded with mechanical closures; flanged, O screw joints etc. can be replaced by welded joints.

The resulting maintenance problem in a system where removal and replacement of a component involves cutting and rewelding is justified if contamination is to be avoided. Wherever such closures are not possible, a steam box should surround the joint. All other connections to the aseptic region of the plant should be steam sealed, including the glands of the valves used to control liquid flow and steam flow in the pipe and to the steam lock. There should be no connection between the sterile and non sterile sections of the plant.

Pipeline should be kept under steam when not in use and should be constructed as a slope to a definite drain point so that stagnant liquid cannot accumulate at any point. The steam is fed at top of the slope and the condensate is allowed to drain through a steam trap at the drain point. The general design should be such that it avoids stagnant regions, dead spaces, pockets, pipe branches and crevices which not only collect stagnant liquid and micro-organisms but are also difficult to sterilize effectively. These areas are also more liable to corrosion.

4.7.2. Materials and components

Suitable grade of stainless steel is one of the commonest construction material used in production scale fermenters. Different formulations of steel with differing mechanical strength, corrosion resistance, ease of fabrication, availability and cost are available and could be selected according to the requirement of the operation. Stainless steel is more reliable than ordinary mild steel due to its high mechanical strength as well as corrosion resistance due to the chromium oxide layer and thus resistance to the oxidizing conditions. Some of its drawbacks are the ease of damage by reducing agents and high cost as well as difficulty to weld. An alloy containing 14% chromium, 4% nickel and 3% molybdenum has given best result so far.

Valves are needed to regulate fluid flow and should be capable of handling hot and cold liquids possibly containing suspended solids and steam. They constitute an infection risk point since they inevitably involve a joint or mechanical closure. Diaphragm valves are widely used in fermentation, but for strictly aseptic conditions, a piston valve with a steam sealed gland is used.

Pumps should be avoided wherever possible. As an alternative the gravitational movement for the flow of fluids can be utilized, as in case of pump(s) there are moving components which increase contamination risk. However, wherever necessary, they could be supplemented with an intermediate sterilization stage. Centrifugal pumps are commonly used in the biological industry with a seal on the rotating drive shaft and for strictly aseptic operation steam sealed piston pumps are commonly utilized.

Furthermore, in order to impart flexibility to the operation the main plant section should be capable of independent sterilization but must be connected through a steam lock to prevent contamination from unsterilized plant getting connected to sterile plant. The valves are protected by circulating steam through their glands. A full scale plant should have a large number of such locks so that sterilization of units and transfer of material around the plant involves hundreds of sequential operations of valves, instruments and pumps, in such cases computerized controls could serve effectively to ensure the precise sequence of operation.

In the case of aerobic biological process the major requirement is perfect sterile air supply. A typical fermentation batch has to be supplied; with hundreds of tons of perfectly microbe free air. The most effective method to achieve this is the utilization of deep fibrous filters for rendering air free of contaminating micro-organisms. The effect of the depth of the pad on the particle removal is logarithmic, i.e. each unit depth of the pad removes the same proportion of the passing particles from the air in an exponential fashion. The pads are routinely cleaned and sterilized by passing steam through it. The simplest example of these filters is the HEPA (high efficiency particulate air filters) made up of the membranous fibrous supports. These filters have got the pores which retain the bacterial particulates from the air, (a pore size of 0.2 μm) and hence resulting in an absolute sterilization of the air. These filter media are made up of high tensile cellulosic fibers, unglazed, ceramics, and porous plastics.

4.7.3. Selection of the fermenter

The selection of the type, size, and mode of operation and the pattern of the fermenter to be used in a particular biological process is based on the following characteristics of the biological process, are determination of choice of fermenter is:

4.7.3.1. Characteristics of the microorganisms to be used

The mode of operation depends substantially on the type and the stability of the microbes stain. The operation conditions are decisively selected by the factor considering whether the strain is aerobic or anaerobic. In the breeding of the aerobic strains adequate amounts of the oxygen is required. Since the solubility of the oxygen in the medium is low therefore it should be available at a constant rate continuously. The size and the shape of the cells also have considerable effect on the design of the fermenter. Spherical cells are usually smaller and less sensitive to shear than the filamentous organisms. The former needs a higher degree of dispersion of the air than the filamentous mycelia. Small dimensions ensure a high surface to volume ratio and a high rate of uptake of substrate and therefore a rapid growth. Aerobic cells with high rates of growth exhibit high rates of oxygen consumption.

Many organisms tend to grow on surfaces. In the case of metabolite-producing organisms of sewage treatment, these properties may be desirable if continuous operation is required. If this property is pronounced than the surface reactors must be used. In general the film formation is not desirable. If cells show a tendency to grow on the surface, the formation of the stagnant region at the surface must be avoided by a suitable fermenter design.

4.7.3.2. Characteristics predetermined by the properties of the medium

The choice of the strain generally determines not only the culture medium but also exerts a pronounced influence on the choice of the reactor. The characteristics of the medium such as physical properties, biokinetics, difficulty in sterilization and rheological behavior are critical for the selection of the reactor. The physical properties of the substrate used generally differ-gaseous (e.g., methane), liquid and water-soluble (e.g., methanol, ethanol) solid and water-soluble (e.g., glucose, lactose) liquid and water-insoluble (e.g., gas-oil and paraffin) and solid and sparingly soluble or insoluble in water (e.g., starch, cellulose) which affect the choice of bioreactor. On the other hand the biokinetic effects of the substrate or the products also affect the choice of reactor. In the case of substrates showing inhibition or repression of growth, the process is carried out either in semi continuous operation with sustained feed of the substrate ("extended culture" or "fed batch culture") or in a continuous culture. In the case of the thermolabile components of the medium there is a need of special measures to be taken up frequently and to incorporate separate sterilization processes for these materials.

The rheological behavior of the medium has very great influence. An increasing viscosity may influence the rheological properties of the medium, which may arise together due to:

- The secretion of highly viscous products, e.g., pollulan and xanthan particularly in batch operation at the end of the formation of product;
- High concentration of substrate; and
- The morphology of the organisms.

When substrate or product is responsible for the high viscosity, the medium frequently has a new-toning behavior. A high apparent viscosity due to the morphology of the organisms is almost always associated with a non-Newtonian behavior depicted by the medium.

4.7.3.3. Characteristics predetermined by the parameters of the biomedical process

A fundamental factor influencing the choice of the fermenter in the cultivation of aerobic organisms is the specific oxygen transfer rate in the medium. In the case of the continuous fermentation the processes are never carried out in the regime of unlimited growth, since here the fermenter tends to be unstable. The rate of growth and rate of product formation are temperature dependent. Consequently, the cultivation and the formation of the product are usually carried out at controlled temperatures. To facilitate the removal of the in-process generated heat from the fermenter to the cooling water, generally the use of thermophilic organisms is desired. As the volume of the fermenter increases, a limit is reached at which the heat produced cannot be removed solely via the cooling jacket.

The pH of the cell cultivation is determined by the optimum pH desired for reaction. The lowest possible pH that suppresses infection by contaminating organisms is preferred.

4.7.3.4. Characteristics predetermined by the site

The choice of the fermenter depends on the production site. A number of factors which are responsible for choice determination are:

Table 4.9: Fermentation based commercial products

Product	Microorganism
Industrial chemicals	
Ethanol (from glucose)	*Saccharomyces cerevisiae*
Ethanol (from lactose)	*Kluyveromyces fragilis*
Citric acid	*Aspergillus niger*
Gluconic acid	*Aspergillus niger*
Acetic acid	*Acetobacter* spp.
Lactic acid	*Lactobacillus delbrueckii*
Amino acids	
L-lysine	*Corynebacterium glutamicum*
MSG	*C. glutamicum*
Glutamic acid	*C. glutamicum*
Vitamins	
Riboflavin	*Ashbya gossypi*
Vitamin B_{12}	*Pseudomonas denitrificans*
Ascorbic acid (L-sorbose)	*Gluconobacter oxidans*
Enzymes	
Amylase	*Aspergillus oryzae*
Cellulase	*Trichoderma reesii*
Invertase	*Saccharomyces cerevisiae*
Lipase	*Saccharomyces lipolytica*
Protease	*Bacillus*
Polysaccharides	
Dextran	*Leuconostoc mesenteroides*
Xanthan gum	*Xanthomonas compestris*
Pharmaceuticals	
Penicillin	*Penicillium chrysogenum*
Cephalosporin	*Cephalosporium acemonium*
Amphotericin B	*Streptomyces nodosus*
Kanamycin	*Streptomyces kanamyceticus*
Neomycin	*Streptomyces fradiae*
Streptomycin	*Streptomyces griseus*
Gramicidin S	*Bacillus brevis*
Polymyxin	*B. polymyxa*
Chloramphenicol	*Streptomyces venezualae* or chemical synthesis
Erythromycin	*Streptomyces erythreus*
Steroidal transformations	*Rhizopus nigricans*

1. Trading facilities for the product as well as the raw material
2. Availability of raw materials and their supply
3. The cost of raw materials and labor (skilled or unskilled)
4. Cost of energy and cooling water
5. Economical use of the byproducts

6. Working and safety regulations

7. Market features (stable sales-single product works or when a variable sales a flexible plant is required)

All these aspects have to be carefully examined before choosing the fermenter. In general depending on the size of the production to be planned, the number of fermenter units should not fall below a minimum. However, the plant should be capable of producing more than one product so that an economical utilization of the same could be assured. Experience proves that although the plant is utilized for a single product, a flexible design comprising of considerable reserves for the flows of materials and drives should be utilized. The correct manipulations of the parameters as well as the choice of the producing strain and media composition are critical considerations for achieving high yield in fermentation.

4.8. FERMENTATION BASED INDUSTRIAL PRODUCTS

4.8.1. Antibiotics

Research efforts made in the field of antibiotics have been rising and falling: following the discovery of penicillin, amazingly no other antibiotic was introduced into the market for quite some time. With the introduction of second-generation lactam type antibiotics, research was revitalized. Therefore that time is considered as the golden era in antibiotic research. Since the discovery of penicillin in 1942, more than 5,500 natural microbial compounds, which display antibiotic activity, have been discovered. Only a relatively small number of these products have been found to be practically useful. About 150 antibiotic compounds are currently being produced exclusively by the fermentation process. These antibiotics have distinct applications in medical, veterinary and agriculture practices.

The term antibiotic appeared as early as 1924 in the French microbiological literature related to antibiotics. The word antibiotic in its retrospective meaning is a biosynthetic product of microbial origin which has the capacity of inhibiting growth, and even distorting other micro-organisms in dilute solutions. Most antibiotics are produced by fermentation, but detailed discussion is beyond the scope of the book. Only a few important antibiotics with their production strategy are discussed here.

4.8.1.1. Tetracycline

It is now over 30 years since tetracycline was discovered as an antibiotic. Biological research till date has been focused on its production organism (morphological and physiological studies, improvement procedures, genetic analysis, etc.), on biosynthetic, metabolic, and genetic controls, on the mechanism of antibiotic action and origin of resistance as well as on various pharmacological aspects of tetracycline application. The basic structure of tetracycline as shown in Fig. 4.21 and chemistry of tetracycline represented in table 4.10.

4.8.1.1.1. Strain improvement and genetics of tetracycline producers

Tetracycline is produced mainly by *S.aureofaciens* and *S. rimosus*. With modern technologies, tetracycline production has increased manifold by utilizing various breeding techniques. A general consideration, the strain improvement technique, i.e. mutation could be utilized. In the case of tetracycline the use of the technique increased the antibiotic titer by 30-500%, depending on the strain, the mutagen and a number of selection steps. The best results were obtained with the mutagens like UV light, ethyleneimine, X-rays, γ-radiation and nitrogen mustards alone or in combinations. Further, by utilizing appropriate selection systems like isolation of prototrophic revertants from auxotrophs, producing revertants of non producing mutants, etc., some good strains for better selection were developed. Hybridoma techniques did not contribute much to the strain improvement effort as compared to mutational selection.

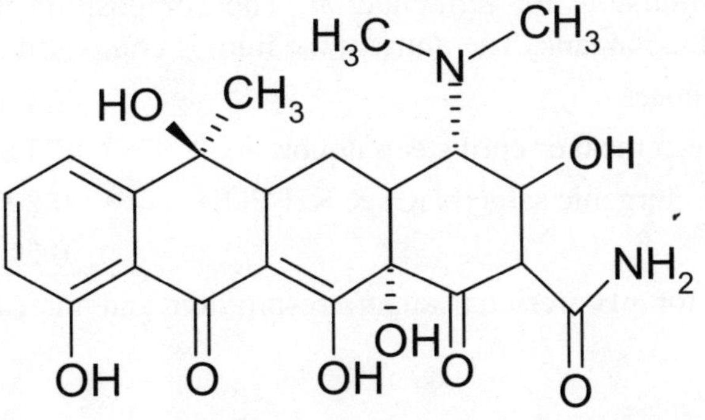

Fig. 4.21: Basic ring of tetracycline

Table 4.10: Chemistry of tetracycline

Name	R^2	R^5	R^6	$R^{6'}$	R^7
Oxytetracycline	H	H	OH	CH_3	Cl
Tetracycline	H	OH	OH	CH_3	H
Demeclocycline	H	H	OH	CH_3	H
Methacycline	H	OH	$=CH_2$	H	H
Doxycycline	H	OH	H	CH_3	H
Minocycline	H	H	H	H	$N(CH_3)_2$

4.8.1.1.2. Fermentation processes

Unlike abundant literature available on medical and technological applications of tetracycline, references on process technology are rather scant. This is surprising as the tetracycline is in the hundred million dollar fraternity. Fermentation technology of five of the principal tetracycline antibiotics has been protected by 33 US patents. Most of the patents reported tetracycline yields up to hundred or thousands of µg/ml of fermenter broth, the existing industrial yields exceed 20,000 µg/ml with, about 200 hours fermentation.

Equipment

The fermentation tanks described previously can be utilized for an appropriate production of tetracyclines. However, for proper growth, a fermenter should provide facility for oxygen supply (0.4-0.4 ~ mol/liter per min.) in a fermenter of 100-150 m^3 working volume. It should have three open turbines 1460-2100 mm in diameter and maximum speed of 40 rpm, and a power input of 300 kW at the axle, which corresponds to 3 kW/m^3 of fermented broth. Variable revolution stirrers are often advantageous, so as to solve the inverse relationship between oxygen transfer into the liquid by the stirrer and the shear stress of the biomass, and they can better cope with foam formation particularly when the stirrer cannot be switched off. The supply of oxygen should be carefully monitored for proper yield of tetracycline.

Preparation of inoculum

For prolonged preservation, the strains for industrial fermenters are maintained either by freeze-drying or at liquid nitrogen temperature as spore stock. A stepwise flow sheet (Fig. 4.22) shows .the preparation of *S. aureofaciens* inoculum.

A temperature of 29°C is suitable for fermentation. The composition of inoculum medium is similar to that used in the production tank. The nutrient medium is composed of:

Carbohydrate: sucrose and maltose	2.5% w/v
Organic nitrogen source: soybean meal or corn steep liquor	1.7% w/v
Buffer: calcium carbonate and inorganic salts (NaCI & KH_2PO_4)	0.2-0.3% w/v
Vegetable oil	0.2% w/v

The culture is monitored for pH, residual sugar, respiration and increase of biomass both in volume and morphology.

Nutrients

Commercially produced strains utilize sucrose (molasses), starch or technical glucose as cheap carbon sources. Being a polysaccharide, starch is particularly suitable for prolonged fermentation of about 200 hours. Organic nitrogen sources include corn-steep, soybean meal, and peanut meal. Calcium carbonate not only helps in maintaining pH, but also binds the formed antibiotic from the heterogeneous phase of complexes insoluble above 1500~g/ml and thus decreases the inhibitory effect of their own products on the product ions. Animal or vegetable lipids are used as antifoaming agents and even as carbon sources. Chloride ions serve as processors of chlortetracycline biosynthesis, while benzyl thiocyanate is used as an inhibitor of undesirable metabolic pathway, particularly in the absence of oxygen.

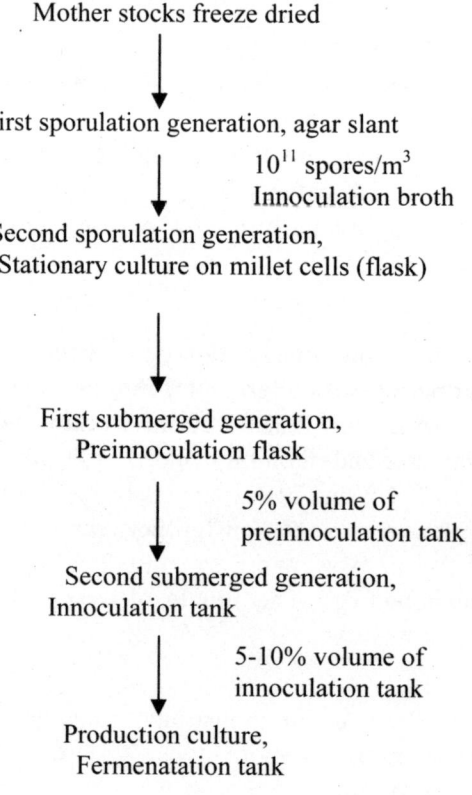

Fig. 4.22: Preparation of inoculum

4.8.1.1.3. Process parameters in production

The sterilization of liquid nutrient broth is undertaken either at 120°C for 40 minutes or at 140°C for 1 min interval (carbon and nitrogen separately). Stirring uses 2.5-5 kW/m^3 medium, revolutions can be varied up to a peripheral velocity of the propeller equal to 500m/min, aeration ranges up to 0.4 medium vol./min, and oxygen over pressure up to 0.1 M psi. The temperature (29±1°C), pH, oxygen content of medium (at least 20% saturation), and CO_2 in outlet air are monitored continuously.

4.8.1.1.4 Product recovery and purification

The major aspect of isolation process focuses around the amphotropic nature of the substances and the possibility of their polymerization and rearrangement. Several cases have been reported with different methods of isolation and purification of various tetracyclines in various patents. Some of them are compiled here and are presented below:

i. Adsorption on diatomaceous earth or active charcoal.

ii. Chromatography or selective extraction.

iii. Extraction from acid or alkaline medium. The most frequently used extraction agent is I-butanol, owing to its suitable partition coefficient and economic availability.

iv. Direct mesh extraction based on solubilization of the antibiotic by acidification, precipitation of Ca^{2+} with ammonium compounds as carriers, and extraction of metabolites with an organic solvent usually with methyl alkyl ketone.

v. Precipitation (dry salt) process is based on precipitating the antibiotic from dilute aqueous solution of aryl azosulfonic acid dyes. Tetracyclines are precipitated as complexes with alkaline earth metal compounds or with primary and secondary alkyl amine.

vi. Solvent extraction of antibiotic with salt, based on salting out (NaCl) of the antibiotic from the aqueous to the organic phase (I-butanol). This method is also suited for refining of a crude product. The preparations are purified by crystallization as salts (e.g., hydrochlorides) or bases. Particularly efficient is crystallization from boiling solvent, such as lower alcohols, ketones or aliphatic ethers of ethylene glycol, which yield non-hygroscopic preparations. The specific crystal surface depends upon temperature, stirring and pH value. The schematic representation of production of Tetracycline showed in Figure 4.23.

4.8.1.2 Penicillin

In 1924 Alexander Fleming's curiosity was aroused by zones of inhibition surrounding mould colonies contaminating a used petridish. On further investigations he concluded that the mould had secreted a compound which has activity against several pathogenic bacteria. He named the lytic filtrate of the mould *P. notatum* as penicillin. Further development of this compound has revolutionized the treatment of bacterial infections and has led to the discovery and served as a model for the development of numerous pharmacologically active compounds produced by fermentation. In 1941, when penicillin manufacturing began in United States, the process was to grow the *P. notatum* on the surface of a simple medium for 5–10 days and to use the liquid underlying the culture, which contained the penicillin in concentration of 10–20 Oxford units per ml (an activity equivalent to 0.006-0.012 mg pure benzyl penicillin sodium salt). A solvent extraction procedure was used to isolate the material for clinical, pharmacological and chemical characterization.

4.8.1.2.1. Process overview

The technology of the manufacturing process is still regarded as highly proprietary in nature by the major commercial firms even though excellent fermentation technology and organisms are available for purchase. Similarly, purification of these compounds is thoroughly described in the literature. The distinguishing aspects of commercially acceptable process are based on operational simplicity and cost effectiveness. This explicitly entails for process optimization and development of better alternative options.

Various penicillins viz., penicillin G and penicillin V are produced by *P. chrysogenum*, provided the appropriate carboxylic side chain is added to the medium in sufficient quantities. Basically, the process involves the cultivation of *P. chrysogenum* in vessels of increasing size up to 200,000 liters beginning with a slant or a vial of frozen vegetative mycelium. At harvest, the batch is filtered to remove the mycelium and the filtrate is extracted and crystallized or precipitated by acidification.

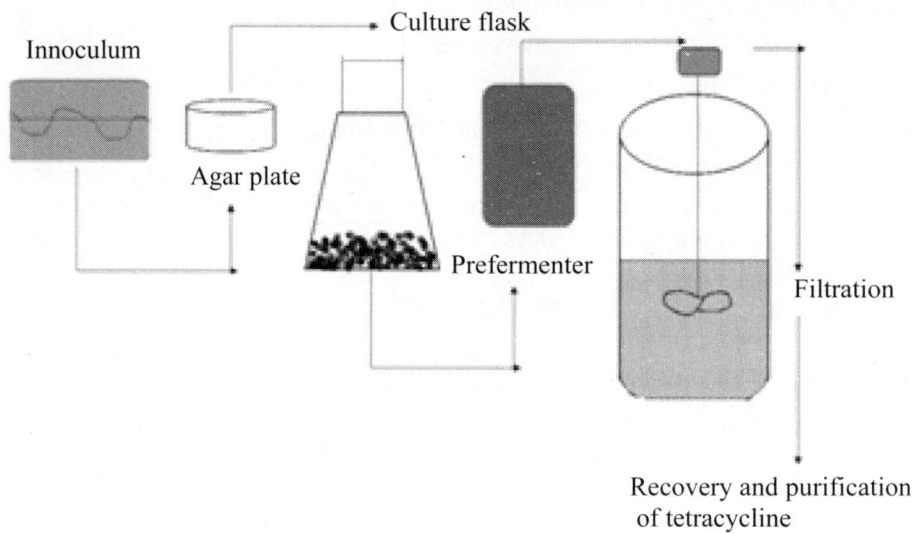

Fig. 4.23: Flow chart of production of tetracycline

4.8.1.2.2. Strain development

Strain maintenance and initial seed

The process begins with lyophilized spores of selected producer strain. Alternatives are to store the master or secondary cell bank in the form of spore suspension in liquid nitrogen or as frozen vegetative material with glycerol and/or lactose as suspending agents at either -70°C or in liquid nitrogen. Frozen spores are inoculated on slants and allowed to sporulate, then transferred to a vegetative culture in Erlenmeyer flask containing a vegetative medium generally of similar composition as of the production medium. The schematic representation of production of penicillins showed in Fig. 4.24.

Mutation

Until the middle 1960's, UV irradiation and nitrogen mustards were the preferred mutagens used in penicillin strain improvement. Table 6.6 lists the various mutagens which were used. In recent years, NTG, a mutagen providing extremely high mutation rate as compared to its lethal effect has become the preferred compound. NTG has a high potential of inducing different mutations. Screening (i.e., examining all members of a mutagenized population) has been the most significant technique for increasing the penicillin yields to date. One approach to improve the efficiency of the procedure is the potency index agar plate technique used for the improvement of high yielding cultures. In this case the zone size was reduced by incorporating penicillinase in agar to reduce the sensitivity to a useful range.

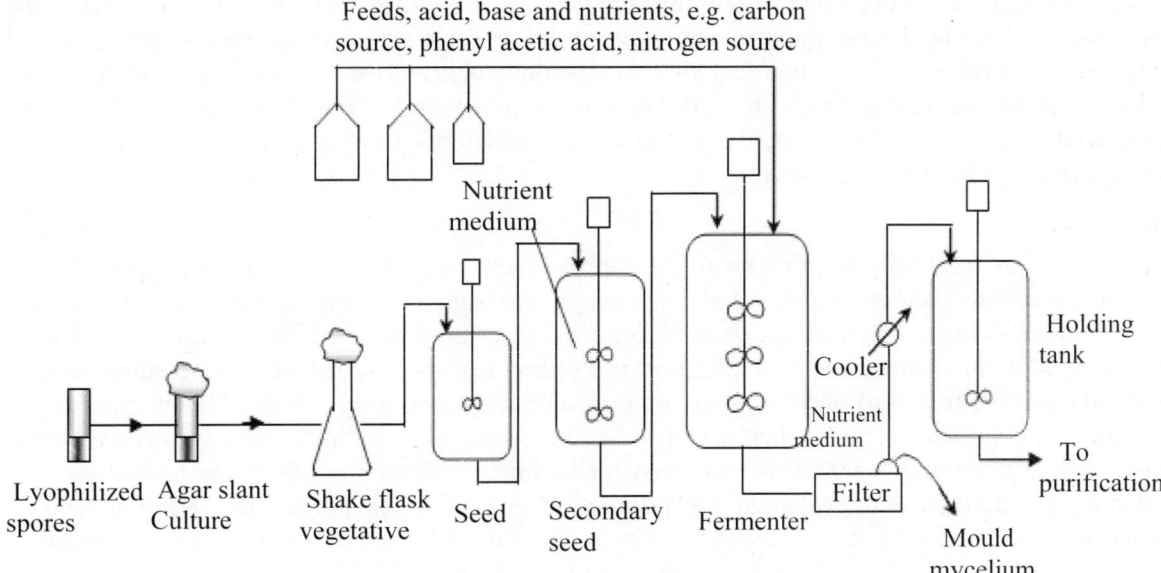

Fig. 4.24: Flow chart of production of penicillin

Table 4.11: List of various mutagens used in the improvement of penicillin yields by *P. chrysogenum*

S.No.	Mutagens	S.No.	Mutagens
1.	Methylbis(2-chloroethyl)amine	5.	Ethyl methanesulfonate
2.	Ultraviolet light irradiation (275 and 253 nm)	6.	X-rays
3.	Nitrous acid	7.	γ -rays
4.	Diepoxybutane	8.	Ethyl amine

Selection

The proven success of the empirical approach has been appreciated widely (mutation and screening for increasing potency) even though it is a tedious procedure. A specific selection procedure designed to identify organisms producing and possessing a desired phenotype (generally by allowing only that group to survive) can greatly increase the effectiveness of the program provided that the trait is selected from the whole population so as to improve the yield. Several different and quite successful selective techniques are described in literature. The improved yield has been achieved largely through the sequential application of the selective procedure involving high concentrations of amino acids, biosynthetic intermediates and amino group analogues. These selective techniques presumably lead to the organisms with the higher levels of amino acids and intermediates. An important contaminant of the high potency broth turned out to be oxidized parahydroxy form of phenyl acetic acid which, when incorporated interferes with the semisynthetic chemistry of the analogs. An interesting selection technique used by Pan Labs involved selection and further evaluation of small colonies from plates with phenylacetic acid used as sole carbon source, except for just enough glucose to produce a small colony.

Thus the small colonies selected were those impaired in terms of the ability to oxidize the side chain precursor. The technique was successful and as a result several commercial users of P14B-4 and its progeny are concerned about interference by p-hydroxy penicillin G. Also this loss of precursor is eliminated. The literature is mainly useful as source of information on approaches which may prove useful in the development of other strains such as those producing cephalosporin and helping the physiologist to understand the organism for which the nutritional environment must be optimized. The strain improvement and selection procedures have promoted development of the linkage between the whole processes.

Genetics

Genetic studies were utilized in two ways to improve penicillin production. First studies with blocked mutants facilitated understanding of the pathways and suggested appropriate selective techniques described previously. Second, the two techniques that have allowed the merging of potentially desirable traits are parasexual breeding and protoplast fusion. The parasexual breeding techniques basically involve fusion of one strain having desirable traits with other strain. The parents are grown together on complete medium, then selected for the presence of both markers, allowed sporulating, and stable diploid spores are then isolated. After various treatments to allow recombination, haploid colonies are derived and evaluated for production and other characteristics. Recombinants with superior yields over the parents have been effectively utilized for industrial strain improvement.

4.8.1.2..3. Fermentation process

Facilities

Production of penicillin G or V by fermentation is carried out in liquid culture. In modern practice the culture volume is typically 40,000-200,000 liter. The process is aerobic, having a volumetric oxygen uptake rate in the range of 0.4-1.0 mMol/lit/min and an RQ of approximately 0.95. Oxygen is supplied by passing air through the culture at a rate of 0.5-1.0 volumes of air (volume of fluid)$^{-1}$ min^{-1} and the air are vigorously purged through fluid using turbine agitators of various designs.

Power introduced to the culture is generally of the order of 1-4 WI^{-1} including that introduced by the air stream. Other fermenter designs, including Waldhof fermenters and air-blown columns, are used, some of which are either more energy efficient than the conventional designs or offer other advantages in terms of capital costs or higher oxygen-transport capacity.

Inoculum development

The main purpose of vegetative cultures and subsequent inoculum development steps is to increase the biomass with a population which can be added to the next stage, such that each step will be reasonably short and large-scale equipment could be used efficiently.

Inoculum development stages are typically conducted at 25°C in shake cultures and agitated vessels. A typical vegetative or seed-stage medium contains an organic nitrogen source, such as corn-steep liquor, and a sufficient concentration of a fermentable carbohydrate, such as 2% (w/v) sucrose or glucose. Calcium carbonate is often included as a buffer at 0.5–1.0% (w/v) concentration level. Other inorganic salts required for proper growth are also incorporated. Lag-phase growth is usually desirable in these stages, and a mass doubling time of about six hours (minimum for typical production strains) is achieved. Criteria for monitoring the inoculum stages include cycle time, change in pH value, residual carbon source concentration, packed cell volume and respiration rate.

4.8.1.2.4. Culture medium

Carbon source

P. chrysogenum can utilize a variety of carbon and energy sources. Various carbon sources used for penicillin production are sucrose, dextrin, and starches. Crude carbohydrates of low purity such as molasses have also been used. Animal and vegetable oils and ethanol inclusion has also been reported. Stoichiometric ratio number of moles of oxygen consumed per kilogram of sugar is constant at 33, regardless of growth rate and that the concentration of glucose after the rapid growth phase remains constant within a range of glucose feed rate to the fermenter. This indicates that under certain conditions the carbon in the fat or glucose is completely combusted for energy production and is not incorporated into cell mass.

Nutrients other than carbon-energy sources

In general the media used in the earlier years of penicillin production and those being used now are quite similar. Table 4.12 presents commonly used media.

Table 4.12: Typical fermentation media for production of penicillin G or V in 1945 and 1967

1945	Concentration	1967	Concentration
Lactose	3-4%	Glucose or molasses (by continuous feed)	10.0% total
Corn steep liquor solids	3.5%	Corn steep liquor solids	4-5%
Calcium carbonate	1.0%	Phenylacetic acid (by continuous feed)	0.5-0.4% total
KH$_2$PO$_4$	0.4%	cod oil (or vegetable oil) antifoam (by continuous feed)	
Lard oil antifoam	0.25%		

Nitrogen source

Until 1975 most industrial processes included corn steep liquor as an organic nitrogen source in the media. This was included due to a marked increase in the yield of penicillin after its addition because it is a component precursor of side chain. Later reports suggested that cottonseed meals could also be a satisfactory substitute for corn steep liquor.

Side chain processor

Recent studies have demonstrated that the side chain attachment is relatively non specific and that relatively high concentrations of phenylactic acid and phenoxyacetic acid (sodium salts) have to be included in the medium or in feeds of the fermenter, if the desired single component penicillin is to be obtained. In order to avoid toxicity of sodium phenyl acetate as well as its deterioration due to hydroxylation by the microorganism, it is fed at a well defined rate continuously throughout the process. More than 90% conversion of phenyl acetic acid into penicillin G side chain has been obtained through continuous feeding of one of its salts to maintain a low residual concentration. The penicillin V precursor, phenoxyacetic acid may be fed in a few large doses. More than 40% of the material can be incorporated into the penicillin V side chain.

Sulfur source

Ammonium sulfate is a common ingredient used in the production media for providing nitrogen and sulfur in the proportions necessary for penicillin synthesis. Sulfur is also provided in significant quantities by the organic nitrogen sources used in media.

Phosphorus source

Phytic acid in corn steep liquor is an important source of phosphorus. Phosphorus may also be added in the form of inorganic salts and can be maintained by feeding inorganic phosphorus salts. A level of phosphate phosphorus of 250 to 500 mg/ml is optimum for penicillin production.

Other nutrients

Inorganic salts of potassium and magnesium as well as additional nitrogen, phosphorus and sulfur are necessary for growth and product formation. Chemically defined media include requirements for phosphorus, sulfur, potassium, magnesium, manganese, zinc, cobalt and copper.

4.8.1.2.5. Recovery of penicillin

Carbon process

The original commercial process of penicillin recovery from the fermentation broth was based upon the adsorption of the product on activated charcoal. The carbon is collected, washed with water and the carbon adsorbate is eluted with 40% acetone. The penicillin is concentrated by distillation or evaporation under vacuum at 15-32°C. The remaining aqueous solution is cooled to 2°C, acidified to pH 2.0-3.0 and the penicillin extracted into amyl acetate from which it is crystallized with excess mineral salts of buffer near neutral pH under vacuum. As higher quantities of penicillin are produced, this approach became impractical because of excessively increased carbon requirements.

Solvent extraction process (industrial standards)

An outline of the current standard process is presented in table 4.13. Solvent extraction forms the basis of isolation and purification.

Table 4.13: Outline of the penicillin purification process

Steps	Purpose	Equipment	Bases
Filtration	Separate mycelia from penicillin	Rotary drum vacuum filter	Size of particles
Extraction	Remove soluble contaminants	Mixer and drum filter	Adsorption of impurities
Crystallization	Further purification and stabilization	Tank and drum filter, settlers, or basket centrifuge	Via addition of Na or K salts
Drying	Stabilization	Horizontal belt filters/warm dry air	Dry solvent vacuum or air

The basic process has changed very little since late 1940s except for the addition of automatic controls and simplifications permitted by broth of higher potency and purity, by increased scale of operation and also by improved design of specific equipment. Typical steps and related yields for the solvent extraction process are presented in table 4.14.

4.8.2. AMINO ACIDS

4.8.2.1. L-lysine

A considerable amount of attention has been focused on the production of amino acids by fermentation process. L-lysine is currently manufactured by a process protected by United States patents.

Table 4.14: Typical yields in penicillin purification

Step	Yield
Holding	95% but losses can even be large if broth is not rapidly chilled or if microbial contamination occurs
Filtration	90-95% based on filtrate assay. 5% of the loss is accounted for by insoluble solids in the broth. Other losses are from degradation and leakage to drain.
Solid extraction	
Single stage	40-90%
Lead-trail	92-96%
Aqueous (back) extraction	95-97%
Crystallization	95%
Drying	95%
Overall	74%

A large number of microorganisms have been identified which produce free extracellular lysine in small quantities. Richard and Haskins (1957) screened some 600 fungi in order to determine their ability to form free, extracellular lysine in submerged culture conditions. However, further investigations revealed some other microorganisms producing a considerable yield of lysine. The yield obtained about 400 μg/ml of extracellular lysine in shaken flasks using strains of *Gliocladium* species and a strain of *Ustilago maydis*.

4.8.2.1.1. Fermentation for production of lysine

Industrial production of lysine is based on a two-step process. Diaminopimelic acid is first produced by microorganisms (*Corynebacterium diphtheriae* and *Mycobacterium tuberculosum*). It is then converted into L-lysine as described by Casida (1964).

New strain development and improvement

Although L-lysine is industrially produced by the above process, some work on mutation and selection principles has yielded novel strains that could alternatively be utilized. Furthermore, the use of mutant strains of *C. glutamicum* has been effectively utilized for production of lysine. It could be inferred that aspartokinase, the first enzyme in the biosynthetic route, is inhibited only when lysine and threonine are present above their respective threshold concentrations. An important feature of the pathway is that lysine does not exert any control over the biosynthetic route from aspartic semialdehyde into lysine. A mutant which did not catalyze the conversion of aspartic semialdehyde to homoserine would grow only in homoserine supplemented medium and so would be described as a homoserine auxotroph. If such an organism were grown in the presence of very low concentration of homoserine, the endogenous level of threonine would not reach the inhibitory concentration of aspartokinase control and aspartate will be converted to lysine. The knowledge of a biosynthetic route allows the geneticist to raise a mutant showing desirable features.

The control of lysine production in *B.flavum* is similar to that as shown for *C. glutamicum*. Lysine analogues (2-aminoethyl)- cysteine (AEC) inhibited growth completely in the presence of threonine which indicates that AEC plus threonine cause feedback inhibition of aspartokinase and deprive the organism of lysine and methionine. Mutants growing in AEC and threonine were isolated by plating the survivors of mutation treatments onto agar containing the two factors. A relatively high proportion of resulting colonies were lysine overproducers.

4.8.2.1.2. Commercial production process

A two-stage process is used for the commercial production of lysine. First step involves the production of diaminopimelic acid and the second involves its conversion into L-lysine.

Step 1: Diaminopimelic acid production

A large number of organisms can produce this acid. The production of diaminopimelic acid utilizing *Corynebacterium diphtheriae* and *Mycobacterium tuberculosum* was also reported. The high yield reported by some lysine-requiring auxotrophs of *E. coli* (A.T.C.C. 12,404). For industrial production, A.T.C.C. 12,404 strain of *E. coli* is utilized.

Inoculum preparation I

The inoculum for production medium could be prepared by growing *E .coli* A.T.C.C., 12,404 for 20 h at 24°C with proper agitation and aeration in a medium of following composition:

Glycerol	0.5%
Corn-steep liquor	0.5%
$(NH_4)_2HPO_4$	0.5%

pH of the medium is adjusted to 7.5 with KOH. The medium is sterilized at a pressure of 20 psi for 30 min.

Instrumental requirement

The fermenter design is quite similar to those mentioned earlier. The fermenter tank however, should be equipped with an agitator and an appropriate air supply device. The temperature should be controlled at 24°C.

Growth medium

One production medium, cited as an example in the patent issued to Casida, contained:

$(NH_4)_2 HPO_4$	4.0%
$CaCO_3$	0.5%
Glycerol	6.0%
Corn-steep liquor	4.0%

The pH of the medium is adjusted to 7.5 with KOH and medium is sterilized. The medium may be seeded with 1 to 5 % of inoculum and incubated at 24°C with agitation and aeration (1% v/v of medium per minute). Traces of soybean oil or DC anti foam-A may be added.

Process control

During fermentation, it is important to maintain the pH in the range of 7 to 7.5. After about 24 h it is necessary to add an alkali, ammonium hydroxide being preferred (but KOH and NaOH are satisfactory), after about 64 hours, it may be necessary to add H_2SO_4. Aeration of broth is an important factor and should be controlled. The temperature should be maintained at 29°C. Optimum yields (about 9 mg/ml) are obtained in about 3 days.

Step 2: Decarboxylation of diaminopimelic acid to L-lysine

The enzyme diaminopimelic acid decarboxylase that converts diaminopimelic acid into lysine is produced by several bacteria, for example strains of *Aerobacter aerogenes* and *E. coli* which do not require lysine for growth. Earlier studies reported that a strain of *A. aerogenes* (now designated as A.T.C.C., 12409), has been found satisfactory particularly for converting diaminopimelic acid into lysine. This organism lacks the enzyme lysine decarboxylase. *A. aerogenes*, A.T.C.C., 12409, may be grown on the same medium and under similar conditions to those favorable for the propagation of inoculum for the mutant strain of *E. coli*. In general, the conversion of diaminopimelic acid to lysine may be carried out at about 24°C; it is completed in approximately 24 h. Furthermore, the addition of 0.004 to about 0.032 molar citric acid and EDTA sodium salt favors the conversion.

Recovery of lysine

After conversion of diaminopimelic acid to lysine, the reaction mixture is filtered and the lysine is absorbed on a cation-exchange resin such as Amberlite IR-120, and eluted with dilute alkali by passing it through a weak cation-exchange resin such as Amberlite IRC-50. Elutes are pooled and dried to crystallize lysine which may be recrystallized for purification. .

4.8.2.2. L-glutamic acid

It is an essential amino acid and could be produced in various ways: by the hydrolysis of wheat glutin, soybean cake or some other protein rich food materials; by cleavage of pyrrolidone carboxylic acid found in stiffens molasses; or by one step fermentation process using single microorganism; or by a two step process involving a-ketoglutaric acid by fermentation followed by conversion by another microbe or by an enzyme process. The schematic presentation was given below in Fig. 4.25.

4.8.2.2.1. Single stage fermentation process for production of glutamic acid

The commercial process is mainly used in Japan where sweet potatoes are employed as chief raw material. It utilizes the strain of *Micrococcus* no.541 for production of glutamic acid. The strain is a biotin auxotroph, requiring 0.5-5 µg per liter of biotin for good yields. The carbon source may be glucose, fructose, sucrose, maltose, xylose or hydrolyzed starch. Nitrogen source contains at least one of the following components: urea, ammonia, ammonium salts, peptones, corn steep liquor, hydrolyzed casein, meat extract or digested soybean meals or fish meal. The pH of the medium should be maintained within a range of 6-9, however, the optimum range is found to be 7.0–4.5. Ammonium ions are essential for growth. The temperature of the fermenter should be maintained within the range of 27–30°C. Proper aeration of culture is essential for good production.

4.8.2.2.2. Production by *Cephalosporium* species

L-glutamic acid is directly produced by a strain of *Cephalosporium*, such as *C. salmosynnematum* RRL 2271, *C. diospyri* A TCC 9066 or *C. acremonium* A TCC 10141. The mould is cultivated in nutrient medium containing a carbohydrate source and urea at pH 4–9 under aerobic conditions. Fermentation is continued until appreciable amount of L-glutamic acid accumulates.

Two- stage process for production of glutamic acid involves:

(i) Formation of α-ketoglutaric acid.

(ii) Conversion of α-ketoglutaric acid into L-glutamic acid, via enzymatic or microbial conversion.

Production of α-ketoglutaric acid by fermentation was utilizing different microorganisms and shown to be highly productive.

Microorganisms being utilized

Although considerable work has been carried out regarding the utilization of an appropriate microorganism involved in the production of α-ketoglutaric acid yet there is a need of work to establish, identify an appropriate mutant strain which should be utilized for production. Table 4.15 indicates various types of microorganisms which are utilized for improved production of α-ketoglutaric acid.

Table 4.15: Various strains producing L-glutamic acid with their respective yields

Strain No.	Name	Approximate yield (%)
--	*Bacterium α-keloglutaricum*	50–60
--	*Bact. succinicum*	13.6
1	*Bacillus megatherium*	20.6
2	*B. natto (var.B. subtilis)*	14.6
3	*Escherichia coli*	40–60
7	*Escherichia coli*	40–60
5,9,12	*E. freundii*	40–60
4	*Aerobacter cloacae*	40–60
44C,11	*Kluyvera citrophila var. α*	40–60
NRRLB-6	*Pseudomonas fluorescens (reptilivora)*	47.90
14	*Serratia marcescens*	49.30

Nutrient requirements

The production medium contains a carbon source, a nitrogen source, minerals, and occasionally some vitamins. The most widely used source of carbon is glucose but some other sources like fructose, sucrose and some organic acids such as acetic acid or succinic acid can also be used. Nitrogen source contains at least one of the following components: urea, ammonia, ammonium salts, peptones, corn steep liquor, hydrolyzed casein, meat extract or digested soybean meals or fish meal. Minerals like magnesium sulfate or potassium acid phosphate may be added to the synthetic or semisynthetic media. Addition of traces of iron enhances the yield. Yeast extract is added in some media as a source of vitamins.

Process parameters

Two organisms utilized for production of α-ketoglutaric acid are *K. citrophila var. α* and *Pseudomonas fluorescens*.

4.8.2.2.3. Production from *Pseudomonas fluorescens*

The growth medium for this bacterial strain (strain B-6) contains glucose, ammonium sulfate, potassium acid phosphate, magnesium sulfate, calcium carbonate (sterilized separately) and ferrous ammonium sulfate. It is dispersed in a 200 ml portion in a 1 liter Erlenmeyer flask, sterilized, cooled, inoculated and incubated at 24°C on a reciprocating shaker. The nitrogen supply has a marked effect on the yield of α-ketoglutaric acid. At 25 μM/ml nitrogen level an incomplete fermentation resulted; whereas at above 50 μM/ml the yield of α-ketoglutaric acid was low or negligible but the rate of fermentation was considerably high. Therefore, 25 μM/ml nitrogen level was used for the production of α-ketoglutaric acid.

4.8.2.2.4. Production from *Kluyvera citrophila* var. α

The medium used for this strain contains fructose, $NH_4H_2PO_4$, $(NH_4)_2SO_4$, KH_2PO_4, $MgSO_4.7H_2O$, NaCl, $CaCO_3$ (sterilized separately), $Fe_2(SO_4)_3. 7H_2O$. The yield of α-ketoglutaric acid was up to 56% from a 10.4 % of glucose solution after 72 h with strain No. 44C of *Kluyvera citrophila* var. α. 50 ml aliquots, of the medium were dispensed in 500 ml flasks, sterilized, inoculated and incubated at 30°C on a reciprocating shaker. For maximum yield nitrogen concentration of 0.05% proved optimum.

Transforming α-ketoglutaric acid to L-glutamic acid

Two methods for conversion of α-ketoglutaric acid into L-glutamic acid have been reported: based on microbial conversion or enzymatic conversion.

Microorganism based conversion

Microorganisms belonging to following genera can accumulate glutamic acid: *Pseudomonas, Xanthomonas, Erwinia, Serratia, Bacillus, Micrococcus, Escherichia, Aerobacter, Hansenula,* etc. Three different media (A_1, A_2 and A_3) are frequently used for these microorganisms for growth and hence conversion to L-glutamic acid. Their compositions are as follows:

Medium A_1

Sodium-α-ketoglutarate	1.0% (as free acid)
Glucose	0.1%
NH_4CI	0.5%
K_2HPO_4	0.1%
$MgSO_4.7H_2O$	0.05%

Medium A_2

Medium A_1 plus 0.01% caseine-tryptic-hydrolysate

Medium A_3

Medium A_1 plus 0.004% caseine-tryptic-hydrolysate plus 0.007% yeast extract. A 1:1 mixture of distilled water and tap water was used in the preparation media. The pH of each medium was adjusted to 7.

Conversion by enzymes

Two enzymatic methods have been developed for converting α-ketoglutaric acid and ammonium ions to glutamic acid, using:

1. A biological catalytic system, containing a reversibly oxidizable and reducible nicotinic acid containing co-enzyme.

2. A water-soluble hydrogen donating reactant.

3. A dehydrogenase system specific for this reactant

The hydrogen donor oxidizes the coenzyme of dehydrogenase and as a result glutamic acid is formed. The reaction proceeds at a pH of 6.0-4.5 and the temperature is 20–45°C. The hydrogen donating reactant may be citric acid, maleic acid, or glucose-6-phosphate.

4.8.3. VITAMINS

Vitamins are essential components of human diet, required for a normal physiological behavior of the body. These products are being produced by microorganisms using the fermentation principles. Various vitamins have been identified till date and their production strategies have been designed. Here, the discussion will be limited only to two, viz., riboflavin (vitamin B_2) and ascorbic acid (vitamin C).

4.8.3.1. Riboflavin

Riboflavin, also known as vitamin B_2 was first isolated from milk and synthesized in 1935. It occurs as an intense yellow colored substance due to the presence of a complete isoalloxazine ring. Chemical structure of riboflavin is shown below. Riboflavin is hygroscopic, sensitive and decomposed by light

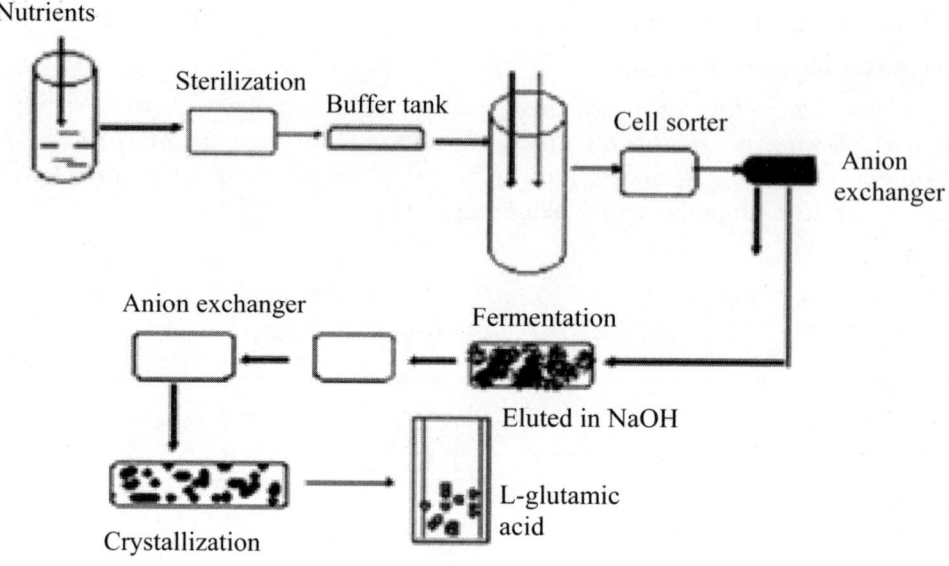

Fig. 4.25: Flow chart of production of L-glutamic acid

(Ultraviolet and visible). It is essential for growth and reproduction in mammals. Riboflavin is produced by several microorganisms including yeasts and bacteria. The most important of these are *Eremothecium ashbyii, Ashbya gossypii,* and certain *Clostridium* species (Table 4.16). The chemical structure of riboflavin was shown in Figure 4.26.

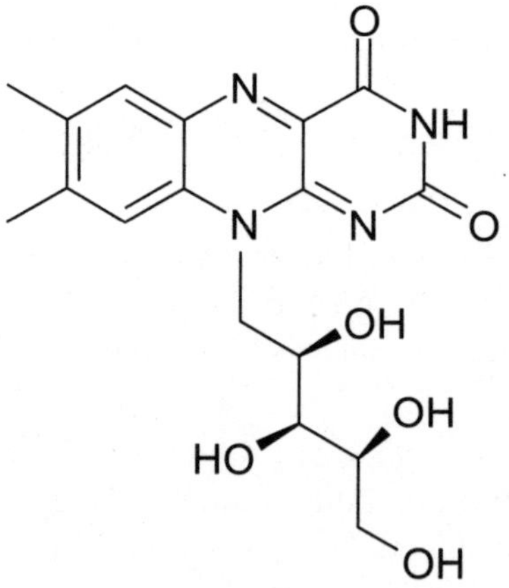

Fig. 4.26: Chemical structure of riboflavin

4.8.3.1.1 Production by *A. gossypii*

A. gossypii is the causative organism of a disease of cotton bolls (especially in South Africa), which produces rotting and staining. It may also infect beans, citrus fruits, coffee, okra and tomatoes. Since the organism is highly pathogenic, it is essential to sterilize all fermentation residues and cultures before they are discarded.

Table 4.16: Various sources of riboflavin

Bacteria	Yeast	Yeast like
Clostridium butyricum	Anascosporogenous	*Ashbya gossypii*
Cl. acetobutylicum	*Candida arborea*	*Eremothecium ashbyii*
Cl. felsineum	*C. flareri*	
Cl. roseum	*Cl. utilis*	
Aerobacter aerogenes	Ascosporogenous:	
A. cloacae	*Hansenula suaveolens*	
Azotobacter chroococcum	*Saccharomyces* sp.	

Nutrient requirement

In order to achieve maximum yield of riboflavin, commercial glucose and sometimes sucrose and maltose are used as the source of carbon. Peptone and animal stick liquor are used as nitrogen source, and corn-steep liquor is used as plant protein source. Biotin, thiamine, and meso-inositol are also required hence are added for the optimum growth of micro-organism.

Stock culture

A. gossypii may be transferred at weekly intervals on a medium containing:

Peptone	0.5%
Yeast extract	0.3%
Malt extract	0.3%
Commercial glucose	1.0%
Agar	2.0%

Incubation temperature 27–30°C

Inoculum development

Pfeifer *et al.*, (1950) described a method for preparing an inoculum for pilot-plant fermentation. A loopful of a 24 h old culture of *A. gossypii* NRRL Y -1056 is placed in 100 ml of the following medium in a 500 ml flask and incubated for 24 h on a reciprocating shaker at 26 to 30°C.

Glucose	2.0%
Peptone	0.5%
Corn-steep liquor	1.0%
Water up to	100 ml.

The pH of this medium before sterilization for 30 min. at 121°C is adjusted and maintained at 6.5. The contents of the flask were used to seed 6 liter of sterilized medium of the following composition contained in a 9 liter glass bottle.

Glucose	2.0%
Corn-steep liquor	1.0%
Animal-stick liquor	0.5%
Water to	6.0 liter

The pH of the medium before sterilization for 45 minutes at 121°C is adjusted to 6.5. The organism is grown for 24 hours with aeration provided by passing sterile air through a perforated tube at the bottom of the bottle. This culture can be used to inoculate 200 or 300 gallons of sterilized medium in a fermenter.

Production

For maximum yield of riboflavin, the following composition of medium is recommended and used:

Glucose	2.0%
Corn-steep liquor	1.4-2.1 %
Animal-stick liquor	1.0%
An anti foam agent,	small amount

The medium is sterilized at pH 4.5 and at 135°C for 5 minutes. An inoculum of 0.5 to 1.0% is used for seeding the fermenters. Sufficient aeration for adequate mixing of the medium but one that does not hamper growth should be provided. An aeration rate of about 0.25 vol. of air per vol. of medium per min. is satisfactory. Fermentation is carried out at 24 to 30°C for 96 to 120 hour. The yields are about 500 to 600 µg/ml. of riboflavin. The fermentation liquor thus produced may be evaporated to syrup and then dried on drum dryers to yield a concentrate containing 2.5% w/v of riboflavin.

4.8.3.1.2. Production by *E. ashbyii*

Riboflavin is produced industrially from *E. ashbyii*, yeast like organism belonging to the *Ascomycetes*. Various patents describe the methodologies for riboflavin production. The methods described production from *E. ashbyii* involves the use of carbohydrate-free media. The medium contains 1-6% of proteinaceous materials, a metabolizable lipid and nutrient such as peptone or a combination of salts (0.05%, KH_2PO_4, 0.07% $MgSO_4$. $7H_2O$), 0.107% NaCI and 0.01% $FeSO_4.7H_2O$). In carrying out production, the following procedure is illustrative of the procedure.

The medium is adjusted to an initial pH of 5.5 to 7:5 and dispensed in containers to give a depth of 0.5 inch, sterilized at 20 psi for 45 minutes, cooled to 30°C, and inoculated with 0.7% of an active culture of *E. ashbyii*. During production, the temperature is maintained between 20 and 34°C and the medium is aerated with 1.5 to 2 Cu ft of sterile air/ min/sq. ft of mesh surface. At the end of 50 to 90 h, the conversion is completed. The dried residue contains 200 to 6000 µg/g of riboflavin.

It has been reported that riboflavin can be produced fro from citrus molasses, using *E. ashbyii* NRRL 1363. The molasses were clarified by settling followed by decantation. The inoculum was prepared by growing the microorganism for 24 h in a sterilized medium containing:

Clarified citrus molasses	1.5%
Yeast extract	0.30%
Peptone	1.0%
pH adjusted to 6.6 to 6.4	

The use of an initial concentration of citrus molasses equivalent to approximate 6.0% reducing sugar, fortified by the addition of a commercial enzymatic yeast hydrolysate at a concentration of 0.3% has been recommended for the production of highest yields of riboflavin. The pH of the production medium is adjusted 6.5-4 before sterilization. This medium is inoculated with 4% by volume of inoculum. Yields of approximately 720 µg/ml of riboflavin can be achieved after 7-9 days of incubation and fermentation at 27°C to 30°C in shaker flasks.

4.8.3.1.3. Production by *Candida* species

It was found that *Candida guilliermondii* grew and produced riboflavin satisfactorily in media containing dextrose, mannose, levulose, or sucrose. Asparagine and glycine are suitable and relatively inexpensive sources of nitrogen for riboflavin production by strain A. T .C.C. 9054.

Table 4.17: Composition of culture medium

Ingredients	g/l	Ingredients	PPM
KH_2PO_4	0.5	Boron	0.01
$MgSO_4.7H_2O$	0.5	Manganese	0.01
$CaCl_2.2H_2O$	0.3	Zinc	0.07
$(NH_4)_2SO_4$	2.0	Copper	0.01
KI	0.1	Molybdenum	0.01
Asparagine	2.0	Iron	0.01
Dextrose	20.0	Biotin	1µg

Most satisfactory results are obtained when the pH is adjusted between 5 to 6 and temperature maintained at 30°C. An increased yield of riboflavin is obtained by adding small amount of sterile potassium cyanide to the medium under vigorous fermentation. The fermentation time was 6-7 days. Recently a method was descried for producing riboflavin from *C. flareri*. The method briefly consists of fermentation under aerobic conditions at 30°C for about 7 days using other suitable *Candida* species, in a medium containing a fermentable sugar, an assimilable source of nitrogen, non iron salts, biotin and less than 10.3µg of iron/ 100 ml. The preferred species of candida are *C. flareri* and *C. guilliermondia*.

4.8.3.1.4. Recovery of riboflavin

Riboflavin may be recovered from production substrates by a variety of procedures, many of them are patented. In a patented, a procedure for extracting riboflavin with butanol, followed by the use of other solvents, such as petroleum ether and acetone. They used chemical precipitation method, in which a soluble reducing agent and finely divided diatomaceous earth were used. The other method wherein riboflavin was absorbed on fuller's earth, silica gel, or other adsorbent and eluted with an aldehyde, ketone or alcoholic solution of an organic base.

4.8.3.2. Ascorbic acid (vitamin C)

Vitamin C (L-ascorbic acid) has been isolated from lemons, capsicum fruit, adrenals etc. prior to 1930s. In 1933 Reichstein and associates published first synthesis of vitamin C. Industrial production of Vitamin C is based chiefly on Reichstein procedure.

4.8.3.2.1. Reichstein synthesis

In this method D-glucose is hydrogenated chemically to produce D-sorbitol. A deionized enzymatic hydrolysate of starch obtained following the action of mould glucoamylase, is directly hydrogenated in a contemporary method, instead of using crystalline glucose. Non isolated sorbitol thus produced in the form .of 20% or more concentrated solution, is then subjected to biochemical dehydrogenation, by *Acetobacter suboxydans*, to yield L-sorbose. L-sorbose is then isolated and condensed with acetone to form 2,3,4,6-diisopropylidene-L-sorbose (so called diacetonesorbose). This offers protection to L-sorbose from an advanced oxidation. In the above-mentioned step: 2,3,4,6-diissopropylidene-L-sorbose is oxidized to diacetone-2-keto-L-gluconic acid, which after hydrolysis, enolization, and lactonization yields L-ascorbic acid.

4.8.3.2.2. Sorbose fermentation

Initially employed *Acetobacter xylinum* (previously named 'sorbose bacterium' by Bertrand), when used in surface fermentation process yields 40-60% sorbose after about 6 weeks. Other species of *Acetobacter* has also been studied. *A. suboxydans* was discovered and yielded 40-90% sorbose after 7 days of surface fermentation. For the preparation of inoculum, a medium containing 10% sorbitol, 0.5% yeast extract, 1 % glucose, and 3.1% calcium carbonate.

Growth medium for *Acetobacter suboxydans* required an inclusion (apart from assimilable sources of carbon, organic nitrogen and mineral salts) of, pantothenic acid. It does not require riboflavin and biotin. Sorbitol serves as the source of carbon whereas other nutrients are supplied by dried yeast extract (0.1-1.0%), yeast autolysate, or corn steep liquor. Industrial production of sorbose requires cheap materials as corm steep liquor, a decoction of Waste brewers yeast, acidic yeast hydrolysate and alfalfa extract. Generally, 0.3% of corn steep liquor is used but its concentration can be lowered to as low as 0.1 % according to later experiments. Organic sources of nitrogen may be partly replaced by ammonium sulfate, phosphate or nitrate. Cells grown in medium with a high content of organic nutrients show higher growth rate and lower dehydrogenation activity than those grown in less nutrient media. Amounts of phosphate, i.e., 10-50 mg/ml were found to be optimal. It was found earlier that the sorbitol concentration in the medium may be as high as 35%, in such cases the sorbose content attainable per 100ml of the medium is 24g/100ml after complete fermentation. On the production scale sorbitol concentration 20g/100ml; as a rule was used. In such concentration inoculum can be cultivated in the same batch; whenever possible, inoculum used should be collected from the preceding batch at a time when the culture achieves the highest activity. Fresh inoculum is prepared only in the cases of contamination or where decreased activity of the culture is noticed. The amount of inoculum added varies between 5 and 20%. Use of small amount of inoculum extends the duration of fermentation. If media with higher sorbitol concentration are to be used, it is better to begin with the fermentation in a less concentrated medium (e.g., 10-20 g/100ml), and subsequently to enrich it by gradually adding concentrated solution of sorbitol (if necessary with respective nutrients added) until the total amount of sorbitol added corresponds to an initial concentration of 24 g/100 ml of the medium. Intense aeration is required during the preparation of inoculum as well as fermentation. Fermentation may be accelerated by increasing the air pressure in the fermenter. Substitution of air by oxygen under increased pressure substantially shortens the duration of fermentation where *Acetobacter xylinum* and *Acetobacter suboxydans* were used. Some investigators have reported that oxygen content elevated over its usual percentage in the air inhibited the activity of some species, e.g. *Acetobacterium malanogenum*.

Appropriate time to interrupt the sorbose fermentation is when the concentration of reducing sugars, calculated as sorbose, reaches about 96-99% of refractometrically estimated sugars in the solution, the latter is filtered or centrifuged and the clear liquid is then thickened under reduced pressure (at a temperature not exceeding 50°C) for crystallization. Deionization prior to thickening leads to the increased yield. It has been observed that crystallization at pH 3.0 gives an increased yield and better quality of sorbose. Yields have been reported in the range of 70-40% and with previous de ionization as high as 47% of sorbitol used. On the laboratory scale, production of other reducing sugars as D-fructose, 5-keto-D-fructose (2,5-D-threodi-ketohexose) has been also recorded in small amounts as a result of simultaneous metabolism.

Initially sorbose fermentation was carried out in rotating drum with air under pressure of 30 psi over periods of 33-45 h and which yielded approximately 94%. A defoamer 0.04%, octadecanol was sometimes added to the rotating drum. Later conventional type fermenters were developed which were equipped with means like perforated papers for dispersion of air. Because of high toxicity of nickel for *Acetobacter suboxydans*, equipment was constructed in high purity aluminum or nickel free stainless steel. Defoamers employed were 0.1% octadecanol, soyabean oil and liquid portions of cord. Activated charcoal was also recommended for this purpose. Later on cylindrical fermenters equipped with mechanical stirrers and aeration devices, similar to those commonly used in the production of antibiotics were developed.

The problem of sensitivity of commonly used *Acetobacter* to nickel has been studied in detail. Nickel may be present in sorbitol because of use of Raney Nickel present in sorbitol, was removed by using disodium hydrogen phosphate. It can also be removed by using cat exes (cationic exchange resins). Removal of nickel by precipitation with raw protein contained in the nourishing additive e.g. corm steep liquor is preferred. Precipitate formed by boiling is removed by filtration or centrifugation, thereby subsequently reducing the nickel content. Besides these approaches, in laboratory conditions *Acetobacter suboxydans* has been adapted to tolerate concentrations of nickel as high as 600 mg/l of fermentation medium. Normal upper limit for the organism is 10mg/l.

Efforts to simplify Reichsteins synthesis mainly involves finding a process which would allow direct oxidation of sorbose 10, 3 -keto-L-gluconic acid. Initially, direct chemical oxidation of sorbose to 2 - keto-L-gluconic acid gave yields of 15 -20 % because of concomitant side reactions. Newer processes use slow air oxidation, catalyzed by platinum, with stated yields of 60 -65%. A Pfizer patent uses 0.5 -2% solution of sorbose that is oxidized by selected strains of genus *Pseudomonas* in a weakly alkaline medium. The process lasts for 50-70 hours. Another process utilizes a mutant of *Pseudomonas*, for fermentation of 2% solution of sorbose. About 16% conversion of 2 keto-L-idonic acid takes place, 0.4% sorbose remaining in the solution. Japanese patents use selected species of genera *Acetobacter* or *Pseudomonas* for oxidation of up to 5% sorbitol solutions directly to 2 keto-L- idonic acid. This acid may be, if separated from the solution with the help of an annex (anionic exchange resin) or esterified without previous isolation, and converted to L-ascorbic acid.

4.8.3.2.3. Newer processes for vitamin C preparation

Bernhauer's team produced calcium 5-keto-D-gluconate (5 keto L-idonate) and calcium 2, keto-D-gluconate for the first time by fermentation. In this process glucose is converted by biochemical dehydrogenation in the presence of calcium carbonate to calcium 5, keto-D-gluconate. D-gluconic acid is an intermediate product. According to the original procedures calcium 5, keto-D-gluconate was catalytically dehydrogenated to a mixture of calcium-D-gluconate with calcium-L-idonate in a 1:1 ratio. Only L-idonate component of the mixture can be used for further preparation stages of L-ascorbic acid. The D-gluconate processed analog yields isoascorbic acid (a-D-arboascorbic acid) that possesses only about 1/20 of the biological activity of L-ascorbic acid (VI). Therefore, the reduction mixture was to be processed further in order to separate out either hexonate or at least to isolate L-idonate component from the mixture.

Several separation processes have been used, some of which are as under

1. Chemical separation by formation of slightly soluble dibenzyl L-idonic acid and likewise slightly soluble binary salt which consists of cadmium (II) L-idonate and cadmium (II) chloride or bromide.

2. Calcium-D-gluconate present in reduction mixture is dehydrogenated, using a suitable strain of *Acetobacter suboxydans* back to slightly soluble calcium 5, keto-D-gluconate, and this salt is returned into the process while calcium L-idonate remains in the solution. The yields obtained from this relatively simple procedure are not satisfactory.

3. The reduction mixture is directly hydrogenated by bacterial strains capable of selective dehydrogenation of hexanoic acid at position 2. It was found that, in this case, D-gluconate is fIrst dehydrogenated to 2-keto-D- gluconate (2-keto-D-mannolate (VIII) which is totally degraded during further course of the process, while 2- keto-L-idonate (2, keto-L-gulonate)(V) remains in the solution. This simple process of separation directly yielding the intermediate product has the disadvantage of losing one half of the material at the third stage of synthesis.

4.9. ALCOHOL FERMENTATION

Alcohol fermentation is known since ages. Ayurveda also deals with alcoholic preparations from crude drugs. Asavas and aristas are the alcoholic ayurvedic preparations prepared by Dentation of crude drugs. Louis Pasteur, almost a century ago, first reported the yeast-mediated fermentation of sugars for the production of alcohol.

The chemical name of alcohol is ethyl alcohol or ethanol and its chemical structure is CH_3CH_2OH. The term alcohol indicates the source of raw material from which it is manufactured, or to indicate the general purpose for which it is used. For example grain alcohol is alcohol made from grains such as whey, rice; industrial alcohol is ethyl alcohol, used in various industrial purposes. Alcohol finds many applications in the pharmaceutical industry. It is used in the preparation of various formulations.

4.9.1. Raw material

Ethyl alcohol may be produced from frementable sugar by yeast under suitable conditions. Starches and certain carbohydrates may be hydrolyzed to fermentable sugars by some biological or chemical means.

Raw materials for alcohol fermentation may be classified into three categories:

1. Sucrose containing or the saccharine materials; for example, corn, sugar beets, molasses and fruit juices.

2. Starch containing materials such as wheat, rice, corn, malt, barley, rye, oats, sorghum, potatoes, etc.

3. Cellulose containing materials such as wood and waste sulfite liquor.

Various types of raw materials used in alcohol production are listed below:

1. Cellulose pulp; crude ethanol mixtures,   8.Ethyl sulfate

2. Cerelose   9.Ethylene gas

3. Corn syrup   10.Grain and grain products

4. Corn sugar by- products   11.Molasses

5. Citrus waste concentrates   12.Potato and potato products

6. Fermented liquor   13.Sulfite liquor

7. Fruit juices   14. Whey

Molasses and grains are the principal carbohydrate materials used in the production of ethanol by fermentation.

4.9.2. Ethanol from molasses

This is the main source of industrial alcohol. It is a by-product of sugar industry. It is mainly a syrupy substance that is left after the recovery of crystalline sugar from the concentrated juice of sugar cane. It usually contains 44–55% of sugars of which major proportion is represented mainly by sucrose. There are seven steps involved in the production of ethanol from molasses. They are as follows:

1. Selection of yeast
2. Preparation of starter
3. The molasses and its preparation for fermentation
4. Optimization of process parameters
5. Distillation and recovery
6. Yield
7. Purification
8. Storage

4.9.2.1. Selection of yeast

Various strains of *S. cerevisiae* are commonly used, but other yeasts such as *S. anamensis* and *S. pombe* are also employed under certain conditions in the fermentation and production of alcohol.

4.9.2.2. Preparation of starter

After selection of the yeast for the fermentation and its isolation in pure culture, a starter is prepared and the large quantities of starters are used to 'pitch' or inoculate the main mesh. About 10 ml of sterile wort is inoculated from a pure culture of yeast using aseptic technique. After incubation for suitable time period at a temperature 25-30°C, the culture is used to inoculate a flask containing 200 ml of sterile mesh. After incubation, the contents of flask may be used to seed a sterile mesh of about 4-liter capacity. Aeration is used to increase the production of yeast cells. The automatic systems are used for preparing the starter instead of the above method. In these types of system a stock of the pure culture is maintained in the upper drum of the apparatus. Meshes are inoculated using this pure culture.

4.9.2.3. The molasses and its preparation for fermentation

Molasses is the main source of industrial alcohol. Molasses represent a byproduct of sugar industry, the syrup that is left after the recovery of crystalline sugar. It usually contains 44-55% of sugar, mainly sucrose.

Adjustment of concentration of sugar

Higher concentration of sugar inhibits the action of yeast. As a consequence of this, the fermentation time is prolonged, leaving some sugar unutilized. The use of very low sugar concentration on the other hand is uneconomic. A sugar concentration of 10-15% w/v is optimum for alcohol production. In practice 12% w/v sugar concentration is used. Molasses is diluted to desired sugar concentration with water. The sugar concentration is determined by means of Balling hydrometer.

Nutrient substances

Generally, molasses contain most of the nutrient substances required for fermentation; however, ammonium salts such as ammonium sulfate or phosphate have to be added to the mesh to supply nitrogen and phosphorus.

pH of the mesh

The optimum pH for the fermentation is 4.0-4.5. This pH favors the growth of yeast but at the same time it inhibits the growth of many types of bacteria. Sulfuric acid is commonly used to adjust the pH of mesh. Sometimes lactic acid may be used. Lactic acid favors the growth of yeast but inhibits the growth of butyric acid producing bacteria which have some detrimental effect on the development of yeast.

Oxygen tension

Large amount of oxygen is required in the early stages to facilitate the maximum reproduction of yeast cells; it is not required for the bio-production of alcohol. During fermentation carbon dioxide is evolved which creates anaerobic conditions.

Temperature

The mesh is inoculated at a temperature between 14 to 24°C. Heat is evolved during fermentation resulting in an increased temperature of mesh. To maintain suitable temperature of mesh, cooling with sprays on the outside of the tank is maintained. At temperature above 24°C, alcohol evaporates rapidly, favoring bacterial growth, which effectively modulates the temperature.

Time required for fermentation

Fermentation is usually completed in 50 h or less, depending on the temperature, sugar concentration and other factors.

Distillation

The fermented mesh 'beer' is distilled to separate ethyl alcohol and fused oil from other constituents of the mesh. Fractions containing different concentrations of alcohol and slops are separated. The fraction containing 60 to 90% of ethanol is known as 'high wines'. These fractions are concentrated to 95% ethanol concentration level by further distillation fractionation.

Yield

Approximately 90% of the theoretical yield is achieved on the basis of the amount of fermentable sugar. However, the yield of the product could be specifically increased by variation of the process parameters as per the available plant facilities.

Purification

The 95% alcohol is further purified, dehydrated or denatured. The facilities and the processes vary in regard to the starter and the nutrient used for the initiation of the fermentation.

4.9.3. Ethanol from whey

The main constituent of whey is lactose 5%. Lactose fermenting yeasts are used in the production of alcohol from whey. Some yeast most often used in alcohol fermentation is listed below.

Torula cremoris	*Saccharomyces fragilis*	*S. lactis*
Torula sphaerica	*Z. lactis*	*T kefir*
Torula lactosa	*S. anamensis*	*M. lactis*

Torula cremoris is generally used because the rate of lactose fermentation is high as compared to other micro-organisms. 2 % w/w yeast is required for seeding as compared to lactose present in the whey before fermentation. Temperature of 33-34°C is optimum for fermentation. At 37°C the fermentation is more rapid, but the evaporation of alcohol is also more.

4.9.3.1. Production methodology

The whey is heated to boiling, and pH is adjusted to 5.0 by adding acid, followed by filtration of the proteins. The pH of the clarified whey should be 4.4 to 5.2. The pH of the whey mesh is adjusted to a range of 4.7 to 5.0. The fermentation profile and apparatus are schematically presented in figure 4.27. The clear whey is cooled to 34°C and 500 g of *C. pseudotropicalis* added per 1000 liter of whey. Fermentation is carried out at 33-34°C for 44-72 h. The yeast is separated out and alcohol is distilled off. A 90% yield of alcohol is obtained on a laboratory scale and 44% under semiplant conditions.

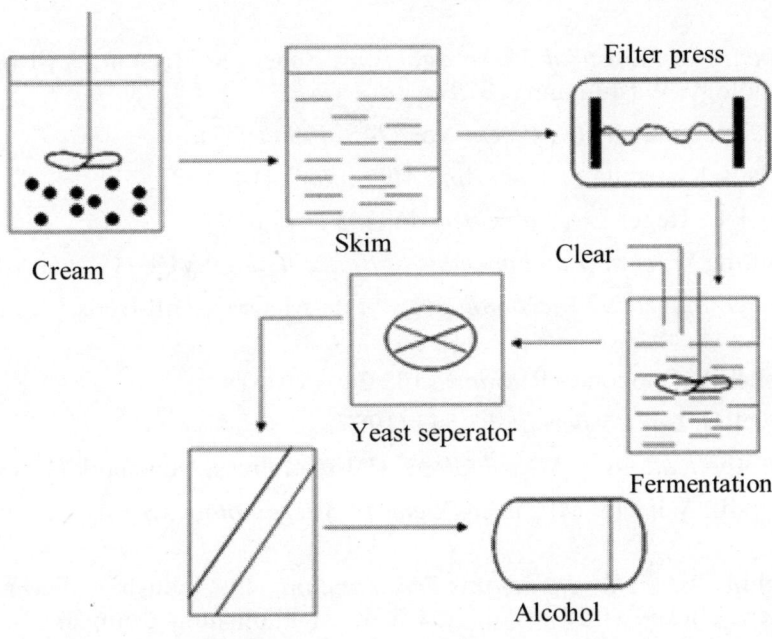

Fig. 4.27: Schematic presentation of fermentation production of alcohol

SUGGESTED READING

- Aharonowitz Y, Cohen G. *Sci Am* 245,140 (1941).
- Asai T, Aida k, Oisho K. *Bull Arg Chern Soc* 21,134 (1957).
- Atkinson B, Mavitana F. *Biochemical Engineering and Biotechnology Hand Book*, Stockton Press, New York (1991).
- Barnhauer K. *Erged Enzym Forsch* 11,151 (1950).
- Brown AG, Butterworth D, Cols M, *et al. J Antibiot* 29, 664 (1976).
- Casida Jr LE. *US Patent* No.2, 771,396 (1956).
- Casida Jr LE. Industrial Microbiology, New Age International (P) Ltd. New Delhi (1964).
- Davis BD. *PNAS* (USA) 35, 1(1949).
- Demain AL. *Science* 214, 947 (1941).
- Fiechter A. *Decherna Monogr* 42,17 (1974).
- Growich Jr J A, Deduck N. *US patent* No. 3, 092,556 (1963).
- Gupta PK. *Elements of Biotechnology*,Rastogi Publication, Meerut (1997).

- Hochfeld WL. *Growth and Synthesis Fermenters*, Bioreactors, and Biomolecular Synbthesisers, Interpharm Press Inc., Buffalo Grove, IL (1944).

- Hockenhull DJD. *The Biochemistry of Streptomycin Production*; In: Progress in Industrial Microbiology, D.J.D. Hockelhull (Ed.), Vol. II, Interscience Publishers, Inc., New York, 131-165(1960).

- Hodgkin DC, Pickworth J, Robertson JH, *et al. Nature* 176,325 (1955).

- Hollaender A. (Ed.) *Genetic Engineering of Micro-organisms for Chemicals*, Plenum Press, London (1942).

- Hopwood DA. *Genetics of Industrial Microorganisms*, Sebek, K., Laskin, A., I (Eds), American Society for Microbiology, Washington (1979).

- Katagiri HI, Imai K, Tochikura T. *US Patent* No. 2746, 799 (1957).

- Nakayama K, Kituda S, Kinoshita S. *JGen Appl Microbio* 7,41 (1961).

- Pfeifer VF, Vojnovick C, Heger EN. *Eng Chem* 46, 443 (1954).

- Prave P, Faust V, Sitting W, *et al. Fundamentals of Biotechnology* VCH, Germany (1947).

- Prescott SC, Dunn CG. *Industrial Microbiology*, 3rd Ed., McGraw-Hill Book Co., Inc., New York (1959).

- Reichstein T, Grussner A, Opperauer R. *Nature* 132,240 (1933).

- Richards M, Haskins RH. *Can J Microbiol* 3,543 (1957).

- Riviere J. *Industrial Applications of Microbiology*, Halstead Press, New York (1946).

- Stanier Y, Ingraham JL, Wheelis ML, *et al. General Microbiology*, 5 Ed, Macmillan Education Ltd., London(1947).

- Sylvester JC, Coghill RD. *The Penicillin Fermentation*; In: Industrial Fermentations, L.A. Underkotler and R.J. Hickey (Eds.), Vol. II, Chemical Publishing Company Inc., New York., 219-263(1954).

- Trehan K. *Biotechnology*, Wiley Eastern Ltd. New Delhi, 17-102(1994).

- Underkotler LA, Hickey RJ. (Ed.), *Industrial Fermentation*, Chemical Publishing Company Inc ., New York (1954).

- Vandamme EJ. (Ed.) *Biotechnology of Industrial Antibiotics*, 1st Ed., Marcel Dekker Inc., New York (1944).

PLANT CELL AND TISSUE CULTURE

5.1. INTRODUCTION

5.2. THE STANDARD TISSUE CULTURE LABORATORY

5.3. CULTURE CONDITIONS AND PREPARATION OF CULTURE MEDIA

5.3.1. Culture conditions

5.3.2. Culture media

5.3.3. Isolation of organs, tissues and cells

5.3.4. Establishment of cultures

5.4. STANDARD CELL CULTURE TECHNIQUES

5.4.1. Subculturing

5.5.2. Growth Curves and Measuring Cell Growth

5.5. TYPES OF CULTURE

5.5.1. Callus culture

5.5.2. Meristem-tip culture

5.5.3. Shoot-tip culture

5.5.4. Flower organ culture

5.5.5. Fruit organ culture

5.5.6. Microspore and anther culture

5.5.7. Dual fungal and plant cell culture

5.5.8. Protoplast culture

5.5.9. Modification through transformative cell culture

5.6. TISSUE CULTURE AND BIOSYNTHESIS OF SECONDARY PRODUCTS

5.6.1. Factors affecting biosynthesis

5.6.2. Indole alkaloids

5.6.3. Tropane alkaloids

5.6.4. Quinoline alkaloids

5.7. APPLICATIONS

5.7.1. To study respiration and metabolism

5.7.2. To study polarity and organ function

5.7.3. Studies of plant diseases and their elimination

5.7.4. Single cell cultures of higher plant cells

5.7.5. Procurement of commercial products

5.7.6. Germplasm storage

5.7.7. Embryo rescue

5.7.8. Somaclonal variation or modification

5.7.9. The production of haploids

5.7.10. Production of artificial seeds

5.7.11. Clonal propagation and micropropagation

5.7.12. Mutant selection

5.7.13. Endosperm culture

5.7.14. Nucellus culture

5.8. CONCLUSIONS

5.1. INTRODUCTION

Tissue culture is an experimental technique through which a mass of cells (callus) is produced from an explant tissue. The callus produced through this process can be utilized directly to regenerate plantlets or to extract or manipulate some primary and secondary metabolites. Plant tissue culture is used as a gross term for protoplast, cell, tissue and organ cultures grown under aseptic conditions. The term **'cell culture'** covers the growth of any cell, be it a microbe or a plant or animal cell. On the other hand **'tissue culture'** refers to the cultivation of a plant or mammalian cell, which normally forms a multicellular tissue. In these cultivation processes the cells used for culture may be isolated from nature or the strains improved by selection, mutation or genetic manipulation.

When grown on agar medium, the tissue forms a callus or a mass of undifferentiated cells. The technique of cell culture is convenient for starting and maintaining cell lines, as well as, for studies pertaining to organogenesis and meristem culture. The liquid suspension cultures are comprised of mixtures of cell aggregates, cell clusters and single cells. Generally, the growth rate of such cultures is much higher than on solidified medium and a better control over the growth of biomass is offered as the cells are surrounded by the nutrient medium, and for the same reason, the cell material could be probably more uniform physiologically. Both callus and suspension cultures can be derived from tissues of most of the species, but the ease of starting the cultures varies with the type of plant and the origin of tissue. A callus and a suspension culture can be induced from any part of the plant. These necessary tissues can be obtained from roots, stem, seedlings, pollen and leaf portions and they usually grow as a mass of undifferentiated cells on enriched solidified medium. Some of the salient features of tissue culture are:

1. The culture of the cells/tissues is carried out in a sterile medium under controlled conditions.

2. Clones generated through tissue culture are identical in terms of size, developmental stage and rate of metabolic activities.

3. The rate of tissue multiplication is rapid within a small area.

4. The clones are capable of performing the transformative activity, which involves biotransformation to produce primary and secondary metabolites in the tissue culture medium.

5.2. THE STANDARD TISSUE CULTURE LABORATORY

A tissue culture laboratory may be a core facility, working in conjunction with other laboratories, or it may be the primary facility for a cell biology laboratory. All the basic cell culture studies can be performed in this facility that would be adequate for cell culture use for most cell and molecular biology laboratories, as well as use by physiologists, biochemists, and others who might occasionally need access to a culture facility. If it is to be a shared core facility, need for the minimizing potential contamination vectors becomes paramount. This is critical not only with regard to bacterial or fungal contamination, but also for possible cross-contamination of cell cultures. Some facilities have an airlock that can serve as a buffer zone and somewhat deterrent to the bacterial and fungal contaminants, largely because in its most minimal configuration, it discourages unnecessary traffic in and out of the primary laboratory. Optimally, the entryway might be large enough to include a sink for hand washing, storage for sterile tissue culture supplies, and even space for a freezer or cell counter. A high-use tissue culture core facility might be designed around a plan such as that shown in Fig. 5.1 When this is not possible, or is impractical, the laboratory should be designed so that cell cultures can be "compartmentalized," that is, primary cell cultures can be handled in a specifically designated hood(s), and kept in an incubator chamber separate from other cell lines being maintained as long-term culture. Cell cultures coming into the laboratory, as frozen vials or as viable cultures, primaries, or established cell lines, should be quarantined in an incubator chamber and handled in a designated hood until they are tested for mycoplasma. Incubators are available as two-gas or three-gas models, this being largely determined by cost and specific needs of the investigators. It is always possible to augment a two-gas incubator chamber when this has not been incorporated into the original design. Insulation is maintained by either a water jacket or an air jacket, with corresponding advantages and disadvantages. The water-jacketed incubator can maintain temperature over a longer period of time should there be a power outage, and this can be a critical feature for some installations. It is much heavier when filled, however, and the level must be maintained by periodic "topping off" and the jacket drained when the incubator has to be moved. The air-jacketed incubator is lighter, has more moving parts to fail, comes up to temperature faster, but will lose heat much faster when the fan goes off (e.g., in case of an electricity shutoff).

More importantly, the interior design and construction, materials used, and ease of assembly and disassembly can determine in part how well the cultures can be maintained free of contamination. Contaminating mold will grow on stainless steel, labeling tape, and even plastic, so shelving and the hardware securing it must be easy to remove and clean when necessary. Copper shelving and interior walls can inhibit the growth of such organisms but it is expensive, and unless all hardware components are of copper construction, one cannot completely inhibit the growth of mold on interior surfaces.

Routine cleaning of stainless steel or aluminum shelves with a disinfectant and ethanol rinse will help to reduce these risks. A disinfectant recommended by incubator supplier should be used. Many excellent disinfectants are volatile and may kill cultured cells as well as contaminants. The chamber should be allowed to equilibrate overnight after a thorough cleaning prior to returning the cultures.

Incubator manufacturers have various proprietary methods of delivering and regulating gas flow into the chamber. Independent of this, the tissue culture laboratory needs a supply of CO_2 and other gas as per need should be delivered to the chamber through pre-filters. In-house supplied gas can be a relatively inexpensive source; it need only be equipped with a miniature regulator to reduce the house gas to a flow rate optimal for the incubator and an in-line 0.2-μm filters to prevent introduction of mold and other potential contaminants that can accumulate on the inner wall of a gas hose. If oxygen based experiments are to be carried out in an incubator that has such a provision, then nitrogen supply should also be made properly into the laboratory.

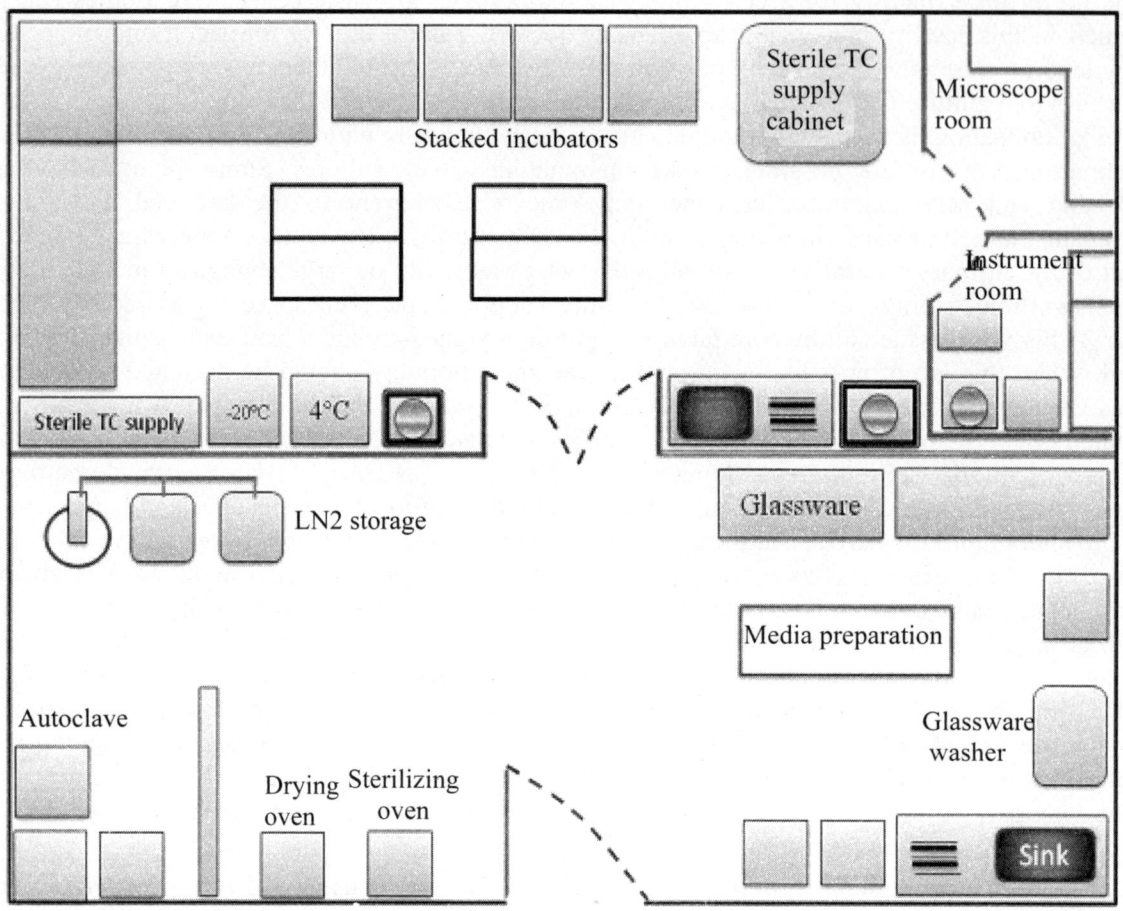

Fig. 5.1: Suggested floor plan for an ideal high-use tissue culture facility or a core

Alternatively, when house gas is unavailable, commercial gas cylinders may be used, the critical point being to maintain an uninterrupted flow of gas. A manifold, connecting two or more supply cylinders with two-stage regulators, can be configured to supply the gas efficiently and economically. Reinforced silicon tubing that can be sterilized by autoclaving should be used to connect the gas source to the incubator. It is important to know if the displays on the incubator control panel are reflecting in fact the actual conditions inside the chamber. For accurate temperature determination, a portable RTD thermometer is recommended. The appropriate thermometer-probe combination can provide accuracy within 0.05°C.

The tissue culture hood can be as simple as an open, laminar flow unit with air passing initially through a HEPA filter and moving parallel to the work surface, exiting at the front of the hood. However, current regulations may require the use of biosafety cabinets, in which HEPA filtered air is circulated within the hood and exhausted through appropriate filters and ductwork to the outside. These hoods are generally available in 4-ft and 6-ft lengths, the latter being somewhat more convenient in terms of workspace. Two people can also work side by side in a 6-ft hood. This is convenient if the experimental protocol requires two people to work together. Larger hoods also may be necessary if large-scale tissue culture work is to be done where many large spinners or roller bottles are handled at the same time. Regardless of the size being used, it is important that the interior of the hood be as free of obstruction as is practical to optimize airflow. Quite frequently one finds the hood being used as a repository for a variety of tissue culture supplies, vacuum units, personal belongings, and other sundry items, leaving little room for work space, thus minimizing airflow and increasing the ever possible risk of contamination. Keep only the minimum necessary equipment in each hood, have one set of dedicated equipment and supplies for each hood, and restrict the use of designated equipments to the assigned hood (e.g., a tube rack, automatic pipettes, or bulb).

No mouth pipetting should ever be done for tissue culture work. Currently available biosafety cabinets have duplex electrical outlets, convenient for plugging in pipetting aids and gas and vacuum valves, and are equipped with UV fixtures. There is little need for gas supply to use a Bunsen burner in this type of hood. In fact, an open flame interrupts the airflow pattern in the hood and decreases barrier efficiency. In addition, an open flame creates a hazardous condition when working with flammable reagents in the hood. Thus, a flame should only be used when essential (e.g., for flaming a coverslip). The only other item of major importance is a vacuum trap, consisting of two 1- or 2-liter Erlenmeyer flasks connected on one end to the vacuum source (house vacuum or pump) and on the other to a small hook attached to the hood. This apparatus should placed on the floor beneath the hood and be emptied regularly. Tubing, preferably silicon or latex should have an inner diameter equivalent to the outer diameter of a Pasteur pipette and should be of sufficient length to facilitate aspirating medium and other reagents. The primary flask (at least) should contain disinfectant and the tubing should be flushed with disinfectant after the work in the hood is completed. All hoods should have biohazard waste containers lined with autoclave bags.

The laboratory should have at least one inverted phase contrast microscope, equipped with 10x, 20x, and 40x objectives. If fluorescent microscopy will be needed, an epifluorescent attachment should be included. A 4x objective is useful for scanning large fields. For detecting mycoplasma, a 100x objective and fluorescence capability is necessary. A spring-loaded marker that screws into the nosepiece of the microscope is useful for marking areas of interest in culture dishes.

The standard tissue culture laboratory should have a reliable source of water for preparing medium. Considerable study has gone into water quality requirements for optimal cell growth, some cell types being far more sensitive to water quality than others. Nonetheless, all cells respond to water quality and it is important to be able to control this as much as possible. Ideally, water supplied by the city or county should first pass through a deionization unit. Often, institutions have a source of deionized water supplied to the laboratories. To this source, the investigator should connect a purification unit, usually in the form of several organic resin cartridges, a charcoal cartridge to remove organic compounds (including those leaching from the previous column), and a final ultrafiltration cartridge, with a 0.2 μm filter attached to the outlet. A still can also be used but this should be a double distillation with potassium permanganate in the first reservoir should be added to remove organic material.

Do not use tap water or water straight from a deionizing column. Liquid nitrogen freezers for long-term storage of cell cultures should be considered necessary for standard tissue culture facility. These can be "portable" units, which can be moved when needed and can hold up to 2,500 vials. This type of unit is filled with NO_2 manually. Alternatively, there are stationary freezers that can hold up to 10,000 vials or more and are filled automatically by a supplied NO_2 source tank. In either case, but particularly the former, it is absolutely necessary to regularly monitor the liquid nitrogen levels.

5.3. CULTURE CONDITIONS AND PREPARATION OF CULTURE MEDIA

5.3.1. Culture conditions

For the successful culture of isolated plant cells and tissues on artificial media, many formulae have been developed. These have been based on the nutritional and hormonal requirements of the whole plants and these serve to suit the nutrition of particular tissues, be they free cells in suspension, somatic embryos or protoplasts. The components of the media are modified and adapted according to the objective of experimental studies of regeneration, micropropagation, cytodifferentiation, experimental androgenesis, and biosynthesis of secondary metabolites or biotransformation of cells. Furthermore, in addition to an appropriate medium, maintenance of temperature, agitation, aeration, an optimum pH is essential for promoting growth or differentiation of cultured cells or tissues.

5.3.2. Culture media

The plant cells and tissues require a proper medium for their growth and development. The nutrient media for plant cell is a well-defined mixture of inorganic salts and typical carbon sources like sucrose and glucose. In majority of cells, supplementary constituents are required which are essentially growth regulators, i.e. indole acetic acid (IAA), kinetin and NAA, vitamins like thiamin and nicotinic acid, amino acids, inositol and sugar alcohol. The various components of tissue culture media essentially involve the following ingredients.

5.3.2.1. Ingredients

Basically a complete media has the following ingredients:

I. Inorganic elements

a) Macro-elements (in mmol/l), e.g., Na, P, K, Ca, Mg, S.

b) Micro-elements (in μmol/l), e.g., Mn, Zn, Cu, MO, Cl, Ni, AI, etc.

II. Organic components

a) Sugar (mmol/l).

b) Vitamins (mmol/l), e.g., thiamin, riboflavine, ascorbic acid, etc.

c) Phytohormones, e.g., auxins, cytokinins, abscisic acid, etc.

III. Complex extract(s): This includes natural plant extracts and other undefined components. (e.g., coconut milk, yeast extract, malt extract, potato extract, tomato juice, casein hydrolysate, etc.).

IV. Water: Demineralized and double distilled water.

V. Agar: As a gelling agent when solid surface is required for growth.

The composition of Murashige and Skoog medium, the most widely used medium, is outlined in table 5.1.

5.3.2.2. Stock-solutions

The word 'medium' refers to the basic culture medium devoid of any organic solution or growth hormones. In the preparation of media, usually a series of stock solutions is employed. Solutions of microelements and vitamins are made in 1000x final concentration and stored in the freezer. Stock solutions of KI can also be prepared. Calcium and magnesium sulfates and phosphates, however should not be combined keeping in view their insolubility and consequent precipitation. Hormones should be dissolved in a little of ethanol and their volume should be made up with water to yield a concentration of 2–3 mM. Alternatively, they can be dissolved in dimethyl sulfoxide. Care should be taken to quantify media components in molar units rather than by weight. This enables the possible the valid comparison and interpretation of concentration effects of equimolar concentration of various constituents.

Table 5.1: Composition of Murashige and Skoog Medium

Compound	Conc. in medium mg/L	Amount in stock solution	Stock vol. ml
NH_4NO_3	1650	8.25g	
KNO_3	1900	9.50 g	
$MgSO_4.7H_2O$	370	1.85g	
KH_2PO_4	170	0.85 g	
KI	0.83	4.18mg	400
$MnSO_4.4H_2O$	22.30	111.50mg	
$ZnSO_4.7H_2O$	8.6	43.00mg	
Myo-inositol	100	0.50g	
$CaCl_2.2H_2O$	440	2.20g	
$FeSO_47H_2O$	27.8	139.25mg	100
$Na2EDTA.2H_2O$	37.3	186.25mg	
$CuSO_45H_2O$	0.025	12.50mg	100
$Na_2MoO_42H_2O$	0.25	12.50mg	10
$CoCl_2.6H_2O$	0.025	12.50mg	100
Nicotinic acid	0.50	25.00mg	10
Pyridoxine-HCl	0.50	25.00mg	10
Thiamin-HCl	0.10	5.00mg	10
Glycine	2.0	100mg	10
Sucrose	30g/L		

5.3.2.3. Preparation of the media

The various steps involved in the preparation of media can be outlined as:

1. Macronutrients are dissolved in 200 ml of distilled water.

2. Micronutrients are dissolved in 200 ml of distilled water in another flask.

3. Vitamins are dissolved in 100 ml of distilled water in a separate flask and stored at refrigerated conditions.

4. Growth hormones are also dissolved separately in 100 ml of distilled water and stored in a cool place.

5. To prepare I liter of the media the above solutions are mixed together

6. Sucrose and amino acids (if any) are added to the medium.

7. The volume of the media is made up to 950 ml by the addition of distilled water.

8. The pH of this solution is adjusted to 5.6 with 0.1M sodium hydroxide solution or 0.1M hydrochloric acid solution as needed.

9. Finally, the volume of this media is made up to 1 liter with distilled water.

10. The prepared media is transferred to conical flasks and the mouths of these flasks are plugged with non-adsorbent cotton. If a solid medium is desired, agar amounting to 2% w/v is added to each flask.

11. The above conical flasks are autoclaved and subsequently used for tissue culture.

5.3.2.4. pH of the media

pH of the media greatly affects the uptake of ingredients, solubility of salts and gelling efficiency of agar. An initial pH of the media prior to autoclaving is measured although it undergoes changes during culture. The pH is maintained and adjusted by using a pH meter with 0.1M NaOH or HCl. Optimum pH depends upon the particular strain of tissue but a pH of 5.6-5.8 is often suitable for maintaining all the salts in a near buffered form. In spite of the initial adjustments, the pH of the medium usually changes after autoclaving and the media composition also gets affected. Normally, plant tissue culture media are poorly buffered, still pH remains stabilized to some extent as the media contains both nitrate and ammonium ions. Further, it is highly desirable to maintain the pH at the optimum value as agar may fail to gel at a low pH.

5.3.2.5. Sterilization of media

Sterilization of media can be carried by autoclaving at 15 psi for 20 minutes. Thermolabile components like certain carbohydrates, vitamins, growth regulators and plant extracts can be conveniently sterilized by micro-filtration and then added aseptically to the sterile medium (after it has been autoclaved but before it has reached the solidification temperature of agar).

5.3.3. Isolation of organs, tissues and cells

As discussed earlier all the manipulations involved in isolating and establishing plant tissue *in vitro* is conducted under aseptic conditions in a transfer chamber or transfer room. The basic necessary tools for plant tissue culture work include transfer loops, microspatulas, scalpels and forceps. These tools may be placed upright in alcohol and flamed and cooled prior to use.

5.3.3.1. Explant preparation

An explant is a detached portion of the plant body which is used in tissue culture to produce callus tissues. The age of explant (i.e., the age of meristematic tissue) plays a vital role in the production of callus. The desired portion is excised from the parent plant and utilized for callus induction. Seeds and grains are also considered to be good sources for preparation of explants. Seeds and grains after surface-sterilization are germinated aseptically in nutrient media by placing them on double layers of pre-sterilized filter paper petri dishes moistened sufficiently with sterile distilled water or on moist cotton plugs in petri dishes or culture tubes. After few days, they germinate into seedlings, which are removed and surface-sterilized. These can then be used as a source of explants.

5.3.3.2. Surface sterilization of explants

In general, to carry out fresh isolation of tissues or organs, the surface sterilization of the plant materials should be modulated and kept at minimum. Commonly used surface sterilizing agents are sodium hypochlorite (1-2%), bromine water (1-2%), hydrogen peroxide (10-12%), mercuric chloride (0.1-1.0%) and silver nitrate (1%). The aerial portion of plants such as bud, leaf and stem sections are sterilized by submerging for 2-3 min in 70% ethanol, followed by 2-3 rinses with sterilized distilled water.

5.3.4. Establishment of cultures

5.3.4.1. *Agar gel culture*

The surface sterilized plant material is aseptically transferred onto solidified nutrient medium in flasks, glass jars or culture tubes and then incubated at 26-28°C in dark. After 3-4 weeks, the callus should be about 5 times the size of the explant. Many tissue explants possess some degree of polarity. Therefore the callus is formed most easily at one surface. In stem segments, callus is formed particularly from the surface which *in vivo* is directed towards the root. The callus often develops more readily from the tissue not in contact with and particularly not immersed in the solidified culture medium. The maintenance of growth in callus tissue by subculture requires the transfer of a piece of

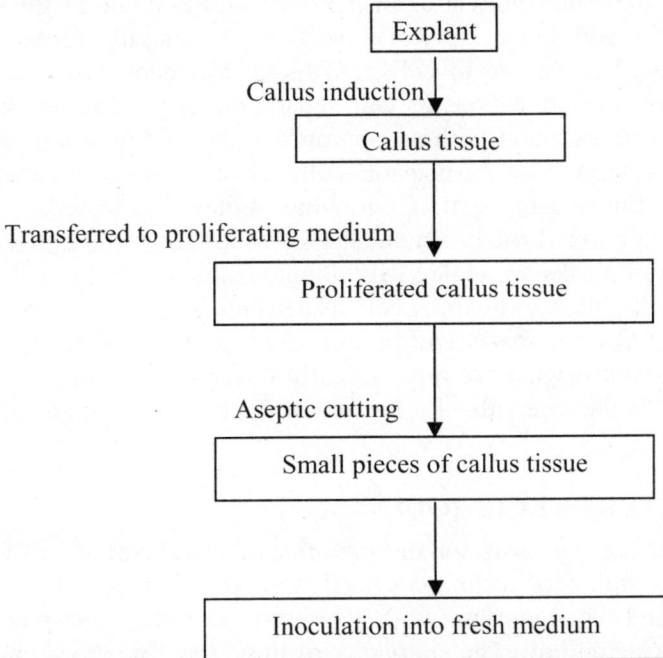

Fig. 5.2: Various stages involved in callus induction, proliferation and sub-culture

healthy tissue every 4 weeks into the flasks containing fresh solidified nutrient medium. Many cultures shall, however, remain healthy and continue a slow rate of growth for much longer periods without subculturing, if the standard incubation temperature of 26°C is lowered to 5–10°C. It has been observed that the growth of many cultures and particularly of those which form chlorophyll is stimulated by low-intensity illumination. Light either on a 12h cycle or continuously, therefore, usually provided in the incubation chambers by fluorescent tubes. The well-developed callus is cut into small pieces with a sterile knife. The pieces of callus are then transferred to another media (the proliferation media), to induce proliferation of callus. In this media the callus tissue multiplies 'more rapidly. 2,4-D, IAA is avoided in the proliferation medium as it induces callus product in most tissues. Instead the callus segments are cultured in the media containing growth hormone like IAA, NAA, 6- benzyl anrtnopurine, and kinetin. IAA induces callus production in the dicots, however high concentration reduces the callus production in monocots.

Sub culture of callus after the proper growth of callus tissues is usually developed as it is transferred to a fresh medium at regular intervals. This transfer of callus tissues facilitates the maintenance of the cells in a viable state. The previously cultured tissues serve as an explant for establishing the secondary culture. This process of culture is also referred to as sub-culture. Generally, this process of sub-culture is practiced at regular intervals of four weeks. All steps involved are represented in a scheme in Figure 5.2.

5.3.4.2. *Suspension culture*

This culture essentially contains homogeneous individual plant cells in its liquid medium. The suspension cultures are generally initiated by transferring an established callus tissue to an agitated liquid nutrient medium in Erlenmeyer culture vessels (30-60 ml medium per 250 ml flasks). The composition of the medium for the establishment of suspension cultures could be the same as defined for callus cultures except for the addition of agar. The soft callus generally forms in a suspension culture without much difficulty. The release of cells and tissue fragments from less friable callus masses and the maintenance of a good degree of cell separation may often be promoted by the presence of a high auxin concentration and with an appropriate balance between yeast extract and auxin or between auxin and kinetin. The suspension cultures are usually incubated at 25°C in darkness or in low intensity fluorescent light. Continuous agitation of flask cultures is most commonly employed by using horizontal rotary orbital shaker which rotates at between 100 and 200 revolutions per minute; the culture flasks are sealed with double aluminum foil or parafilms to reduce evaporation during the process of culture growth. A cell suspension is generally formed within 4 to 6 weeks. The cells grown in cultures are **meristematic** and usually undifferentiated and there is no evidence that cells of shoot or root origins are metabolically different. The suspension cultures are **subcultured** by the transfer at regular intervals of untreated or fractionated aliquots of the suspension to a fresh medium.

5.4. STANDARD CELL CULTURE TECHNIQUES

A few standard techniques that are the basis for the majority of manipulations of cells *in vitro* as discussed here in brief. More complicated techniques needed for special types of culture, the special considerations to be kept in mind when working with a serum-free culture, and preparation of cells for primary culture and large-scale culture. The simplicity of these basic methods makes cell culture an ideal tool.

5.4.1. Subculturing

Subculturing, or "splitting cells," is required in order to periodically provide fresh nutrients periodically and also creating space for continuously growing cell lines. Frequency of subculture and the split ratio, or density of cells plated, depends on the characteristics of each cell or cell line being handled. If cells split too frequently or at low density, the cell line may be lost. If cells are not splited frequently enough, the cells may exhaust the medium and subsequently die, or a different type of cell particular cell line, it should be used consistently for that cell line, with only minor variations when it is absolutely essential. Different subculture strategies can therefore be selected for different properties in the cell lines carried.

Subculture involves removing the growth media, washing the plate, disassociating adhered cells, usually enzymatically (e.g., with trypsin, although some cells may be removed by repeated pipetting or gentle scraping), and re-suspending the cells into fresh media. If this process involves the use of serum and the split ratio is high (e.g., 1:100), it is usually not necessary to remove the residual enzyme. If the culture is maintained in serum free media, however it is necessary to neutralize the enzyme by using an appropriate protease inhibitor, such as soyabean trypsin inhibitor. There are other

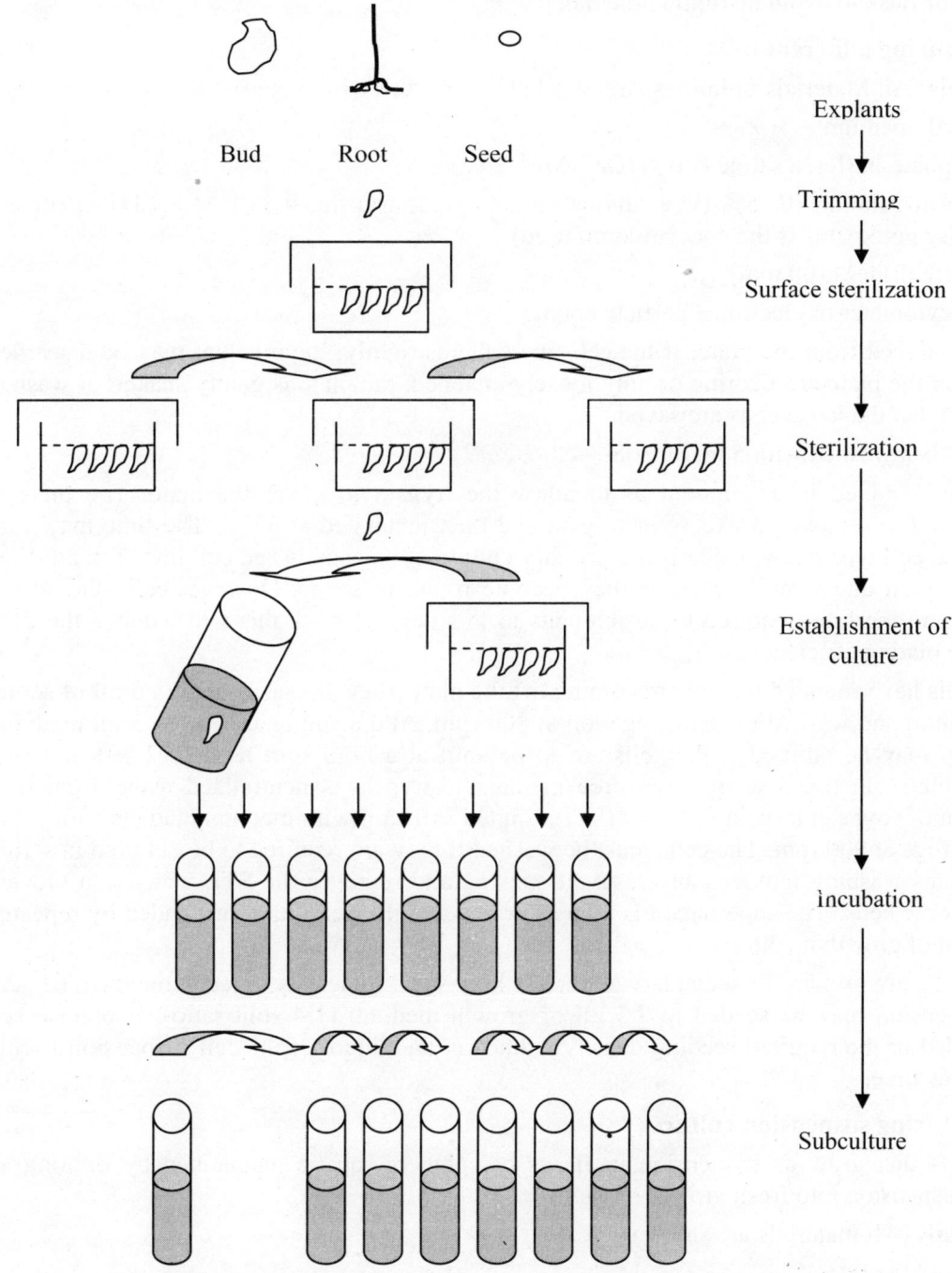

Fig. 5.3. Outline of the basic procedure in plant tissue culture

considerations that may require the use of different methods. For example, if the cell line is grown at a very low split ratio, it is advisable to wash the cells after enzyme treatment even if serum is present. All solutions added to the dishes/flasks with adherent cells should be added by pipetting along the side of the dish or flask to avoid disrupting the monolayer.

5.4.1.1. Subculturing adherent cells

Materials (All Materials/Solutions Are Sterile Unless Otherwise Noted)

1. Growth medium

2. Phosphate-buffered saline (PBS) (Ca^{2+}/Mg^{2+} free)

3. Trypsin solution (0.05% (w/w) tissue culture grade trypsin, 0.53 mM EDTA; (unless otherwise noted, this is the concentration used)

4. Culture dishes (100 mm)

5. Hemcytometer or electronic particle counter

1. Medium is removed from the plate. If the cell line adheres tightly, the medium may be discarded but when cells in the plate are floating or only loosely attached, the plate is gently shaken or washed with a pipette so that the loose cells are saved.

2. The cells are then washed with 5 ml of PBS.

3. Then trypsin is added in an amount as to allow the trypsin to cover the plate. The plate is subsequently tilted to remove an excess of trypsin and then incubated at 37°C. The time may vary depending on the cell type and whether it is a primary culture or an established cell line. The attached cell can be observed under microscope as they become round in shape. However cells should not trypsinized beyond the time required to detach cells to this degree, since this will damage the cells and may reduce plating efficiency.

4. When the cells have rounded up and are coming off the plate, they are suspended in 5 ml of serum containing medium and washed by centrifugation at 800 rpm. And again resuspend in 5 ml medium. [This wash step may be omitted if the cells are to be split at a high split ratio (> 1:50) in serum containing medium]. In the case of serum-free media, the trypsin is neutralized using 1 ml of a 1mg/ml solution of soybean trypsin inhibitor (STI), diluted to 10 ml with medium, and centrifuged in a clinical centrifuge at 900 rpm. The cells must be washed if they are required to be cultured in serum free medium. This washing removes any residual enzyme and removes the STI, which can prevent attachment of some cells. The supernatant is then aspirated and the pellet is resuspended by repeated pipetting in 5 ml of growth medium.

5. In case the cells are primary or secondary cultures a high seeding density is recommended, i.e., 2.5 ml of cell suspension may be seeded to 7.5 ml of growth medium (1:4 split ratio). If precise cell counts are needed or the required seeding density is known, an aliquot of the cell suspension should be counted at this time.

5.4.1.2. Subculturing suspension cultures

Cultures of cells that grow as suspension in flasks or spinners can be maintained by diluting an aliquot of the suspension into fresh growth medium.

Materials (All materials are sterile)

1. Flasks (75 cm^2)

2. Growth medium

3. Hemocytometer or electronic particle counter

Procedure

1. The flask is held upright and the cell suspension is pipetted up and down two or three times to disperse clumps if any.

2. An aliquot is removed for counting or in case precise counts are not required, transfer 200μl to 1 ml of the suspension is transferred to a fresh flask containing 10 ml of growth medium. If a split ratio is less than 1:10, the appropriate volume of cell suspension is placed in a 15 ml conical tube, diluted to 10 ml with medium, and centrifuged at 900 rpm for 3 to 4 min. Pellet is re-suspended into fresh growth medium. The aliquot that contains the appropriate number of cells is transferred into the number of flasks needed. In this way, the dilution of fresh medium with exhausted medium components or carrying over toxic cell metabolites or proteases is avoided.

5.5.2. Growth curves and measuring cell growth

5.5.2.1. Growth profile

Cell culture

The various stages of growth exhibited by the plant cell culture are to a great extent similar to those of the microorganisms. The various stages of growth are indicated in Figure 5.4 which can be enumerated as following:

1. **Lag phase**: Here following subculture into the fresh medium, the cell regains ability of division and the tissue shows slow growth.

2. **Exponential phase**: This stage involves rapid cell division. The duration of this stage varies according to the cell and its nutrient regime. In majority of the cases it is a short one and lasts for only 3-4 generations.

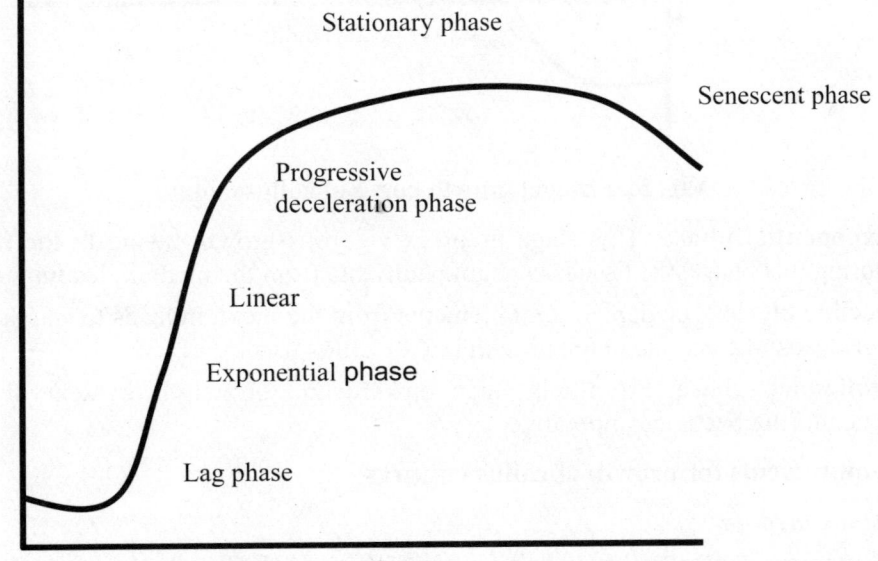

Fig. 5.4: Model growth curve of single cell culture

3. **Linear phase**: The growth in this phase follows a linear pattern with respect to time.

4. Progressive deceleration phase: In this stage the rate of cell division tends to decline with the aging of the culture.

5. Stationary phase: During this phase the rate of production of cell equals the rate of their death.

6. Senescent phase: During this phase the cells are dying.

Callus culture

The growth profile for the callus to a great extent is similar to that of cells suspension culture and presented in Figure 5.5. The various stages of growth recorded are:

1. **Lag phase**: Following inoculation of an explant, there is a lag time before the growth of cells. undergo cell division. Then a few cells start to divide and the tissue resumes its growth, albeit a slower one.

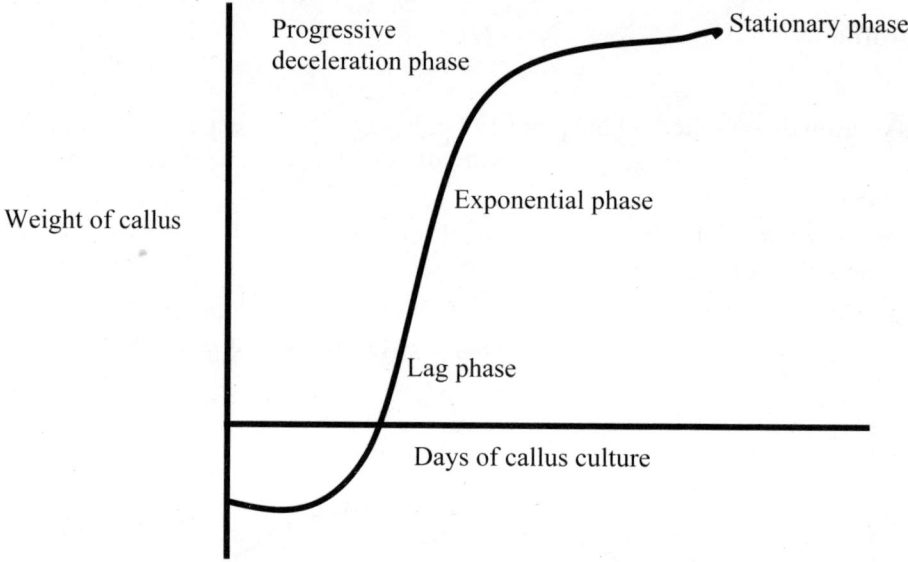

Fig. 5.5: Model growth curve of callus culture

2. **Exponential phase**: This stage involves vigorous growth owing to the rapid cell division. During this phase, the tissues consume nutrients from the medium leading to their depletion.

3. **Decline phase**: The depletion of elements from the medium leads to starvation of some cells. This leads to a decline in the growth rate of callus tissue.

4. **Stationary phase**: From this stage onwards no growth is evident. For further growth subculturing becomes imperative.

5.5.2.2 Requirements for growth of callus cultures

The pH of the medium

The pH of medium is often adjusted to an initial value of pH 5.5-6.0. However, the optimum acidity depends upon the particular strain of tissue employed, usually pH of the medium drifts toward neutrality from more acid or alkaline conditions during growth period. Studies have also indicated that the tissues could change the pH of the medium in the areas of the medium they occupy and grow. For example Tobacco tissues from the hybrid (*Nicotiana glauca x Nicotiana langsdorfil*) grow best in media with initial pH averaging 5.0 to 5.4 and final pH 5.5 to 5.9. Similarly, com endosperm grows best between pH 6.0 and 7.0. It was observed that regardless of the initial pH, the pH of the medium at the end of the growth period is drifted towards pH 6.0. Thus, when graphs indicated growth of cultures on originally more acid or alkaline media, it was observed that growth actually occurred when the final pH values were close to 6.0.

Temperature

The optimum temperature for growth of callus cultures varies with the strain of tissue. However, temperature of the growth room is generally maintained at 26° ± 1°C. The temperature requirement variability is best exemplified by tobacco hybrid (*N. glauca x N .langsdorffii*) that grows best between 28°C and 32°C while sunflower crown gall tissue grows the best between 24°C and 28°C.

Light

In general, the tissue cultures are maintained in light or dark environment. When chlorophyll production by callus in the light is undesired, the tissues are grows best in darkness. Intensity of light and length of darkness have also been identified to have some effect on the growth as well.

Inorganic nutrition

The nutritional requirement of callus tissues has been discussed earlier. However, after much precise work other media for specific tissues have also been developed. The proper balance of mineral and the concentrations of both minor and major elements in the media are usually critical for optimum growth of specific tissues. However, the isolated cell masses could tolerate a wide range of concentrations of the ingredients in media.

Carbohydrate nutrition

An isolated callus tissue, in order to grow *in vitro* needs an outside source of carbon. Though freshly isolated tissues, in some cases, may remain alive for months but eventually they die if an organic carbon source is not provided. Commonly utilized sources of carbon include dextrose, levulose, mannose, sucrose, maltose, cellobiose, dextrin, pectin, starch, etc. Tissues from sunflower and tobacco grow more on dextrose, levulose, sucrose, maltose, cellobiose, pectin or dextrin. The concentration of sugars and polysaccharides are determent and optimal for growth. Often a concentration range 0.5-2% has been found to be optimum. Alcohol and organic acids alone are generally not good sources of carbon. However, in the presence of 2% w/v sucrose all species could grow more or less on media containing methanol, ethanol, glycerol, erythritol or mannitol, however the growth is very poor.

Nitrogen nutrition

In order to ascertain growth of the tissues, sources and concentrations of nitrogen present in the media are important. Many organic and inorganic compounds have been tested as nitrogen sources for tissues of many species. Nitrate, nitrogen often promotes excellent growth of the tissues. Among the nitrogen compounds tested as the sources of nitrogen, only aspartic acid and urea have been found to be effective. Arginine, aspartic acid, glycine, proline and threonine are to a little extent at a concentration of 0.002M.Urea as the sole source of nitrogen favorably promotes the growth of sunflower crown gall tissue. Amino acids in concentrations from 0.256 to 0.00006 M as source of nitrogen have been tested but they failed to turn out as a good source. Moreover, with ammonia, alanine, glycine, arginine, asparagine and aspartic acid good to poor growth resulted. Good growth has also been observed with casein hydrolysate, peptone and yeast extract. Aspartic acid, alanine and glutamic acid permitted growth appreciably at 0.064M concentration. Transamination studies carried out to study the effect of the amino acids suggested that the amino acids are converted to the keto acids during transamination. Some studies have indicated that the optimal concentration of inorganic nitrogen is 8mM. The pH also influences the utilization of nitrate and ammonia.

Vitamins and growth substances

Many callus tissues synthesize vitamins and growth substances to meet their requirements. Thus, additional requirements are limited to few vitamins either alone or in combination with other metabolites. Vitamin B_{12} was found to be most beneficial for callus from white spruce, pantothenic acid for *Crataegus*, p-amino benzoic acid for *Jerusalem antichoke* and ascorbic acid for *Juniperus*.

The requirements for growth nutrients vary with the isolate and species. The growth hormones employed include auxins, cytokinins and gibberellins and are listed in Table 5.2.

Table 5.2: The commonly used auxins and cytokinins

Auxins	Cytokinins
Indole-3-butyric acid (IBA)	Benzyl amino purine (BAP)
Napthaleneacetic acid (NAA)	Isopentenyl adenine (2 IP)
p-Chlorophenoxyacetic acid (p-CPA)	Furfurylaminopurine (FAP)
Naphthoxyacetic acid (NOA)	N-Methylaminopurine (MAP)
Trichlorophenoxyacetic acid (2 4 5- T)	
Oichlorophenoxy acetic acid (2 4 -D)	
Indole acetic acid (IAA)	

Requirements of callus may be of three types:

1. Some species grow indefinitely on media without any addition of IAA;

2. Certain species or strains of tissues require IAA in varying concentrations as a supplement;

3. The habituated strains of tissue require added IAA during the first few weeks or months in culture and following transfer, synthesize their own requirements.

The presence of antibiotic also affects growth of callus tissue. The growth of sunflower tissue was found to be stimulated by penicillin. Streptomycin, terramycin and bacitracin stimulated growth of Rumex tissue. In contrast polymyxin and chloramphenicol inhibited the tissue growth while terramycin has been found be toxic to marigold tissue of crown gall origin.

Nucleic acids, purines and pyrimidines

Depending on the species and concentration of the nucleic acids, certain purines and pyrimidines may inhibit or stimulate the growth of the callus tissue. The growth of *Rumex virus* tumor tissue was improved by ribonucleic acid (RNA) at concentrations from 0.2 to 0.8 mg and impaired by deoxyribonucleic acid (DNA). Presence of adenine, adenosine and adenylic acid inhibited the callus growth. Guanine, uracil, xanthine and hypoxanthine showed some beneficial effect. However, uric acid has been found to be toxic. The RNA has been found to be a good source of nitrogen for tobacco tissue but not for marigold tissue however DNA could not serve as a good nitrogen source for either of the tissues.

Complex extracts

To induce continued growth in certain tissues various plant and animal extracts have been employed in addition the supplements like basic mineral salts and sucrose. These include yeast extract, malt extract, tomato, and other, vegetable juices, casein hydrolysate and various liquid endosperms including those from horse chest nuts, coconuts, and corn. Malt extract is recorded to be beneficial for pure tissue culture whereas casein hydrolysate has been shown to stimulate growth of many species including normal sunflower stem callus and carrot callus.

5.5.2.3. Growth determination

There are various techniques available which can be used to measure culture growth. They are discussed in the following paragraphs.

Cell number

This method furnishes the most accurate information about cell growth as it involves direct counting of cells. This method, however, demands a high percentage of countable single cells. But plant cell suspension mostly comprises of cell clumps of varying sizes. Thus, for determination of cell numbers an additional step for disruption of cell clumps into single cells is required. This disadvantage can be circumvented by the treatment of cells with pectinase, a macerating enzyme or chromic trioxide before counting. Nevertheless, the entire process becomes lengthy.

Packed cell volume

This method gives very quick results however; they are more or less rough approximations only. The method involves the centrifugation of a known volume of suspension culture for the deposition of the cells at the bottom of the tube. Following settlement, the total volume of packed cells is measured. The concentration of cells in the culture can be calculated in terms of percentage with reference to the total volume of suspension.

Fresh and dry weights

This is the most widely used method for growth determination. During the linear phase, plant cells synthesize cell wall material and starch from available carbohydrates. As the cell enters the progressive deceleration and stationary phases, all the available carbohydrates are metabolized by the cells. Accumulation of starch is thereby stopped. Therefore, there is a decline in the dry weight corresponding to the metabolism of accumulated starch. But at this stage a progressive increase in fresh weight is observed as the cells are larger and they trap culture medium on the filter bed.

Nutrient uptake studies

Analysis of growth medium for nutrients like sucrose, glucose, fructose, nitrate, inorganic phosphates, etc. indicates if a particular component is limiting at any stage in the culture cycle. Carbon conversion efficiency of cell suspension culture can be calculated from the data of carbohydrate analysis and biomass measurements.

Cell viability measurements

The term viability refers to the capacity of a cell or organism to live and grow. When it comes to measuring viability, measuring some parameters of metabolic activity is more reliable and informative than the growth measurements. Based on these metabolic functions, the viability tests can be categorized as follows:

(I). Cytoplasmic streaming

This is a nondestructive assay method. A serious limitation of the method is that, it can only be applied to cell suspensions, protoplasts and single clumps of cells through which light can pass. Even in single cells and protoplasts, the observation of cytoplasmic streaming is hampered by large vacuoles.

(II). Measuring membrane integrity

This can be applied to virtually all types of cultured plant material. However, an erroneous interpretation may be drawn if there is a lack in homogeneity in tissue composition. There is always a possibility that different cell types in the tissue would leak electrolytes at different rates. Also, typically the conductance of distilled water containing a tissue sample that is employed for assessing electrolyte leakage may give some clumping and misleading results. Thus, electrolyte loss is measured only from cells having a contact with the water.

Another approach of stain exclusion assays is limited to cell suspensions and protoplasts or small clumps of cells through which light can pass. Also, a possibility of misinterpretation exists in the presence of dead cells which have lost their cytoplasm. These cells are not stained and they may be considered as alive. Some dyes (like phenosafranine) are bound to cell walls of *Zea mays* and thereby any exclusion or cytoplasmic binding could be hindered.

(III). Measuring biochemical activity

This is performed by the reduction of 2,3,5-triphenyl tetrazolium chloride (TTC) and fluorescein diacetate (FDA) stains. TTC is water soluble and gives a colorless solution. Within a live cell it is reduced to water insoluble red formazan by dehydrogenase activity or mitochondrial electron transport chain. In a dead cell, mitochondrial activity would be absent and TTC would remain unreduced. Thus, in a TTC solution a live tissue will turn red whereas dead tissue will not change color. This assay can be quantified by extraction of red precipitate from the tissue with ethanol and measuring its absorbance spectrophotometrically.

FDA is a nonpolar, nonfluorescent molecule. It enters plant cells where esterases remove the acetate moiety. The resulting fluorescence is retained in the cell owing to its polar nature and is unable to cross plasmalemma. Dead cells have limited esterase activity and have leaky membranes as well. As a result they would produce less fluorescein in comparison to live cells and the fluorescence produced would not be retained. Thus, after exposure to FDA, live cells will fluoresce whereas dead cells will not. In comparison to TTC reduction, FDA is faster and can be visualized within cells microscopically. Therefore, in addition to general viability assay it can be utilized to determine the number of live cells in a population.

5.5. TYPES OF CULTURE

5.5.1. Callus culture

Callus culture is a mass of cells or tissue resulted subsequent to initiation and continued proliferation of the undifferentiated parenchyma cells from parent tissue on a clearly defined semisolid media. This is observed when an explant from a differentiated tissue is cultured on a medium. The quiescent (non-dividing) cells undergo changes to achieve meristematic state.

This phenomenon of mature cells reversion back to the meristematic state leading to the formation of callus growth is called **dedifferentiation**. Moreover, the cells from callus are capable of generating into whole plant, a phenomenon referred to as redifferentiation. These two typical characters are components of **cellular totipotency**.

These cultures present a convenient mode for the long term maintenance of cell lines; as such culture can be maintained for extended periods *via* subculturing at 2-4 weekly intervals. Cell suspension is usually derived from the callus culture and the plant regeneration is often initiated from them as well.

Callus is frequently formed *in vivo* as a result of wounding at the cut edge of a stem or a root that follows invasion by the microorganisms or damage by the insect feeding. The callus formation is

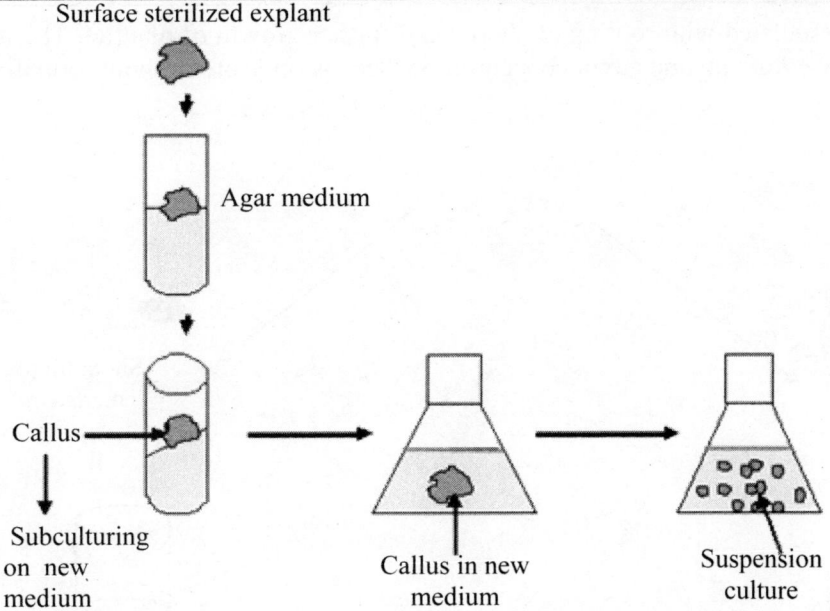

Surface sterilized explant

Agar medium

Callus

Subculturing
on new
medium

Callus in new
medium

Suspension
culture

Fig. 5.6: Callus culture and initiation of suspension culture

controlled by the endogenous auxin and cytokinin. *In vitro* callus formation on the explant of the parent tissue can be induced by incorporating the above mentioned plant growth regulators into growth medium. Organogenesis can be initiated and regulated in the callus culture by manipulation of the ratio of auxin and cytokinins. With a few exceptions, a high ratio of cytokinin to auxin results into the shoot formation whereas a high ratio of auxin to cytokinin gives rise to the root formation. There are a number of plant tissue culture media documented in the literature that facilitate callus formation. One such media is that of Murashige and Skoog. Other techniques involved in the induction of organogenesis proceed *via* selection of a suitable inoculums and control of physical environment.

5.5.2. Meristem-tip culture

Meristem is the mass of undifferentiated parenchyma cells found at the extreme tip of the shoot and root systems. They have the totipotency to regenerate into plantlets. In meristem-tip culture organized apex of the shoot from a selected donor plant is excised for subsequent *in vitro* culture. The culture conditions are manipulated to permit only for organized outgrowth of the apex directly into a shoot, without the intervention of any adventitious organs. The meristem tip is excised by sterile dissection under the microscope and is often kept less than 1 mm in length. The excised portion excludes any differentiated provascular or vascular tissues and contains the otical dome and a limited number of youngest leaf primordial. The most widely used media for meristem culture are MS medium and White,s medium. A diagrammatic representation of shoot tip (or meristem culture) in micropropagation is given in Figure 5.7.

In stage I, the culture of meristem is established. Addition of growth regulators namely cytokinins (kinetin, BA) and auxin (NAA or IBA) will support the growth and development. In stage II, shoot development along with axillary shoot proliferation occurs. High levels of cytokoinins are required for this purpose.

Stage III is associated with rooting of shoots and further growth of plantlet. The root formation is facilitated by low cytokinin and auxin concentration. This is opposite to shoot formation since high

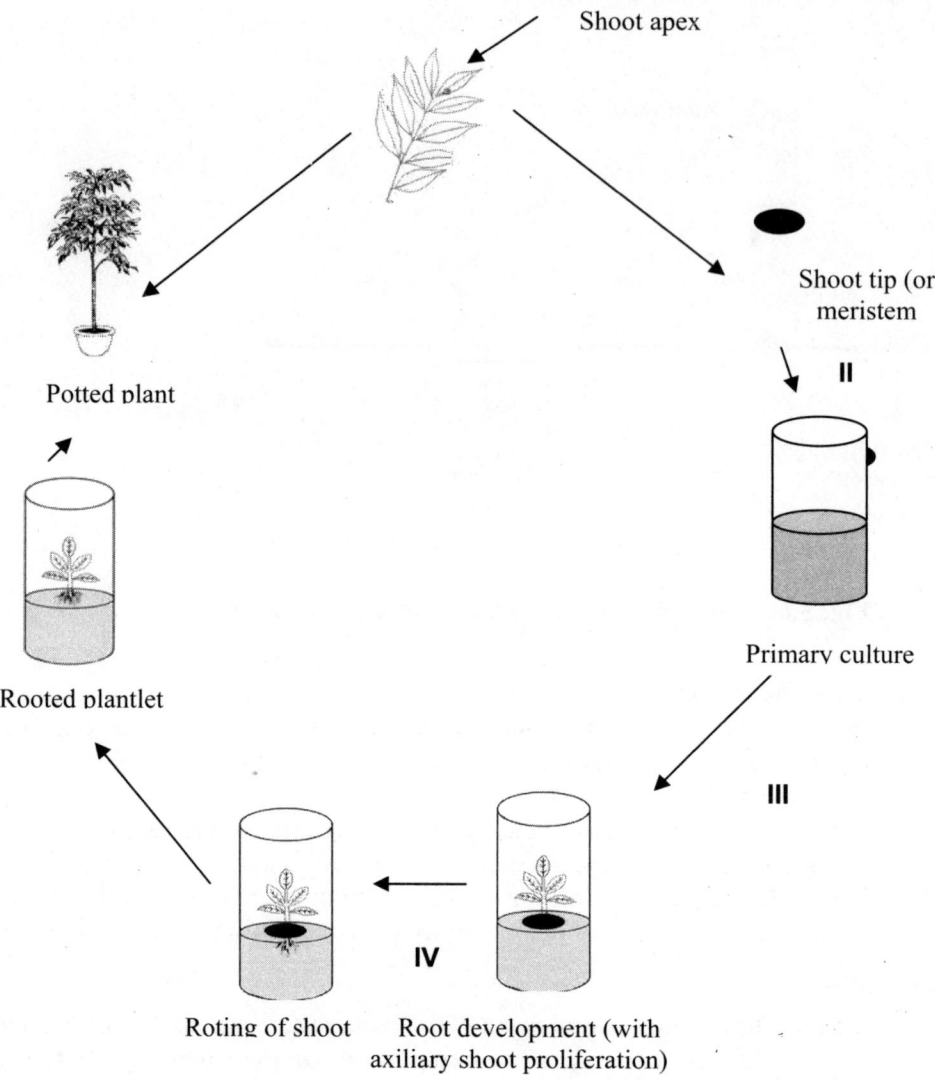

Fig.5.7: Diagrammatic representation of shoot tip and meristem tip culture

levels of cytokinins are required (in stage II). Consequently, stage II medium and stage III medium should be different in composition. Some of the advantages of the meristem culture are given below:

1. Viral, bacterial and fungal pathogen free stock for the propagation can be effectively prepared even from the infected donor plants. This is possible because terminal region of the shoot meristem that is used for culture is unlikely to contain pathogenic particles.

2. *In vitro* clonal propagation with maximal genetic stability is possible since plantlets production through adventitious organogenesis or any callus tissue formation can be avoided.

3. The meristem tip is sufficiently small and the tissue is homogeneous. Thus, it provides a practical propagule for cryopreservation and other techniques for of culture storage.

4. This technique preserves precise arrangements of cell layers necessary for micropropagation of chimeral material. In a typical chimera, the surface layers of the developing meristem are from different genetic background. It is only their contribution in a particular arrangement that elicits desired characteristics to the plant organ.

5. These cultures are usually acceptable for international transport as they comply with quarantine requirements and regulations.

5.5.3. Shoot-tip culture

The shoot apex or shoot-tip consists of the apical meristem and one to three adjacent leaf primordia, whereas the apical meristem refers only to the portion of the shoot apex lying distal to the youngest leaf primordium. Although true meristem culture has been widely employed to eliminate virus infestation, but the small size of this explant (80–100μm) limits its utility. Thus, usually virus eradication is achieved using the shoot apex, which includes the meristem and 2-3 primordial leaves. This method is widely used with both monocot and dicot species.

Table 5.3: A selected list of somaclonal variants obtained from different crop species with their morphological characters

Crop	Character(s)
Rice	Flowering period particle size; plant height; leaf length; shape and colour frequent of fertile seed; sterility mutants.
Wheat	Plant height; tiller number; grain colour; seed storage protein.
Maize	Reduced pollen fertility and male sterility twin stock from a single node
Sugarcane	High sugar yield; increased stalk length; diameter weight and density.
Barley	Increased grain yield; leaf shape; heading date; ash content.
Oats	Plant height; heading date; morphology and fertility
Soyabean	Variable height; maturity; seed protein and oil content
Potatoe	High yield; growth habit; maturity and morphology.
Tomatoe	Dwarf habit; easy flowering; orange fruit colour.
Carrot	Higher carotene content
Pineapple	Foliage density; eat color; width and spine formation
Brassica	Multiple branching stem; altered leaf; slow growth; failure to flower or delay in flowering; large pollen grains.
Tobacco	Increased yield; plant height; leaf number, shape, width and yield; type of inflorescence and yield.

Some of the crop species that have been freed of viruses by this technique include horse raddish, soyabean, sweet potato, cauliflower, sugar cane and rhubarb. There are no reports of variant plant types resulting from this explant in culture. As the plants are derived from a preexisting shoot meristem, the true genetic type and agronomic and phenotypic characters are maintained.

Asexual reproduction using shoot tip or axillary bud explant, generates plants that are genetically identical to the stock plant. On the other hand, in plants arising from callus culture or suspension culture cells, the somatic embryo or shoot meristem develops adventitiously. These plants thereby exhibit a variety of culture-induced changes termed as **somaclonal variations**. Somaclonal variation is the genetic variability observed in plants derived from a callus intermediate.

The adaptation of this procedure to transformation studies can eliminate many of the present restrictions relating to species and variety that arise due to the lack of an appropriate *in vitro* regeneration method. Transformed plants can be obtained using shoot apex explant in co-cultivation with *Agrobacterium tumefaciens*.

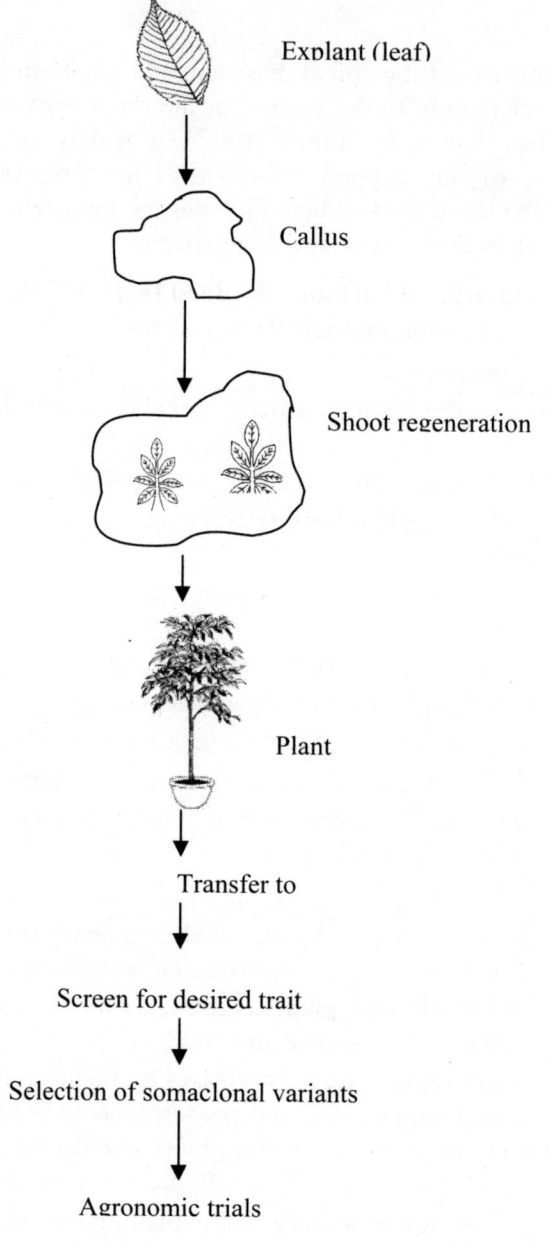

Explant (leaf)

Callus

Shoot regeneration

Plant

Transfer to

Screen for desired trait

Selection of somaclonal variants

Agronomic trials

Fig. 5.8: A diagrammatic representation of isolation of somaclones without *in vitro* selection

5.5.4. Flower organ culture

Flower formation in tissue culture has been observed in several plant species and is reported to arise from a variety of explant sources. There are varieties of factors that contribute to flower induction in nature. It is assumed that various factors are mainly responsible for *in vitro* flowering. Reasons for studying flower formation in tissue culture include:

1. It provides a model system for studying whole flower development from an excised part of the flower (e.g., ovary culture).

2. It provides an opportunity for conducting microbreeding.

3. It provides a source of biochemicals and pharmaceuticals.

Thus, by using appropriate plants like **Amaranthus** there is a possibility of completing an entire life cycle of a plant. This leads to a model system useful in studying microclimates or nutritional effects on the vegetative and reproductive processes of the plant.

5.5.5. Fruit organ culture

The culture of fruit tissues as whole organ or isolated tissue sections has been carried out with various species. Whole, isolated ovaries have been successfully cultured to give rise to mature fruits (e.g., strawberry). Usually when an isolated portion of the fruit tissue is introduced into a sterile environment, it immediately loses structural integrity and degenerates into a rapidly dividing callus mass. Loss of structural integrity is associated correspondingly with an alteration of physiology that is subsequently reflected in the production of an altered metabolism. Thus at times, it is not possible to make a meaningful study of fruits development using callus derived from fruit tissues.

At present, the use of fruit culture is to serve as a bioassay system to study fruits maturation events within a controlled environment. The reports of these studies can then be extrapolated for the improvement of field grown crops. A large quantity of extractable plant biochemical's and pharmaceuticals are derived from flowers and fruits. Seemingly, with an improvement in the present status of fruit culture technology, edible products from cultured fruits would be one of the possible future perspectives.

5.5.6. Microspore and anther culture

Microspore culture offers a powerful alternative to the protoplast culture as a single cell culture method. In microspore culture a true haploid cell system is utilized. Haploids are sporophytes with half chromosome number. For successful microspore culture the following factors have been appreciated and identified which play an important role:

1. Growth profile of donor plant;
2. Genotype of donor plant;
3. The pretreatment;
4. The developmental stage of microspore;
5. The culture medium and the conditions during culture growth.

Various steps involved in anther and microspore culture are outlined in figures 5.9 and 5.10 respectively. Microspore culture is usually preferred over the anther culture even though the former has been successful in some species only.

The haploid production using isolated pollen grains involves following steps:

1. Dissected pollen grains are taken in a beaker containing liquid medium, they are skewed with the help of a glass rod or syringed piston;

2. The suspension is then filtered through a millipore nylon filter and the filtrate is collected which contains only microspores;

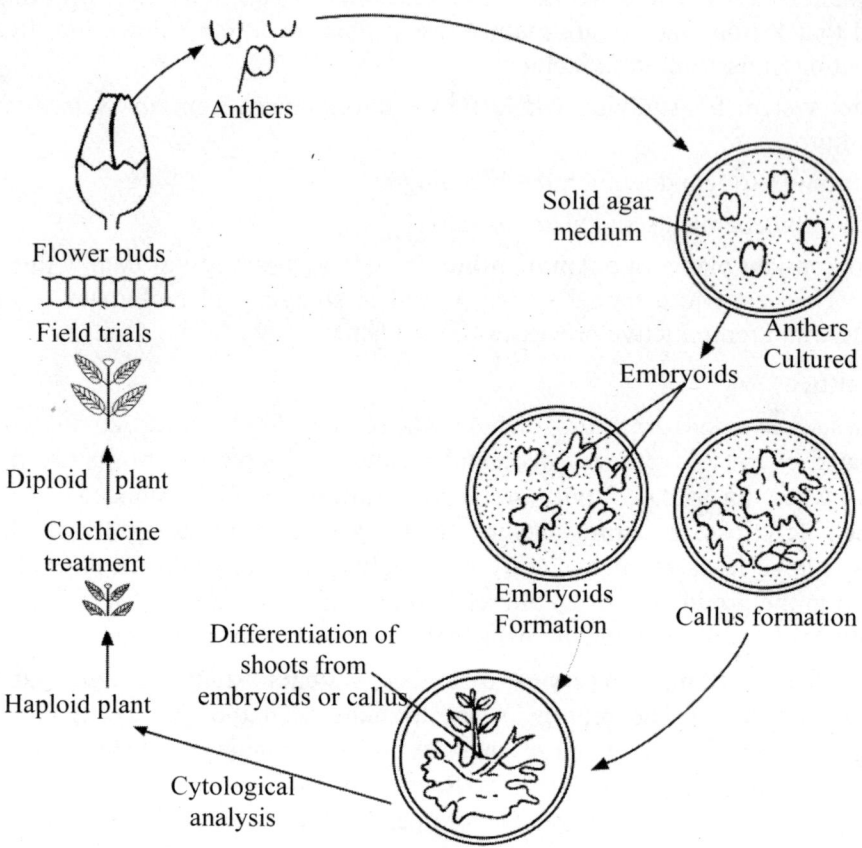

Fig. 5.9: Various steps involved in the production of haploid plants from anther culture

3. Microspores containing filtrate is centrifuged at 1000 rpm for 5 minutes;

4. The pellet is resuspended in a fresh medium;

5. Microspore suspension is used as an inoculum and transferred on a solid/liquid medium maintained at 25°C for 10–15 h.

Microspores may develop directly into embryos within 15 days. In anther as well as microspore culture spontaneously doubled haploids are also generated hence requiring no colchicine treatment. Similarly, haploids can be produced from female gametophytes. Haploid production with gymnosperms has been successful. Zamia, Ephedra and Cycads are some representative examples of this class. Nevertheless, the results were found to be promising and now haploids could be obtained from cultured ovaries in a few crop species like tobacco, barley and wheat. The haploid production technology seems to be possible with a number of plant species and thereby holds great potential to be an effective tool in plant species modifications.

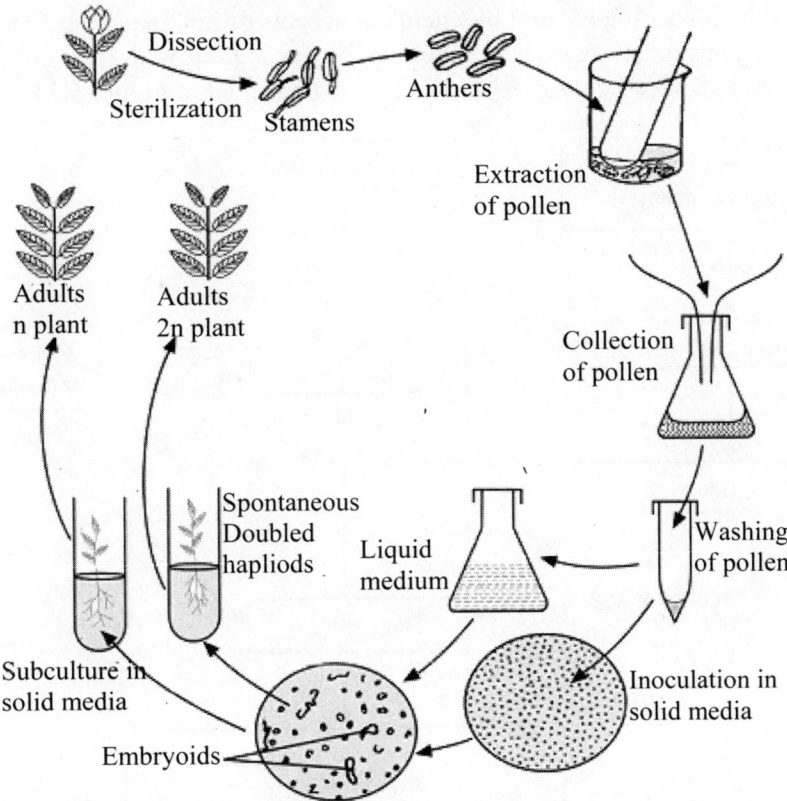

Fig. 5.10: Various steps involved in the production of haploid plants using isolated pollen grains

Some of the inherent advantages of microspore culture are:

1. The large somaclonal variations associated with protoplast selection in protoplast culture are largely eliminated.
2. A more synchronized embryo development facilitates accurate mutation and selection methods.
3. A high plant regeneration frequency (more than 80%) can be readily obtained.
4. The entire sequence from microspore isolation to plantlet development takes place in as little as 4 weeks time.

5.5.7. Dual fungal and plant cell culture

Success with combined fungal-plant cultures has been variable, especially in terms of establishing cultures that may be maintained in a balanced state for prolonged periods. But, undoubtedly such cultures are of immense utility for studying cell-cell interactions. Callus culture provides the host tissue that can be maintained in an undifferentiated state with the help of supplements and nutrients in a controlled environment. The tissue is axenic and cell population is nearly homogeneous. By judicious manipulation of growth conditions tissue differentiation can be affected and from sterile tissue, a plant similar to that of the intact plant can be obtained.

The interaction between pathogen and its host plant involves complex recognition and response mechanisms. Studies have indicated that some resistance genes can operate in callus tissue and thus tissue culture can be exploited for programs that could be utilized for screening of disease resistance.

Investigation of the physiological and biochemical aspects of host-pathogen interaction and operation of resistance mechanisms at the cellular level can be carried out with dual cultures. The protocol for the dual fungal and plant cell culture is schematically presented in Figure 5.11

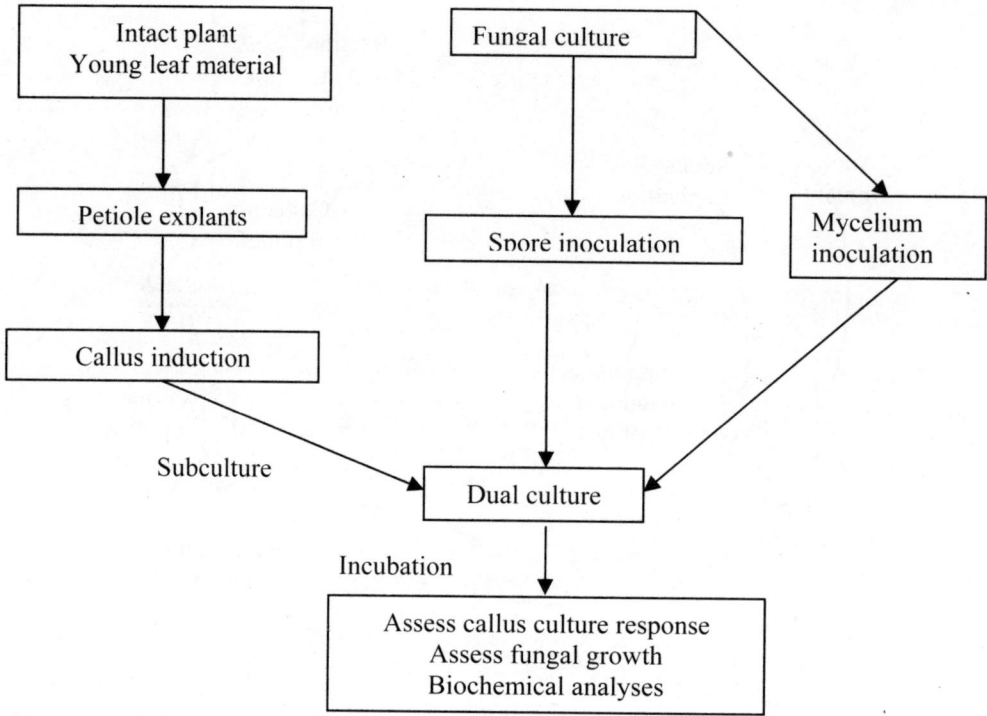

Fig.5.11: Summary protocol for dual fungal and plant cell cultures

5.5.8. Protoplast culture

A protoplast is a cell without a cell wall. They contain all the normal cell organelles plus nucleus. The nucleus expresses totipotency through conversion of the protoplast to the regenerated plant. Cell wall of a plant cell can be decomposed and removed by the treatment of the lytic enzymes like cellulose and pectinase. Studies conducted with the regenerating plantlets from the protoplast culture indicated that all the clones generated from the protoplasts are not identical but exhibit some variation in their characters. This type of variation is referred to as somaclonal variation or **somatic variation**.

The salient features of protoplast culture are:

1. The somatic protoplasts are prone to fuse with one another, thereby leading to the formation of somatic hybrids. These somatic hybrids can be used for regeneration of plantlets having new characters, the ones that are not found in their parents.

2. The isolated protoplasts have tendency to take up the foreign gene from culture. Following this uptake, protoplast undergoes genetic modification. 'This feature can be exploited for crop improvement in agriculture.

3. The protoplasts are also capable of engulfing larger particles such as isolated cell organelles present in culture. For genetic manipulation of crops isolated chloroplasts, mitochondria, nucleus and chromosomes can be added to the protoplast culture (Fig. 5.12)

4. Protoplasts can also utilize in the establishment of cybrids through the fusion of protoplasts.

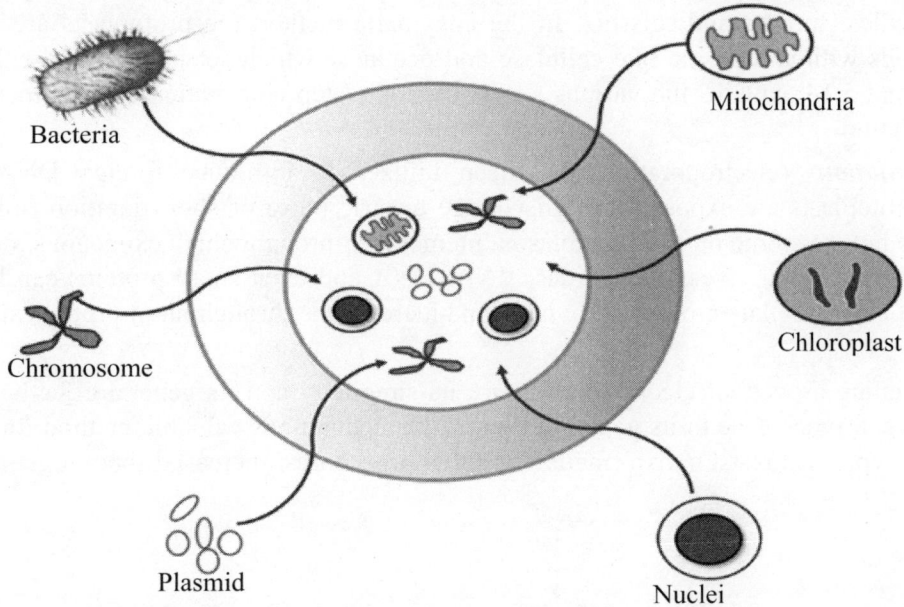

Fig. 5.12: Various biological components that can be taken up by isolated protoplasts

5. The plants regenerated from protoplasts are referred as somatic variants, show some variations in their character as discussed earlier. These somatic variants are used in crop improvement.

The above mentioned applications are only possible if isolated protoplasts have the element of totipotency. With the passage of time protoplasts synthesize new cell walls around themselves. These cells are cultured in a medium for the plantlet regeneration. This property of the plant cells is referred to as totipotency. If the isolated protoplasts lack their totipotency, the protoplast technology fails to give its beneficial results.

5.5.8.1. Applications of protoplast culture

The protoplast can be utilized for a variety of studies including the following:

1) Uptake of exogenously supplied materials like bacteria, algae, virus and macromolecules like DNA.
2) For physiological investigations and the ultra structural studies.
3) For transformation assessments
4) The isolation of subcellular components like nuclei, vacuoles and chromosomes.

In its simplest form the protoplast is used as the starting point in the manipulation for genetic (somaclonal) variation following the mass generation of the plants. The source of protoplasts can be of whole plant or tissue culture. Leaves, *in vitro* grown shoots or callus/cell suspension culture give high yields of the protoplasts.

5.5.8.2. Methods of isolation of protoplasts

The two methods commonly used in preparation of plant protoplasts from cultured plant tissues are mechanical and enzymatic method. In the mechanical method, removal of cell wall is facilitated by the aid of needles, forceps and scissors. In the enzymatic method the protoplasts are prepared by treating the cells with an enzyme like cellulase and pectinase which selectively digest the cell wall. Figures 5.13 and 5.14 explains the various stages of single step enzymatic isolation method used in protoplast isolation

Electromanipulation- (electroporation) has been utilized to introduce foreign DNA into plant protoplasts. Protoplasts are exposed to high voltage electric pulse of short duration (micro or milli seconds). This induces some pores in the plasma membrane, through which exogenous molecules and macromolecules including dyes, nucleotides, RNA, DNA and even small proteins can be taken up. Such electric fields stimulate protoplast division and increase the throughput of protoplast derived cell colonies.

The outstanding aspects of electroporation are its simplicity and its general effectiveness with a wide range of cell types. Due to its general efficacy the technique is valuable method for introducing DNA into cell types that resist transformation by other procedures. Increased shoot regeneration.

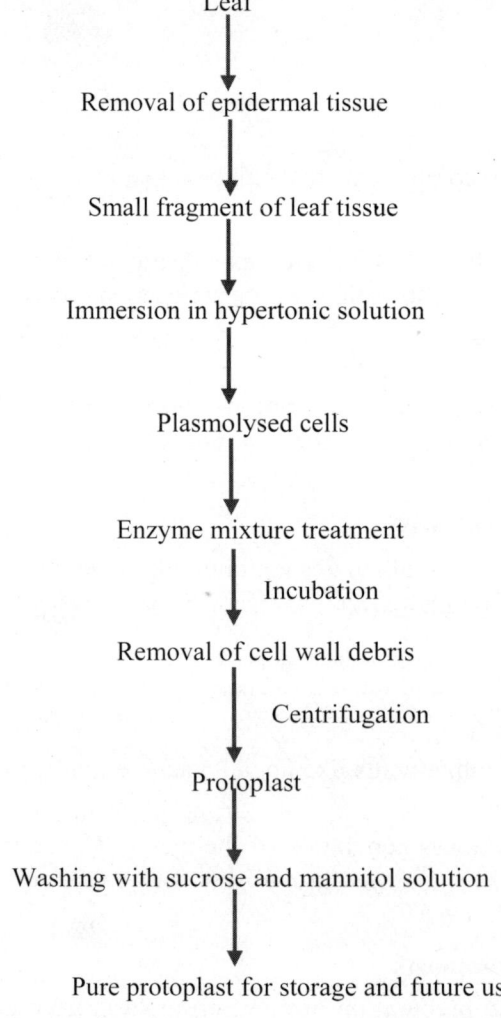

Fig. 5.13: Stages of single step enzymatic isolation method of protoplast isolation from leaf tissues

capability through the influence of low voltage electric impulse on auxin metabolism has been reported in such colonies.

*Microinjection-*Another important and effective technique particularly applicable to animal cells is microinjection. This technique of introducing DNA into plants is sufficiently well developed and can be more generally adapted. One of the methods developed for protoplast microinjection involves the use of low melting point agarose, both for holding protoplasts during microinjection and for their subsequent culture.

Protoplasts are useful for microinjection only on the day of their preparation, and possibly on the following day, because after this period of time cell wall reformation starts, making needle penetration difficult. Alternatively, the time available for microinjection can be extended by delaying cell wall reformation by holding the protoplasts at a lower temperature.

5.5.8.3. Protoplast fusion

Protoplast fusion is of great significance for hybridization between species and genera, which are not amenable to crossing by conventional method of sexual hybridization.

Techniques of protoplast fusion

1. Spontaneous fusion: Enzymatic degradation of cell walls is performed during isolation of protoplasts. During this process some of the protoplasts lying in close proximity may undergo fusion to produce homokaryons or heterokarones which contain 2–40 nuclei. If protoplasts are prepared from actively dividing cells, the frequency of multinucleate fusion bodies is more. But this spontaneous fusion is intraspecific. Another approach of inducing spontaneous fusion is by bringing protoplasts into intimate contact using micropipettes and micromanipulators. It has been observed that protoplasts isolated from young leaves are more prone to spontaneous fusion.

2. Induced fusion: Induced fusion is of great utility when fusion of protoplasts from two different species (intersepcific fusion) or from two different sources of same species has to be achieved. In this technique a fusogen is employed for inducing fusion. Inactivated sendai virus is often used in animals for fusion induction, whereas in plants the inducing agent brings the protoplasts together and this is followed by adherence to one another and finally lead to fusion of plant protoplasts.

1. Sodium nitrate treatment: In this method the isolated protoplasts are suspended in an aggregation mixture comprising of 5.5% sodium nitrate in 10% sucrose solution and incubated at 35°C to induce fusion. To improve the frequency of fused protoplasts, centrifugation of the mixture followed by resuspension of the pellet and incubation for additional cycles can be opted. As the final step liquid medium is used to replace the mixture and protoplasts in this mixture are incubated once again and finally protoplasts are plated on a solid medium.

2. Treatment with calcium ions at high pH: In this method protoplasts in a fusion inducing solution ($0.05M$ $CaCl_2.2H_2O$ in $0.4M$ mannitol at pH 10.5) are subjected to centrifugation for 30 min. The fusion of 20–50% protoplasts is completed after it is incubated at 37°C for 40–50 min. However, in some cases high pH may be toxic and a constraint in its application.

3. Polyethylene glycol (PEG) treatment: This approach has several advantages including low cytotoxicity, high fusion frequency and reproducibility. Agglutination of protoplasts can perform by any of the following methods:

a) When the quantity of protoplast is sufficient, protoplasts suspended in 1 ml. of culture medium is added to 1 ml. of PEG solution (56%). The tube is shaken for 5 sec and protoplasts is allowed to sediment for 10 min. Protoplasts are then washed with growth medium and observed for successful agglutination and fusion

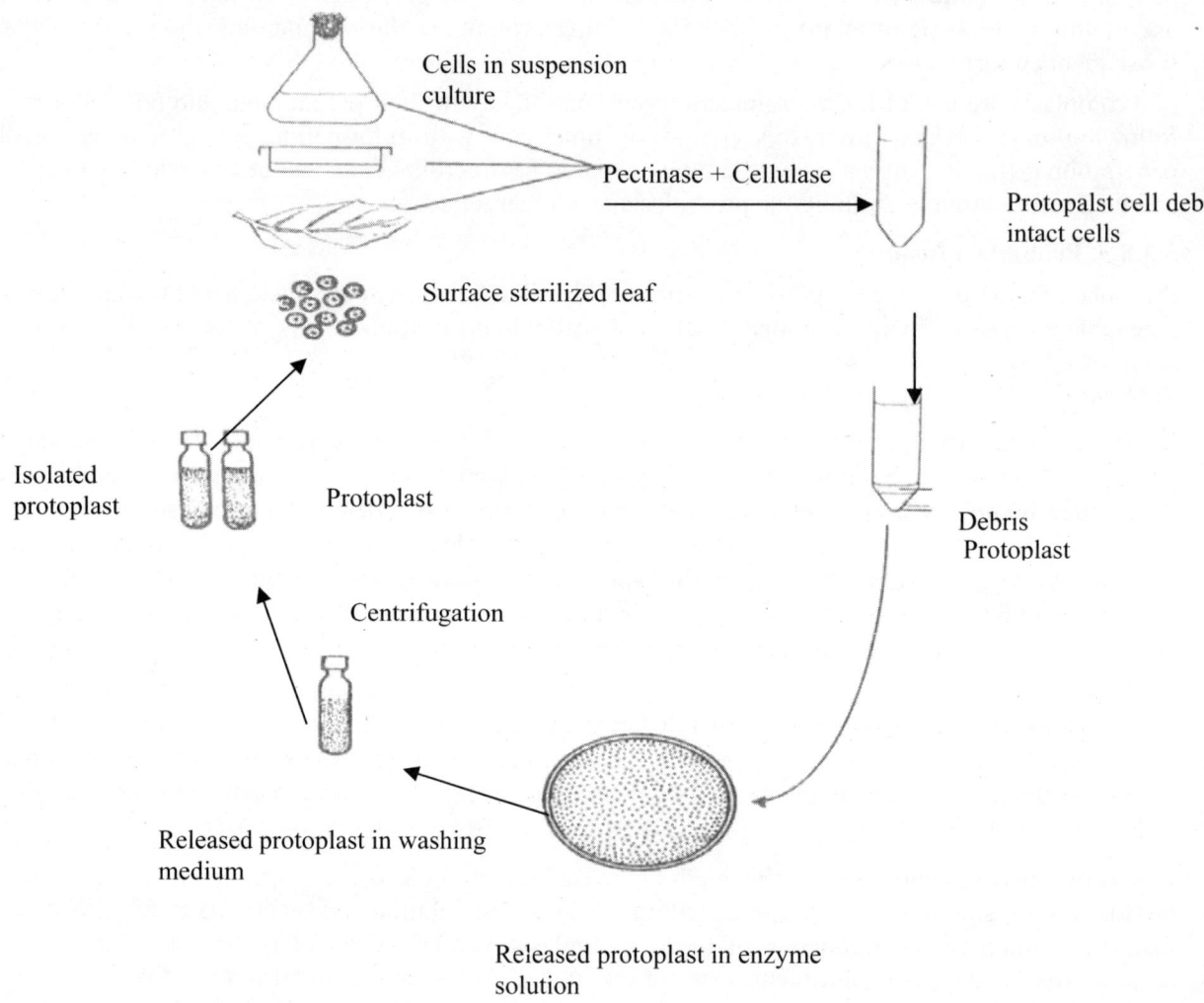

Fig. 5.14: Schematic presentation of enzymatic isolation of plant protoplast

b) When the amount of available protoplasts is small i.e., in microquantities, drop cultures are preferred. In which the two types of protoplasts are taken and mixed in equal quantities. 4–6 microdrops or 100μl. of each are transferred to petri plates and allowed to settle for 5–10 min. at room temperature. From the periphery in each plate 2–3 microdrops or 50 μl of PEG is added and incubated at room temperature (24°C) for 30 min. Once the agglutination of protoplasts is complete, protoplasts are gradually washed and then the PEG is replaced by culture medium to facilitate the growth of fused protoplasts.

4. Electric fusion: In this approach protoplasts are placed in culture cell containing electrodes and a potential difference is applied. This induces the protoplasts to line up between the electrodes. Fusion of protoplasts is subsequently achieved by application of a short square wave electric shock.

5.5.8.4. Selection of fused protoplasts

The protoplasts population after fusion treatment comprises of a mixture of parental types heterokaryons and homokaryons. Heterokaryons are potential source of future hybrids and are only 0.5-10% in composition. Selection of heterokaryons or calli derived from the same has been attempted by employing these methods:

1) Growing hybrids on a medium in which the parent protoplasts fail to grow e.g., the hybrids *Nicotiana glauca* x N. *longsdorfi*.

2) Selection of hybrids in the form of green callus which represents only hybrid cells, e.g., hybrids of *Petunia parodii* x *P. inflorata. Datura innoxia* x *Atropa belladonna.*

3) Labeling of protoplasts of two parents by different fluorescent agents, e.g., hybrids of genus Nicotiana.

In theory, the protoplast fusion technique promises to open up the potential 'gene pool' of a plant to every other living cell. However, in practice few technical problems are confronted. One of the major problems encountered is due to the diminishing capacity of a cell culture to regenerate plants over a time period. This causes difficulties in cell selection techniques, because by the time selection and testing stages are completed, and selected cells may fail to regenerate. These problems are to be sorted out so that the protoplast and somatic cell fusion techniques can be exploited for obtaining improved and desirable chemical products and biochemicals from plants.

5.5.9. Modification through transformative cell culture

Gene transfer can be achieved in plants by protoplast fusion or by DNA mediated transformation which could be achieved by the use of *Agarobacterium. Agrobacterium* is a genus of Gram-negative bacteria and uses horizontal gene transfer and cause tumors in plants. *Agrobacterium tumefaciens* is the most commonly studied species in this genus which caused crown gall disease which is characterized by tumor like growth or gall at the junction between root and shoot in infected plant by transferring tumor inducing T-DNA from bacterial tumor inducing Ti plasmid between itself and plants. For this reason *Agrobacterium tumefaciens* has become a potential vector for plant improvement by genetic engineering. A closely related species *A. rhizogenes* which induces root tumors is also utilized for the genetic transformation of plants. For the successful transformation *agarobacterium* should recognize and invade the suitable host and integrate T-DNA into it. In addition the tumorus property` of crown gall tissue shows overgrowth in the culture media devoid if growth hormones and synthesis of opines (an unusual amino acid which is not found in normal tissue). The type of opine produces is determined by bacterial strain as it is the sole source of energy in bacteria.

5.5.9.1. Tumour inducing principle and Ti plasmid

Ti plasmids have four regions in common- (i) Region A, comprising T-DNA is responsible for tumour induction, so that mutations in this region lead to the production of tumours with altered morphology (shooty or rooty mutant galls). Sequences homologous to this region are always transferred to plant nuclear genome, so that the region is described as T-DNA (transferred DNA).
(ii) Region B is responsible for replication.
(iii) Region C is responsible for conjugation

(iv)Region D is responsible for virulence, so that mutation in this region abolishes virulence. This region is therefore called virulence region and plays a crucial role in the transfer of T-DNA into the plant nuclear genome. The components of this Ti plasmid have been used for developing efficient plant transformation vectors.

The T-DNA consists of the following regions
(i) An one region consisting of three genes (two genes tms and tms2 representing 'shooty locus' and one gene tmr representing 'rooty locus') responsible for the biosynthesis of two phytohormones, namely indole acetic acid or lAA (an auxin) and isopentyladenosine 5'-monophosphate (a cytokinin).

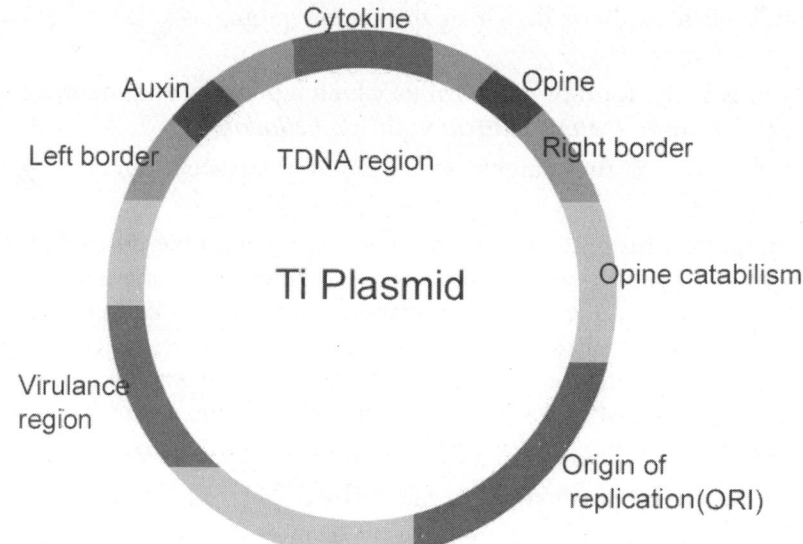

Fig. 5.15: Ti Plasmid structure

Incorporation of T -DNA into the nuclear DNA

These genes encode the enzymes responsible for the synthesis of these phytohormones, so that the incorporation of these genes in plant nuclear genome leads to the synthesis of these phytohormones in the host plant. The phytohormones in their turn alter the developmental programme, leading to the formation of crown gall.
(ii) An OS region responsible for the synthesis of unusual amino acid or sugar derivatives, which are collectively given the name opines. Opines are derived from a variety of compounds (e.g. arginine + pyruvate), that are found in plant cells. Two most common opines are octopine and nopaline. For the synthesis of octopine and nopaline, the corresponding enzymes octopine synthase and nopaline synthase are coded by T- DNA.

The transfer of T -DNA proceeds with the formation of nick at the Ti plasmid DNA at two specific sites each between third and fourth base of the bottom strand of 25bp repeat. At the loci of nick DNA synthesis initiates in the right hand 25bp repeat sequence in 5'-3' direction. As a result a single T -DNA strand is displaced. This T-DNA single strand then forms a complex with *vir* E protein and consequently transported to plant nucleus. The *vir* D operon that encodes for endonuclease expresses the enzyme that produces the nicks in the border sequences. Several other *vir* B operons may guide and direct T -DNA transfer extracellularly.

Additionally the genes which are located on *Agrobacterium* chromosomes also help in virulent activities. These genes characteristically synthesize and secrete glucons, cellulose, fibrils and cell-surface proteins. There are some active loci which play a more general role in the virulence of *Agrobacterium* and as a result *Agrobacterium* mediated gene transfer.

Disarmed plasmid Ti-derivative as plant vectors

In genetically engineered plant cell Ti-plasmid is a natural vector as it can transfer its DNA from the bacterium to the plant genome. But the wild type Ti-plasmids are not suitable as general gene vectors because due to the effects of oncogenes in the T -DNA they cause disorganized growth of the recipient plant cells.

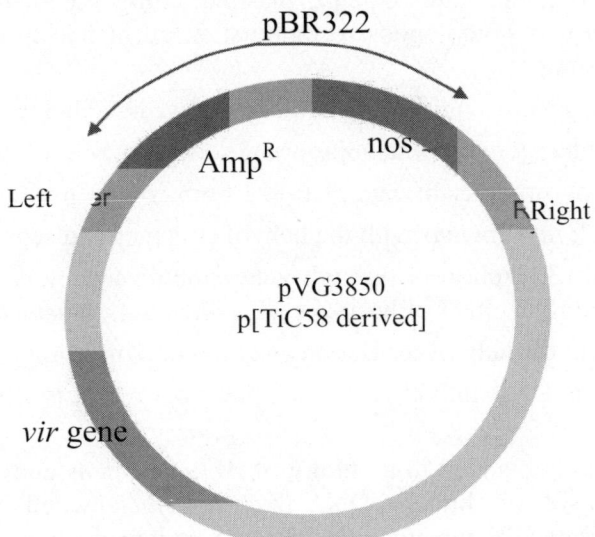

Fig.5.16: Structure of the Ti-plasmid pGV3850, in which the T-DNA has been disarmed

The tumor cells resulting from integration of normal T -DNA have proven to be recalcitrant to attempts to induce regeneration, either into normal plantlets or into normal tissue which can be grafted onto healthy plants. However, it was also observed that tobacco callus transferred with wild-type Ti-plasmid could rarely regenerate into shoots. On grafting these shoots onto healthy plants, some of the grafted shoots were found to be fertile and produced seed that developed into apparently normal plants. But these plants lacked opine and almost all the T- DNA had been deleted from them.

The observations made above indicate that for efficient regeneration of plants, the vectors used should be the ones in which the T -DNA has been disarmed by making it non-oncogenic, and this can be achieved by simply deleting all of its oncogenes (Figure 5.16).

Transfer of foreign DNA into T-DNA

Large size of wild-type Ti plasmids renders them unsuitable as experimental gene vectors. Large size means that it is impossible to find adequate unique restriction sites in the T-region, and other procedures are also cumbersome. In an attempt to alleviate this problem intermediate vectors (IV) have been developed. In IV (a vector) the T-DNA has been subcloned into conventional small plasmid vectors of *E. coli*, standard procedures can then be employed to insert the desired DNA into the T -region of such vector. The IV, vector containing foreign DNA in the T-region, can be transferred to *A. tumefaciens* by conjugation. Since IVs are conjugation-deficient, conjugation ought to be brought about by a helper vector (a conjugation-proficient plasmid which can mobilize the IV).

The whole process of transfer proceeds with a typical 'triparental' mating. In these matings three bacterial strains are mixed together. They are:

1. The *E. coli* carrying the conjugation-proficient helper plasmid,

2. The *E .coli* strain carrying the recombinant IV,

3. The recipient *Agrobacterium*.

During the course of the incubation the helper plasmid transfers recombinant IV to the *E. coli* strain which is subsequently mobilized and transferred to *Agrobacterium*. The *Agrobacterium* recepient frequently receives both the IV and the helper plasmid. Following the introduction of vector IV into *Agrobacterium, in vivo* it is homologous recombination event that inserts vector IV into a resident nonrecombinant Ti plasmid.

The process essentially involves genetic engineering strategy as discussed below:

1. Identification and isolation of target gene from appropriate source.

2. Construction of intermediate plasmid vector e.g., pBR 322 from *coli* E1 plasmids.

3. Isolation of Ti plasmid from *A. tumefaciens* with the help of enzymes and separation of T-DNA.

4. Insertion of T -DNA in PBR 322 plasmid through gene cloning technique thus formation of a shuttle vector capable of replicating in either of hosts, i.e., *E. coli* and *A. tumefaciens*.

5. Cutting of cloned T -DNA with the help of restriction enzymes and insertion of foreign DNA.

6. Insertion of so formed chimeric DNA into *E. coli*. The uptake by *E. coli* is affected in the presence of calcium chloride solution.

7. Transformed *E. coli* cells are then added to a culture of *A. tumefaciens* and incubated for a few hours. This results into the-transfer of chimeric DNA to *A. tumefaciens* cells through cytoplasmic factors of *E. coli*. The transformed *A. tumefaciens* cells are endowed with terramycin resistance acquired through *E. coli* pBR 322 plasmid.

8. Selection of transformed *A. tumefaciens* by culturing in a kanamycin containing medium. .

9. The selected transformed cells are then used to infect the culture plant cells whose genome is to be manipulated for improvement.

10. Regeneration of plantlets from modified plant tissue using standard tissue culture techniques.

5.5.9.2. *A. rhizogenes* and Ri-plasmids

A. rhizogenes, incites a disease which is known as hairy root disease, in dicotyledonous plants. A large plasmid, the Ri (root inducing) plasmid, is responsible for pathogenicity and induction of opine synthesis. The Ri plasmids are thus analogous to Ti plasmids. They have been of interest for vector development as opine-producing root tissue. Ri T -DNA is transmitted sexually by these plants and affects a variety of morphological and physiological traits but generally does not appear to be deleterious. Therefore, Ri plasmids are apparently equivalent to disarmed Ti-plasmid1 Thus, many principles of the disarmed Ti-plasmids and Ri-plasmids are similar. An intermediate vector co-integrating system has been developed and applied to the study of modulation in transgenic legumes, *Lotus corniculation*.

Agrobacterium containing both a Ri plasmid and a disarmed Ti plasmid can frequently co-transfer both plasmids, and this fact has been exploited. The Ri plasmid induced hairy root .disease in recipient *Arabidopsis* and carrot cells, served as a transformation marker for the co-transferred recombinant T -DNA, and also allows regeneration of intact plants. With this plasmid combination there was no need of incorporation of drug resistance marker on the T -DNA.

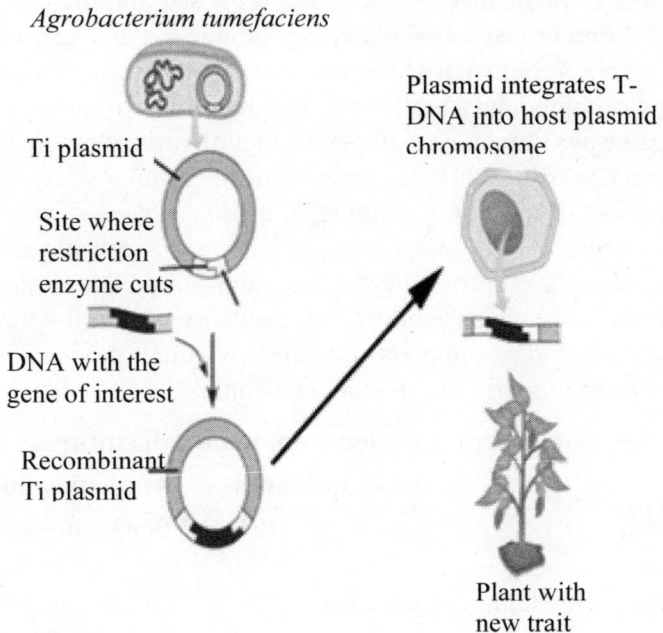

Fig. 5.17: Modification of plant through transformative cell culture

5.6. TISSUE CULTURE AND BIOSYNTHESIS OF SECONDARY PRODUCTS

Attention has been diverted towards exploration of possibilities of tissue culture as a tool for the purpose of micropropagation particularly in horticulture and agriculture. The potential for synthesis of chemicals by plants is enormous. It covers a wide range of compounds of pharmaceutical value as well as complex food materials. Growing research in practical tissue culture technology provides with

Table 5.4: Natural product yields from cell cultures and whole plants

Natural product	Species	Cell culture yield	Whole plant yield
Anthraquinones	*Morinda citrifolia*	900 nmol/g dry wt.	Root 110 nmol/g dry wt.
Anthraquinones	*Cassia tora*	0.34% fresh wt.	0.209% seed dry wt.
Ajmalicine & serpentine	*Catharanthus roseus*	1.3% dry wt.	0.26% dry wt
Diosgenin	*Dioscorea deltoidea*	25 mg/g dry wt.	20 mg/g dry wt. tuber
Ginseng saponins	Panax ginseng	0.38% fresh wt.	0.3-3.3% fresh wt.
Nicotine	*Nicotiana tabacum*	3.4% dry wt.	2-5% dry wt.
Thebaine	*Papaver bracteatum*	130 mg/g dry wt.	1400 mg/g dry wt. leaf and 3000 mg/g
Ubiquinone	*Nicotiana tabacum*	0.5 mg/g dry wt.	16 mg/g dry wt. leaf

the opportunity of biosynthesis of a variety of natural products using tissue culture. The various compounds which have been modulated synthesized and modified Include alkaloids, anthraquinones, plant phenolics and volatile oil, etc. The production of chemicals using plant tissue cultures has attained a remarkable status are summarized in Table 5.4.

Tissue cultures of a number of plant species have been proposed and the cell extracts have been analyzed for biosynthesis of different classes of secondary products. Plant cell suspension culture is especially regarded as a suitable system particularly for the production of photochemicals. Plant secondary metabolites are the compounds which are not required for normal plant growth and development by metabolic pathways common to all plants. Out of various products, medicinals are of great value for their effective use in health care. Narcotic from *Cannabis*, opium and heroin from Papaver, stimulants, i.e. caffeine from *Coffea arabica, Camellia synensis* (tea) and anthraquinone from *Cassia podocarpa*, are some of the compounds which can be considered as a group of the natural products. Similarly analgesics, antifertility agents, anti-microbial, cardiovascular and anti-malarial drugs are other compounds which could be derived from natural source. A comparative account of yields from cell culture and whole plants of different natural products is presented in table 5.4. Different substances as hitherto reported from plant cell cultures are tabulated in table 5.5.

Table 5.5: Substances reported from plant cell cultures

Alkaloids	Allergens	Anthraquinones	Antileukaemic agents
Antitumor agents	Antiviral agents	Aromas	Benzoquinones
Cardiac glycosides	Carbohydrates (including Oianthrones Polysaccharides)	Chalcones	Dianthrones
Lipids	Latex	Naphthoquinones	Nucleic acids
Nucleotide	Oils	Opiates	Organic acids
Peptides	Perfumes	Phenols	Pigments
Enzymes	Plant growth regulators	Enzyme inhibitors	Proteins
Flavonoids	Flavones	Steroids and its derivatives	Flavors (including sweeteners
Furanocoumarins	Tannins	Hormones	Sugars
Terpenes terpenoids	Insecticides	Vitamins	

Product biosynthesis has been related to three basic levels of cellular organization, i.e. cell suspension, callus and organ explants. A careful survey of literature reveals that cell culture is the best technique wherein modification in biosynthetic compounds can be affected. It has been noticed that secondary product from intact plants are produced at generally higher level as compared to their production from tissue cultures. Explanted materials of an alkaloid producing plants cultured *in vitro* have been found to attain capacity to synthesize alkaloid identical to that alkaloid in the intact plant. In some of the cases altered biosynthesis or metabolisms have been noticed particularly in the case of cell suspension culture or callus culture. *Atropa* callus produces tropane alkaloids, when the roots are differentiated whereas no such compounds are synthesized in non differentiated callus tissue. Thus, it was suggested that during culture process the production of metabolites is mainly dependent on organ differentiation. Therefore, potential for production of secondary metabolites is not lost; however, due to some unknown reasons they are not expressed or produced. There are reports regarding organogenesis in the form of roots in *Dioscorea deltoidea* and *Bulbils* and *Agar wighii* capable of producing metabolites particularly sapogenins. High yields of indole alkaloids are reported in tissue culture of *Rauwolfia serpentina*. Plant natural products and cells cultured *in vitro* could be produced through different metabolic pathways or synthesis generally referred to as biotransformation which could be used as a route to the synthesis of the novel products not found in the parent plants. Compounds like diosgenin, saponin, etc., were produced in culture in quantities comparable or even higher than in the intact plant. With the advancement in the knowledge of biochemistry and biology of cell culture there have been reports on cell culture(s) claiming for reasonably higher yields of the compounds such as anthraquinone, diosgenin, nicotine, thebaine.

The cell suspensions are ideal as they can be grown in simple bioreactors and could provide opportunities for scale up.

5.6.1. Factors affecting biosynthesis

Various factors which could affect the biosynthetic process, its rate and as a consequence the yield may typically include origin of tissue, media formulations, carbon sources, incorporation of plant growth regulators and precursor feed. Amino acids particularly tryptophan, phenylalanine and ornithine can be used as precursor. Feeding of phenyalanine to the culture of *Capsicum frutiscence* and 4-hydroxy-2-quinoline to the culture of *Butea graveolanice* for obtaining better yield of alkaloids are the classical examples of precursor feed based amelioration and biotransformations. The effect of addition of precursors during the course of alkaloid synthesis by suspension *C. Jxture* technique particularly in the case of *Solanaceous* plants and of *Catharanthus roseus* and *Cinchona ledgeriana* has been investigated. The concentration level at which the precursor is added to the media is critical as at one concentration, it may respond as an initiator and promoter of biosynthesis while turns to be inhibitor at another (higher) concentration.

The presence of amino acids was found to be toxic when added to the culture media in concentration more than 2mM causing cell death. However, accumulation of number of indole and quinoline derivatives has been reported. Cell culture techniques offer exciting opportunities in the production of various novel compounds. Cells in culture can be channeled into particular biochemical pathways as exemplified by the production of rutacultin by tissue cultures of *Ruta graveolens*. However, the process was found to be prohibitive and nonadaptive on the basis of Gost factor. Production of medicinal alkaloids such as opiates and indole using cell cultures of *C. roseus* has been of prime interest in the research of modern times. Some of the alkaloids such as ajmalicine, reserpine, vinblastine, vincristine and vincanine are derived from the precursor tryptophan. The commercial production is however, not appreciable due to poor yield.

Furthermore, the poor yields of secondary metabolites appear to be due to:

1. Differences between young, dispersed and rapidly dividing cells, akin to meristem tissue

2. Nature of slow-growing cells in organized mass

3. Variation in product formation as a function of time in culture repressing or dormancy of desired biosynthetic pathway, and

4. Non-excretion of products from cultured cells.

To overcome these problems, development of hairy root cultures, immobilized cell systems and techniques to encourage excretion of desired products into medium are being attempted. However, examples do exists that show that callus and suspension culture can synthesize secondary metabolite with yields that are comparable to the intact plant. In some cell lines the rate of production of secondary metabolites was found to be exceedingly higher to that found in the intact plant, e.g., jatrorrhizini from berberis, shikonin from *Lithospermum*, berberine from *Coptis* and rosamarinic acid from *Coleus*.

Table 5.6: Some pharmaceutically significant metabolites produced by plant tissue-culture

Compound	Plant species	Culture type
Ajmalicine	*Catharanthus roseus*	Suspension
Anthraquinones	*Cassia angustifolia*	Cell
Atropine	*Atropa belladonna*	Hairy root
Berberine	*Coptis japonica*	Cell & suspension
Caffeine	*Coffea Arabica*	Cell
Cardenolides	*Digitalis purpurea*	Cell & suspension
Codeine	*Papaver somniferum*	Suspension
Digoxin	*Digitalis lanata*	Suspension
Diosgenin	*Dioscorea compositae*	Cell
Hyoscyamine	*Hyoscyamus niger*	Suspension
Indole alkaloids	*Ipomoea violacea*	Cell & suspension
Morphine	*Papaver somniferum*	Suspension
Nicotine	*Nicotiana tabacum*	Suspension
Papain	*Carica papaya*	Cell
Quinine and Quinidine	*Cinchona ledgericna*	Root culture
Reserpine	*Rauwolfia serpentine*	Suspension
Rosamarinic acid	*Coleus blumei*	Cell & Suspension
Tropane alkaloids	*Datura innoxia*	Suspension
Vinblastine	*Catharanthus rose us*	Cell
Xanthotoxin	*Ruta graveolens*	Suspension

From a biotechnological point of view, suspension cultures are the most appropriate systems for the production of secondary metabolites on an economical scale. The productivity of metabolites synthesized by cell culture is a function of the amounts of metabolite in the cells and of growth rate of cells. A majority of the secondary metabolic activities are repressed in cultured cells and thus it becomes difficult to produce useful secondary products using them. Some of the pharmaceuticals that have been successfully isolated from plant tissue cultures are listed in table 5.6.

Sometimes cell cultures have been reported to produce compounds which are not found as normal constituents of that species. For example, unusual ether lipids, 1(3),2 diacylglycero 3(1)-O-4'-(N,N,N-trimethyl) homoserines have been isolated from algae cultures of *Chlorella fuscq*. Some other promising commercial products include a new CNS-active indole alkaloid percine and a new anti-inflammatory lignin.

Large scale production of bio-mass containing useful secondary metabolites has been achieved, however due to economical constraints the tissue culture technique is limited only to a few constituents only. To date more than 30 classes of compounds have been identified to be produced by plant cell cultures in appreciably high quantities, some of the classic examples are digitalis glycosides, diosgenin-derived steroid hormone precursors, shikonin, rosamarinic acid, opium alkaloids (codeine and morphine), ginsenosides, ajmalicine and other indole alkaloids, including vinblastine and vincristine and possible complex mixtures such as rose and jasmine oil. Furthermore, Mitsui petrochemical industries of Japan have been producing shikonin (a red colored phenolic naphthoquinone compound used as a dye and astringent) from cell cultures of *Lithospermum erythrorhizon*. A German pharmaceutical company is producing digitalis glycosides by biotransformation in cell cultures.

5.6.2. Indole alkaloids

Several important drugs, such as ajmalicine, phytostigmine, reserpine, vincristine and vinblastine belong to the class of molecules referred to as indole alkaloids. These alkaloids are found in plant family *Apocynaceae, Loganiaceae, Rubiaceae,* and *Fabaceae* out of these' vincristine and vinblastine are complex dimeric mono terpene indole alkaloids. They are used as antineoplastic agents. Although extensive work has S been undertaken to produce these compounds using classical plant tissue culture techniques but the efforts have so far failed. Only by the induction of differentiated surface cultures *via* the addition of phytohormone benzyladenine into the growth media vindoline production has been demonstrated. The media alteration however, to some extent has been reported to be instrumental in modulation of the yield. The alteration of media typically included addition of sucrose as a carbon source and some phytohormones. Bioregulators, like dimethylaminoethyl-I-2,4-dichlorophenyl ether on incorporation have been reported to increase the ajrnalicine content by 270-570% and the production of catharanthine by 82-146%.

In another approach transformed *C. roseus* cells with *Agrobacterium tumefaciens* produced tumorous cell lines was able to produce ajmalicine 0.060mg/g fresh weight. Such, modifications are referred as crown gall culture and reported to produce monomeric units catharanthine however failed to synthesize vindoline. Another report relating with the transformation of *C. roseus* cell with a mild *A. rhizogenes* which resulted in production of hairy root culture showed a 20 fold increase in cell mass over 28 day growth period. The cultures have been reported to synthesize high yields of a variety of monomeric indole alkaloids including catharanthine, ajmalicine and vindolinine.

5.6.3. Tropane alkaloids

Tropane alkaloids which occur in plants of *Solanaceae, Convolvulaceae* include several important pharmaceuticals most notably scopolamine, hyoscyamine (Fig.5.18), atropine and cocaine. The plants from Solanaceae family are highly responsive to cell culture techniques and plants producing these alkaloids have been studied extensively. Plants from these species synthesize biologically active compounds mainly in their roots. Therefore, attempts have been made to produce crown gall culture. *A. rhizogenes* to form hairy root culture exhibited a 20 fold increase in cell with an alkaloid content of 0.68% of the dry weight, wherein hyoscyamine and scopolamine were present in a comparable ratio of whole intact plant) Another solanaceous species, *A. belladonna* on transformation is with *A. rhizogenes* produced a hairy root culture with around 60 fold increase in cell mass over a 28 day growth period and synthesized scopolamine at 0.02% of the dry weight, whereas the content of hyoscyamine was estimated to be 0.371% as dry weight. The results with crown gall culture of *H.muticus, S. japonica* also exhibited increased production of tropane alkaloids in hairy root culture as compared with normal culture or suspension culture.

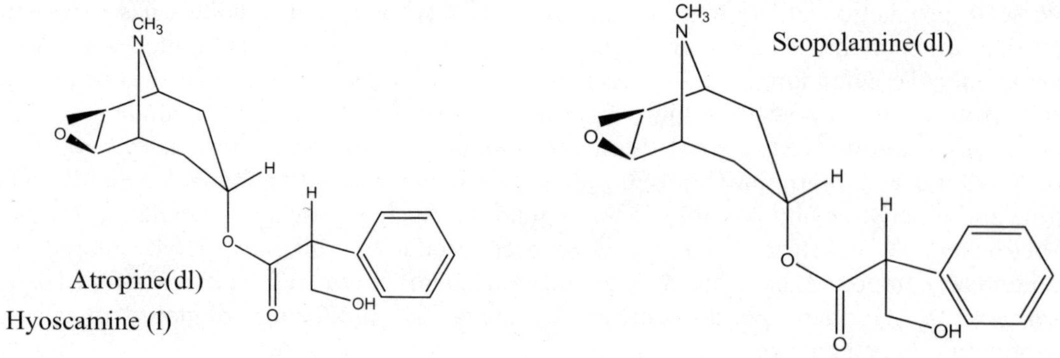

Fig. 5.18: Representative examples of tropane alkaloids

5.6.4. Quinoline alkaloids

The alkaloids mainly quinidine and quinine (Fig. 5.19) are of particular importance in treatment of malaria and in restoring normal "heart rhythms. These are the contents belonging to the family *Rutaceae*, where commercial source of quinine and quinidine is *Cinchona*. The cell culture and production of these alkaloids was experimented and revealed that cell suspension and callus culture failed to produce significant quantity of the either alkaloids whereas differentiated shoot systems demonstrated to possess bio-synthesizing capacity. The transformation of this species using *A. tumefaciens* to form hormone independent undifferentiated cell suspension culture (i.e., crown gall culture) exhibited promising results. The average quinoline alkaloid content of these cells was 5-6 times greater than previously studied untransformed form. The most recent reports on hairy root culture *C. ledgeriana* transformed with *A. rhizogenes* indicated 2-3 times alkaloid content of most of the products of dark grown crown gall cells, with the methoxylated quinoline, in quinine and quinidine yielding up to 50–70% of total alkaloids.

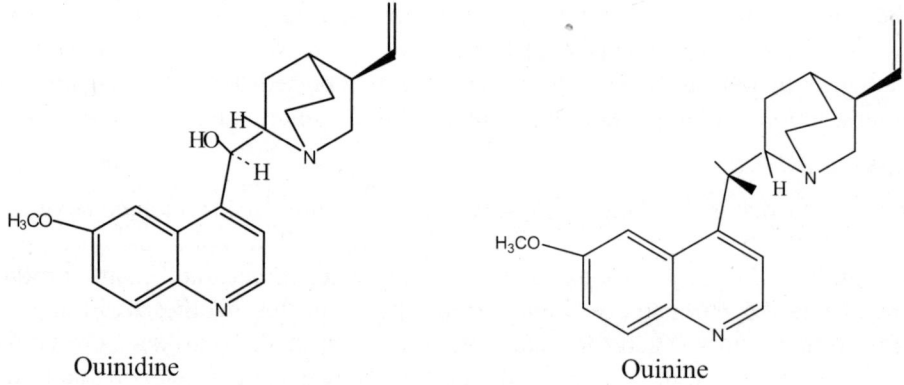

Ouinidine   Ouinine

Fig. 5.19: Representative examples of quinoline alkaloids

5.7. APPLICATIONS

There are immense possibilities for basic studies using plant tissue culture methods. This technology can be exploited for the procurement of commercial products as well. Details of the specific applications are discussed below:

5.7.1. To study respiration and metabolism

Studies of respiration of, whole pieces of callus tissue, homogenates and cellular fraction provide means of separating normal and diseased growth. For example, enzymatic differences in tissue of crown gall and normal origins exist even after growth in culture for extended periods. A reduction in respiratory levels in crown gall tissue culture has also been noted. There was an apparent increase maintained in endogenous auxins synthesis by crown gall tissue culture. C^{14} labeled fructose, sucrose and glutamine absorption and their incorporation into the alcohol insoluble fraction by crown gall tissues of *Parthenocissus* were lower than in normal tissue culture.

An increment in oxygen uptake by Rumex tissue has been demonstrated when 2-4-D, IAA and 2,3,5- triiodobenzoic acid and colchicine were used at concentrations from 0.001 to 1 mg/liter, and decreased on their incorporation at higher concentrations. The secretion of a α-amylase enzyme by this tissue accounted for the utilization of starch. The metabolism involved in cell enlargement of cultured tobacco pith parenchyma and transformations of carbohydrates by carrot tissue have also being studied and described. Tissue on IAA media in comparison to those on media lacking auxin displayed a rise in respiratory rate, an increment in ascorbic acid oxidase activity, a rise in intact cells to oxidize -SH groups of cysteine and glutathione within 72 hours, increase in invertase and pectin methyl esterase activity and a decrease in peroxidase activity. Changes in the media composition were followed by an increase or decrease in respiration and ascorbic acid oxidase activity. Phenylthiourea at critical concentrations inhibited ascorbic acid oxidase activity and the growth, whereas a large respiratory increase of auxin was permitted. Changes in the composition of the medium altered different phases of metabolism that control cell enlargement, or growth.

The oxidative and phosphorylative activities of cytoplasmic particles from crown gall and normal tissue cultures of tomato were studied and found to be qualitatively similar but quantitatively different. Both tissues had relatively constant respiratory activity during the active period of growth of tissues, but this activity period of growth of tissues decreased as growth leveled off. Crown gall tissue gave a lower activity profile than normal tissue on a dry weight basis however the values were comparable on nitrogen basis.

5.7.2. To study polarity and organ function

Isolated tissues are useful for conducting studies related to polarity and organ function. Three major types of proliferations developing in isolated tissues, viz. of unorganized parenchyma, of specialized cambial layer or that of organized growing points have been described. These may develop in fresh explants or in established cultures. Variations in these types of proliferation may be observed in a variety of tissues from many species. For instance, proliferation from a fresh stem or carrot section commonly occurs as a layer of new growth over the cut surface. Proliferation may also occur from preexisting cambia or from diffused cambia scattered in the tissue. Isolated tissue often produces root or bud meristems. Various types of proliferation have been observed in established strains of tissue as well. Cultures originally parenchymatous may develop vascular bundles, with phloem and xylem, after several transfers, and eventually root and stem primordia may be developed.

Sustained efforts have been made to clarify cell growth, cell division, callus differentiation and organ formation in terms of growth substances and balances of common metabolites. Interactions between lAA and adenines were found to be related to bud formation in tobacco callus. IAA prevented and adenine promoted the process of bud formation. Concentrations were found to be critical and the adenine-IAA ratio determined quantitatively for the degree of bud formation. The tobacco callus cells enlarged enormously without dividing when supplied with auxin alone. In the presence of auxin, cell division resulted by contact with vascular stem tissue, or by adding coconut milk or malt extract. Kinetin was isolated from DNA and was noted to be highly active in promoting cell division in the tobacco callus.

The callus tissue masses may or may not change morphologically and/or physiologically with change in time. Tissue changes, if recorded, have been correlated with auxin requirements (habituation), with pigment formation and with varied sucrose concentration or light conditions. Similarly, for growth substances such as coconut milk or 2,4-D, IAA modifications in rate of growth and firmness of tissue mass were observed. Nutritional requirements differ depending on the length of time in culture as in insect gall tissue and normal tissue, whereas crown gall tissues are remarkably constant in nutritional and growth substance requirements.

5.7.3. Studies of plant diseases and their elimination

A comparison of normal and diseased tissues of various plants can be made by tissue culture. The possibility of growing crown gall tissue *in vitro* has been demonstrated. The gall tissue was found to be more growth substance active than normal tissue Detailed study has been performed to clarify the pathological nature and physiological differences between normal and gall tissue.

Tissues of gall of genetic origin were among the first grown *in vitro*. Galls of virus origin established in tissue cultures have been examined for nutritional requirements and metabolism. Callus tissues infected with tomorrow mosaic virus (TMV) and other viruses have been examined to clarify virus infection and multiplication. The amount of virus in the tobacco callus cultures varied depending on the strain of host tissue and nutritional and physical environments. The amount of virus in tobacco tissue cultures was influenced by growth substances. The number of tobacco tissue pieces artificially infected with TMV exhibited dependence on the type and number of injuries caused and induced at inoculation time. Depending on the concentration, nucleic acids, purines, pyrimidines and analogs influenced the growth of TMV infected tobacco tissue and the infectivity of the TMV. Plants free from pathogens can be raised from the existing infective plants. Since the pathogens infect almost all the portions of plants except the growing buds, disease-free plants can be raised through the meristem and callus culture method. Alternatively meristems can be treated with heat shocks to inactivate the virus. Virus infection can also be eliminated through repeated sub-culturing.

5.7.4. Single cell cultures of higher plant cells

Over the years tissue culture methods have expanded from organ culture to cell culture. It is now even possible to isolate and grow single cells of higher plants. But the critical question remains whether all the cells in a callus tissue mass are similar or not and If variation of cells exists, what are their types that make up the mass. Single cell clones are a valuable means to study similarities and differences between normal cells and various kinds of diseased cells. Single cell clones of tissue from marigold crown gall tissue have shown constant differences in growth rate, texture and color. Some clones with varied media developed shoots or roots in culture. Single cell clones of tissue derived from isolated single cells of tobacco crown gall teratomas were developed into masses of tissue of morphologically abnormal structures. These structures were typical of the teratoma cultures from which they were derived. Single cell clones of tobacco (N. tabacum x N.glutinosa) callus tissue demonstrated considerable variation in growth rate, morphology, color, texture and nutrient requirements. The amount of TMV in respective clones also varied greatly after 4 successive monthly passages of inoculated clones in virus- free liquid, shake cultures. Furthermore, it was observed that young largely meristematic single cell clones of the hybrid tobacco tissue were more resistant to TMV infection and subsequent multiplication of TMV than were older cultures (containing largely enlarging or senescent cells). When a single cell clone of *N. tabacum* was infected with a mixture of TMV strains, a single mild strain of TMV was selected. This mild strain multiplied in the tissue culture whereas the other strains in the mixture were lost. Single cell clones of tissue reisolated from two parent single cell clones of the hybrid tobacco tissue, maintained differences in growth rates which were observed between the two parent clones. The clone reisolates from a single parent displayed differences in color and consistency.

Phylloxera gall and normal grape stem tissues have also been used to establish their respective single cell clones. The clones varied in color, growth rate, texture and the ability to grow on media with various combinations of casein hydrolysate, growth substances and other nitrogen and carbon compounds as substitutes for coconut milk. The growth of the single cell clones coming from the gall and normal grape stem tissues was influenced by the type and concentration of sugar.

The single cell methods have enabled to carry out many new studies that were previously impossible. Single cell clones may be further evaluated for additional chemical, morphological, genetical and pathological similarities and differences. Clarification of the mechanism of virus infection and multiplication and location of the virus in the cell may be carried out. In a similar fashion, mutation of cells, the process of habituation, action of chemical growth regulators and of pathogenic agents (other than virus) may be further delineated. The possibility of developing an entire plant from a single cell (as from cells in mixed cultures) is also high. All the more, the somatic cells growing in microculture provide a simple experimental method for carrying out detailed cytological studies of both normal and diseased cells. This material is free of artifacts that are common, with killed and stained preparations. The physical and chemical microenvironments can be controlled to observe the effects over a prolonged time period, e.g., for metabolites, growth substances, toxic materials and disease incidents.

5.7.5. Procurement of commercial products

Commercial products like cardiac glycosides, morphinone alkaloids, essential oil and original rubber can be procured by exploiting tissue culture which otherwise are to be obtained from plants] But in spite of the fact that plant cell cultures can accumulate sufficiently high concentration of secondary metabolites to render its production viable to the commercial use, compounds at these levels are not of great commercial importance. Commercially significant plant products are either not found in cell cultures or even if present they are only in very small concentrations. Interestingly, cardiac glycosides are found only in morphologically differentiated cell cultures with concentration of only 1 mg/l suspension. Even morphine and codeine are found in about 1.5 mg/gm dry weight in the cell cultures of *Papaver* species.

The technical problems encountered in quantitative recovery of useful products in cell culture are:

1. Several metabolites are released in cell vacuoles and not in the medium, thus they are in a way locked and not available.

2. To release the product continuously, the viability of the cells must remain unaltered.

Since time immemorial, the plants have been utilized as an inexhaustible source of medicinal extracts, with the latest techniques the active constituents of these extracts have been isolated and characterized, their phyto-therapeutic activities verified and the dose-response relationships have been specified. Conventionally, the plants from which important pharmaceuticals are obtained are grown on large scale plantations. Nevertheless, if a factory-type production of biomedicinals could be possible, it would undoubtedly be of interest and shall attract the pharmaceutical industry. An interesting alternative for controlled production of plant constituents, like secondary metabolites is the tissue culture technique. The technique of plant tissue cultures can offer possible solution to some of the problems surfacing due to current rate of extinction and decimation of floras and ecosystems.

5.7.6. Germplasm storage

Generally most of the plants are stored in the form of seed or as growing plants. But some seeds fail to develop into plants while others fail to retain their originality. This limitation can be successfully eliminated to raise identical clones by employing tissue culture technique. The plant materials can be collected and stored in a minimal medium with low light intensity and low temperature without any appreciable loss in its viability. This helps in reducing the growth rate of plant tissue meanwhile the totipotency of tissue is retained. Thus, a large number of individual tissues can be stored in a limited area. This type of storage is referred to as germplasm storage. The sub-culturing of these tissues can be performed at regular intervals of one year. Germplasm can be stored in the form of seeds, buds, protoplasts, shoot tips, etc. The germplasm in the growing stage is used for, storage of tissues. Their growth is suspended by any of these techniques:

1. Addition of hormones or other chemical retardant;
2. Lowering temperature;
3. Reduction in oxygen concentration.

Out of this storage at low temperature using liquid nitrogen i.e. cryopreservation is the most effective method. Whenever required, germplasm can be used following rapid thawing.

5.7.7. Embryo rescue

In some plants, normal fertilization occurs but the ovule fails to develop into a mature seed. In such instances, the fertilized egg on immature embryo is removed from the immature fruits and cultured in the tissue culture medium. The individuals so generated are hybrids, which show a few new characters. This process of embryo culture is also referred to as embryo rescue and can be used for embryo culture, ovule culture and ovary culture In the cases where it is not feasible to excise embryos due to small size whole ovules can be cultured. Even if ovules cannot be excised whole ovaries may be cultured.

5.7.8. Somaclonal variation or modification

Generally, the clones released through tissue culture bear uniformity in their characters but at times few clones show variations. These variant clones express new characters which were absent in their parent cells. The formation of variant clones from the cultured callus tissues is called **somaclonal variation**. The somaclonal variants can be desirable or undesirable. Desirable variants are useful in crop improvements whereas the undesirable ones are not. A variety of somaclonal variants have been raised from plants like sugarcane, maize, rice and other cereals. The regenerated variant clones are tested for their resistance to herbicide, temperature and heavy metals. The resistant clones are further tested for their productivity.

5.7.9. The production of haploids

The haploid plants are characterized by having only a single set of chromosomes in their cells. Production of haploids is relatively easy when anther, ovule or pollen grain culture is established in the medium. These haploid plants are employed in improving the field and agricultural crops. The detection and selection of recessive mutants for a few characters can be performed with haploid plants. Pollen incompatibility can be removed by mentor pollen technology.

5.7.10. Production of artificial seeds

An artificial seed is a synthetic seed which is made up of a somatic embryo surrounded by the nutrient medium and this as a whole protected by a thin synthetic membrane. In comparison to natural seeds, these artificial seeds are smaller in size. They are identical and contain only the somatic embryos of a known strain. They can be stored even for a period of one year without any appreciable loss in viability. The seeds are encapsulated in a synthetic membrane made up of polyoxyethylene, sodium alginate or polyacrylamide gel. The pattern of germination in artificial seeds is similar to that of natural seeds and can be directly sown in the soil but unlike natural seeds they do not need hardening in green house. High cost of production seems to be the only limitation.

5.7.11. Clonal propagation and micropropagation

Clonal propagation involves propagation through cell, tissue or organ culture. Its advantages are rapid multiplication of superior clones, maintenance of genetic uniformity and multiplication of sexually derived sterile hybrids. Shoot tips or axillary buds are utilized for propagation on culture media without the intervention of callus phase.

Micropropagation is the most commonly used technique both at the research level and commercial level. It can be employed for the mass production of plants including nursery stock species, ornamental vegetables and field crops. The method as such enables large scale production of selected genotypes. It provides a process which could effectively eliminate pathogens of viral and bacterial origin. It is desirable that the micropropagation system should produce a large number of uniform plants which are genotypically and phenotypically the same as the plant from which they are produced. A most suitable technique is one that involves multiplication through axillary buds. This method produces genetically stable plants under sterile conditions where minimum possible stress is imposed on the growing plants. The method allows for easy manipulation and strict control over environmental and nutritional levels. However, the main disadvantage of this method is meager possibilities for physiological experimentation because the plants produced are generally juvenile in nature, which tend to suffer epicuticular wax(s) removal/reduction. Palisade cell layer is smaller with larger mesophyll air sacs and disrupted stomatal physiology. Micropropagation is practised in four main stages.

1. Selection and sterilization of elite plants;
2. Establishment of axillary buds and culture;
3. Multiplication in culture; and
4. Rooting of *in vitro* plants and transfer to compost.

1. Selection of elite plants: Plants apparently free from any disease, stress or surface blemishes are selected. This material is preferably grown in environmentally controlled growth cabinets or clean glasshouses and should have been tested for the presence of any specific virus using sophisticated diagnostic tests like ELISA. The selected elites are washed with 70% ethanol containing 4–5 drops of surface-active agents in 100 ml solution, followed by 2% chloros and 4 drops of surfactant per 100 ml of solution at room temperature. Using a clean sharp blade, axillary buds of the desired variety are excised and stored in distilled water until enough buds have been collected. In a laminar flow bench a maximum of 20 buds are kept in a sterile test tube, filled up to the brim with ethanol solution and left immersed for 1-1.5 minutes. The ethanol is decanted off and the tube refilled with chloros solution. Agitation is provided at 120 strokes/min for 12min using a arbitrary hand wrist action shaker. The chloros rinse is washed of decanted off with sterile water 3 times and stored in sterile and distilled water.

2. Establishment of axillary buds and culture: Axillary buds are taken out in an empty sterile petri dish. Up to 4 buds are placed in a 50 ml petri dish containing medium I (M&S medium) and all essential medium components and nutrients. The base of bud is stuck firmly but not buried in the medium. The petri dish is sealed in such a way that adequate gaseous exchange is ensured. This is transferred to room temperature in an incubator for 1-2 weeks/months.

3. Multiplication in culture: When a shoot appears, the apical part is cut and the cuttings and internodal cuttings are transferred to a sterile jar containing appropriate medium in such a way that basal portion of stem is embedded (not buried) in the medium.

4. Rooting of *in vitro* plants and transfer to compost: The *in vitro* plant is pieced into 5 mm fragments and transferred into a fresh appropriate medium, left for 5 days until some sturdy roots are visible. Each plant is removed carefully from the jar and then transferred into damp compost in 50 mm pots. The high humidity is maintained for 12-24 hours. Then the pots are placed in a glass house under shade protected from light until they are approximately 70 mm high and have begun to lose their juvenile nature or character. They can then be transferred to larger pots or to the field.

5.7.12. Mutant selection

Mutant selection is an important tool effectively utilized in crop improvement. Cells are subjected to mutagenic treatments and subsequently mutants are selected. Selection of mutant cells is usually performed by addition of toxic substances to cells followed by isolation of resistant cells. In this manner cell lines resistant to these toxic substances can be efficiently selected. By exploiting this approach, cell lines resistant to antibiotics, amino acid analogs and fungal toxins have been isolated. Alternatively indirect selection can also be performed. For example, nitrate reductase deficient cell lines can be selected as chlorate resistant cells. On similar lines cell cultures of Nicotiana were selected, for resistance against herbicides like sodium chlorate, sulfometuron and amitrol. Cell lines of potato resistant to 5-methyltryptophan were selected and these cultures permitted the accumulation of free phenylalanine, tryptophan and tyrosine.

In haploids only one set of chromosomes is present and thereby even the recessive mutations are expressed immediately. Thus, the desirable mutants can be isolated among haploids derived in culture. Pollens can be grown as single cells on solid medium and a larger population can be screened in the laboratory and thereby precluding the phase of initial growth of plants in the field.

5.7.13. Endosperm culture

Tissue culture techniques are utilized for endosperm culture. Endosperm is triploid in its chromosome constitution. It supplies nutrition to the developing embryo. Triploid plants are useful for production of seedless fruits of banana, watermelon, etc. Production of trisomics for cytogenetic studies has also been reported. Triploids are generally obtained by crossing colchicine-induced tetraploids with diploids and this is followed by rescue of triploid embryos. Strong cross ability barriers at times preclude production of triploids from 4x X 2x crosses and in such cases endosperm culture may be used as an alternative strategy for triploid production.

The various steps involved in the endosperm culture are:

1. Aseptic dissection of immature/mature seeds;

2. Excision of endosperms along with embryos;

3. Culturing of excised endosperms on a suitable medium;

4. Removal of embryos after initial callus growth;

5. Embryogenesis or shoot bud differentiation of the callus;

6. Development of shoots and roots;

7. Establishment of complete triploid plants.

5.7.14. Nucellus culture

In some plant like citrus, adventative embryos develop from nucellar cells. In such cases nucellus from pollinated flowers can also be utilized for micropropagation. It can be grown on White's medium supplemented with casein hydrolysate to obtain callus. This callus may give rise to pseudobulbils differentiating into embryoids. These embryoids eventually develop into seedlings. Nucellus obtained from unfertilized ovules is also capable of developing embryoids. The seedlings obtained from the nucellar tissue are of parental type. Thereby they are important for maintaining purity of horticultural stocks.

5.8. CONCLUSION

It is obvious that the past few decades have seen considerable efforts in the use of plant cell cultures in bioproduction, bioconversion or biotransformation and biosynthetic studies. The potential commercial production of pharmaceuticals by cell culture techniques depends upon detailed investigations into the biosynthetic sequences. Recent advances in sensitive analytical techniques, particularly of enzyme assay and radioimmunoassay, have enabled biogenetic investigations within plant cell cultures to proceed at a faster rate than before. The potential use of cell cultures in the production of valuable secondary products is being viewed with a great sense of optimism and enthusiasm by biotechnologists. The key to commercially promising production of biomedicinals is clearly the induction and selection of high yielding cell lines. Recent advances in plant biotechnology offer several mechanisms for unlocking the diverse and potentially profitable synthetic capabilities of cultured plant cells.

Some of the major advantages expected from tissue culture systems over the conventional cultivation techniques are given below:

1. Availability of uniform plant material at all times and manageable under regulated and reproducible conditions.

2. Synthesis of those chemical compounds which are otherwise impossible or too difficult to synthesize chemically.

Further, the compounds from tissue cultures may be more easily purified because of simpler extracts and absence of significant amounts of pigments.

3. Production of natural compounds under controlled environmental conditions independent of soil conditions and changes in climate.

4. Biogenesis of the secondary metabolites can be studied. By supplying labelled precursors to the cell cultures, the metabolic pathways involving the desired compound can be traced.

5. They offer an opportunity to attempt envisaged biotransformation or bioconversion reactions. It is expected that specific modification of chemical structures of certain compounds may be achieved more easily in cultured plant cells in comparison to micro-organisms or chemical synthesis.

6. The technique provides completely controlled conditions to elucidate growth and physiology of cells and to study host-parasite interaction at cellular level.

7. The cells of most tropical and temperate plants may be multiplied to yield specific metabolites produced by them.

8. Cellular totipotency, the unique propensity of plant cells, can be revealed. All living cells, irrespective of their totipotency level can potentially give rise to whole plants. It offers efficient, safe and economical methods of plant propagation.

9. The cultured cells can generally be maintained free from microbial contamination and insect attack.

10. Cells can be immobilized and then used for various biotransformations and biochemical reactions.

At times, plant germplasm may be stored in tissue cultures at refrigerated temperature more economically and safely than by conventional methods. The feasibility of growing single cells and protoplast fusion of completely unrelated species has opened up new avenues for plant improvement.

SUGGESTED READING

- Anderson PG (Ed.) *Plant Tissue Culture and its Agricultural Applications*, Butterworths, Stoneham, Massachussets (1986).

- Barz W, Reinhard E and Zenk MH (Eds.) *Plant Tissue Culture and its Biotechnological Applications,* Springer-Verlag, Berlin and New York (1977).

- Bengochen T and Dodds JH, *Plant Protoplasts: A Biotechnological Tool for Plant Improvement*, Chapman and Hall, London, New York (1986).

- Bhojwani SS and Razdan MK, *Plant Tissue Culture: Theory and Practice*, Elsevier, Amsterdam (1983).

- Dixon RA, (Ed.). *Plant Cell Culture: A Practical Approach, IRL*, Oxford and Washington DC (1985).

- Evans DA, Sharp WR, Amrnirato PV, and Yamada Y, (Eds.) *Handbook of Plant Cell Cultures*, New York (1984).

- George EF and Sherrington PD, *Plant Propagation by Tissue Culture, Exegetics Ltd.*, Reading (1984).

- Green CE, Somers DA, Hackett WP and Biesboer DD, (Eds.) *Plant Tissue and Cell Culture*, Liss, New York (1987).

- Gupta PK, *Elements of Biotechnology*, Rastogi Publications, Meerut (1997).

- Hartman HT and Kester DE, *Principles of Tissue Culture for Micropropagation*, Prentice Hall, New Jersey (1983).

- Ingram DS and Hegelson JP, (Eds.) *Tissue Culture Methods for Plant Pathologists*, Blackwell Scientific, U.K (1980).

- Mather J and Moore In: *The Encyclopedia of Bioprocess Technology: Fermentation, Biocatalysis, and Bioseparation* (M. Flickinger and S. Drew, eds.), John Wiley, New York, (in press) (1998).

- Moore A, Donahue CJ, Hooley J, Stocks DL, Bauer KD, and Mather JP, Cytotechnology 17(1),11(1995).

- Moore A, Mercer J, Dutina G, Donahue C, Bauer K, Mather JP, Etcheverry T and Rhyll T *Cytotechnology,* 23,47(1997).

- Murashige T, *Ann. Rev. Plant Physiol*, 25,135(1974).

- Orly J and Sato G, *Cell*,17(295),305(1979).

• Parks DR, Bryan VM, Oi VT, Herzenberg LA, *Proc Natl Acad Sci USA*,76,1962(1979).

• Pollard JW and Walker JM, (Eds.) *Methods in Molecular Biology Volume 6, Plant Cell and Tissue Culture*, Humara Press, Clifton, New Jersey, (1990).

• Sharp WR, Larsen OP, Paddock EF and Raghavan V, (Eds.) *Plant Cell and Tissue Culture*, Ohio State University Press, Ohio (1979).

• Thorpe TA, (Ed.) *Frontiers of Plant Tissue Culture*, IAPTC, Calgray (1978).

• Thorpe TA, (Ed.) *Plant Tissue Culture: Methods and Applications in Agriculture*, Academic, don and New York (1981).

• Tsien R, *Annu. Rev. Neurosci*,12,227 (1989).

• White PR, *A Handbook of Plant Tissue Culture*, Jacques Cottel Pennsylvania (1963).

• Withers LA and Alderson PG, (Eds.) *Plant Cell Culture and its Agricultural Applications*, Butterworths, UK(1986).

• Yeoman MM, (Ed.) *Plant Cell Culture Technology*, Blackwell Scientific, Oxford (1986).

6

ANIMAL CELL, TISSUE AND ORGAN CULTURE

6.1. INTRODUCTION

Animal cell culture refers to the maintenance and propagation of animal cells in a suitable nutrient medium. Various laboratories are interested in the commercial production of a variety of pharmaceutically important macromolecules such as hormones, enzymes, antibodies, interferons and cytokines etc. Besides these categories of products, the animal cell culture technique has been successfully established in a number of scientific fields, particularly in diagnostic virology, in the analysis of oncogenics, aging research, in determination of cytostatic substances, in amniocentesis, gene mapping and in cell-cycle related events. The developments have been possible because of the feasibility of *in vitro* cultivation of animal cells and their bio- products.

Before going into the details of the biotechnological aspects, it is necessary to know a few commonly used terms. The culture produced by the cell or tissue taken from an organism is termed as **primary culture**, and the term 'cell line' refers to the sequence of culture obtained from the first sub-cultivation of the primary culture. This differs from cell strain derived from a clone of cells with specific stable properties like having marker chromosomes, marker enzymes, antigens, etc. By culture alteration one can produce continuous **(permanent)** cell lines. This has the potential for an unlimited sub-cultivation *in vitro*. In the present state of our knowledge, it is impossible to determine the moment when the transition to continuous cell line has taken place. However, generally it takes at least 70-fold sub-cultivation (passage) at intervals of about 3 days. The result of culture alteration was formerly called transformation; however, this term should be restricted to those cases in which the alteration can be ascribed unambiguously to foreign genetic materials.

Cell culture has become an indispensable technology in many branches of life sciences. It provides the basis for studying the regulation of cell proliferation, differentiation and product formation in carefully controlled conditions, with processes and analytical tools which are scalable from the level of the single cell to excess of 10 kg wet weight of cells. Cell culture has also provided the means to define almost the entire human genome, and to dissect the pathways of intracellular and intercellular signaling, which ultimately regulate gene expression. From its ancestry in developmental biology and pathology, this discipline has now emerged as a tool for molecular geneticists, immunologists, surgeons, bioengineers, and manufacturers of pharmaceuticals, while still remaining a fundamental tool to the cell biologist, whose input is vital for the continuing development of the technology.

Cell culture has matured from a simple, microscope driven, observational science to a universally acknowledged technology with roots set as deep in industry as they are in academia. It stands among microelectronics, avionics, astrophysics and nuclear engineering, as one of the major bridges between fundamental research and industrial exploitation and in the current climate; perhaps the more commercial aspects will ensure its development for at least several more decades. The prospects for genetic therapy and tissue replacement are such that the questions are rapidly becoming ethical, as much as technical, as new opportunities arise for genetic manipulation, whole animal cloning and tissue transplantation.

6.2. BIOLOGY OF CELLS IN CULTURE

6.2.1. Origin and characterization

The list of different cell types which can be grown in culture is extensive and includes representatives of most major cell types, and has significantly increased in recent years, due largely to the improved availability of selective media and specialized cell cultures through commercial sources such as Clonetics. The use of markers that are cell type specific has made it possible to determine the lineage from which many of these cultures were derived, although the position of the cells within the lineage is not always clear. During propagation, a precursor cell type will tend to predominate, rather than a differentiated cell. Consequently a cell line may appear to be heterogeneous, as some cultures, such as epidermal keratinocytes, can contain stem cells, precursor cells, and mature differentiated cells. There is constant renewal from the stem cells, proliferation and maturation in the precursor compartment, and terminal and irreversible differentiation in the mature compartment. Other cultures, such as dermal fibroblasts, contain a relatively uniform population of proliferating cells at low cell densities (about 10^4 cells/cm^2) and an equally uniform, more differentiated, non-proliferating population at high cell densities (10^5 cells/cm^2). This high-density population of fibrocyte-like cells can re-enter the cell cycle if the cells are trypsinized or scraped (or 'wounded' by making a cut in the monolayer) to reduce the cell density or create a free edge. Most of the cells appear to be capable of proliferation, and there is little evidence of renewal from a stem cell compartment.

Culture heterogeneity also results from multiple lineages being present in the cell line. The only unifying factors are the selective conditions of the medium and substrate, and the predominance of the cell type (or types) which can survive and proliferate. This tends to select a common phenotype but, due to the interactive nature of growth control, may obscure the fact that the population contains several distinct phenotypes only detectable by cloning. Nutritional factors like serum, Ca^{2+} ions, hormones, cell and matrix interactions, and culture density, can affect differentiation and cell proliferation. Hence, it is not only essential to define the lineage of cells being used, but also to characterize and stabilize the stage of differentiation, by controlling cell density and the nutritional and hormonal environment to obtain a uniform population of cells, which will respond in a reproducible fashion to given signals.

As the dynamic properties of cell culture (proliferation, migration, nutrient utilization, product secretion) are sometimes difficult to control, and the complexity of cell interactions found *in vivo* can be difficult to recreate *in vitro,* there have been numerous attempts to either retain the structural integrity of the original tissue, using traditional organ culture, or to recreate it by combining propagated cells of different lineages in organotypic culture. Among the most successful examples of the latter are the so-called skin equivalent models, where epidermal keratinocytes are co-cultured with dermal fibroblasts and collagen in filter well inserts or some similar mechanical support. The result is a synthetic skin suitable for grafting and is now being evaluated for tests of irritancy and inflammation.

6.2.2. Differentiation

As propagation of cell lines requires that the cell number increases, culture conditions have evolved to favour maximal cell proliferation. It is not surprising that these conditions are often not conducive to cell differentiation where cell growth is severely limited or completely abolished. Those conditions which favour cell proliferation are low cell density, low Ca^{2+} concentration (100–600 mM), and the presence of growth factors such as epidermal growth factor (EGF), fibroblast growth factor (FGF), and platelet-derived growth factor (PDGF). High cell density (> $1x$ 10^5 cells/cm^2), high Ca^{2+} concentration (300-1500 mM), and the presence of differentiation inducers, hormones such as hydrocortisone, paracrine factors such as IL-6 and KGF, and nerve growth factor, retinoids, and planar polar compounds, such as dimethyl sulfoxide, will favour cytostasis and differentiation. The role of serum in differentiation is complex and depends on the cell type and medium used. While a low serum concentration promotes differentiation in oligodendrocytes, a high serum concentration causes squamous differentiation in bronchial epithelium. In the latter case, this is due to transforming growth factor B (TGFB) released from platelets. Because of the undefined composition of serum and the ever-present risk of adventitious agents such as viruses, controlled studies on selective growth and differentiation are best conducted in serum-free media.

The establishment of the correct polarity and cell shape may also be important, particularly in epithelium. Many workers have shown that growing cells to high density on a floating collagen gel allows matrix interaction, access to medium on both sides and, particularly, to the basal surface where receptors and nutrient transporters are expressed. The plasticity of the substrate can facilitate a normal cell shape and normal polarity of the interactive ligands in the basement membrane. Different conditions may be required for propagation and differentiation and hence an experimental protocol may require a growth phase for expansion and to allow for replicate samples, followed by a non-growth maturation phase to allow for increased expression of differentiated functions.

6.3. CHOICE OF MATERIALS

6.3.1. Cell type

The cell type chosen will depend on the question being asked. For some processes, such as DNA synthesis, response to cytotoxins, or apoptosis, the cell type may not matter, provided the cells are competent. In other cases a specific process will require a particular cell type, for example surfactant synthesis in the lung will require a fresh isolate of type II pneumocytes or a cell line, such as NCI-H441, which still expresses surfactant proteins. A reasonable first step would be to determine from the literature whether a cell line exists with the required properties.

6.3.2. Source of tissue

6.3.2.1. Embryo or adult?

In general, cultures derived from embryonic tissues survive and proliferate better than those from the adult. This presumably reflects the lower level of specialization and higher proliferative potential in the embryo. Adult tissues usually have a lower growth fraction and a higher proportion of non-replicating specialized cells, often within a more structured and less readily disaggregated extracellular matrix. Initiation and propagation are more difficult, and the lifespan of the culture often shorter. Embryonic or fetal tissue has many practical advantages, but it must be remembered that in some instances the cells will be different from adult cells and it cannot be assumed that they will mature into adult-type cells unless this can be confirmed by appropriate characterization.

Examples of widely used embryonic cell lines are the various 3T3 lines primitive mouse mesodermal cells and WI-38, MRC-5, and other human fetal lung fibroblasts. Mesodermally derived cells (fibroblasts, endothelium, and myoblasts) are on the whole easier to culture than epithelium, neurons, or endocrine tissue. This selectivity may reflect the extensive use of fibroblast cultures during the early development of culture media and the response of mesodermally derived cells to mitogenic factors present in serum. Selective media have been designed for epithelial and other cell types, and with some of these it has been shown that serum is inhibitory to growth and may promote differentiation. Primary culture of epithelial tissues, such as skin, lung, and mammary gland, is routine in some laboratories, and prepared cultures are available commercially (for example, Clonetics; Promocell).

6.3.2.2. Normal or neoplastic?

Normal tissue usually gives rise to cultures with a finite lifespan, while cultures from tumours can give rise to continuous cell lines. However, there are several examples of continuous cell lines (BHK-21 hamster kidney fibroblasts, MDCK dog kidney epithelium, 3T3 fibroblasts) which have been derived from normal tissues and which are non-tumorigenic. Normal cells generally grow as an undifferentiated stem cell or precursor cell, and the onset of differentiation is accompanied by a cessation in cell proliferation, which may be permanent. Some normal cells, such as fibrocytes or endothelium, are able to differentiate and still de-differentiate and resume proliferation and in turn re-differentiate, while others, such as squamous epithelium, skeletal muscle, and neurons, once committed to differentiate, appear to be incapable of resuming proliferation.

Cells cultured from neoplasms, such as B16 mouse melanoma, can express at least partial differentiation, while retaining the capacity to divide. Many studies of differentiation have taken advantage of this fact and used differentiated tumours such as hepatomas and human and rodent neuroblastomas, although whether this differentiation is normal are not known.

Tumour cells can often be propagated in the syngeneic host, providing a cheap and simple method of producing large numbers of cells, albeit with lower purity. Where the natural host is not available, tumours can also be propagated in animals with a compromised immune system, with greater difficulty and cost, but similar advantages. Many other differences between normal and neoplastic cells are similar to those between finite and continuous cell lines as immortalization is an important component of the process of transformation

6.3.3. Subculture

Freshly isolated cultures are known as primary cultures until they are subcultured. They are usually heterogeneous and have a low growth fraction, but are more representative of the cell types in the tissue from which they were derived and in the expression of tissue-specific properties. Subculture allows the expansion of the culture (it is now known as a cell line), the possibility of cloning, characterization and preservation, and greater uniformity, but may cause a loss of specialized cells and differentiated properties unless care is taken to select the correct lineage and preserve or reinduce differentiated properties. The greatest advantage of subculturing a primary culture into a cell line is the provision of large amounts of consistent material suitable for prolonged use.

6.3.3.1. Finite or continuous cell lines

After several subcultures a cell line will either die out (finite cell line) or 'transform' to become a continuous cell line. It is not clear in all cases whether the stem line of a continuous culture pre-exists or arises during serial propagation. Because of the time taken for such cell lines to appear (often several months) and the differences in their properties, it has been assumed that a mutation occurs, but the pre-existence of immortalized cells, particularly in cultures from neoplasm, cannot be excluded.

Complementation analysis has shown that senescence is a dominant trait, and immortalization is the result of mutations and/or deletions in genes such as p53. The activity of telomerase is higher in immortal cell lines and may be sufficient to endow the cell line with an infinite lifespan. The appearance of a continuous cell line is usually marked by an alteration in cytomorphology (giving cells that are smaller, less adherent, more rounded, and with a higher ratio of nucleus to cytoplasm), an increase in growth rate (population doubling time can decrease from 36-48 h to 12-36 h), a reduction in serum dependence, an increase in cloning efficiency, a reduction in anchorage dependence (as measured by an increased ability to proliferate in suspension as a liquid culture or cloned in agar), an increase in heteroploidy (chromosomal variation among cells) and aneuploidy (divergence from the donor, euploid, karyotype), and an increase in tumorigenicity. The resemblance between spontaneous *in vitro* transformation and malignant transformation is obvious but nevertheless the two are not necessarily identical although they have much in common. Normal cells can 'transform' to become continuous cell lines without becoming malignant, and malignant tumours can give rise to cultures which 'transform' and become more (or even less) tumorigenic, but acquire the other properties listed above. Transformation *in vitro* is primarily the acquisition of an infinite lifespan. Simultaneous or subsequent alterations in growth control can be under positive control by oncogenes or negative control by tumour suppressor genes.

The advantages of continuous cell lines are their faster growth rates to higher cell densities and resultant greater yield, their lower serum requirement and general ease of maintenance in commercially available media, and their ability to grow in suspension. Their disadvantages include greater chromosomal instability, divergence from the donor phenotype, and loss of tissue-specific markers. A number of techniques, including transfection or infection with viral genes (such as E6 and E7 from human papilloma virus, and SV40T) or viruses (such as Epstein-Barr virus, EBV) have been used to immortalize a wide range of cell types. The retention of lineage-specific properties is variable.

6.3.3.2. Propagation in suspension

Most cultures are propagated as a monolayer attached to the substrate, but some, including transformed cells, haematopoietic cells, and cells from ascites, can be propagated in suspension. Suspension culture has advantages, including simpler propagation (subculture only requires dilution, no trypsinization), no requirement for increasing surface area with increasing bulk, ease of harvesting, and the possibility of achieving a 'steady state' or biostat culture if required.

6.3.4. Selection of medium

Regrettably, the choice of medium is still often empirical. What others used previously for the same cells, or what is currently being used in the laboratory for different cells, often dictates the choice of medium and serum. For continuous cell lines it may not matter as long as the conditions are consistent, but for specialized cell types, primary cultures, and growth in the absence of serum, the choice is more critical. There are two major advantages of using more sophisticated media in the absence of serum: they may be selective for particular types of cell, and the isolation of purified products is easier in the absence of serum. Nevertheless, culture in the presence of serum is still easier and often less expensive, though less controlled. Two major determinants regulate the use of serum-free media:

(a) Cost. Most people do not have the time, facilities, or inclination to make up their own media and serum-free formulations, with their various additives, tend to be much more expensive than conventional media.

(b) Requirements for serum-free media are more cell type specific. Serum will cover many inadequacies revealed in its absence. Furthermore, because of their selectivity, a different medium may be required for each type of cell line. This problem may be particularly acute when culturing tumour cells where cell line variability may require modifications for cell lines from individual tumours. In the final analysis the choice is often still empirical: read the literature and determine which medium has been used previously. If several media have been used, as is often the case, test them all, with others added if desired (Table 6.1).

Table 6.1: Commonly used media

Medium	Properties
RPMI 1640	No Ca^{2+}, low Mg^{2+}; designed for lymphoblastoid and useful for other adherent and non-adherent cell lines. Unsuitable for calcium phosphate transfection.
MEM/Hanks' salts	Classic broad specificity medium; low HCO_3 for use in air.
MEM/Earles' salts	Classic broad specificity medium; high HCO_3 for use in 5% CO_2.
F12	Large number of additional constituents (trace elements, copper, iron, additional vitamins, nucleosides, pyruvate, lipoic acid), but at low concentrations; suitable for cloning.
DMEM/F12	50:50 mixture of DMEM and F12; suitable for primary cultures and serum-free with appropriate supplementation.
L15	Bicarbonate-free; buffers in the absence of CO_2.
MCDB 153	One of a series of serum-free media; suitable for growth of keratinocytes.

Measure the growth (population doubling time (PDT) and saturation density), cloning efficiency, and expression of specific properties (differentiation, transfection efficiency, cell products, etc.). The choice of medium may not be the same in each case, for example differentiation of lung epithelium will proceed in serum, but propagation is better without. If possible, include one or more serum-free media in the panel to be tested, supplemented with growth factors, hormones, and trace elements as required (Fig. 6.1). Once a medium has been selected, try to keep this constant for as long as possible. Similarly, if serum is used, select a batch by testing samples from commercial suppliers and reserve enough to last six months to one year, before replacing it with another pre-tested batch. Testing procedures are as described above for media selection. To develop and optimize nutrient formulations for a broad range of cell types and applications, it is useful to classify cell culture-based applications as follows:

- cells as research and diagnostic tools to investigate normal and aberrant cell function;
- cells as biological factories to produce medicines for human or veterinary therapy; and
- cells as therapeutic products for ex vivo therapy or tissue engineering use.

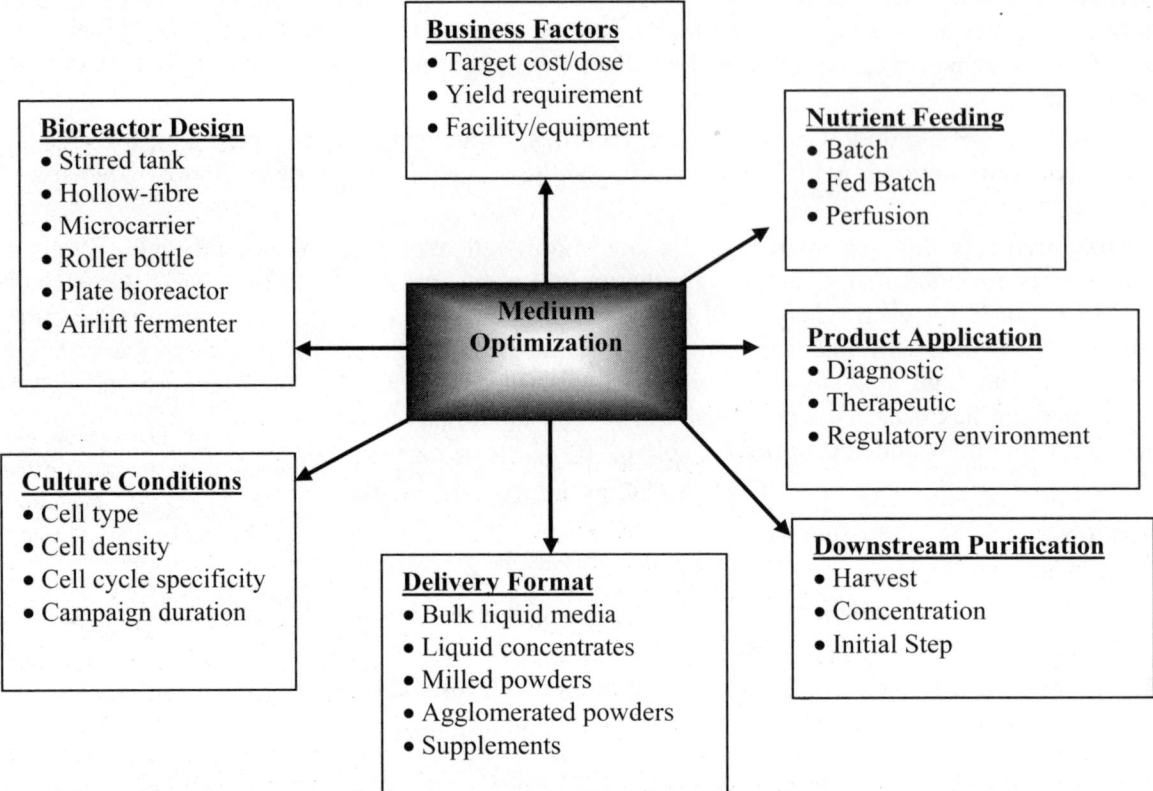

Fig. 6.1: Integrated nutrient medium optimization. Effective nutrient medium optimization for biopharmaceutical production applications cannot effectively focus exclusively on biochemical composition. Integration of formulation design optimization within process development through incorporating inputs from bioproduction, bioreactor engineering, downstream purification, regulatory affairs and business perspectives results in technical and economic superiority

6.3.5. Gas phase

The composition of the gas phase is determined by:

• The type of medium (principally its sodium bicarbonate concentration)

• Whether the culture vessel is open (petri dishes, multiwell plates) or sealed (flasks, bottles)

• The amount of buffering required

Several variables are in play, but one major rule predominates and three basic conditions can be described. The rule is that the bicarbonate concentration and carbon dioxide tension must be in equilibrium. The three conditions are summarized in Table 6.2. It should be remembered that carbon dioxide/bicarbonate is essential to most cells, so a flask or dish cannot be vented without providing carbon dioxide in the atmosphere. Prepare medium to about pH 7.1-7.2 at room temperature, incubate a sample with the correct carbon dioxide tension for at least 0.5 h in a shallow dish, and check that the pH stabilizes at pH 7.4. Adjust with sterile 1 M HC1 or 1 M NaOH if necessary. Oxygen tension is usually maintained at atmospheric pressure, but variations have been described, such as elevated for organ culture and reduced for cloning melanoma and some haematopoietic cells.

Table 6.2: Relationship between CO_2 and bicarbonate

Type of Vessel	Buffer capacity	HCO_3^-	Gas phase	HEPES
Closed	Low	4 mM	Air	-
Open or closed	Moderate	26 mM	5% CO_2	-
Open or closed	High	8 mM	2% CO_2	20 mM

6.3.6. Culture system

Originally, tissue culture was regarded as the culture of whole fragments of explanted tissue with the assumption that histological integrity was at least partially maintained. Now 'tissue culture' has become a generic term and includes organ culture, where a small fragment of tissue or whole embryonic organ is explanted to retain tissue architecture, and cell culture, where the tissue is dispersed mechanically or enzymatically, or the cells migrate from an explant, and the cells are propagated as a suspension or attached monolayer. Cell cultures are usually devoid of structural organization, have lost their histotypic architecture and often the biochemical properties associated with it, and generally do not achieve a steady state unless special conditions are employed. They can, however, be propagated, expanded, and divided into identical replicates. They can be characterized and a defined cell population preserved by freezing, and they can be purified by growth in selective media, physical cell separation, or cloning, to give a characterized cell strain with considerable uniformity.

Organ culture will preserve cell interaction and retain histological and biochemical differentiation for longer than cell culture. After the initial trauma of explanation and some central necrosis, organ cultures can remain in a steady state for a period of several days to years. However, they cannot be propagated easily, show greater experimental variation between replicates, and tend to be more difficult to use for quantitative determinations. Purified cell lines can be maintained at high cell density to create histotypic cultures and different cell populations can be combined in organotypic culture, simulating some of the properties of organ culture.

6.3.6.1. Substrate

The nature of the substrate is determined largely by the type of cell and the use to which it will be put. Polystyrene which has been treated to make it wettable and give it a net negative charge is used almost universally. In special cases (culture of neurons, muscle cells, capillary endothelial cells, and some epithelial cultures) the plastic is pre-coated with fibronectin, collagen, gelatin, or poly-L-lysine (which gives a net positive charge). Glass may also be used, but must be washed carefully with a non-toxic detergent.

6.3.6.2. Scale

Culture vessels vary in size from microtitration (30 mm^2, 100–200 µl) up through a range of dishes and flasks to 180 cm^2, and roller bottles and multisurface propagators for large-scale culture. The major determinants are the number of cells required (5 X 10^4 to 10^5/cm^2 maximum for most untransformed cells, 10^5 to 10^6/cm^2 for transformed), the number of replicates (96 or 144 in a microtitration plate), and the times of sampling: a 24-well plate is good for a large number of replicates for simultaneous sampling, but individual dishes, tubes, or bottles are preferable where sampling is carried out at different times. Petri dishes are cheaper than flasks and good for subsequent processing, e.g., staining or extractions. Flasks can be sealed; do not need a humid carbon dioxide incubator, and give better protection against contamination. Volume is the main determinant for suspension cultures. Sparging (bubbling air through the culture) and agitation will become necessary as the depth increases. Where a product is required rather than cells, there are advantages in perfusion systems, which can be used to culture cells on membranes or hollow fibres. These supply nutrients across the membrane, and the product is collected either from the cell supernatant or the medium, depending on the molecular weight, which will determine the partitioning of the product on either side of the membrane. Perfusion is also useful for time lapse studies, where cells are monitored on a microscope stage by a video camera and for pharmacokinetic modeling where the duration and concentration of a test compound can be regulated precisely.

6.4. PROCEDURES

6.4.1. Substrate

Most laboratories now utilize disposable plastics as substrates for tissue culture. They are optically clear, prepared for tissue culture use by modification of the plastic to make it wettable and suitable for cell attachment, and come sterilized for use. On the whole they are convenient and provide a reproducible source of vessels for both routine and experimental work. Some more fastidious cell types, such as bronchial epithelium, vascular endothelium, skeletal muscle, and neurons require the substrate to be coated with extracellular matrix materials such as fibronectin, collagen or laminin. Most matrix products are available individually (Becton Dickinson, Life Technologies, Sigma, Biofluids) or combined in Matrigel (Becton Dickinson), extracellular matrix produced by the Engelberth Holm Swarm sarcoma cell line. Alternatively, the substrate may be coated with extracellular matrix by growing cells on the plastic and then washing them off with 1% Triton X in ultra pure water.

Matrix coating can be carried out in three ways:

(a) By wetting the surface of the plastic with the matrix component(s), incubating for a short period (usually ~ 30 min), then removing the surplus and using the plastic with adsorbed matrix within seven to ten days (stored at 4°C if not used immediately).

(b) By wetting the plastic and removing the surplus matrix material and allowing the residue to dry.

(c) By adding collagen or Matrigel and allowing it to gel. Wet or dry coating is used mainly for propagation, while gel coating is used to promote differentiation of cells growing on or in the gel.

6.4.2. Medium

Most of the commonly used media (see Table 6.1) are available commercially, presterilized. For special formulations or additions it may be necessary to prepare and sterilize some of the constituents. In general, stable solutions (water, salts, and media supplements such as tryptose or peptone) may be autoclaved at 120°C (100 kPa or 1 atmosphere above ambient) for 20 min, while labile solutions (media, trypsin and serum) must be filtered through a 0.2 μm porosity membrane filter (Millipore, Sartorius, Pall Gelman). Sterility testing should be carried out on samples of each filtrate. Where an automatic autoclave is used care must be taken to ensure that the timing of the run is determined by the temperature at the centre of the load and not just by drain or chamber temperature or pressure which will rise much faster than the load. The recorder probe should be placed in a package or bottle of fluid similar to the load and centrally located.

6.4.3. Cell culture

6.4.3.1. Primary cultures

The first step in preparing a primary culture is sterile dissection followed by mechanical or enzymatic disaggregation. The tissue may simply be chopped to around 1 mm^3 and the pieces attached to a dish by their own adhesiveness, by scratching the dish, or by using clotted plasma. In these cases cells will grow out from the fragment and may be used directly or subcultured. The fragment of tissue, or explant as it is called, may be transferred to a fresh dish or the outgrowth trypsinized to leave the explant and a new outgrowth generated. When the cells from the outgrowth are trypsinized and reseeded into a fresh vessel they become a secondary culture, and the culture is now technically a cell line.

Primary cultures can also be generated by disaggregating tissue in enzymes such as trypsin (0.25% crude or 0.01-0.05% pure) or collagenase (200-2000 U/ml, crude) and the cell suspension allowed to settle on to, adhere, and spread out on the substrate. This type of culture gives a higher yield of cells though it can be more selective, as only certain cells will survive dissociation. In practice, many successful primary cultures are generated using enzymes such as collagenase to reduce the tissue, particularly epithelium, to small clusters of cells which are then allowed to attach and grow out. When primary cultures are initiated, all details of procedures should be carefully documented to form part of the provenance of any cell line that may arise and be found to be important. A sample of tissue, or DNA extracted from it, should be archived to be available for DNA fingerprinting or profiling for authentication of any cell lines that arise.

6.4.3.2. Subculture

A monolayer culture may be transferred to a second vessel and diluted by dissociating the cells of the monolayer in trypsin (suspension cultures need only be diluted). This is best done by rinsing the monolayer with PBS lacking Ca^{2+} and Mg^{2+} (PBSA) or PBSA containing 1 mM EDTA, and removing the rinse, adding cold trypsin (0.25% crude or 0.01-0.05% pure) for 30 sec, removing the trypsin, and incubating in the residue for 5-15 min, depending on the cell line. Cells are then resuspended in medium, counted and reseeded.

6.4.3.3. Growth curve

When cells are seeded into a flask they enter a lag period of 2–24 h, followed by a period of exponential growth (the 'log phase'), and finally enter a period of reduced or zero growth after they become confluent ('plateau phase'). These phases are characteristic for each cell line and give rise to measurements which should be reproducible with each serial passage: the length of the lag period, the population doubling time (PDT) in mid-log phase, and the saturation density at plateau, given that the environmental conditions are kept constant. They should be determined when first handling a new cell line and at intervals of a few months thereafter. It is an important element of quality control to be able to demonstrate that the same seeding concentration will yield a reproducible number of cells at subculture, carried out after a consistent time interval, without necessarily performing a growth curve each time.

The determination of the growth cycle is important in designing routine subculture and experimental protocols. Cell behaviour and biochemistry changes significantly at each phase and it is therefore essential to control the stage of the growth cycle when drugs or reagents are added or cells harvested. The shape of the growth curve can also give information on the reproductive potential of the culture where differences in growth rate (PDT) adaptation or survival, and density limitation of growth (level of saturation density in plateau) can be deduced from the shape of the curve. However it is generally recognized that the analysis of clonal growth is easier, and less prone to ambiguity and misinterpretation.

6.4.3.4. Feeding

Some rapidly growing cultures, such as transformed cell lines like HeLa, will require a medium change after three to four days in a seven day subculture cycle. This is usually indicated by an increase in acidity where the pH falls below pH 7.0. Medium can also deteriorate without a major pH change, as some constituents, like glutamine, are unstable, and others may be utilized without a major pH shift. It is therefore recommended that the medium is changed at least once per week.

6.4.3.5. Contamination

The problem of microbial contamination has been greatly reduced by the use of laminar airflow cabinets. The risk of contamination can also be reduced by use of antibiotics, but this should be reserved for high-risk procedures, such as primary culture, and cultures should be maintained in the absence of antibiotics so that chronic, cryptic contaminations are not harboured. Check frequently for contamination by looking for a rapid change in pH (usually a fall, but some fungi can increase the pH), cloudiness in the medium, extracellular granularity under the microscope, or any unidentified material floating in the medium. If a contamination is detected, discard the flask unopened and autoclave. If in doubt, remove a sample and examine by phase microscopy, Gram's stain, or standard microbiological techniques.

Mycoplasma

Cultures can become contaminated by *mycoplasma* from media, sera, trypsin, imported cell lines, or the operator. Mycoplasma is not visible to the naked eye, and, while they can affect cell growth, their presence is often not obvious. It is important to test for mycoplasma at regular intervals (every one to three months) as they can seriously affect almost every aspect of cell metabolism, antigenicity, and growth characteristics. Several tests have been proposed, but the fluorescent DNA stain technique of Chen is the most widely used, although it is less sensitive than the PCR-based and culture methods (Fig. 6.2).

6.4.3.6. Cross-contamination

Its severity is often underrated, and consequently it still occurs with a higher frequency than many people admit. A significant number of cell lines, including Hep-2, KB, and Chang liver, are still in regular use without acknowledgement of their contamination with HeLa. Many other cell lines are cross-contaminated with cells other than HeLa. Many more cross-contaminations are yet to be detected.

To avoid cross-contamination:

• Do not share bottles of media or reagents among cell lines

• Do not return a pipette, which has been in or near a flask or bottle containing cells, back to the medium bottle; use a fresh pipette

• Do not share medium among operatives

• Handle one cell line at a time

6.4.3.7. Instability and preservation

Early passage cell lines are unstable as they go through a period of adaptation to culture. However, between about the 5th and 35th generation (for human diploid fibroblasts; other cell types may be different) the culture is fairly consistent. As the culture will start to senesce, as it gets older, finite cell lines should be used after the period of adaptation but before senescence. As continuous cell lines can be genetically unstable they should only be used continuously for approximately three months, before stock replacement. Some cell lines, such as 3T3 and other mouse lines which are immortal but not transformed, can transform spontaneously, and should not be propagated for prolonged periods.

Validated and authenticated frozen stocks of all cell lines should be maintained to protect against cell line instability, and to give insurance against contamination, incubator failure, or other accidental loss. Animal cell culture is a precise discipline. Beware of those who say it is not, or it is 'magic', or due to 'green fingers'; they are not controlling all the variables. Consistency can be achieved, and the following chapters are intended to indicate how best to control conditions within the present limitations of our knowledge.

6.5. DESIGN AND EQUIPMENT FOR THE CELL CULTURE LABORATORY

6.5.1. Laboratory design

Perhaps one of the most under-rated aspects of tissue culture is the need to design the facility to ensure that good quality material is produced in a safe and efficient manner. Most tissue culture is undertaken in laboratories that have been adapted for the purpose and in conditions that are not ideal (Fig. 6.3). However, as long as a few basic guidelines are adopted this should not compromise the work.

There are several aspects to the design of good tissue culture facilities. Ideally work should be conducted in a single use facility which, if at all possible, should be separated into an area reserved for handling newly received material (quarantine area) and an area for material which is known to be free of contaminants (main tissue culture facility). If this is not possible work should be separated by time with all manipulations on clean material being completed prior to manipulations involving the 'quarantine material'. Different incubators should also be designated. In addition, the work surfaces should be thoroughly cleaned between activities. All new material should be handled as 'quarantine material' until it has been shown to be free of contaminants such as bacteria, fungi and particularly mycoplasma. Conducting tissue culture in a shared facility requires considerable planning and it is essential that a good technique is used throughout to minimize the risk of contamination occurring.

6.5.2. Microbiological safety cabinets

A microbiological safety cabinet is probably the most important piece of equipment since, when operated correctly, it will provide a clean working environment for the product, whilst protecting the operator from aerosols. In these cabinets operator and/or product protection is provided through the use of HEPA (high efficiency particulate air) filters. The level of containment provided varies according to the class of cabinet used. Cabinets may be ducted to atmosphere or re-circulated through a second HEPA filter before passing to atmosphere.

Environmental monitoring with Tryptose Soya Broth agar settle plates inside the cabinet for a minimum of four hours should be a good indicator of how clean a cabinet is. There should be no growth of bacteria or fungi on such plates.

In most cases a class II cabinet is adequate for animal cell culture. However each study must be assessed for its hazard risk and it is possible that additional factors, such as a known virus infection or an uncertain provenance, may require a higher level of containment.

6.5.3. Centrifuges

Centrifuges are used routinely in tissue culture as part of the subculture routine for most cell lines and for the preparation of cells for cryopreservation. By their very nature centrifuges produce aerosols and thus it is necessary to minimize this risk. This can be achieved by purchasing models that have sealed buckets. Ideally the centrifuge should have a clear lid so that the condition of the load can be observed without opening the lid. This will reduce the risk of the operator being exposed to hazardous material if a centrifuge tube has broken during centrifugation. Care should always be taken not to over-fill the tubes and to balance them carefully. These simple steps will reduce the risk of aerosols being generated. The centrifuge should be situated where it can be easily accessed for cleaning and maintenance. Centrifuges should be checked frequently for signs of corrosion.

6.5.4. Incubators

Cell cultures require a strictly controlled environment in which to grow. Specialist incubators are used routinely to provide the correct growth conditions, such as temperature, degree of humidity and CO_2

levels in a controlled and stable manner. Generally they can be set to run at temperatures in the range 28°C (for insect cell lines) to 37°C (for mammalian cell lines) and set to provide CO_2 at the required level (e.g., 5-10%). Some incubators also have the facility to control the O_2 levels. Copper-coated incubators are also now available. These are reported to reduce the risk of microbial contamination within the incubator due to the microbial inhibitory activity of copper. The inclusion of water bath treatment fluid in the incubator water trays will also reduce the risk of bacterial and fungal growth in the water trays. However, there is no substitute for regular cleaning.

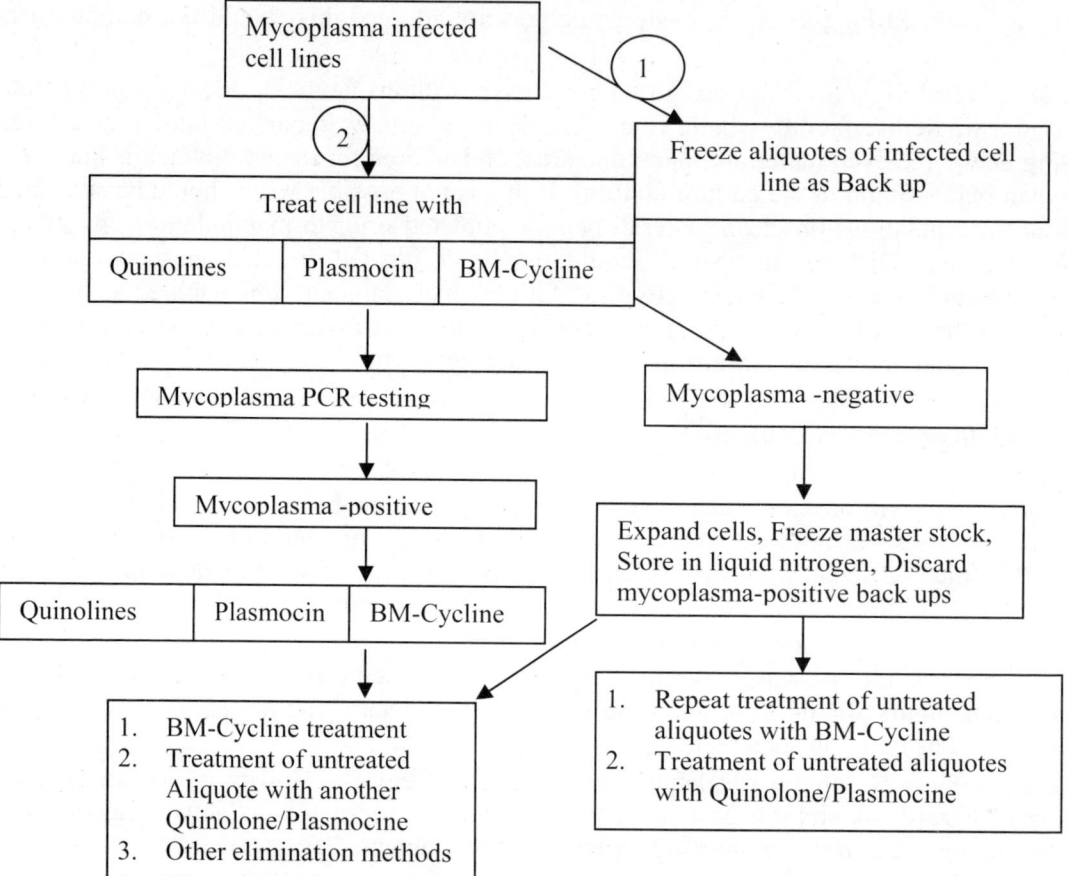

Fig. 6.2: Scheme for mycoplasma eradication. Different antibiotics can be used to treat mycoplasma-contaminated cell lines with a high rate of expected success. We recommend (1) cryopreservation of original mycoplasma-positive cells as backups and (2) splitting of the growing cells into different aliquots. These aliquots should be exposed singly to the various antibiotics. Post treatment mycoplasma analysis and routine monitoring with a sensitive and reliable method (e.g., by polymerase chain reaction [PCR]) are of utmost importance

6.5.5. Work surfaces and flooring

In order to maintain a clean working environment the laboratory surfaces including benchtops, walls and flooring should be smooth and easy to clean. They should also be waterproof and resistant to a variety of chemicals (such as acids, alkalis, solvents and disinfectants). In areas used for the storage of materials in liquid nitrogen, the floors should be resistant to cracking if any liquid nitrogen is spilt.

In addition, the floors and walls should be continuous with a covered skirting area to make cleaning easier and reduce the potential for dust to accumulate. Windows should be sealed. Work surfaces should be positioned at a comfortable working height.

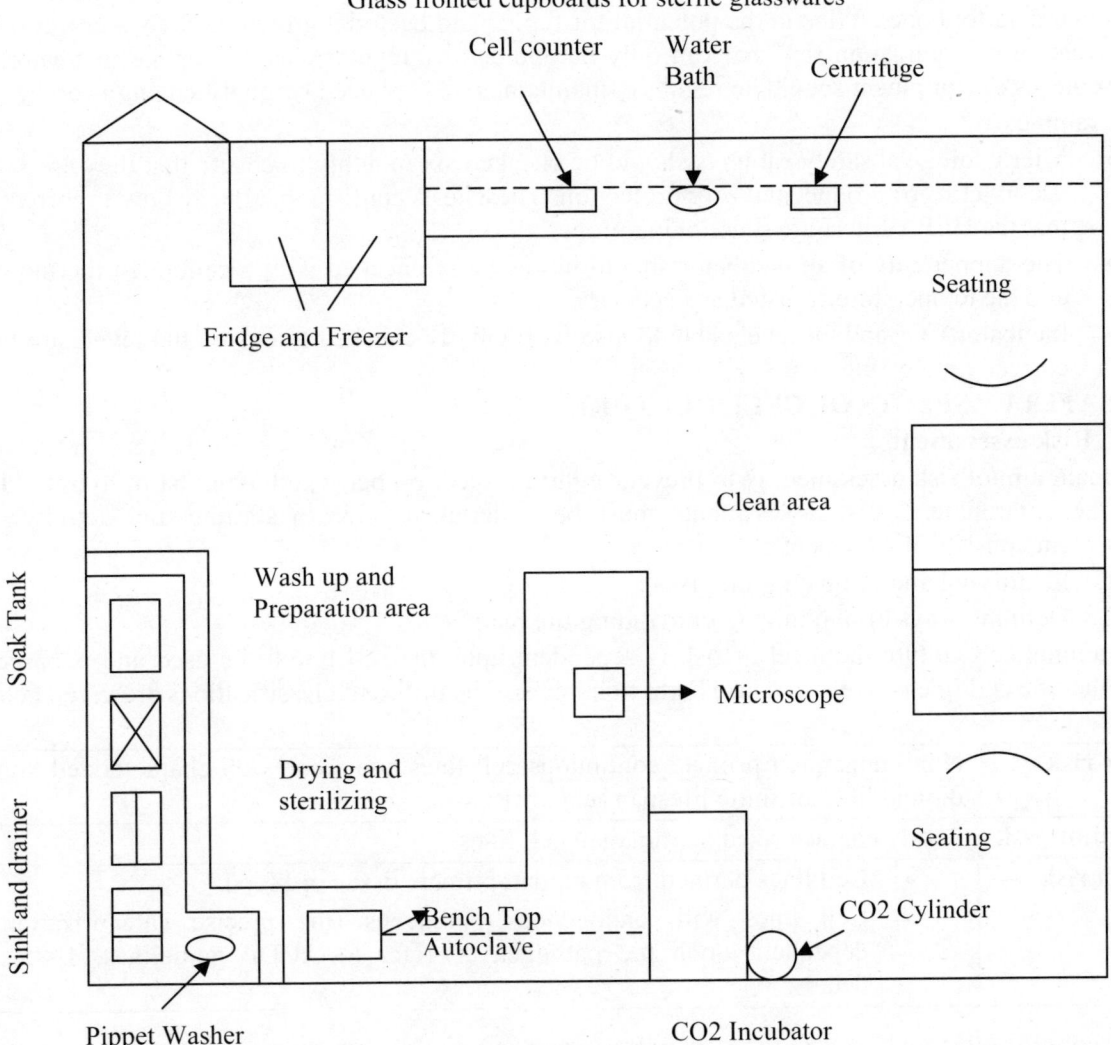

Fig. 6.3: Plan for a cell culture laboratory

6.5.6. Plasticware and consumables

Almost every type of cell culture vessel, together with support consumables such as tubes and pipettes, are commercially available as single use, sterile packed, plasticware. The use of such plasticware is more cost effective than recycling glassware, enables a higher level of quality assurance and removes the need for validation of cleaning and sterilization procedures. Plastic tissue culture flasks are usually treated to provide a hydrophilic surface to facilitate attachment of anchorage dependent cells.

6.5.7. Care and maintenance of laboratory areas

In order to maintain a clean and safe working environment tidiness and cleanliness are key factors. Obviously all spills should be dealt with immediately. Routine cleaning should also be undertaken involving the cleaning of all work surfaces both inside and outside of the microbiological safety cabinet, the floors and all other pieces of equipment e.g., centrifuges. Humidified incubators are a particular area for concern due to the potential for fungal and bacterial growth in the water trays. This will create a contamination risk that can only be avoided by regular cleaning of the incubator. All major pieces of equipment should be regularly maintained and serviced by qualified engineers.

For example:

- Microbiological safety cabinets should be checked six monthly to ensure that they are safe to use in terms of product and user protection. These tests confirm that the airflow is correct and that the HEPA filters are functioning properly
- The temperature of an incubator should be regularly checked with a calibrated thermometer and the temperature adjusted as necessary
- Incubator CO_2 and O_2 levels should also be regularly checked to ensure the levels are being correctly maintained

6.6. SAFETY ASPECTS OF CELL CULTURE

6.6.1. Risk assessment

The main aim of risk assessment is to prevent injury, protect property and avoid harm to individuals and the environment. Risk assessments must be undertaken prior to starting any activity. The assessment consists of 2 elements:

1. Identifying and evaluating the risks.
2. Defining ways of minimizing or avoiding the risk.

For animal cell culture the level of risk is dependent upon the cell line to be used and is based on whether the cell line is likely to cause harm to humans. The different classifications are given below:

Low risk	Non human/non primate continuous cell lines and some well characterized human diploid lines of finite lifespan (e.g., MRC-5).
Medium risk	Poorly characterized mammalian cell lines.
High risk	- Cell lines derived from human/primate tissue or blood. - Cell lines with endogenous pathogens (the precise categorization is dependent upon the pathogen) – refer to ACDP guidelines, 1985, for details.

A culture collection, such as ECACC will recommend a minimum the containment level required for a given cell line based upon its risk assessment. For most cell lines the appropriate level of containment is Category 2. However, this may need to be increased to Category 3 depending upon the type of manipulations to be carried out and whether large culture volumes are envisaged. For cell lines derived from patients with HIV or HTLV Category 3 containment is required.

Containment is the most obvious means of reducing risk. Other less obvious measures include restricting the movement of staff and equipment into and out of laboratories. Good laboratory practice and good bench techniques such as ensuring work areas are uncluttered, reagents are correctly labeled and stored, are also important for reducing risk and making the laboratory a safe environment in which to work. Staff training and the use of written standard operating procedures and risk assessments will also reduce the potential for harm.

6.6.2. Disinfection

Methods designed for the disinfection/decontamination of culture waste, work surfaces and equipment represent important means for minimizing the risk of harm.

The major disinfectants fall into four groups and their relative merits can be summarized as follows:

Hypochlorites

- Good general purpose disinfectant
- Active against viruses
- Corrosive against metals and therefore should not be used on metal surfaces, e.g. centrifuges
- Readily inactivated by organic matter and therefore should be made fresh daily
- Should be used at 1000 ppm for general use surface disinfection, 2500 ppm in discard waste pots for washing pipettes, and 10,000 ppm for tissue culture waste and spillage

NB: When fumigating a cabinet or room using formaldehyde all the hypochlorites must first be removed as the two chemicals react together to produce carcinogenic products.

Phenolics

- Not active against viruses
- Remains active in the presence of organic matter

Alcohol (e.g., ethanol, isopropanol)

- Effective concentrations 70% for ethanol, 60–70% for isopropanol
- Their mode of activity is by dehydration and fixation
- Effective against bacteria. Ethanol is effective against most viruses but not non-enveloped viruses
- Isopropanol is not effective against viruses

Aldehydes (e.g. glutaraldehyde, formaldehyde)

- Aldehydes are irritants and their use should be limited due to problems of sensitization
- Glutaraldehyde may be used in situations where the use of hypochlorites is not suitable, e.g. cleaning of centrifuge bowls or materials constructed of stainless steel that may be attacked or corroded by using hypochlorite solutions.

6.6.3. Waste disposal

Any employer has a 'duty of care' to dispose of all biological waste safely. Given below is a list of ways in which tissue culture waste can be decontaminated and disposed of safely. One of the most important aspects of the management of all laboratory-generated waste is to dispose of waste regularly and not to allow the amounts to build up. The best approach is 'little and often'. Different forms of waste require different treatment.

- **Tissue culture waste** (culture medium) - Inactivate overnight in a solution of hypochlorite (10,000 ppm) prior to disposal to drain with an excess of water
- **Contaminated pipettes** should be placed in hypochlorite solution (2500 ppm) overnight before disposal by autoclaving and incineration
- **Solid waste** such as flasks, centrifuge tubes, contaminated gloves, tissues etc. should be placed inside heavy duty sacks for contaminated waste and autoclaved prior to incineration. If at all possible waste should be incinerated rather than autoclaved

6.7. CRYOPRESERVATION AND STORAGE OF CELL LINES

6.7.1. Cryopreservation of cell lines

The aim of cryopreservation is to enable stocks of cells to be stored to prevent the need to have all cell lines in culture at all times. It is invaluable when dealing with cells of limited life span. The other main advantages of cryopreservation are:

- Reduced risk of microbial contamination
- Reduced risk of cross contamination with other cell lines
- Reduced risk of genetic drift and morphological changes
- Work conducted using cells at a consistent passage number (refer to cell banking section below)
- Reduced costs (consumables and staff time)

There has been a large amount of developmental work undertaken to ensure successful cryopreservation and resuscitation of a wide variety of cell lines of different cell types. The basic principle of successful cryopreservation is a slow freeze and quick thaw. Although the precise requirement may vary with different cell lines as a general guide cells should be cooled at a rate of −1°C to –3°C per minute and thawed quickly by incubation in a 37°C water bath for 3-5 minutes. If this and the additional points given below are followed then most cell lines should be cryopreserved successfully.

1. Cultures should be healthy with a viability of >90% and no signs of microbial contamination.

2. Cultures should be in log phase of growth (this can be achieved by using pre-confluent cultures i.e. cultures that are below their maximum cell density and by changing the culture medium 24 hours before freezing).

3. A high concentration of serum/protein (>20%) should be used. In many cases serum is used at 90%.

4. Use a cryoprotectant such as dimethyl sulphoxide or glycerol to help protect the cells from rupture by the formation of ice crystals. The most commonly used cryoprotectant is DMSO at a final concentration of 10%, however, this is not appropriate for all cell lines e.g., HL60 where DMSO is used to induce differentiation. In such cases an alternative such as glycerol should be used.

6.7.2. Ultra-low temperature storage of cell lines

Following controlled rate freezing in the presence of cryoprotectants, cell lines can be cryopreserved in a suspended state for indefinite periods provided a temperature of less than -135°C is maintained. Such ultra-low temperatures can only be attained by specialized electric freezers or more usually by immersion in liquid or vapor phase nitrogen. The advantages and disadvantages can be summarized as follows:

Storage in liquid phase nitrogen allows the lowest possible storage temperature to be maintained with absolute consistency, but requires the use of large volumes (depth) of liquid nitrogen and sealed glass ampules. Both of these requirements create potential hazards. There have also been documented cases of cross contamination by virus pathogens via the liquid nitrogen medium. For these reasons ultra-low temperature storage is most commonly in vapor phase nitrogen.

For vapor phase nitrogen storage, the ampules are positioned above a shallow reservoir of liquid nitrogen, the depth of which has to be carefully maintained. A vertical temperature gradient will exist through the vapor phase, the extremes of which will depend on the liquid levels maintained, the design of the vessel, and the frequency with which it is opened. Temperature variations in the upper regions of a vapor phase storage vessel can be extreme if regular maintenance is not carried out.

All liquid nitrogen storage vessels should include alarms that at least warn of low liquid nitrogen levels. This is particularly true of vapor phase storage systems. The bulk liquid nitrogen storage vessel should not be allowed to become less than half full before it is resupplied. This will ensure that at least one delivery can be missed without catastrophic consequences.

Table 6.3: Comparison of ultra-low temperature storage methods for cell lines

Method	Advantages	Disadvantages
Electric Freezer (-135ºC)	• Ease of maintenance • Steady temperature • Low running costs	• Requires liquid nitrogen back-up • Mechanically complex • Storage temperatures high relative to liquid nitrogen
Liquid Phase Nitrogen	• Steady ultra-low (-196ºC) temperature • Simplicity and mechanical reliability	• Requires regular supply of liquid nitrogen • High running costs • Risk of cross-contamination via the liquid nitrogen
Vapor Phase Nitrogen	• No risk of cross-contamination from liquid nitrogen • Low temperatures achieved Simplicity and reliability	• Requires regular supply of liquid nitrogen • High running costs • Temperature fluctuations between - 135ºC and - 190ºC

Inventory control

All ultra-low temperature storage vessels will include a racking / inventory system designed to organize the contents for ease of location and retrieval. This should be supported by accurate record keeping and inventory control incorporating the following:

- Each ampule should be individually labeled, using "wrap around", liquid nitrogen resistant labels with identity, lot number and date of freezing
- The location of each ampule should be recorded ideally on an electronic database or spreadsheet, but also on a paper storage plan
- There should be a control system to ensure that no ampule can be deposited or withdrawn without updating the records

6.7.3. Safety considerations

General safety issues

It is important that staffs are trained in the use of liquid nitrogen and associated equipment including the storage vessels, which need to be vented safely, and containers, which may need to be filled. As with all laboratory procedures personal protective equipment should be worn at all times whilst handling nitrogen, including a full-face visor and thermally insulated gloves in addition to a laboratory coat. Proper training and the use of protective equipment will minimize the risk of frostbite and other minor incidents.

Risk of asphyxiation

The single most important safety consideration is the potential risk of asphyxiation due to the high levels of nitrogen that can lead to oxygen depletion. This is critical since oxygen depletion can very rapidly cause loss of consciousness, without warning.

Consequently liquid nitrogen refrigerators should be placed in well-ventilated areas in order to minimize this risk. Large volume stores should have low oxygen alarm systems.

Preventative measures

- Use oxygen alarms set to 18% oxygen (v/v)
- Staff training – staff should be trained to evacuate the area immediately on hearing the alarm and not return until the oxygen is back to normal (~ 20% v/v)
- Staff should work in pairs when handling liquid nitrogen
- Prohibit the use of nitrogen outside of normal working hours
- Mechanical ventilation systems should be installed if at all possible

6.8. AUTHENTICATION OF CELL LINES

6.8.1. Authentication techniques

Whatever the scope of work to be carried out it is important to know that the work is being conducted using the correct reagents. This is no less important for cell cultures, since if cell cultures are not what they are reported to be then work can be invalidated and resources wasted. There is now considerable evidence of gross cross-contamination of cell lines, in particular with HeLa where up to 16 lines were offered to ECACC with DNA profiles identical to HeLa. These include Hep 2, WISH, INT 407, Chang liver and Giradi heart. To minimize the risk of working with contaminated cell lines it is advisable to obtain cells from a recognized source such as a culture collection that will have confirmed the identity of the cells as part of the banking process. Tests used to authenticate cell cultures include iso-enzyme analysis, karyotyping/ cytogenetic analysis and more recently molecular techniques of DNA profiling. Whilst most of the techniques above are generalized tests and are applicable to all cell lines additional specific tests may also be required to confirm the presence of a product or antigen of interest.

6.8.2. Iso-enzyme analysis

Iso-enzymes are a series of enzymes present in different species that have similar catalytic properties but differ in their structure. By studying the iso-enzymes present in cell lines it is possible to identify the species from which the cell line was derived. The technique is also used as a means of excluding the possibility of gross cross-contamination of the cell line with another culture of a different species.

The principles upon which iso-enzyme analysis is based are:

- Each iso-enzyme has multiple gene loci coding for different polypeptides with identical enzyme activity (e.g., lactate dehydrogenase, LD)
- Electrophoretic migration rates change dependent on sub-unit composition e.g., LD has five possible iso-forms (LD 1-5)
- Different species have different combinations of these iso-forms
- Using a typical panel of 4 iso-enzymes a composite picture is built up enabling the species of origin to be determined by the use of reference tables

6.8.3. DNA fingerprinting

DNA fingerprinting enables the following:

- Identification of individual cell lines from the same species
- Confirmation of the identity of cell banks compared to reference master stocks
- Detection of cross-contamination

6.8.4. Multi locus DNA fingerprinting

- Probes cross-hybridize with most common species
- Has the disadvantage that the profiles require visual interpretation and comparison with other samples can be subjective

6.8.5. Multiplex - PCR (STR) DNA profiling

- Uses a set of primers recognizing micro-satellites using PCR and automated DNA sequencing techniques
- Primers are species specific and are used only for human cell lines
- Produces a color-coded banding pattern, that translates into a digital code that can easily be stored on a database and compared to other stored profiles

6.9. CHARACTERISTICS OF CELLS IN CULTURE

6.9.1. Source of cells

A major choice has to be made when establishing a cell culture as to whether cells are obtained directly from animal tissue or from a culture collection. The choice will depend upon what the objective of the project is and the nature of the experiments planned. Isolation directly from tissue offers a means of culturing cells close to their state in vivo. However, the isolation process is far more demanding and troublesome compared to establishing a culture from a cell sample that could be obtained from a culture collection. Most culture laboratories prefer to use cell lines from collections because they are well characterized in terms of growth, origin and genetic traits.

6.9.2. Cells from tissue: a primary culture

A primary culture is established when the cells taken directly from animal tissue are added to growth medium. Primary cultures are often established from embryonic tissue because the cells are more easily dispersed and have a superior growth potential. The structure of a tissue is highly ordered and comprises a range of cell types as shown for the cross-section of the epidermis. The objective of establishing a primary culture is to select a single cell type from this ordered structure. The original methods developed for tissue culture by Harrison and Carrel involved the maintenance of tissue fragments (or explant) on a solid surface and supplied with suitable nutrients. However, such cultures are of greater use if the individual cells are separated out before culture. This is done by fragmenting tissue with forceps and scissors followed by treatment with a proteolytic enzyme such as trypsin or collagenase. The proteolytic action of the enzymes disaggregates the tissue into individual cells after which the cells are isolated by low-speed centrifugation. The time that the cells are in contact with the degradative enzymes should be minimized otherwise membrane damage may occur. Cells can be bathed in trypsin for 10–20 minutes. Longer exposure times are undesirable because breakdown of the protein components of cell membranes could occur. Collagenase degrades collagen and is less harmful to cell membranes. This technique works well for most tissues although some modifications to the general procedure may be necessary to ensure the maximum yield of a particular cell type. One of the major difficulties and reasons for failure at this stage is that the cell population becomes contaminated with bacteria or fungi. To avoid this problem it is important to maintain aseptic techniques throughout the process of establishing the surfaces should be swabbed with 70% alcohol. When the cells in a primary culture stop growing a new culture may be established by inoculating some of the cells into fresh medium. This is called subculturing or passaging.

A secondary culture is established after the first passage of the primary culture. The term 'cell line' is applied to the cell population that can continue growing through many subcultures. However it should be noted that the greatest chance of genetic alteration occurs in the first few passages following the primary culture as cells adapt to a new chemical environment. The chick embryo fibroblasts for example may grow for around 30 passages before becoming senescent. The passage number of a culture is often recorded as the number of subcultures from the primary source.

6.9.3. Cell types

Animal cells are usually defined by the tissue from which they have derived and have characteristic shapes that can be observed and recognized easily through a light microscope. Figure 6.4 illustrates the morphology of the cells commonly grown in culture. These are derived from five main types of animal tissue.

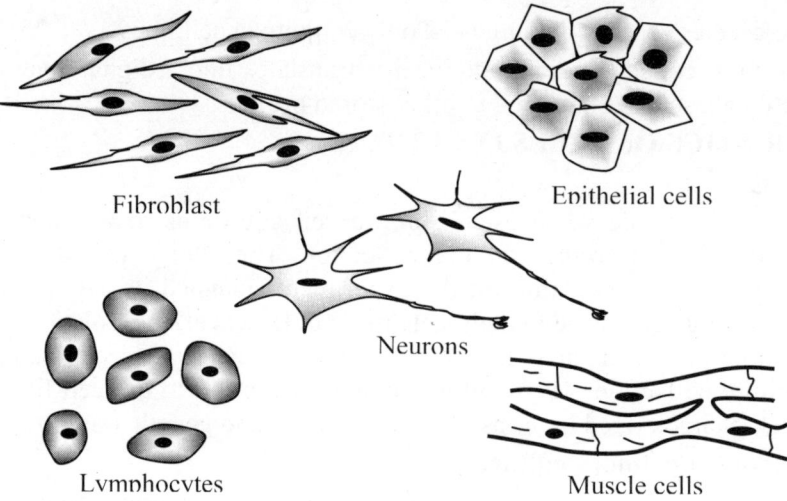

Fig. 6.4: Cell types commonly used in culture

■ Epithelial tissue consists of a layer of cells which cover organs and line cavities; examples include skin and the lining of the alimentary canal. The epithelial cells grow well in culture as a single cell monolayer and have a characteristic cobble-stone appearance.

■ Connective tissue forms a major structural component of animals, consisting of a fibrous matrix and including bone cartilage. The tissue contains fibroblasts which are amongst the most widely used cells in laboratory cultures. Fibroblasts are bound to the fibrous protein collagen in the connective tissue. The cells are spherical when first dissociated by trypsin from the tissue but elongate to a characteristic spindle-shape on attachment to a solid surface. Fibroblasts have excellent growth characteristics and have been the 'favorite' cells for establishing cultures. Fibroblast and epithelial cells adapt relatively easily to culture and have growth rates with a doubling time of 18–24 hours.

■ Muscle tissue consists of a series of tubules formed from precursor cells which fuse to form a multinucleate complex and which also contain the structural proteins (actin and myosin). The precursor cells are myoblasts which are capable of differentiation to form myotubes—a process that can be observed in culture. Figure 6.4 shows the myoblast alignment that occurs during the process.

■ Nervous tissue consists of characteristically shaped neurons which are responsible for the transmission of electrical impulses and supporting cells, such as glial cells. Neurons are highly differentiated and have not been observed to divide in culture. However, the addition of nerve growth factor to cultures of neurons may cause the formation of cytoplasmic outgrowths called neurites.

Some of the characteristics of nerve cells can be observed with neuroblastomas which are tumor cells that undergo cell growth in culture.

■ Blood and lymph contain a range of cells in suspension. Some of these will continue growth in a culture suspension. These include the lymphoblasts which are white blood cells and are used extensively in culture because of their ability to secrete immune-regulating compounds.

6.10. Animal cell culture and technology

6.10.1. Selection of a particular cell type

The primary culture will almost certainly contain a variety of different cell types with differing growth capacities. However, for most experimental work it is important to isolate a single cell type from the culture population. There are several ways this can be achieved.

■ Allow the cells to grow. Fast-growing cell types may assume dominance in a population. For example, fibroblasts have relatively short population doubling times and may outgrow other cells after a few generations (called 'fibroblast overgrowth').

■ Control the composition of the growth medium. The addition of specific growth factors or known growth inhibitors may allow selective growth of certain cell types.

■ Separate cells by using gradient centrifugation: The cells sediment to an equilibrium position equivalent to their own density—a process called isopycnic sedimentation. The gradients can be formed by nontoxic, high-molecular-weight material such as colloidal silica as developed by Pharmacia in their formulations 'Ficoll' and 'Percoll'. This method is particularly effective for the isolation of certain cell types in sterile medium, for example lymphocytes from blood. Cell separation by a simple gradient centrifugation process is shown in Figure 6.5.

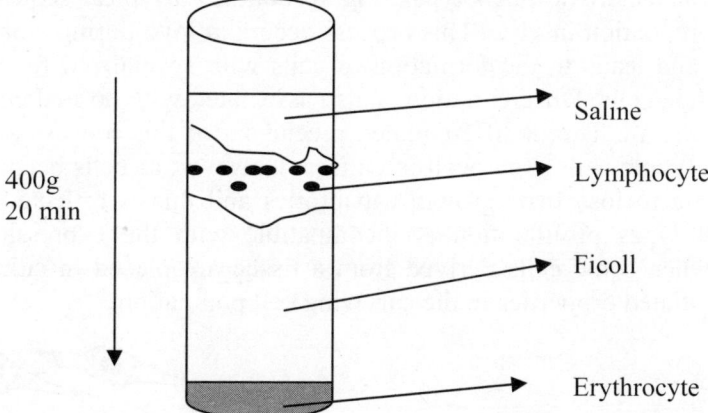

Fig. 6.5: Separation of cells by density gradient centrifugation

6.10.2. Normal cell

In the 1960s, 'normal' mammalian cells were required as hosts for the production of human vaccines in order to ensure the safety of these products. In order to meet this requirement, a number of characteristics of 'normal' animal cells were defined by Hayflick and Moorhead following their work with human embryonic cells:

■ A diploid chromosome number (e.g., 46 chromosomes for human cells). This indicates that no gross chromosomal damage has occurred;

■ Anchorage dependence: The cells require a solid substratum for attachment and growth. Growth continues until a confluent monolayer of cells is formed on the substratum;

■ A finite lifespan: This is a reflection of the intrinsic growth potential of the cells;

■ Nonmalignant: The cells are not cancerous. This can be shown by the inability of the cells to form a tumor following injection into immuno-compromised mice.

6.10.3. Anchorage-dependence

Anchorage-dependence is the requirement of cells for a solid substratum for attachment before growth can occur. At the laboratory scale this substratum can be provided by the solid surface of Petri dishes, T-flasks, or Roux bottles which are made of specially treated glass or plastic. The interaction between the cell membrane and the growth surface is critical and involves a combination of electrostatic attraction and van der Waal's forces. Cell adhesion occurs by divalent cations (usually Ca^{2+}) and basic proteins forming a layer between the solid substratum and the cell surface. In most cases the cell-surface interaction is provided by a range of nonspecific proteins which form a 2.5 nm-thick layer on the substratum prior to cell attachment. Figure 6.6 outlines the process of cell attraction to the substratum and the involvement of various proteins in cell-surface bonding. Serum-derived glycoproteins (e.g., fibronectin) can provide a surface coating conducive to cell attachment. Conditioning factors are released by cells into the medium and help in forming a bond between cell surface glycoproteins and the substratum. The density of the electrostatic charge on the solid substratum is also critical in maximizing cell attachment. A negative charge is provided on glass surface containers by alkali treatment. Tissue culture-grade plasticware consists of sulfonated polystyrene with a surface charge of 2–5 negatively charged groups per nm^2. Culture systems are also available for the large-scale production of anchoragedependent cells. The culture of differentiated cells Differentiation is a process whereby cells slowly change their characteristics to become specialized cells with characteristic phenotypes. Figure outlines a typical sequence of changes that occurs during cell differentiation in vivo. This process occurs in vivo during embryo development or during wound healing and leads to the formation of cells with specialized function (differentiated) such as neurons or muscle cells. Differentiation is also associated with normal cell replacement, as is necessary in the bloodstream. The undifferentiated precursors of this process are called stem cells. Most stem cells or embryonic cells grow well in culture. However, as cells become more specialized (differentiated) they tend to lose their growth capabilities and this is reflected by poor growth in culture. For most cell types proliferation is incompatible with the expression of differentiated properties. However, when some cells derived from a tissue are placed in culture there can be an apparent loss in differentiated properties in the surviving cell population.

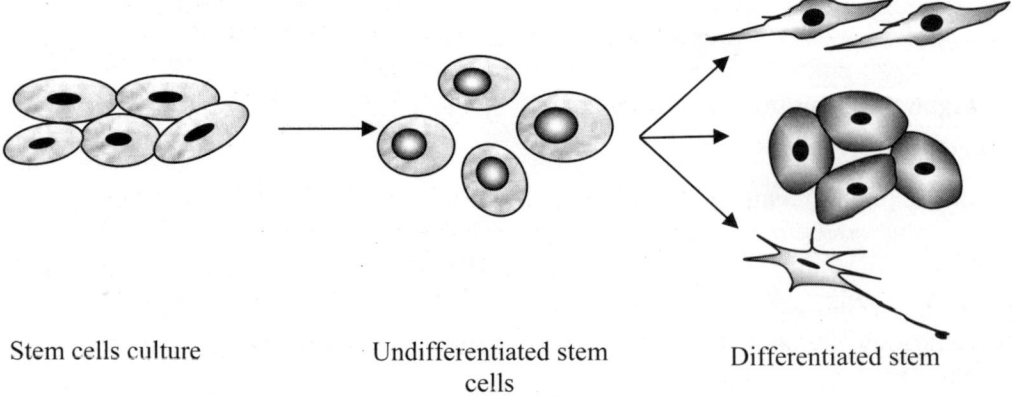

Stem cells culture   Undifferentiated stem cells   Differentiated stem

Fig. 6.6: Cell differentiation

Some explanation can be offered for this:

■ Selective outgrowth of undifferentiated cell types: These include fibroblasts and epithelial cells that may be obtained from non-growing animal tissue;

■ Adaptive response of cells to the culture media: Tumor cells are, in most cases, undifferentiated and have good growth characteristics. However, there are also some differentiated tumor cells which have proved extremely valuable. For example, neuroblastomas are fast-growing tumor cells which have been used to study response effects with nerve growth factor. Differentiated tumor cells retain the phenotypic characteristics of normal differentiated cells but are also able to grow in culture. Although growth of most differentiated cells is poor, the following factors may allow some differentiated properties of normal cells to be maintained in culture.

■ Hormones and growth factors: There are a number of media formulations containing selective components that can maintain the differentiated state of specific cell types, for example keratinocytes, hepatocytes and nerve cells.

■ Chemical agents: Solvents such as dimethyl sulfoxide (DMSO) may allow the maintenance of a differentiated state by an effect on membrane fluidity.

■ Cell interactions: Contact between cells may allow the formation of gap junctions and allow metabolites to synchronize the expression of differentiation within a cell population. This may also play a part in the arrest of growth when a cell population has covered an available growth surface (defined as 'confluence').

■ Interaction with the growth surface: Collagen has been found to be essential for maintaining the polarity of hepatocytes in relation to the attachment surface. Cell polarity is governed by an asymmetrical distribution of ion currents (particularly Ca^{2+}). This allows one end of the cell to be functionally distinct from the other. Some culture systems have been extremely valuable in investigating the metabolic changes that are associated with differentiation. However, growth in these cultures is either nonexistent or can be prolonged only for a short period (weeks).

6.11. CELL CULTURE AND MAINTENANCE

For establishing a primary culture, the source of the cell lines is required with markers, the number of passages, the feeding conditions, the survival rate, the growth rate, the plating efficiency, morphology, density of a monolayer, and sterility. The methods used for setting up a culture are generally based on a combination of the following:

- Mechanical comminution of a tissue;
- Chemical breakdown by chelating agents such as EDTA; and
- Treatment with enzymes.

The most common enzymes used for this purpose are a crude trypsin preparation with chymotrypsin trace activities, elastase, DNAse, etc. Enzymes such as collagenase, pronase, and hyaluronidase have not found the same broad use but still are important in combination with trypsin. After such pretreatments, the cover-slip method can be used for fibroblasts in order to supply a fragment of tissue between microscope slides with plasma or medium. On incubation, an exuberant growth of cells takes place. The grown cells can be removed from the glass support and transferred into a monolayer culture. Organs with small proportions of connective tissue (liver, kidneys) can be perfused with an enzyme-EDTA mixture and subsequently be broken down immediately after they have been dissected out or even in situ. After mechanical dissection, pieces of tissues or individual cells can then be transferred to culture bottles. Even embryonic and cancer-like tissues are susceptible to mild processes, since they contain weak matrix. For other differentiated tissues, more intensive methods are necessary in order to degrade intercellular materials (fiber proteins, mucopolysaccharides). Treatments with oncogenic chemicals, transformation by viruses, or the fusion of the primary cells with cancer cells are suitable process options for the deliberate conversion of diploid primary cells into continuous cells.

6.11.1. Cultured cells and cell lines

The cultured cells are classified mainly as:

1. Precursor or stem cells or master cells are capable of proliferation, but they need stimulant or inducing conditions; till then they remain undifferentiated. On stimulation under appropriate conditions some or all of the cells mature and differentiate. These cells are referred to as totipotent or pluripotent. The stem cells exhibit varied levels of stemness, e.g., totipotent stem cells can generate cells, capable of producing entire blood cellular components and immune system. They can be differentiated from pluripotent cells which are less general, yet can be differentiated into several types, such as

2. Committed precursor cells; and

3. Differentiated, matured cells.

The cell culture therefore may be perceived as a mass of culturing cells under the state of equilibrium between the multipotent stem cells, undifferentiated but committed precursors and mature differentiated cells. The equilibrium as such could shift depending upon the environmental conditions as under high serum concentration in medium and growth factors, a low density cell mass will promote proliferation of the cells while under low serum concentration in the presence of appropriate hormone a high density cell mass may promote differentiation. Further, the cell types in a particular culture are determined by the source of culture. The concept can be clarified with the help of following example;

1. Cell lines of embryo origin may contain relatively more stem cells (precursor cells) capable of cell renewal.

2. Similarly, the cultures from tissues undergoing continuous renewal *in vivo* i.e., intestinal epithelial, epidermis, haemopoietic and vaginal endometrium possess stem cells even though they are derived from adults.

3. Some of the tissues that renew under stress conditions include fibroblasts, muscles and glia. These cells contain basically committed precursors which have very short (limited) culture life span. Using anyone of these cells derived from primary explant it is possible to develop respective cell lines. After first subculture, the primary culture becomes cell line in itself which can be propagated and sequentially subcultured several times. It is interesting to note that every successive cell culture process provides proliferating population component predominantly and at the same time it may be observed that non-proliferating slowly growing cells get diluted out.

The cell lines may be propagated for a limited number of generations beyond which they may die off or give rise to continuous cell lines. The latter are aneuploids with larger amount of variation in chromosome number while the finite cell lines are often euploid with little variation particularly in the number of chromosomes. The process by which a culture transforms and gives rise to a continuous cell line is termed as *in vitro* transformation. This transformation may be induced by viruses or some chemical reactions. Furthermore, this term (transformation) is implied for continuous cell line due to the reason that the culture undergoes not only morphological and kinetic alterations but the cell lines are more frequently accompanied with an increased tumorogenicity. They exhibit malignant transforming properties reflected in their characteristics as reduced serum requirements, reduced density with limitation of growth, or aneuploid.

6.11.2. Maintenance of culture cell lines

During the process of culturing owing to differentiation and proliferation the medium is largely consumed and the substrate is inhabited or colonized by growing cells and requires subculturing. Obviously, the heterogeneous primary cultures containing various types of cells generate homogenous cell lines on subculturing. Such cultures are referred to as cell lines, which can be propagated, characterized, preserved and stored. The phrase cell line defines the presence of several cell lineages which may be similar or distinct. A particular cell lineage may have specific properties which are well identified and distinctive in bulk of the cells. This cell lineage is referred to as cell strain. The cell strain or line may be finite or continuous depending upon whether the life span is limited or immortal in culture. Finite cell lines may extinct following 20-80 population propagation.

Maintenance of adherent cell lines

Most of the primary cultures are continuous cell lines that grow in the form of mono layers requiring continual albeit periodic change of medium irrespective of the situation whether cells are proliferating or not. The adherent cell line subculturing involves:

1. Removal of medium;

2. Dissociation and segregation of cells in the monolayer using trypsin or other enzymes.

   Highly proliferative cell lines sucha as HeLa are subcultured once per week; likewise, media are replaced once every four days. Slow growing cells are subcultured once every 2, 3, or 4 weeks while medium is changed weekly between subcultures. The factors and steps involved in the maintenance of cell lines are presented in Figure 6.7.

6.11.3. Cloning of cell lines

From a heterogeneous culture pure cell lines can be produced by employing cloning technique. However, cloning seems to be successful in the isolation of variants in continuous cell lines because most of the cultures have a finite life span. The mutants or variants may typically be biochemical mutants and strains with marker chromosomes. A method based on dilution cloning has been described by Puck and Marcus (1955). In this method trypsinized individual cells are seeded at low density in multi-well dishes or in Petri dishes or plastic bottles. The seeded cells are incubated until colonies are formed. The colonies are isolated and propagated independently as a well identified clone of cells.

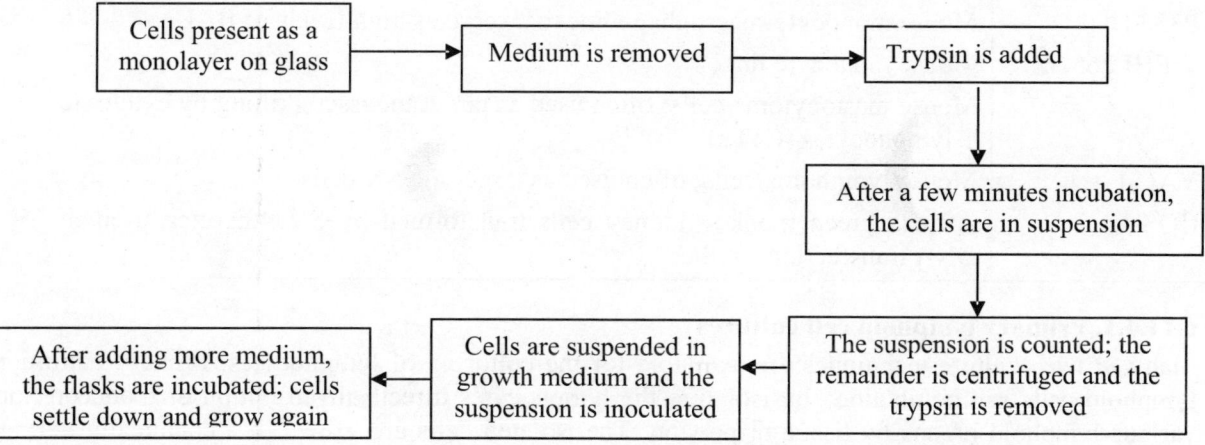

Fig. 6.7: Maintenance of a cell line

6.11.4. Cell-culture system

A variety of cells can be cultured by using anyone of the above methods. For example, bone marrow cells and leukocytes are directly collected from patient or animal, and could directly be inoculated to a culture medium. Some different cell cultures and cell lines used in immunological research include primary lymphoid cells, cloned lymphoid cell lines, and hybrid cells.

Table 6.4: Cell lines commonly used in immunological research

Cell line	Description
L929	Mouse fibroblast cell line; often used in DNA transfection studies and to assay tumor necrosis factor (TNF)
SP2/0	Non-secreting mouse myeloma; often used as a fusion partner for hybridoma secretion
PX63-Ag8.653	Non-secreting mouse myeloma; often used as a fusion partner for hybridoma secretion
MPC II	Mouse IgG2a-secreting myeloma
P3X63Ag8	Mouse IgG I-secreting myeloma
MOPC 315	Mouse IgA-secreting myeloma
J558	Mouse IgA-secreting myeloma
ABE-8.1/2	Mouse pre-B cell lymphoma
70Z/3	Mouse pre-B lymphoma; used to study early events in B-cell differentiation Mouse B-cell lymphoma that expresses membrane IgM and IgD and can be activated with mitogen to secrete IgM
LBRM-33	Mouse T -cell lymphoma that secretes high levels of IL-2 after mitogen activation
CTLL-2	Mouse T -cell lymphoma that secretes high levels of IL-2 after mitogen activation
C6VL	Mouse thymoma expressing CD3 and CD4
Pu 5-1.8	Mouse monocyte-macrophage line
P338 DI	Mouse monocyte-macrophage line that secretes high levels of IL-1
WEHI 265. I	Mouse monocyte line
P815	Mouse mastocytoma cells; often used as target to. assess killing by cytotoxic T lymphocytes (CTLs)
YAC-I	Mouse lymphoma cells; often used as target for NK cells
COS-I	African green monkey kidney cells transformed by SV 40; often used in DNA transfection studies

6.11.4.1. Primary lymphoid cell cultures

Many *in vitro* culture techniques are available for the culturing of lymphocytes. Primary culture of lymphoid cells can be obtained by isolating the lymphocytes directly from lymph or blood or from various lymphoid organs by tissue dispersion. The isolated cells are grown in a chemically defined nutrient medium consisting of sodium chloride, carbohydrates, proteins, vitamins, trace elements and other nutrients to which various serum supplements are also added. In some cultures, serum-free media are employed. This is because, the *in vitro* culture techniques require 10-100 folds more specific cells than *in vivo,* so that, the immunologists can assess the functional properties of minor subpopulations of lymphocytes. For example, functional differences between D4$^+$ T helper cells and CD4$^+$ T cytotoxic cells could be studied precisely with the help of cell culture techniques. These techniques have also been used as diagnostic tool for identifying various cytokines involved in the activation, growth and differentiation of various cells of the immune system.

6.11.4.2. Cloned lymphoid cell lines

Tumor cells or normal cells mutated with chemical carcinogens or viruses are multiplied indefinitely in suitable nutrient cultures. Because of growing nature, the multiplication of the specific defined cells is very fast. Unlike normal mammalian cell growth, these highly proliferating cells are referred to as cell lines.

The first cell line (the mouse fibroblast L cells) was cultured in the 1940s from mouse connective tissue, mutated chemically by exposing to methylcholanthrene over a period of 120 days. Similarly, cell-lines can be obtained directly from culturing infected cells like HeLa cells derived by cultured human cervical cancer cells.

Various techniques are available for ensuring whether a cell line is derived from a single parent cell or not. Such a cloned cell line possesses a population of genetically identical cells that can be grown indefinitely in suitable culture (Table 6.4). In other cases the cell line can be obtained by transformation of normal lymphoid cells by viruses such as Abelson's murine leukemia virus (A-ML V), Simian virus-40 (SV -40), Epstein-Barr virus (EBV) and human T -cell leukemia virus (HTLV - 1).

6.11.4.3. Hybrid lymphoid cell lines

Hybridoma cells are obtained by somatic-cell hybridization. In brief during the hybridization, due to fusion of normal B or T lymphocytes with tumor cells in presence of polyethylene glycol after random loss of some chromosomes a hybridoma is formed, consisting of single nucleus with mixed chromosomes from each of the fused parent cells (Fig. 6.8).

The transformed hybridoma cells are competent to express the antibody genes of the normal B or T lymphocytes with rapid growth characteristics. These hybridoma cells are cultured in defined nutrient media to propagate the antibody secretion with a single antigenic specificity called monoclonal antibody as it is derived from a single clone. .

6.11.5. Whole embryo culture

The whole embryo culture technique is well exemplified and represented by the work on embryonic development by Spratt (1947). A 40 hours old embryo was used. The technique involved preparation of well-defined suitable medium. One ml aliquots of medium were added to sterile watch glasses placed on moist cotton wool pads in pertidishes, incubated hence at 38°C for 40-45 hours to provide a dozen embryos. Alcohol wiped egg cells were broken in a sterile evaporating dish containing nearly 50 ml of chick saline. A circular cut was made with the help of scissors into the allantoin membrane around the blastoderm. The blastoderm was transferred to a petri dish containing BSS. The adherent allontoin with the help of a forcep and embryo was microscopically observed for any damage. The blastoderm was then transferred over the top of the medium in the watch glass after spreading on agar gels. Excess of BSS was removed and culture was incubated at 37±0.5°C.

6.11.5.1. Culture of mammalian embryo or ova

Two to eight celled fertilized ova have been cultured. The embryos were observed to develop up to blastocytes. The developed blastocytes or embryo can be re-implanted to give rise to healthy animals.

The media used for mammalian embryo culturing varied from 100% serum to simple Krebs ringer solution supplemented with 1% of white egg yolk or bovine albumin. The embryo can be cultured in pre-implantation state or at the post implant stage; however, in the post implantation stage a special care is needed in the removal of embryo in an undamaged form.

6.11.5.2. Flask culture methods

The flask culture technique is mainly used to establish and maintain a strain of fresh explant tissue. The flasks possess excellent optical properties or microscopic examination. The flask made up of glass or polystyrene should have a wide neck for convenient handling of explants. The method is critically endowed with following advantages:

1. Tissue can be maintained for months or even for years in the same flask.

2. A scale up or handling of large amount of culture and tissue is possible.

The culture flask techniques are mainly of two types: thick clot cultures and thin clot cultures. The technique essentially involves 3 steps, i.e. preparation of flask cultures, renewal of medium and transfer of culture.

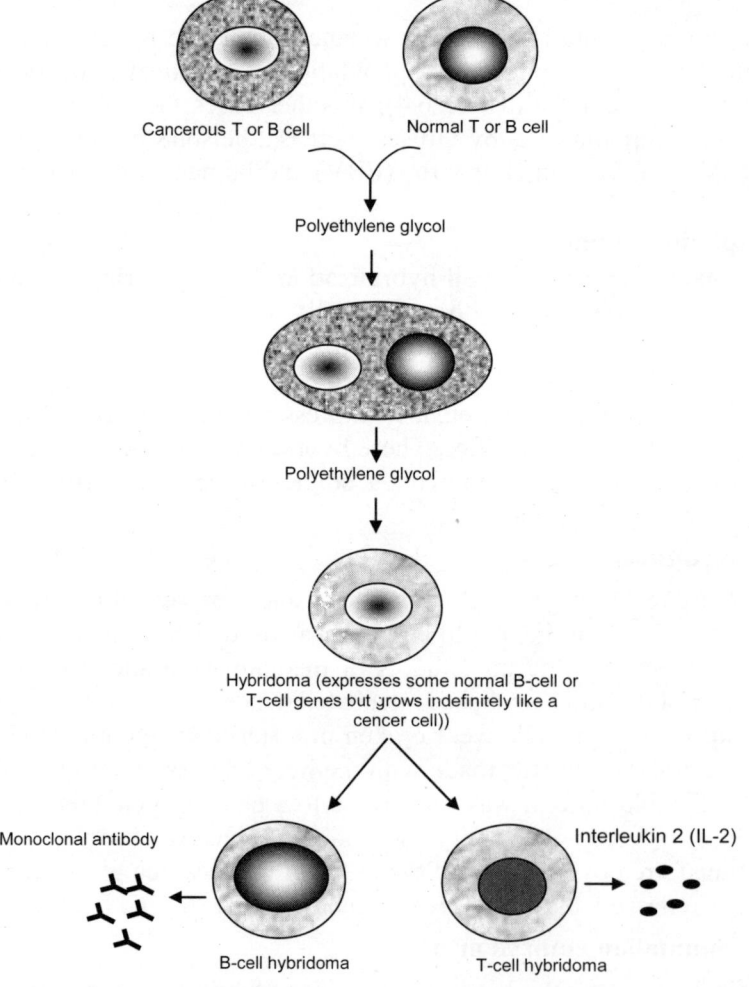

Fig. 6.8: Somatic cell hybridization

Preparation of flask cultures

Up to 6 carrel flasks (d-3 .5) are placed in a rack after flaming their necks and pointing to the right, a drop of the plasma is placed on the floor of the flask and carefully spread in the form of a circle. With the help of a spatula desired number of explants are transferred to the flask to the plasma and clotting is allowed, after plasma clots and explants get fixed up in position, extra medium is added for thick clots measuring up to 1.2 ml of diluted plasma and for thin clots 1.2 ml of diluted serum in place of plasma. The flasks are gassed.

Renewal of medium

The renewal of medium may be undertaken periodically where old fluid is drawn off with the help of a pipette while 1.2 ml of fluid medium is added as a replacement, followed by supply of gas.

Transfer of culture

The culture grown in a flask needs to be removed, cut into pieces when it is to be transferred where the pieces serve for re-plantation as usual.

6.11.5.3. Test-tube culture

Test tubes can be conveniently used for the purpose of tissue culture where large number of cultures could be prepared. The tubes can be placed on a stationary rack or roller drums. The tissue culture technique suffers from poor optical properties for microscopy and high risk of contamination. The method however, is the same as for flasks. But tissues may be grown on the test tube without growing over plasma clots. The feeding, patching renewal of medium, transfer of culture and other steps are similar to those used in case of other primary explantation techniques.

6.11.6. Organ cultures

Organ culture technique employs culturing of organ pieces *in vitro* with an objective of viability. It is essential that tissue chosen should be undamaged. This necessitates careful handling; hence the method is much more sensitive and sophisticated than tissue culture. The basic media used are more or less the same as those used for tissue culture.

6.11.6.1. Organ culture on agar

Solidified agar is used for organ culture. The agar media typically consist of 7 parts of I % agar solution, 3 parts of chick embryo extract and 3 parts of horse serum. Media with or without serum may also be used. This method has advantage that support liquefies and no additional support is required. The embryonic organs are found to grow well on these media.

6.11.6.2. Culture of embryonic organs

The culture of embryonic organs is easier as compared to the culture from adult. Embryo organs can be cultured using plasma clots, agar substrates or fluid media methods.

6.12. MEASUREMENT OF VIABILITY AND CYTOTOXICITY

Any scientific analysis depends solely on the methods of quantifying experimental data. Routine culturing of cell lines also requires quantification of the cell number/density to enable optimum cell culturing. Methods available for cell growth can be divided in two subgroups:

1. Direct method: Cell numbers are directly determined by either counting them on electronic particle counter or by using a counting chamber.
2. Indirect method: Measurement of DNA content or protein content related to cell number to determine the biomass.

6.12.1. Direct methods for quantification

Commonly, the improved Neubauer haemocytometer is used which was originally used for counting blood cells. It is the cheapes andsimplest method for counting. The haemocytometer is a modified microscope slide with two polished surfaces/chamber of known depth, which displays a precisely ruled grid, etched out on a silver base. The grid consists of nine primary squares, 1 mm each side (area 1 mm^2) having two to three closely spaced lines (2.5 mm apart). These lines determine the limits of the cell to be counted-whether inside or outside. The primary square consists of more lines which are basically to keep sight and assessment of the cell counted. The plane of the grid lies 0.1 mm below two ridges, which support the coverslip. Also there is a depression on the outer edge of each polished surface where the cell suspension is added; this is to be drawn by capillary action.

Cells per ml = $100 \times 5 \times$ dilution $\times 10^{-4}$

The cell concentration per ml of suspension can be calculated simply by

$C = n/v$, where C is the cell concentration, n the number of cells counted, v the volume (ml) represented the grid.

Measurement by electronic particle counter

Cells in suspension can be counted accurately and rapidly using a coulter counter. Electronic particle counter consists of two electrodes separated by a small orifice. If a potential is applied to the electrodes, current will pass between them through the buffer in the orifice. The amount of current will be dependent on the conductance (dielectric constant) of the buffer. Cells are suspended in an electrolyte and a metered volume of the suspension is pulled through a narrow aperture that carries a nominal current. As the cells pass through the orifice, it produces a fluctuation in the pulse. The pulse is amplified and the pulse within a prefixed threshold is counted and displayed on an oscilloscope.

Cell size can also be determined as the amplitude is directly proportional to cell volume. The size of the change in current flow depends on the size of the particle and the difference in the dielectric constant or conductivity. Cell clusters can also create a pulse. Such an error can be eliminated by adjusting the threshold of the pulse amplitude.

Cell viability by dye exclusion method

This method is used to count the number of cells by mixing an aliquot of cell suspension with a colored dye that is visible under the microscope. The dye should be membrane lipid insoluble, for example 0.4 % erythrocin B or trypan blue. Only the cells with damaged plasma membrane will take up the dye. The viable cells will exclude the dye, hence the name. Hence we can correctly assess the number of cell that has not taken up the dye, and therefore percent viability can be easily calculated.

Cytotoxicity assay

Four kinds of nonradioactive cell growth and cytotoxic assays are being routinely used. They are:

1. Cell or colony counter;
2. Macromolecular dye-binding assays;
3. Metabolic impairment;
4. Membrane integrity,

An ideal assay would be simple, rapid, sensitive, reproducible, quantitative, inexpensive, objective and reliable. Cell and colony counters are slow and time consuming, subject to individual discrepancies in methodology. Cell count enumerates morphologically intact cells but fail to discriminate between live and dead cells.

Dye-binding assays are definitely more reliable and sensitive for growth and cytotoxicity. They are simple and rapid but require a spectrophotometer and a 96-well plate. They can indicate cell killing and growth inhibition.

Metabolic impairment assays measure the enzyme decay kinetics following toxic insults. They are more unreliable and complex than dye-binding assays. The success of these experiments relies heavily on reproducibility under identical conditions which are difficult to achieve in biological reactions. Deviations in experiments may cause serious errors their advantage is that they are capable of distinguishing normal cells from the cells having altered cellular metabolism.

Membrane integrity assays measure the ability of the cell to impermeat extracellular molecules. It can either be colorimetric or fluorescent, similar to dye-binding assays. They provide a surrogate index of the viability of the cells by their ability to exclude the dye, but cells can slowly accumulate the molecule. Hence extra caution should be taken while designing experimental protocols.

6.12.1. Indirect methods for quantification

MTT assay

This can be put under membrane integrity assay as well as colorimetric assay. Tetrazolium salts have been extensively used to localize dehydrogenase enzyme activity. These salts do not react with dehydrogenase per se but with their products NADH and NADPH. These methods are developed to estimate cell number based on the cellular contents of enzyme or substarte and subsequent extraction of the dye. A yellow-colored water-soluble salt 3-(4,5-dimethylthiazole-2-yl),2,5-diphenyl tetrazolium bromide [MTT] reacts with the mitochondrial dehydrogenase enzymes of live cells, which reduces them to purple colored insoluble formazone crystals which are precipitated in the immediate vicinity. Dehydrogenase content is consistent among cells of a specific type and the amount of formazone reduced is proportional to the cell number. Different cell types may have varied amount of dehydrogenase. Culture conditions may alter the enzyme content and activity.

Once a cell line has been established there is an urgent need to characterize it so as to confirm its species and tissue of origin, and also to determine the differentiated status of the cell within the lineage. To begin with, a complete record of the species and tissue of origin needs to be recorded. The species of origin can be confirmed by cytogenetics, isoenzymology, karyotyping and immunological methods.

6.12.2. Characterization of cultured cells

Cytogenetics

There is need to verify that the cells are derived from the particular species. Chromosome content and analysis is species specific and is a reliable method of species characterization. The correlation of chromosomal structure with heredity and variation is termed cytogenetics.

Karyotype

Karyotype is the collective term used to describe the chromosome number, size and shape. Primary cell lines retain diploid chromosomes and also the chromosomes of the donor. Lines from individuals with cytogenetic abnormalities have been extensively used for mapping genes, not merely to individual chromosomes but also to specific regions on chromosomes.

Isoenzymplogy

Enzymes that exist in multiple forms in animal tissue and in different molecular forms catalyzing the same reaction are called isoenzymes.

Immunological test

This test depends on the specificity of antigen-antibody reaction. Species-specific antigens can be detected by immunofluorescence.

Intraspecies contamination

Once the species has been characterized, the next logical step is to characterize the tissues of origin. A number of techniques have been used for this:

Recombinant DNA methods: It is possible to directly determine an individual's genotype by typing the genes themselves. For many genes there are slight variations between individuals of a species and such molecular difference in the DNA of a particular genes are called polymorphism. The presence of dissimilar arrangements of DNA bases means that each individual's DNA is cleaved at slightly different sites by restriction enzymes, generating distinct lengths of restriction fragments. DNA probes can be used to detect polymorphisms in a technique known as restriction fragment length polymerization (RFLP). Cellular DNA is digested with restriction with restriction enzymes and the fragments of DNA are separated by agarose gel electrophoresis. The DNA is then transferred to a membrane by southern blotting and the DNA on the membrane is 'melted' to form single strands. The membrane is then exposed to radioactivity labeled DNA probes. These probes are prepared using highly repetitive nucleotide sequences (so-called satellite DNA). These radioactive probes will react with the DNA fragments, which contain complementary nucleotide sequences, and they are detected by autoradiography. This process is called DNA fingerprinting.

High-resolution two-dimentional electrophoresis: The different proteins in the cell can be separated on the basis of isoelectric point and molecular weight using isoelectric focusing in the presence of urea in one dimension and electrophoresis in the presence of sodium dodecyl sulfate (SDS) in the second dimension. This process separates the proteins according to isoelectric point and also according to their size. By this method one can resolve a number of proteins simultaneously.

Allozyme analysis: Every individual belonging to the same species expresses different alleles for a given enzyme locus. Allelic isoenzymes are reffered to as allozymes. This analysis is like a genetic signature for that cell line.

Blood group antigen and HL-A: This involves the determination of the antigens present on the surface of the cell. Blood group antigens are present on normal human epithelium in primary culture and on some continuous epithelial lines. The use of anti-human A, B or AB typing antiserum can be used to type these cell lines. The major histocompatibility antigens (or major histocompatibility complex-MHC) are highly variable antigens which are responsible for the immunological individuality of each person. These antigens are present on the plasma membrane of nucleated cells and are responsible for the fact that tissue transplanted from one individual to an unrelated individual will be recognized as foreign and will be rejected by the recipient's immune system. In man, the histocompatibility antigens are referred to as the human lymphocyte antigen (HLA) system. The genes coding for the HLA antigens are on chromosome 6 and occupy 4 loci (designated A, B, C and D) along the chromosomes. The genes at any locus are not always the same, and the different forms of each gene are called alleles.

6.13. PHARMACEUTICAL APPLICATIONS

The most important commercial utilization of animal cell cultures at the present time is still the multiplication of viruses for the manufacturing of vaccines, which offers considerable technological advantages over conventional production, e.g., in incubated eggs. In addition to this, a series of substances are on the verge of being manufactured on a large scale using cell culture technique.

Viruses require a living substrate for their multiplication. Previously, duck embryos or organ cultures from animal nerve and kidney tissues were used for the manufacture of virus vaccines. Such explants consist of different types of cells with different demands on the medium and have the disadvantage that comprehensive sterility tests must be carried out before they could be used. Furthermore, tissues from kidneys of wild apes frequently contain simian viruses (SV-5, SV-40) or their constituents. Side reactions after the administration of such vaccines are also not infrequent. The setting up of characterized cell cultures under sterile conditions therefore provides a decisive advantage.

The polio vaccines have been produced by the replication of the virus on simian kidney cells. After attachment to the support, the primary cells are grown for 7 to 8 days with no change of medium, which leads to a ten folds increase in their number. In this phase, sterility tests and chromosome analysis can be carried out on aliquots. Three days after infection by polio virus, the culture becomes ready for the preparation of vaccine by concentration, chromatography method (Sepharose-6B & DEAE-Sephadex) and inactivation (formaldehyde). Similar processes have been used for the production of rabies vaccine via dog kidney cells. Human diploid fibroblasts have also been successfully grown with cellulose fiber micro carriers using suspension culture techniques. The polio titer yield from this technique has been more than polio titers from cultures monkey kidney cells.

Cell surface antigens are produced on a large scale for several purposes. They are used to raise antibodies against themselves, which may then be used for therapeutic and diagnostic purposes. However, the efforts put into the production of antigens by cell culture techniques have suffered some setback by the dramatic advances in recombinant DNA technology, which makes it possible to synthesize them on a large scale. Anti-lymphocyte serum (ALS) is an immune serum that is used as an alternative for proliferation inhibiting medicaments after organ transplantation in order to suppress the immune defense. Surface antigens from cultivated continuous human lymphoma or leukemia cell lines leading to the synthesis of far more specific antibodies can be used as an alternative to ALS.

Carcinoembryonic antigen (CEA) is a tumor associated glycoprotein used for diagnosis and monitoring of cancer patients. CEA is expressed in significant amounts during embryonic life, especially by the fetal colon. In healthy adults the antigen is expressed in small amounts (< 2.5 ng/ml) in normal colonic mucosa and in serum saliva, feces and colon lavages. CEA can be detected in relatively high concentrations (> 20ng/ml) in the sera of patients with metastatic colonic cancer and in moderate to low levels in the sera of patients with primary lesions of various cancers. Low levels of CEA were also found in the case of various non-malignant inflammatory diseases, particularly those of the liver, lung, pancreas and bowel. In current clinical practice, CEA serum levels are used for monitoring cancer patients for their response to therapy and for an early detection of recurrences.

Many cell types are involved in an immune response. Besides B-cells, the antibody producing cells, and T -cells which are responsible for the cell-mediated immunity, macrophages, T -helper cells and many others from parts of a complex network where they communicate *via* several dozens of soluble factors (cytokines), particularly Iymphokines (lymphocyte-derived) and monokines (macrophage-derived). There are three techniques by which Iymphokines can be produced with the help of T -helper cells: Stimulation of lymphocytes from buffy coat or spleen cells by non-specific stimulators such as plant lectins, using certain continuous tumor cell lines, and synthesis by immortalized lymphocytes that have been obtained by hybridoma techniques. An alternative method of producing Iymphokines is the production of monoclonal **T -T hybridoma** which secretes distinct Iymphokines. By adapting the hybridoma technology for T cells, one can select T hybridomas which may serve as constant sources for the production of uniform and well defined Iymphokines. Similarly, B cells growth factor (Iymphokines) is primarily produced and secreted by activated T -cells. The growth factor stimulates and regulates the proliferation of B cells in culture and can maintain continuous growth of human B- cells. One of the putative uses of this factor might be the establishment of monoclonal B-cell lines which secrete specific antibodies. These antibodies could be used for passive immunization or *in vivo* immuno-diagnostics. A factor interleukin-2 (formerly 'T -cells growth factor') is attracting current interest. Its synthesis triggers antigen-specifically *in vivo* but once synthesized it has an antigen-nonspecific proliferative and differentiating action upon cytotoxic T cells (CTL) which, in turn communicate with natural killer (NK) cells *via* interferon-γ. Since CTL and NK cells are the most important in cellular immunity, interleukin-2 shows great promise as an agent through which the immune response can be regulated by direct application in certain immune deficiency diseases or indirectly by growing antibodies and using them for the intermediate suppression of unwanted responses.

Animal cell cultures have been crucial for the mass-production of certain proteins. These fall into two classes: monoclonal antibodies obtained from hybridoma cells, which are mainly used for analytical and separation purposes and require only a modest degree of purification; and secondly, proteins for therapeutic use, e.g., growth factors, immunomodulators or hormones produced in recombinant cell-lines. These proteins often have to undergo posttranslational modification e.g., correct glycosylation, which cannot be performed in recombinant microorganisms.

Today, the antiviral action of interferons is well understood and interferon therapy is about to become routine in viral diseases like herpes zoster and viral encephalitis. The bulk of α-interferon is being obtained by a process from buffy coats (leukocyte pellets) which are available as a waste product from blood banks. The leukocytes can be brought into suspension (10^7 cells/ml) and induced to secrete interferon with newcastle-disease or sendai virus. Human β-interferon is usually produced by cultivation and induction of human primary fibroblast cells, e.g. FS4 cells but alternatively it can be done with recombinant mammalian cell lines (e.g., mouse L-cells).

The species specificity of many polypeptidal hormones makes it necessary to develop highly productive strains of human origin of which, however, only a few have been described. Thus calcitonin secreting cell lines from thyroid tumors ceased their growth after a few months. A cell line 'Be Wo' (ATCC No. CCL 98) from a placental tumor efficiently secretes human chorionic gonadotropin (HCG). It represents the only bulk producing source for a human hormone that has been established *in vitro*. A cell line from kidney carcinoma secreting erythropoietin has not acquired the same importance since the optimum conditions for cultivation are yet to be worked out. However, the availability of both human insulin and human growth hormone from recombinant technology has discouraged corresponding attempts to establish human cell lines for *in vitro* production purposes.

The production of enzymes by using cell culture is not a familiar strategy although a few homologous enzymes can be produced by cell culture techniques. Plasminogen activator urokinase, from continuous line of porcine kidney cells (LLC-PKI; ATCC, No. CL 101) has been patented by the Lily Research Laboratories. Another example is the Bowes melanoma cell line. The enzyme is mainly expressed during cell growth phase rather than from stationary culture cells. The production of enzymes has to be a 2-step operation with initial growth to about 70% confluency in the presence of serum followed by a change in serum-free conditions for the final period of growth after which the enzyme is harvested. To increase the enzyme yield, means of amplifying enzyme expressions, using a serum-free medium have been suggested for continuous harvesting of the enzyme. The stimulation of stationary phase cells can be improved by the inclusion of number of mitogenic lectins (15-20 fold increase of enzyme yield).

6.13.1. Cell culture models for examining intestinal absorption of peptides

The absorption of peptides across cellular barrier mainly occurs by two general pathways namely paracellular and transcellular. In most cases it is the molecular size of the peptide that screens up their intestinal, brain or liver absorption through paracellular route. Obviously, the chief route for peptide absorption is transcellular, either passive or non-passive. Cell culture techniques allow estimation of intestinal absorption of peptides. The passive diffusion has been observed to be low, because a major fraction of peptide degrades by enzymatic reactions. These findings were substantiated using caco-2 culture model. A small number of peptides have been observed to undergo low level of non-saturable, bidirectional diffusion across monolayers. Thus, using this particular character, cell culture model could be utilized for examining the physicochemical properties. The significance of hydrogen bonding in passive diffusion across caco-2 cell monolayer has been established and it appears that hydrogen bonding has inverse relation to the corresponding permeability across caco-2 monolayers.

Similarly, intestinal absorption of di and tri-peptides including cephalosporin antibiotics is facilitated by di-peptide transport/carrier system. The presence of the latter has been confirmed by using the enzymatically stable cephalosporin. The absorption of cephalosporin is typically pH-dependent, with a maximum uptake at pH.6. In another study, it was established that uptake of cephalexin in caco-2 monolayers is inhibited competitively by various types of peptides and similar findings were observed *in vivo*. Likewise, using caco-2 cell monolayer carrier system for cepharidin has been discovered, to be γ-GTP, located on this artificial plasma membrane. Another route for transporting peptides across the GI barriers is active intestinal absorption of peptides either by fluid phase or receptor mediated endocytosis. Horseradish peroxide in combination with caco-2 cell culture has been used to elucidate absorption mechanism of proteins following fluid phase endocytosis. The receptor mediated endocytosis of transferrin has been examined using caco-2 cell line and receptor binding in transferrin was found to be polarized to the basal side of the caco-2 cell membrane. These examples suggest that a near approximation of qualitative and quantitative aspects in nature could be achieved in regard to absorption of protein drugs following oral administration using *in vitro* cell lines techniques.

6.13.2. Cell culture model for examining peptide absorption in the BBB

DSIP (Delta sleep inducing peptide) peptides are known to cross blood brain barrier (BBB) via passive diffusion pathway and vasopressin *via* apical to basolateral route. The cell culture technique allows studying the effect of conformation of structure of proteins on their invasive BBB permeability. In general, the hydrophilic nature of the peptide presents major obstacle to passive diffusion across BBB. In an attempt to increase diffusion of peptides through the BBB the functional groups of peptide have been modified to be more lipophilic. The substitution of D-alanine at position 4 of DSIP by a glycine residue increases the lipophilicity of the analogue which has higher permeability profile across primary culture BMC (bovine milk casein). Studies evaluating carrier-mediated transport across cultured BMC are somewhat limited. Moreover, cell culture study could establish selective carrier system for AVP which is saturable in nature. However, carrier mediated transport of AVP (arginine, vasopressin) was found to be in the basolateral to apical direction suggesting that it cannot be utilized for successful delivery of peptide to the brain. Similarly, carrier systems for the apical to basolateral transport of both glucose and biotin have been identified using cell culture technique. Such carrier holds promise in peptides transport promotion across the BBB. However, the confirmation of the contribution remains to be established. Using cell culture technique it was found that epiratide, a cationic adrenocorticotropic hormone (ACTH) is transported across primary culture bovine BMC through endocytosis pathway. This has inspired the designing of chimeric peptides consisting of β-endorphin and cationized albumin. The resulting system showed significantly higher permeability across the BBB suggesting that cationization may be a viable method for the enhanced transport of peptides and proteins across the BBB. Thus, using cell culture strategies towards improvisation of BBB, the permeability profile of proteins could be studied *in vitro*.

6.13.3. Cell culture models for examining hepatic absorption of peptides

Like the epithelial intestinal barrier and endothelial BBB, the tight junctions on the sinusoidal and canalicular membrane of hepatocytes limit the passive cellular clearance of peptides. Therefore, passive diffusion of peptides must occur through interactions with the plasma membranes of the hepatocytes. Cell culture study, can be used for the determination of cellular engineering. Smaller lipophilic peptides undergo passive clearance by hepatocytes. Most peptides are absorbed through receptor mediated endocytosis. This has been successfully studied and confirmed using cell culture technique. Various cell culture techniques for receptor mediated uptake are shown in Table 6.5.

6.13.4. Strategies of foreign gene expression

Several eukaryotic genes have been incorporated into *E. coli* for high expression of the respective proteins. However, the proteins accumulate in the cell as insoluble inclusion bodies, and need to be dissolved by the application of some chaotropic agent such as urea or guanidine-HCl.

Table 6.5: Representative receptor and transport systems expressed in various cell culture models

Receptor and Transporter	Caco-2	BMEC	Hepatocytes
Amino acid	+	+	+
Angiotensin II		+	+
Asialoglycoprotein			+
Atrial natruiretic factor		+	
Bile acid (taurocholate)	+		+
Biotin	+,-	+	-
Cobalamine (vit.B12)	+		
Choline		+	
Dipeptide	+		+
Epidermal growth factor	+		+
Ferritin			+
Folate	+		
Glucose (Na-dependent)	+	+	+
Immunoglobulin A			+
Insulin		+	+
Insulin-like growth factor 1		+	
Low density lipoprotein	+	+	+
Methyldopa	+		
Monocarboxylic acid		+	
Nucleotide		+	
P-glycoprotein	+	+	+
Peptide YY	-		
Phosphate	+		
Spermidin	-		
Transferrin	+	+	+
Tissue plasminogen activator			+
Vasoactive intestinal peptide (VIP)	+		+
Vasopressin		+	+

Note: BMEC is brain micro vessel endothelial cells, either functional or biochemical, of the various receptor and transport system listed. (+) indicates studies showing expression and (-) indicate studies that did not show expression.

This induces refolding of the proteins as per their specific structural configuration and is a very difficult task. Most of the proteins of pharmaceutical interest (e.g., growth factors, hormones, and serum proteins) are fortunately soluble and secretory proteins. Therefore an alternative host *Saccharomyces cerevisiae* might be an appropriate system for the expression of secretory proteins. This system, however, suffers from low expression levels and altered pattern glycosylation.

Meanwhile, animal cell culture techniques have altered research focus in biotechnology. These allow the production of many biologicals using reactive proteins and cloning of genes such as expression of interferons, hepatitis-B surface antigen (HBsAg), tissue type plasminogen activator and herpes simplex glycoprotein. In many cases, tumor cell lines are used which overproduce proteins of therapeutic value. In some other cases, gene engineering is used for improvisation of production via introduction of cloned genes into animal cells. The processes of gene expression and animal cells culture essentially involve gene engineering, followed by cloning and transfection of cloned gene in to the cultured cell line with the help of appropriate means. It's under optimized culture condition need to be incorporated for optimum expression of protein of interest. It also involves removal and processes in most situations as they are used in culture technology that operates at batch level.

The choice of cell line is critical. Let us consider a case of cloned immunoglobulin-G (IgG) for regulation of expression in a tissue specific manner. It is the first example of an expression system based on an enhancer sequence. The promoter could be substituted by viral promoter and enhancer, yet sequence that had an intragenic restricted expression to lymphoid cells may also be used. So the restriction sequence limits the choice of cell line as in the stated case it is only feasible in lymphoid cells. Here, availability of such a cellular culture may not be a problem, but other cell line specific problems could crop up. These problems are mainly related to availability, as well as *in vitro* culture feasibility.

6.13.5. Eukaryotic and prokaryotic cultures and secondary metabolites

Bio-transformations are chemical transformations which are catalyzed by microorganisms or their enzymes. Enzymatically catalyzed bio-transformations are superior to chemically catalyzed ones because of:

Reaction specificity: Only one type of reaction takes place and hence no side reactions occur;

Regiospecificity: Biotransformation is specific in relation to the position of the reaction in substrate molecule;

Stereospecificity: Only one enantiomer can be selectively or at least preferentially transformed out of a racemic mixture;

Mild reaction conditions: Biotransformation can be carried out under mild conditions of temperature (less than 40°C); pH (in vicinity of 7); and in aqueous solutions;

Lowering of activation energy: This permits accessibility to relatively non activated positions in the substrate molecule for selective transformation under mild conditions. Biotransformation can be carried out by growing cells, stationary cells, spores or immobilized cells or enzymes. Cell culture can successfully be applied in biotransformation in two ways e.g., growing cells and stationary cells;

Growing cells: In this technique substrate to be transformed is added during growth phase of cells at a most favorable moment determined experimentally. This method is simple and used for screening of desired enzymatic activity in cells. But good conversions are often achieved in the stationary phase;

Stationary cells: Cells of biomass are harvested by centrifugation or filtration after cultivation in growth media. These are resuspended in transformation medium and substrate is added. Buffers are used to maintain optimum pH. Certain nutrients are also added to maintain viability for long period, growth and biotransformation can take place independently while growth inhibiting effects of substrate or products are eliminated. Biotransformation of certain important classes of compounds is discussed here.

6.13.5.1. Steroids

Steroids in the form of hormones as androgen, progesterone, estrogen, glucocorticoid and mineralocorticoid, perform central functions in human metabolism. Their natural structures and derivatives also exhibit important pharmacological activities as anti-inflammatory, anabolic, sedative, cytostatic and contraceptive effects. Hormone antagonists have been also obtained from hormones by chemical modifications.

Diosgenin (from root of Mexican yam *Dioscorea composita*), stigmasterol (from soyabean) and deoxycholic acid (from animal bile) serve as starting material for chemical synthesis of steroidal structures. But chemical synthesis requires many steps and the process is very lengthy. For example, the anti-inflammatory compound cortisone when synthesized from deoxycholic acid requires 31 steps for completion (Fig. 6.9). Similarly, nine steps are required for displacing I2-α,hydroxy group to form keto function in position 11.

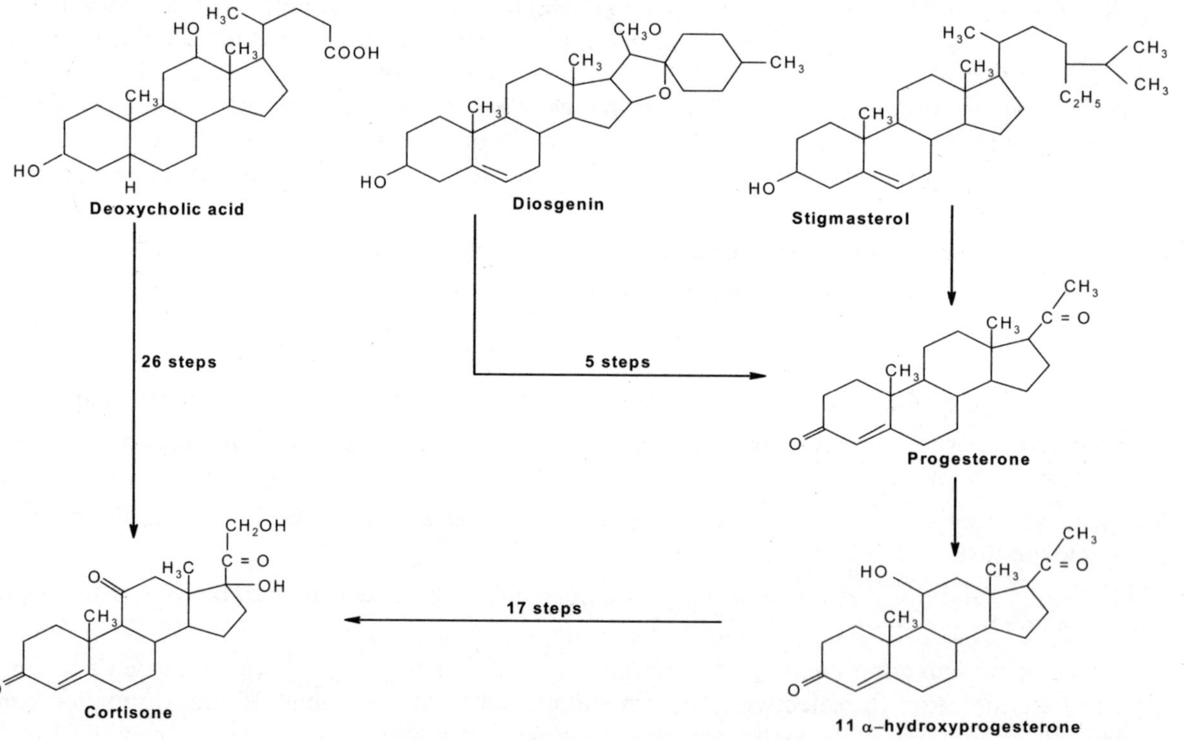

Fig. 6.9: Production of cortisone from natural sterols

But investigators in Upjohn Company effected considerable simplification of the synthesis of these hormones. Hydroxyl group into the 11 α position of progesterone was introduced with *Rhizopus arrhizus* or *Rhizopus nigricans* in yields more than 85%. This made available the important corticosteroid hormones with characteristics oxygen function in position 11 from the cheap natural products stigmasterol or diosgenin. Introduction of a hydroxyl group on 11β position was also achieved with *Cunninghamella blakesleeana* by which hydrocortisone was obtained directly from

Reichstein's compounds. These results made biotransformation an important technical method. Chemical modifications in steroids which can be attempted through bio-transformation are:

1. 11α-Hydroxylation

Cultures of the fungus *Aspergillus ochraceus* can be used for 11α hydroxylation of progesterone with substrate concentration of 50 g/l of culture broth. Other suitable strains of fungi also affect biotransformation. But with *Aspergillus ochraceus* very small amount of the byproduct 6 β, 11α-dihydroxyprogesterone is formed. A number of other steroid structures can be hydroxylated at 11α-position with high regio and stereo- specificity.

2. 11β Hydroxylation

Reichstein's substance S and its analogues can be hydroxylated at 11β-position with *Cunninghamella blakesleeana* but paralleled 6β hydroxylation and its subsequent oxidation to 11 ketones also occur, which can be partially suppressed enzymatically so that the reaction rate is modulated.

Fungus *Curvularia lunata* also carries out 11β-hydroxylation and is more frequently used; nevertheless it performs unwanted hydroxylation at 7α, 9α and 14α positions. Use of 17-acetate of Reichstein's substance S avoids these side reactions as sporty-filling ester residue exerts protective effect on the rear(a) side of substrate against undesirable attack without affecting the 11 hydroxylation of the front (β) side. Similar screening effects are possible by substituting the 16 α position. In the β hydroxylation of the D-homo analog of Reichstein's substance S to D-homohydrocortisone with an anti-inflammatory action, the altered linkage blocks position 14.

3. 16α Hydroxation

Strains of *Streptomyces* sp. have been utilized for the 16α hydroxation for the synthesis of Triamcinolone (an inflammation inhibiting agent) (Fig. 6.10).

4. Hydroxylation at other positions

Hydroxylation at other positions has been found useful in the production of new steroid structures with varied or new pharmacological activities. Hydroxylation at any position of steroid can be carried out using very diverse strains of fungi or more rarely with species of bacteria.

Broad systemic investigations have made possible the development of an enzyme-substrate model which permits approximate predictions of the type of attack in mono and dihydroxylations according to the position of a polar group of the substrate for enzymatic action process. Non-polar substrates often undergo introduction of two hydroxyl groups which can likewise be used for preparative purposes.

5. 1,2-Dehydrogenation

Prednisone, prednisolone, triamcinalone, 6-methylprednisolone, dexamethasone formed by the dehydro-genation of the corresponding 1,2 saturated structures possess significantly enhanced anti-inflammatory activity. This has led to the development of method of 1,2 dehydrogenation using *Bacillus sphaericus, Bacterium cyclooxydans* and *Arthrobacter simplex (Corynebacterium)* at technical scale.

Using *Arthrobacter simplex (Corynebacterium)* in special process substrate concentrations up to 500 mg of hydrocortisone per liter of culture broth can be converted to prednisolone in yields of over 90% in five days. The substrate is added in micronized form without a solvent and hence process has been termed as pseudo-crystallofermentation.

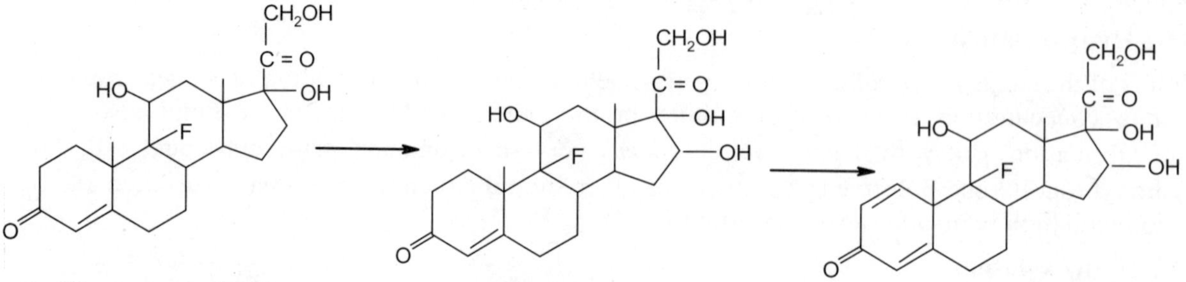

Fig 6.10: 16α-Hydroxylation of 9α-fluorohydrocortisone by *Streptomyces* sp

6. Ester saponification and oxidation of hydroxyl groups

The wide distribution of hydrolyzing enzymes in microorganisms often couples ester saponification some other microbiological reaction in one step fermentation which can be used in practice when *Flavobacterium **dehydrogenans*** is used to transform triolone diacetate into Reichsftein's compound S, the acetate groups in positions 3 and 21 are hydrolyzed off before the oxidation of 3 β -hydroxy-5-ene system to 3-keto-4~ene structure takes place (Fig. 6.11). If the pH is kept constant carefully at 6.6 in the corresponding 3β, 17α,21 tri-acetate, the 17α ester group is retained which leads to the 17-acetate of Reichstein's substance S, an advantageous starting material for the commercial preparation of hydrocortisone.

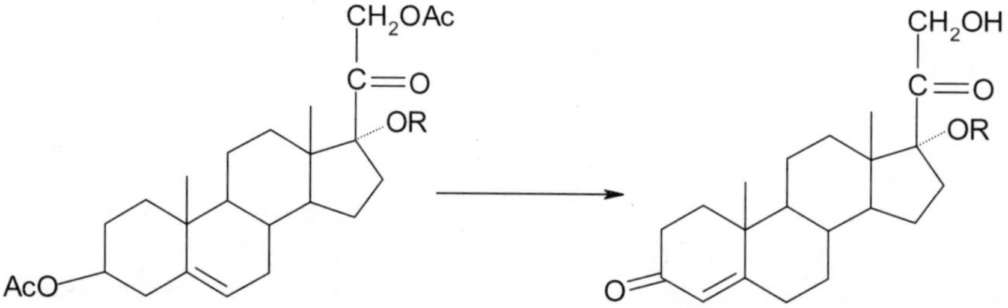

R=H Triolone diacetate   Reichstein's substances S
R=H Triolone triacetate   17-acetate of Reichstein's substances

Fig. 6.11: Coupled saponification and oxidation of triolone acetates by *Flavobacterium dehydrogenans*

7. Reduction of keto group

Reduction of 17-keto group is utilized in the production of testosterone from androst-4-ene,3,17 dione (Fig.6.12). The process utilizing yeast was the first steroid transformation for which a patent was granted. Additionally, if a chiral or prechiral diketones are taken as substrates, then microbial reduction can selectively form four possible enantiomers. The introduction of first center of asymmetry by enzymatic reaction made it possible to synthesize steroids economically for the first time.

One of the two equivalent keto groups of secodione can be stereospecifically and regiospecifically reduced to secolone which doubles the yield by eliminating the formation of racemate. An excellent application of the procedure lies in the manufacture of D-norgesterol, an important contraceptive.

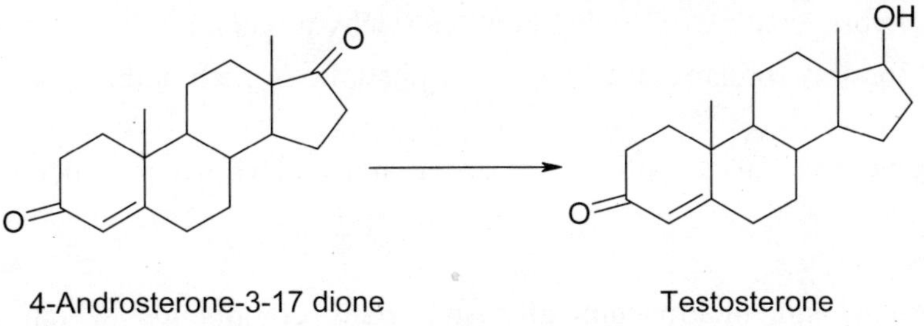

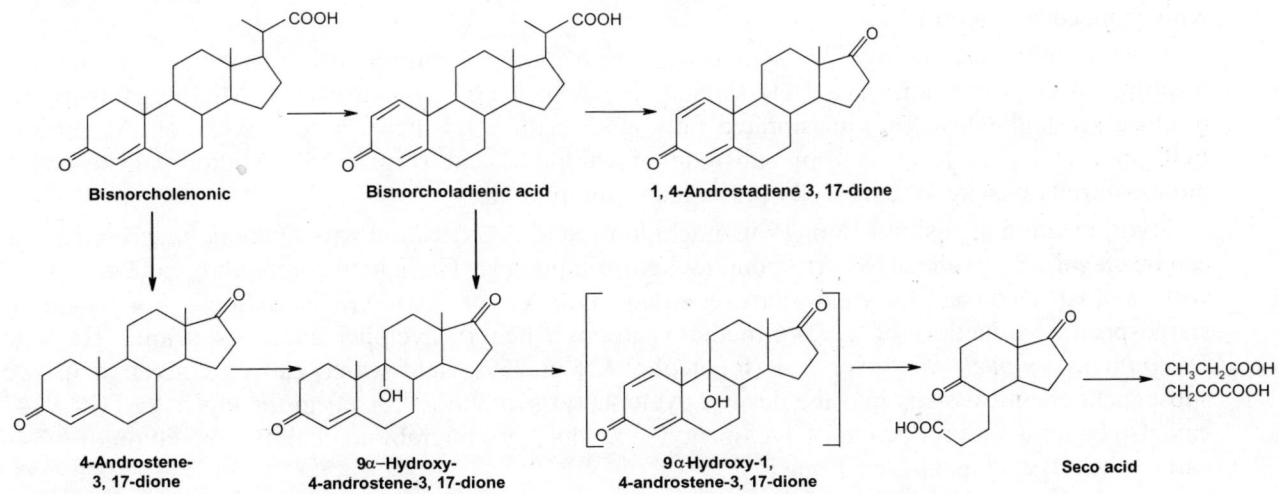

4-Androsterone-3-17 dione   Testosterone

Fig. 6.12: Stereoselective reduction of 4-androstene-3, 17 -dione to testosterone

8. Sterol side-chain degradation

Several possibilities exist for suppressing the undesirable degradation of steroid skeleton and side chain can be degraded alone by microbial degradation. These possibilities can be unraveled from elucidation of enzymatic reaction mechanism. Various strategies which could possibly be employed for the purpose are schematically shown in Figure 6.13.

One possibility is the inhibition of formation of 9α-hydroxy adrostene-1, 4, diene 3,17 dione which is unstable and initiates total degradation. Sterol side chain degradation permits the use of cholesterol as a starting material for steroids. Besides cholesterol stigmasterol, sitosterol and mixture of sterols containing compesterol, stigmasterol, siboester can be used with equivalent possible potentials. These products are obtained on large scale at low cost from soyabean and til oil. Optimized procedures have been developed for the large scale production and technical manufacture of androstene-4-ene-3,17 dione and androstene-I,4-diene 3,17 dione. These require special media additives and substrate. Yields of more than 80% of 17-ketosteroids are obtained with suitable mycobacteria in fermentation times of 3-4 days when substrate concentration is kept at several grams per liter.

Fig. 6.13: Pathway of enzymatic degradation in steroids

9. Miscellaneous biotransformations

Various other types of reactions in microbiological biotransformation of steroids include:

1. Oxidation: It involving aromatization of ring A during dehydrogenation of 19 norsteriods; oxidation of pregnan-20-ones to testolactone structure and epoxidation of double bonds.

2. Reduction: It includes hydrogenation of double bond and dehydrogenation.

3. Hydrolytic reactions (possibly oxidative): Cleavage of phenolic 3-methylethers as well as cleavage of glycosides.

4. Glycosidation of the glycosides at phenolic 3-OH group and 16-OH group is included in this class of biotransformation.

6.13.5.2. Prostaglandins

Prostaglandins are lipoidal and pharmaceutically important compounds which occur in low concentration in nature and require expensive purification methods for isolation. Initial total syntheses were generally limited because of production of racemic mixtures as even simplest prostaglandins possess 3 to 5 centers of chirality (Fig.6.14).

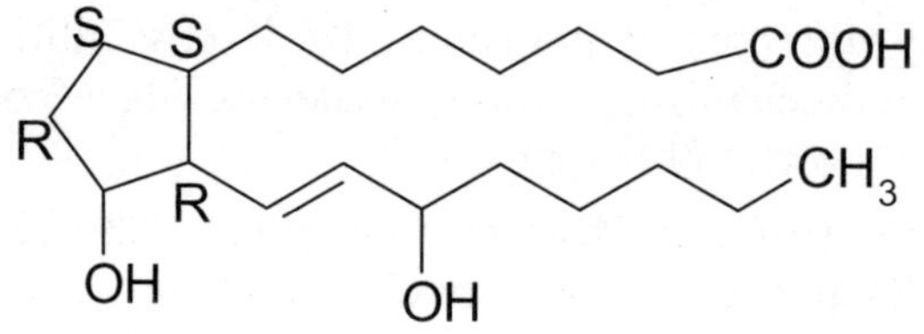

Fig. 6.14: Structure of prostaglandins

Pure chiral structures can be obtained by following ways:

1. By initiating biogenesis with incorporation of native constructional units;

2. By chemical synthesis using an enzymatic (generally microbial) reaction step to introduce the first chirality which directs the subsequent pathway of chemical synthesis to the desired enantiomers;

3. Microbial transformation of native or synthetic prostaglandins to obtain new types of structures with changed action profiles.

Prostaglandins are biologically synthesized from essential fatty acids by enzymatic cyclization resulting in the formation of a cyclopentane ring with α and co-side chains. Microorganisms can produce prostaglandins from unsaturated fatty acids with a 1,4-diene system oxidation. Mixture of PGE and PGE2 is formed from substrate arachidonic acid (Fig. 6.15). Microorganism-driven biotransformations are schematically presented in figure 6.16.

Hydroxylation at position 18 or 19 in arachidonic acid is carried out with *Ophiobolus graminis* and can be chemically oxidized to corresponding keto compounds: These keto compounds can be cyclized with animal enzymes to yield corresponding hydroxy or oxo-PGE structures. For example, stereospecific reduction of a 2-(6-methoxycarbonyl hexyl) cyclopentane-1,3,4 trione [I] with *Diplodascus uninucleatus* gives a 4 (R)-alcohol [2] in 75% yield which can be converted in two subsequent chemical steps into the desired cyclopentyl synthon [3]. *Aspergillus niger* A TCC 9142 can also be used for production of cyclopentyl synthon[3] by microbiological hydroxylation of a 2-(6 carboxyhexyl) cyclopent-2-en-1 one [4].

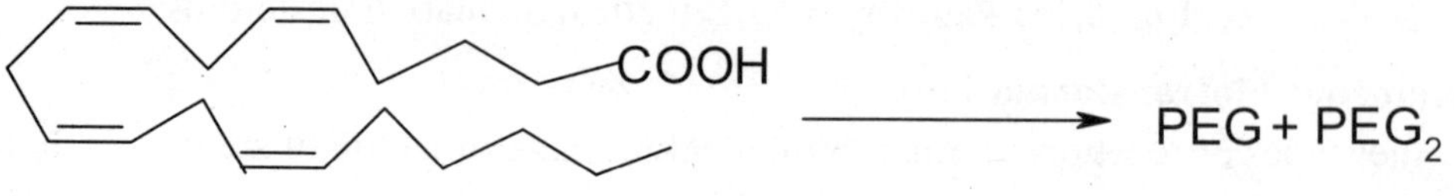

Fig. 6.15: Arachidonic acid as prostaglandin precursor

Yield is 67% but optical purity of the product is poor. Lithium cuparate of a (+)-3(s)-indooct-l-en-3-ol [6] is used as octenyl synthon for introduction of ro-side chain. This chiral alcohol can also be obtained from the corresponding 3-ketone [7] similarly 2-(6 methoxycarboxylhex-cis-2 enyl) cyclopentane-I,3,4-trione can be used as cyclopentyl synthol to start preparation of PGE2.

In another synthetic pathway, the reduction of 15 keto group leads to a keto structure with racemic 11 hydroxy group *via* the undermentioned pathways:

a. *Flavobacterium* sp. NRRLB-3874 gives the transdiol in 30% yield;

b. *Pseudomonas* sp. NRRLB-3875 gives the transdiol [II] in 24% yield;

c. *Rhodotorula glutinis* gives onl'1 a d,l-transdiol;

d. *Flavobacterium* sp. NRRLB-5641 gives a mixture of cis-diols.

The bioconversions are presented schematically in figures 6.16. An active compound sulprostane has been synthesized with the avoidance of racemate by specific reduction of an analogous conjugated keto group with *Kloeckera Jensenii* sp.

Biotransformation can also be initiated and employed in selective resolution of racemates by the saponification of esters of the 11-hydroxy group; an intermediate stage of this synthesis *Saccharomyces sp.*1375-143 hydrolyzes the acetate, propionate or isobutyrate of the R form steriospecifically giving 52% yields of R-alcohol.

The 3(R)-acetoxy-5(R)-hydroxycyclopent-l-ene can be obtained to a maximum yield of 11.5% by careful control of saponification which is also a desirable prostaglandin synthon. The corresponding pure cis-diacetate gives with *Bacillus subtilis* a 56% yield of the 3(s)-acetoxy-5(s)-hydroxy product, which is converted chemically into a lactone with the desired absolute configuration. Although optical purity of up to only 35% is obtained, still the lactose is considered to be an important intermediate in various prostaglandin synthesis.

One of the most interesting applications of biotransformations is that they can be used in the synthesis of artificial biotransformation also. For example, *Saccharomyces cerevisiae* A TCC 4 I 25 has been used in 15 keto reduction of 9, 15-diketo-1 1-deoxyprostanic acid. Another example is of *Trechispora brinkmanii* CMI 80439 which being used in reduction of 15 dehydroprostaglandins. Besides synthesis, interconversions like reduction of nat PGE_1 to $PGF_{1\alpha}$ and nat PGE_1 to $PGF_{1\alpha}$ by baker's yeast have also been carried out. Here 9-keto group was reduced to a 9(S)-~H group without the formation of the 9(R) byproduct. When methyl ester is used in this process, saponification takes place prior to keto reduction. When racemic mixtlire of PGEl and PGEz is taken both enantiomers are reduced to nat PGE_1 to $PGF_{1\alpha}$, nat $PGF_{2\alpha}$ and nat $PGF_{1\beta}$ and $PGF_{2\beta}$, but side reactions limit maximum yield to 10%.

PGA2 can be transformed into 15 hydroxy-9 oxo prosta-5, 13 dienoic acid by the hydrogenation of 10,11-double bond with *Cephalosporium* sp. NRRL 5499. *Dactylium dendroides* NRRL 2572 gives as a by-product 9,15-dioxaprost-5-enoic acid and 9,15-dioxoprosta-5,8-dienoic acid. An analogous 18-hydroxylated product is formed in addition to 10, 11-dihydrocompound by *Cunninghamella blakesleeana*. 10, 11-double bond can be reduced while hydrolyzing ester group by *Corynespora cassiicola* 1M I 560007. *Pseudomonas* and *Streptomyces* species can also perform this in case of 15-epiprostaglandin A_2. Interestingly, structures of new types have been obtained by microbial β oxidation of natural and synthetic prostaglandins. *Pencillium* sp. M8904 converts prostaglandins 8_2 and A_2 into tetramer structures and attacks only a side chain forming various by-products. *Mycobacterium rhodochrons* UC6I76 can also perform oxidative degradation to tetranor or dinor structures. A summary of these biotransformations is presented in Table 6.6.

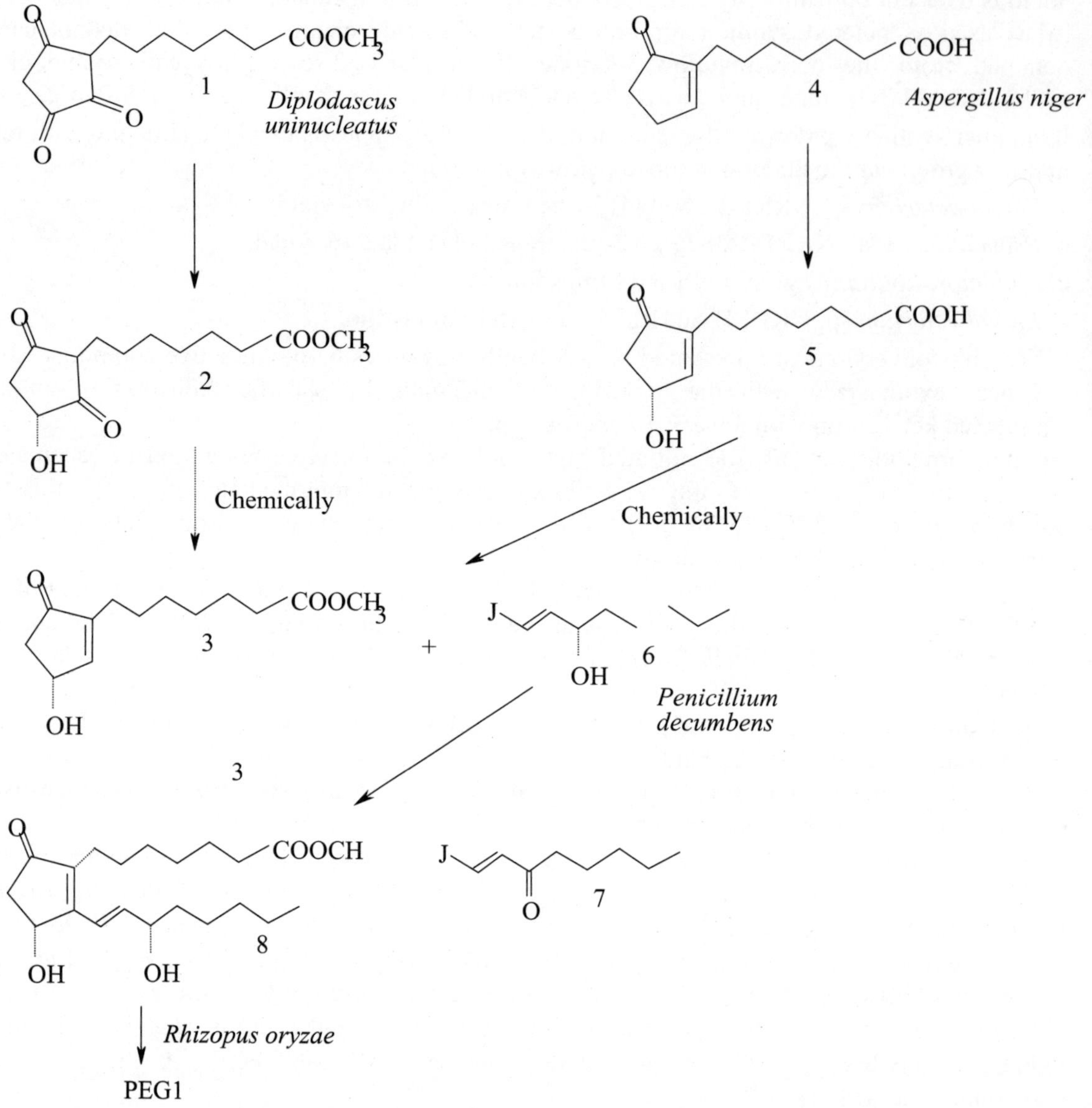

Fig. 6.16: Synthesis of PGE₁ with the aid of microbiological reaction steps

Table 6.6: Hydroxylation in prostaglandins

PGF2a	Streptomyces UC 5761	18-0H; 19-0H
PGE2	Streptomyces UC5761	18-OH; 19-OH
PGEA2	Streptomyces sp.	17-OH : 18-OH; 19-OH
Various prostaglandins	Streptomyces sp.	17-OH : 18-OH; 19-OH; 20-OH
d,1-prost-13-enoic acid	Microascus trigonosporus	18-OH; 19-OH

6.13.6. Miscellaneous products

6.13.6.1. Dihydroxyacetone

Dihydroxyacetone is an important agent in cosmetic preparations for promoting suntan. *Acetobacter* species, particularly *Acetobacter suboxydans* oxidize glycerol regioselectively to give dihydroxyacetone. Optimum concentration of glycerol is 110g/l and yield is 82% after 72 hours. *Gluconobacter melanogenus* also performs the same reaction and the rate of conversion can be increased at least three fold by enriching the aeration flow with pure oxygen.

6.13.6.2. L-Maleic acid and L-tartatic acid

L-Maleic acid is used in the treatment of liver diseases and as an additive to infusion solution. It is an important intermediate in tricarboxylic acid cycle. *Brevibacterium ammoniagenes* cells immobilized in polyacrylamide gel or *Brevibacterium flavum* cells immobilized in carrageenan have been used for the production of L maleic acid by asymmetric addition of water to fumaric acid. Immobilized cells are treated with bile extract for suppressing the undesirable by-product synthesis of succinic acid. Enzyme responsible is fumarase of which highest activity and the longest half life (160 days at 37°C) were observed with *B flavum* immobilized in carrageenan.

L-tartaric acid production involves initial oxidation of maleic acid to cis-epoxysuccinic acid by hydrogen peroxide (H_2O_2) and then asymmetric hydrolysis of epoxide by using microorganisms *Nocardia tartaricus* or *Achromobacter tartarogenes* cells immobilized in polyacrylamide gel as biocatalysts.

6.13.6.3. Sugar transformations

Although many sugar transformations have been studied, three processes particularly important from technical application point of view are discussed here.

a. Isomerization of glucose to fructose to enhance sweetening effect has been carried out by using *Bacillus coagulans* immobilized with glutaraldehyde; *Streptomyces phaeochromogenes* immobilized in poly-acrylamide and *Achromobacter missouriensis* immobilized on cellulose fibers. Use of *Bacillus coagulans* makes possible conversion of 1000 Kg glucose to a mixture of 45% fructose and 55% glucose per Kg of biocatalyst. Transforming enzyme present in the microbes is glucose isomerase.

b. Hydrolysis of raffinose to sucrose and galactose by α-galactosidase to increase yields of sucrose from beet sugar molasses. Mycelial pellets formed naturally by *Mortierella vinacea* var *raffinoseutilizer* are rich in α-galactosidase and have been used for continuous hydrolysis of raffinose.

c. Lactose in skimmed milk has been hydrolyzed by cells of *Lactobacillus bulgaricus, Escherichia coli,* and *Kluyveromyces lactis* showing high β-galactosidase activity and immobilized on polyacrylamide gel to produce lactose free milk products. Products formed are glucose and galactose. This process is also useful in utilization of whey.

6.13.6.4. Hycanthone and oxamniquine

Drug hycanthone is active against *Schistosoma mansoni*. The activity is enhanced by selective hydroxylation of an aromatic methyl group with *Aspergillus sclerotiorum*. The more potent drug formed is Hycanthone. Oxamniquine, a schistosomacidal drug is produced from corresponding methyl compound by *Aspergillus sclerotiorum*.

6.13.6.5. Biotransformations of antitumor drugs

Biotransformations have also been employed for many antitumor drugs. Reductive cleavage of glycosides, reduction of ketone groups in anthracyclines, hydrolysis of amine moiety of bleomycin, regioselective hydroxylation in **withaferrin A** and in aromatic rings of acromycin (acronin) and vinblastine, N-demethylation in D-tetrandrine and vindoline, the formation of ether derivatives and the dimerization of vindoline and the opening of quinone ring in lapachol are some of the representative examples. Unfortunately these and other bio-transformations have not led to development of products with significantly enhanced activity or reduced toxicity.

6.13.6.6. Oxidation of naphthalene

Pseudomonas putida degrades naphthalene by reductive dihydroxylation to give cis 1 ,2-dihydroxy-1,2-dihydronaphthalene. Cis isomer formed is an important precursor for pesticides. Trans 1,2-dihydroxy-1,2- dihydronaphathalene is formed by *Nocardia* sp. NRRL 3385. Subsequent oxidation proceeds through several steps to salicylic acid, however its production by this method is insignificant even with the most suitable strain *Corynebacterium renale* ATCC 15070.

6.14. CELL CULTURE AND ANIMAL BIOTECHNOLOGY

Many types of animal cells can now be grown in culture. These include tumour cells, steroid-producing; adrenal cells, ACTH-secreting pituitary cells, growth hormone- and prolactin-secreting cell; from pituitary tumour, pigmented melanoma cells, teratoma cells capable of differentiation *in vitro,* and neuroblastoma cells. Functionally differentiated cells from tumours can be readily cultured. Pigmented cells and cartilage cells have been cultured since the early 1920s. Cancerous mast cell lines producing serotonin and heparin have also been raised. Chick myoblasts are known to proliferate and fuse to form muscle straps. Rat myoblasts cannot only fuse in culture but also repair injury in crushed muscle (Sato and Rifkin, 1982). Whereas cells of bacteria and yeasts can be grown freely suspended in deep suspension cultures, those of mammals can only be grown in industrial-scale cultures in multiple low-productivity roller bottles. This is because the mammalian cells require attachment to a suitable surface and consequently the surface area available limits the maximum cell numbers. This kind of limitation can now be overcome by growing mammalian cell cultures on microcarriers such as beads of anion exchange resin. By employing conventional conditions of medium, serum, and oxygen, and using suitable beads as carriers, Thilly *et al.*, (1982) have grown certain mammalian cells to densities as high as 5×10^6 cells/min. By substituting fructose for glucose, they have been able to control the overproduction of lactate, which in many cell cultures uses an abnormal lowering of the pH, thus limiting the growth of the cells.

During the last few decades, various types of additives have been used to protect freely suspended animal cells in culture from agitation and aeration damage. These include pluronic polyols, various derivatized celluloses and starches, protein mixtures, polyvinyl-pyrrolidones, dextrans, and, more recently, polyethylene glycol (PEG) and polyvinyl alcohol. Damage of suspended cells in agitated and/or aerated bioreactors is usually due to the interactions of cells with bubbles and the rearrangement at gas-liquid interfaces. In bubble-column reactors, cell injury appears to be due to shear forces generated either by film drainage around bubbles (such as in unstable foams), or by bubble breakup. In agitated bioreactors, cultures of suspended cells appear to suffer damage by the following two fluid mechanical mechanisms:

(1) Formation of a gas phase due to bubble breakup, either because of direct sparging or because of gas entrainment.

(2) Cell damage occurs in the absence of a gas phase (and, therefore, the absence of bubbles) only at very high agitation rates by stress in the bulk turbulent liquid. With this second mechanism, cell damage correlates with eddy sizes similar to or smaller than the cell size (9–15 μm).

Regardless of whether cells are damaged in viscometric well-defined laminar flows, or due to bubble breakup and film drainage, or due to interactions with eddies, damage is caused by shear forces acting on the cells through the surrounding fluid layer (boundary layer), which is always in a state of laminar flow. Cell damage occurring in such cases may therefore be referred to as either shear or fluid-mechanical damage.

All additives that protect freely suspended cells from fluid-mechanical injury must either decrease the fragility of the cells or affect the forces on the cells due to their interactions with gas-liquid interfaces. Serum permits better cell growth in agitated and/or aerated cultures in a dosage-dependent fashion. Low serum or serum-free cultures are more susceptible to fluid-mechanical damage. Concentrations up to 10% of foetal bovine serum (FBS) tend to reduce cell death and allow growth of cells at substantially higher agitation rates in bioreactors with surface aeration where cell damage is due to air entrainment and bubble breakup. The protective effect of FBS appears to be largely physical, but it can vary depending on the design and operational characteristics of the bioreactor and the cells in question.

The non-ionic surfactants Pluronie F68 and F88 block copolymer glycols of poly (oxyethylene)-poly (oxypropylene)-poly (oxyethylene) protect cells from fluid-borne mechanical damage in agitated and aerated bioreactors. Several investigators have used these surfactants as medium additives in static, agitated and/or aerated cell cultures. For long, derivatized celluloses have been used for suspension cell culture technology; methyl celluloses (MCs) have not been unequivocally established as reliable shear protectants. MCs and other derivatized celluloses have been frequently included as media additives (in combination with serum, various protein mixtures and other defined additives) in the cultivation of a large variety of cells. It is not known whether these derivatized celluloses are indeed needed as shear-protection additives in most formulations of modern serum-free media, since control experiments to demonstrate their shear-protection effect are lacking.

The use of MCs (in combination with other shear-protecting additives such as serum, yeast extract or protein hydrolysates) has been somewhat restricted to the cultivation of insect cells. It seems that both the MCs and dextran increase the shear robustness of these insect cells through a biological mechanism. The effect of MCs as additives to protect animal cells from shear damage in agitated, bubble-column or otherwise mixed cultures may be cell-type, MC-grade, and MC-make dependent. In addition, MCs may elicit biological responses from cells, either positive or negative; these responses appear to be also cell-type and MC-grade and MC-make dependent. Several protein mixtures (in addition to serum) and a protein have been used as shear protectants for the cultivation of various cells. Again, their protective effect is not definitely established and there is a lack of proper control experiments. Bovine serum albumin (BSA), a major component of bovine serum, is a widely used additive in serum-free media, and has been frequently used as a shear protectant. It may be an effective additive against fluid-mechanical damage of hybridoma cells in an airlift bioreactor, although it has no effort on the cells in static or spinner cultures.

While several options are available regarding shear-protecting additives, it is not clear if the use of these additives is suitable for all cell culturing and processing needs. For each cell type, the physiological and/or product expression effects of an additive must be assessed carefully under both static and bioreactor growth conditions. If there are no obvious detrimental effects, the effect of the additive on cell aggregation must be evaluated, in case cell aggregation is an undesirable processing property. The effect of the additive on a possible modification of the cell culture protein product as well as on the purification of this product also has to be assessed. Most additives may complicate membrane, adsorption, precipitation, and chromatographic processes. So, on the basis of a combination of chemical structure, molecular mass and protective-effect concentration, some additives may be more advantageous than others from the DSP (down streaming processing) point of view.

SUGGESTED READING

- Andersson LC, Jokinen M, Gahmberg CG. *Nature* 278, 364 (1979).
- Andersson LC, Nilsson K., Gahmberg CG. *Int J Cancer* 23, 143 (1979).
- Barnes D, Sato G. *Anal Biochem* 102, 255 (1980).
- Berdichevsky F, Gilbert C, Shearer M. *et al., J Cell Sci* 102, 437 (1992).
- Bodnar AG, Ouellette M, Frolkis M. *et al.*, *Science* 279, 349 (1998).
- Boyce ST, Ham RGJ. *Invest Dermatol* 81 (Suppl 1), 33s (1983).
- Capek KA, Hanc O, Tadra M. (Eds.) *Microbial Transformation of Steroids*, Akademia Press, Prague (1966).
- Chambard M, Verrier B, Gabrion J. *et al.*, *J Cell Biol* 96, 1172 (1983).
- Courtenay VD, Selby PJ, Smith IE. *et al.*, *Br J Cancer* 38, 77 (1978).
- Davis JM. (ed.) *Basic cell culture: a Practical Approach.* IRL Press at Oxford University Press, Oxford (1994).
- Doyle A, Griffiths JB, Newall DG. (Eds.) *Cell and Tissue Culture: Laboratory Procedures.* Wiley, Chichester (1990).
- Dulbecco R, Freeman G. *Virology* 8, 396 (1959).
- Eagle H. *Science* 130, 432 (1959).
- Fogh J, Wright WC, Loveless JD. *J Natl Cancer Inst* 58, 209 (1977).
- Fonken GS, Johnson RA. (Eds.) *Chemical Oxidation with Microorganisms*, Marcel Dekker, New York (1972).
- Frame MC, Freshney RI, Vaughan PF. *et al.*, *Br J Cancer* 49, 269 (1984).
- Freshney MG. In *Culture of hematopoietic cells* R. I. Freshney, I. B. Pragnell, and M. G. Freshney(Eds.) Wiley-Liss, New York p. 265 (1994).
- Freshney RI. *Culture of epithelial cells* Wiley-Liss, New York (1992).
- Freshney RI. *Freshney's culture of animal cells, a multimedia guide.* Wiley-Liss, New York (1999).
- Freshney RI. *Nature,* 356 (2000).
- Freshney RI. *Culture of animal cells: a manual of basic technique,* 4th edn. Wiley- Liss, New York (2000).
- Freshney RI, Freshney MG. (Ed.) *Culture of immortalized* cells. Wiley-Liss, New York (1994).
- Friend C, Scher W, Holland JG. *et al.*, *Proc Natl Acad Sri* USA, 68, 378 (1971).
- Gallagher R, Collins S, Trujillo J. *et al.*, *Blood* 54, 713 (1979).
- Gaush CR, Hard WL, Smith TF. *Proc Soc Exp Biol Med* 122, 931 (1966).
- Gey GO, Coffman WD, Kubicek MT. *Cancer Res* 12, 364 (1952).
- Ghigo D, Priotto C, Migliorino D. *et al.*, *J Cell Physiol* 174, 99 (1998).
- Giard DJ, Aaronson SA, Todaro GJ. *et al.*, *J Natl Cancer Inst* 51, 1417 (1973).
- Gillis S, Watson J. *J Exp Med* 152, 1709 (1980).
- Gluzman Y. *Cell* 23, 175 (1981).
- Graham FL, Smiley J, Russell WC. *et al.*, *Gen Virol* 36, 59 (1977).

- Grander D. *Med Oncol* 15, 20 (1998).
- Green H, Kehinde O. *Cell* 1, 113 (1974).
- Greene LA, Tischler AS. *Proc Natl Acad Sci USA* 73, 2424 (1976).
- Hall EA, *Biosensors* Open University Press, Milton Keynes (1990).
- Ham RG. *Proc Natl Acad Sci USA* 53, 288 (1965).
- Hopkinson J. *Biotechnology* 3, 225 (1985).
- Jacobs JP, Jones CM, Bailie JP. *Nature* 227, 168 (1970).
- Jizuka H, Naito A, *Microbial Transformation of Steroids and Alkaloids*, University of Tokyo Press, Tokyo (1967).
- Kieslich K, Steroid Conversions; In: *Economic Microbiology-Microbial Enzymes and Transformation*, Vol. V, 369 (1980).
- Knowles BB, Howe CC, Aden DP. *Science* 209, 497 (1980).
- Lechner JF, McClendon IA, Laveck MA. *et al., Cancer Res* 43, 5915 (1983).
- Leibovitz A. *Am J Hyg* 78, 173 (1963).
- Macpherson I, Stoker M. *Virology* 16, 147 (1962).
- McCormick C, Freshney RI. *Br J Cancer* 82, 881 (2000).
- Meyers RA. *Molecular Biology and Biotechnology*, VCH Publishers, Inc., New York, 110 (1995).
- Moore GE, Gerner RE, Franklin HA. *J Am Med Assoc* 199, 519 (1967).
- Nicosia RF, Ottinetti A. *In Vitro* 26, 119 (1990).
- North JR. *Trends in Biotechnology* 3, 180 (1985).
- Peehl DM, Ham RG. *In Vitro,* 16, 526 (1980).
- Pereira-Smith OM, Smith J. *Proc Natl Acad Sci USA* 85, 6042 (1988).
- Puck TT, Marcus PI. *Proc Natl Acad Sci USA* 41, 432 (1955).
- Spier R, Hennessen W. (Eds.) *Developments in Biological Standardization*, Vol. 66, Academic Press, San Diego, CA (1985).
- Raff MC, Miller RH, Noble M. *Nature* 303, 390 (1983).
- Rooney SA, Young SL, Mendelson CR. *FASEB J* 8, 957 (1994).
- Sasaki M, Honda T, Yamada H. *et al., Cancer Res* 54, 6090 (1994).
- Sattler CA, Michalopoulos G, Sattler GL *et al., Cancer Res* 38, 1539 (1978).
- Schaller F, Schubert F. *Biosensors* Elsevier, Amsterdam (1992).
- Speirs V, Ray KP, Freshney RI. *Br J Cancer* 64, 693 (1991).
- Sporn MB, Roberts AB. *Cancer Res* 43, 3034 (1983).
- Spratt NTJ, *Science* 106, 452 (1947).
- Thomson AA, Foster BA, Cunha GR. *Development* 124, 2431 (1997).
- Vlodavsky I, Lui GM, Gospodarowicz D. *Cell* 19, 607 (1980).
- Yevdokimova N, Freshney RI. *Br J Cancer* 76, 261 (1997).

THERAPEUTIC CARBOHYDRATES AND BOTANICAL DRUGS

7.1. THE GLYCOME

Somewhat analogous to the genetic code, the glycome (the sugar code) defines the interactions between cell-coating sugars and proteins along with about how they recognize each other. The sugars (Saccharides) are most complex of the three main classes of biopolymers-proteins, nucleic acids and sugars. Each monosaccharide building block has several attachment sites, so that sugars can be built in a variety of linear or branched fashions. For example, glucose and mannose can be linked to form a disaccharide in up to 80 different ways. Microarray techniques offer the possibility of high-throughput analysis and have been investigated in a series of reports (Fukui *et al.*, 2002; Wang *et al.*, 2002: Flitsch and Ulijn, 2003).

One best-known example of sugar-protein interaction is the action of the human blood-group antigens A, B and O. The difference between these three antigens lies in a single carbohydrate unit in an oligosaccharide sequence on the surface of red blood cells. When different blood types are mixed, any 'foreign' A, B or O antigen is recognized by highly specific sugar-binding proteins (agglutinins) that make blood agglutinate or clot. A few other types of sugar-recognizing proteins include those activated to adhere to sugars in immune responses, lectins that cross link cell-surface sugars and antibodies that are specific to certain sugars. Microarrays have been widely employed for understanding gene expression and protein interactions. They are also suitable for studying the glycome. By attaching complex sugars to a microarray plate, the compounds can be quickly and easily screened to work out their specific interactions with proteins. The problem is how to link the sugar under study to the microarray surface.

Fukui *et al.* (2002) devised a method based on the fact that the reducing end of all oligosaccharides has an aldehyde that reacts with an amino lipid to form a so-called neoglycolipid by covalent conjugation. The neoglycolipids can then be immobilized by spotting them into arrays on nitrocellulose membranes. Using highly specific antibodies to probe for certain carbohydrate sequences, Fukui *et al.* (2002) obtained structural information on the oligosaccharides present. Wang *et al.* (2002) showed that carbohydrates could also be spotted directly on single nitrocellulose-coated glass slides without the need for covalent conjugation.

Each of the above two techniques has some drawbacks; in the neoglycolipid approach, the first monosaccharide unit is lost on binding to the nitrocellulose membrane, and the Wang *et al.* (2002) method provides little control over the orientation of the immobilized polysaccharide. An exciting new development is the use of cycloaddition reactions–a class of simple, selective chemical reactions in which a ring structure is formed (Houseman and Mrksich, 2002; Fazio *et al.*,2002). Houseman and Mrksich (2002) used a specific cycloaddition, the Diels-Alder reaction and showed that a series of ten different monosaccharides could be specifically detected by five different lectins. Fazio *et al.*(2002) exploited cycloaddition between azides (which contain an N_3 group) and alkynes. In a simple cycloaddition reaction, "complex" sugars attach to a microtitre plate. The alkyne group at the end of a hydrocarbon chain (attached to the plate) is a natural tether for azidoethyl glycoside, whose terminating N_3 group binds to the alkyne, forming a ring The above works reveal the potential for sugar-microarray technology, which should permit systematic and high-throughput analysis of protein-sugar interactions and enzyme-inhibition screening, similar to the analysis being developed for nucleic acids and proteins (Flitsch and Ulijn, 2003).

7.2. GLYCOBIOLOGY FOR DRUG DEVELOPMENT

Researchers on genomics and proteomics have tended to neglect the various ways in which proteins are "tweaked" through the attachment of sugars. Carbohydrates determine the three-dimensional structures of proteins; these structures are inherently linked to their function and their efficacy as therapeutics. In contrast to some of the other chemical tags employed by cells (e.g., phosphates and lipids), carbohydrates show an enormous diversity of structures, can confer cell-type specificity, which are crucial components of cell-to-cell signaling. At the same time, they are the most difficult biological molecules to analyze and synthesize, and break rapidly in the bloodstream. Despite these challenges, recent technological advances have prompted some biotechnology companies to pursue "new carbohydrate-based products".

In contrast to nucleic acids and proteins, carbohydrates can form branching structures –a relatively simple set of sugars can form a huge number of complex structures. For instance, the nine common monosaccharides found in humans could be assembled into more than 15 million possible tetrasaccharides, all of which are relatively simple glycans. Different cell types express different complements of glycosylating enzymes, and have different sets of proteins that can be glycosylated. Glycosylation serves a wide variety of purposes in complex organisms (Dove, 2001).

The process of glycosylation begins when the protein is targeted to the glycosylation pathway during translation of messenger RNA (mRNA) into protein. During translation, the ribosome is attached to the endoplasmic reticulum (ER), and the nascent protein is fed into the lumen of the ER where some glycosylation enzymes attach sugars to specific parts of the protein. Other such enzymes then either add more sugars to these core structures, or partially trim the structures back so that new sugars can be added to a different part of the growing carbohydrate structure. Glycosylation continues into the Golgi apparatus, which sorts the new proteins, distributing them to their final destinations in the cell. In human cells, sialic acid is usually added to the tips of the carbohydrates branches, serving as a final cap important for a variety of glycoprotein functions.

Carbohydrates significantly affect protein structure and protein function. They are used as tags to sort proteins in the Golgi apparatus, either targeting them to specific compartments within the cell or directing them to the cell surface. Once on the cell membrane, glycoproteins (and glycolipids) interact with receptors on other cells to convey various messages. Cells of the immune system use the glycans on the cells that they encounter to identify everything from bacterial invaders to fellow leukocytes (Dove, 2001).

In view of the importance of carbohydrates, any defects in their metabolism can produce disastrous consequences. In Gaucher's and Fabry's diseases, inherited mutations in carbohydrate-processing enzymes cause glycolipids to accumulate, damaging the kidneys, heart, and brain. The inability to form certain glycoproteins results in another set of inherited diseases called congenital disorders of glycosylation, which can produce symptoms ranging from chronic diarrhoea to serious neurological problems.

Besides relatively rare genetic diseases, sugars play crucial roles in some common health problems. Injured tissues stimulate endothelial cells to express selectins, glycoproteins that induce leukocytes in the bloodstream to infiltrate damaged tissue and mount an inflammatory response. However, this inflammation process can sometime get out of control. In surviving stroke and heart attack patients, for example, blood flow is briefly cut off from a tissue, and then restored. As the blood starts to flow again, selectins in the affected tissue recruit leukocytes from the bloodstream, leading to a strong inflammatory response. The resulting tissue damage (reperfusion injury) is typically more severe than that sustained by the initial interruption of blood flow. Modulation of the glycan-mediated signal from the selectins might help mitigate the damage. Carbohydrates are important for tumor development because cancer cells change their surface glycoprotein expression to evade the immune system. By cloaking themselves with the right assortment of glycoproteins, the tumor cells can invade other tissues without being identified as aliens (Dove, 2001).

The potential of carbohydrate-based therapies has so far been hampered by certain technical problems. In the absence of high-throughput methods for analyzing and synthesizing carbohydrates, detailed knowledge of the structure and function of each carbohydrate moiety could be elucidated through extremely labour-intensive experiments. Indeed, even the nomenclature of carbohydrates is rather confusing. Whereas molecular biologists use simple alphabetic codes to describe the nucleic acid or protein sequences they study, glycobiologists have been stuck and have to use the complete, clumsy chemical names of the complex carbohydrates.

Unlike DNA and proteins, no technology has been developed to allow carbohydrates to be "sequenced" conveniently techniques. Instead, sugar structures must be solved by a combination of chromatography and mass spectrometry, procedures requiring much technical skill. Glycoproteomics is at least an order of magnitude more difficult than proteomics.

Usually a glycoprotein is isolated from a chromatography gel, and the carbohydrate groups are then released from the protein by chemical or enzymatic treatment. The mixture of carbohydrates can then be subjected to high-performance liquid chromatography (HPLC) to separate out individual carbohydrates. Finally, individual carbohydrates are studied by chemical digestion and mass spectrometry–techniques that give precise structural information about such small molecules as monosaccharides (Dove, 2001).

Glycobiologists must also contend with the heterogeneity of sugar structures within a sample. For example the human prion protein can carry one of 52 different sugar structures at one site on the protein; this makes it very difficult to analyze, because if you've got 'x' amount (of sample), you've got 'x' divided by 52 of any one carbohydrate. Obtaining sufficient quantities of a given glycan for analysis is a major problem when studying glycoproteins present in low concentrations in cells. Once a carbohydrate structure is solved, duplicating the structure artificially is also very difficult. Cells that can glycosylate proteins generate a diverse array of carbohydrate structures, and the production of a specific glycoprotein *in vivo* cannot be controlled.

The digestive system can effectively break down most naturally occurring carbohydrates, and any therapeutic carbohydrates may have to be injected directly into the bloodstream. Glycosidases in the blood can reduce a carbohydrate-based drug's half-life to just a few minutes, depending on its structure. Carbohydrate based drugs such as heparin; the world's best-selling prescription drug and the *Haemophilus influenzae* type B (Hib) vaccine have avoided this pharmacokinetic pitfall because their structures are not readily recognized by the body's normal glycosidases. But other carbohydrate-based therapeutics may not fare so well.

Indeed, carbohydrates also present a major drug delivery problem for ordinary protein therapeutics, most of which must be correctly glycosylated to function. Glycosylation also affects protein breakdown; thus proteins lacking terminal sialic acid residues on their sugar groups are usually targeted by the immune system and are rapidly degraded. Some work is underway to improve the glycosylation of medically useful glycoproteins. Strategies are being developed to drastically cut the cost of protein production, for both pharmaceutical and industrial uses. Some companies contemplate using enzymes to add sugars to protein *in vitro* for significantly improving the yield of usable protein from fermentations.

7.2.1. Synthesizing sugars

Improved means of synthesizing carbohydrates for further study and drug development are emerging; these approaches fall into four major categories: one pot synthesis is a direct descendant of traditional organic chemistry techniques, in which successive reactions are carried out in a single test tube to produce the final carbohydrate product. In solid-phase synthesis, the initial sugar groups are bound to beads or surfaces, allowing them to be isolated and moved easily at each step of the process; enzymatic processes use glycosylating enzymes, extracted from cells, to carry out the reactions. Finally, novel biological systems, in which carbohydrates are produced in genetically modified animal, yeast, or bacterial cells have been developed.

An automated system based on advances in solid-phase synthesis has been developed that may eventually be used as oligopeptide and oligonucleotide synthesizers (Plante *et al.,* 2001). This general procedure is based on an application which builds on monosaccharide molecules. Carbohydrates will play an increasingly important role in future drug development. Besides heparin and the Hib vaccine, some other successful carbohydrate-based drugs include the influenza antivirals, Tamiflu and Relenza and the antibiotics erythromycin and vancomycin (Dove, 2001).

Biotechnology companies are also now turning to glycosylation, which can be a major problem in protein production. Amgen (Thousand Oaks, CA), for instance, discards about 75% of the erythropoietin it produces because the protein is not correctly glycosylated. Like many other therapeutically important proteins, erythropoietin fails to function properly if it lacks the right sugar groups.

Carbohydrates are increasingly being targeted as potential new medicines. Carbohydrate-based antibiotics are well established in medicine. Pathogenic bacteria often use glycoprotein receptors on the surfaces of host cells to colonize a tissue. New antibiotics might act to prevent this attachment. Some oligosaccharide may be designed that is identical or mimics the docking molecule on the host cell to thwart the ability of the microorganism to colonize. As carbohydrates are well tolerated by the human digestive system, carbohydrate-based medicines may have fewer side effects than traditional antibiotics for treating gastrointestinal infections. As many intracellular pathogens also require sugars, glycosylation is itself an attractive target for novel antivirals.

7.2.2. Targeting cancers

One class of carbohydrate-based cancer treatments is based on alerting the immune system to the tumor's glycan disguise. Anti-cancer vaccines are being developed that stimulate an immune response against the carbohydrate antigens found on tumor cells. Although these antigens are normally tolerated by the immune system, there is evidence that chemically modified glycans and adjuvants may boost immunity, causing tumors to be held in check or possibly even eliminated (Fig. 7.1).

Besides helping cancer evade the immune system, glycans help orchestrate normal and pathological immune responses. Many autoimmune diseases are driven by a process called the Th1 response, in which the immune system initiates a chain reaction of inflammatory signals. Use of glycoconjugates to initiate compensatory anti-inflammatory Th2 responses is therefore being contemplated: a large number of studies have been done in three different animal models in which the glycoconjugates appeared to be therapeutic. Adjuvants for improved vaccines are being developed and it is hoped to use similar carbohydrate-based drugs to modulate a wide range of immune responses. While many companies plan to target glycosylation and carbohydrates for drug development, sugars will continue to present a bigger challenge than DNA or proteins. Yet, for companies, glycobiology is an area that is ripe for potential therapeutic intervention.

7.3. OLIGOSACCHARIDE SYNTHESIS AND GLYCOENZYMES THERAPEUTICS

Oligosaccharides, other carbohydrates, and glycoenzymes are important in living organisms. The functions of oligosaccharides in the form of glycoconjugates in biological systems; these include fertilization, embryogenesis, neuronal development, cell proliferation and metastasis (Varki, 1993). Pharmaceutical companies are greatly interested in oligosaccharide synthesis in view of the potential application of these biomolecules as therapeutics. But this potential is limited because the complex structure of oligosaccharides makes classical chemical synthesis difficult as any manipulations of protecting-groups are needed to control the stereospecificity and the regiospecificity of the products which are complicated, tedious and hinder the efficient production of oligosaccharides, required for biological testing (Zopf and Roth, 1996; Crout and Vic, 1998).

It is possible to synthesize oligosaccharides enzymatically by controlling the regio- and stereo-specificity of the reaction. Two main classes of enzymes used are the glycosyltransferases and the glycosidases. This approach is superior to traditional chemical synthesis in the regio- and stereo-selectivity that can be achieved without the need for protecting functional groups. However, the limited availability of glycosyltransferases, the high cost of their substrates, and the poor yields from the synthetic reactions mediated by the glycosidases limit their use in the large-scale production of oligosaccharides (Perugino *et al.,* 2004). A much better approach is to use glycosynthases, which are specifically mutated glycosidases that efficiently synthesize oligosaccharides but do not hydrolyze them (Henrissat and Davies, 2000; Sears and Wong, 2001).

Glycosynthases have been used in obtaining high yields of a variety of oligosaccharides by means of commercially available glycosyl donors. More and more novel glycosynthases are being produced to enhance the potential applications of these biocatalysts. About ten glycoside hydrolases (GH), belonging to seven different GH families from bacteria, eukaryotes and archaea, have been successfully modified as efficient glycosynthases (Malet and Planas, 1998; Jakeman and Withers, 2002). Almost each different glycosynthase produces a specific type of product. Thus, by using the appropriate glycosynthase we can synthesize any oligosaccharide of interest.

Endo glycosynthases have proven particularly valuable tools for the synthesis of not only complex oligosaccharides but also polysaccharides. They have been produced from *Bacillus licheniformis, Humicola insolens* and barley. One glucansynthase from barley has been exploited in the production of compounds that show antibacterial, antiviral and antitumour activity (Maeda and Chihara, 1971; Perugino *et al.,* 2004). Although glycosynthase-catalysed reactions give very high yields because manipulation of the enzymes precludes hydrolysis of the products, the reactions usually require either large quantities of mutant enzyme or extended incubation times. Certain mutants of glycosynthases show much improvement in enzymatic activity and lead to better product yields, reduced reaction times and enhanced synthetic repertoire.

Solid-phase oligosaccharide synthesis has attracted focus because immobilization of the sugar significantly improves the recovery of the product (Seeberger and Haase, 2000). This approach has high potential in the exploitation of glycosynthases in large-scale oligosaccharide synthesis. Also, the idea of engineering glycosidases for producing oligosaccharides has been further extended by a novel strategy on retaining glycosidases–two β-glycosidases from *Agrobacterium* sp. have been found to efficiently synthesize thioglycosides (Jahn *et al.,* 2003). Certain mutants (of acid/base catalyst) from *Agrobacterium* sp. and *Cellulomonas fimi* could be reactivated in the presence of glucoside donors and SH-sugars used as acceptors. These mutant enzymes named thioglycoligases, proved effective in the preparation of thioglycosides. They are particularly valuable as targets for the pharmaceutical industry (Witczak, 1999). Recent advances in the synthesis of oligosaccharides have underscored their potential as therapeutics. Chemical synthesis on polymer supported carbohydrates or the use of whole microorganisms as cell factories represent notable advances in this context (Endo and Koizumi, 2000). Large-scale chemical synthesis of oligosaccharides is, however, constrained by control of the stereo- and regio-chemistry of bond formation.

Synthesis of oligosaccharides by the glycosynthase enzymes, which do not hydrolyze the products and use inexpensive sugars, is a better alternative to scaling up of oligosaccharide production. It seems certain that the ready availability of glycosidases and their high biodiversity will enhance their utility and potential applications in the near future.

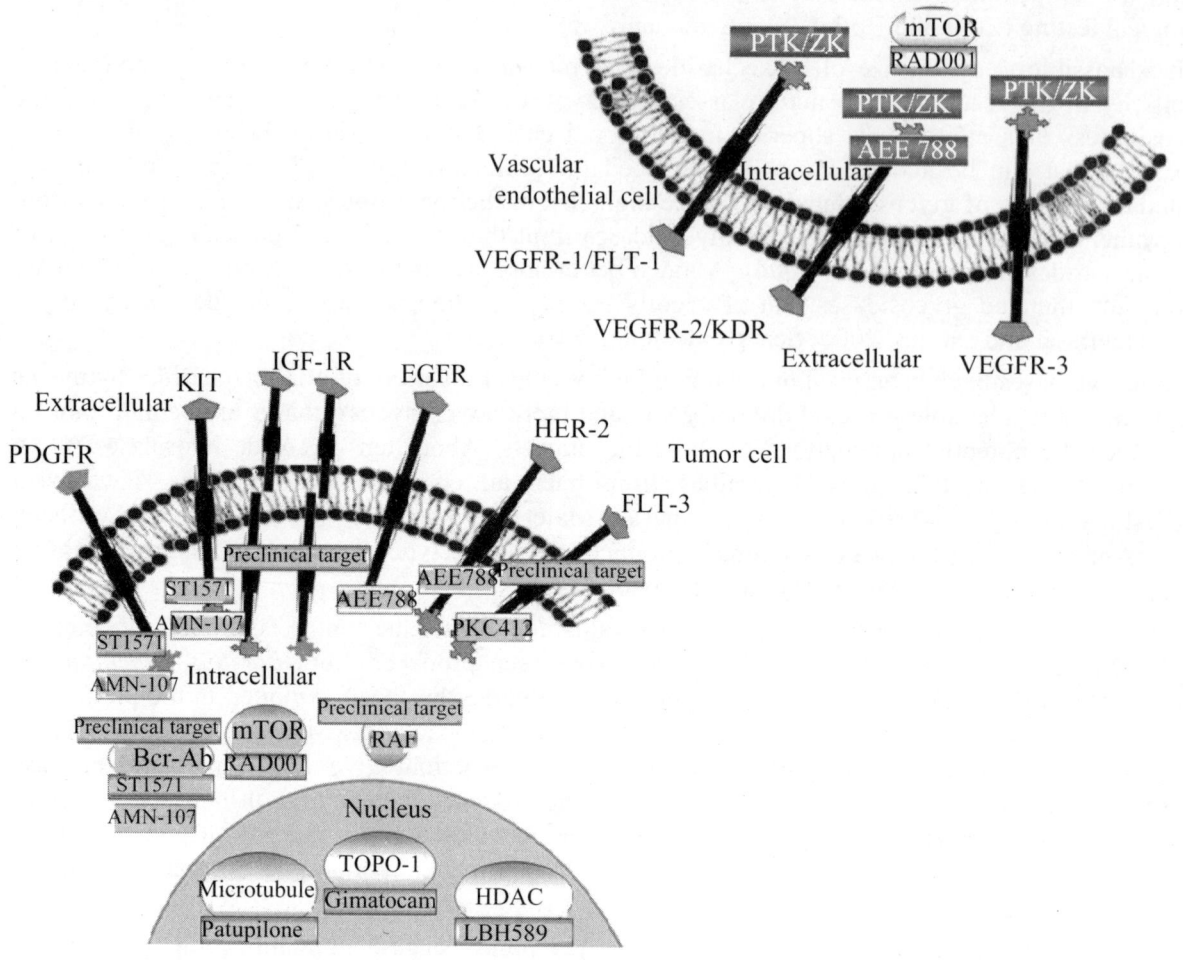

Fig. 7.1: Targeting cancer through multiple pathways

7.4. HUMANIZING PROTEIN GLYCOSYLATION THROUGH GM YEAST

The application of recombinant DNA technology has greatly improved the availability of therapeutic proteins. For expressing biologically active recombinant proteins, prokaryotic-cell and mammalian-cell culture systems have been employed as the primary hosts, but more recently, certain eukaryotic-yeast expression systems have also been developed. The proteins expressed need to be glycosylated with saccharides structures that are native (or at least not antigenic) to humans. Choi *et al.* (2003) achieved such glycosylation by synthesizing a hybrid N-linked oligosaccharide in yeast (*P. pastoris*) expression host. This yeast has served extensively as the host cell for large-scale production of secreted recombinant proteins. Many proteins of pharmaceutical importance are N-glycosylated, and so require an expression host that yields N-linked oligosaccharides that are structurally and functionally identical to the human counterpart.

However, although glycosylation is essential for many therapeutically important proteins, it is also a serious disadvantage of yeast-expression systems because in yeast N-glycosylation usually involves glycans having many mannose residues (hyperglycosylations) (Bretthauer and Castellino, 1999;

Gemmill and Trimble, 1999). This necessitates extensive genetic alterations of the glycosylation pathway in yeast strains so as to overcome the aberrant non-human nature of yeast protein-glycosylation (Bretthauer, 2003).

Choi *et al.* (2003) described the use of combinatorial genetic libraries to alter the N-glycosylation pathway in *P. pastoris* to yield N-linked oligosaccharides with hybrid structures similar to the intermediates of mammalian-protein N-glycosylation. This development has aroused hopes of producing complex human glycans in yeasts. Choi *et al.* (2003) and Hamilton *et al.* (2003) have shown that N-glycosylation pathways in *P. pastoris* can be extensively re-engineered without abolishing the viability of host cells. Hirose *et al.* (2002) have reported mannosyl phosphorylation in several expressed recombinant proteins from *P. pastoris.* As this probably alters structural or functional features of the glycoprotein, it can be considered in genetic engineering of *P. pastoris.* These researches contribute greatly to the 'humanization' of N-linked oligosaccharide pathways in fungal hosts.

7.5. GLYCOENGINEERING OF CYTOKINE HORMONES

Erythropoietin (EPO), thrombopoietin (Mpl ligand), and leptin exemplify structurally related cytokines, hormones and growth factors (Type 1 cytokines) those bind to specific but structurally related surface receptors on their respective target cells (Nicola and Hilton, 1998). The Type I cytokines also include interleukins, hematopoietic growth factors, such as EPO and Mpl ligand, as well as metabolic cytokines, such as growth hormone, prolactin and leptin. Each family member binds to the extracellular domains of a receptor dimer, thereby changing receptor conformation and triggering intracellular signalling. The specific binding sites of a Type I cytokine molecule to its receptor are determined by the tertiary conformation of specific peptide sequences, but the binding affinity tends to be affected by oligosaccharides that are covalently bound to asparagine (N-linked glycans) in those parts of the molecule that are not directly involved in receptor binding (Koury, 2003). Besides their effects on receptor binding, these oligosaccharides also affect the metabolic clearance of the cytokine. Elliott *et al.* (2003) have shown increased *in vivo* activities and their durations by engineering hyperglycosylations of recombinant human (rh) EPO, Mpl ligand and leptin. The successful use of the hyperglycosylated recombinant human erythropoietin (rhEPO) in patients suggests that this glycoengineering technique could be gainfully applied not only to other recombinant proteins being used as therapeutic agents but also to growth factors, hormones and cytokines.

The rhEPO, an effective and widely used therapeutic agent, has been produced by bioengineering. Modification of the rhEPO protein by glycoengineering has further increased abundance of N-glycosylation, which augments its erythropoietic activity *in vivo* by decreasing its metabolic clearance.

7.6 BOTANICAL DRUGS, THERAPEUTICS AND NUTRACEUTICALS

Plant biotechnology and medicine are being increasingly influenced by the idea of growing crops for health rather than for food or fiber. Novel botanical therapeutics (Table 7.1) includes plant-derived pharmaceuticals, multicomponent botanical drugs, dietary supplements, functional foods and recombinant proteins produced in plants. Many of these products can complement conventional pharmaceuticals in the treatment, prevention and diagnosis of diseases (Rates, 2001; Cordell, 2000; Raskin *et al.,* 2002).

Since times immemorial, people have been using herbs and other plants for healing. Plant products (particularly from seed plants) have been used to cure and prevent diseases throughout history, but more commonly in the 20th century when synthetic-chemistry-dominated pharmaceutical industry and replaced natural extracts with synthetic molecules some of which had no obvious connection to natural products. But the benefits of modern drugs have been felt largely in developed countries while developing countries continue to depend on ethno botanical remedies as their primary medicines.

Table 7.1: Categories of botanical therapeutics (Raskin *et al.,* 2002)

Therapeutics	Description	Examples
Drugs	Pharmaceuticals with single active ingredient from plants	Vinblastine. taxol, aspirin
Botanical drugs	Clinically validated and standardized phytochemical mixtures	None in the USA, several in clinical trial
Dietary supplements/ nutraceuticals	A plant component with health benefits	Garlic, echinacea extract
Functional/medicinal foods	A food engineered or supplemented to provide health benefits	Canola oil, golden rice, edible vaccine
Recombinant proteins	Pharmaceutical protein expressed in or isolated from plants	Several undergoing clinical trials

7.6.1. Single ingredient drugs

Plants have been an important source for the extraction of novel pharmacologically active drugs (Table 7.2). In the 1970s, about 25% of all drugs dispensed in the USA contained compounds derived from flowering plants, with an even greater proportion of phytochemicals used as drugs worldwide (Farnsworth, 1988). About 16% of drugs dispensed in the USA came from microbial and animal sources. The strongest recent impact of plant-derived drugs has been felt in the antitumour area where taxol, vinblastine, vincristine and camptothecin have enhanced the efficacy of chemotherapy against some deadly cancers.

Recent advances in combinatorial chemistry and computational drug design (Schreiber, 2000; Clark and Pickett, 2000; Adang and Hermkens, 2001) have lessened the importance of natural products in drug discovery. But according to Gentry (1993) and Mendelson and Balick (1995), many valuable plant-derived natural products still remain undiscovered or unexplored for their pharmacological activity. One major obstacle in using plants in pharmaceutical discovery, despite the great diversity of compounds they synthesize, is the lack of reproducible activity for >40% of plant extracts (Cordell, 2000). Further, the biochemical profiles of plants harvested at different times and locations vary. The current focus on high throughput drug discovery favors single compounds over mixtures and so is not compatible with complex plant extracts in which valuable bioactive molecules tend to be masked or obscured by pigments and polyphenols. It can take several months to isolate and structurally characterize a natural product from a plant extract. Various kinds of stress, locations, climates, physical and chemical elicitors, qualitatively and quantitatively modify the content of bioactive secondary metabolites (Shu, 1998; Ebel and Cosio, 1994; Facchini, 2001).

In the West, treatment of complex diseases has generally been based on the concept of using a single golden molecular bullet. This approach suffered a setback when problems of resistance to antimicrobial and anticancer drugs manifested. The multifactorial nature of many complex diseases, e.g., diabetes, heart disease and cancer, needs to be realized. Many such diseases cannot be attributed to a single genetic or environmental change but arises from a combination of genetic, environmental or behavioural factors (Kibertis and Roberts, 2002).

In contrast to the Western custom, traditional medicinal systems of the East have believed that complex diseases are best treated with complex combinations of botanical and non-botanical remedies properly adjusted to the individual patient and to the specific stage of the disease. This approach emphasizes the mutually potentiating effect of different components of complex medicinal mixtures. Conceivably, plants have adapted a similar strategy in their biochemical warfare with their own pathogens. Hsiang and Lewis (2000) showed that plants could produce families of structurally and functionally diverse antimicrobial compounds that act together to prevent the development of resistance.

The future of botanical drugs critically rests on two factors, sustaining a favorable regulatory environment and developing technologies for the efficient discovery, development and manufacture of botanical drugs. Today, most of the botanical drugs being developed come from ethnobotanical sources and have traditional medicinal uses. The difficulties in working with complex extracts and relatively small size of companies developing botanical drugs preclude heavy investments on new botanical drugs. Besides the creative and innovative technologies needed for new botanical drug discovery, manufacturing such drugs faces a challenge not encountered by the modern pharmaceutical industry: The process should involve 'seed-to-pill' and 'batch-to-batch' standardization of complex phytochemical mixtures-a challenge not encountered by chemical synthesis or single compound extraction processes. Since environmental and genetic factors might dramatically affect the biochemical compositions of plant extracts, production of botanical drugs will require genetically uniform monocultures of source plants grown in standardized conditions conducive to biochemical consistency and to optimize safety and efficacy in every crop. It is unlikely that field-grown plants can meet the quality standards for botanical drugs (Raskin *et al.*, 2002)

7.6.2. Botanical nutraceuticals

Many herbal dietary supplements or plant-derived materials provide health benefits. Some leading examples of plants as sources of nutraceuticals include *Allium sativum* (garlic), *Trigonella foenum-graecum* (fenugreek), *Silybum marianum* (milk thistle), *Panax ginseng* (ginseng), *Serenoa repens* (saw palmetto), *Aegle marmelos*, and *Azadirachta indica*. Whereas botanical drugs must undergo rigorous tests before they are marketed, the botanical supplements are generally exempted from strict regulatory standards, provided that the disease prevention, curing or detection claims are not made. In the same way, botanical cosmetic supplements (cosmeceuticals) (e.g., aloe extract) added to cosmetic and personal hygiene products attract relaxed regulatory control as a trade off for the absence of disease cure or prevention claims. Cosmeceuticals represent a relatively small segment of the total botanical supplement market.

Although the general public in Europe and North America is greatly attracted to the use of botanical supplements as natural and safe alternatives to conventional synthetic pharmaceuticals, actually there is very little scientific evidence behind this belief (Glaser, 1999). Although botanical supplements are sometimes blamed for weak efficacy, low safety, and potential interactions with prescribed drugs (Izzo and Ernst, 2001), data from clinical trials with the common botanical supplements suggest that most are at least mildly effective against a specific indication (Ernst, 2002; Kroll, 2001). It is conceivable that botanical supplements and functional foods may be potentially promising for a proactive preventive strategy that follows genetic identification of a medical risk (Raskin *et al.*, 2002).

7.6.3. Functional and medicinal foods

Raskin *et al.* (2002) defined and restricted functional foods to only those crops that are engineered or selected to deliver certain health benefits above and beyond those normally present in the natural crops. This definition excludes those botanical functional foods, which are produced by fortification, e.g. orange juice fortified with calcium.

Table 7.2: Some economically important plant pharmaceuticals or their precursors (Balandrin *et al.*, 1993; Raskin *et al.*, 2002)

Name	Alkaloid type	Source	Therapeutic use
Atropine[a], hyoscyamine, scopolamine	Tropane	*Solanaceous* spp.	Anticholinergic
Capsaicin	Phenylalkylamine	*Capsicum* spp.	Topical analgesic
Codeine, morphine	Opium	*Papaver somniferum*	Analgesic, antitussive
Colchicines	Isoquinoline	*Colchicum autumnale*	Antigout
Emitine	Isoquinoline	*Cephaelis ipecacuanha*	Antiamoebic
Galanthamine	Isoquinoline	*Leucojum aestivum L.*	Cholinesterase inhibitor
Nicotine	Pyrrolidine	*Nicotiana spp.*	Smoking cessation therapy
Pilocarpine	Imidazole	*Pilocarpus jaborandi*	Cholinergic
Quinine, quinidine	Quinoline	*Cinchona*	Antimalarial, cardiac depressant
Reserpine	Indole	*Rauwolfia serpentina*	Antihypertensive
Tubocurarine	Bis-benzyl isoquinoline	*Strychnos toxifera*	Skeletal muscle relaxant
Vinblastine, Vincristine	Bis-indole	*Catharanthus roseus*	Antineoplastic
Terpenes and steroids			
Artemisinin	Sesquiterpene lactone	*Artemisia annua*	Antimalarial
Diosgenin[a], stigmasterol[a],	Steroids	*Dioscorea spp.*	Contraceptives
Taxol, and other taxoids[a]	Diterpenes	*Taxus brevifolia*	Antineoplastic
Glycosides			
Digoxin, digitoxin,	Steroidal glycosides	*Digitalis* spp.	Cardiac tonic
Sennosides	Hydroxy anthracene glycodides	*Cassia angustifolia*	Laxative
Other and mixtures			
Ipecac	Mixture of ipecac alkaloids and other components	*Cephaelis ipecacuanha*	Emetic

[a]Most often used as precursors in chemical synthesis of final product

The best examples of engineered functional food are golden rice, healthy plant oils from modified oil crops, edible vaccines and plants with higher levels of essential vitamins and nutrients. Golden rice was engineered with two plant genes from *Narcissus pseudonarcissus* and one bacterial gene from *Erwinia uredovora* to synthesize β-carotene, a precursor of vitamin A, at quantities sufficient to reduce vitamin-A deficiency, which affects over 20 million children worldwide (Potrykus, 2001). The health-related goals of plant oilseed engineering are to enhance the content of healthy fatty acids while reducing unhealthy fatty acids in the four most important oilseed crops viz., soybean, oil palm, rapeseed and sunflower. Genetic engineering helped reduce levels of *trans*-unsaturated fatty acids and the ratio between omega-6 and omega-3 unsaturated fatty acids in some vegetable oils (Walmsley and Arntzen, 2000), thereby lowering the risk of heart disease (Bonetta, 2002). Plant-produced oral vaccines have proved highly effective as boosters to increase the immunity of humans to hepatitis B (Kong *et al.,* 2001; Thelen and Ohlrogge, 2002; Liu, 2001).

Some other notable advances in functional plant foods relate to increasing vitamin E content, selecting high lycopene or vitamin C tomatoes, metabolic engineering of legumes and tomatoes for enrichment in bioflavonoids, known for their antioxidant, anticancer and estrogenic properties; and possible uses of thioredoxin to decrease allergenicity of foods (Shintani and DellaPenna, 1998; Barber and Barber, 2002; Forkmann and Martens, 2001; Buchanan *et al.*, 1997). Consumers should, however, know that none of the genetically engineered plant derived functional foods selected, bred and marketed for high content of therapeutically active molecules such as isoflavones, antioxidants, folic acid and pigments are advertised and labeled as such in the USA. For proper labeling, we need effective technologies for characterizing pharmacologically active compounds in foods. Once the various scientific, regulatory and public acceptance issues are solved, the marketing of plant-based functional foods will receive a strong boost and functional foods with proven health benefits will lead to greater acceptance of crop genetic engineering that is now controversially used for crop protection (Raskin *et al*., 2002).

7.6.4. Recombinant proteins

Recombinant proteins such as antibodies, vaccines, regulatory proteins and enzymes constitute a rapidly growing segment of today's pharmaceutical industry. Several proteins are in clinical development and there is a shortage of industrial capacity to manufacture future recombinant drugs (Garber, 2001). Plants (such as tobacco) are promising biopharming systems for commercial production of pharmaceutical proteins (Table 7.2). Advantages of plants in this context are low cultivation cost, high biomass production, relatively fast 'gene to protein' time, low capital and operating costs, excellent scalability, eukaryotic post-translational modifications (i.e. glycosylation, folding, and multimeric assembly), low risk of human pathogens and endotoxins and a fairly high protein yield (Raskin *et al.,* 2002). Plants can be readily transformed by particle bombardment, electroporation, *Agrobacterium* or infection with modified viral vectors (Fischer and Emans, 2000).

Most major groups of human pharmaceutical proteins have been raised in several crops and model systems (e.g. maize, rice, wheat, soyabean, tomato, mustard, rape seed, tobacco and Arabidopsis), using stable nuclear and plastid transformations, as well as transient expression systems such as viruses. The highest yield of recombinant protein in plants is that achieved by chloroplast expression, but plastid expression suffers from the lack of glycosylation and correct folding of multimeric proteins whereas viral expression is problematic for complex proteins and could possibly introduce safety hazards. Seeds (corn) and tubers (potatoes) are excellent long-term storage compartments for recombinant proteins before purification, but have lower protein yield.

Two approaches can reduce the cost of downstream purification of plant produced proteins: oleosin-fusion technology for heterologous proteins produced in oilseeds, and rhizo- and phyllo-secretion platforms involving continuous, non-destructive recovery of a target protein from plant exudates (Borisjuk *et al.,* 1999; Hodgson, 1993; Raskin *et al.,* 2002). Although there is no plant-produced protein drug on the market today, some are in clinical trials. It is likely that plants will provide substantial benefits and savings for protein manufacturing over the alternative systems. Some companies are keenly interested in commercializing recombinant protein manufacturing in plants, with special emphasis on pharmacological applications (Hodgson *et al.,* 1993).

It appears that in the coming years, plants will attract increasing focus as valuable sources of human health products, in view of the unique properties of phytochemicals based on the (1) enormous power of plants to synthesize mixtures of structurally diverse bioactive compounds with multiple and mutually potentiating therapeutic effects; (2) their low-cost and highly scalable protein and secondary metabolite biomanufacturing capacity; (3) diminishing return of the single NCE (new chemical entity) approach to drug discovery and disease treatment and prevention; (4) cost limitation on the chemical synthesis of complex bioactive molecules; and (5) general belief that because of the history of human use and co-evolution of plants and humans, phytochemicals provide a safer and better approach to disease treatment and prevention (Raskin, 2002).

The growing popularity of botanical therapeutics could conceivably add more value to world agriculture than the more conventional application of plant biotechnology for yield enhancement. Crops that are likely to benefit the most include tobacco and corn as the major recombinant protein manufacturing crops along with several minor crops and medicinal plants that may become sources of future botanical therapeutics. Farmers that switch over to growing crops for health, rather than calories, may profit from greater margins and higher values enjoyed by the health industry and, consequently also our planet could become greener (Raskin *et al.,* 2002).

7.6.5. Vitamin E enriched plants

As vitamin E has been hailed as a panacea for such age-related diseases as cardiovascular disease and Alzheimer's disease, its demand has increased greatly and has, in turn, intensified research to increase vitamin E production from plant sources, and to bioengineer plants for enhanced vitamin E content (Grusak and DellaPenna, 1999; Ajjawi and Shintani, 2004).

Vitamin E comprises a group of potent antioxidant compounds known as tocols, especially α-tocopherol. Animals and humans harbour a highly specific protein that binds to α-tocopherol and ensures its preferential absorption and distribution throughout the body. Indeed α-tocopherol is the most potent form of vitamin E.

7.6.6. Plant sources of vitamin E

Plants are the primary sources of dietary vitamin E, oilseeds being the richest source, having total tocol levels ranging from 330 to 2,000 µg per gram of oil (Grusak and DellaPenna, 1999). Green vegetables are other good sources.

The enzymes, which catalyze the later steps of the tocopherol biosynthetic pathway such as tocopherol cyclase and the γ-tocopherol methyltransferase (γ-TMT), are important in determining tocopherol composition. Van Eenennaam *et al.*(2003) succeeded in over expressing the genes encoding γ-TMT and BMPQMT in soybean seeds so as to improve this important dietary source of vitamin E. Like many other oilseeds, soybeans do not accumulate α-tocopherol (the most potent form of vitamin E) but instead accumulate precursor tocopherol species (e.g., γ-tocopherol) with much lower vitamin E activity. But the over expression of the two-tocopherol methyl-transferases resulted in a 95% conversion of these inferior forms of vitamin E to α-tocopherol, which translated to a fivefold increase in vitamin E activity.

Expression of recombinant proteins in transgenic plants has been exploited for production of pharmaceuticals and industrial enzymes. Achieving high levels of expression depends on several factors such as genetics, metabolism and tissue processing during manufacturing. Molecular factors such as promoters, preferred codon usage, RNA stability factors and specific sub-cellular location are also crucial (Hood, 2004).

7.6.7. Engineering of vitamin C synthesis

Vitamin C (ascorbic acid or ascorbate) forms an essential part of the human diet. Most of our daily requirement of this vitamin comes from fruits and vegetables. Agius *et al.* (2003) identified a novel enzyme expressed in strawberry fruit that increases ascorbate concentration about two fold when expressed in the model experimental plant *Arabidopsis thaliana*. The results point to the feasibility of engineering ascorbate synthesis in plants by manipulating a pathway that normally plays a minor role.

Ascorbate functions in both plants and animals as an enzyme cofactor. In dioxygenases, for example, it is involved in the synthesis of hormones and of hydroxyproline, a constituent of collagen. Many of the symptoms of scurvy are related to impaired collagen synthesis (Halliwell, 1999; Smirnoff, 2003). Ascorbate is also an antioxidant that confers protection against reactive oxygen species, and could therefore help in preventing several diseases (e.g. cancer) and slow down ageing. In plants, ascorbate seems to function as an effective antioxidant. Low-ascorbate mutants are more sensitive to oxidative damage from ozone and high salinity (Smirnoff, 2001). It may also protect chloroplasts against photo-oxidative stress. This makes ascorbate an attractive target for metabolic engineering, with a view to increasing the nutritional value of fruits and vegetables, and to improve the stress resistance of crops.

Agius *et al.* (2003) identified a gene that encodes a D-galacturonic acid reductase (*GalUR*) quite similar to aldo-ketose reductases. It mediates the conversion of D-galacturonic acid to ascorbate in strawberry. Pectin, a polymer of D-galacturonic acid (in methylated and unmethylated form), is hydrolyzed during strawberry fruit ripening, and could be used as a source of D-galacturonic acid for ascorbate synthesis.

Expression of D-galacturonic acid reductase in *A. thaliana* increases leaf ascorbate content up to threefold, pointing to the potential of this gene for engineering ascorbate biosynthesis. Adding methyl D-galacturonic acid to *A. thaliana* cell suspension cultures effectively increases their ascorbate content (Davey *et al.*, 1999) indicating that *A. thaliana* has a reductase that can catalyze this reaction. At least one gene whose product resembles strawberry D-galacturonic acid reductase is found in *A. thaliana*. So far, attempts to engineer the D-mannose/L-galactose pathway by over expression of various pathway enzymes have failed. The ability to engineer ascorbate may enhance our understanding of how ascorbate helps to control reactive oxygen species and increases stress resistance (Smirnoff, 2003).

7.7. BIOPHARMING

Biopharming represents an experimental application of biotechnology involving the use of genetically engineered plants to produce pharmaceutical proteins and chemicals. In general companies engaged in biopharming do not disclose the types of chemicals that are being developed and rather treat this information as confidential, but in rare cases, the information has been disclosed. Plants have been engineered to produce contraceptive, potent growth hormones, a blood clotter, blood thinners, industrial enzymes and vaccines. Corn has been the most popular biopharm plant, followed by soybean, tobacco and rice. Hundreds of biopharm products are now in the pipeline, and numerous open-air field trials have already been conducted in unidentified locations in some countries.

There is some concern that if food becomes contaminated, these substances might possibly harm human health. Plants process proteins differently than animals or humans. This points to the possibility that a plant-produced "human" protein could be perceived as foreign by the body and elicit an allergic reaction, including life-threatening anaphylactic shock. In fact corn-grown industrial enzymes (trypsin and antitrypsin) are already known to be allergens. Trypsin corn was grown on hundreds of acres throughout the Corn Belt in 2002 .According to Giddings *et al.* (2001), "Biopharmaceuticals usually elicit responses at low concentrations and may be toxic at higher ones. Many have physiochemical properties that might cause them to persist in the environment or bioaccumulation in living organisms, possibly damaging non-target organisms."

7.7.1. Biopharm corn

In the USA, 500,000 bushels of soybeans destined for human consumption had to be quarantined due to contamination by corn genetically engineered to produce a pharmaceutical chemical. The corn was genetically modified to produce a protein not proven safe for human consumption, by ProdiGene, a leading biopharmaceutical company based in Texas. The biopharm corn was grown in a test plot in Nebraska. When ordinary soybeans were planted in 2002 in the same field, corn seeds from the test crop sprouted (Hickley, 2002). It is suspected that volunteer corn plants from previous year's biopharm field trial may have cross-pollinated with conventional corn surrounding the field. ProdiGene was forced to destroy 155 acres of conventional corn that may have been contaminated with the firm's biopharm crop (Hickley, 2002).

Recently, the Biotechnology Industry Organization (BIO) announced that its members would voluntarily stop growing pharmaceutical crops in several large corn producing states of USA so to reduce the chance of accidental contamination of food or animal feed. The grocery industry has expressed concerns that this proposal may not be able to prevent accidental contamination of food crops. Some trade groups want only non-food crops such as tobacco to be genetically engineered to produce drugs and industrial chemicals (Hickley, 2002).

7.7.2. Crop biopharming

In biopharming, corn and tobacco are being manipulated with recombinant DNA techniques to produce high-value-added pharmaceuticals. Such a genetic modification enables biopharming to make old plants to do new things economically. The plants being photosynthetic require only water and carbon dioxide as primary raw materials. The energy for the manufacturing process comes from the sun, increasing the acreage of a crop which requires much less capital than doubling the capacity of a factory; this makes biopharmed drugs less expensive than those produced industrially.

And yet, the biopharming technology is highly controversial because of the food industry's fears that gene transfer or 'volunteer' biopharmed plants in the field might contaminate the food supply with vaccines, drugs, or other products, thereby necessitating costly recalls and raising tricky liability issues. The food industry's concerns to protect our systems of food production and distribution are understandable but seem to be excessive and misplaced (Miller, 2003). In nature, gene flow is ubiquitous. Crop plants do have wild relatives somewhere on the earth, and some gene flow can occur if the two populations are grown close together. Although genes could be transferred from a crop that has been modified to synthesize a pharmaceutical, it is likely to occur only if the gene(s) involved confers some selective advantage on the recipient-an event that should be uncommon with biopharming, where most often the added gene (which directs the synthesis of large amounts of substances intended for nonagricultural purposes) will actually confer a selective disadvantage on the modified plant. In other words, plants that acquire the ability to produce the pharmaceutical would not compete successfully and proliferate.

Canola, the genetically improved rapeseed is an exceptional example of a critical need to segregate crops. The original rapeseed oil was quite harmful when ingested because of high levels of erucic acid. Through conventional plant breeding, low erucic acid genetic varieties of rapeseed were developed and canola oil is now widely consumed. But as high erucic acid rapeseed oil still is used as a lubricant and plasticizer, the high- and low-erucic acid varieties of rapeseed plants have to be carefully segregated in the field and thereafter. This can be done routinely and easily by farmers and processors.

In March 2003, the US Department of Agriculture (USDA) announced stringent new rules for biopharmed crops as demanded by the food industry and the radical environmental lobby. These new rules, according to Miller (2003), impose classical, highly prescriptive 'design' standards that do not take into account the actual risks of a given situation, but dictate one-size-fits-all requirements. The new rules are outlined below.

- Double the buffer zones, from a half-mile to a mile that biotechnology companies must maintain between their specialty corn and ordinary corn.

- Land used to grow biopharmed corn must lie fallow for a year; this appears an anti-environmental requirement because the absence of plant cover in a fallow promotes soil erosion.

- Separate planting, storage, and harvesting equipment be set aside for biopharmed crops, this rule can spell excessive and unnecessary expense.

By and large, the sophistication of modern agriculture "enables us to safely cultivate crops for food and for new pharmaceuticals, and to ensure that the two streams do not meet at least in a manner likely to cause injury, it appears that even in a worst-case scenario the likelihood of consumers suffering injury would be very low. Genetically modified plants for food and fiber have already been grown worldwide on more than 100 million acres annually. More than 60% of processed foods in the United States contain ingredients derived from recombinant DNA organisms. Not a single mishap has resulted in injury to any person or ecosystem. Such an enviable safety record of traditional agriculture, including the production of medicines points to the predictability and safety of recombinant DNA technology and its products (Miller, 2003).

7.7.3. Molecular farming of drugs in plants

High-value recombinant proteins can be produced on a large scale in plants. Several efficient plant-based expression systems are available and >100 recombinant proteins have already been produced through these. Avidin was commercially produced from transgenic maize (Hood *et al.*, 1997). Several plant-derived biopharmaceutical proteins currently in late stages of commercial development include antibodies, vaccines, human blood products, hormones and growth regulators (Fischer and Emans, 2000; Giddings, 2001). For these products, plants are more practical, safer and cheaper systems than microbial or animal cells or transgenic animals (Twyman *et al.*, 2003). However, certain constraints hinder the widespread use of plants as bioreactors. Quality and homogeneity of the final product and the challenge of processing plant-derived pharmaceutical macromolecules under good manufacturing practice conditions are crucial as also biosafety aspects.

One chief merit of transgenic plants for molecular farming is the comparatively low cost of large-scale production. Recombinant proteins have been estimated to be produced in plants at 2-10% of the cost of microbial fermentation systems and at 0.1% of the cost of mammalian cell cultures (Giddings, 2001; Twyman *et al.*, 2003). Another merit of plants as a production system for pharmaceutical proteins is their greater safety than both microbes and animals; this is because they generally lack human pathogens, oncogenic DNA sequences, and endotoxins. The protein synthesis pathway in plants is generally similar to that in animals, but there are some differences in post-translational modifications, particularly with respect to glycan-chain structure: plant-derived recombinant human proteins tend to have certain carbohydrate groups that are absent in mammals, but they lack the terminal galactose and sialic acid residues found on many native human glycoproteins. Even small differences in glycan structures can change the distribution, activity or longevity of recombinant proteins as compared with their native counterparts, and this can render such proteins immunogenic when administered to humans. Certain changes in the glycosylation pathway are needed to produce proteins with typical human glycan structures in plants (Warner, 2000). Two strategies for humanizing the glycan structures of recombinant human glycoproteins are: (i) the use of purified human β-galactosyl transferase and sialyl transferase enzymes for the *in vitro* modification of plant-derived recombinant proteins; and (ii) expression of human β (1,4)-galactosyltransferase in transgenic plants to produce recombinant antibodies with galactose-extended glycans (Bakker *et al.*, 2001).

7.8. MAXIMIZING YIELDS

One important consideration that determines the commercial viability of molecular farming is to have adequate recombinant protein yields, which can depend on the crop species used for production. Another relates to the expression technology that can help to achieve maximum yields of recombinant protein in any given species (Twyman *et al.*, 2003).

7.8.1. Protein targeting

The targeting of recombinant proteins to oil bodies or the plasma membrane is one way to facilitate isolation and purification. Another is sub-cellular targeting to increase the yield of recombinant proteins because the compartment in which a recombinant protein accumulates strongly influences the interrelated processes of folding, assembly and post-translational modification (Schillberg *et al.*, 2002). The secretory pathway seems to be a better compartment for folding and assembly than the cytosol, and is therefore advantageous for high-level protein accumulation (Schillberg *et al.*, 1999). Because many plant-derived recombinant proteins being developed happen to be human proteins, which can pass through the endomembrane system, this principle is applicable to antibodies and other proteins.

High levels of protein expression can occur when transgenes are introduced into the chloroplast or the nuclear genome. Chloroplast-based molecular farming has been well studied in tobacco. Human growth hormone, human serum albumin, cholera and tetanus toxin fragments, and thermostable xylanase have been successfully produced in tobacco chloroplasts (Twyman *et al.*, 2003). The chloroplast transgenic system give high yields and chloroplasts also offer biosafety advantages in terms of transgene containment, owing to maternal inheritance. But a disadvantage of this system is the inability of chloroplasts to carry out several post-translational modifications, including glycosylation. Also, biosafety concerns have arisen from the recent demonstration of horizontal gene transfer from the chloroplasts of transplastomic plants to bacteria (Kay *et al.*, 2002).

7.8.2. Species choice

Molecular farming can be practised in leafy species, seeds of legumes and cereals, fruit and vegetable crops, in fiber and oil crops. Tobacco has been one of the most widely chosen crops for the commercial production of recombinant proteins. Its merits include the well-established technology for gene transfer and expression, high biomass yield, prolific seed production and the existence of a large-scale processing infrastructure (Twyman *et al.*, 2003). Being neither a food nor a feed crop, tobacco is not likely to contaminate either the food or feed chains. And certain low-alkaloid varieties can be used for the production of pharmaceutical proteins; since these metabolites are often absent from tobacco cell suspensions, these suspensions can also be used to produce recombinant proteins. Other possible leafy crops for molecular farming may include alfalfa, soyabean and lettuce, of which alfalfa and soyabean fix atmospheric nitrogen and so reduce the need for chemical fertilizers. These legumes are used to produce recombinant antibodies (Khoudi *et al.,* 1999). Lettuce is also being tried as a production host for edible recombinant vaccines. But a major disadvantage of leafy crops is that recombinant proteins are synthesized in an aqueous environment and are sometimes quiet unstable, resulting in low yields. Also some biosafety concerns relate to the potential exposure of herbivores to pharmaceutical products expressed in leaves, and the leaching of recombinant proteins into the environment (Twyman *et al.,* 2003).

Unlike leafy crops, the expression of proteins in seeds allows long-term storage, even at room temperature. Antibodies expressed in seeds usually remain stable for a few years at ambient temperatures with no detectable loss of activity. But the overall yields of recombinant proteins in seed crops are lower than in leafy crops. The specific expression of recombinant proteins in seeds reduces exposure to herbivores and other non-target organisms. Some different crops attempted for seed-based production (Hood, 2002) include cereals (rice. wheat and maize) and legumes (pea and soyabean).

Expression of proteins in fruit and vegetable crops is sometime preferred because the edible organs can be consumed as uncooked, unprocessed or partially processed material, which makes them ideal for the production of recombinant subunit vaccines, nutraceuticals and antibodies designed for topical application. Potatoes constitute the system of choice for vaccine production (Tacket *et al.,* 2000) and have been used for the production of glucanases, diagnostic antibody-fusion proteins and proteins from human milk (Chong, 1997). Tomatoes have been used for the production of a rabies vaccine candidate, and to produce antibodies, although yields have been very low. Bananas are also good vehicles for edible vaccine. Use of fibre and oil crops (flax, cotton, and oilseed rape) can potentially offset the costs of recombinant protein production to some extent by secondary revenues from alternative products. Both fibre and oil tend to interfere with downstream processing so the above merit holds good mainly for proteins that do not need to be extensively purified.

7.8.3. Other plant-based systems

Plant-cell-suspension cultures have been used to produce recombinant proteins (Fischer *et al.,* 1999) and are particularly advantageous for the production of therapeutic proteins, which require sterile and defined production conditions (Doran, 2000). Indeed, a wide panel of recombinant antibodies has been expressed in tobacco and rice-cell-suspension cultures, including full-size immunoglobulins, Fab fragments, signal chains, biospecific antibody fragments and fusion proteins (Torres *et al.,* 1999; Twyman *et al.,* 2003). Target proteins can be secreted and captured from the culture supernatant, or they are released from the cells by disruption or mild enzymatic digestion (Twyman *et al.,* 2003).

Transgenic plants are promising vehicles for large-scale production of safe, pure and highly efficacious therapeutic proteins that are indispensable for the production of a wide range of biopharmaceuticals, including monoclonal antibodies (MAbs), enzymes, blood proteins and novel types of subunit vaccines for preventing infectious diseases (Peterson and Arntzen, 2004). MAbs and other biopharmaceuticals are some of the fastest growing classes of therapeutics, with >200 products now under clinical evaluation (Fischer *et al.,* 2003; Peterson and Arntzen, 2004). These products are intended to treat serious and chronic diseases such as arthritis, cancer, infection, inflammation and cardiovascular diseases.

Twelve therapeutic MAbs have been approved by the United States Food and Drug Administration. All these complex multi-subunit proteins are being produced in mammalian cell culture facilities. Seven plant-derived antibodies or antibody derivatives have reached advanced stages of product development (Ma *et al.,* 2003). It has been predicted that about 70 therapeutic

MAbs would be in the market by 2008, requiring production of >10 metric tons of MAbs annually. This will call for an unprecedented demand for additional manufacturing capacity for MAbs. In the face of the looming shortage in manufacturing capacity, plant-based biopharmaceuticals could be a cost-effective alternative to traditional cell-culture production of these therapeutic proteins. In fact, plant biotechnology may well provide an efficient, high capacity alternative to traditional cell-culture production (Peterson and Arntzen, 2004).

Examples of the proteins being produced in plants include *Streptococcus mutans* surface protein antigen A, hepatitis B surface antigen, *E. coli* heat-labile enterotoxin, human collagen, α-interferon and rabies virus glycoprotein (Sala *et al.*, 2003). Some plants that have been used for pharmaceutical protein production include tobacco, carrot, tomato, maize, potato, soyabean and rice.

There are several advantages of using plants to produce pharmaceutical proteins. Plants, particularly crop species, potentially offer highly cost-effective and efficient production for pharmaceuticals. Protein production in plant cells appears to be safer than traditional techniques because of the lack of contamination with extraneous viral or bacterial materials, mammalian pathogens and other animal cell culture contaminants. Still, it is important to critically evaluate the comparative biosafety and risk factors for plant based versus traditional production systems, before using plant systems.

The current focus on *L. lactis* is on the food-grade production of metabolites involved in flavour, texture and health (de Vos and Hugenholtz, 2004). *L. lactis* and other LAB have small genomes of ~2-3 Mb, many of which have either been fully sequenced or are being sequenced now. *L. lactis* has been exploited for producing large amounts of protein or peptide ingredients and therapeutic proteins (Kuipers *et al.*, 1997). This and other LAB have also been used in the production of glucose activated sugars, diacetyl, ethanol, acetaldehyde, and homoalanine.

Efficient rerouting of the glycolytic highway and its uncoupling of other catabolic pathways has been found to result in the high level production of both natural and novel end products in LAB. Knowledge of the main metabolic routes in LAB, in combination with the existing efficient genetic tools, the complete genome sequences and developing high-throughput genomics approaches should stimulate novel and rapid advances in the efficient design and practical evaluation of new metabolic engineering strategies aiming at the overproduction of relevant metabolites in these industrial bacteria (de Vos and Hugenholtz, 2004).

SUGGESTED READING

- Adang AE, Hermkens PH. *Curr Med Chem* 8, 985 (2001).
- Agius F, Gonzalez-Lamothe R, Cabaillero JL, *et.al. Nat Biotechnol* 21, 177 (2003).
- Ajjawi I, Shintani D. *Trend in Biotech* 22,104 (2004).
- Bakker H, Bardor M, Molthoff JW, et al. *PNAS* (USA) 98, 2899 (2001).
- Barber NJ, Barber J.*Prostate Cancer Prostatic Dis* (USA) 5, 6 (2002).
- Bonetta. L. *Na. Med* 8, 95 (2002).
- Borisjuk NV, Borisjuk LG, Logendra S, *et al. Nat Biotechnol* 17, 466 (1999).
- Bretthauer RK. *Trends in Biotech* 21,459 (2003).
- Bretthauer RK, Castellino FJ. *Biotechnol Appl Biochem* 30,193 (1999).
- Buchanan BB. *PNAS* (USA) 94,5372 (1997).
- Choi BK, Bobrowicz P, Davidson RC,*et al. PNAS* (USA) 100,5022 (2003).
- Chong DKX. *Transgenic Res* 6,289 (1997).

- Clark DE, Pickett SD. *Drug Discov Today* 5, 49 (2000).
- Cordell GA. *Phytochemistry* 55, 463(2000).
- Crout DH, Vic G. *Curr Opin Chem Biol* 2, 98 (1998).
- Daniell H. *Trends in Plant Biol* 6,226 (2002).
- Davey MW, Gilot C, Persiau G, etal. *Plant Physiol* 121,535(1999).
- de Vos WM, Hugenholtz J. *Trends in Biotech* 22,72 (2004).
- Doran PM. *Curr Opin Biotechnol* 11,199 (2000).
- Dove A. *Nat Biotechnol* 19, 913 (2001).
- Ebel J, Cosio EG. *Int Rev Cytol* 148,1 (1994).
- Elliott S, Lorenzini T,Asher S, *et al. Nat Biotechnol* 21,414 (2003).
- Endo T, Koizumi S. *Curr Opin Struct Biol* 10,536 (2000).
- Ernst E. *Ann Intern Med* 136, 42 (2002).
- Facchini PJ. *Annu Rev Plant Physiol Plant Mol Biol* 52,29 (2001).
- Farnsworth NR. Screening plants for new medicines. In *Biodiversity* Wilson, E.O. (ed.) 83-97, National Academy Press, Washington, D.C. (1988).
- Fazio F, Bryan MC, Blixt O, *et al. j Am Chem Soc* 124, 14397 (2002).
- Fischer R, Twyman RM, Schillberg S. *Vaccine* 21, 820 (2003).
- Fischer R, Drossard J, Commandeur U, *et al. Biotechno Appl Biochem* 30,101 (1999).
- Fischer R, Emans N. *Transgenic Res* 9, 279 (2000).
- Flitsch SL, Ulijn RV. *Nature* 421, 219 (2003).
- Forkmann G, Martens S. *Curr Opin Biotechnol* 2, 155 (2001).
- Fukui S, Feizi T, Galustian C, *et al. Nat Biotechnol* 20,1011 (2002).
- Garber K. *Nat Biotechnol* 19,184 (2001).
- Gemmill TR, Trimble RB. *Biochim Biophys Acta* 1426, 227 (1999).
- Gentry AH. *ACS Sympos Series* Washington, DC. *Amer Chem Soc* 534, 13 (1993).
- Giddings G. *Curr Opin Biotechnol* 12,450 (2001).
- GlaserV. *Nat Biotechnol* 17, 17 (1999).
- Grusak MA, DellaPenna D. *Plant Mol Biol* 50, 133 (1999).
- Halliwell B. *Trends Biochem Sci* 24, 255(1999).
- Hamilton SR, Bobrowicz P, Bobrowicz B, *et al. Science* 301,1244 (2003).
- Henrissat B, Davies GJ. *Plant Physiol* 124, 1515 (2000).
- Hickley E. *Global Pesticide Campaigner* 12, 16 (2002).
- Hirose M, Kameyama S, Ohi H. *Yeast* 19, 1191 (2002).
- Hodgson J. *Biotechnology* 11, 887 (1993).
- Hood EE, Witcher DR, Maddock S, *et al. Mol Breed* 3,291 (1997).
- Hood EE. *Enzyme Microbial Technol* 30, 279 (2002).
- Hood E E. *Trends in Biotech* 22, 53 (2004).
- Houseman BT, Mrkisch M. *Chem Biol* 9, 443 (2002).
- Hsiang P, Lewis K. *PNAS* (USA) 97,1433 (2000).
- Izzo AA, Ernst E. *Drugs* 61, 2175 (2001).
- Jahn M, Marles J, Warren RAJ, *et al. Angew Chem Int Ed Engl* 42, 352 (2003).
- Jakeman DL, Withers SO. *Can J Chem* 80, 866 (2002).
- Kay E,Vogel TM, Bertolla F, *et al. Appl Environ Microbiol* 68,3345 (2002).
- Khoudi H, Laberge S, Ferullo JM, *et al. Biotechnol Bioeng* 64, 135 (1999).

- Kibertis P, Roberts L. *Science* 296, 685 (2002).
- Kong Q, Richter L, Fang Yang Y, *et al. PNAS* (USA) 98,11539 (2001).
- Koury MJ. *Trends in Biotech* 21, 462(2003).
- Kroll DJ. *J Herbal Pharmacotherapy* 1, 3(2001).
- Kuipers OP, Ruyter PGGA de, Kleerebezem M, *et al.Trends in Biotech* 15,135 (1997).
- Liu K. In *Proc World Conf Oilseed Processing Utilization* Cancun, Mexico, 12-17 November 2000, 84-89 (2001).
- Ma J K, Drake PM, Christou P. *Nat Rev Genet* 4,794 (2003).
- Maeda YY, Chihara GL. *Nature* 229,634 (1971).
- Malet C, Planas A. *FEBS Lett* 440,208 (1998).
- Mendelson R, Balick MJ. *Econ Bot* 49,223(1995).
- Miller HI. *Nature Biotech* 21, 480 (2003).
- Nicola NA, Hilton DJ. *Adv Protein Chem* 52, 1 (1998).
- Perugino G, Trincone A, Rossi M, *et al. Trends Biotechnol* 22, 31(2004).
- Peterson RKD, Arntzen C J. *Trends Biotech* 22,64 (2004).
- Plante OJ, Palmacci ER, Seeberger PH. *Science* 291,1523 (2001).
- Potrykus I. *Plant Physiol* 125,1157 (2001).
- Raskin I., Ribnicky, DM, Komarnytsky S, *et al. Trends Biotech* 20,522 (2002).
- Rates S M K. *Toxicon* 39, 603 (2001).
- Sala F, Manuela Rigano M, Barbante A, *et al.Vaccine* 21,803 (2003).
- Schillberg S, Zimmermann S, Voss A, et. al. *Transgenic Res* 8,255 (1999).
- Schillberg S, Emans N, Fischer R. *Phytochem Rev* 1,45 (2002).
- Schreiber SL. *Science* 287,1964 (2000).
- Sears P, Wong CH. *Science* 291, 2344 (2001).
- Seeberger PH, Haase WC. *Chem Rev* 100, 4349 (2000).
- Shintani D, DellaPenna D. *Science* 11 2098 (1998).
- Shu YZ. *J Nat Prod 61*, 1053 (1998).
- Smirnoff N. *Phil Trans R Soc Lond* 355, 1455 (2001).
- Smirnoff N. *Nat Biotechnol* 21, 134 (2003).
- Tacket CO, Mason HS, Losonsky G, *et al. J infect Dis* 182, 302 (2000).
- Thelen JJ, Ohlrogge JB. *Metab Eng* 4,12 (2002).
- Torres E, Vaquero C, Nicholson L, *et al. Transgenic Res* 8, 441 (1999).
- Twyman RM, Stoger E, Schillberg S, *et al. Trends Biotech* 21, 570 (2003).
- Varki A. *Glycobiology* 3, 97 (1993).
- Eenennaam VAL, Lincoln K, Durrett TP, *et al. Plant cell* 15, 3007 (2003).
- Walmsley AM, Arntzen CJ. *Curr Opin Biotechnol* 11, 126 (2000).
- Wang D, Coscoy L, Zylberberg M, *et al. PNAS* (USA) 99, 15687 (2002).
- Wang D, Liu S, Trummer BJ, *et al. Nat Biotechnol* 20, 275 (2002).
- Warner TG, Metabolic engineering glycosylation: biotechnology's challenge to the glycobiologist in the new millennium. In: *Carbohydrates in Chemistry and Biology,* Ernst, B. *et al. (*Eds) 1043-1064, Wiley-VCH, Weinheim (2000).
- Witczak ZJ. *Curr Med Chem* 6,165 (1999).
- Zopf D, Roth S. *Lancet* 347, 1017 (1996).

8

CELL REPLACEMENT, STEM CELLS, CLONING AND REGENERATIVE MEDICINE

8.1. NUCLEAR TRANSPLANTATION AND CELL REPLACEMENT THERAPY

Half a century ago, Briggs and King (1952) showed that normal hatched tadpoles could be obtained by transplanting the nucleus of a blastula cell to the enucleated eggs of *Rana pipiens*. Since then two general principles have emerged from work in amphibian and mammals: (i) Conservation of the genome during cell differentiation-a small percentage of adult or differentiated cells have totipotent nuclei, and a much higher percentage of cells committed to one pathway of cell differentiation have multipotent nuclei; and (ii) the remarkable reprogramming capacity of cell, especially egg and cytoplasm. The eventual identification of reprogramming molecules and mechanisms could facilitate a route towards cell replacement therapy in humans. The work paved the way to a direct test of the genetic equivalence of somatic cell nuclei in development and cell differentiation.

Briggs and King (1952) noted surprisingly that, whereas blastula nuclei supported normal tadpole development in up to 40% of all tests, gastrula nuclei were much less successful. Already in early development, nuclei were found to undergo some change restricting their ability to substitute for a zygote nucleus, and this loss of developmental capacity was heritable (Smith, 1965). It emerged that nuclear transplantation from gastrulae and later stages usually resulted in chromosome damage, whereas nuclei from blastula cells were not much damaged, probably owing to the slowing cell cycle as cells differentiate and to other changes in the course of cell specialization.

Fischberg *et al.* (1958) achieved successful nuclear transfer in another frog, *Xenopus*. Several publications described the developmental capacity of nuclei transplanted from the endoderm lineage using donors from blastulae up to the intestinal epithelium of feeding larvae, confirming the conclusion of Briggs and King (1952) that the ability of transplanted nuclei to promote normal development declines as development progresses. The main conclusion was totally different-some normal development could be obtained from nuclei of even the most differentiated cells pointing to the possibility that the process of cell differentiation may not necessarily require any stable change to the genetic constitution of a cell and may depend on changes in the expression and not on the content of the genome (Gurdon and Byrne, 2003). Although, an adult animal could not be obtained by nuclear transplantation from the cell of an adult frog, the multipotent properties of nuclei from many different adult organs, e.g., lung, heart, and liver, were demonstrated when Laskey and Gurdon (1970) found that 1-2% of transplanted nuclei from all these adult sources resulted in nuclear transplant embryos that reached feeding larval stages.

8.1.1. Mammals

One major problem in achieving somatic cell nuclear transfer in mammals is the much smaller size of the mammalian egg as compared to the larger volume of an amphibian egg (Gurdon and Byrne, 2003). Development of appropriate micromanipulation techniques that could handle, enucleate and fuse a very small mammalian egg with a single somatic cell eased this difficulty in mammals (Lin, 1971).

Bromhall (1975) was the first to report development to the morula stage following mammalian nuclear transfer; he used both microinjection and Sendai virus induced fusion to transfer labeled rabbit morula cell nuclei into enucleated rabbit eggs. Embryos were produced that arrested during cleavage, but a few did reach the morula stage. McGrath and Solter (1984) obtained live mice after transferring a zygote donor nucleus into an enucleated zygote. But no successful development occurred when they used donor cell nuclei from later developmental stages. The primary problem with early murine nuclear transfer experiments may have been that they transferred donor nuclei into enucleated zygotes rather than into unfertilized eggs (Gurdon and Byrne, 2003).

Willadsen (1986) used electro fusion or Sendai virus to fuse cells of 8 to 16 cell-embryos into enucleated eggs of sheep and obtained two healthy cloned sheep. Nuclear transfer using embryonic donor cell nuclei was also later successful in rabbits, pigs, mice, cows and monkeys (Sims and First, 1994). Cloning technology started attracting much interest in the mid 1990s with exciting practical applications (Campbell *et al.*, 1996; Wilmut *et al.*, 1997). Nuclear transfer was carried out with the nuclei of an established cell line, originating from a day 9 embryo that had differentiated *in vitro*. These cells were induced to enter a quiescent state before electro fusing them into enucleated sheep eggs. These nuclear transfers resulted in two healthy cloned sheep (Campbell *et al.*, 1996). In 1997, the same technique was used with nuclei of cultured adult mammary gland cells and a single cloned sheep "Dolly" was produced (Wilmut *et al.,* 1997). Since then many other mammals have been cloned from adult donor cell nuclei and include cows, goats and pigs.

In general, the efficiency of mammalian nuclear transfer experiments is quite similar to that obtained in amphibian. Less than 1% of all nuclear transfer from adult or differentiated cells results in seemingly normal offspring although some developmental and physiological abnormalities occur in a small proportion of the foetuses obtained (Gurdon and Byrne, 2003). Many of these abnormalities are not inherited.

8.1.2. Nuclear programming

Complete nuclear programming occurs in only a small percentage of nuclear transfer from differentiated cells. The causative agent is change of cytoplasm and this point to the possibility of identifying molecules having reprogramming activity (Rossant, 2002). Conceivably, this information might be used to improve the efficiency of reprogramming by egg cytoplasm. Some day it may also be possible to use molecules derived from eggs to convert adult somatic cells directly into multipotent embryonic cells for the purpose of cell replacement (Gurdon and Byrne 2003).

Although somatic cell nuclei transplanted to enucleated eggs undergo rapid morphological changes, changes in gene expression have not been recorded before the 5000-cell blastula stage in amphibian (5 h) or before the 4-cell stage in mice (36 h), when new zygote gene expression starts. Two principles emerging from the work on nuclear transplantation are the conservation of the genome during cell differentiation and the ability of cell cytoplasm to reprogram gene activity and hence to redirect cell differentiation. These principles are indispensable in the context of reproductive and therapeutic cloning; if either condition did not prevail, cloning would not be possible (Gurdon and Byrne 2003). Reproductive cloning means the production of adult animals by transplantation of somatic cell nuclei to eggs. It is of potential value in animal husbandry, and for the preservation of rare genetic stocks (Cibelli *et al.*, 2002).

Therapeutic cloning, on the other hand, involves the production by nuclear transfer of cells for replacement; it may have many potential benefits if applied to humans. It can provide donor cells of the same genetic constitution to the recipient, avoiding the need for immune-suppression that is usually required when donor and recipient are not genetically matched. Therapeutic cloning may be expected to follow the route of deriving embryonic stem cells from nuclear transplant embryos and could ease the supply of such cells to a recipient in need of replacement cells (Gurdon and Byrne 2003).

8.1.3. Stem cells

A long cherished goal of modern biomedicine has been to repair damaged organs. Stem cells have the potential to form a wide variety of different cell types and are considered to be essential to this endeavor. But the results of some recent studies have cast doubts on the plasticity of adult stem cells;

also there are strong ethical problems associated with deriving pluripotent embryonic stem cells from human embryos. An alternative approach is to stimulate the damaged organ to regenerate or heal itself. Adoption of this strategy has successfully demonstrated that the heart of the adult zebra fish *Danio rerto* – a model for vertebrate development – can regenerate (Scott and Stainier, 2002).

Mammals including humans show very few examples of regeneration; most notably the ability of liver hepatocytes to regenerate damaged liver tissue. Regenerative capacities are broader in animals such as the salamander, newt, hydra and flatworm. Flatworms can generate an entirely new animal from a small fragment of tissue. Regeneration of fins, spinal cord and retina is known to occur in the zebra fish (Scott and Stainier, 2002). To find out whether the adult zebra fish heart also has the capacity for regeneration, the apex of the ventricle, representing roughly 20% of its volume was surgically removed. Whereas mouse hearts subjected to similar damage induced by freezing do not regenerate, this experiment revealed that while at first initial fibrin deposits formed at the wound site in zebra fish hearts, further scarring and collagen deposition characteristic of damaged mammalian hearts did not occur. Instead, cardiomyocytes, the specialized muscle cells of the heart infiltrated the injured area and sealed off the wound. Remarkably, 60 days after surgery the zebra fish hearts appeared fairly normal.

The idea that life can exist at physical and chemical extremes thought previously to be well beyond the capabilities of life has tremendous implications for fields as dissimilar as biodiversity and biotechnology. The environmental space of life on earth defines for humans the minimum limits for life. Stem cells are undifferentiated cells that divide to multiply and to produce more specialized cell types. There are many cases in botany and zoology in which one daughter cell maintains the stem cell characteristic while the other daughter differentiates. For example, in early division of embryos of the nematode *Caenorhabditis elegans*, the time taken by different daughter cells to divide is very different. Conceivably some similar cell division pattern may underlie the development mathematical patterns in plants.

The cell proposal predicts that floral meristems growing spirally and dividing asymmetrically will produce dexter and sinister arrangements in equal proportion. Randomness is expected in binary systems in which no bias exists (Klar, 2002). Stem cells are believed to function by dividing to generate an identical daughter cell and a cell that becomes more specialized. This confers upon stem cells the unique ability to perpetuate itself while continually replenishing tissues throughout the life of an organism. This ability involves a distinctive asymmetry in their division, such that when a stem cell divides, it gives rise to both an exact copy to itself and a new type of cell that is destined to differentiate into mature cells of the tissue.

One strong hurdle in the study of how stem cells divide has been their elusive nature. Because these cells are rare and physically resemble their differentiated daughter cells they cannot be easily recognized in a tissue. The identity of stem cells in most tissues continues to be debated. Embryonic stem cells are well characterized but they exist before tissues form. This identity crisis has been resolved in a few cases, e.g., neuroblasts and germ line stem cells (GSCs) in *Drosophila* and ventricular zone progenitor cells in the brains of mammalian embryos (Lin, 2002). In flies, a neuroblast divides asymmetrically to renew itself and to produce a smaller ganglion mother cell which in turn generate specific nerve cells. In fly ovaries, germ line stem cells are always in contact with a subset of signaling "cap" cells and these stem cells also divide asymmetrically. Such oriented asymmetric division also occurs in germ line stem cells in the fly testis. Yamashita *et al.,* (2003) observed stem cell division in fly testis, confirming the orientation and asymmetry of division (Lin, 2003).

8.2. STATUS OF HUMAN EMBRYONIC STEM CELLS IN EUROPE

In Europe there are four different policies relating to the application of stem cells in humans. United Kingdom permits the generation and use of human embryonic stem (ES) cells as well as therapeutic cloning with certain restrictions. The Netherlands permits the generation and use of human ES cells but forbids therapeutic cloning. In Germany, the generation of new human ES cell line and therapeutic cloning are forbidden but, under exceptional conditions, the use of existing human ES cell lines is allowed for research only. Ireland and Austria forbid all generation and use of human ES cells and therapeutic cloning. In the light of these different models, the European Union (EU) Research Commissioner has framed guidelines for the funding of human ES cell research. The generation of new embryos solely for the purpose of producing new human ES cell lines is not permitted. But a compromise permits scientists to create new human ES cell lines (Gruss, 2003).

Stem cell research is progressing so rapidly that new discoveries may enable us to avoid some of the current ethical problems. For instance, the sacrifice of surplus embryos is usually invoked by opponents to the generation of new cell lines; the ethical issue here is whether the death of supernumerary embryo is more important than its death for its later use for the benefit of seriously ill patients. Some recent but surprising results suggest that there may be new ways of generating stem cells. ES cells from mice can differentiate, in culture condition, into oocyte like cells that are potential recipients for nuclear transfer, this could not only reduce the need for oocyte donations but should also allow the generation of patient specific stem cells that would not be rejected by the patient's immune system (Gruss, 2003).

In England, a stem cell line from human embryonic cells has been successfully cloned by a team at King's College London. This feat can usher in an era of much cheaper and readily available stem cells. The team used 58 embryos to generate three stem cell populations, out of which two were lost early but the third could be saved. The success has been attributed to the use of donated embryos that had been screened for genetic disorder, rather than discarded embryos from in vitro fertilization procedures. The first human ES cell lines were created in 1998. Only nine lines were available across the world and they are extremely expensive. ES are extremely useful because they carry the potential to develop into any type of cell in the body. Cell replacement therapy can effectively treat disease such as diabetes and Parkinson's – the major difficulty has been to produce enough cells to treat even one patient. An additional ES cell line can go a long way in greatly increasing the number and availability of these cells.

Although there has been some progress in understanding how extrinsic signaling regulates stem cell self-renewal, very little is still known about how cell autonomous gene regulation controls this process. In *Drosophila* ovaries, GSCs divide asymmetrically to produce daughter GSCs and cystoblasts, the latter of which develop into germ line cysts. GSCs can readily be distinguished from their differentiation daughters by their position in the ovary and by their morphology. Further, differentiating daughters of GSCs develop into germ line cysts that form a linear array of egg chambers according to their birth order; this makes it easy to trance GSC division. Although GSCs themselves come from primordial germ cells (PGCs) which are initially made in the posterior region of the embryo, during subsequent embryogenesis PGCs migrate to the embryonic gonads, where they proliferate without differentiation during larval development. Eventually, they become GSCs at the larval/ pupal transition (Lin, 2004).

Wang and Lin (2004) showed that removing the translational repressor Nanos (Nos) from either GSCs or their precursors, the primordial germ cells (PGCs), causes both cell types to differentiate into germ line cysts. Thus, Nos is essential for both establishing and maintaining GSCs by preventing their precocious entry into oogenesis. These functions seem to be achieved by repressing the translation of differentiation factors in PGCs and GSCs. The Nos is a family of translation repressors that has evolutionary conserved function in PGC migration and survival during early embryogenesis. Still the function of Nos in PGC proliferation, GSC establishment and oogenesis is mostly unexplored. It is continuously needed for both the establishment and self-renewal of GSCs and it does this by preventing PGCs and GSCs from prematurely entering the oogenic pathway. Translational regulation maintains the fate of stem cells and their precursors by preventing the precocious activation of differentiation pathway.

8.3. GERM LINE STEM CELLS

The testis cell transplantation method is a powerful approach to study the biology of the male germ line stem cell and its microenvironment – the stem cell niche. In mice germ line stem cells have been studied in great detail as they can be identified at about seven days of gestation as a group of about 100 PGCs arising from embryonic ectoderm. Over the next few days, PGCs give rise to about 20,000 cells while migrating to the genital ridges. In females they undergo meiosis and become oocytes – this ends their stem cell potential. In males, they enter foetal seminiferous tubules, become gonocytes and stop dividing (Brinster, 2002). Unlike oocytes, gonocytes retain their stem cell potential. Following birth, the gonocytes migrate to the seminiferous tubule basement membrane where they differentiate into spermatogonial stem cells (SSCs). These SSCs share two characteristics with other adult stem cell: they can both self renew and provide daughter cells which differentiate into one or more terminal cell types. Stem cells traditionally have been defined by function and unequivocal identification is based on their abilities to regenerate the appropriate system of the body. Transplantation assays have been developed fully only for hematopoietic stem cells (HSCs) and SSCs; stem cells of other self renewing systems are tentatively identified by such characteristics as morphology, surface markers, and the ability to differentiate into two or more cell types (van der Kooy and Weiss, 2000; Spradling *et al.*, 2001).

For testis cell transplantation, the basic procedure involves harvesting testis cells from a fertile male and microinjecting the cell suspension into seminiferous tubules of an infertile recipient in which colonies of donor-derived spermatogenesis are established. In rats, the differentiation and meiotic process that begins with division of a single stem cell theoretically can produce 4096 spermatozoa, although as a result of apoptosis the efficiency does not exceed 50 %. In the adult human male this process generates about 1000 spermatozoa each time the heart beats, and every sperm contains a different complement of paternal genes, thereby generating the male half species diversities (Brinster, 2002).

The assay provides a powerful mechanism to study the biology of the stem cell. These studies are otherwise difficult because only about 1 in 5000 mouse testis cells is a stem cell and they have no distinguishing morphological or biochemical characteristics. Purification and characterization of the stem cell have been facilitated by use of specific antibodies and fluorescence – activate cell sorting, followed by transplantation of selected cell population (Shinohara *et al.*, 2000). Stem cell transplantation also enables study of the stem cell niche (Shinohara *et al.*, 2001). Stem cells compete for niches and the number of both stem cells and available niches increases with age and testis growth. The interaction between stem cell and niche, particularly the signals that determine whether a cell will remain self-renewing or differentiate, deserves study.

Testis cell transplantation is also a useful approach to determine the role of the germ cell and Sertoli cell in natural or induced defects of spermatogenesis. Germ cell defects may be corrected by genetic modification of the stem cell during the transplantation procedure. Fertility in mice with functional stem cells and a Sertoli cell defect already has been restored by microinjecting a viral vector with a corrective gene into the seminiferous tubules (Kanastu-Shinohara *et al.*, 2002).

Using testis cell transplantation, the immense regenerative capability of the spermatogenesis process has been revealed by experiments in which fewer than 200 transplanted stem cells, less than 1% of the number present in a normal wild type testis, restored fertility in a mouse with a stem cell defect (Ogawa *et al.*, 2000). This efficiency and the generation of normal spermatogenesis after testis cell transplantation between rats that are not immunologically compatible points to the potential clinical application of the technique in animals and human. Spermatogonical stem cells happen to be the only cells in the postnatal animal that undergo self-renewal throughout life and transmit genes to subsequent generations. Ability to cryopreserve culture and transplant these unique cells provides a powerful system to study stem cell biology, preserve individual genomes and modify germ lines (Brinster, 2002).

8.4. CONTROL OF STEM CELL FATE BY SYNTHETIC SMALL MOLECULES

While stem cells may be of help in the treatment of certain degenerative diseases such as Parkinson's disease and diabetes (Kim *et al.*, 2002), hurdles such as host rejection, control of stem cell fate and availability of stem cells need to be crossed before their therapeutic potential is realized. Stem cell differentiation is controlled by both intrinsic regulators and the extracellular environment and is typically controlled *ex vivo* by cell culture manipulation with "cocktails" of growth factors, signaling molecules, and/or by genetic manipulation. Small cell permeable molecules e.g., retinoic acid (RA) are extremely useful in inducing differentiation of various progenitor cells such embryonic stem cells (ESCs), neural stem cells (NSCs) and mesenchymal stem cells (MSCs) (Ding *et al.*, 2003). Since the action of RA is pleiotropic there is need to identify other small molecules that permit precise regulation of stem cell self renewal and differentiation as well as the dedifferentiation of lineage – committed cell, which could eventually facilitate therapeutic applications of stem cells (Rosania *et al.*, 2000).

Ding *et al.* (2003) attempted to identify small molecules that induce the selective differentiation of stem cells to neurons. Mouse and human ESCs (Zhang *et al.*, 2001) are able to differentiate *in vitro* into neural progenitor cells which can further mature into neurons and glial cells. Since kinases may have an important role in these processes, in view of their involvement in many cell cycle and development events, combinatorial libraries of heterocyclic compounds designed around many kinases directed molecular scaffolds were screened. From these libraries, small molecules were discovered that induce neuronal differentiation in pluripotent murine embryonic carcinoma (EC) cells and ESCs.

A high throughput phenotypic cell based screen of kinase directed combinatorial libraries led to the discovery of TWS 119, a 4,6 di-substituted pyrrolopyrimidine that can induce neurogenesis in murine ESCs. The target of TWS 119 was shown to be glycogen synthase kinase-3β (GSK-3β). This study provides evidence that GSK-3β is involved in the induction of mammalian neurogein ESCs. This and similar other molecules are expected to enhance the understanding of molecular mechanisms that control stem cell fate and may ultimately prove useful for *in vivo* stem cell biology and therapy (Moon *et al.*, 2002; Aubert *et al.*, 2002).

The isolation of pluripotent human embryonic stem cells (HESCs) from the inner cell mass of blastocyst – stage embryos has generated hopes for the possible use of these cells in therapeutic transplantation in view of the following reasons: (i) while remaining undifferentiated, these cells appear to have an unlimited capacity to propagate in culture condition (Thomson *et al.,* 1998; Reubinoff *et al.*, 2000; Hochedlinger and Jaenisch, 2003); (ii) differentiation can be induced to raise cells of the three embryonic germ layers. When the cells are transferred to non adherent plates in the laboratory they undergo differentiation to form embryoid bodies (EBs) (Itskovitz–Eldor *et al.*, 2000). Alternatively, they can differentiate in vivo by injection into severe combined immune-deficient (SCID) mice in which they develop into teratoma (germ cell tumors that can contain several different types of tissue). Unfortunately, none of these protocols has yielded pure cell lines suited for therapeutic use: rather, a mixture of cell types has resulted. The primary goal of laboratories working with HESCs is to direct their differentiation and purify specific cell types, e.g., neurons, trophoblasts, endothelial cells, cardiomyocytes, hematopoietic precursors and hepatocyte like cells have been successfully developed (Drukker and Benvenisty, 2004).

The current sources for transplantable cells are adult– and fetal–derived cells. But HESCs derivatives are more suitable for clinical applications in view of the relative ease with which HESCs can be maintained in culture conditions and availability of a wide range of genetic manipulation techniques for HESCs. Genetic manipulation and gene targeting in mouse embryonic stem cells (MESCs) has greatly advanced the study of mammalian development and disease. This raises the hope that similar advances in the manipulation of HESCs e.g. transfection by chemical reagents, electroporation and infection by viral vectors will also be crucial in cell therapy and in the analysis of human embryogenesis, provided that several critical issues like bio-safety are addressed before using HESC derivatives in the clinic. The transplanted cells must contain only purified differentiated cells. Any cell can potentially cause tumors. Transplanted cells must undergo rigorous screening to exclude the chance of infectious agents from the cell lines or feeder cells being transferred to the patient. It is also possible that transplanted HESC derivatives may be destroyed by the patient immune system. To allow their clinical use, differentiation protocols for HESCs have to be developed and safety standards need to be met. The cells should improve symptoms without adverse side effects and their immune rejection must be overcome. Profiling of the immune antigens expresses molecules of the major histocompatibilty complex. Drukker and Benvenisty (2004) proposed methods of overcoming the rejection of human embryonic stem cells after transplantation. HESCs carry the potential as the ultimate cell source for regenerative medicine. However, to exploit this potential, the immune rejection processes that can develop following transplantation of HESCs to unmatched patients need to be carefully analyzed and studied. The most important molecules, which activate rejection, are the MHC molecules (Gould and Auchincloss, 1999) some of which do express at low levels on HESCs. Therefore, rejection of HESCs derivatives because of allo-recognition by the immune system can pose a grave threat to clinical use of these cells. To circumvent rejection, the cell may possibly be transplanted into immune privileged sites where immune responses tend to be restricted (Drukker and Benvenisty, 2004).

8.5. FUSION

Sperm and eggs fuse together selectively, not randomly with any other cell type (Fig. 8.1). Some viruses express fusion proteins that enable them to penetrate mammalian cells. Cells transformed by polyoma virus can fuse spontaneously are repaired by the fusion into each cell of single nucleus, undifferentiated cell (myoblasts) with other cells *in vivo*. Fusion has long been known to be advantageous for specialized cell types and primitive organisms; the new surprise now is that stem cells derived from adults might use fusion as a mechanism to change their fate. Some recent findings in tissue culture have shown that embryonic stem cells can fuse either with the precursors of neuronal cells or with adult bone marrow cells; this has started a new debate and spawned the important idea that fusion could be a promising means by which some cells might be 'reprogrammed' for a different function in adulthood (Blau, 2002).

The new work suggests that cell fusion may well be a mechanism that induces adult bone marrow-derived cells to change their morphology and activate new genes. Fusion of stem cells might also possibly serve as a means of supplying cells with new genes, such as tumor suppressor genes, or of correcting that continues to function throughout our lives. Conceivably much more damage occurs in differentiated tissues than was believed previously because bone marrows derived cells gain access to the injured cells and restore them-at least up to a point. Beyond that point, when the balance between damage and repair shifts and fusion cannot cope with the demand, disease manifests itself. Cell fusion has long been known to result in effective reprogramming of cells.

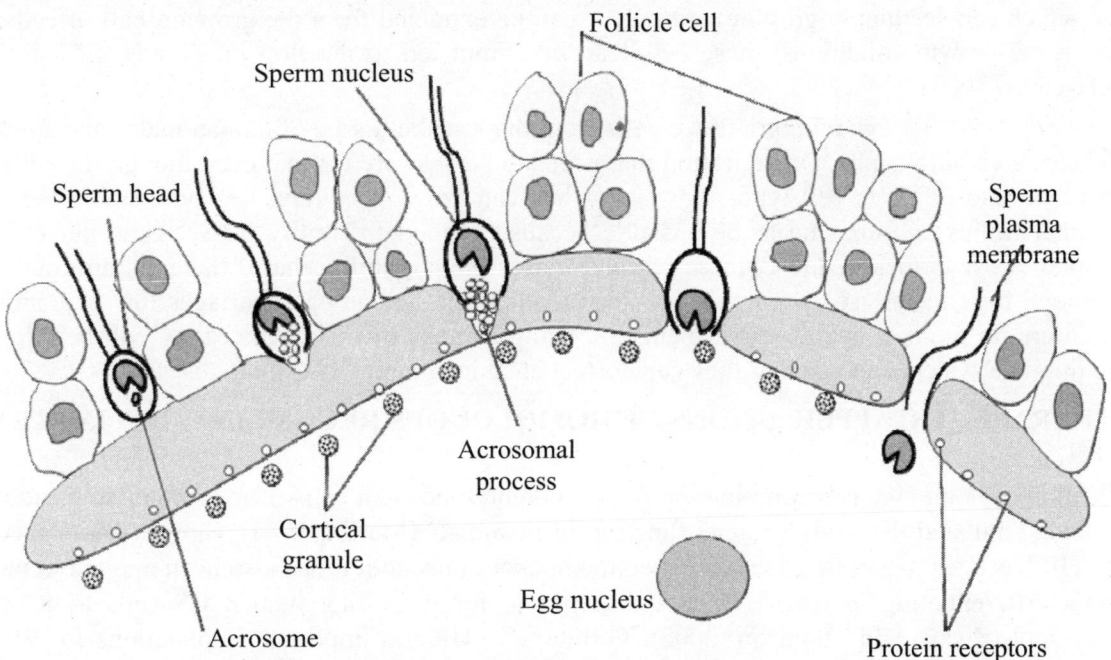

Fig: 8.1 Schematic representation of fusion of sperm with oocyte

Differentiation is not fixed and irreversible; the phenotype of a differentiated cell is plastic, dynamic and determined by the balance of regulators at any given time. The discoveries of genetic reprogramming in different cell systems have changed our concept of differentiation: it is now viewed as an active rather than passive process. Understanding its underlying mechanism should allow increased efficiency of fusion, which might lead, for instance, to the rescue of muscle cells in muscular dystrophies.

When the signals and underlying mechanisms are better understood, adult bone marrow derived cells could be genetically engineered to deliver genes to specific targets, making possible a new form of gene therapy. The fusion that takes place when sperm meets egg, the beginning of life, may also underlie a process of repair in adulthood that helps to maintain life (Blau, 2002).

In China, scientists have reprogrammed human cells by fusing them with rabbit eggs emptied of their genetic material. They have also extracted stem cells from the resulting embryo (Dennis, 2003). These derived stem cells could provide biomedical researchers with an alternative to stem cell lines extracted from human embryos, provided that these cells show the same ability as human embryonic stem cells to grow indefinitely in culture (Chen *et al.*, 2003). This work is likely to revive debate on the ethics of cross species reprogramming. But having the data available for public discussion should help both the researchers and regulators to decide what kind of cross-species work needs to be perused.

Reprogramming of adult cells to revert to the embryonic state can potentially help in growing new cells and tissues to replace those lost to aging and disease. Using an individual's own cells, in therapeutic cloning, could eliminate problems associated with the immune system rejecting the cell therapy. To re-program an adult cell, it can either be fused with, or have its nucleus injected into a de-nucleated egg. The reconstituted cell is then coaxed into dividing as if it were an embryo, with all memory of its previous life as a liver, skin or kidney cell erased. After about a week, embryonic stem cells – which can seemingly grow indefinitely – can be extracted from the growing ball of cells. By changing the growth conditions, these cells can be stimulated to develop into many different cell types (Dennis, 2003).

Chen *et al.* (2003) have reprogrammed cells from the foreskin tissue of human males and from the facial skin of an old woman. One question that needs to be answered is that even though the cells can differentiate into different cell types, how long they can grow in culture, i.e., how stable they are. Many interspecies hybrids tend to be unstable because of incompatibility between the nucleus and mitochondria. Nevertheless, the Chinese research raises the possibility that if the cells turn out to be safe enough for clinical use, they could provide a solution to human egg shortages for programming in the future. In the meanwhile, experiments are being planned to see whether they will be tolerated by the immune system and whether they can correct an animal model of human disease.

8.6. THERAPEUTIC APPLICATIONS OF HOMOLOGOUS RECOMBINATION IN STEM CELLS

Application of homologous recombination (HR) to embryonic stem cells of mouse has tremendously aided and stimulated the study of gene function in mammals (Martin, 1981; Thomas and Capecchi, 1987). HR has been most often used to generate knockout mice, but it has also been applied in mouse ES cells differentiating *in vitro*. HR is indispensable for exploiting human ES cells as a useful research tool (Zwaka and Thomson, 2002). Furthermore HR has important implications for ES cell based transplantation and gene therapies. The differences between mouse and human ES cells have hampered development of HR in human ES cells. Very often high stable transfection efficiencies in human ES cells have not been achieved and in particular, electroporation protocols that work well for mouse ES cells, work only poorly in human ES cells (Eiges *et al.*, 2001). In contrast to murine ES cells, human ES cells cannot be cloned efficiently from single cells; this makes it difficult to screen for rare recombination events. Zwaka and Thomson (2002) reported an electroporation approach, based on the physical characteristics of human ES cells, that they used to target HPRT1, the gene encoding hypoxanthine phosphoribosyltransferase 1 (HPRT1) and POU5F1, the gene encoding octamer binding transcription factor 4 (Oct4 also known as POU domain, class 5 transcription factor 1) (Pesce and Scholer, 2001). As the HPRT1gene is found on the X chromosomes, a single HR event completely abolishes the function in XY cells. HPRT1 deficient cells are selected on the basis of their resistance to 2-amino-6-captopurine (6-TG) and so the frequency of homologous recombination events can be easily estimated (Albertini, 2001).

Zwaka and Thomson (2002) successfully achieved targeting ratios for both HPRT 1 and Oct4 quite comparable to those observed for mouse ES cells, suggesting that although successful transfection strategies differ between human and mouse ES cells, the frequency of HR itself is probably similar. However, it has still not been determined whether this similarity of rates between human and mouse ES cells holds true for genes not expressed in ES cells. HR in human ES cells is important both for elucidating gene function *in vitro* and for modifying specific ES cell-derived tissues for therapeutic applications in transplantation medicine. For therapeutic applications, controlled modification of specific genes should prove useful for purifying specific ES cell-derived differentiated cell types from a mixed population, for changing the antigenicity of cells, and for endowing cells with novel properties (such as viral resistance) to fight specific diseases. HR in human ES cells might also be used for new approaches combining therapeutic cloning with gene therapy (Rideout *et al.*, 2002). Modifying specific genes for *in vitro* studies will be crucial for enhancing our understanding of the pathogenesis of those diseases for which mouse models are unsuitable. Indeed, HR and human ES cells are of considerable value for understanding the function of any human gene; this approach should be particularly important for those genes that differ in clinically significant ways from the corresponding mouse genes (Zwaka and Thomson, 2002).

Till hitherto, tissue engineers have used materials derived from living organisms, which suffer from problems of batch variations and customization. So, most engineers have a cherished desire to substitute synthetic materials for living tissues. The synthetics can be tailor made for specific studies. Some work has been done using synthetic polymers that form 3-D matrices with micrometer scale pores. Some researchers interested in developing materials for biomedical tissue engineering, use poly(lactide-co-glycolide), which forms a sponge-like structure with pores 100-200 μm in diameter (Shea *et al.*, 1999). Others are turning to systems based on amino acids that assemble into protein fibers of their own accord. Upon mixing with water, these fibers form gels with a nano-scale structure that more closely matches that of a living tissue. Self-assembly yields nano-fibers having architecture similar to that of fibrils in the extracellular matrix.

In fact, Samuel Stupp of the University of Chicago, for instance, has used a matrix made from self-assembling of nanofibers to coax neural stem cells into becoming neurons (Abbott, 2003). S. Zhang of the Massachusetts Institute of Technology has weaved nanofibers of self-assembling peptides into a mesh with just the right porosity to slowly distribute nutrients and other necessary biological molecules to embedded liver stem cells. In this environment, the stem cells continued to divide to reproduce themselves and differentiated into mature liver cells (Semino *et al.*, 2003).

8.6.1. Cloning

HESCs are potentially important in regenerative medicine and as a window on early human embryology. Embryonic stem cells show two remarkable properties. First, they can proliferate in an undifferentiated but pluripotent state, and hence can self-renew. Second, they can differentiate into many specialized cell types. HESCs are derived from the early human blastocyst (5 days post-fertilization) from a region of the embryo called the inner cell mass (ICM). As with mouse embryonic stem cells (MESCs), HESCs show the following basic characteristics: (i) The cells are karyotypically normal, (ii) they survive and proliferate *in vitro* indefinitely under well–defined tissue culture conditions, (iii) many of the cells recover after freezing and thawing, (iv) they differentiate into a variety of cell types *in vitro* and *in vivo* and (v) scientists can derive or reproduce HESCs by using effective culture conditions (Brivanlou *et al.*, 2003).

The issue of ES cells is generally thought to be linked to that of cloning but in reality this is not so. ES cells are usually isolated from excess embryos employed in *in vitro* fertilization procedures. Although these cells are clones of one another, they have not been cloned by any scientist. Neither their creation nor their use necessarily involves nuclear transfer. Different tumor cells can be used as donors for nuclear transfer into enucleated oocytes. Resultant blastocysts were explanted in culture to produce ES cell lines. The tumorigenic and differentiation potential of these ES cells was assayed *in vitro* by inducing teratomas in SCID mice, and *in vivo* by injecting cells into diploid or tetraploid, blastocysts to generate chimeras and entirely ES-cell-derived mice, respectively (Fig. 8.2).

But scientists do need to have continued access to new lines of stem cells for research because the currently approved human ES cells have all been cultured in the presence of mouse cells–called "feeder cells"–that seem to supply the required growth factors. It is possible that contamination from mouse viruses or proteins could make such cells unsuitable for introduction into humans for therapeutic purposes. Fortunately, it is now possible to grow and differentiate human ES cells without the mouse feeder cells. According to Kennedy (2003), it is not wise to restrict work with human ES cells. For therapeutic purposes, adult stem cells (those isolated from embryos in which tissues have already undergone some differentiation) may be used instead. Such cells generate tissues of their own type and possibly others by a process called "trans-differentiation". Furthermore, ES cells are useful progenitors for some tissues but not for others. This warrants a continuing need for ES cells, especially if tissues made in culture are to be used to remedy certain human diseases and disorders. For that embryonic cell lines derived from persons with the genetic constitution corresponding to those conditions will be needed. In this context the problem with the existing cell lines is their lack of genetic diversity–another reason for abolishing the ban on raising new lines.

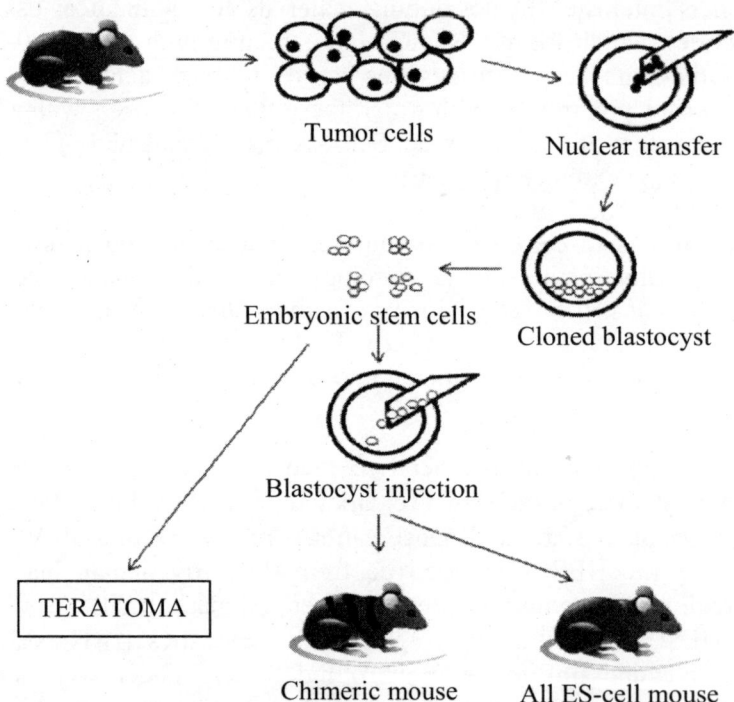

Fig. 8.2: Two-step cloning procedure to produce mice from cancer cells

Currently known culture conditions allow the maintenance of HESCs for many passages in the undifferentiated state (Thomson *et al.*, 1998; Reubinoff *et al.*, 2000).Genes have been successfully transfected and later expressed in HESCs. Human retroviral vectors (such as lentiviruses) and biochemical strategies can potentially transfect HESCs. *In vitro* HESCs do differentiate into various (but not all) cell types that derive from the three embryonic germ layers. Cultured HESCs form neurons and skin cells (indicating ecto dermal differentiation); blood, muscle, cartilage, endothelial cells, and cardiac cells (indicating meso dermal differentiation); and pancreatic cells (indicating endo dermal differentiation) (Schuldiner *et al.*, 2000; Zhang *et al.*, 2001; Levenberg *et al.*, 2002; Brivanlou *et al.*, 2003). Also, HESCs form embryonic bodies containing all three germ layers. Thus, HESCs possess an *in vitro* differentiation potential similar to that of MESCs.

Ethical reasons argue against the implantation of HESCs with human embryos as hosts. There is need for designing improved assays for understanding the biology of HESC differentiation as a prerequisite for their use in regenerative medicine. While it is relatively easier to design *in vitro* assays, *in vivo* assays are more difficult to design. Work on model systems suggests, for instance, that marked HESCs may be transplanted into defined tissue environments in discrete regions of nonhuman adults or fetuses to test for their ability to be incorporated into these tissues. Human fetal and adult neuronal and hematopoietic stem cells have been transplanted into mouse embryos and their contribution to a variety of organs has been reported (Verfaillie, 2002).

8.6.2. Mammalian somatic cell cloning

Willadsen (1986) first cloned lambs from embryonic cells. His work aroused great interest in nuclear transplantation in animal breeding. In 1997, Wilmut produced the first mammal cloned from a somatic cell and Campbell (1999) discussed the enormous potential of somatic-cell cloning in changing selection strategies in farm-animal species besides the possibility of using nuclear transfer for genetically modifying cells that could simplify the production of transgenic animals (McCreath *et al.*, 2000). Indeed, cloning could be a potent tool for saving some endangered mammals (Loi *et al.*, 2001, 2003).

However, although sheep cloning methods for somatic cells are now a routine, the rate at which viable clones are produced is fairly low in most mammalian species. Furthermore, all clones suffer from some common abnormalities particularly in the placenta. There occurs considerable early mortality of somatic cell clones; the founder mammalian clone, Dolly the sheep, died in February 2003 at the young age of six years. According to Loi *et al.* (2003), mammalian somatic cell cloning and the early nuclear-transfer data from amphibians have much in common. They suggested that the only way to improve nuclear reprogramming is to modify the chromatin structure of somatic cells before nuclear transfer, to provide the oocyte with a chromosomal structure that is more compatible with the natural reprogramming machinery of the oocyte.

Successful cloning of adult mammals not only overturned previous ideas regarding the restricted developmental plasticity of somatic cells but also raised exciting prospects for human regenerative medicine (Colman and Kind, 2000). Somatic cloning, together with genetic modification, can potentially make it possible to produce human therapeutics as well as xenograft tissues and organs from livestock. However, restoration of nuclear totipotency in differentiated somatic cells following nuclear transfer, to produce healthy cloned animals, is quite inefficient and prone to epigenetic errors. The high rates of mortality throughout development make somatic cloning unacceptable. Resort to embryonic cloning can alleviate these problems (Wells *et al.*, 2003). Adoption of animal cloning and transgenesis in agriculture is much more challenging than biomedical applications because they require greater biological efficiency at reduced cost to be economically viable.

Oback *et al.* (2003) achieved blastocyst development rates superior to *in vitro* fertilization (IVF) and were able to double the rate of production of cloned offspring but even then, only about 9% of zona-free-somatic-cell-cloned bovine embryos transferred to recipients resulted in viable calves at weaning. Such a low cloning efficiency contrasts with the figure of 40% bovine IVF embryos that typically develop into healthy calves (Kruip and den Daas, 1997).

8.6.3. Donor cell type embryonic versus somatic cells

The degree of donor cell differentiation seems to affect cloning efficiency. A higher proportion of transferred cloned embryos reconstructed from less differentiated embryonic blastomeres or (murine) ES cells (pluripotent cells derived from embryonic blastomeres) result in viable offspring as compared with somatic cell clones. Although cloning from embryonic cells is more efficient than using somatic cells, the supply of blastomeres from embryos is limiting. To increase the probability of ES cell isolation from a selected embryo, an initial round of embryonic cloning creates more blastomeres for culture (or fetuses to be aborted in early gestation, if ethically acceptable, for embryonic germ cell derivation). Isolated blastomeres or short-term blastomere cultures can prove useful for small-scale cloning applications, but long-term ES cell lines are necessary for genetic modification by homologous recombination and large-scale cloning (Wells *et al.*, 2003). In fact, based on donor cell type, three broad categories of nuclear transfer can be recognized: blastomere cloning, ES cell cloning (collectively, both are referred to as embryonic cloning), and somatic cloning.

Cloning with F1 mouse ES cells results in up to about 20% of transferred embryos reaching adulthood, as compared with only about 3% in the case of commonly used somatic donor cells (fibroblasts and cumulus cells) and <0.03% for terminally differentiated cell types (B or T lymphocytes) (Jaenisch *et al.*, 2002). Also, candidate gene expression profiling has revealed that all ES-cell-derived blastocysts faithfully express key embryonic genes and related sequences present in the pluripotent cells of the early embryo, whereas 38% of cumulus-cloned blastocysts failed to re-activate these genes (Bortvin *et al.*, 2003). It seems likely that blastomeres also retain an epi-genotype compatible with early embryonic development without the need for extensive reprogramming (Wells *et al.*, 2003).

Efficient cloning facilitates rapid dissemination of superior genotypes from elite-nucleus breeding flocks and herds, directly to commercial producers, by the transfer of frozen-thawed cloned embryos. This can generate substantially higher profits than from conventional breeding schemes (Nicholas and Smith, 1983). Small numbers of genetically superior animals can also be produced for natural breeding. Effective cloning strongly depends on proper identification of superior genotypes in the population. These individuals are either selected on the basis of the phenotypic performance of their offspring following progeny testing or from clonal family testing in which a few clones are produced at first and their performance are tested in different environments before large-scale release. In those clonal lines that perform favorably, the remaining animals may be used for breeding. Genetic-marker-assisted selection (MAS) has high predictive value for livestock production characteristics and so can not only aid in the direct selection of adults but also help in selecting pre-implantation-stage embryos produced within the nucleus population. Cloning from MAS embryos reduces the genetic lag between the nucleus and commercial populations by three-generation intervals (equivalent to six years in cattle) as compared with cloning of progeny-tested adults (Williams and Wilmut, 1999; Georges, 2001; Brophy *et al.*, 2003; Wells *et al.*, 2003).

In primary somatic cell cultures raised from farm animals, random transgenesis using well-established transfection protocols can be readily achieved (Brophy *et al.*, 2003), but involves a risk of introducing undesirable genetic and phenotypic changes. These problems may be avoided by applying homologous-recombination technology (i.e., gene targeting) for the controlled, precise modification of the genome, either to introduce, functionally delete, or subtly change target genes and their regulatory sequences. Homologous recombination has been achieved at a small number of target loci in somatic cells from sheep (McCreath *et al.*, 2000) and pigs (Harrison *et al.*, 2002). But one problem of gene targeting in livestock with primary somatic cells is their limited lifespan, with many selected clonal cell lines becoming senescent before they can be used for nuclear transfer.

As compared with somatic cells, ES cells have the distinct advantage of markedly higher recombination. This, along with their greater *in vitro* lifespan allows several cycles of gene targeting. ES cells, isolated from genetically elite embryos, can serve as universal donor cells for all gene-targeting purposes, thereby facilitating the application of highly sophisticated tools for precise genetic modification, to enhance not only livestock productivity but also human health and sustainable agriculture (Wells *et al.*, 2003).

Some genetic errors can appear even in surviving clones. These errors could be some point mutations or chromosomal anomalies derived from the donor cells, or errors originating after artificial activation and embryo culture. Normal mammalian embryos can be mixoploid (Slimane-Bureau and King, 2002), i.e., have cells with either diploid or aneuploid chromosomal constitutions - and still develop to blastocysts. Following embryo transfer, severe genetic abnormalities can result in pregnancy failure or in a congenital defect; more-subtle errors can still permit normal development.

Chromosomal abnormalities tend to increase by long-term cell culture. ES cells show a much slower mutation rate. Unfortunately, however, mutations in ES cells usually result from chromosome loss and reduplication rather than from mitotic recombination as in somatic cells; this generates the risk that multiple recessive genetic traits are uncovered (Cervantes *et al.*, 2002). If the lost chromosome happens to be a sex chromosome the situation becomes further complicated. Nuclear cloning perpetuates genetic aberrations that occur in the donor genome. An alternative cloning method is tetraploid embryo complementation: it increases the chances of generating karyotypically normal animals from ES cells (Eggan *et al.*, 2001).

According to Wells *et al.* (2003), embryonic cloning may ultimately prove more useful than somatic cloning for agricultural applications in view of the following factors: (1) Embryonic donor cells show greater cloning efficiency, reduced animal production costs and fewer animal welfare issues; all these merits enhance commercial and ethical acceptance of the technology. (2) Cloning from embryonic cells, especially when coupled with MAS, rapidly propagates the most recent genetic gains made in nucleus breeding herds as compared with adults. (3) ES cells are better suited to easy gene targeting; (4) Nuclear cloning might even become redundant if the entire animal can be raised directly from a group of pluripotent ES cells complemented by suitable helper-cells to establish the placenta.

Death of the terminally ill Dolly on 14th February 2003 raised many biological questions, such as how ageing occurs in clones (Williams, 2003; Gurdon and Colman, 1999). The work on Dolly had led to the coining of the term 'therapeutic cloning'. The possibility of producing nuclear-transfer embryo-derived cell lines for autologous cell and gene therapy carries enormous potential for human medicine. The molecular mechanisms of nuclear reprogramming are now being studied critically with a focus on the isolation of key remodeling factors in several animal models (Burns *et al.*, 2003). All this work can contribute greatly to improving somatic cell cloning. It has emerged that only occasionally can totipotency be fully restored in a somatic-cell nucleus, allowing normal embryonic, foetal and postnatal life (Loi *et al.*, 2003). Enhanced understanding of nuclear reprogramming mechanisms should enable scientists to reprogram nuclei of differentiated cells *in vitro* at least partially before their transfer into enucleated oocytes (Loi *et al.*, 2002). This in turn may prove helpful in making somatic-cell transplantation more reliable and efficient.

8.7. TISSUE ENGINEERING – REGENERATIVE MEDICINE

Modern biotechnological approaches have prepared the ground not only for tissue and organ replacement but also for the continuous and controlled release of therapeutic agents to the host. Cell microencapsulation aims to overcome the present difficulties relating to whole organ graft rejection and, consequently, the requirements for the use of immunomodulatory protocols or immunosuppressive drugs. Cell encapsulation, or bio-artificial organs, can be used for enclosing bioactive materials within some polymeric membrane, which allows the entry of nutrients and oxygen and the exit of therapeutic proteins products. As this membrane is semi-permeable it prevents high molecular weight molecules, antibodies and other immunologic moieties from coming into contact with the encapsulated cells and destroying them as foreign invaders (Orive *et al.*, 2004).

It is highly desirable that only biocompatible materials that do not interfere with cell homeostasis be applied within capsules to help in survival of the enclosed cells. Also, the polymers used for allo- and xenotransplantation differ: xenotransplantation requires a much tighter membrane. The capsules should be sufficiently stable mechanically to permit exchange of nutrients and metabolic waste (Orive *et al.*, 2004). The material of choice for making capsule is sodium alginate (composed of mannuronic and guluronic (G) dimers) and poly-L-lysine (PLL) as the poly-anion and poly-cation, respectively.

Also for avoiding graft rejection, only highly purified and biocompatible polymers must be selected in view of the fact that a reduction in endotoxin content and the elimination of proteins are essential. Live cells and their secretory products may have a role in the biological acceptance of the encapsulated cells, as well as the graft site and the adopted transplant procedure.

Careful choice of encapsulated cells is a must for any successful biomedical application. Many different cell sources have been immobilized or immuno-isolated. Not all cells are suitable for encapsulation. Those that proliferate following encapsulation can eventually fill the entire capsular space leading to lowered efficacy of therapeutic diffusion. So the long-term viability of encapsulated cells is often adversely affected (Chang and Bowie, 1998). In contrast, cells, which do not proliferate after encapsulation (e.g. myoblasts), continue to deliver therapeutic products for longer periods of time. Finally, thanks to genetic engineering, genes can now be used as templates, cells as reactors to secrete the final product and capsules as immune-isolation vehicles for drug delivery *in vivo* (Orive *et al.*, 2004). But the use of genetically modified cells will need to be balanced in respect of safety and stability of gene expression.

8.7.1. Engineering of growing tissues

Engineering of new tissues has addressed various problems relating to tissue reconstruction or replacement by using selective cell transplantation on polymer scaffolds. Functional biologic prostheses are created by entrapping dissociated cells into synthetic biodegradable polymer substrates that deliver the cells to the appropriate site, define a space for tissue development and direct the gross size and shape of the engineered tissue (Alsberg *et al.*, 2003). This strategy has succeeded with skin, bone, and cartilage but not for the regeneration of tissues capable of growing over time. While regenerating new tissues and organs may bring within our reach routine replacement of lost tissues and organs, these engineered tissues must also grow in concert with the changing needs of the body over time. One example of a growing tissue is the epiphyseal growth plate involved in bone elongation during development through the process of endochondral ossification. This process involves the deposition of osteoid matrix on top of calcified cartilage and its subsequent mineralization (Weiss, 1987). The process becomes compromised in certain multiple disease and injury states (Beers *et al.*, 1999). Alsberg *et al.* (2003) hypothesized that a growing tissue might be engineered by presenting appropriate growth stimuli from the cell transplantation scaffold. They tested this hypothesis in the context of engineering growing bony tissues by the co-transplantation of osteoblasts and chondrocytes. The multiplication of transplanted cells has to be promoted if one is to engineer a growing tissue *in vivo*, and one required growth stimulus for most mammalian cell types is an appropriate adhesive substrate (Peppas and Langer, 1994). Hoping that provision of a high density of adhesive ligands to transplanted chondrocytes from the polymeric delivery vehicle might promote their multiplication, Alsberg *et al.* (2003) covalently coupled synthetic peptides containing the arginine-glycine-aspartic acid (RGD) cell adhesion sequence to the alginate polymer chains used to form the hydrogel delivery vehicle to meet this requirement. This approach allows one to specify the mechanism of cell-material adhesion and an appropriate density of RGD ligands promotes the proliferation of various cell types *in vivo* (Alsberg *et al.*, 2003). Although much work has been done to regenerate bone and cartilage tissues separately and together, a growing bony tissue has not been made. It is possible to regenerate a tissue structurally and functionally similar to a growth plate by providing growing cartilage anlagen with transplanted chondrocytes, similar to that in long-bone development, as a template for subsequent bone formation by co-transplanted osteoblasts. Chondrocytes and osteoblasts were co-trasplanted on hydrogels modified with an RGD-containing peptide sequence to promote cell multiplication. New bone tissue was formed that grew in mass and cellular number by endochondral ossification in a manner similar to normal long bone growth. Transplanted cells organized into structures that morphologically and functionally resembled growth plates. These engineered tissues proved useful in treating diseases and injuries of the growth plate, testing the effect of experimental drugs on growth-plate function and development, and investigating the biology of long-bone growth. This concept of promoting the growth of engineered tissues could prove valuable in engineering of several tissue types by way of the transplantation of a small number of precursor cells. Indeed, the work of Alsberg *et al.* (2003) may have valuable therapeutic applications and could serve as a model system to study bone formation.

This promising approach to tissue engineering, transplantation of a small number of cells and growing the tissue *in vivo*, may lessen or remove current difficulties in the *in vitro* engineering of large tissue masses for subsequent transplantation that are related to a lack of vascularity and large-scale cell death. Also it may promote the utilization of small numbers of stem cells for the regeneration of various tissues in the body (Alsberg *et al.*, 2003).

8.7.2. Biomaterial scaffolds

The extracellular matrix of cells in living tissues provides a scaffold for organizing the tissues whose 3D geometry is the outcome of both cell-matrix and cell-cell interactions. Matrix scaffold contains several proteins and their constituent biologically active adhesive motifs (Hynes, 1999; Holmes, 2002). Transient or persistent biologically active adhesive or anti-adhesive interactions maintain the architecture of adult tissues. As many of the molecular cues responsible for tissue organization during development are absent in the adult animal, the presence or absence of tissue-organizing cues in the extracellular matrix is involved in the tissue regenerative capacity. Such molecular cues are also critical for some specialized cellular functions such as axonal regeneration (Fournier and Strittmatter, 2001).

In the biomedical field, a pressing need for tissue repair has stimulated the development of biomaterial scaffolds that can be used in artificial tissues and for such transplantable devices as biosensors. Biomaterial scaffolds form components of cell-laden artificial tissues and transplantable biosensors. Some of the most promising new synthetic biomaterial scaffolds are composed of self-assembling peptides that can be modified to contain biologically active motifs. Materials ranging from spider silks to extracellular matrix proteins exemplify biomaterial scaffolds. Although naturally occurring biomaterial scaffolds such as collagen can be chemically modified to confer desirable properties, nature is still the ultimate and the best material engineer; however, the need for designing flexibility is motivating human material engineers. Self-assembling peptides, organic polymers, inorganic materials or mixed co-polymer combinations can be used to create synthetic biomaterial scaffolds. Biomaterial promotion of multi-dimensional cell-cell interactions and cell density are crucial for proper cellular differentiation and for subsequent tissue formation (Holmes, 2002).

With the emergence of cell-based therapy as an alternative therapeutic approach to many diseases, diseases resistant to small-molecule drug treatment are attracting attention for being treated with certain types of naturally derived animal products such as collagen-based biological scaffolds, their derivatives and bio-compatible co-polymers, as scaffolds for cell attachment (Ellis and Yannas, 1996). The potential problem with all animal-derived biomaterials is that they can carry dangerous pathogens such as transmissible spongiform encephalopathy (TSEs), which can cross species barriers during disease transmission (Scott *et al.*, 1999). A recent appearance of prion-mediated spongiform encephalopathy, which has been accompanied by the cross-species transfer of the prions to humans, underscores this concern.

Unlike natural materials, synthetic biomaterials minimize the risk of carrying biological pathogens or contaminants; they are also attractive for applications in controlled drug release, tissue repair and tissue engineering. Several synthetic biomaterials show *in vivo* biocompatibility and can be designed to meet specific needs. Promising biomaterials, composed of spontaneously self-assembling oligopeptides, have been discovered recently (Schachner, 2000). The constituents of these biomaterial scaffolds are self-complementary amphiphilic oligopeptides having regular repeating units of positively charged residues (lysine or arginine) and negatively charged residues (aspartate or glutamate), separated by hydrophobic residues (alanine or leucine). The self-complementary amphiphilic peptides contain 50% charged residues and are characterized by their periodic repeats of alternating ionic hydrophilic and uncharged hydrophobic amino acids (West *et al.*, 1999).

Holmes *et al.* (2000) and Schachner (2000) have studied cell attachment, differentiation, neurite outgrowth and the formation of functional synapses by primary and cultured neuronal cells on peptide matrix scaffolds. As these neuro-laden matrix scaffolds can be readily transported between different environments, neuron/matrix cultures are potentially important for use in transplantation. So, neuron and/or peptide-matrix cultures established in tissue culture could be gainfully used for transplantation.

8.8. TISSUE ENGINEERING AND REPAIR

Tissue engineering is defined as the application of principles and methods of engineering and life sciences for the development of biological substitutes so as to restore, maintain or improve tissue function (Langer and Vacanti, 1993). Recent focus on using biomaterials for tissue engineering applications has been on the importance of the physical properties and dimensionality of biomaterials in hollow organ (e.g., bladder) and bone tissue engineering. Some breakthroughs in these areas bring out the importance of those biomaterials that mimic the natural geometry of cell-cell and cell-biomaterial scaffold interactions (Homles, 2002). The availability of stem cell precursors for making neo-tissue together with an understanding of factors governing cellular differentiation into desired neo-tissue types is crucial for successful neo-tissue construction (Atala, 2000; Hutmacher, 2000). Oberpenning *et al.* (1999) successfully transplanted a tissue-engineered neo-organ bladder in dogs by making a neo-organ scaffold from a mixed-polymer synthetic biomaterial. This scaffold was seeded with autologous urothelial and smooth muscle donor cells, which were collected from host animals and then separated and expanded in culture into urothelial and smooth muscle cell pools. Biodegradable poly-glycolic acid (PGA) coated with the copolymer poly-DL-lactide-co-glycolide

(PLGA) was used to make the neo-organ bladder scaffold. The cell-seeded neo-organs were transplanted into dogs whose bladder was partly removed. The dogs that received cell-seeded neo-organ bladder transplants showed normal function for urine retention, uro-dynamic bladder compliance and histological architecture for up to 11 months after transplantation. The animals appeared to recover completely.

For bone-tissue engineering (Petite *et al.,* 2000), three-dimensional cell-cell interactions and cellular density are crucial for proper cellular differentiation leading to the formation of mature bony tissue, another requirement being careful selection and treatment of the precursor cells used for seeding the biomaterial scaffold. Another promising target for tissue engineering is cartilage regeneration-cartilage, being a vascular, heals poorly. Transplantation of chondrocytes seeded on biomaterial scaffolds has proven promising for cartilage regeneration (Suh and Matthew, 2000).

Other refinements in tissue engineering include the use of stem cells, cell pre-selection and growth factor pre-treatment of cells that are used for seeding scaffolds. These cell-culture technologies, combined with improved processes for defining the dimensions of peptide-based scaffolds, might lead to further improvements in tissue engineering. Novel peptide-based biomaterial scaffolds seeded with cells seem to have considerable promise for tissue repair and other medical applications (Hynes, 1999; Holmes, 2002).

Biomedical researchers are designing improved biomaterial scaffolds by constructing mixed materials containing inorganic molecules or metal-binding groups, which could lead to biomaterials with greater tensile strength. In this context, abalone shell, a highly tensile but hard natural material that contains a mixture of organic and inorganic materials, is a good example (Dan, 2000). Biomineralized scaffolds form the physical basis for bone repair and other hard tissue repairs. Xu *et al*. (2001) have made self-assembling mono layers derived from a combinatorial peptide library. The peptides in this library were selected for their ability to fold into six-stranded amphiphilic beta-sheets. Monolayer self-assembly of these amphiphilic peptides occurs at air-water interfaces. These results point to the exciting possibility of creating laminated biomaterials composed of sheets of defined organic proteins and inorganic minerals (Holmes, 2002).

8.8.1. Bioreactors

3D tissue structures can be generated by the association of cells (autologous or allo-geneic) with porous scaffolds serving as the template for tissue development and which later degrade or become reabsorbed. Culturing of 3D cell-scaffold constructs (Butler *et al*., 2000) in the laboratory under conditions that support efficient nutrition of cells can prove beneficial in the development of functional grafts for the treatment of lost or damaged body parts (i.e., functional tissue engineering). In some cases, 3D tissues are engineered *in vitro* to make non-implantable structures to be used as external organ support devices when a compatible donor is not readily available (Mazariegos *et al*., 2002). It is a more difficult task, however, to generate 3D tissues *ex vivo*.

Ex *vivo* engineering of living tissues can have high potential impact on many biomedical applications. Some major hurdles in the production of functional tissues and their clinical use stem from lack of good understanding of the regulatory role of specific physicochemical culture parameters on tissue development as well as the high manufacturing costs of the few engineered tissue products that are commercially available. Bioreactors are devices in which biological and/or biochemical processes develop under closely monitored and tightly controlled environmental and operating conditions (pH, temperature, pressure, nutrient supply and waste removal). Processing in bioreactors is highly reproducible. By enabling reproducible and controlled changes of specific environmental factors, bioreactor systems can be the appropriate technological means to unravel underlying mechanisms of cell function in a 3D environment. They can also potentially improve the quality of engineered tissues. By automating and standardizing tissue manufacture in controlled, closed systems, bioreactors reduce production costs and so facilitate a wider use of engineered tissues (Martin *et al.*, 2004).

Bioreactors are widely used in industrial fermentation processing, waste water treatment, food processing and production of such pharmaceuticals and recombinant proteins as antibodies, growth factors, vaccines and antibiotics. Some representative bioreactors for tissue engineering applications include spinner-flask bioreactors for the seeding of cells into 3D scaffolds and for subsequent culture of the constructs; rotating-wall vessels; hollow-fiber bioreactors which are used to enhance mass transfer during the culture of highly metabolic and sensitive cell types such as hepatocytes; direct perfusion bioreactors in which medium flows directly through the pores of the scaffold used for seeding and/or culturing 3D constructs; and bioreactors that apply controlled mechanical forces, e.g., dynamic compression, to engineered constructs, used as model systems of tissue development under physiological loading conditions, and to generate functional tissue grafts (Jasmund and Bader, 2002; Sodian *et al.*, 2002; Martin *et al.*, 2004).

8.8.2. Artificial heart

An exciting new initiative, known as Living Implants from Engineering (LIFE) was started in 1999 with a view to growing artificial human organs (such as heart) in the laboratory. It was hoped that LIFE would rival the Human Genome Project in scale and in its potential to revolutionize medical practice. The grand project is still largely unfunded and is functioning mostly as a weak coalition of researchers. But this does not undermine the enormous clinical promise of tissue engineering.

Tissue-engineered skin grafts have already won marketing approval from the US Food and Drug Administration and implants of lab-grown cartilage are undergoing clinical trials. But these exemplify fairly simple tissues-growing complex organs such as the heart is a much greater challenge. Some researchers have adopted a simpler approach rather than attempt to create the highly complex heart focusing on growing some of its component parts-patches of cardiac muscle, valves, or coronary blood vessels. There is a pressing clinical need for heart tissue. Patients requiring a transplant have to wait a few years for a donated organ, and even then, because of immunological rejection and other complications, donated hearts do not last for more than decade.

In tissue engineering a scaffold is first made on which tissue can grow. Some cells are then placed into it. The inoculated scaffold is placed in a suitable 'bioreactor' that provides nutrients and oxygen. When the cells have multiplied to fill the scaffold, the structure is removed from the bioreactor and implanted into the body. In 1995, the above basic principle was elegantly demonstrated to the world as images of a 'human' ear made from scaffold-grown cartilage protruding from the back of a mouse (Zandonella, 2003). But heart tissue is more difficult to grow. Adult cardiac muscle cells usually do not divide so the scaffold has to be inoculated with cells from another source. One possibility is to use skeletal-muscle cells that do proliferate. Researchers are also interested in the potential of stem cells extracted from adult bone marrow, or from a few-day old human embryos, both of which can differentiate into cardiac muscle cells if given the right stimuli. Indeed, it may be possible to repair small areas of damaged cardiac muscle by injecting stem cells or skeletal-muscle cells directly into the tissue. Ongoing clinical trials involving patient's own skeletal muscle cells have shown some muscle contraction.

Direct injection of cells may perhaps repair small areas of damage. Repairing large areas of dead tissue will require the lab-grown patches of muscle. For their three dimensional growth, cells need a scaffold that is accepted by the body and which degrades over time into harmless components. One may possibly use either collagen, which provides mechanical support for natural tissues, or synthetic, biodegradable polymers such as poly (L)-lactic acid. To increase the chances of attachment of seeded cells, the polymers may be coated with cell adhesion proteins; or they may be designed to release cell-signaling molecules. Another idea is to make scaffolds that carry specific instructions for controlling tissue formation, analogous to the signals that control embryological development (Zandonella, 2003).

In a project already a scaffold made of chains of elastin polypeptides, a bio-molecule that provides elastic properties to some of our tissues, has been designed. Keeley *et al.* (2002) experimented with different molecules to crosslink the polypeptide chains and created structures ranging from a delicate mesh to an elastic band. For a patch of heart muscle, the ideal scaffold is something having the properties of both – allowing cells to burrow into the matrix but providing as much strength and elasticity as a beating heart (Keeley *et al.*, 2002; Zandonella, 2003).One major challenge is how to grow 3D structures that contain more than a few layers of muscle cells. Most bioreactors are unable to supply enough nutrients and oxygen to the growing tissue. Whereas human heart muscle can be up to 2 centimeters thick, growth in a bioreactor typically ceases once the tissue is about 100 micrometers, or 4–7 cell layers thick.

One way to sidestep this problem is to drop the use of scaffolds and instead grow single layers of cells that are then sandwiched into slabs of tissue like a layered cake. This is being attempted by using cardiac-muscle cells from newborn rats-these cells can divide. The cells are grown on polymer surfaces that allow the intact cell layers to detach when the culture temperature is lowered (Shimizu *et al.*, 2000). Four of these sheets have been laid on top of each other and fused. They were then implanted under the skin of immune-deficient rats. When the skin was opened six months later, the engineered cardiac tissue was beating and blood vessels had permeated it (Zandonella, 2003).

It is also hoped that tissues could be grown on scaffolds interweaved with artificial capillaries. Some workers are using the body itself as a bioreactor. By growing tissues in the body cavity of the rat, an environment has been created that duplicates the conditions for the development of normal tissues. It is, of course, easier to grow a patch of heart muscle than making it actually pump blood. The heart is a powerful muscle and engineered tissue needs to be equally vigorous. Eschenhagen *et al.* (2002) have made cylindrical patches of cardiac muscle using cardiac-muscle cells from newborn rats. But instead of seeding the cells on a scaffold, they are mixed into a collagen gel and cast in a cylindrical mould. After a few days the tissue patch is transferred to a stretching device that subjects it to an exercise that simulates the heart's contractions. Implantation of the tissues into rats showed that the cardiac cylinders contract much more vigorously than un-stretched tissues (Eschenhagen *et al.*, 2002).

Niklason *et al.* (1999) have grown functional arteries by seeding a tubular scaffold with muscle cells from a cow's aorta. When the growth filled the scaffold, the tube's interior was inoculated with endothelial cells forming the smooth lining of blood vessels. Throughout the procedure, fluid was flown through the tubes to simulate the mechanical stresses that blood vessels must face. When implanted into miniature pigs, these tissue-engineered arteries functioned well for over three weeks (Niklason *et al.*, 1999).

It is very difficult to grow heart valves because of their complex architecture of cells and extracellular matrix that continuously remodels itself to respond to fluid flow in the heart. Tissue-engineered versions would be a boon for children born with defective valves because mechanical implants have to be successively replaced as the heart grows. In some cases, the problem is identified during pregnancy; in these a sample of foetal tissue may be taken to grow valves that would be ready for implantation shortly after birth, which would subsequently grow along with the heart. Researchers at the Children's Hospital Boston seeded a biodegradable scaffold with endothelial and muscle cells taken from arteries in the necks of lambs. Fluid was passed through the growing tissue to mimic the conditions experienced by a working valve. After implantation into the same lambs, which donated the cells, the valves continued to grow and survived for up to five months (Hoerstrup *et al.*, 2000).

After the valves, muscle, coronary blood vessels and other parts have been made, the parts will have to be assembled together into a functioning organ. The best approach may be to grow the parts all at the same time in a complex, multi-chamber bioreactor, and to make them grow in a coordinated fashion. Even if it proves impossible to successfully address this enormous challenge, tissue engineered heart components might benefit many patients who would otherwise need a replacement heart to live without transplant, thanks to careful running repairs. Tissue engineering can potentially allow damaged areas of the heart to be healed as the damage occurs (Zandonella, 2003).

8.8.3. Clinical xenotransplantation

The technology of clinical xenotransplantation has generated an extended conflict between individuals, society and the other concerned stakeholders– xenotransplantation involves the transplantation of organs, tissues or cells from another species (usually pigs) to humans. There are millions of individuals each year that could benefit from a transplant but there is acute shortage of human organs that can be transplanted. In the USA alone the gap between organs available and organs needed each year exceeds 50,000. If pigs could be used as donors, there would, in principle, be an unlimited supply of organs, tissues and cell (Bach and Ivinson, 2002). One formidable problem here is that of rejection of pig organs by non-human primates. Another is that the promise of xenotransplantation has given rise to a new ethical dilemma. As with all mammals, pigs harbor many viruses or ghosts of viruses, some active, some latent and others represented only by a partial genetic sequence embedded in the pig genome. Possibly pig endogenous retroviruses (PERVs) could be transmitted to a human xenotransplant recipient. Under specific *in vitro* conditions, PERVs can infect human cells and van der Laan *et al.* (2002) demonstrated that PERVs carried in xenotransplanted tissue are transcriptional active and infectious across the pig-mouse species barrier. In view of the possibility that PERVs could be transmitted to a human xenotransplant recipient, it is also possible that such an infection could be passed on from a patient to close contacts and even to the general population. There is considerable disagreement on the magnitude of such a risk (Daar *et al.*, 1998), but many agree that the risk is high enough to arouse serious concern.

As for genetically modified crops or food, so also for xenotransplantation several countries in Europe have imposed a moratorium. Meanwhile, the US FDA has shown some willingness to entertain protocols for xenotransplantation and has allowed certain trials of cellular xenotransplantation (Bach *et al.*, 2001). But a meaningful informed public engagement is warranted on the pros and cons of xenotransplantation (Bach and Ivinson, 2002). Informed representatives of the public should participate actively and meaningfully in the decision about whether and under what conditions society is exposed to the risk of xenotransplantation. It is just as unethical to foist a particular medical risk on a patient as to expose the public to a risk without first considering their opinion.

8.8.4. Human reproduction and neurodegenerative diseases

As research on human embryos and embryonic stem cells can greatly enhance understanding of human reproduction and development and also stimulate regenerative medicine, informed consent is particularly important because of the diverse opinions and strong emotions that surround these issues.

Whereas some potential donors consider all such research to be unacceptable; others support some forms of research (Lo *et al.*, 2003). A donor might accept infertility research but have reservation about stem cell lines, patenting, or commercial products (Radin, 1996; Kimbrell, 1997).

In the USA, the requirement of informed consent for the research use of anonymous biological materials that cannot be linked to the donor can be waived off. But some people still consider as wrong or offensive using gametes or embryos for certain kinds of research without consent, even after identifiers have been removed (Feinberg, 1988; Lo *et al.*, 2003).The consent of the woman or couple in the assisted reproductive technology (ART) program is essential for research with frozen embryos remaining after completion of infertility treatment.

If stem cell lines are created, it is the donor's genetic material that is propagated indefinitely. Lo *et al.* (2003) suggested that gamete donors' wishes should be determined and respected; also that informed consent from both oocyte and sperm donors should be obtained for an embryo to be used in research (NIH, 1994). There is certainly a need to encourage broad public discussion to evolve guidelines for informed consent that protect donors while allowing important research to proceed.

Although there is some therapeutic potential of early embryonic stem cell research to treat presently intractable diseases, the approach faces strong ethical, regulatory and patent challenges. There exists a wide gap between researchers and patients. While researchers are enthusiastic about the potential of therapeutic embryonic stem cell cloning, regulators and opponents are equally keen to prevent further research in this area. In the UK, the House of Lords allowed a government panel to issue licenses for therapeutic cloning research, but the Judicial Office of the House of Lords has permitted the anti-embryo research group Pro-Life Alliance to challenge the current regulatory system. A judgment in favor of the challenge could seriously affect Britain's stem cell research.

In the USA, there is a ban on public funding on most aspects of such research. But it is hoped that a ban may turn into a moratorium with the prospect eventually of some research. The US President's Council on Bioethics is slowly moving towards that recommendation. This Council unanimously supports a ban on cloning to produce a human baby but there is no such unanimity on therapeutic cloning. The majority of the Council supports a moratorium of two to six years on research cloning, but some of its members are opposed to such a move (Nigel, 2002).

Meanwhile, efforts are underway to discover potentially therapeutic stem cells from sources other than early embryos, which most people would find ethically preferable. Results suggest there may be alternatives to work with embryos. Recent research at the University of Minnesota points to the growth of stem-like cells from mesenchymal cells derived from the bone marrow of mice, rats and humans. But many scientists are skeptical about the therapeutic potential of cells derived from older animals. While many aspects of embryonic stem cells are still being debated, the first patent to cover human cloning was granted by the US Patent and Trademark Office in April 2001, registered to the University of Wisconsin, with financial interest shared by the private company Biotransplant in Massachusetts. This patent covers a 'method of producing a cloned mammal' and even refers specifically to the use of human embryo cells.

While in Europe the European Patent Office has banned patents involving human cloning, there are no such bans in the US. In the US, government research on stem cells is highly restricted but industry-funded research is not regulated. Both action and inaction may spell serious consequences, either for the embryo or for patients who might be helped by embryonic stem cell-based therapy. For patients suffering from multiple sclerosis, Parkinson's disease, leukemia or cancer, the ethical debate is meaningless. What they urgently need is a solution, which may come from stem cells (Nigel, 2002).

Human ES cells are not protected from the immune system. As the cells differentiate, they express increasing levels of the markers the body uses to distinguish between native and foreign cells. A patient's immune system seems to reject transplanted tissues derived from ES cells. Those hoping to use the ES cells to treat various maladies will have to find ways to reconcile the body's defense system with the transplanted cells.

Even though ES cells are not invisible to the immune system, there may be some potential avenues around the problem of transplant rejection, such as genetically altering ES cells so that MHC proteins would not be expressed, build up a cell bank (like a blood bank) of cells with a range of MHC profiles, or use nuclear transfer techniques-better termed cloning-to create genetically matched ES cells for individual patients (Vogel, 2002).

Each of these approaches has its drawbacks. No ES cell line bank could possibly have a match for all patients. Genetically altering ES cells to develop a "universal donor" cell that would not express MHC proteins is technically difficult and could leave the resulting tissue even more susceptible to infections and turn two things MHC molecules help the body fight against. The cloning by using nuclear transfer techniques is highly controversial and too expensive. Yet, the relatively low levels of MHC expression might at least mean that tissues derived from ES cells would be less prone to rejection than today's whole-organ transplants (Vogel, 2002). The medical potential, risks and ethics of studying human embryonic stem (ES) cells have attracted much recent debate. Proponents believe that these cells have enormous potential for treating serious disorders such as Parkinson's disease, diabetes and spinal cord injuries. But for those who oppose the use of cells derived from human embryos, stem cells from adults offer an ethically acceptable alternative.

Kim *et al.* (2002) generated a specific class of neurons from cultured mouse ES cells and used them to reverse symptoms of Parkinson's disease in rats. They showed that ES cells could generate specialized therapeutically effective cell types. Jiang *et al.* (2002) extracted highly versatile cells from the bone marrow of adult mice, rats and humans. ES cells (and mouse multi potent adult progenitor cells, MAPCs) need growth factor for growth; other cultured cells do not. This may be a unique feature of pluripotent stem cells (Table 8.1).

Stem cells are essential building blocks of multi-cellular organisms and have two defining properties: (1) they can produce more stem cells and (ii) they can generate specialized cell types such as nerve, blood, or liver cells in various different forms depending on when and where they are produced during development, and also on their versatility. Pluri-potent stem cells can give rise to all cell types. ES cells are found in very early mammalian embryos. These cells proliferate indefinitely in culture and retain the potential to differentiate into virtually any cell type when coaxed. In principle, ES cells could generate large quantities of any desired cells for transplantation into patients (Orkin and Morrison, 2002).

Those stem cells that are taken from tissues of adults or older embryos show a restricted development and proliferative potential. These are exemplified by blood forming (hematopoietic) stem cells, which produce all types of blood cells *in vivo* but proliferate little in culture and probably do not make cells of other tissues. Those opposed to using human ES cells suggest that pluripotent adult stem cells could help us in achieving medical benefits without ethical pain. Besides ethical issues, there are technical obstacles to the use of ES cells. First, these cells can come only from very early embryos and may not be immunologically compatible with most patients requiring cell transplants. This means that researchers will have either to raise many more ES-cell lines or to customize ES cells on a patient-by-patient basis by 'therapeutic cloning'. Second, undifferentiated ES cells form benign tumors containing a mixture of tissue types, after being transplanted. Thus ES cells have to be properly differentiated into the appropriate cell type in culture before transplantation (Orkin and Morrison, 2002). Moreover, it is conceivable that specialized cells derived from cultured ES cells may not actually function within tissues after transplantation (Lumelsky *et al.*, 2001).

The disadvantages of ES cells could possibly be avoided by identifying a pluripotent adult stem cell that proliferates indefinitely in culture, as achieved by Jiang *et al.* (2002). Pittenger *et al.* (1999) had earlier indicated that there exists a population of mesenchymal stem cells in bone marrow that can form muscle, cartilage, bone and fat. Using a similar approach, Jiang *et al.* (2002) cultured non-hematopoietic bone marrow cells and isolated a population that they called multipotent adult progenitor cells (MAPCs).

Single mouse MAPCs proliferated indefinitely in culture and differentiated into many specialized cell types. Upon injection into mouse blastocyst-stage embryos, individual MAPCs contributed to developing tissues. Upon being injected intravenously into adult mice, they gave rise to several blood and epithelial cell types. But there is some possibility that the MAPCs might have fused with blastocyst cells (Terada *et al.*, 2002; Ying *et al.*, 2002). Table 8.1 shows there are both similarities and important differences between MAPCs and ES cells. Conceivably, MAPCs might represent some rare pluripotent stem cells that persist from the embryo into adult life.

MAPCs appear to have a potential in treating diseases irrespective of their origin; however, although they can generate many specialized cell types, it is not clear whether those cells function normally and could be used to treat animals (as Kim *et al.* used ES-cell derived neurons). Such experiments are being contemplated by isolating MAPCs from the bone marrow of a patient, and transplanting the progeny of these cells back to the same patient without risk of rejection (Orkin and Morrison, 2002).

Table 8.1 Comparison of embryonic stem (ES) cells and the multipotent adult progenitor cells (MAPCs)

Property	ES cells	MAPCs
Origin	Embryo	Adult bone marrow
Growth potential	Indefinite	Indefinite
Differentiation into most cell types	Yes	Yes
Requirement of growth factor LIF	Yes	Yes (for mouse)
Stability of chromosome integrity	Moderate	High
Expression of marker protein	High	Very low
Contribution to germ cells	Yes	Not known
Production of blood cells on transplantation	No	Yes
Possibility of auto-transplantation	No	Yes

8.8.5. Restorative neurology

Damage caused from stroke and Parkinson's disease may now be amenable to repair by using immortalized neural precursor cells, seeded in a biodegradable polymer scaffold or directly injected in the injured brain (Steindler, 2002).In pursuit of regenerative medicine, Park *et al.* (2002) integrated materials science and stem cell biology to generate novel tissue-engineering capabilities for extensive

CNS injuries. Ourednik *et al.* (2002) described humoral augmentation of a single population of sick neurons in an animal model of Parkinson's disease.

The therapeutic potential of neural stem cells (NSCs) for CNS diseases comes partly from the fact that upon transplantation, NSCs are attracted to neurodegenerative environments, where they tend to replace dead or dysfunctional cells (Ourednik *et al.*, 1999, 2002; Bjorklund and Lindval, 2000). If NSCs are genetically engineered *ex vivo* to over express specific therapeutic molecules, they can deliver those substances to the desired targets (Snyder *et al.*, 1995).

Ourednik *et al.* (2002) pursued the idea of whether NSCs can "rescue" dysfunctional neurons in the brains of aged mice. Their study focused on a neuronal cell type with stereotypical projections that is commonly compromised in the aged brain–the dopaminergic (DA) neuron. Unilateral implantation of murine NSCs into the midbrains of aged mice, in which the presence of stably impaired but non apoptotic DA neurons was increased by treatment with 1-methyl-4-phenyl-1,2,3,6-tetrahydropyridine (MPTP), was found to be associated with bilateral reconstitution of the mesostriatal system. Functional assays paralleled the spatiotemporal recovery of tyrosine hydroxylase (TH) and dopamine transporter (DAT) activity, which, in turn, mirrored the spatiotemporal distribution of donor-derived cells. Many DA neurons in the mesostriatal system were found to be "rescued" host cells. Undifferentiated donor progenitors spontaneously expressing neuro protective substances provided a plausible molecular basis for this finding.

NSCs have been previously used for neuronal replacement and gene therapy. The work of Ourednik *et al.,* (2002) suggests a third mechanism by which therapeutic outcomes might be achieved: an inherent, constitutive capacity of NSCs (even in lieu of neuronal differentiation) to create host environments that are fairly rich in trophic and/or neuroprotective support to rescue imperiled host cells. The implications for CNS repair are that one very probably needs to provide a variety of cell types –not just neurons, but also undifferentiated progenitors or glia to serve as "chaperones" (as seen in development)—to promote optimal recovery and a reconstructed organ. Dissecting the molecular determinants of this reciprocal intercellular signaling may suggest new treatment approaches to progressive neurodegenerative diseases (Lowenstein and Castro, 2001; Ourednik *et al.,* 2002).

Certain "stem-like" cells (e.g. Cl7.2) of mouse can insinuate themselves within established and compromised rodent CNS structures and circuits, migrate to injured areas, show diverse lineage potential, release neurohumoral factors, and generally reconstitute neural circuitry in models of neurological disease (Reynolds and Weiss, 1992; Richards *et al.*, 1992). It is this C17.2 cell line that was used in the new studies of Park *et al.* (2002) and Ourednik *et al.* (2002). This line is appropriately described to as "stem-like" because the starting cell population (neonatal mouse cerebellar external granular layer cells) was immortalized by retrovirus-mediated transduction of avian Myc (v-Myc), producing a clonal multipotent progenitor cell line (Fig. 8.3). These are therefore, special transformed cells that are remarkably plastic. Although they do not satisfy the defining criteria of normal stem cells, they do offer enormous insights into the integration and fate of cells that may eventually be used as therapeutics for human diseases (Steindler, 2002). Hypoxia-ischemia (HI) is a common cause of neurological disability. It damages the nervous system through loss of cerebral parenchyma and of the cells and connections found there. HI acts as a prototype for major abnormalities of the brain and other organs characterized by extensive tissue loss (Sharp, 1995).

NSCs are self-renewing primordial cells that can give rise to differentiated progeny within all neural lineages in all regions of the neuraxis; they exist in embryonic and foetal germinal zones where they participate in CNS (central nervous system) organogenesis. Cells with stem like qualities can be isolated from the mammalian CNS at all ages, propagated in culture, and re-implanted into abnormal CNS regions, where they replace lost neural cells and deliver therapeutic gene products as integral members of the host parenchyma (Gage; 1998; Akerud *et al.*, 2001). Stem cells from the CNS can serve as a prototype for solid organ-derived stem cells (Park *et al.*, 2002).

The response of endogenous and transplanted NSCs to HI-induced cerebral degeneration has been traced (Park *et al.*, 2002). Although NSCs engraft within regions of HI injury in the severely affected regions, large amounts of parenchyma are irretrievably lost; this limits the ability of grafts to reconstitute cerebrum and re-form connections. The core of the infarct changes rapidly to a cystic cavity. Stem cells need intrinsic organization and a template to guide restructuring. Also many of them fail to survive if located more than a few hundred micrometers from the nearest capillary. To address this problem, Park *et al.*, implanted bridges made of NSCs seeded upon poly glycolic acid (PGA) based scaffolds into the evolving infarction cavity resulting from unilateral ligation of the right common carotid artery followed by hypoxia. Strong reciprocal interactions between exogenous implant and injured host brain occurred spontaneously, resulting in considerable reduction in parenchymal loss and the reconstitution of anatomical connections.

This work demonstrated that parenchymal loss was greatly reduced, as intricate meshwork of many highly arborized neurites of both host- and donor-derived neurons emerged, and some anatomical connections were reconstituted. The NSC scaffold complex altered the trajectory and complexity of host cortical neuritis. Reciprocally, donor-derived neurons apparently elicited directed, target-appropriate neurite outgrowth (extending axons to the opposite hemisphere) without specific external instruction, induction or genetic manipulation of host brain or donor cells. These "bio-bridges" appeared to unveil or augment a constitutive reparative response by promoting reciprocal interactions between NSC and host; these included promoting neuronal differentiation, enhancing the elaboration of neural processes, fostering the re-formation of cortical tissue, and promoting connectivity. Inflammation and scarring were also reduced, facilitating reconstitution (Park *et al.*, 2002). This work has important implications for tissue engineering and regenerative medicine (Nerem and Sambanis, 1995; Putnam and Mooney, 1996; Vacanti and Langer, 1999).

Park *et al.* (2002) used a postnatal mouse hypoxic-ischemic model of severe cerebral palsy, to combine biomaterials science and stem cell biology for the first time in brain repair. They generated a massive cortical lesion by a common carotid ligation-hypoxic atmosphere protocol. Such a severe ischemic event causes much tissue damage. Scaffolding, such as the poly glycolic acid (PGA) biodegradable polymer used, provided a support system in which a multipotent neural precursor cell could possibly integrate with a very hostile environment and ultimately contribute to CNS tissue reconstitution (Fig. 8.3). The group turned to biomaterials science in a new approach to rebuilding a cerebral hemisphere. Such artificial extracellular biopolymer matrices as PGA have been used in various tissue-engineering models and are well-suited to CNS applications in view of their malleability, their loss of mechanical strength over a few weeks in the body, and the likelihood that they could provide a scaffold for young cells to ease themselves into a post-injury disturbed environment containing many growth-inhibitory molecules. Hopefully, once neural progenitor cells embedded within a PGA matrix have been transplanted into the injured CNS, they may establish some synaptic interconnectivity with the host. At the same time, the bio-matrix facilitates diffusion of nutrients and neovascularization. Vascular infiltration of the cell seeded-scaffold takes place. The PGA dissolves and the C17.2 cells differentiate into neuronal and glial phenotypes, with the neurons both receiving and giving rise to axonal connections (Park *et al.*, 2002).

According to Steindler (2002), a syrinx that forms in syringomyelia after, for example, contusive spinal-cord injury in humans may be particularly amenable to a repair mechanism involving the type of cell-seeded scaffold used by Park *et al.* (2002). Clinical trial of foetal human neural tissue grafts as therapy for human spinal-cord injury has shown that the foetal tissue helps to fill such a cavity (Wirth *et al.,* 2001). A scaffold seeded with neural stem cells may be a good alternative. If a cell-seeded biodegradable scaffold could inhibit monocyte infiltration and scar formation in the injured human CNS, as it probably does in the animal model described by Park *et al.,* (2002) and also promotes synaptogenesis and the formation of functional connections on and from new neurons, this would be a great advancement in restorative neurology.

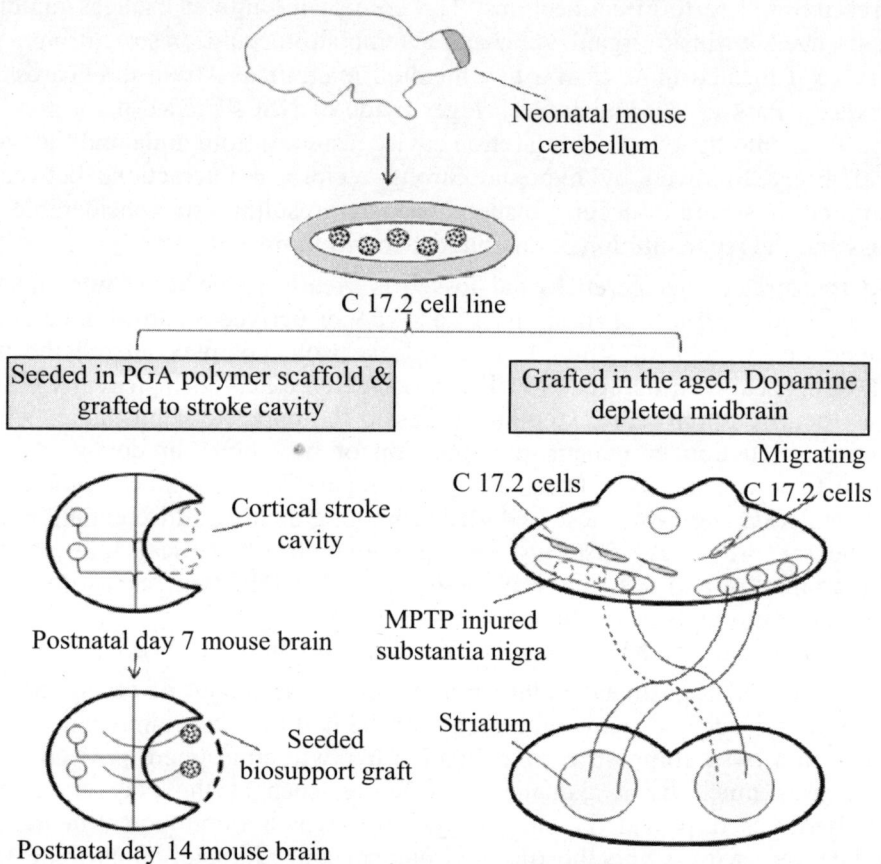

Fig. 8.3: Immortalized cerebellar precursor cells for stroke repair and dopamine neuron rescue. (I) the C17.2 cell line was generated by V-myc-immortalization of neonatal mouse cerebellar precursor this line has been previously used to "chase" tumor cells, replace lost cells in the injured cerebral cortex, help ameliorate some of the behavioral deficits following spinal cord injury, and replace lost cerebellar neurons in a mutant mouse. (II) Seeding a biopolymer scaffold with C17.2 cells and transplanting them to a cortical stroke cavity 7 days after a hypoxic-ischaemic event in postnatal mice resulted in space-occupation, integration within the damaged hemisphere, and the appearance of connections to and from cells in the graft site. (Ill) Grafts of C17.2 cells within the dopamine neuron-injured midbrain of adult mice that have a "chaperone" effect on the rescuing of dopamine neurons in this rodent MPTP model of Parkinson's disease. In addition to an apparent neurotrophic rescue of the injured dopaminergic neurons and their nigrostriatal axonal projections, C17.2 cells also gave rise to small numbers of newly-generated dopamine neurons, and migrated to disparate CNS sites

Arvidsson *et al.* (2002) attempted self-repair by indigenous "brain marrow" stem cell populations without experimental coercion, also in a rodent model of stroke (Steindler and Pincus, 2002). But these cells did not survive and stroke induced reactive neurogenesis in the adult rodent led to the death of about 80% of "new" neurons within two weeks of the ischaemic events this underscores the need for alternative approaches to provide an environment suitable for long-term cell survival and integration, the work of Park *et al.* (2002) is important in this context.

Ourednik *et al.* (2002) described an intriguing chaperone effect of the C17.2 stem-like cell population for rescuing tyrosine hydroxylase expression by injured cells in the midbrain substantia nigra of aged mice injured with 1-methyl-4-phenyl 1,2,3,6-tetrahydropyridine (MPTP). Grafting studies had shown that C17.2 cells engineered to release glial cell line-derived neurotrophic factor (GDNF, a well-established neuroprotective molecule for midbrain dopamine neurons) in mice injured with 6-hydroxydopamine (6-OHDA) prevented the loss of substantia nigra dopaminergic neurons in this model of Parkinson's disease. The "rescue" probably occurred from protective effects of the released GDNF on dopamine axon terminals within the striatal graft site and its retrograde transport back to the nigral neurons in the midbrain.

Transplantation of non-engineered C17.2 cells in the vicinity of the MPTP injured dopamine neurons in the midbrain generated some new dopaminergic neurons, but most of the tyrosine hydroxylase (the rate-limiting enzymes in dopamine synthesis) was produced by "rescued" host cells—a "chaperone" effect. Although ES cells readily generate neurons *in vitro*, directing their differentiation into specific neuronal subtypes is difficult however, mechanisms that regulate neuronal specification during development can be applied to ES cells *in vitro*; this can create new ways of generating cells for therapy.

The marked capacity of ES cells to divide indefinitely *in vitro* without transformation and their ability to generate all types of differentiated progeny of the embryo make these cells well suited for generating spare cells for the treatment of degenerative diseases. However, although ES cells can potentially produce a large variety of cell types *in vitro,* they appear to have a bias for certain lineages. For example, they seldom produce endodermal cells. Their ability to readily generate neural cells, however, has aroused much hope that they may serve as a good source of replacement neurons for patients with central nervous system (CNS) injuries and diseases (Bjorklund and Lindvall, 2000; Tropepe *et al.*, 2001*;* Wichterle *et al.*, 2002).

In some neurodegenerative diseases, such as amyotrophic lateral sclerosis (ALS) and Parkinson's disease, there occurs a selective loss of certain classes of neurons; that is why both are now major targets for the development of stem-cell-based therapies. Unfortunately, ES cells do not always generate the types of neuron one would wish, and finding ways to steer the differentiation of ES cells into specific neuronal subtypes is a major challenge, Two recent studies have raised hopes that this challenge can be overcome; methods have been suggested to generate homogeneous populations of specific neurons from ES cells, Wichterle *et al.* (2002) reported results with possible implications for ALS. Neuralizing ES cells makes them behave almost identically to neural plate cells during normal embryonic development; further treatments can yield the major classes of spinal cord neurons, including perfect motor neurons, from ES cells. Kim *et al.* (2002) mimicked developmental cues to induce ES cells to form dopamine neurons the cells affected in Parkinson's disease. Hynes (1999) had earlier characterized the steps involved in the generation of dopaminergic midbrain neurons during development. Kim *et al.* (2002) developed suitable protocols for the generation of dopaminergic neurons from both foetal neural stem cells and ES cells. Aided by these and other similar findings, Kim *et al.* (2002) could develop a protocol that produces a very highly enriched culture of dopamine neurons whose electrophysiological properties are similar to those of their *in vivo* counterparts. These cells were then transplanted to the striatum of animals in which a Parkinson-like lesion had been induced by selectively killing the midbrain dopamine neurons. The rationale for this experiment was that these transplanted neurons might integrate into the striatum and release dopamine, thereby replacing the lost input from the midbrain dopamine neurons (Cassidy and Frisco, 2002).

The experimental animals registered a marked recovery effect in behavioral tests. Indeed, it even appears that the loss of neurons may be overcompensated, as the animals showed signs of higher than normal dopamine release. This finding suggests that the number of cells that are transplanted should not be higher than needed. While dopamine neuron transplants derived from ES cells have provided some encouraging results in the rodent Parkinson's disease model (Kim *et al.*, 2002), the rescue of at-risk dopaminergic neurons would certainly be a major breakthrough in the case of Parkinson's disease (Steindler, 2002). Ourednik *et al.* (2002) found that not only did the C17.2 cells rescue midbrain dopaminergic neurons in MPTP lesioned animals but also D-amphetamine-evoked rotational behaviour regressed in a functional assay.

These findings have strong potential biotechnological and translational applications. Immortalized neural stem cells may have a role in rescuing dysfunctional neurons in Parkinson's disease. Finding the molecular determinants of reciprocal intercellular signalling may also suggest new treatment approaches to progressive neurodegenerative diseases. Biotechnology should take due notice of stem cell-seeded therapeutic biomatrices (Steindler, 2002).

Some concerns over the use of immortalized, transformed cells for replacement therapies or for neuroprotective or trophic support of at-risk neuronal populations arise from the fact that transformed stem or progenitor cell populations may be involved in some cancers, e.g., leukaemia. In fact, Ignatova *et al.* (2002) have pointed to some connection between neuropoiesis and gliomagenesis in the human brain. Yet the C17.2 cells seem to differentiate upon transplantation into the CNS, and have not been reported to form tumors.

8.8.6. Durable blood vessels

Producing stable or durable blood vessels has posed a formidable challenge for tissue engineering in regenerative medicine, No doubt some genes can be introduced into vascular cells to enhance their survival and proliferation, but these manipulations can cause cancer. Koike *et al.* (2004) showed that a network of long-lasting blood vessels can be formed in mice by co-implantation of vascular endothelial cells and mesenchymal precursor cells; this bypasses the requirement for risky genetic manipulations. These networks are stable and functional for about a year *in vivo*.

To make stable vessels, human umbilical-vein endothelial cells (HUVECs) and 10T1/2 mesenchymal precursor cells were first seeded in a three-dimensional fibronectin-type I collagen gel. The 10T1/2 cells differentiate into mural cells through heterotypic interaction with endothelial cells. For observing the engineered vascular networks *in vivo,* Koike *et al.* (2002) implanted the 3D constructs into mice. The gene for enhanced green fluorescent protein (EGFP) was introduced for tracking the implanted HUVECs.

Initially, the HUVECs formed long, interconnected tubes with many branches that showed no evidence of perfusion but later they connected to the mouse's circulatory system and became perfused. There was a rapid increase in the number of perfused vessels in the first fortnight followed by stabilization whereas the number of non-perfused vessels decreased and then disappeared, By contrast, constructs prepared from HUVECs alone showed minimal perfusion and disappeared after

60 days. Labelling for *in vivo* microscopy confirmed that 10T1/2 cells had been incorporated into the vessel wall.

8.8.7. Mutant (cancer) stem cells and cancer

Some indications point to the possibility that the capacity of stem cells to replicate indefinitely may also be the source of the mutant cells that give rise to cancerous tumors and maintain their growth. Cancer stem cells have been identified in leukemia's, and in breast and brain cancers. It seems possible that the mutations leading to cancer development could originate in the body's small supply of naturally occurring stem cells—cancer stem cells resemble these normal stem cells in several ways. Both types are self-renewing, i.e., when they divide, one of the daughter cells differentiates into a particular cell type that eventually stops dividing, but the other daughter retains its stem cell properties, including the ability to divide in the same way again (Marx, 2003).

Cancer stem cells, which make up only a small proportion of the total tumor cell population, happen to be the only tumor cells that can keep tumors growing. To cure cancer completely, it may therefore be feasible to design therapies that target cancer stem cells but without destroying the vital stem cells needed to maintain tissues such as the bone marrow and intestinal lining. More importantly, however, the new findings generate some caution and suspicion against using stem cells for organ repair. Because some cancers are sustained by only a few cells that otherwise resemble normal stem cells, this might explain why many cancers are so hard to eradicate, and it has prompted researchers to rethink about cancer treatments. It seems likely that some initial mutations that give rise to leukemia arise in normal stem cells, causing them to take the wrong developmental pathway.

Although the cells of solid tumors are more difficult to isolate and study than those of the haematopoietic system, there are indications that solid tumors also contain stem-like cells. It appears that mutant stem cells can seed brain tumors also; some brain cancers, ranging from slow-growing astrocytomas to highly aggressive medulloblastomas and glioblastomas, contain small numbers of self-renewing cells with stem cell-like properties. They can differentiate, at least in lab cultures. All these qualities suggest that the different types of tumors probably derive from a common stem cell population.

Preliminary evidence suggests that the proportion of stem cells in a tumor may determine how deadly it is. Fast-growing medulloblastomas and glioblastomas have many more putative tumor stem cells than do astrocytomas. An extremely aggressive breast cancer has been found to contain about 25% stem cells (Marx, 2003). Gene expression patterns in colon cancer cells are fairly similar to those in colon stem cells. However, even though there is growing evidence that some cancers arise in stem cells, the issue is not finally settled. But the proponents of the idea give two more arguments. Whereas stem cells already have the ability to self-renew, more mature cells would somehow have to regain it if they were to turn cancerous. Second, especially in organs such as the skin and colon lining, where older cells continue to die and slough off, stem cells may be the only ones that persist long enough to accumulate the several mutations needed to produce full-fledged cancers. Cancer development is long-term; we cannot have a cancer develop in a cell that is short-lived (Marx, 2003).

Many current cancer therapies kill dividing cells. Rather surprisingly, stem cells are mostly quiescent; they seem to wake up to divide only occasionally. This implies that they may escape the cell-killing effects of standard therapies. Researchers may have to seek methods to wipe out cancer stem cells. Beyond the implications for cancer therapy, there are concerns about efforts to use stem cells to treat other diseases. Many potential applications require that stem cells be forced to divide to produce enough cells to replace damaged tissue, and that might facilitate the accumulation of potentially cancer-causing mutations. Perhaps it may be possible to exploit modern methods of marker analysis and cell sorting so as to identify and then eliminate cells bearing dangerous mutations.

SUGGESTED READING

- Abbott A. *Nature* 424, 870 (2003).
- Akerud P, Canals JM, Snyder EY, *et al. J Neurosci* 21, 8108 (2001).
- Albertini RJ. *Mutat Res* 489, 1 (2001).
- Alsberg E, Anderson KW, Albeiruti A, *et al. PNAS* (USA) 99, 12025 (2003).
- Amit M, Carpenter MK, Inokuma MS, *et al. Dev Biol* 227, 271 (2000).
- Arvidsson A, Collin T, Kirik D, *et al. Nat Med* 8, 963 (2002).
- Atala AJ. *Endourol* 14, 49 (2000).
- Aubert J, Dunstan H, Chambers I, *et al. Nat Biotechnol* 20, 1240 (2002).
- Bach FH, Ivinson AJ. *Trends in Biotech* 20, 129 (2002).
- Bach FH, Ivinson AJ, Weeramantry C. *Am J Law & Medicine* 27, 283 (2001).
- Beers MH, Berkow R, Burs M. (Eds.) *The Merck Manual of Diagnosis and Therapy* 17th   Ed. Merck, Rahway, NJ (1999).
- Bjorklund A, Lindvall O. *Nat Neurosci* 35, 37 (2000).
- Blau HM. *Nature* 419, 437 (2002).
- Bortvin A, Eggan K, Skaletsky H, *et al. Development* 130,1673 (2003).
- Briggs R, King TJ. *PNAS (USA)* 38, 455 (1952).
- Brinster RL. *Science* 296, 2174 (2002).
- Brivanlou AH, Gage FH, Jaenisch R, *et al. Science* 300, 913 (2003).
- Bromhall JD. *Nature* 258, 719 (1975).
- Brophy B. *Nat Biotechnol* 21, 157 (2003).
- Burns KH, Viveiros MM, Ren Y, *et al. Science* 300, 633 (2003).
- Butler DLJ. *Biomech Eng* 122, 570 (2000).
- Campbell KH. *Semin Cell Dev Biol* 10, 245 (1999).
- Campbell KH, McWhir J, Ritchie WA, *et al. Nature* 380, 64 (1996).
- Cassidy R, Frisen J. *Current Biology* 12, R705 (2002).
- CEC (Commission of the European Communities). Report on human embryonic stem cell research. Office of Publications for the EU, Luxembourg (2003).
- Cervantes RB. *PNAS* (USA) 991, 3586 (2002).
- Chang PL, Bowie KMM. *Adv Drug Deliv Rev* 33, 31 (1998).
- Chen Y, He XZ, Liu A, *et al. Cell Research* 13, 251 (2003).
- Cheung VG, Conlin LK, Weber TM, *et al. Nat Genet* 33, 422 (2003).
- Cibelli JB, Lanza RP, Campbell KH, West MD. (Eds.) *Principles of Cloning.* Academic, San Diego (2002).
- CIHR (Canadian Institutes for Health Research). Human pluripotent stem cell research: Recommendations for CIHR-funded research (2002).

- Colman A, Kind A. *Trends in Biotech* 18, 192 (2000).
- Daar AS, Salomon DR, Ferguson RM, *et al. Nature* 392, 11 (1998).
- Dan N. *Trends in Biotech* 18, 370 (2000).
- Dennis C. *Nature* 424, 711 (2003).
- Ding S, Wu TYH, Brinker A, *et al. PNAS (USA)* 100, 7632 (2003).
- Drukker M, Benvenisty N. *Trends in Biotech* 22, 136 (2004).
- Eggan K, Akutsu H, Loring J, *et al. PNAS (USA)* 22, 6209 (2001).
- Eiges R, Schuldiner M, Drukker M, *et al. Curr Biol* 11, 514 (2001).
- Ellis DL, Yannas LV. *Biomaterials* 17, 291 (1996).
- Eschenhagen T, Didie M, Heubach J, *et al. Transplant Immunol* 9, 315 (2002).
- Feinberg J. *Harmless Wrongdoing,* Oxford Univ Press, New York (1988).
- Fournier AE, Strittmatter SM. *Curr Opin Neurobiol* 11, 89 (2001).
- Gage FH. *Nature* 392(Suppl), 18 (1998).
- Georges M. *Theriogenology* 55, 15 (2001).
- Gould DS, Auchincloss H Jr. *Immunol Today* 20, 77 (1999).
- Gruss P. *Science* 301, 1017 (2003).
- Gurdon JB, Byrne JA. *PNAS* (USA) 100, 8048 (2003).
- Cheung VG, Conlin LK, Weber TM, et al. *Nat Genet* 33, 422 (2003).
- Gurdon JB, Colman A. *Nature* 402, 743 (1999).
- Harrison PM, Kumar A, Lang N, et al. *Nucleic Acids Res* 30, 1083 (2002).
- Hochedlinger K, Jaenisch R N. *Engl J Med* 349, 275 (2003).
- Hoerstrup SP, Sodian R, Daebritz S, *et al. Circulation* 102 (Suppl3), 44 (2000).
- Holmes TC. *Trends in Biotech* 20, 16 (2002).
- Hutmacher DW. *Biomaterials* 21, 2529 (2000).
- Hynes RO. *Trends Cell Biol* 9, 33 (1999).
- Ignatova TN, Kukekov VG, Laywell ED, *et al. Glia* 39, 193 (2002).
- Itskovitz-Eldor J, Schuldiner M, Karsenti D, *et al. Mol Med* 6, 88 (2000).
- Jaenisch R, Eggan K, Humpherys D, *et al. Cloning Stem Cells* 4, 389 (2002).
- Jasmund I, Bader A. *Adv Biochem Eng Biotechnol* 74, 99 (2002).
- Jiang M, Milner J. *Oncogene* 21, 6041 (2002).
- Kanatsu-Shinohara M, Ogura A, Ikegawa M, *et al. PNAS* (USA) 99, 1383 (2002).
- Keeley FW, Bellingham CM, Woodhouse KA. *Phil Trans R Soc Lond B Biol Sci* 357, 185 (2002).
- Kennedy D. *Science* 300, 865 (2003).
- Kim JH, Auerbach JM, Rodriguez G, *et al. Nature* 418, 50 (2002).
- Kimbrell A. *The Human Body Shop: The Cloning, Engineering, and Marketing of Life* Regnery Publishing, Washington, DC (1997).
- Klar AJS. *Nature* 417, 595 (2002).

- Koike N, Fukumura D, Gralla O, *et al. Nature* 428, 138 (2004).
- Kruip TAM, den Daas JHG. *Theriogenology* 47, 43 (1997).
- Langer R, Vacanti JP. *Science* 260, 920 (1993).
- Laskey RA, Gurdon JB. *Nature* 228, 1332 (1970).
- Levenberg S, Golub JS, Amit M, *et al. PNAS* (USA) 99, 4391 (2002).
- Lin H. In: *Stem Cells Handbook.* Sell S (Ed) Humana Press, Totowa, NJ 57 (2004).
- Lin H. *Nat Rev Genet* 3, 931 (2002).
- Lin H. *Nature* 425, 353 (2003).
- Lin TP. In: *Methods in Mammalian Embryology* Freeman, San Francisco (1971).
- Lo B, Chou V, Cedars MI, *et al. Science* 301, 921 (2003).
- Loi P, Ptak G, Barboni B, *et al. Nat Biotechnol* 19, 962 (2001).
- Loi P, Clinton M, Barboni B, *et al. Biol Reprod* 67, 126 (2002).
- Loi P, Fulka J, Ptak G. *Trends in Biotech* 213, 471 (2003).
- Lowenstein PR, Castro MG. *Physiol Behav* 73, 833 (2001).
- Lumelsky N, Blondel O, Laeng P, *et al. Science* 292, 1389 (2001).
- Martin GR. *PNAS* (USA) 78, 7634 (1981).
- Martin I, Wendt D, Heberer M. *Trends in Biotech* 22, 80 (2004).
- Marx J. *Science* 301, 1308 (2003).
- Mazariegos GV, Patzer II J F, Lopez RC, *et al.* J *Am J Transplant* 2, 260 (2002).
- McCreath KJ, Howcroft J, Campbell KHS, *et al. Nature* 405, 1066 (2000).
- McGrath J, Solter D. *Science* 226, 1317 (1984).
- Moon RT, Bowerman B, Boutros M, *et al. Science* 296, 1644 (2002).
- Nerem RM, Sambanis A. *Tissue Eng* 1, 3 (1995).
- Nicholas FW, Smith C. *Anim Prod* 36, 341 (1983).
- Nigel W. *Current Biology* 12, R473 (2002).
- NIH (National Institutes of Health). Report of the Human Embryo Research Panel. National Institutes of Health, Bethesda, MD (1994).
- Niklason LE, Gao J, Abbott WM, *et al. Science* 284, 489 (1999).
- Oback B, Wiersema AT, Gaynor P, *et al. Cloning Stem Cells* 5, 3 (2003).
- Oberpenning F, Meng J, Yoo JJ, *et al. Nat Biotechnol* 17, 149 (1999).
- Ogawa T, Dobrinski I, Avarbock MR, *et al. Nature Med* 6, 29 (2000).
- Orive G, Hernandez RM, Gascon AR, *et al. Trends in Biotech* 22, 87 (2004).
- Orkin SH, Morrison SJ. *Nature* 418, 25 (2002).
- Ourednik J, Ourednik V, Lynch WP, *et al. Nat Biotechnol* 20, 1103 (2002).
- Ourednik V, Ourednik J, Park KL, *et al. Clin Genet* 56, 267 (1999).
- Park KL, Teng YD, Snyder EY. *Nat Biotechnol* 20, 1111 (2002).
- Peppas NA, Langer R. *Science* 263, 1715 (1994).

- Perugino G, Trincone A, Rossi M, Moracci M. *Trends in Biotech* 22, 31 (1994).
- Pesce M, Scholer HR. *Stem Cells* 9, 271 (2001).
- Petite H, Viateau V, Bensaïd W, *et al. Nat Biotehnol* 18, 959 (2000).
- Pittenger MF, Mackay AM, Beck SC, *et al. Science* 284, 143 (1999).
- Putnam AJ, Mooney DJ. *Nat Med* 2, 824 (1996).
- Radin MJ. *Contested Commodities* Harvard Univ Press, Cambridge MA (1996).
- Reubinoff BE, Pera MF, Fong CY, *et al. Nat Biotechnol* 18, 399 (2000).
- Reynolds B, Weiss S. *Science* 255, 1707 (1992).
- Richards LJ, Kilpatrick TJ, Bartlett PF. *PNAS* (USA) 89, 8591 (1992).
- Rideout WM, Hochedlinger K, Kyba M, *et al. Cell* 109, 17 (2002).
- Rosania GR, Chang YT, Perez 0, *et al. Nat Biotechnol* 18, 304 (2000).
- Rossant J. *Nature* 415, 967 (2002).
- Schachner M. *Nature* 405, 747 (2000).
- Schuldiner M, Yanuka O, Itskovitz-Eldor J, *et al. PNAS* (USA) 97, 11307 (2000).
- Scott IC, Stainier DYR. *Science* 298, 2141 (2002).
- Scott MR, Will R, Ironside J, *et al. PNAS* (USA*)* 96, 15137 (1999).
- Semino CE, Merok JR, Crane GG, *et al. Differentiation* 71, 262 (2003).
- Sharp FR. *Ann Neurol* 34, 322 (1995).
- Shea LD, Smiley E, Bonadio J, *et al. Nat Biotechnol* 17, 551 (1999).
- Shimizu T,Yamato M, Isoi Y, *et al. Circ Res* 90, e40 (2002).
- Shinohara T, Avarbock MR, Brinster RL. *Dev Biol* 220, 401(2000).
- Shinohara T, Orwig KE, Avarbock MR, *et al. PNAS (USA)* 98, 6186(2001).
- Sims M, First NL. *PNAS* (USA) 91, 6143 (1994).
- Slimane-Bureau WC, King WA. *Cloning Stem Cells* 4, 319 (2002).
- Smith LD. *PNAS* (USA) 54, 101 (1965).
- Snyder EY, Taylor RM, Wolfe JH. *Nature* 374, 367 (1995).
- Sodian R, Lemke T, Fritsche C, *et al. Tissue Eng* 8, 863 (2002).
- Spradling A, Drummond-Barbosa D, Kai T. *Nature* 414, 98 (2001).
- Steindler DA. *Nat Biotechnol* 20, 1091 (2002).
- Steindler DA, Pincus DW. *The Lancet* 359, 1047 (2002).
- Suh JK, Matthew HW. *Biomaterials* 21, 2589 (2000).
- Terada N, Hamazaki T, Oka M, *et al. Nature* 416, 542 (2002).
- Thomas KR, Capecchi MR. *Cell* 51, 503 (1987).
- Thomson JA, Itskovitz-Eldor J, Shapiro SS, *et al. Science* 282, 1145 (1998).
- Tropepe V, Hitoshi S, Sirard *C, et al. Neuron* 30, 65 (2001).
- Vacanti JP, Langer RS. *Lancet* 354(Suppl 1), S32 (1999).
- Van der Kooy D, Weiss S. *Science* 287, 1439 (2000).

- Vander Laan LJ, Lockey C, Griffeth BC, *et al. Nature* 407, 90 (2002).
- Verfaillie CM. *Nat Immunol* 3, 314 (2002).
- Vogel G. *Science* 297, 175 (2002).
- Wang Z, Lin H. *Science* 303, 2016 (2004).
- Weiss L. (Ed.) *Histology: Cell and Tissue Biology* Elsevier, New York 212 (1987).
- Wells DN, Oback B, Laible G. *Trend in Biotech* 21, 428 (2003).
- West MW, Wang W, Patterson J, *et al. PNAS* (USA) 96, 11211 (1999)
- Wichterle H, Lieberam I, Porter J, *et al. Cell* 110, 385 (2002).
- Willadsen SM. *Nature* 320, 63 (1986).
- Williams N. *Current Biology* 13, R209 (2003).
- Wilmut I, Schnieke AE, McWhir J, *et al. Nature* 385, 810 (1997).
- Wirth ED 3rd, Reier PJ, Fessler RG, *et al. J Neurotrauma* 18, 911 (2001).
- Williams JA, Wilmut I. *Anim Sci* 68, 245 (1999).
- Xu G, Wang W, Groves JT, *et al. PNAS* (USA) 98, 3652 (2001).
- Yamashita YM, Jones DL, Fuller MT. *Science* 301, 1547 (2003).
- Ying QY, Nichols J, Evans EP, *et al. Nature* 416, 545 (2002).
- Zandonella C. *Nature* 421, 884 (2003).
- Zhang SC, Wernig M, Duncan ID, *et al. Nat Biotechnol* 19, 1129 (2001).
- Zwaka TP, Thomson JA. *Nat Biotechnol* 21, 319 (2002).

RECOMBINANT DNA TECHNOLOGY

9.1. INTRODUCTION
    9.1.1. Historical perspective
    9.1.2. An outline of molecular cloning by rDNA technology
9.2. MOLECULAR TOOLS IN rDNA TECHNOLOGY
    9.2.1. Cutting and joining DNA
    9.2.2. Major classes of restriction endonucleases- DNA cutting enzyme
       9.2.2.1. Restriction endonclease nomenclature
       9.2.2.2. Recognition sequences for type II restriction endonucleases
    9.2.3. DNA ligase
       9.2.3.1. Homopolymer tailing
       9.2.3.2. Linker and adaptor
       9.2.3.3. Problems with ligation
    9.2.4. Vectors – The cloning vehicle
       9.2.4.1. Choice of vector is dependent on insert size and application
       9.2.4.2. Plasmid DNA as a vector
          9.2.4.2.1. Nomenclature of plasmids
          9.2.4.2.2. pBR322- The most common plasmid vector
          9.2.4.2.3. Methods of gene transfer
             9.2.4.2.3.1. Transformation: transfer of recombinant plasmid DNA to a bacterial host
             9.2.4.2.3.2. Electroporation
             9.2.4.2.3.3. Conjugation
       9.2.4.3. Vectors for cloning large pieces of DNA
          9.2.4.3.1. Bacteriophage lambda (λ) as a vector
             9.2.4.3.1.1. Bacteriophage λ vectors permit efficient construction of large DNA libraries
          9.2.4.3.2. Hybrid plasmid/phage vectors
          9.2.4.3.3. Artificial chromosome vectors
          9.2.4.3.4. Yeast artificial chromosome (YAC) vectors

9.3. RECOMBINANT SELECTION

9.3.1. Blue-white screening

9.4. AMPLIFICATION AND PURIFICATION OF RECOMBINANT PLASMID DNA

9.5. SOURCES OF DNA FOR CLONING

9.6. CREATING AND SCREENING DNA LIBRARIES

9.6.1. Making a gene library

9.6.1.1. Genomic library

9.6.1.2. cDNA library

9.6.2. Screening by DNA hybridization

9.6.3. Screening by immunological assay

9.6.4. Screening by protein activity

9.7. Analysis of clone

9.7.1. Characterization based on mRNA translation *in vitro* genes

9.7.2. Gcl electrophoresis

9.7.3. Restriction mapping

9.7.4. Restriction fragment length polymorphism (RFLP)

9.7.5. Blotting techniques

9.7.6. DNA sequencing

9.7.6.1. Maxam–Gilbert (chemical) sequencing

9.7.6.2. Sanger–Coulson (dideoxy or enzymatic) sequencing

9.7.6.3. Electrophoresis and reading of sequences

9.7.6.4. DNA sequencing by primer walking

9.7.6.5. Chromosome walking in DNA sequencing

9.7.6.5.1. Chromosome jumping

9.8. EXPRESSION SYSTEMS

9.9. PRODUCTION AND PURIFICATION OF rDNA PRODUCTS

9.10. ANALYSIS OF rDNA PRODUCTS

9.1. INTRODUCTION

Recombinant DNA technology primarily involves the manipulation of genetic material (DNA) to achieve the desired goal in a predetermined way. The key or cornerstone of most molecular biology technologies is the gene. To facilitate the study of genes, they can be isolated and amplified. There are many diverse and complex techniques involved in gene manipulation. One method of isolation and amplification of a gene of interest is to clone the gene by inserting it into another DNA molecule that serves as a vehicle or vector that can be replicated in living cells. This combination of two DNAs of different origin is referred to as a recombinant DNA molecule. Although genetic processes such as crossing-over technically produce recombinant DNA, the term is generally reserved for DNA molecules produced by joining segments derived from different biological sources. The recombinant DNA molecule is transferred in a host cell, either prokaryotic or eukaryotic. The host cell then replicates (producing a clone), and simultaneously the vector with its foreign piece of DNA also replicates. The foreign DNA thus becomes amplified in number, and following its amplification can be purified for further analysis.

9.1.1. Historical perspective

Recombinant DNA technology was developed from discoveries in molecular biology, nucleic acid enzymology and the molocular genetics of both bacterial viruses (bacteriophage) and bacterial extrachromosomal genetic elements (plasmids). The present day DNA technology has its root in the experiments performed by Boyer and Cohen in 1973. In there experiments, they successfully recombined two plasmids (*pSC* 101 and *pSC* 102) and cloned the new plasmid in *E.coli*. Plasmid *pSC*101 possesses a gene resistant to antibiotic tetracycline while *pSC*102 contains a gene resistant to another antibiotic kanamycin. The newly developed recombined plasmid when incorporated into the bacteria exhibited resistance to both the antibiotic- tetracycline and kanamycin. The synthesis of many experimental observations into recombinant DNA technology occurred between 1972 and 1975, through the efforts of several research groups working primarily on bacteriophage lambda (λ).

9.1.2. An outline of molecular cloning by rDNA technology

The basic procedure of molecular cloning involves a series of steps. The basic principle of recombinant DNA technology is reasonably simple, and broadly involves the following steps.

- The DNA fragments to be cloned are generated by using restriction endonucleases.
- The fragments produced by digestion with restriction enzymes are ligated to other DNA molecules that serve as vectors. Vectors can replicate autonomously (independent of host genome replication) in host cells and facilitate the manipulation of the newly created recombinant DNA molecule.
- The recombinant DNA molecule is transferred to a host cell. Within this cell, the recombinant DNA molecule replicates, producing dozens of identical copies known as clones. As the host cells replicate, the recombinant DNA is passed on to all progeny cells, creating a population of identical cells, all carrying the cloned sequence.
- The cloned DNA segments can be recovered from the host cell, purified, and analyzed in various ways.
- Therapeutic protein from the cells can be obtained by cloning the gene for a particular protein of interest and allowing its expression in appropriate host cells commonly referred to as expression vector/host system.

9.2. MOLECULAR TOOLS IN rDNA TECHNOLOGY

9.2.1. Cutting and joining DNA

Two major categories of enzymes are important tools in the isolation of DNA and the preparation of recombinant DNA: restriction endonucleases and DNA ligases. Restriction endonucleases recognize a specific, rather short, nucleotide sequence on a double-stranded DNA molecule, called a restriction site, and cleave the DNA at this recognition site or elsewhere, depending on the type of enzyme. DNA ligase joins two pieces of DNA by forming phosphodiester bonds.

9.2.2. Major classes of restriction endonucleases- DNA cutting enzyme

There are three major classes of restriction endonucleases. Their grouping is based on the types of sequences recognized, the nature of the cut made in the DNA, and the enzyme structure. Type I and III restriction endonucleases are not useful for gene cloning because they cleave DNA at sites other than the recognition sites and thus cause random cleavage patterns. In contrast, type II endonucleases are widely used for mapping and reconstructing DNA *in vitro* because they recognize specific sites and cleave only at these sites (Table 9.1).

In addition, the type II endonuclease and methylase activities are usually separate, single subunit enzymes.

Although the two enzymes recognize the same target sequence, they can be purified separately from each other. Some type II restriction endonucleases do not conform to this narrow definition, making it necessary to define further subdivisions. The discussion here will focus on the "orthodox" type II restriction endonucleases that are commonly used in molecular biology research.

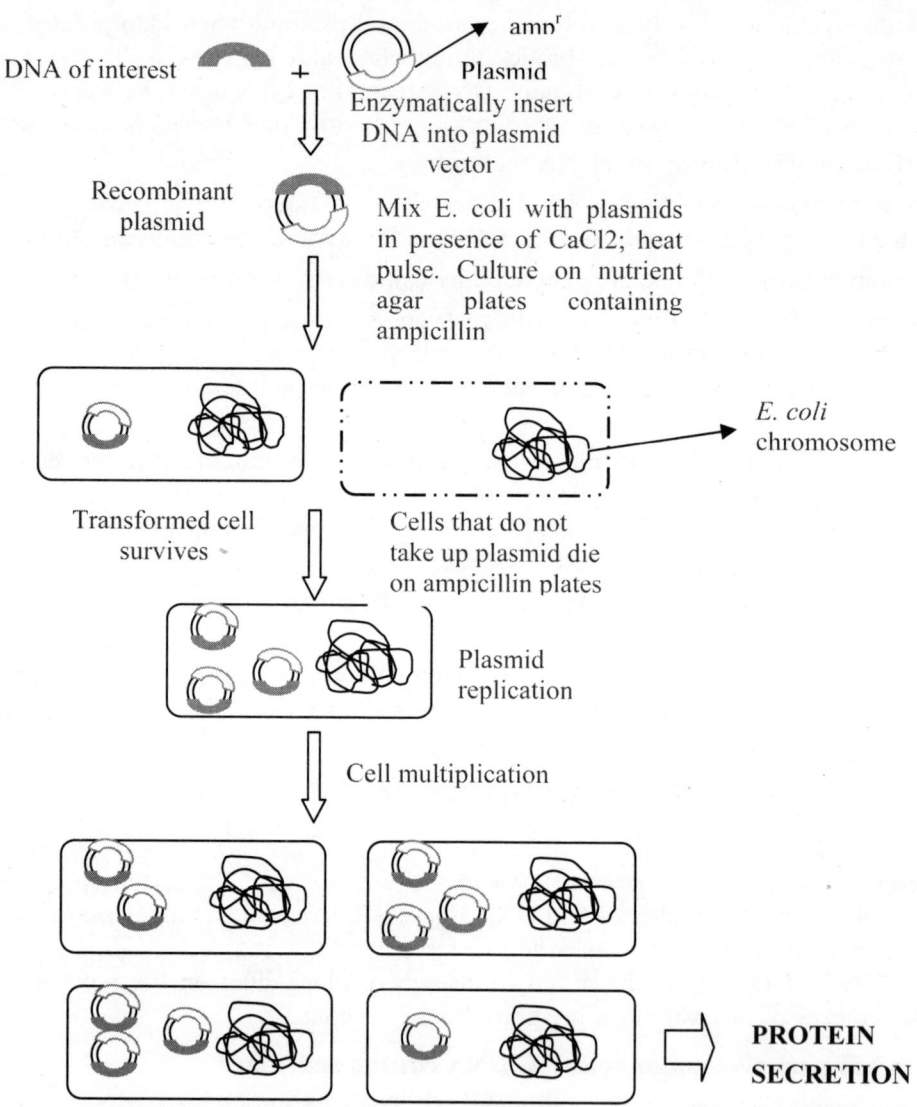

DNA of interest   +   amp^r
                                            Plasmid
                                   Enzymatically insert
                                   DNA into plasmid
                                        vector

Recombinant
plasmid   Mix E. coli with plasmids
                                   in presence of CaCl2; heat
                                   pulse. Culture on nutrient
                                   agar   plates   containing
                                   ampicillin

                                                    E. coli
                                                    chromosome

Transformed cell   Cells that do not
survives   take up plasmid die
                        on ampicillin plates

                                   Plasmid
                                   replication

                        Cell multiplication

                                                    PROTEIN
                                                    SECRETION

Colony of cells, each containing copies of the same recombinant plasmid

Fig. 9.1: Protein production by rDNA technology- A fragment of DNA to be cloned is first inserted into a plasmid vector containing an ampicillin-resistance gene (*amp^r*), such. Only the few cells transformed by incorporation of a plasmid molecule will survive on ampicillin-containing medium. In transformed cells, the plasmid DNA replicates and segregates into daughter cells, resulting in formation of an ampicillin resistant colony. These colonies finally secrete the required protein

Table 9.1: Recognition sequence of some restriction endonucleases

Enzyme	Recognition site	Type of cut end
EcoRI	G↓ A-A-T-T-C C- T- T-A-A ↑G	5' phosphate extension
BamHI	G ↓G- A- T- C- C C – C- T- A- G ↑G	5' phosphate extension
PstI	C – T- G- C- A ↓G G ↑A- C- G- T- C	3'hydroxyl extension
Sau3AI	↓ G- A- T- C C- T- A- G ↑	5' phosphate extension
PvuII	C- A- G↓C- T- G G- T- C↑G- A- C	Blunt end
HpaI	G- T- T↓A- A- C A- G- G↑T- T- G	Blunt end
HaeIII	G- G↓C- C T- T ↑G- G	Blunt end
NotI	G↓ C- G- G- C- C- G- C C C- C- C- G- G- C↑G	5' phosphate extension

9.2.2.1. Restriction endonuclease nomenclature

Restriction endonucleases are named by a standard procedure, with particular reference to the bacteria from which they are isolated. The first latter (in italics) of the enzyme indicates the genus name, followed by the first two letters (also in italics) of the species, then comes the strain of the organism and finally a Roman numeral indicating the order of discovery. For example, *Hin*dIII (pronounced "hindee-three") was discovered in *Haemophilus influenza* (strain d). The *Hin* comes from the first letter of the genus name and the first two letters of the species name; d is for the strain type; and III is for the third enzyme of that type. *Sma*I is from *Serratia marcescens* and is pronounced "smah-one," *Eco*RI (pronounced "echo-r-one") was discovered in *Escherichia coli* (strain R), and *Bam*HI is from *Bacillus amyloliquefaciens* (strain H). Over 3000 type II restriction endonucleases have been isolated and characterized to date. Approximately 240 are available commercially for use by molecular biologists.

9.2.2.2. Recognition sequences for type II restriction endonucleases

Each orthodox type II restriction endonuclease is composed of two identical polypeptide subunits that join together to form a homodimer. These homodimers recognize short symmetric DNA sequences of 4–8 bp. Six base pair cutters are the most commonly used in molecular biology research. Usually, the sequence read in the 5′→3′ direction on one strand is the same as the sequence read in the 5′→3′ direction on the complementary strand. Sequences that read the same in both directions are called palindromes (from the Greek word *palindromos* for "run back"). Figure 9.3 shows some common restriction endonucleases and their recognition sequences. Some enzymes, such as *Eco*RI, generate a staggered cut, in which the single-stranded complementary tails are called "sticky" or cohesive ends because they can base pair through hydrogen bond to the single stranded complementary tails of other DNA fragments. If DNA molecules from different sources share the same palindromic recognition sites, hence both will contain complementary sticky ends (single-stranded tails) when digested with the same restriction endonuclease. Other type II enzymes, such as *Sma*I, cut both strands of the DNA at the same position and generate blunt ends with no unpaired nucleotides when they cleave the DNA.

Table 9.2: Major classes of restriction endonuclease

Class	Abundance	Recognition	Composition	Use in recombinant DNA research
Type I	Less common than type II	Cut both strands at a nonspecific location > 1000 bp away from recognition site	Three-subunit complex: individual recognition, endonuclease, and methylase activities	Not useful
Type II	Most common	Cut both strands at a specific, usually palindromic, recognition site (4–8 bp)	Endonuclease and methylase are separate, single-subunit enzymes	Very useful
Type III	Rare	Cleavage of one strand only, 24–26 bp downstream of the 3′ recognition site	Endonuclease and methylase are separate two-subunit complexes with one subunit in common	Not useful

Restriction endonucleases exhibit a much greater degree of sequence specificity in the enzymatic reaction than is exhibited in the binding of regulatory proteins, such as the Lac repressor to DNA. For example, a single base pair change in a critical operator sequence usually reduces the affinity of the Lac repressor by 10- to 100-fold, whereas a single base pair change in the recognition site of a restriction endonuclease essentially eliminates all enzymatic activity. Like other DNA-binding proteins, the first contact of a restriction endonuclease with DNA is nonspecific. Nonspecific binding usually does not involve interactions with the bases but only with the DNA sugar–phosphate backbone. The restriction endonuclease is loosely bound and its catalytic center is kept at a safe distance from the phosphodiester backbone. Nonspecific binding is a prerequisite for efficient target site location. For example, *Bam*HI moves along the DNA in a linear fashion by a process called "sliding." Sliding involves helical movement due to tracking along a groove of the DNA over short distances (<30–50 bp). This reduces the volume of space through which the protein needs to search to one dimension. However, the "random walk" nature of linear diffusion gives equal probabilities for forward and reverse steps, so if the distances between the nonspecific binding site and the recognition site are large (>30–50 bp), the protein would return repeatedly to its start point. The main mode of translocation over long distances is thus by "hopping" or "jumping." In this process, the protein moves between binding sites through three-dimensional space, by dissociating from its initial site before re-associating elsewhere in the same DNA chain. Because of relatively small diffusion constants of proteins, most rebinding events will be short range "hops" back to or near the initial binding site. In the example of *Bam*HI, once the target restriction site is located, the recognition process triggers large conformational changes of the enzyme and the DNA (called coupling), which leads to the activation of the catalytic center. In addition to indirect interaction with the DNA backbone, specific binding is characterized by direct interaction of the enzyme with the nitrogenous bases. In the presence of the essential cofactor Mg^{2+}, the enzyme cleaves the DNA on both strands at the same time within or in close proximity to the recognition sequence (restriction site). The enzyme cuts the DNA duplex by breaking the covalent, phosphodiester bond between the phosphate of one nucleotide and the sugar of an adjacent nucleotide, to give free 5′-phosphate and 3′-OH ends. Type II restriction endonucleases do not require ATP for their nucleolytic activity. Although there are a number of models for how this nucleophilic attack on the phosphodiester bond occurs, the exact mechanism by which restriction endonucleases achieve DNA cleavage has not yet been proven experimentally for any type II restriction endonuclease.

9.2.3. DNA ligase

The study of DNA replication and repair processes led to the discovery of the DNA-joining enzyme called DNA ligase. DNA ligases catalyze formation of a phosphodiester bond between the 5′-phosphate of a nucleotide on one fragment of DNA and the 3′-hydroxyl of another (Fig. 9.2). This joining of linear DNA fragments together with covalent bonds is called ligation. Unlike the type II restriction endonucleases, DNA ligase requires ATP as a cofactor. Because it can join two pieces of DNA, DNA ligase became a key enzyme in genetic engineering. If restriction-digested fragments of DNA are placed together under appropriate conditions, the DNA fragments from two sources can anneal to form recombinant molecules by hydrogen bonding between the complementary base pairs of the sticky ends. However, the two strands are not covalently bonded by phosphodiester bonds. DNA ligase is required to seal the gaps, covalent bonding of the two strands and regenerating a circular molecule. The DNA ligase most widely used in the lab is derived from the bacteriophage T4. T4 DNA ligase will also ligate fragments with blunt ends, however the reaction is less efficient and higher concentrations of the enzyme are usually required *in vitro*. To increase the efficiency of the reaction, researchers often use the enyzme terminal deoxynucleotidyl transferase to modify the blunt ends by homopolymer tailing.

9.2.3.1. Homopolymer tailing

The complementary DNA stands are joined by annealing. This particular mechanism is used in homopolymer tailing. For example, if a single-stranded poly(dA) tail is added to DNA fragments from one source, and a single stranded poly(dT) tail is added to DNA from another source, the complementary tails can form hydrogen bonds (Fig. 9.3). Recombinant DNA molecules can then be created by ligation. The homopolymer extension (by adding 10-40 residues) can be synthesized by using terminal deoxy nucleotidyltransferase (of calf thymus).

9.2.3.2. Linker and adaptor

Linker and adaptor are chemically synthesized, short, double stranded DNA possessing multiple cloning site (also called the polylinker region) which has a number of unique target sites for restriction endonucleases. Cutting of the circular plasmid vector with one of these enzyme result in a single cut, creating a linear plasmid. A foreign DNA molecule, referred to as the "insert," cut with the same enzyme, can then is joined to the vector in ligation reaction. They can be ligated to blunt ends of any DNA molecule and cut with specific restriction enzyme to produce DNA fragments with sticky ends.

Adaptor contains preformed sticky or cohesive ends. They are usefull to be ligated to DNA fragments with blunt ends. The DNA fragments held to linker or adaptors are finally ligated to vector DNA molecule.

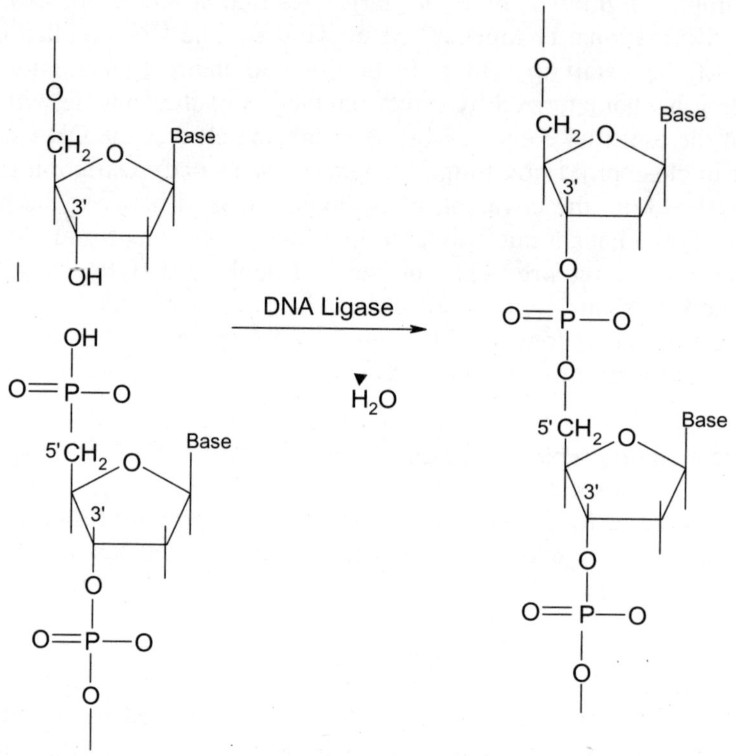

Fig. 9.2: DNA ligases catalyze formation of a phosphodiester bond between the 5′-phosphate of a nucleotide on one fragment of DNA and the 3′-hydroxyl of other nucleotide

9.2.3.3. Problems with ligation

Ligations of the insert to vector are not 100% productive, because the two ends of a plasmid vector can be readily ligated together, which is called self-ligation. The degree of self-ligation can be reduced by treatment of the vector with the enzyme alkaline phosphatase. Alkaline phosphatase is an enzyme which removes the terminal 5′-phosphate. When the 5′-phosphate is removed from the plasmid it cannot be recircularized by ligase, since there is nothing with which to make a phosphodiester bond. But, if the vector is joined with a foreign insert, the 5′-phosphate is provided by the foreign DNA. Another strategy involves using two different restriction endonuclease cutting sites with noncomplementary sticky ends. This inhibits self-ligation and promotes annealing of the foreign DNA in the desired orientation within the vector.

9.2.4. Vectors – The cloning vehicle

Vectors are the DNA molecules, which can carry a foreign DNA fragment to be cloned. The ideal characteristics of cloning vectors are that they:

(i) Can independently replicate themselves and the foreign DNA segments they carry are also replicated

(ii) Contain a number of unique restriction endonuclease cleavage sites that are present only once in the vector

(iii) Carry a selectable marker (usually in the form of antibiotic resistance gene or genes for enzymes missing in the host cells) to distinguish host cells that carry vectors from host cells that do not contain a vector; and

(iv) Should relatively easy to recover from the host cell. There are many possible choices of vector depending on the purpose of cloning.

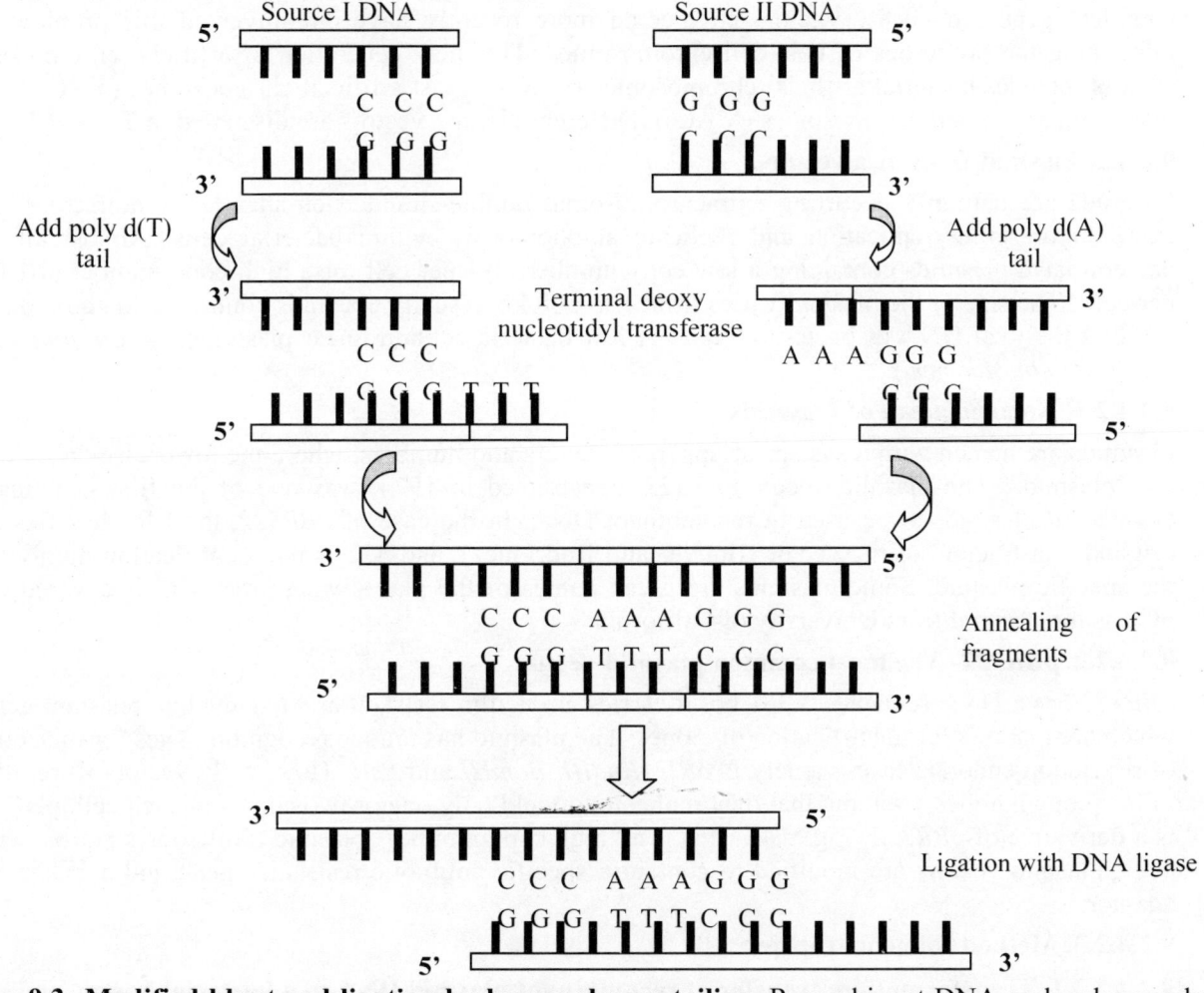

Fig. 9.3: Modified blunt end ligation by homopolymer tailing. Recombinant DNA molecules can be formed from DNA cut with restriction endonucleases that leave blunt ends, such as *Sma*I. Without end modification, blunt end ligation is of low efficiency. The efficiency is increased through using the enzyme terminal deoxynucleotidyl transferase to create complementary tails by the addition of poly(dA) and poly(dT) to the cleaved fragments. These tails allow DNA fragments from two different sources to anneal. "Source 1" DNA and "source 2" DNA are then covalently linked by treatment with DNA ligase to create a recombinant DNA molecule. Note that the *Sma*I site is destroyed in the process

The greatest variety of cloning vectors has been developed for use in the bacterial host *E. coli.* Thus, the first practical skill generally required by a molecular biologist is the ability to grow pure cultures of bacteria.

9.2.4.1. Choice of vector is dependent on insert size and application

The classic cloning vectors are plasmids, phages, and cosmids, which are limited to the size insert they can accommodate, taking up to 10, 20, and 45 kb, respectively (Table 9.2). The feature of plasmids and phages and their use as cloning vectors will be discussed in more detail in later sections. A cosmid is a plasmid carrying a phage λ *cos* site, allowing it to be packaged into a phage head. Cosmids infect a host bacterium as do phages, but replicate like plasmids without lysing host cells. Mammalian genes are often greater than 100 kb in size, so originally there were limitations in cloning complete gene sequences. Vectors engineered more recently have circumvented this problem by mimicking the properties of host cell chromosomes. This new generation of artificial chromosome vectors includes bacterial artificial chromosomes (BACs), yeast artificial chromosomes (YACs), and mammalian artificial chromosomes (MACs). Different cloning vectors are discussed in Table 9.3.

9.2.4.2. Plasmid DNA as a vector

Plasmids are naturally occurring extrachromosomal double-stranded circular DNA molecules that carry an origin of replication and replicate autonomously within bacterial cells. Almost all the bacteria have plasmids containing a low copy number (1-4 per cell) or a high copy number (10-100 per cell). The size of the plasmid varies from 1 to 500 kb. Usually plasmids contribute to about 0.5 to 5.0% of the total DNA of bacteria. (**Note**: A few bacteria contain linear plasmids e.g. *Streptomyces sp, Borella burgdorferi*).

9.2.4.2.1. Nomenclature of Plasmids

Plasmids are named with a system of uppercase letters and numbers, where the lowercase "p" stands for "plasmid." The plasmid vector *pBR322*, constructed in 1974, was one of the first genetically engineered plasmids to be used in recombinant DNA. In the case of *pBR322*, the BR identifies the original constructors of the vector (Bolivar and Rodriquez), and 322 is the identification number of the specific plasmid. Some plasmids are given names of the places where they are discovered e.g. pUC is the plasmid from University of California.

9.2.4.2.2. *pBR322*- The most common plasmid vector

pBR322 has a DNA sequence 4,361 bp. It carries ampicillin resistant and tetracycline resistant genes which are markers for identification of clones. The plasmid has unique recognition sites for the action of restriction endonucleases namely *EcoRI, HindIII, BamHI* and *PstI*. These early vectors were often of low copy number, meaning that they replicate to yield only one or two copies in each cell. pUC19, is a derivative of *pBR322* (Fig. 9.4). This is a "high copy number" plasmid (500 copies per bacterial cell). Plasmid vectors are modified to contain a specific antibiotic resistance gene and a linker and adaptor.

9.2.4.2.3. Methods of gene transfer

9.2.4.2.3.1. Transformation: transfer of recombinant plasmid DNA to a bacterial host

The ligation reaction mixture of recombinant and nonrecombinant DNA described in the preceding section is introduced into bacterial cells in a process called **transformation**. The traditional method is to incubate the cells in a concentrated calcium salt solution to make their membranes leaky. The permeable "competent" cells are then mixed with DNA to allow entry of the DNA into the bacterial cell. Alternatively, a process called electroporation can be used that drives DNA into cells by a strong electric current. Since bacterial species use a restriction-modification system to degrade foreign DNA lacking the appropriate methylation pattern, including plasmids, the question arises: why don't the transformed bacteria degrade the foreign DNA? The answer is that molecular biologists have cleverly circumvented this defense system by using mutant strains of bacteria, deficient for both restriction and modification, such as the common lab strain *E. coli* DH5α. Successfully transformed bacteria will carry either recombinant or nonrecombinant plasmid DNA. Multiplication of the plasmid DNA occurs within each transformed bacterium. A single bacterial cell placed on a solid surface (agar plate) containing nutrients can multiply to form a visible colony made of millions of identical cells. As the host cell divides, the plasmid vectors are passed on to progeny, where they continue to replicate. Numerous cell divisions of a single transfomed bacteria result in a clone of cells (visible as a bacterial colony) from a single parental cell. This step is where "cloning" got its name. The cloned DNA can then be isolated from the clone of bacterial cells.

Table 9.3: Principal features and applications of different cloning vector systems

Vector	Basis	Size limits of insert	Major application
Plasmid	Naturally occuring multicopy plasmids	≤ 10 kb	Subcloning and downstream manipulation, cDNA cloning and expression assays
Phage	Bacteriophage λ	5–20 kb	Genomic DNA cloning, cDNA cloning, and expression libraries
Cosmid	Plasmid containing a bacteriophage λ *cos* site	35–45 kb	Genomic library construction
BAC (bacterial artificial chromosome)	*Escherichia coli* F factor plasmid	75–300 kb	Analysis of large genomes
YAC (yeast artificial chromosome)	*Saccharomyces cerevisiae* centromere, telomere, and autonomously replicating sequence	100–1000 kb (1 Mb)	Analysis of large genomes, YAC transgenic mice
MAC (mammalian artificial chromosome)	Mammalian centromere, telomere, and origin of replication	100 kb to > 1 Mb	Under development for use in animal biotechnology and human gene therapy

9.2.4.2.3.2. Electroporation

The uptake of free DNA can be induced by subjecting bacteria to a high voltage electric field in the presence of DNA .this procedure is called electroporation, a term that is a contraction of the descriptive phrase "electric field–mediated membrane permeabilization".

The experimental protocols for electroporation are different for various bacterial species. For *E.coli*, the cells (-50 microliters[µl]) and DNA are placed in a chamber fitted with electrodes (Fig.9.5A), and a single pulse of approximately 25 micofarads,2.5 kilovolts, and 200 ohms is administered for about 4.6 milliseconds(ms).this treatment yields transformation efficiencies of 10^9

transforms per microgram of DNA for small plasmids (-3 kb) and 10^6 for large plasmids (-136 kb). Similar conditions are used to introduce BAC vector DNA into *E.coli*. Thus, electroporation is an effective way to transform *E.coli* with plasmid(s) set of electroporation conditions can be found for nearly all bacterial species; this procedure has become standard for transforming many different type of bacteria.

Very little is known obout the mechanism of DNA uptake during electroporation (Fig.9.5B). It has been deduced, along the lines of the explanation of chemically induced transformation, that transient pores are formed in the cell wall as a result of the electroshock and that, after contact with the lipid bilayer of the cell membrane, the DNA is taken into the cell.

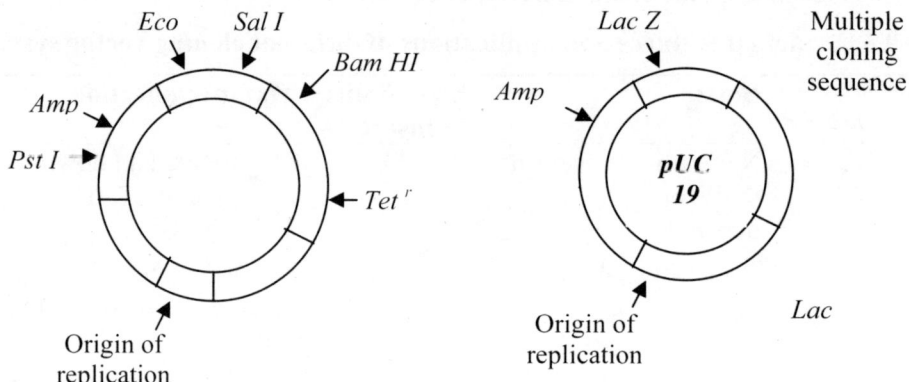

Fig. 9.4: Genetic map of cloning vectors *pBR 322* and *pUC 19*

9.2.4.2.3.3. Conjugation

For some bacteria, the natural system of transmitting plasmids from one strain to another has been used to transport a plasmid – insert DNA construct from a donor cell to a recipient cell that is otherwise not readily transformed. Some plasmids are genetically equipped to form cell-to-cell junctions through which plasmid DNA is transferred from one cell to another. Effective contact between a donor cell and a recipient cell depends on plasmid gene that encodes conjugative functions. Moreover, the mechanical transfer of DNA requires plasmids that encode mobilizing functions. Most of the plasmids that are used for recombinant DNA research lack conjugative functions, and therefore, they cannot be passed to recipient cells by conjugation. However, some nonconjugative plasmid cloning vectors can be mobilized and transferred if the conjugative functions are supplied by a second plasmid in the same cell. In other words, by introducing a plasmid with conjugative function into a bacterial cell that carries a mobilizable plasmid cloning vector, it is possible to transfer the plasmid cloning vector to a recipient cell that is difficult to transform by other means.

The typical experimental protocol for this procedure entails mixing three strains together. When the cells are close to each other, the conjugative plasmid, which in this case is also mobilizable, can be self-transferred to the cell with the mobilizable plasmid cloning vector. Then, with the help of the conjugative plasmid, the plasmid cloning vector is transferred to a target recipient cell. All possible combinations of plasmid transfer occur among the cells, but the genetic features of the strains and plasmids are designed to select for the target recipient cells that receive the cloning vector. For example, one possible selection procedure uses a helper cell (*E.coli*) that maintains a conjugative, mobilizable plasmid with a tetracycline resistant gene and cannot grow on minimal growth medium and carries the non-conjugative mobilizable plasmid cloning vector that has a kanamycin resistant gene; and a recipient cell (*Pseudomonas putida*) that can grow on minimal growth medium, has no incompatible plasmid, and is sensitive to both, tetracycline and kanamycin (Fig 9.6). After the conjugations are allowed to occur, the cells are allowed to grow briefly on growth medium in the absence of antibiotics before being transferred to minimal growth medium with kanamycin. Under the latter growth conditions, only the targeted recipient cells that have acquired the plasmid cloning vector can grow. Neither helper nor donor cells can grow on minimal medium nor do the recipient cells that did not receive a plasmid from a donor cell grow in the presence of kanamycin. Occasionally, the targeted recipient cell may receive both types of plasmids. However, this rare event can be detected by replica plating on to minimal medium with both tetracycline and kanamycin. Colonies that are formed in the presence of both the antibiotics acquire two different plasmids, and those that grow only when kanamycin is present have the cloning vector. Since the transfer of plasmid DNA requires conjugation among three bacterial strains, the process has been designated tripartite mating.

9.2.4.3. Vectors for cloning large pieces of DNA

9.2.4.3.1. Bacteriophage lambda (λ) as a vector

Bacteriophage lambda (λ) has been widely used in recombinant DNA since engineering of the first viral cloning vector in 1974. Phage λ vectors are particularly useful for preparing genomic libraries, because they can hold a larger piece of DNA than a plasmid vector. Today many variations of λ vectors exist. Insertion vectors have unique restriction endonuclease sites that allow the cloning of small DNA fragments in addition to the phage λ genome. These are often used for preparing cDNA expression libraries. Replacement vectors have paired cloning sites on either side of a central gene cluster. This central cluster contains genes for lysogeny and recombination, which are not essential for the lytic life cycle (Fig. 9.7).

The central gene cluster can be removed and foreign DNA is inserted between the "arms." All phage vectors used as cloning vectors have been disarmed for safety and can only function in special laboratory conditions. A typical strategy for the use of a phage λ replacement vector is depicted in Fig. 9.8. The recombinant viral particle infects bacterial host cells, in a process called "transduction." The host cells lyse after phage reproduction, releasing progeny virus particles. The viral particles appear as a clear spot of lysed bacteria or "plaque" on an agar plate containing a lawn of bacteria. Each plaque represents progeny of a single recombinant phage and contains millions of recombinant phage particles. Most contemporary vectors carry a *lacZ'* gene allowing blue-white selection.

9.2.4.3.1.1. Bacteriophage λ vectors permit efficient construction of large DNA libraries

Vectors constructed from bacteriophage λ are about a thousand times more efficient than plasmid vectors in cloning large numbers of DNA fragments. For this reason, phage λ vectors have been widely used to generate DNA libraries, a comprehensive collection of DNA fragments representing the genome or expressed mRNAs of an organism. Two factors account for the greater efficiency of phage λ as a cloning vector: infection of *E. coli* host cells by λ virions occurs at about a thousand fold greater frequencies than transformation by plasmids, and many more λ clones than transformed colonies can be grown and detected on a single culture plate. When a λ virion infects an *E. coli* cell, it can undergo a cycle of lytic growth during which the phage DNA is replicated and assembled into more than 100 complete progeny phage, which are released when the infected cell lyses (see Fig. 9.7). If a sample of λ phage is placed on a lawn of *E. coli* growing on a petri plate, each virion will infect a single cell. The ensuing rounds of phage growth will give rise to a visible cleared region, called a *plaque*, where the cells have been lysed and phage particles released. A λ virion consists of a head, which contains the phage DNA genome, and a tail, which functions in infecting *E. coli* host cells. The λ genes encoding the head and tail proteins, as well as various proteins involved in phage DNA replication and cell lysis, are grouped in discrete regions of the ≈50-kb viral genome. The central region of the λ genome, however, contains genes that are not essential for the lytic pathway.

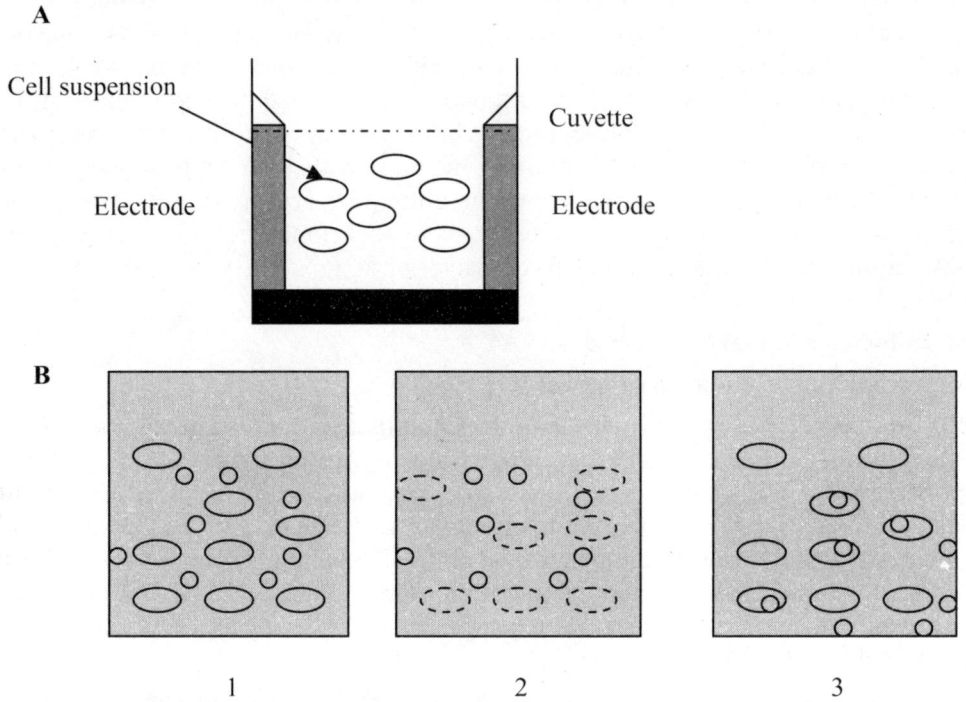

Fig. 9.5: Electroporation. A. Electroporation cuvette with a cell suspension between two electrodes. B. (1) Cells and DNA in suspension in a electroporation cuvette prior to administration of high-voltage electric field (HVEF) pulses. (2) HVEF pulses induce openings in the cells (dashed lines) that allow entry into the cells. (3) After HVEF pulsing, some cells acquire exogenous DNA, and HVEF- induced openings are resealed

Removing this region and replacing it with a foreign DNA fragment up to ≈25 kb long yields a recombinant DNA that can be packaged *in vitro* to form phage capable of replicating and forming plaques on a lawn of E. coli host cells. *In vitro* packaging of recombinant λ DNA, which mimics the *in vivo* assembly process, requires preassembled heads and tails as well as two viral proteins. It is technically feasible to use λ phage cloning vectors to generate a genomic library, that is, a collection of λ clones that collectively represent all the DNA sequences in the genome of a particular organism. However, such genomic libraries for higher eukaryotes present certain experimental difficulties. First, the genes from such organisms usually contain extensive intron sequences and therefore are too large to be inserted intact into λ phage vectors. As a result, the sequences of individual genes are broken apart and carried in more than one λ clone (this is also true for plasmid clones). Moreover, the presence of introns and long intergenic regions in genomic DNA often makes it difficult to identify the important parts of a gene that actually encode protein sequences.

Thus for many studies, cellular mRNAs, which lack the noncoding regions present in genomic DNA, are a more useful starting material for generating a DNA library. In this approach, DNA copies of mRNAs, called complementary DNAs (cDNAs), are synthesized and cloned in phage vectors. A large collection of the resulting cDNA clones, representing all the mRNAs expressed in a cell type is called a cDNA library.

9.2.4.3.2. Hybrid plasmid/phage vectors

One additional feature of phage vectors is that the technique of packaging *in vitro* is sequence independent, apart from the requirement of having the cos sites separated by DNA of packagable size (38--51 kb). This has been exploited in the construction of special vectors that contain plasmid sequences joined to the cos sites of phage λ. Such vectors are referred as cosmids. They are relatively small (4--6 kb) and hence can accommodate cloned DNA fragments up to some 47 kb in size. As they lack phage genes, they behave as plasmids when introduced into *E. coli* by the packaging/infection mechanism of λ (Fig. 9.9). Cosmid vectors therefore offer an apparently ideal system as a highly efficient and specific tool for introducing the recombinant DNA into the host cell, with a cloning capacity nearly twofold greater than the best λ replacement vectors. However, they also suffer from disadvantages, and often the gains of using cosmids instead of phage vectors are offset by losses in regard to ease of use and further processing of cloned sequences. Hybrid plasmid/phage vectors in which the phage functions are retained and expressed and utilised to an extent are known as phagemids.

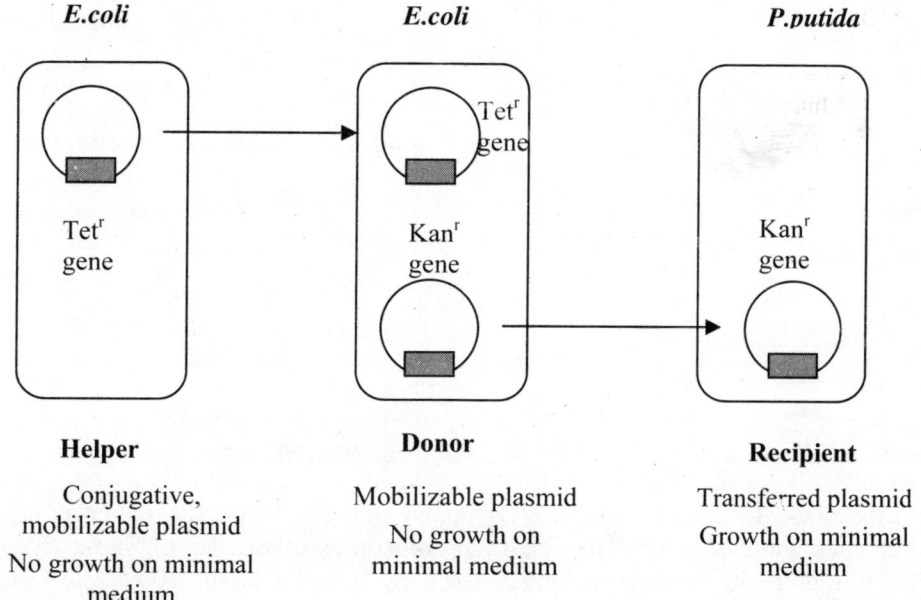

Fig. 9.6: Tripartate mating. A helper cell self-transfers a conjugative, mobilizing plasmid with a tetracycline resistance (Tet^r) gene to a donor cell. The plasmid cell from the helper cell provides conjugative functions for the donor cell's non-conjugative, mobilizable plasmid with a kanamycin resistance (Kan^r) gene and tansports the latter plasmid into recipient cell. Unlike the recipient cells, neither helper nor the donor cells grow on minimal growth medium. The selection strategies identify cells that are resistant to Kanamycin and are able to grow on minimum medium. In this example the cloning vector is transferred from *E.coli* to *P.putida*

One such series of vectors is known as λ ZAP family, produced especially by Stratagene. Features of these phagemids include the potential to excise cloned DNA fragments *in vivo* as part of a plasmid. This automatic excision appears to be useful in that it removes the need to subclone the inserts from λ into plasmid vectors for further manipulation. Hybrid plasmid/phage vectors have been developed to overcome the inherent size limitation of the M13 cloning system and are now widely used for applications such as DNA sequencing and the production of probes for use in hybridisation studies. These vectors are essentially plasmids that contain the fl (M13) phage origin of replication. When cells containing the plasmid are superinfected with phage, they produce single-stranded copies of the plasmid DNA and secrete them into the medium as M13-like particles. Vectors such as pEMBL9 or pBluescript can accept DNA fragments of up to 10 kb.

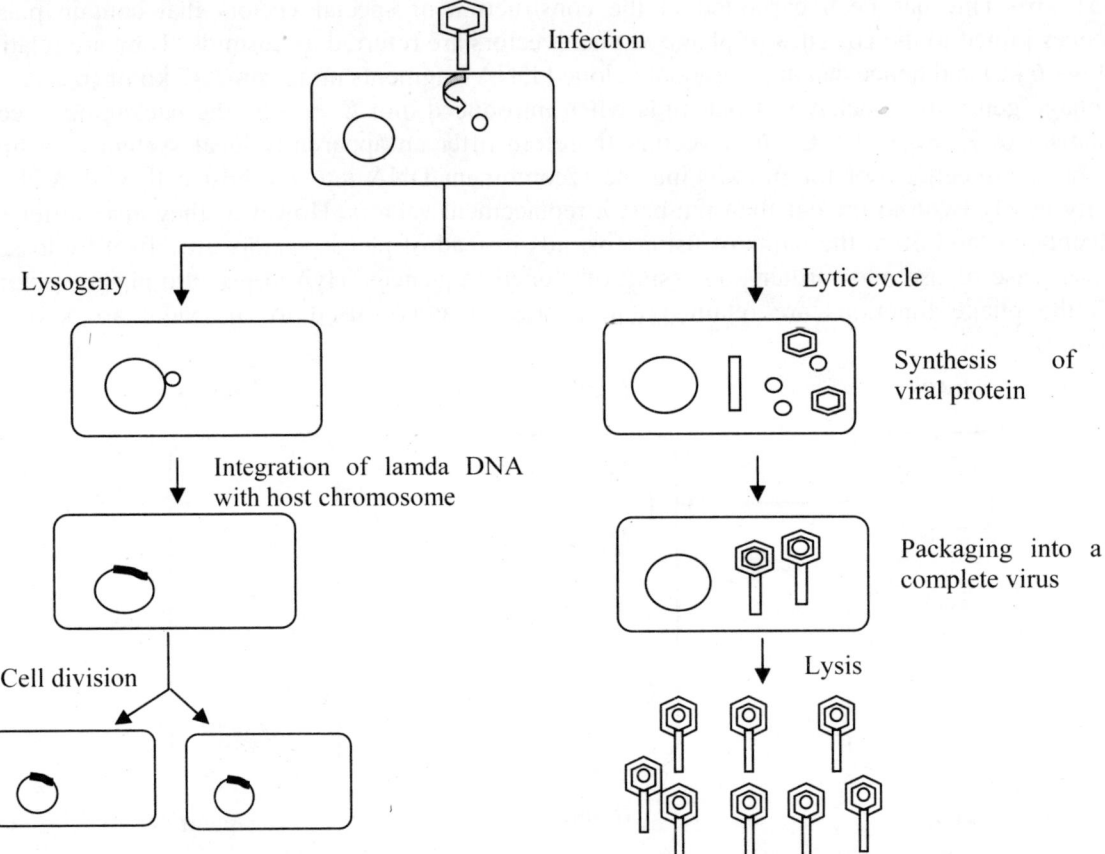

Fig. 9.7: Life cycle of bacteriophage λ. Lysogeny occurs when the bacteriophage λ genome becomes integrated into the host chromosome; otherwise the lytic cycle is initiated, resulting in the production and release by lysis of about 100 bacteriophage particles about 20 minutes after infection

9.2.4.3.3. Artificial chromosome vectors

Bacterial artificial chromosomes (BACs) and yeast artificial chromosomes (YACs) are important tools for mapping and analysis of complex eukaryotic genomes. Much of the work on the Human Genome Project and other genome sequencing projects depends on the use of BACs and YACs, because they can hold greater than 300 kb of foreign DNA. BACs are constructed using the fertility factor plasmid (F factor) of *E. coli* as a starting point. The plasmid is naturally 100 kb in size and occurs at a very low copy number in the host. The engineered BAC vector is 7.4 kb (including a replication origin, cloning sites, and selectable markers) and thus can accommodate a large insert of foreign DNA. The characteristics of YAC vectors are discussed below. Immediately after the construction of the first YAC in 1983, efforts were undertaken to develop a mammalian artificial chromosome (MAC). From there on, it took 14 years until the first prototype MAC was described in 1997. Like YACs, MACs rely on the presence of centromeric sequences, sequences that can initiate

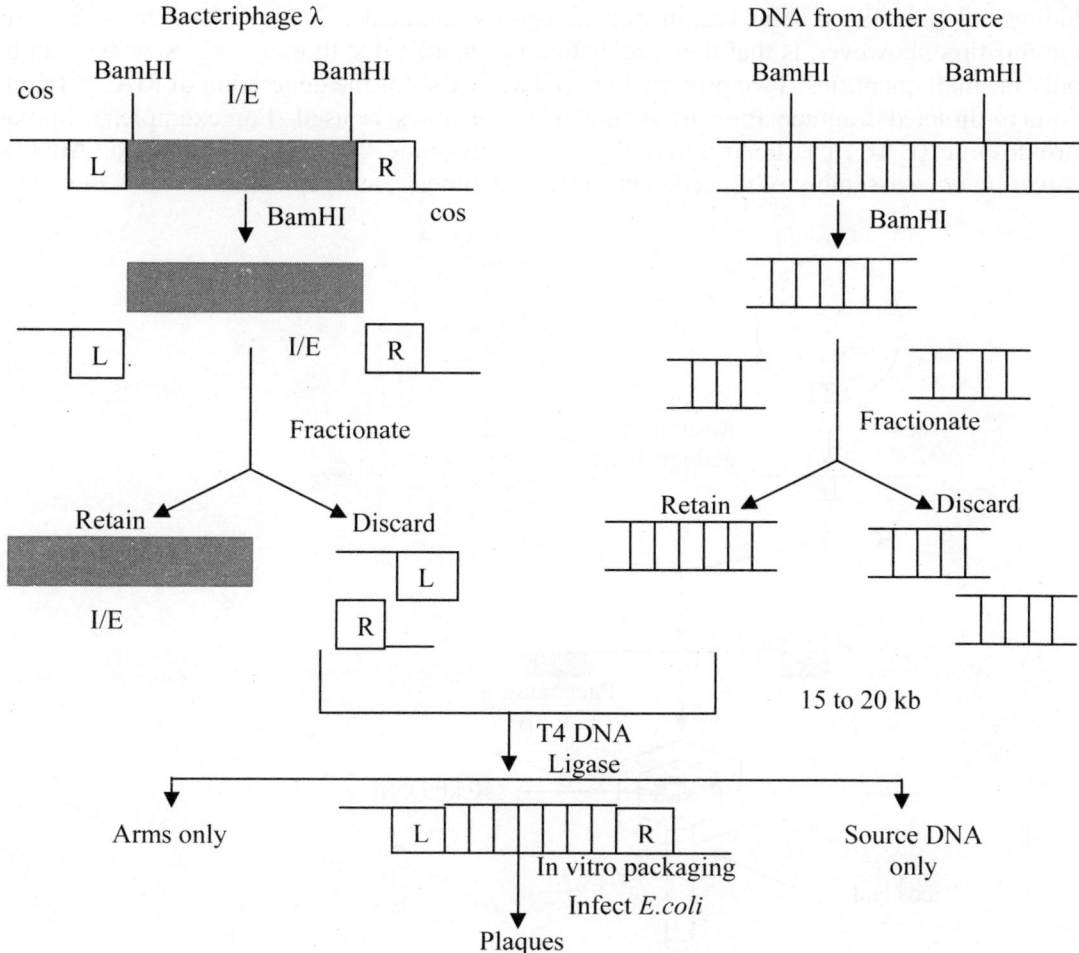

Fig. 9.8: Bacteriophage λ cloning system. Bacteriophage λ is engineered to have two BamHI sites that flank the integration/excision region (I/E), For cloning, the source DNA is cut with BamHI and fractionated by size to isolate the size that are about 15 to 20 kb long. The bacteriophage λ DNA is also cut with BamHI and fractionation removes the I/E segment. The left (L) and right (R) armsplus the 15- to 20-kb source DNA molecules are mixed with T4 DNA ligase. The ligation reaction will produce a number of different DNA molecules including ligated source DNA only; combined L and R arms only; and molecules that have a source DNA molecule flanked by L and R arms. The later molecules are packaged in bacteriophage heads in vitro and infective particles are formed after addition of tail assemblies. The recombined bacteriophage λ are perpetuated by infection of *E.coli*. Some 50-kb source DNA ligated products may be packaged into heads but since this DNA lacks both a functional origin of replication and cos ends, it cannot be perpetuated. Other ligation products are either too small or too large to be packaged

DNA replication, and telomeric sequences. Their development is considered an important advance in animal biotechnology and human gene therapy for two main reasons. First, they involve autonomous replication and segregation in mammalian cells, as opposed to random integration into chromosomes (as for other vectors). Second, they can be modified for their use as expression systems of large genes, including not only the coding region but all control elements. A major drawback limiting application at this time, however, is that they are difficult to handle due to their large size and can be recovered only in small quantities. Two principal procedures exist for the generation of MACs. In one method, telomere-directed fragmentation of natural chromosomes is used. For example, a human artificial chromosome (HAC) has been derived from chromosome 21 using this method. Another method involves *de novo* assembly of cloned centromeric, telomeric, and replication origins *in vitro*.

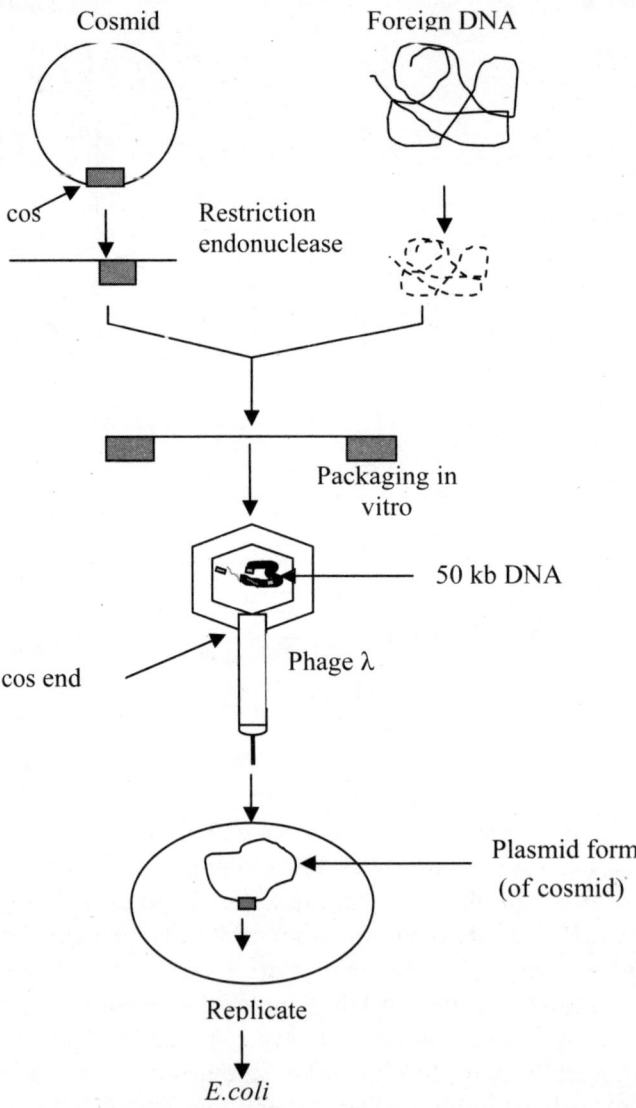

Fig. 9.9: Cosmids vectors accommodate cloned DNA fragments up to some 47 kb in size. As they lack phage genes, they behave as plasmids when introduced into *E. coli* by the packaging/infection mechanism of λ

BACs and **YACs** can be used to clone very long pieces of DNA. The use of a BAC or YAC vector can reduce the number of clones needed to produce a workable genomic library for a particular organism, and this is a desirable outcome in itself. The cloning large pieces of DNA are useful as physical mapping of genomes is made simpler, due to obviously fewer sequences which can fit together in a correct order. For large-scale DNA sequencing projects BAC- or YAC-based cloning is further useful if an ordered strategy is employed.

A further advantage of cloning long stretches of DNA stems from the fact that many eukaryotic genes are much larger than the 47 kb or so that can be cloned using cosmid vectors in *E. coli*. Thus, with plasmid, phage, and cosmid vectors it may be impossible to isolate the entire gene. This makes it difficult to determine gene structure without using several different clones, which is not the ideal way. The use of BAC or YAC vectors can alleviate this problem and can enable the structure of large genes to be determined by providing a single DNA fragment to work from. Let us consider using a YAC vector to clone DNA fragments. In practice, cloning in YAC vectors is similar to other protocols. The vector is prepared by a double restriction digest, which releases the vector sequence between the telomeres and cleaves the vector at the cloning site.

Thus, two arms are produced, as is the case with phage vectors. Insert DNA is prepared as very long fragments (a partial digest with a six-cutter may be used) and ligated into the cloning site to produce **artificial chromosomes**. Selectable markers on each of the two arms ensure that only correctly constructed chromosomes will be selected and propagated.

9.2.4.3.4. Yeast artificial chromosome (YAC) vectors

Yeast, although a eukaryote is a small single cell that can be manipulated and grown in the lab much like bacteria. YAC vectors are designed to act like chromosomes. Their design would not have been possible without a detailed knowledge of the requirements for chromosome stability and replication, and genetic analysis of yeast mutants and biochemical pathways. YAC vectors include an origin of replication (autonomously replicating sequence, ARS), a centromere to ensure segregation into daughter cells, telomeres to seal the ends of the chromosomes and confer stability, and growth selectable markers in each arm (Fig. 9.10). These markers allow for selection of molecules in which the arms are joined and which contain a foreign insert. For example, the yeast genes *URA3* and *TRP1* are often used as markers. Positive selection is carried out by auxotrophic complementation of a *ura3-trp1* mutant yeast strain, which requires supplementation with uracil and tryptophan to grow. *URA3* encodes an enzyme that is required for the biosynthesis of the nitrogenous base uracil (orotidine-5'-phosphate decarboxylase). *TRP1* encodes an enzyme that is required for biosynthesis of the amino acid tryptophan (phosphoribosylanthranilate isomerase).

YAC vectors are maintained as a circle prior to inserting foreign DNA. After cutting with restriction endonucleases *Bam*HI and *Eco*RI, the left arm and right arm become linear, with the end sequences forming the telomeres. Foreign DNA is cleaved with *Eco*RI and the YAC arms and foreign DNA are ligated and then transferred into yeast host cells (Fig. 9.11). The yeast host cells are maintained as spheroplasts (lacking yeast cell wall). Yeast cells are grown on selective nutrient regeneration plates that lack uracil and tryptophan, to select for molecules in which the arms are joined bringing together the *URA3* and *TRP1* genes.

9.3. RECOMBINANT SELECTION

What needs to be included in the medium for plating cells so that non transformed bacterial cells are not able to grow at all? The answer depends on the particular vector, but in the case of *pUC*18, the vector carries a selectable marker gene for resistance to the antibiotic ampicillin.

The multiple cloning site resides in the coding region. If the *lacZ'* region is not interrupted by inserted DNA, the aminoterminal portion of β-galactosidase is synthesized. Importantly, an *E. coli* deletion mutant strain is used (e.g. DH5α) that harbors a mutant sequence of *lacZ* that encodes only the carboxyl end of β - Ampicillin, a derivative of penicillin, blocks synthesis of the peptidoglycan layer that lies between the inner and outer cell membranes of *E. coli* (Table 9.4). Ampicillin does not affect existing cells with intact cell envelopes but kills dividing cells as they synthesize new peptidoglycan. The ampicillin resistance genes carried by the recombinant plasmids produce an enzyme, β-lactamase, which cleaves a specific bond in the four-membered ring (β -lactam ring) in the ampicillin molecule that is essential to its antibiotic action. If the plasmid vector is introduced into a plasmid free antibiotic-sensitive bacterial cell, the cell becomes resistant to ampicillin. Nontransformed cells contain no pUC18 DNA, therefore they will not be antibiotic-resistant, and their growth will be inhibited on agar containing ampicillin. Transformed bacterial cells may contain either nonrecombinant pUC18 DNA (self ligated vector only) or recombinant pUC18 DNA (vector containing foreign DNA insert). Both types of transformed bacterial cells will be ampicillin-resistant. galactosidase (*lacZ'* ΔM15). Both the plasmid and host *lacZ* fragments encode.

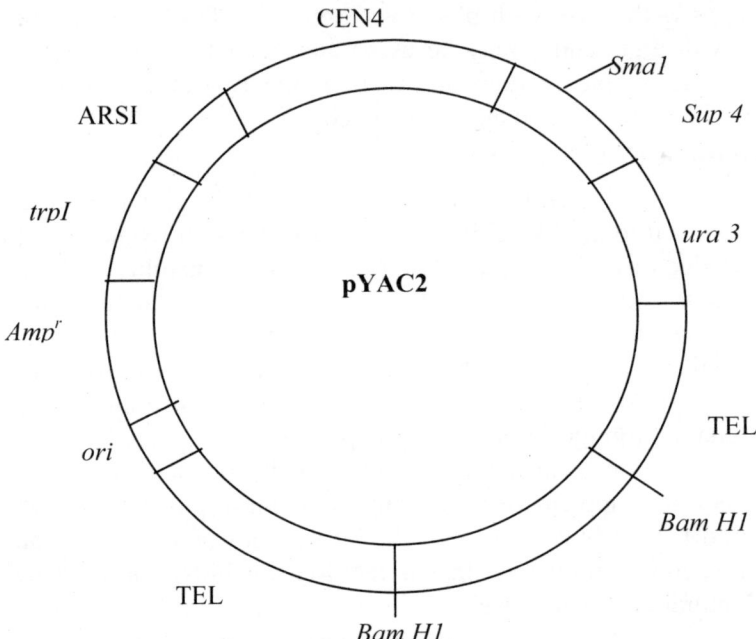

Fig. 9.10: Map of the yeast artificial chromosome vector pYAC2. This carries the origin of replication and ampicillin resistance gene (AMP^r) from pBR322, and yeast sequences for replication (ARS1) and chromosome structure (centromere, CEN4; and telomeres, TEL). The TEL sequences are separated by a fragment flanked by two BamHI sites. The genes trp1 and ura3 may be used as selectable markers in yeast. The cloning site SmaI lies within the sup4 gene

9.3.1. Blue-white screening

To distinguish nonrecombinant from recombinant transformants, blue-white screening or "*lac* selection" (also called α-complementation) can be used with this particular vector. Bacterial colonies are grown on selective medium containing ampicillin and a colorless chromogenic compound called

X-gal, for short (5-bromo-4-chloro-3-indolyl- β -d-galactoside). *pUC*18 carries a portion of the *lacZ* gene (called *lacZ '*) that encodes the first 146 amino acids for the enzyme β-galactosidase nonfunctional proteins. However, by α-complementation the two partial proteins can associate and form a functional enzyme. When present the enzyme β -galactosidase catalyzes hydrolysis of X-gal, converting the colorless substrate into a blue-colored product (Fig. 9.12).

Table 9.4: Some commonly used antibiotics and antibiotic resistance genes

Antibiotic	Mode of action	Resistance
Ampicillin	Inhibits bacterial cell wall synthesis by disrupting peptidoglycan cross-linking	β-Lactamase (*amp^r*) gene product is secreted and hydrolyzes ampicillin
Tetracycline	Inhibits binding of aminoacyl tRNA to the 30S ribosomal subunit	*tet^r* gene product is membrane bound and prevents tetracycline accumulation by an efflux mechanism
Kanamycin	Inactivates translation by interfering with ribosome function	Neomycin or aminoglycoside phosphotransferase (*neo^r*) gene product inactivates kanamycin by phosphorylation

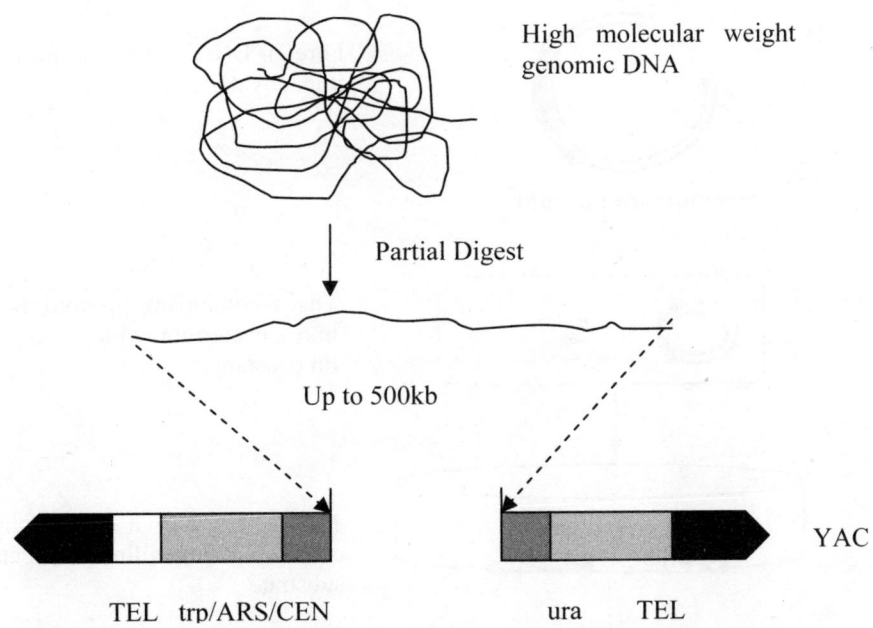

High molecular weight genomic DNA

Partial Digest

Up to 500kb

TEL trp/ARS/CEN

ura TEL

YAC

Fig. 9.11: Cloning in a YAC vector. Very large DNA fragments (up to 500 kb) are generated from high-molecular-weight DNA. The fragments are then ligated into a YAC vector that has been cut with *Bam*HI and *Sma*I (S). The construct contains the cloned DNA and the essential requirements for a yeast chromosome: telomeres (TEL), an autonomous replication sequence (ARS), and a centromere region (CEN). The *trp* and *ura* genes can be used as dual selectable markers to ensure that only complete artificial chromosomes are maintained

9.4. AMPLIFICATION AND PURIFICATION OF RECOMBINANT PLASMID DNA

Further screening of positive (white) colonies can be done by restriction endonuclease digest to confirm the presence and orientation of the insert. When a positive colony containing recombinant plasmid DNA is transferred aseptically to liquid growth medium, the cells will continue to multiply exponentially. Within a day or two, a culture containing trillions cf identical cells can be harvested. The final step in molecular cloning is the recovery of the cloned DNA. Plasmid DNA can be purified from crude cell lysates by chromatography using silica gel or anion exchange resins that preferentially bind nucleic acids under appropriate conditions and allow for the removal of proteins and polysaccharides. The purified plasmid DNA can then be eluted and recovered by ethanol precipitation in the presence of monovalent cations. Ethanol precipitation of plasmid DNA from aqueous solutions yields a clear pellet that can be easily dissolved in an appropriate buffered solution.

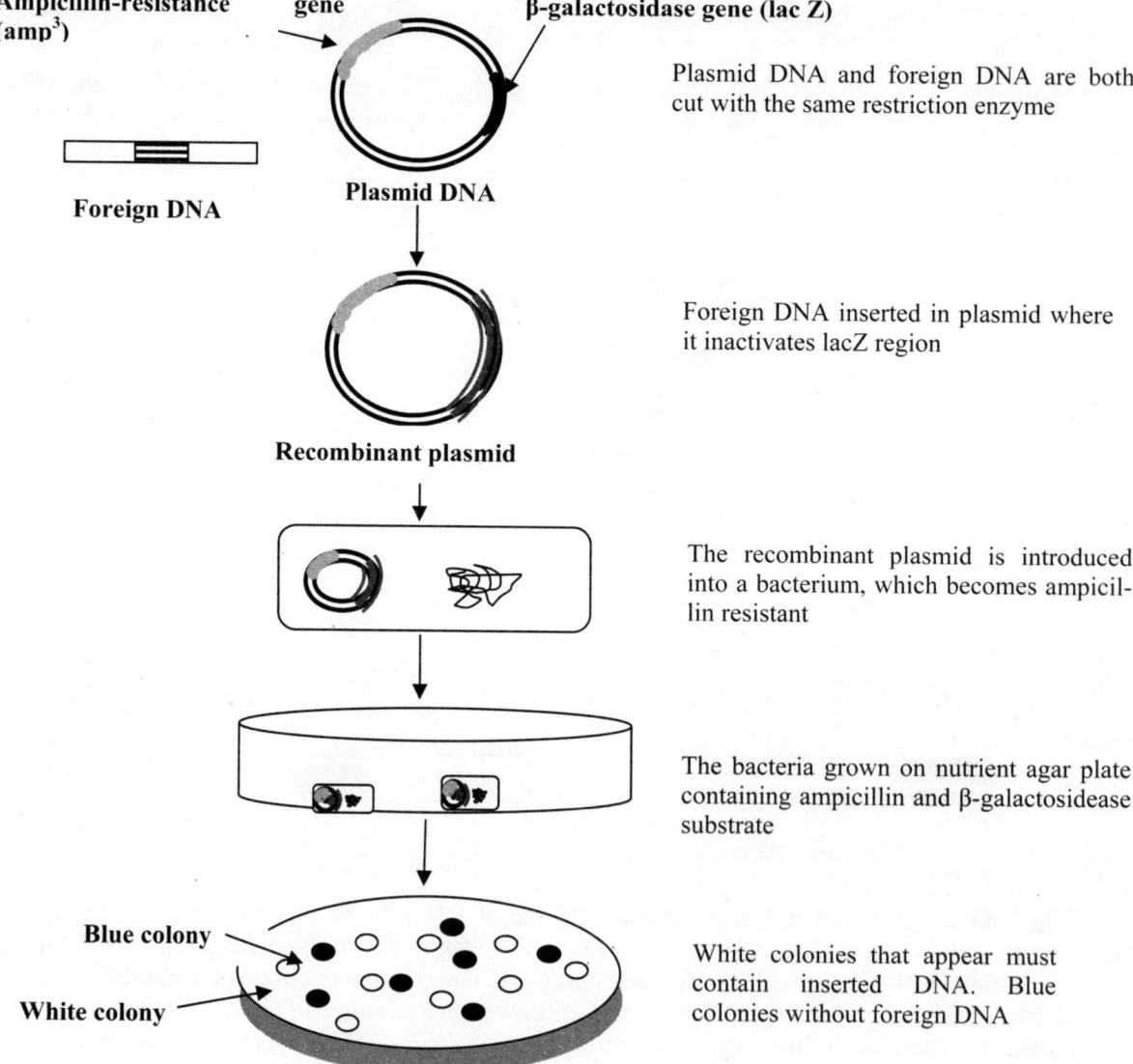

Fig. 9.12: Blue-white screening

9.5. SOURCES OF DNA FOR CLONING

The cloning that has been described so far will work for any random piece of DNA. But since the goal of many cloning experiments is to obtain a sequence of DNA that directs the production of a specific protein, we need to first consider where to obtain such DNA. Sources of DNA for cloning into vectors may be DNA fragments representing a specific gene or portion of a gene, or may be sequences of the entire genome of an organism, depending on the end goal of the researcher. Typical "inserts" include genomic DNA, cDNA, polymerase chain reaction (PCR) products, and chemically synthesized oligonucleotides. When previously isolated clones are transferred into a different vector for other applications, this is called "subcloning."

9.6. CREATING AND SCREENING DNA LIBRARIES

9.6.1. Making a gene library

One of the fundamental objectives of molecular biology is the isolation of gene that encodes protein for industrial, agricultural and medical applications. In prokaryotic organisms the structural gene forms a continuous coding domain in the genomic DNA, whereas, in eukaryotes, the coding regions (exons) of structural genes are separated by noncoding regions (introns). Consequently, different cloning strategies have to be used for cloning prokaryotic and eukaryotic genes. In a prokaryote, the desired sequence (target DNA, or gene of interest) is frequently a minuscule portion (about 0.02%) of the total chromosomal DNA. The problem, then, is how to clone and select the targeted DNA sequence. Vectors are used to compile a library of DNA fragments that have been isolated from the genomes of a variety of organisms. This collection of fragments can then be used to isolate specific genes and other DNA sequences of interest. DNA fragments are generated by cutting the DNA with a specific restriction endonuclease. These fragments are ligated into vector molecules, and the collection of recombinant molecules is transferred into host cells, one molecule in each cell. The total number of all DNA molecules makes up the library. This library is searched, that is screened, with a molecular probe that specifically identifies the target DNA. Once prepared the library can be perpetuated indefinitely in the host cells and is readily retrieved whenever a new probe is available to seek out a particular fragment. Two main types of libraries can be used to isolate specific DNAs: genomic and cDNA libraries.

9.6.1.1. Genomic library

A genomic library contains DNA fragments that represent the entire genome of an organism. The first step in creating a genomic library is to break the DNA into manageable size pieces (e.g. 15–20 kb for phage λ vectors), usually by partial restriction endonuclease digest. Under limiting conditions, any particular restriction site is cleaved only occasionally, so not all sites are cleaved in any particular DNA molecule. This generates a continuum of overlapping fragments. The second step is to purify fragments of optimal size by gel electrophoresis or centrifugation techniques. The final step is to insert the DNA fragments into a suitable vector. In humans, the genome size is approximately 3×10^9 bp. With an average insert size of 20 kb, the number of random fragments to ensure with high probability (95–99%) that every sequence is represented is approximately 106 clones for humans. The maths actually works out to 1.5×10^5 (i.e. $(3 \times 10^9 \text{ bp})/(2 \times 10^4 \text{ bp})$) but more clones are needed in practice, since insertion is random. Bacteriophage λ or cosmid vectors are typically used for genomic libraries. Since a larger insert size can be accommodated by these vectors compared with plasmids, there is a greater chance of cloning a gene sequence with both the coding sequence and the regulatory elements in a single clone.

9.6.1.2. cDNA library

The principle behind cDNA cloning is that an mRNA population isolated from a specific tissue, cell type, or developmental stage (e.g. embryo mRNA) should contain mRNAs specific for any protein expressed in that cell type or during that stage, along with "housekeeping" mRNAs that encode essential proteins such as the ribosomal proteins, and other mRNAs common to many cell types or stages of development. Thus, if mRNA can be isolated, a small subset of all the genes in a genome can be studied. mRNA cannot be cloned directly, but a cDNA copy of the mRNA can be cloned. Because a cDNA library is derived from mRNA, the library contains the coding region of expressed genes only, with no introns or regulatory regions. The latter point becomes important for applications of recombinant DNA technology to the production of transgenic animals and for human gene therapy.

9.6.2. Screening by DNA hybridization

The presence of a target nucleotide sequence in a DNA sample can be detected by using a DNA probe. This procedure called hybridization depends on the formation of stable complementary base pairs between the probe and the target sequence. DNA hybridization is feasible because double-stranded DNA can be converted into single-stranded DNA by heat or alkali treatment. Heating DNA breaks the hydrogen bonds that hold the base together (denaturation) but does not affect the phosphodiester bonds of the DNA backbone. If the heated solution is rapidly cooled, the strand remains single stranded. However, if the temperature of a heated DNA solution is lowered slowly, the double stranded, helical conformation of DNA can be reestablished because of the base pairing of complementary nucleotides (renaturation). The process of heating and slowly cooling double-stranded DNA is called annealing. When DNA from different sources with some shared (homologous) sequence are mixed, heated to 100°C, and slowly cooled, there will be formation of some hybrid DNA molecules among the annealed products, that is, double stranded DNA in which the stands come from different sources.

In general, for a DNA hybridization assay, the target DNA is denatured and the single strands are irreversibly bound to a matrix, e.g., nitrocellulose or nylon. The binding process is often carried out at high temperature. Then the single strands of a DNA probe, which are labeled with either a radioisotope or another tagging system, are incubated with the matrix bound DNA sample. If the sequences of nucleotide in the DNA sample, base pair, i.e., hybridization, occurs (Fig. 9.13). The hybridization can be detected by autoradiography or other visualization procedures depending on the nature of the probe or label. If the nucleotide sequence of the probe does not base pair with a DNA sequence in the sample, then no hybridization occurs and the assay gives a negative result. Generally, probe range in length from 100 to more than 1,000bp, although both larger and smaller probes can be used. Depending on the condition of hybridization reaction, stable base requires a match of > 80% with a segment of 50 bases.

There are at least two possible sources of probes for screening a genomic library. First, cloned DNA from a closely related organism (a heterologous probe) can be used. In this case, the conditions of the hybridization reaction can be adjusted to permit considerable mismatch between the probe and the target DNA to compensate for the natural differences between the two sequences. Second, a probe can be produced by chemical synthesis. The nucleotide sequence of a synthetic probe is based on the probable nucleotide sequence that is deduced from the known amino acid sequence of the protein encoded by the target gene.

Genomic DNA libraries are often screened by plating out the transformed cells on the growth medium of a master plate and then transferring samples of each colony to a solid matrix such as nitrocellulose or nylon membrane, lysing breaking) the cells, deproteinizing and denaturing the DNA, and binding the DNA to the matrix. At this stage, a labeled probe is added and, if hybridization occurs, the signals are detected on an auradiogaph. The colonies from the master plate that correspond to the samples containing hybridized DNA are then isolated and cultured (Fig. 9.14). Because most libraries are created by partial digestions, a number of colonies may give a positive response to the probe. The next task is to determine which clone, if any, contains the complete sequence of the target gene. Preliminary analyses, which use the results of gel electrophoresis and restriction endonuclease mapping reveal the length of each insert and identify those inserts that are the same and those that share overlapping sequences. If an insert in any one of the clones is large enough to include the full gene, then the complete gene can be recognized by DNA sequencing because it will have start and stop codons and a contiguous set of nucleotides that code for the target protein. Alternatively, a gene can be assembled by using overlapping sequences from the different clones.

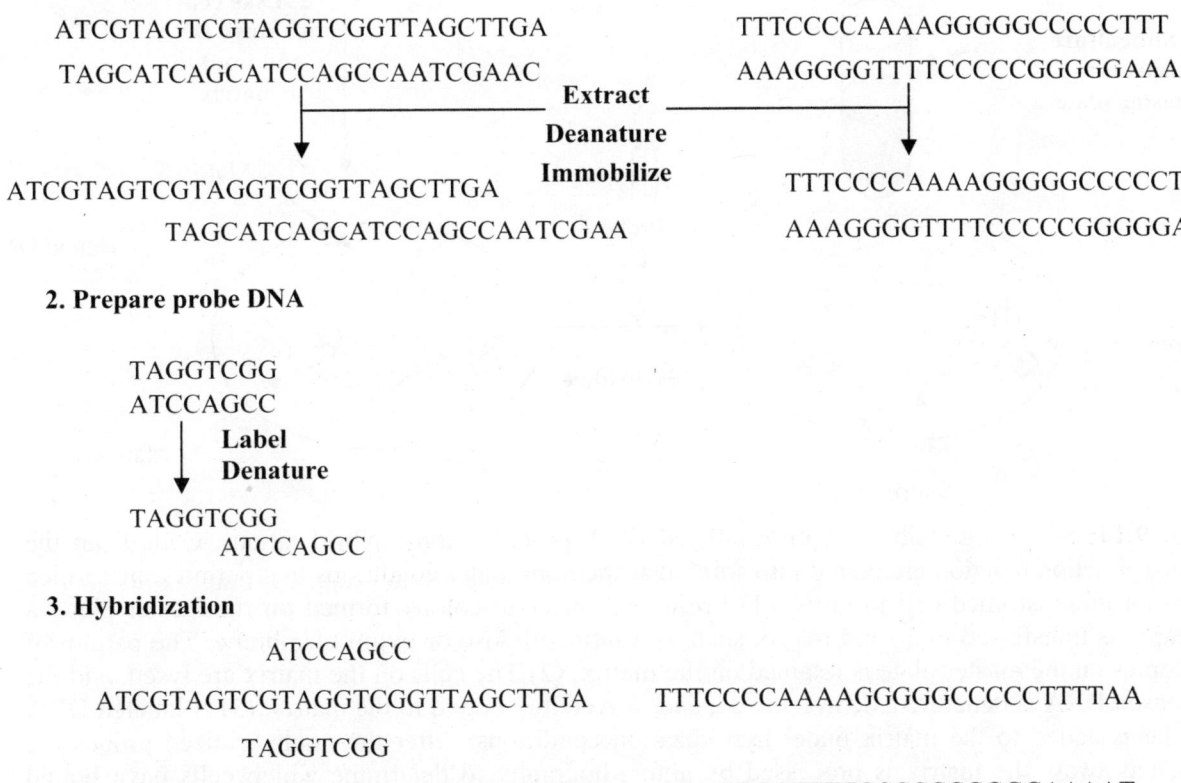

Fig. 9.13: DNA hybridization. (1) The DNA of samples containing the putative target DNA is denatured and the single strands are kept apart, usually by binding them to a solid support, such as nitrocellulose and nylon membrane. (2) The probe, which is usually 100 to 1000 bp in length is labeled, denatured and mixed with the denatured putative target DNA under hybridization conditions (3) After the hybridization reaction, the membrane is washed to remove unhybridized probe DNA and assayed for the presence of labeled tag. If the probe does not hybridize, no label is detected. The asterisk (*) denote the labeled tag (signal) of the probe DNA

Unfortunately, there is no guarantee that the complete sequence of a target gene will be present in a particular library. If the search for an intact gene fails, then another library can be created with a different restriction endonuclease and screened with either the original probe or probe derived from the first library.

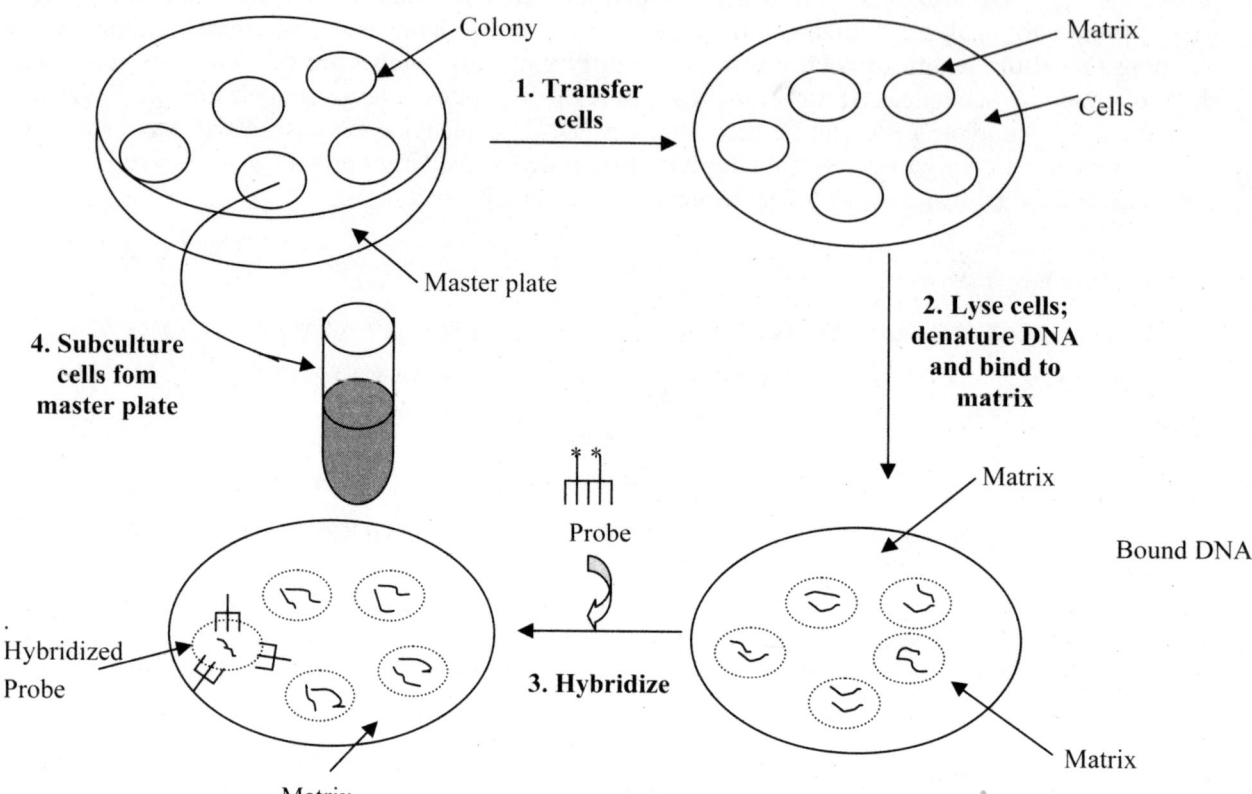

Fig. 9.14: Screening a library with a labeled DNA probe (colony hybridization). Cells from the transformation reaction are plated into solid agar medium under conditions that permit transformed but not untransfomed cell to grow. (1) From each discrete colony formed on the master plate, a sample is transferred to a solid matrix such as a nitrocellulose or nylon membrane. The pattern of colonies on the master plate is retained on the matrix. (2) The cells on the matrix are lysed, and the released DNA is denatured, deproteinized, and irreversibly bound to the matrix. (3) A labeled DNA probe is added to the matrix under hybridization conditions. After the nonhybridized probes are washed away, the matrix is processed by autoradiography to determine which cells have bound labeled DNA. (4) A colony on the master plate that corresponds to the regions of a positive response on the X-ray film is identified. Cells from the positive colony on the master plate subcultures because they may carry the desired plasmid-cloned DNA construct. The asterisk (*) denote the labeled tag (signal) of the probe

9.6.3. Screening by immunological assay

Alternative methods are used to screen a library when a DNA probe is not available. For example, when a cloned DNA sequence is transcribed and translated, the presence of the protein, or even part of it, can be determined by an immunological assay. Technically, this procedure has much in common with a DNA hybridization assay. All the clones of the library are grown separately on master plates.

A sample of each colony is transferred to a known position on a matrix, where the cells are lysed and the released proteins are attached to the matrix. The matrix with the bound proteins is treated with a

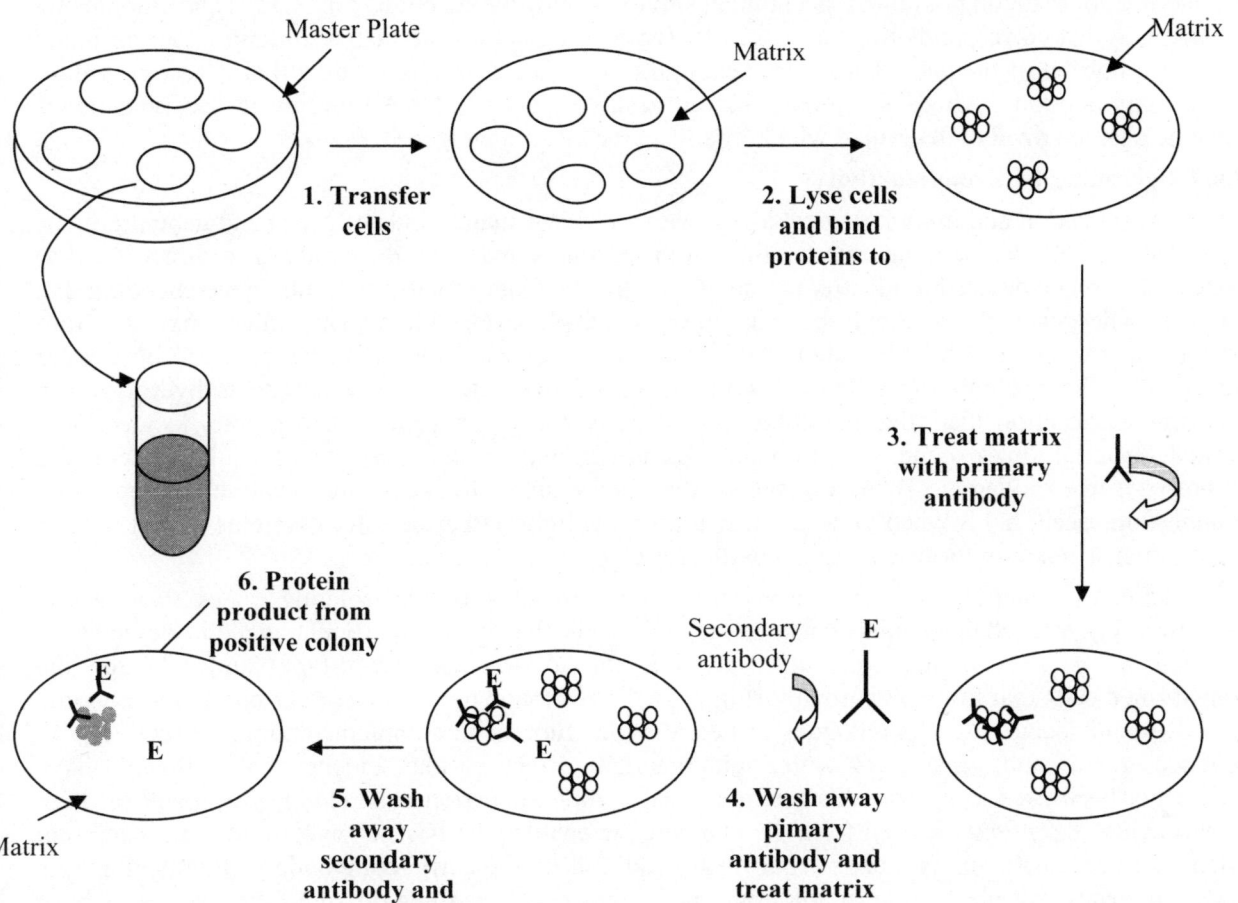

Fig. 9.15: Immunological screening of a gene library (colony immunoassay). Cells from the transformation reaction are plated into solid agar medium under conditions that permit transformed but not untransfomed cell to grow. (1) From each discrete colony formed on the master plate, a sample is transferred to a solid matrix such as a nitrocellulose or nylon membrane. (2) The cells on the matrix are lysed, and the released proteins are bound to the matrix. (3) The sample is treated with a primary antibody that binds to the target potein only. (4) Unbound primary antibodies are washed away, and the matrix is treated with secondary antibody that binds only to the primary antibody. (5) Any unbound secondary antibody is washed away, and a colorimetric reaction, which can occur only if the secondary antibody is present, is carried out. (6) A colony on the master plate that corresponds to a positive response on the matrix is identified. Cells from the positive colony on the master plate are subcultured because they may carry the plasmid-insert DNA construct that encode the protein which binds to the primary antibody

primary antibody that specifically binds with the target protein (antigen), any unbound antibody is washed away. The matrix is then treated with a secondary antibody that is specific for the primary antibody. In many assay system, the secondary antibody has an enzyme, such as alkaline phosphatase, bound to the enzyme. After the matrix is washed, a colorless substrate is added. If the secondary antibody has bound to the primary antibody, the colorless substrate is hydrolysed by the enzyme that produces a colored compound that accumulates at the site of the reaction (Fig. 9.15). The colonies on masterplate that corresponds to positive results (colored spots) on the matrix contain either an intact gene or a portion of the gene that is large enough to produce a protein product that is recognized by the primary antibody. After detection by immunoassay of genomic DNA libraries, the positive clones must be characterized to determine which, if any, carry a complete gene.

9.6.4. Screening by protein activity

DNA hybridization and immunological assays work well for many kinds of genes and gene products. If the target gene produces an enzyme that is not normally made by the host cell, a direct (*in situ*) plate assay can be devised to identify members of a library that carry the particular gene encoding that enzyme. The genes for α- amylase, endoglucanase, β-glucosidase and many other enzymes from various organisms have been isolated in this way. In some cases, the cells of a genomic library are plated onto the medium supplemented with a specific substrate; if the substrate is hydrolyzed, a colorimetric reaction identifies the colonies that carry the target gene. For example, to identify a cloned bacterial lipase gene, transformed cells are grown in the presence of trioleoglyceol and fluorescent dye rhodamine B. As a result of the hydrolysis of the substrate, positive colonies have orange fluorescent halos when viewed under ultraviolet light. Other detection systems do not rely on a colorimetric reaction for discovering a particular gene.

Functional (genetic) complementation is another useful way for isolating genes that encode enzymes. The procedure entails transforming host cells that have a particular genetic defect with plasmids of a DNA library constructed from a normal organism (wild-type) and selecting the transformed cells that function normally (Fig. 9.16). The cloned gene may come from either the same or a different species, i.e., homologous or heterologous functional complementation, respectively. In practice, *E.coli* and yeast cells with mutations that affect various biochemical pathways have frequently been used as a host cells for functional complementation gene cloning. In many of these experiments, the protein derived from the cloned gene enables the host to grow on minimal medium; whereas gowth of the mutant cells requires the addition of a specific compound to the medium. As well, the genes that play a role in antibiotic biosynthesis, root nodulation, and other processes have been isolated in this way.

9.7. Analysis of cloned genes

Once clones are identified by techniques such as hybridization or immunological screening, more detailed characterisation of the DNA can be conducted. There are many ways of tackling this, and accordingly the choice of approach depends on what is already known about the gene in consideration, and on the ultimate aim of the experiment.

9.7.1. Characterization based on mRNA translation *in vitro*

In some cases the identity of a particular clone may require confirmation. This is particularly applicable when the plus/minus methods of screening are used, as the results of such a process are usually somewhat ambiguous and cannot offer a definitive identification. If the desired sequence codes for a protein, and the protein has already been characterised, it becomes possible to identify the protein product by two methods based on translation of mRNA *in vitro*. The two classical methods are known as hybrid-arrest translation (HART) and hybrid-release translation (HRT, sometimes called hybrid-select translation). Although these techniques are no longer being used popularly in gene analysis, they do illustrate how a particular problem can be approached when two different variations of a similar theme exist, and constitute a central part of good scientific method. A comparison of HART and HRT is shown in Fig. 9.17. Both HART and HRT rely on hybridising cloned DNA fragments to mRNA prepared from the cell or tissue type from which the clones have been originally derived. In hybrid arrest, the cloned sequence blocks the mRNA and prevents its translation when placed in a system containing all the components of the translational machinery. In hybrid release, the cloned sequence is immobilised and used to select the clone-specific mRNA from the total mRNA preparation. This is then released from the hybrid and translated *in vitro*. If a radioactive amino acid (usually [^{35}S]methionine) is incorporated into the translation mixture, the proteins synthesised from the mRNA(s) are labeled which can be detected by autoradiography or fluorography after SDS polyacrylamide gel electrophoresis. In hybrid arrest, however one protein band should be absent; whilst in hybrid release there should be a single band. Thus, hybrid release gives a conclusive result than hybrid arrest and is the preferred method of identification.

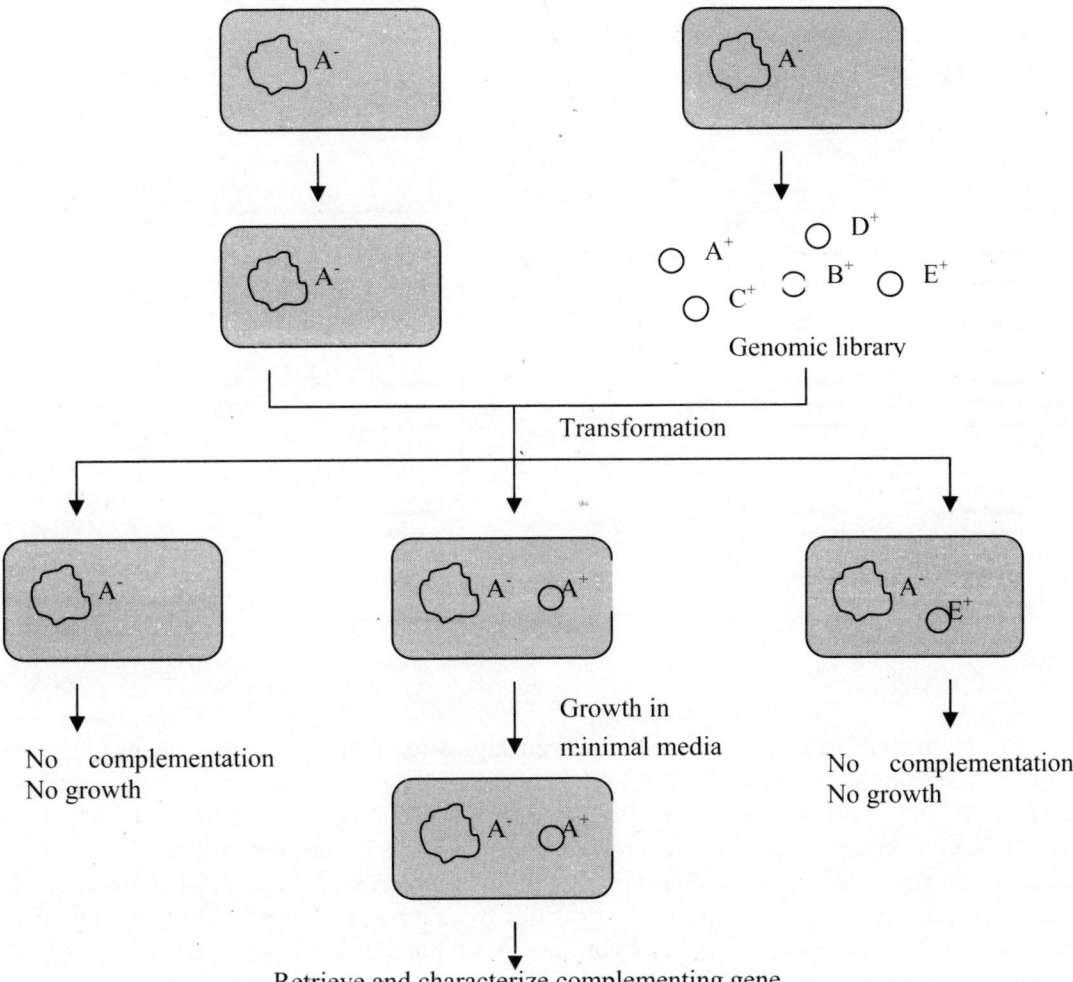

Fig. 9.16: Gene cloning by functional complementation. Host cells that are defective in a certain function, say A$^-$, are transformed with plasmids from a genomic library derived from cells that are normal with respect to function A$^-$, i.e. A$^+$. Transformed cells that carry a gene that confers the A$^+$ function are identified, and the insert of the vector is studied to characterize the gene that corrects the defect in the mutant host cells

9.7.2. Gel electrophoresis

The technique of gel electrophoresis is vital to the genetic engineer, as it represents the main way by which nucleic acid fragments may be visualised directly. The method relies on the fact that nucleic

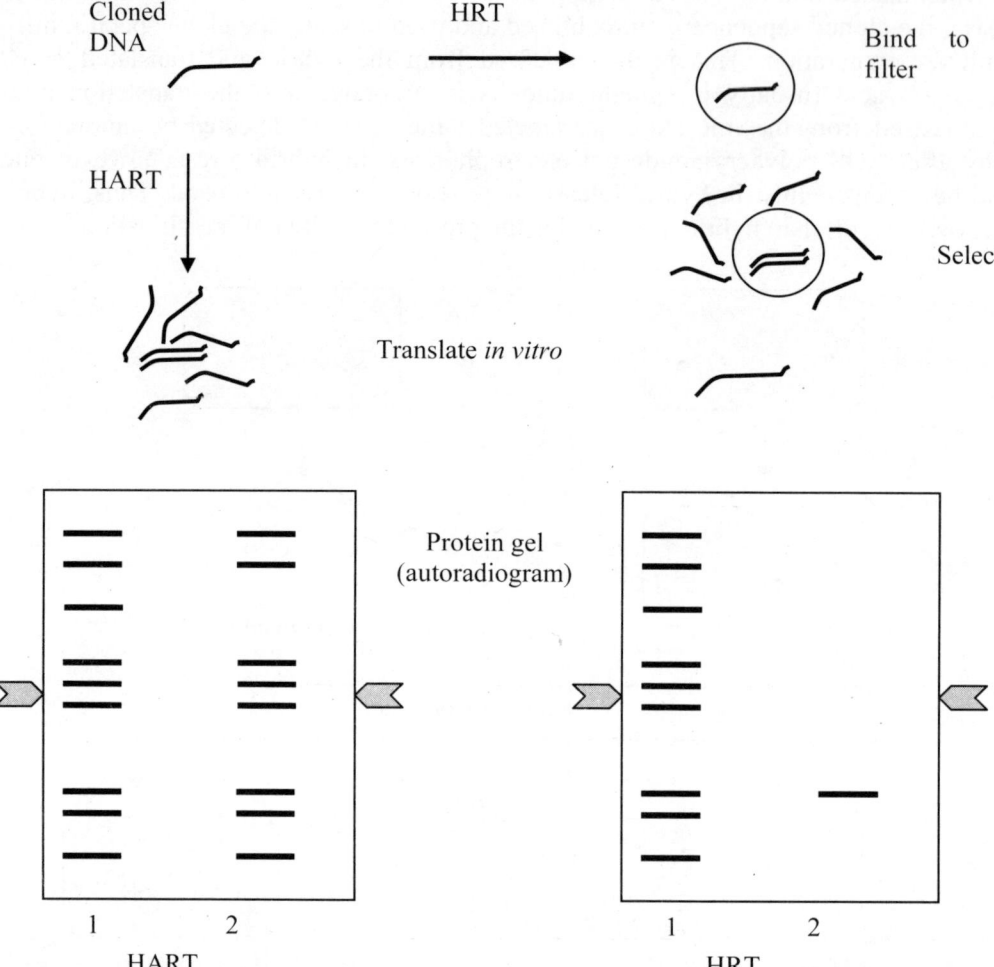

Fig. 9.17: Hybrid-arrest and hybrid-release translation to identify the protein product of a cloned fragment. In hybrid arrest (HART) the cloned fragment is mixed with a preparation of total mRNA. The hybrid formed effectively prevents translation of the mRNA to which the cloned DNA is complementary. After translation *in vitro*, the protein products of the translation are separated on a polyacrylamide gel. The patterns of the control (lane 1, HART gel) and test (lane 2, HART gel) translations differ by one band because of the absence of the protein encoded by the mRNA that has hybridized with the DNA. In hybrid release (HRT) the cloned DNA is bound to a filter and used to select its complementary mRNA from total mRNA. After washing to remove unbound mRNAs and releasing the specifically bound mRNA from the filter, translation *in vitro* generates a single band (lane 2, HRT gel) as opposed to the multiple bands of the control (lane 1, HRT gel). In both cases the identity of the protein (and hence the gene) can be determined by examination of the protein gels. The protein band of interest is arrowed

acids are polyanionic at neutral pH; that is, they carry multiple negative charges because of the phosphate groups on the phosphodiester backbone of the nucleic acid strands. This means that the molecules migrate towards the positive electrode when placed in an electric field. *As the negative charges are distributed evenly along the DNA molecule, the charge/mass ratio remains constant; thus, mobility turns to be dependent on fragment length.* The technique is carried out using a gel matrix, which efficiently separates the nucleic acid molecules according to size. The type of matrix used for electrophoresis has important consequences on the degree of separation achieved, which is dependent on the porosity of the matrix. Two gel types are commonly used namely agarose and polyacrylamide. Agarose is extracted from seaweed and can be purchased as a dry powder that is melted in buffer at an appropriate concentration, normally in the range 0.3–2.0% (w/v). On cooling, the agarose sets to form the gel. Agarose gels are usually run in the apparatus shown in Fig. 9.18, using the submerged agarose gel electrophoresis (SAGE) technique.

Polyacrylamide-based gel electrophoresis (PAGE) is sometimes used to separate small nucleic acid molecules; in applications such as DNA sequencing, as the pore size is relatively smaller than that achieved with agarose. Electrophoresis is carried out by placing the nucleic acid samples in the gel and applying a potential difference across it.

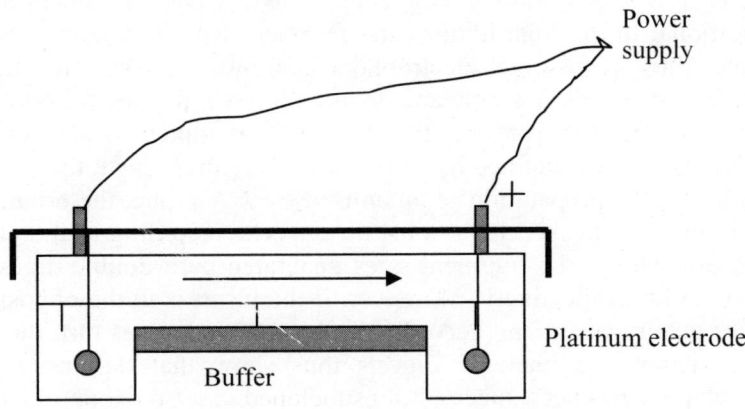

Fig. 9.18: A typical system used for agarose gel electrophoresis. The gel is just covered with buffer; therefore, the technique is sometimes called *submerged agarose gel electrophoresis* (SAGE). Nucleic acid samples placed in the gel will migrate towards the positive electrode as indicated by the horizontal arrow

This potential difference is maintained until a marker dye (usually bromophenol blue, added to the sample prior to loading) reaches the end of the gel. The nucleic acids in the gel are usually visualised after staining the gel with an intercalating dye ethidium bromide and examining under uv light. Nucleic acids appear as orange bands, which can be photographed to provide a document. The data can be used to estimate the sizes of unknown fragments by construction of a calibration curve using standards of known size, as migration is inversely proportional to the $\log_{10}$ of the number of base pairs. This is particularly useful in the restriction mapping. In addition to its use in the analysis of nucleic acids, PAGE is useful extensively in the analysis of proteins. The methodology however differs from that is used for nucleic acids, but the basic principle remains the same. One common technique is SDS-PAGE, in which the detergent SDS (sodium dodecyl sulphate) is used to denature multisubunit proteins and cover the protein molecules with negative charges. In this way the inherent charge of the protein is masked, and the charge/mass ratio becomes constant. Thus, proteins can subsequently be separated according to their size in a similar way as DNA molecules.

9.7.3. Restriction mapping

After the clone of interest has been isolated, the analysis often begins with the creation of a restriction map. The restriction map for cloned fragments is obtained essentially before additional manipulations are carried out. This is particularly important where phage or cosmid vectors are used to clone relatively large pieces of DNA. If a restriction map is available, smaller fragments can be isolated and used for various procedures, including subcloning into other vectors, the preparation of probes for chromosome walking, and DNA sequencing.

The restriction mapping provides a compilation of the number, order, and distance between restriction endonuclease cutting sites along a cloned DNA fragment. In addition, restriction mapping plays an important role particularly in characterizing DNA, mapping genes, and diagnostic tests for genetic diseases. To construct a restriction map, a cloned DNA fragment is cut by co-incubation/digestion with restriction endonucleases and loaded on to an agarose gel for electrophoresis. The lengths of the DNA fragments can be determined by comparing their position in the gel relative to reference DNAs of known lengths in the gel. A DNA fragment migrates a distance that is inversely proportional to the logarithm of the fragment length in terms of base pairs over a limited range in the gel. Thus, agarose gel electrophoresis allows the restriction fragment lengths to be determined. The pattern of cutting in single and double digests indicates the relationship that exists between the two sites. Assume, for example, that we have attempted to subclone a cDNA into a plasmid vector. A positive clone is obtained by blue-white screening. Since the recombinant plasmid DNA is desired and used for the preparation of an antisense RNA probe, the orientation of the insert in the plasmid vector should be checked for it must be correct. According to the plasmid map, if the insert is in the desired orientation, the fragment sizes generated by a double digest with EcoRI and HindIII will be 4.5 and 1.3 kb, respectively. Moreover, if the insert is in the opposite orientation, the order of restriction sites gets reversed and accordingly the fragment sizes turn out to be 3.5 and 2.3 kb. The results of restriction endonuclease digests thus show that the insert is in the correct orientation, and that a template has been successfully subcloned *in vitro* (riboprobe preparation).

9.7.4. Restriction fragment length polymorphism (RFLP)

Mark Skolnick, Ray White, David Botstein, and Ronald Davis in 1980 created a restriction fragment length polymorphism (RFLP, pronounced "rif-lip") marker map of the human genome. A RFLP is defined by the existence of alternative alleles associated with restriction fragments that differ in size from each other. RFLPs are visualized by digesting DNA from different individuals with restriction endonucleases, followed by gel electrophoresis to separate fragments according to size, then Southern blotting, and hybridization using a labeled probe that identifies the locus under investigation (Fig. 9.19).

A RFLP is demonstrated whenever the Southern blot pattern obtained with one individual is different from the one obtained with another individual. These variable regions do not necessarily occur in genes, and the function of most of them in the human genome is unknown. Figure 9.20 shows identified fragments of DNA by southern blotting.

9.7.5. Blotting techniques

Following identification of clones and preparation of restriction map, the information remains insufficient to provide much of an insight into the fine structure of the cloned fragment and hence the gene that it contains. Ultimately, the aim may be to obtain the gene sequence, but it may be that it is not appropriate to begin sequencing straight away. If, for example, a 20 kb fragment of genomic DNA has been cloned in a λ replacement vector, and the area of interest is only 2 kb in length, then much effort would unnecessarily be wasted by sequencing the entire clone. In many experiments, it is therefore essential to determine which parts of the original clone contain the regions of interest. This can be performed by using a variety of methods based on blotting nucleic acid molecules onto membranes and then subsequently hybridising with specific probes. Such an approach is an extension of clone identification by colony or plaque hybridisation, with the refinement the information about the structure of the clone is obtained

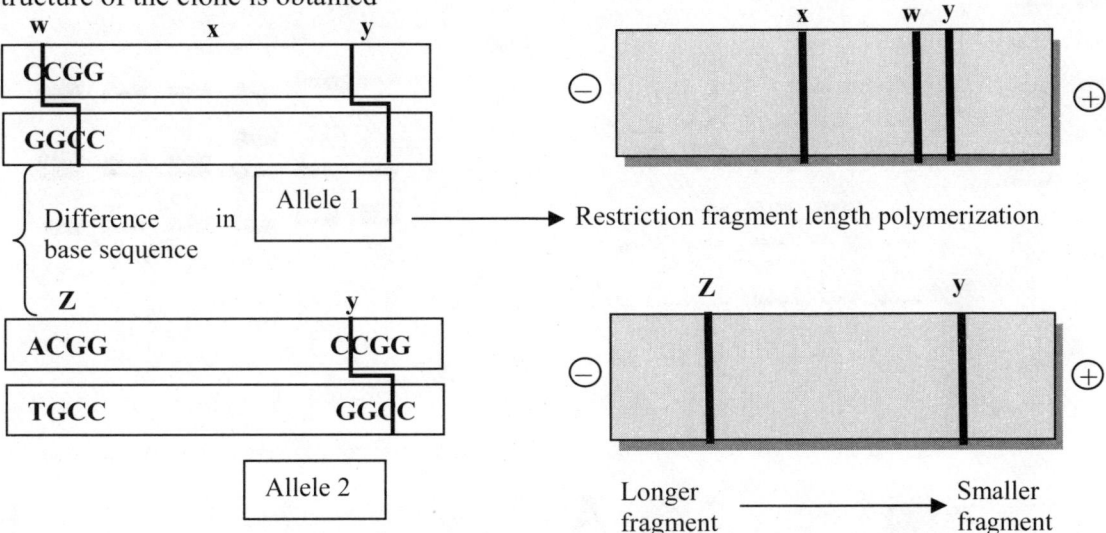

Fig. 9.19: Schematic presentation of RFLP using model alleles (1) and (2). Allele (1) was fragmented into three parts and allele (2) in two parts by same restriction endonuclease followed by gel electrophoresis. Different fragments on the basis of size can be separated and identified by southern blotting

The first blotting technique was developed by Ed Southern, and after him known as Southern blotting. In this method fragments of DNA, generated by restriction digestion, are subjected to agarose gel electrophoresis. A typical blotting apparatus setup is shown in Fig. 9.21.

The separated fragments are then transferred to a nitrocellulose or nylon membrane by a 'blotting' technique. Although other methods such as vacuum blotting and electroblotting have been devised, the original method as such still is being used extensively because it is simple and inexpensive. Blots are often set up with available options, and precarious-looking versions of the blotting apparatus are commonly used in many laboratories. When the fragments are transferred from the gel and bound to the filter, it becomes a replica of the gel. The filter is then hybridised with a radioactive probe in a similar way as colony or plaque filters. In general hybridisation, the key is the availability of a suitable probe.

After hybridisation and washing, the filter is exposed to X-ray film and an x-ray autoradiograph is prepared (Fig. 9.22). The latter provides information on the structure of the clone. An example of the use of Southern blotting in clone characterisation is shown in Fig. 9.23. Although Southern blotting is a very simple technique, it has many applications and has been an invaluable method in gene analysis. The same technique can also be used with RNA, as opposed to DNA, and in this case the method is known as Northern blotting. It is most useful in determining hybridisation patterns in mRNA samples and can be used to determine which regions of a cloned DNA fragment will hybridise to a particular mRNA. However, it is more often used as a method of measuring transcript levels during expression of a particular gene.

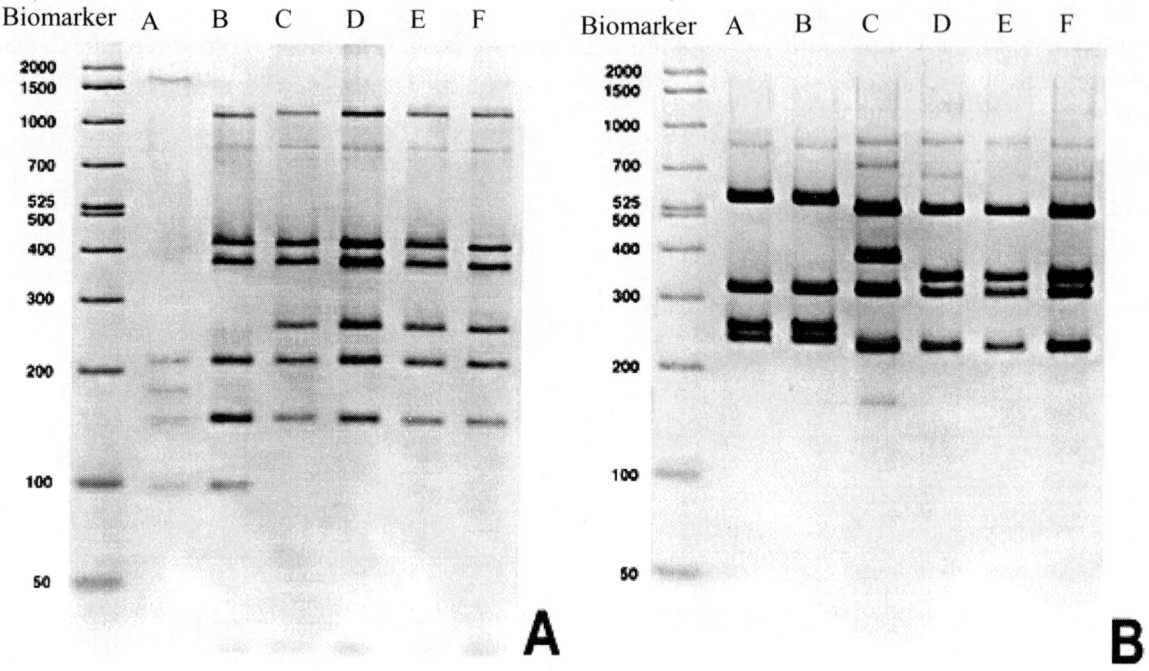

Fig. 9.20: Typical representation of RFLP

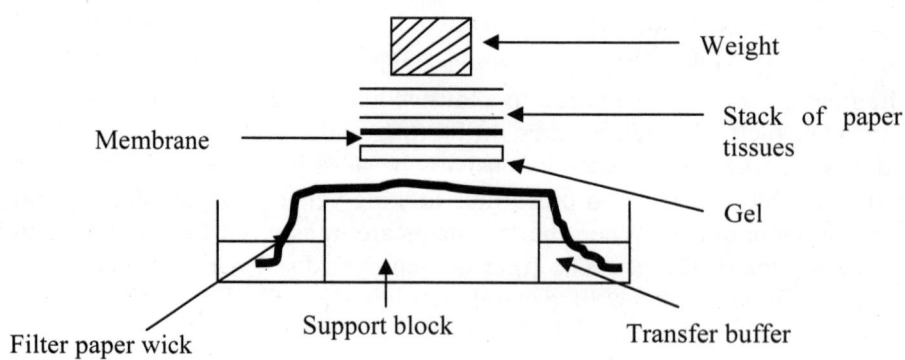

Fig. 9.21: Blotting apparatus. The gel is placed on a filter paper wick and a nitrocellulose or nylon filter placed on top. Further sheets of filter paper and paper tissues complete the setup. Transfer buffer is drawn through the gel by capillary action, and the nucleic acid fragments are transferred out of the gel and onto the membrane

Further variations on the blotting theme are available and reported. If nucleic acid samples are not subjected to electrophoresis but are spotted onto the filters, hybridisation can be carried out as for Northern and Southern blots. This technique is known as **dot blotting** and is particularly useful in obtaining quantitative data used in the study of gene expression. In some variants of the apparatus the nucleic acid is applied in a slot rather than as a dot. Not surprisingly, this is called **slot blotting**! The technique Western blotting, however involves the transfer of electrophoretically separated protein molecules to membranes. Often used with SDS-PAGE (polyacrylamide gel electrophoresis under denaturing conditions), Western blotting can identify proteins specifically, provided an appropriate antibody target protein is available. The membrane with the proteins fixed in position is probed with the antibody to detect the target protein in a similar way to immunological screening of plaque lifts from expression libraries. Sometimes, Western blots can be a useful measure to quantitate a particular protein in the cell at any given time. By comparing with other data (such as amount of mRNA, and/or enzyme activity) it is possible to build up a picture of the expression and metabolic control of the protein.

9.7.6. DNA sequencing

Determining the sequence of bases in DNA remained a labor-intensive process until 1977 which could be applied only to very short sequences, such as the template region for tRNA. Moreover, with the development of techniques for rapid, large-scale DNA sequencing, today's molecular biologists determine the order of bases in DNA as a matter of course. DNA sequencing is used as the ultimate characterization method once a gene has been cloned or amplified by PCR. Although a sequence on its own is of limited value, it is necessary for more informative analyses of the cloned gene. DNA sequencing is used to identify genes, determine the sequence of promoters and other regulatory DNA elements that control expression or reveal the fine structure of genes and other DNA sequences, confirm the DNA sequence of cDNA and other DNA synthesized in vitro (for example, after in vitro mutagenesis to confirm the mutation). They also help deduce the amino acid sequence of a gene or cDNA from the DNA sequence. With the advent of automated DNA sequencing technology, large genome sequencing projects are yielding information very fast about the evolution of genomes, the location of coding regions, regulatory elements, and other sequences, and the presence of mutations that may give rise to genetic diseases .

9.7.6.1. Maxam–Gilbert (chemical) sequencing

An identified and defined target fragment of DNA is required as the starting material. This need not be cloned in a plasmid vector; this lends the technique to be applicable to any DNA fragment. The DNA is radiolabelled with ^{32}P at the 5' ends of each strand, and the strands are denatured, separated, and purified to give a population of labeled strands for the sequencing reactions (Fig. 9.24).

The next step is a chemical modification of the bases in the DNA strand. This is done in a series of four or five reaction tubes with different specificities (Table 9.5), and the reaction conditions are so chosen that, on an average, only one modification gets introduced into each copy of the DNA molecule.

9.7.6.2. Sanger–Coulson (dideoxy or enzymatic) sequencing

Although the end result is similar to that obtained by the chemical method, the Sanger--Coulson procedure however differs totally from that of Maxam and Gilbert. In this case a copy of the DNA to be sequenced is produced by the Klenow fragment of DNA polymerase initiated synthesis through copying the template strand. The template for this reaction is typically a single-stranded DNA, and a primer to provide free 3☐ terminus for DNA polymerase to begin synthesising of the copy. The production of nested fragments results by the incorporation of a modified dNTP in each reaction. These dNTPs lack a hydroxyl group at the 3' position of deoxyribose, which is necessary for chain elongation and further propagation of strand. Such modified dNTPs are known as dideoxynucleoside triphosphates (ddNTPs).

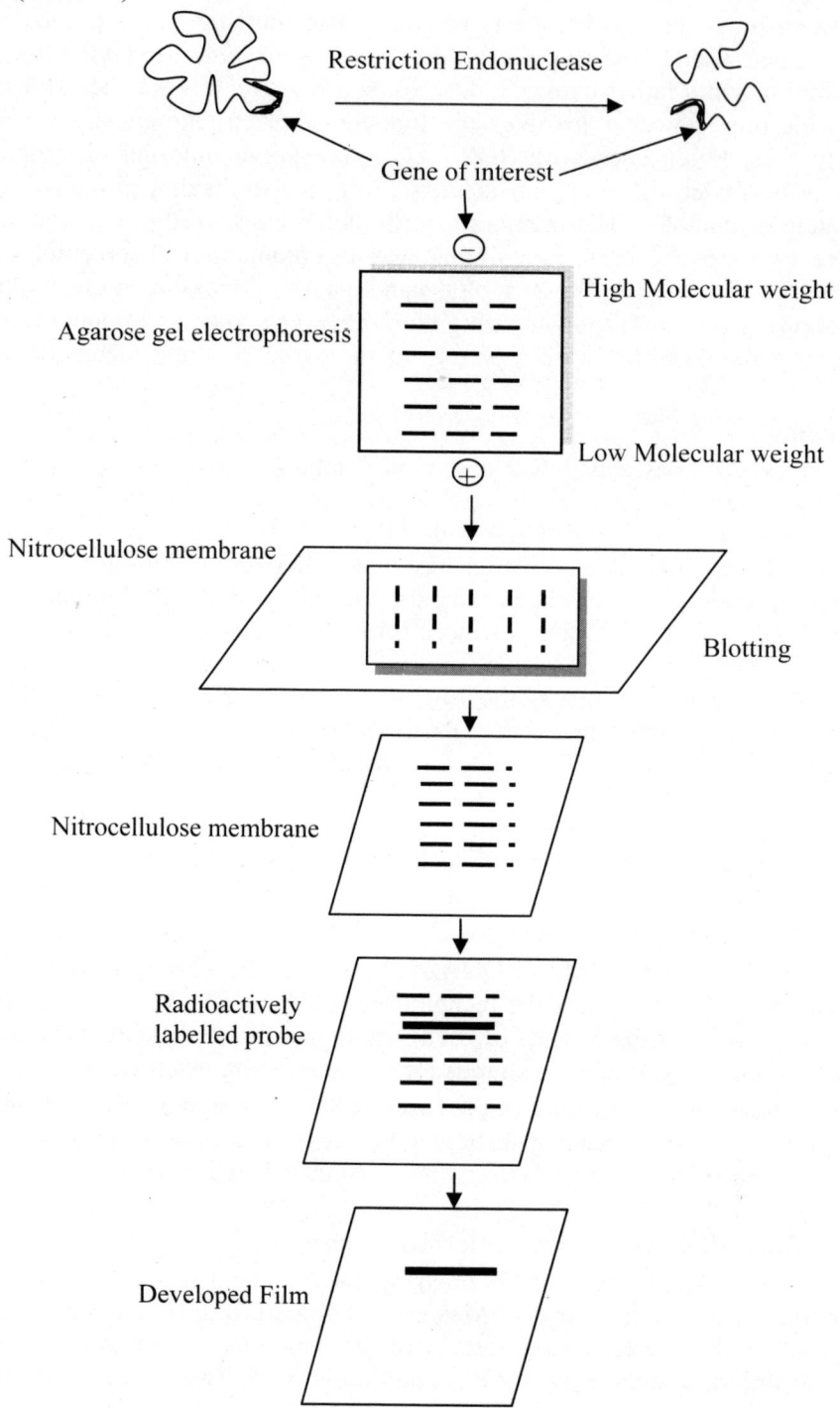

Fig. 9.22: Southern blotting

(a) Gel   **(b) autoradiograph**

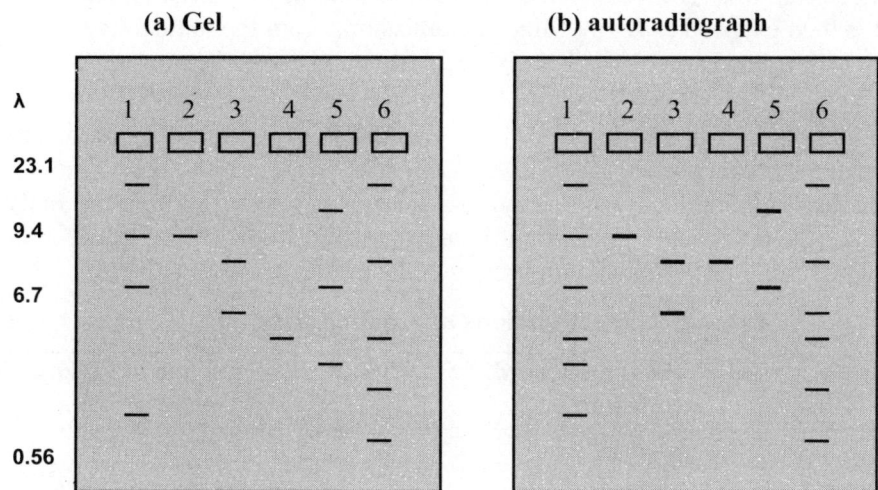

Fig. 9.23: Southern blotting. A hypothetical 20 kb fragment from a genomic clone is under investigation. A cDNA copy of the mRNA is available for use as a probe. (*a*) Gel pattern of fragments produced by digestion with various restriction enzymes; (*b*) autoradiograph resulting from the hybridisation. Lanes 1 and 6 contain λ *Hind*III markers, sizes as indicated. These have been marked on the autoradiograph for reference. The intact fragment (lane 2) runs as a single band to which the probe hybridises. Lanes 3, 4, and 5 were digested with *Eco*RI (E), *Pst*I (P), and *Bam*HI (B). Fragment sizes are indicated under each lane in (*a*). The results of the autoradiography show that the probe hybridises to two bands in the *Eco*RI and *Bam*HI digests; therefore, the clone must have internal sites for these enzymes. The *Pst*I digest shows hybridisation to the 7 kb fragment only. This might, therefore, be a good candidate for subcloning, as the gene may be located entirely on this fragment

The four ddNTPs (A, G, T, and C forms) are included in a series of four reactions, each of which contains the four normal dNTPs. The concentration of the dideoxy form is such that it will be incorporated into the growing DNA chain infrequently. Each reaction, therefore, produces a series of fragments terminating at a specific nucleotide, and the four reactions thus proceeding together will provide a set of nested fragments. The DNA chain is labelled by including a radioactive dNTP in the reaction mixture. This is usually [α-35s] dATP, which enables more sequence to be read from a single gel than the ^{32}P-labelled dNTPs that were used previously. The generation of fragments for dideoxy sequencing is more complicated compared to those generated by chemical sequencing and usually involves subcloning into different vectors. Many plasmid vectors are now available, and some of them can be used directly for DNA sequencing experiments.

9.7.6.3. Electrophoresis and reading of sequences

The DNA fragments generated in sequencing reactions are separated by PAGE. For the standard lab procedure (small-scale nonautomated), a single gel system is used. The gels usually contain 6–20% w/v polyacrylamide and 7 M urea, which acts as a denaturant to reduce the effects of DNA secondary structure. This is important because fragments that differ in length by only one base are being separated. The gels are very thin (0.5 mm or less) and are run at high-power settings which cause them to heat up to 60–70°C. This also helps to maintain denaturing conditions. Sometimes two different samples are loaded onto the same gel at different times to maximize the amount of sequence information obtained through gel pattern comparison.

After the gel has been run, it is removed from the apparatus and may be dried onto a paper sheet to facilitate handling. It is then exposed to X-ray film. The emissions from the radioactive label sensitize the silver grains, which turn black when the film is developed and fixed. The result is known as an autoradiograph (Fig. 9.26).

Reading the autoradiograph is straightforward -- the sequence is read from the smallest fragment upwards. Using this method, sequences of up to several hundred bases may be read from single gels. The sequence data are then compiled and studied using a computer, which can perform analyses such as translation into amino acid sequences and identification of restriction sites, regions of sequence homology, and other structural motifs such as promoters and control regions.

Table 9.5: Specifications of reaction tube

Content of the reaction tube	Size of the primer and extension	Prime and sequence of extension
ddATP +	Pimer+3	Pimer-dGdCddA
four dNTPs	Pimer+7	Pimer-dGdCdTdCdGddA
	Pimer+8	Pimer-dGdCdAdTdCdGdAddA
ddATP +	Pimer+2	Pimer-dGddC
four dNTPs	Pimer+5	Pimer-dGdCdAdTddC
ddATP +	Pimer+1	Pimer-ddG
four dNTPs	Pimer+6	Pimer-dGdCdAdTdCddG
ddATP +	Pimer+4	Pimer-dGdCdAddT
four dNTPs	Pimer+9	Pimer-dGdCdAdTdCdGdAdAddT

9.7.6.4. DNA sequencing by primer walking

For very long pieces of DNA (~5,000 bp), double stranded plasmid DNA sequencing protocol that do not require restriction endonuclease mapping and subcloning have been developed, With these protocols, plasmid DNA containing the target DNA is purified and annealed with a synthetic oligonucleotide (primer) that base pairs with one of the strands of the vector near the insertion site of the cloned DNA. The dideoxynucleotide sequencing reactions are carried out to determine the identity and order of the first 250 to 350 nucleotides of the insert DNA, On the basis of this analysis, a second primer that is designed to hybridize to a region about 300 nucleotides away from the binding site of the initial primer is chemically synthesized and then used to determine the sequence of the next 250 to 350 nucleotides of the insert DNA. In a similar manner, a third primer binding site is selected, another oligonucleotide is synthesized, and the sequence of the next 250 to 350 bases is determined (Fig. 9.27). The "primer walking" (primer extension) strategy proceeds until the entire cloned DNA is sequenced. Different initial primers, one for the strand at one end of the insert and the other for the opposite strand at the other end of the insert, enable sequencing of both the strands. False priming of DNA synthesis can give erroneous and ambigious results. This situation may arise if the primer binds to more than one region within the target DNA. To avoid this problem, the primers used for this procedure are generally at least 24 nucleotide long. In addition, stringent annealing conditions are used which do not permit spurious binding of the primer to similar but nonidentical sequences. Primer walking has been used to sequence pieces of DNA that has been cloned into the bacteriophage λ (~20 kilobase pair [kb]) or a cosmid vector (~ 45 kb).

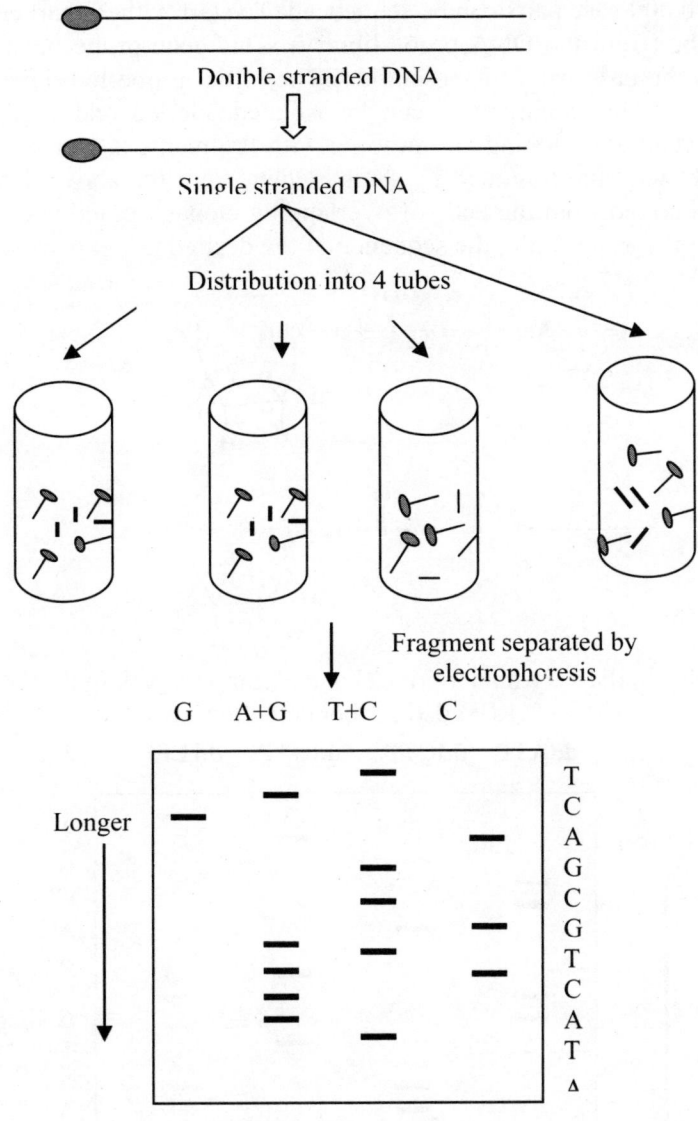

Bands on autoradiograph

ATACTGCGACT   Sequence strand
TATGAGGCTGA   Complementary strand

Fig. 9.24: Maxam Gilbert method for DNA sequenceing

9.7.6.5. Chromosome walking in DNA sequencing

Chromosome walking is a DNA base sequencing method in which the chromosome is analyzed by extending one tip to reach the other. The technique basically involves systematically moving along the chromosome from a known location to an unknown location, and thus determining the DNA sequence. The method involved in chromosome walking is shown in Fig.9.28 (A). A DNA fragment with approximately 40,000 base pairs can be sequenced. To start with, a marker is used to identify the appropriate gene probe (from the DNA probe library). This gene probe must have a section of the base pair identical to the base pairs of the marker. The initial probe hybridizes only with the clone containing fragment A. This fragment A can be isolated, cloned and used as a probe to detect fragment B. This procedure of cloning and probing with fragments is repeated again and again until fragment D hybridizes with the fragment E. As is evident from the above description, chromosome walking uses probes derived from the ends of overlapping clones to facilitate a walk along the DNA sequence. In the process for this walk, the sequence of the desired target gene can be identified.

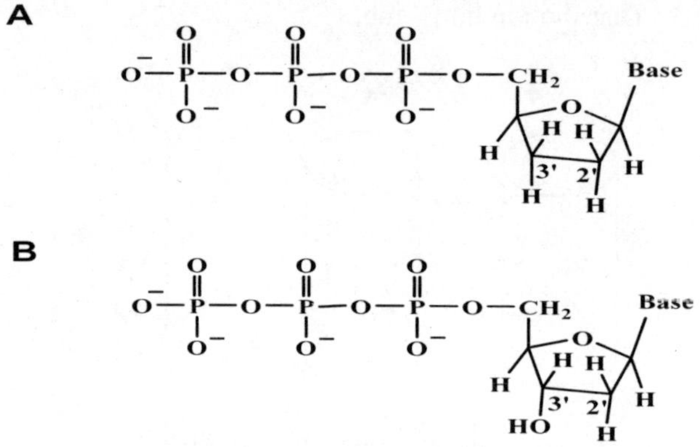

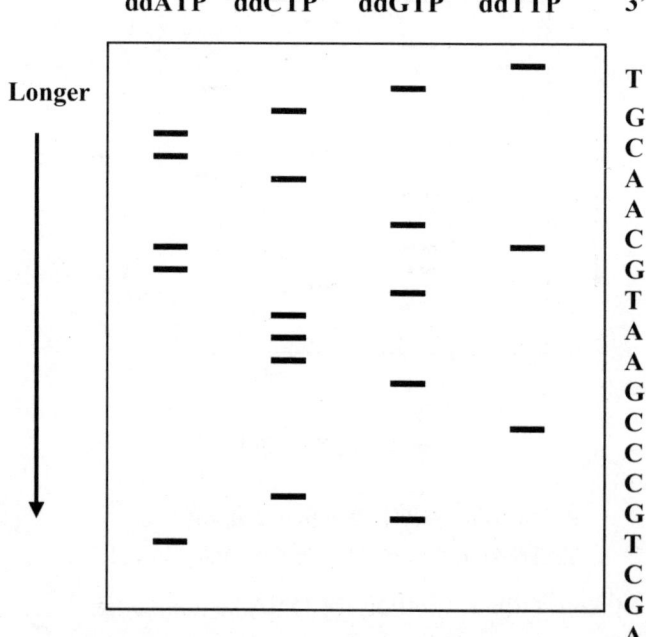

Fig. 9.25: (A) dideoxy nucleotide- 2' and 3' carbons lack hydroxyl groups,
(B) deoxvribonucleotide

Fig. 9.26: Simulated autorediograph of a dideoxynucleotide DNA sequencing gel. Each lane of the gel was loaded with the contents of one of the four reaction tubes, which contained ddATP, ddCTP, ddGTP or ddTTP. By convention, the bands of the autoradiograph are read from the bottom to the top. In this example, the esults of the sequence determination ae shown on the right

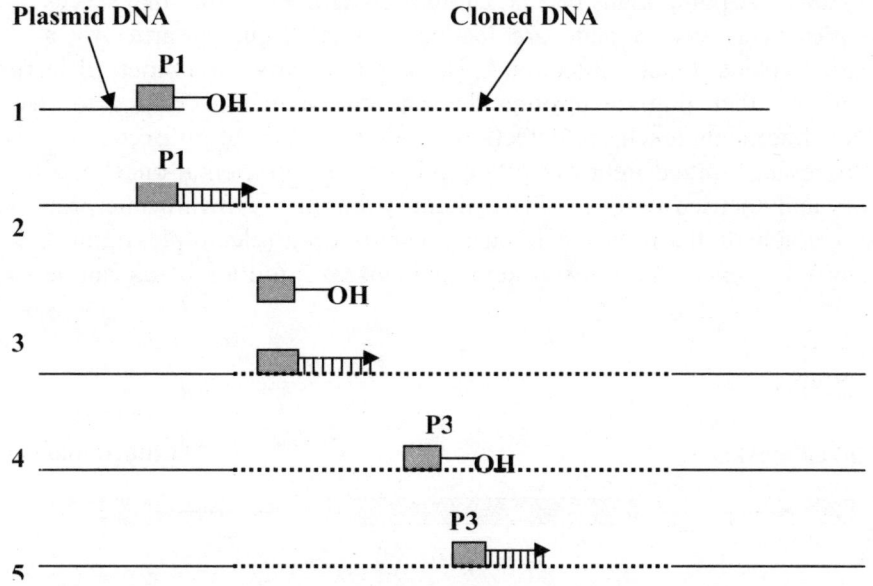

Fig. 9.27: DNA sequencing by primer walking. 1. DNA sequencing is initiated with a pimer (P1) that is complementary to a site on a plasmid near the point of intersection of the cloned DNA. 2. Based on the segment of the cloned DNA that has just been sequenced, a second primer (P2) that is complementary to a stretch of about 20 nucleotides near the end of that segment is synthesized. 3. P2 is used to sequence the next segment of the cloned DNA. 4. Based on the segment of the cloned DNA that has just been sequenced, a third primer (P3) that is complementary to a stretch of about 20 nucleotides near the end of that segment is synthesized. 5. P3 is used to sequence the next segment of the cloned DNA. 6. Based on the segment of the cloned DNA that has just been sequenced, a fourth primer that is complementary to a stretch of about 20 nucleotides near the end of that segment is synthesized. The process is successively synthesizing and using new primers continues until the entire insert is synthesized

9.7.6.5.1. Chromosome jumping

An improved strategy of chromosome walking is chromosome jumping. Many regions of DNA that are difficult to be cloned by walking can be jumped. The procedure involves the circularization of large genomic fragments generated by the digestion of endonucleases. This is followed by cloning of the region lowering the closure of the fragment. By this approach, the DNA sequences located at far off places can be brought together and cloned. A chromosome jumping map can be constructed in this manner and used for long distance chromosome walks (Fig. 9.28 B).

Automated DNA sequencing

In 1986, Leroy Hood and Lloyd Smith automated Sanger's method. In this new sequencing technology, radioactive markers are replaced with fluorescent ones. Each ddNTP terminator is tagged with a different color of fluorophore typically red, green, blue, or yellow. Thus, instead of having to run four separate sequencing reactions, the reactions can be combined into one tube. The first automated sequencer made use of a polyacrylamide gel to resolve the samples, a laser to excite the dye molecules as they reach a detector near the end of the gel, and a computer to read the results as a DNA sequence. In this system each automated sequencer is able to produce 4800 bases of sequence per day. The current automated systems replace the old-style gel with arrays of tiny capilliaries, each of which acts as a "lane." A pump loads special capillaries with a polymer that serves as a separation matrix. DNA samples in a 96-well plate are loaded into the capillary array by a short burst of electrophoresis, called "electrokinetic injection." The capillary array is immersed in running buffer and the DNA fragments then migrate through the capillary matrix according to size, smallest to largest. As the DNA fragments reach the detection window, a laser beam excites the dye molecules causing them to fluoresce. Emitted light from 96 capillaries is collected at once, spectrally separated into the four colors and focused onto a CCD camera. Computer software interprets the pattern of peaks to produce a graph of fluorescence intensity versus time (electropherogram), which is then converted to the DNA sequence. With this system, as many as 2 million bases can be sequenced in a day.

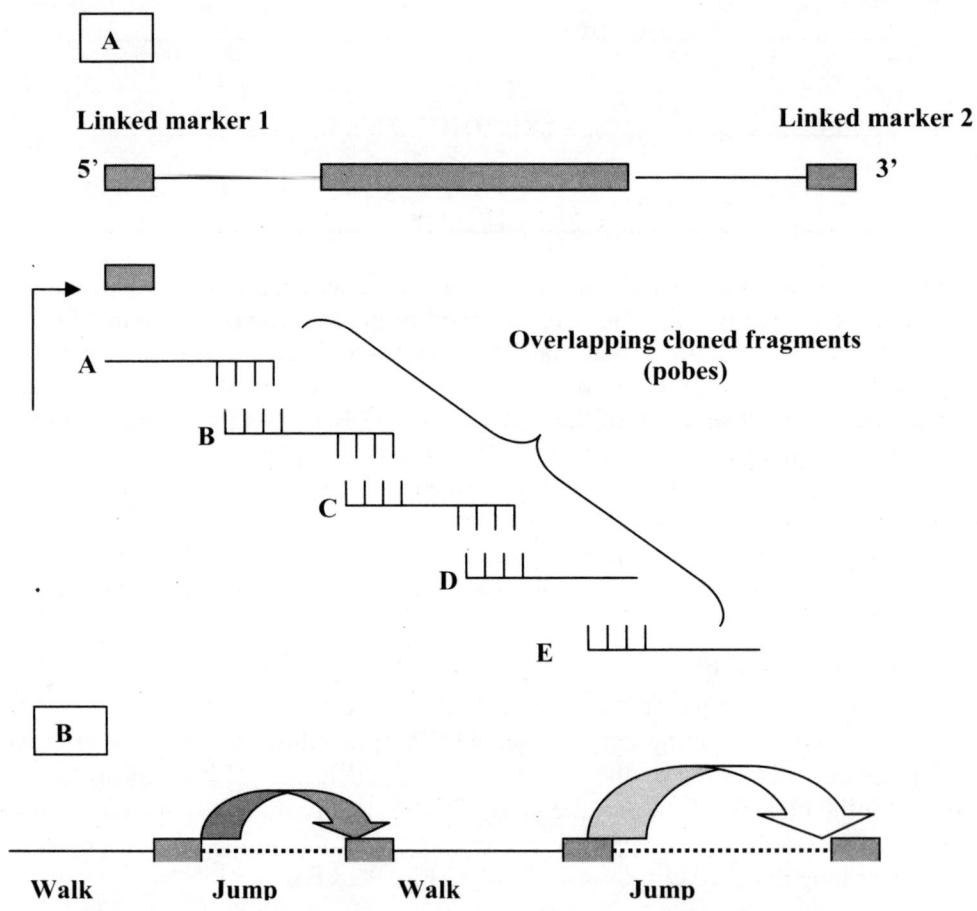

Fig. 9.28: A.Chromosome walking B. Chromosome jumping

The development of rapid methods for DNA sequencing, has meant that this task has now become routine practice in most laboratories where cloning is often carried out. Sequencing a gene provides much useful information about coding sequences, control regions, and other features such as intervening sequences. Thus, full characterisation of a gene will inevitably involve sequencing, and a suitable strategy must be devised inorder to enable this to be achieved most accurately and efficiently. The complexity of a sequencing strategy depends on a number of factors, the main one being the length of the fragment that is to be sequenced. Most manual sequencing methods enable about 300--400 bases to be read from a sequencing gel. If the DNA is only a few hundred base pairs long, it can probably be sequenced in a single step. However, it is more likely that the sequence will be several kilobase pairs in length; thus, sequencing is more complex. There are basically two ways of tackling large sequencing projects. Either a random or 'shotgun' approach is used, or an ordered strategy is devised in which the location of each fragment is explored prior to sequencing.

In the shotgun method, random fragments are generated and sequenced. Assembly of the complete sequence depends on sufficient overlap between the sequenced fragments to enable computer matching of sequences from the generated raw data. An ordered sequencing strategy is therefore more efficient than a random fragment approach. There are several possible ways of generating defined fragments for sequencing. Examples include (1) isolation and subcloning of defined restriction fragments and (2) generation of a series of subclones in which the target sequence has been progressively deleted by nucleases. If defined restriction fragments are used, the first requirement is of a detailed restriction map of the original clone. Using this, suitably sized fragments can be identified and subcloned into a sequencing vector such as M13 or pBluescript. Each subclone is then sequenced, usually by the dideoxy method. Both strands of the DNA should be sequenced independently, so that any anomalies can be spotted and re-sequenced if so needed. The complete sequence is then assembled by using a suitable computer software package. This becomes easier if overlapping fragments have been isolated for subcloning, as the regions of overlap enable adjoining sequences to be identified easily. By devising a suitable strategy and paying careful attention to detail, it is possible to derive accurate sequence data from most cloned fragments.

The task of sequencing a long stretch of DNA is not trivial, but it is now such an integral part of gene manipulation technology that most gene cloning projects involve sequence determination at some point. The technology has improved greatly to the point where entire genomes are being sequenced.

9.8. EXPRESSION SYSTEMS

Prokaryotic (bacteria) or eukaryotic (yeast, mammalian cell culture) systems are generally used as a host for the production of usable quantities of the desired rDNA product. Most of the rDNA products approved by FDA are being produced using these systems. Bacteria such as Escherichia coli are widely used for the expression of rDNA products. They offer several advantages due to high level of recombinant protein expression, rapid growth of cell and simple media requirement. However, there are some limitations such as intracellular accumulation of heterologous proteins, the potential for product degradation due to trace of protease impurities and production of endotoxin. Yeast such as *Saccharomyces cerevisiae*, *Hansenulla polymorpha* and *Pichia pastoris* are among the simplest eukaryotic organisms. They grow relatively quickly and are highly adaptable to large-scale production. These organisms do not produce endotoxin. They are capable of glycosylating proteins up to a certain extent like mammalian cells. Mammalian systems such as Chinese hamster ovary (CHO) cell and baby hamster kidney (BHK) cell systems are often the choice for production of human therapeutic proteins. The CHO and BHK cell systems are an ideal choice as these are capable of glycosylating the protein at the correct sites. However, cost of production of the products using these systems is high because of slow growth and expensive nutrient media. The choice of expression system can influence the character, quantity and cost of a final product. Recent advances have been made in producing therapeutic proteins by using transgenic animals. Transgenic milk production is currently most feasible. The advantages of this system include high expression levels and volume output, low capital investment, low operational costs and reproducible production facility, i.e. inbreeding could pass an animal's ability to produce transgenic protein to its offspring. Despite the attractiveness of this system, a number of issues remain to be solved before it is broadly accepted by the industries and regulatory authorities. These include variability of expression levels and characterization of the exact nature of the post-translational modification in the mammary systems. The use of genetically engineered plants to produce valuable proteins is increasing slowly. The system has potential advantages of economy and scalability. However, variation in product yield, contamination with agrochemical and fertilizer, impact of pest and disease, and variable cultivation conditions should also be considered. Plant cell culture system combines the advantages of whole plant system as well as animal cell culture. Although no recombinant products have yet been produced commercially using plant cell culture, several companies are investigating the commercial feasibility of such a production system.

9.9. PRODUCTION AND PURIFICATION OF rDNA PRODUCTS

Recombinant DNA (rDNA) technology has made a revolutionary impact in the area of human healthcare by enabling mass production of safe, pure and effective rDNA expression products. Currently there are several categories of rDNA products. The first step is isolation of the identified gene that is responsible for expression of the desired product. After isolation and characterization of the human gene, it is inserted into small circular pieces of DNA called plasmid. The recombinant plasmid is inserted into bacterial yeast or cultured animal cell. Clones of transformed host cell are isolated and those that produced the protein of interest in the desired quantities are preserved under suitable condition as a master cell bank. The cell banks are characterized and properly maintained for use in subsequent transformation procedures. The cell bank should be periodically tested for cell viability, genetic and phenotypic stability. As manufacturing needs arise, cells from working cell can be scaled up to produce the product in roller bottles and/or fermentors. Fermentors are generally used for growth of *E. coli* or yeast. Mammalian cells are often grown in roller bottles. Inoculation of host cells that contained an expression vector is added to defined volume of medium in either fermentors or roller bottles. The cells are allowed to grow until the nutrients in the medium are depleted or excreted by the products reaching inhibitory levels. By providing a balanced mixture of nutrients and/or chemicals to neutralize accumulating growth inhibitor, product yield in the medium or cell density can be improved. At the end of the run, the host cells are harvested and the recombinant product is isolated from culture medium or cells. The following points should be considered for production of rDNA products:

(1) Plasmid instability is a major problem in continuous and large-scale fermentation, since these cultures go through many generations. The resulting effects are lower productivity and an increase in production cost, because of the build-up of non-productive plasmid free cells. Mathematically structured and unstructured kinetic models of plasmid stability have been developed, which are ultimately useful for design of recombinant processes.

(2) High level expression of rDNA products in different host systems can often result in aggregation and accumulation of inclusion bodies. Under appropriate conditions, the rDNA products may get deposited in inclusion bodies in approximately 50% or more of the total cell protein. The rDNA protein is highly pure, stable and compact. Recovery of soluble, active rDNA protein from the inclusion body requires the following steps to be carried out:

(a) Isolation of the inclusion body from cell–cell disruption and centrifugation.

(b) Solubilization of the inclusion body protein using a chactrope (denaturant).

(c) Under reducing conditions (to separate all disulphide bonds).

(d) Recovery of active protein by removal of denaturant under conditions that allow the protein to adapt its native configuration.

(e) Undesired disulphide bonds, if present in the structure, need to be re-oxidised under controlled condition, achieving their correct configuration present in native structure.

(3) The cell bank should be periodically tested for cell viability, genetic and phenotype stability. When eukaryotic cells are used for production, distinguishing genetic, phenotypic and immunological markers of the cell will be useful in establishing the identity of the cells. Likewise, when microbial cultures are used, specific phenotypic features which form a basis for identification should be identified and described.

(4) Traditional small-scale fermentors are used for expansion of cells in suspension culture. The presence, extent and nature of any microbial contamination in the culture vessels must be thoroughly examined at suitable stages during production. All the systems associated with fermentors must be validated before being routinely used.

(5) Unintended variability in culture during production may lead to changes which cause alteration in the product. Such variations might result in differing yield of the products.

(6) The steps in a production process should be validated to ensure that the process intermediates are within specifications. Any assay used during process validation must itself be validated, before the process validation is commenced. Purification is an important aspect in the production of rDNA products.

The overall goal of purification is to bring as much product with as little loss as possible. A general purification process is presented in Fig. 9.29. In case the desired product is intracellular, fermentation is followed by harvesting of cells. This step is normally achieved by centrifugation or filtration. The cells are disrupted or lysed and cell debris is removed by centrifugation, leaving behind a dilute solution of crude desired product.

If mammalian or yeast system is used, the desired product can be obtained directly from the medium. Nowadays, ultrafiltration has become the method of choice for concentration of products. There are several different methods which can be used for purification of rDNA products, however only chromatographic purification methods are generally preferred and used (Table 9.6). A combination of two to four different chromatographic techniques is generally employed in a typical downstream processing procedure. Gel filtration and ion exchange chromatography are the most common. Affinity chromatography is employed wherever possible, as it has high biospecificity and one can achieve a high degree of purification. Appropriate attention needs to be given to the validation of the purification process such as column loading capacity and column regeneration.

The purification process must be validated to ensure that it is adequate to remove extraneous substances such as chemicals used in the process if any, purification, column contaminations, endotoxin, residual cellular proteins and viruses. The reproducibility of the purification process with respect to its ability to remove specific contaminants should also be determined. Further, columns should also be validated for possible leaching of legends (e.g. dye, affinity legends, etc.) throughout the expected lifespan of the column. The evidence of purity of the purified product should be established.

Physico-chemical, biological and immunological characterizations of purified product should also be obtained using a wide range of analytical tests. Characterization tests of products may include mainly amino acid composition, peptide mapping, electrophoretic assays (SDS–PAGE, Western blot, isoelectric focusing), HPLC, immunoassay, endotoxin test, potency determination test, etc. An overview of production process of a rDNA product is shown in Fig. 9.30.

9.10. TRANSGENIC ANIMALS

The first transgenic animals carrying foreign DNA in somatic and germ cells were produced in 1976 by exposing mouse embryos to infectious retrovirus. This feat was soon followed by the technique of microinjecting recombinant DNA into a pro-nucleus of a zygote to produce transgenic animals. In these early experiments mice were the animals of choice. Attention was later given to farm animals.

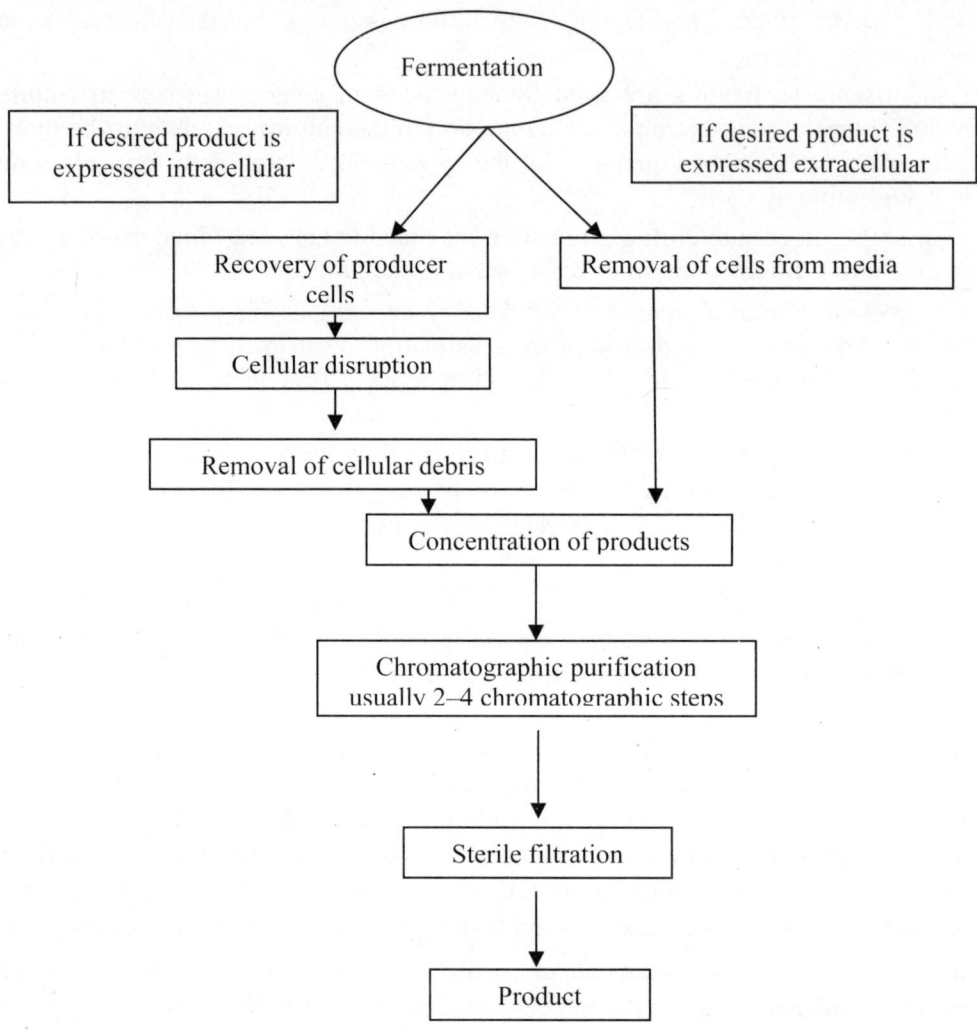

Fig. 9.29: A general schemes for purification of rDNA

By now, gene transfer has been carried out successfully in many classes of animals such as mammals, birds, fish, insects, and worms. Success of genetic engineering in domestic animals depends not only on the identification of relevant genes, but also on proper understanding of the regulation of the alien genes in transgenic animals. For instance, any attempt to use farm animals for molecular farming (i.e., for producing valuable human proteins) requires a better knowledge of basic mechanisms of gene regulation. Also it is sometimes difficult or even risky to extrapolate the findings on mouse to larger animals. Transgenic mice have been used for the analysis of the immune system. Several transgenic mice expressing genes concerned with the immune system have been produced. Transgenic expression of immunoglobulin heavy and/or light chain genes of different specificities have facilitated better understanding of the processes involved in B-cell development such as allelic exclusion of immunoglobulins and B-cell tolerance. Transgenic mice expressing interleukin genes have been used to learn the modes of action of these important growth and differentiation factors in the context of the mouse immune system. Transgenic mice expressing interleukin genes with specificities directed against mouse self-components have been greatly helpful in unraveling the mechanisms involved in the tolerance of B-lymphocytes.

Table 9.6: Chromatographic purification methods used for rDNA products

Reversed phase chromatography
- o   Size exclusion chromatography
- o   Hydrophobic interaction chromatography
- o   Charge transfer chromatography
- o   Ion exchange chromatography
  - • Anion
  - • Cation
- o   Affinity chromatography
  - • Chemical
  - • Dye/ligand
  - • Monoclonal antibodies
  - • Metal chelate

There exists an enormous diversity of T-cell receptor specificities. This enables the immune system to mount a specific immune response to virtually any given antigen encountered by the host. The diversity is produced by somatic rearrangements of distinct germline gene segments during T-cell development and the addition of N regions. Thymocyte precursors from the bone marrow colonize the thymus and soon proliferate and rearrange their T-cell receptor loci. Rearrangement and expression of these loci are determined in relation to time with lymphocytes expressing certain specific receptor loci appearing sequentially during thymic development. Transgenic mice carrying functionally rearranged T-cell receptor genes have advanced our knowledge of T-cell development and of thymic positive and thymic negative selection processes.

Transfer of alien genes into the germline of cattle opens up revolutionary prospects for the modification of animal production traits, including the composition of milk. The mammary gland of a cow or buffalo is an efficient vat for the production of specific proteins, lipids, and sugars. Man is now contemplating to introduce changes in these constituents, especially in proteins, with a view to exploiting the farm animals for producing some human proteins needed for the treatment of diseases. The gene transfer methodology has opened up new vistas for the production of novel proteins in milk. Milk protein genes may be selected and cloned and the sequences governing tissue specific hormonally induced expression in the mammary gland may be identified. Studies with three genes, viz., bovine beta lactoglobulin, rat beta casein, and whey acidic protein of mouse and rat, suggest that beta casein genes can direct the production of novel proteins in the milk of transgenic mice, sheep, rabbits, and pigs. These proteins were biologically active and usually co migrated with authentic proteins. The transfer of recombinant DNA by microinjection into embryonal pro-nuclei is a novel approach for manipulation and in turn production of traits in domestic animals. Historically, the genetic potential associated with such traits as wool growth, milk yield, and body weight has been improved by selective breeding whereby elite animals are used as the breeding stock. This classical approach has several limitations, especially the barrier to inter specific crossing which precludes the transfer of some desired gene from one species to another. The successful transfer of recombinant DNA into mouse embryos by microinjection into pro-nuclei of one-celled embryos has been achieved. This technique can be used to alter the growth of mice. It is now possible to alter the genetic properties of animals without resorting to conventional breeding. It is also possible to transfer small pieces of the genome instead of the entire chromosome. The first transgenic pigs and sheeps were reported in 1985 and even cattle have now come in this category. Indeed, most, if not all, major domestic animal species can be genetically modified by this technology. Some of the systems amenable to genetic manipulation include the endocrine system, the biochemical pathways the structural proteins of textile fibres and milk, and the immune system, By altering the concentration of the circulating growth hormone in transgenic mice, their growth rate and final body size can be significantly increased comparable success has, however, not been achieved in cattle, pigs or other large animals.

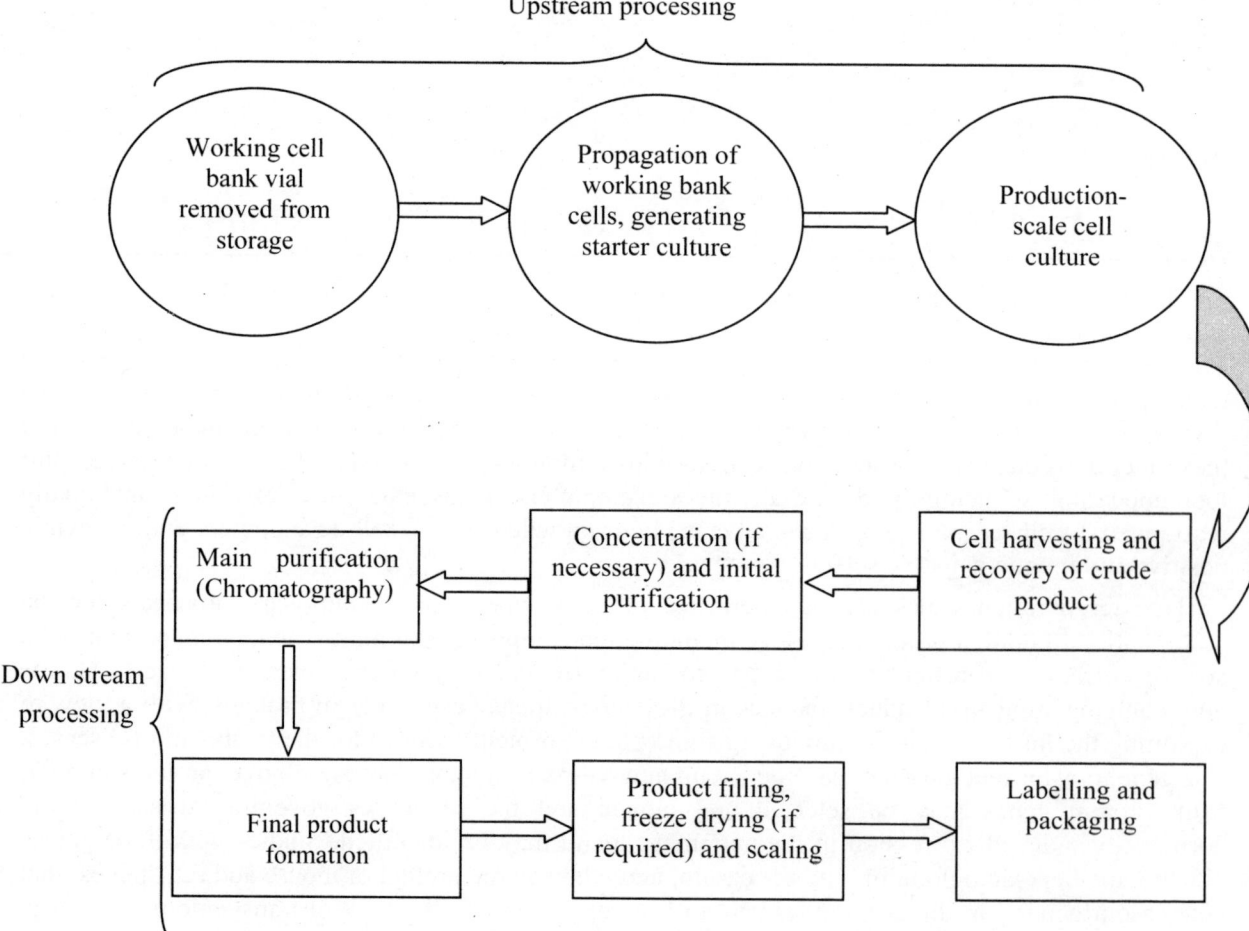

Fig. 9.30: Overview of the production process for a biopharmaceutical product

9.11. GLOBIN GENE SWITCHING

Some work has been done on gene switching mechanisms in animals, especially on the human beta-globin locus using transgenic mice. In humans, a developmental switch occurs during embryonic development. At 8 weeks of development alpha- and gamma-globins are produced. The alpha-globins are also expressed in the adult, but the gamma-genes are turned off at birth and beta-globins persist only at a low level. This switch only occurs in humans and is of particular interest since diseases caused by mutations in the beta-globin gene can only be detected at birth. The locus control region (LCR) has been identified as particularly important in controlling switching of globin genes. The LCR contains DNA hypersensitive sites, which are present in erythrocytes at all times during development, and the LCR can influence chromatin structure over long distances. 100–150 Kb of DNA downstream of the LCR can be affected as can 30 kb upstream. When the LCR region and the beta-globin gene are used to produce transgenic mice, beta-globin is always expressed at high levels independently of the site of integration. In contrast, if the beta-globin coding region is introduced on its own, expression is erratic, its levels vary between mice, and levels of beta-globin are generally low. The LCR probably contains some isolating element. In this way, any gene inserted with the LCR is independent of its new surroundings and is not affected by endogenous positive and negative control elements. The relative distance between the genes and the LCR seems to be important for gene expression and a competitive interaction occurs, so that the balance between alpha- and beta-globins can be maintained. The impaired balance may result thalssaemia.

9.12. ANIMAL BIOREACTORS

Transgenic animals designed to produce useful drugs or proteins have potential as a new industry. The American company Transgenic Sciences has produced transgenic mice, which secrete human growth hormone in their milk at levels of up to 0.5 mg per litre. Unlike cattle and pigs carrying a foreign growth hormone construct, these mice have shown no adverse effects due to the expression of the transgene. This may be because the gene has been targeted so that it is expressed only in the mammary glands. Cattle and pigs expressing extra copies of growth hormone are often infertile. The company has plans to scale up the production of growth hormone by introducing the gene into rabbits. Rabbits have a short gestation period and a high concentration of protein in their milk. Human growth hormone may conceivably be produced in rabbits at much less cost than in the bacterial cultures used at present.

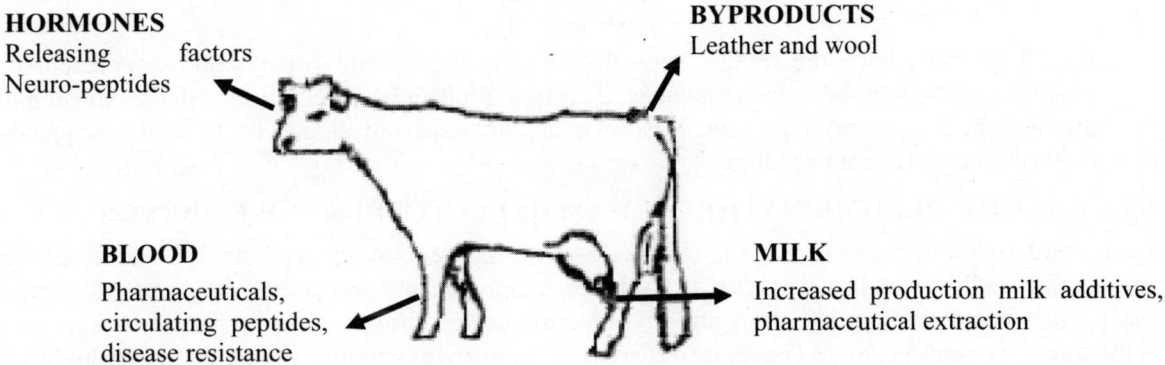

Fig. 9.31: Areas of possible investigation of domestic livestock, using the transgenic technology

9.13. MAMMALIAN GENOME

Until 1976, our concept of the mammalian genome was that genes are encoded in continuous arrays of nucleotides, organized in simple loci containing only those genes corresponding to known alleles. It was also thought that genomic DNA was quite stable, changing slowly one base at a time so as to produce the kind of single amino acid substitutions that distinguish, for instance, normal from sickle-cell hemoglobin. This concept also supposed that genes do not easily move, especially during the lifetime of a somatic cell. Now we know that genes are not encoded in continuous sequences. They are not represented in simple loci reflective of their phenotype; rather, their loci are very complex, laced with extra copies of cryptic pseudogenes. Genomic DNA does not change slowly but does so much more quickly, by inserting and deleting fairly large segments of DNA. Furthermore, DNA is not stable, and genes do move. In fact, genes not only move during evolution (as, for example, the globin and immunoglobulin genes) but they also move during somatic development (for example, in the immune system). The existence of interrupted genes of mammals is an established fact now. Genetic loci consist of large arrays of related gene sequences, some of which encode active genes, whereas others encode inactive or pseudogene copies. The beta-globin locus of the mouse provides the best example of this situation; in this, there are at least seven β-like genes spread over approximately 50 kb of genomic DNA. At one end (3'-end) are found the β-globin major and minor genes that are expressed in the adult red cell. At the 5'-end, the most distal gene, Y2, is an embryonic gene, expressed only in the nucleated red cells that appear in yolk sac of the embryo. The remaining four β-like sequences are the pseudogenes. These later closely resemble the β-globin genes but, having undergone alterations, they cannot encode a coherent globin polypeptide, chain. Pseudogenes are not translated and also appear not to be transcribed either in embryonic or adult erythrocytes.

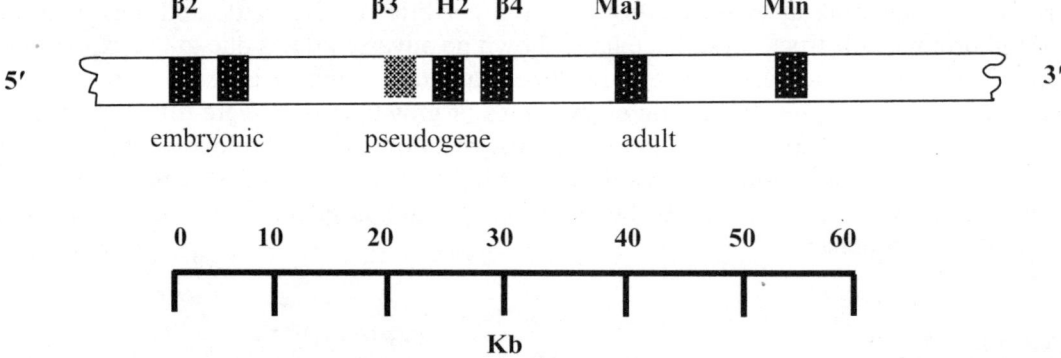

Fig. 9.32: Sketch of the mouse beta-globin gene locus. The filled regions represent the positions of beta-globin-like sequences. The two adult genes, beta-globin major and minor, are shown. The embryonic gene is shown on the left-hand side. The beta-like sequences between the genes are pseudogenes

9.14. GENETIC RECOMBINATION IN MAMMALIAN CELLS AND EMBRYOS

In the mid-1970s, it became possible to integrate foreign genetic material stably into the genome of mammalian cells in such a way that it could be expressed and transmitted to their offspring. This early work was done in mouse cells and involved the use of viruses, e.g., the mouse leukaemia virus, which acts as gene vectors. These are retroviruses and their genome is made of two molecules of single-stranded RNA. When a cell is infected, the reverse transcriptase synthesizes a complementary DNA molecule that becomes integrated into the cellular DNA as a 'provirus'. The later behaves like an episome, and causes the disease.

Another virus that is sometimes used in the foregoing approach is SV40 which has a dsDNA molecule associated with histones. The SV40 DNA has been hybridized with non-viral DNA such as that of *E. coli* plamids, and recombinant DNA molecules have been constructed which may be used as vectors for introducing genes into mammalian cells. Yet another approach is to mix the DNA fragment containing the gene with a carrier DNA, followed by precipitating it with calcium phosphate. The precipitate tends to penetrate at least some cells, and the transferred gene is often expressed and passed on to the offspring. This technique also has been applied mostly to mouse cells.

Alien genes are also being introduced into embryonic cells with a view to following their fate in the transgenic (i.e., young transformed) animals. This kind of work has been done in eggs and embryos of the mouse. The desired gene can be microinjected into the egg by means of a fine glass micropipette, either before or after its fertilization. Before the injection, the envelope of the egg may be dissolved by treatment with proteolytic enzymes. The gene should be injected into the nucleus to increase the chances of its integration and expression. Using this approach, the gene for the herpes virus thymidine kinase has been successfully inserted into mouse cell genome, either alone or along with the gene for β-globin of human haemoglobin. The use of embryonic stem (ES) cells for the genetic manipulation of mice has several advantages over microinjection techniques. More precise genetic modifications are possible using ES cells, and cells carrying the required modification can be selected before being introduced into the host blastocyst. Some recent work has enabled transgenic rather than chimaeric mice to be produced by using ES cells, Tetraploid mouse embryos can divide and implant but cannot survive to produce a viable foetus. Manipulated ES cells can be aggregated with tetraploid embryos and then implanted into a host animal. The tetraploid cells die leaving the ES cells to take over and form an entirely ES-derived embryo. The only remaining contribution of the tetraploid embryos is in the extra embryonic membranes. Some of these embryos mature but no live young are produced. Certain mutations can also be introduced into ES cells, using positive and negative enrichment strategies.

9.15. FERRYING GENES INTO MAMMALIAN CELLS

Certain genetic defects in cultured mammalian cells are amenable to alleviation by the introduction of normal genes. Some methods currently used to move genes or gene products into mammalian cells include chromosome-mediated transfer, liposomes, microinjection, calcium phosphate-mediated transfer, and viral vectors. A widely used method is the calcium co-precipitation technique with dominant selectable markers. Eukaryotic viral vectors are also quite effective in ferrying DNA into cells, facilitating expression of alien genes. This method has several prospects in medicine, e.g., the development of recombinant poxviruses expressing the antigens of hepatitis B virus or poliovirus. Another promising development related to the potential of retroviral recombinants to move genes into hematopoietic cells. This method utilizes the patient's own tissue and eliminates allogenic rejection. Retroviral vectors have good potential as tools for somatic gene therapy. These vectors have a wide tissue and host range and are capable of transducing fairly long pieces (up to 7 kbp) of genetic material.

Much success has been achieved in the microinjection of genes into embryonic cells. All the foregoing techniques can be used for various types of tissue culture experiments. However, only microinjection and retroviruses are effective in inserting functional genes into whole, intact animals. An observed drawback of the procedures for the introduction of alien genetic material into mammalian cells is that the newly introduced DNA fails to integrate into the host genome by homologous recombination, as happens in yeast. Instead, this DNA tends to integrate randomly diverse, unpredictable regions of the host chromosomes. This has potentially undesirable consequences as the introduced DNA could inactivate some essential gene, or it might produce some position effect aberrations.

9.16. GENE TRANSFER INTO MAMMALIAN SOMATIC CELLS

Direct gene transfer into mammalian somatic tissues *in vivo* is a developing technology with potential application for human gene therapy. The current strategy for this approach is to first identify the mutant gene(s) causing a genetic defect, then to supplement the defective somatic tissues with the correct functional gene(s). Direct transfer of functionally active foreign genes into mammalian somatic tissues or organs *in vivo* is a good strategy for gene therapy. Genetically engineered retroviral vectors have been used successfully to infect live animals, affecting foreign gene expression in liver, blood vessels, and mammary tissues. Recombinant adenovirus and herpes simplex virus vectors have been utilized effectively for *in vivo* gene transfer into lung and brain tissues, respectively. Direct injection or particle bombardment of DNA has been demonstrated to provide a physical means for *in situ* gene transfer, while carrier-mediated DNA delivery techniques have been extended to target specific organs for gene expression. These technological developments in conjunction with the initiation of careful human gene therapy trials have marked a milestone in developing new medical treatments for various genetic diseases and cancer. Various *in vivo* gene transfer techniques should also provide new tools for basic research in molecular and developmental genetics.

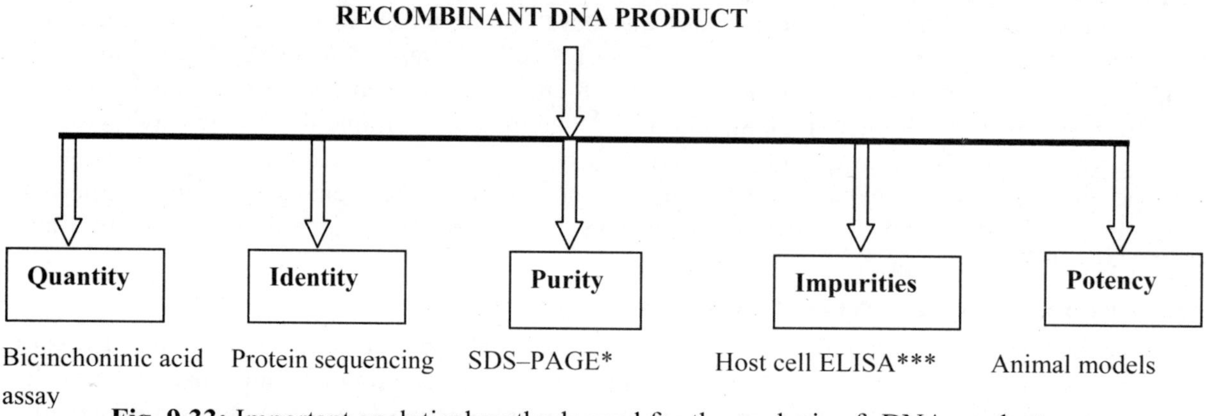

Fig. 9.33: Important analytical methods used for the analysis of rDNA products

9.17. ANALYSIS OF rDNA PRODUCTS

Analytical methods play a vital role in the determination of identity, purity and potency of rDNA products with respect to their evaluation as safe and efficacious medicine for human use. A summary of the analytical methods used in analysis of products is illustrated in Fig. 9.34 and described briefly in the following section. Bicinchoninic acid and Bradford method are generally used for the determination of protein concentration in rDNA product. These methods are important as they give the protein concentration of the product which is used in other assays.

Protein sequencing provides structural information. Amino acid analysis is used to identify rDNA products based on their amino acid composition. Peptide mapping is used to compare protein structure of the product with that of the reference standard and to confirm lot-to-lot consistency of primary structure. Electrophoretic assays (sodium dodecylsulphate polyacrylamide gel electrophoresis, Western blot and isoelectric focusing) are most powerful tools used to evaluate rDNA product purity, identity, homogeneity and stability. More recently, capillary electrophoresis has generated considerable interest as a complementary technique in the analysis of rDNA products. These assays can also be used for detecting molecular or chemical changes in the molecule due to denaturation, aggregation, oxidation, deamidation, etc. Chromatographic method, *viz*; reverse phase-HPLC, size exclusion chromatography and hydrophobic interaction chromatography are used in the determination of purity of the product as well as the level of known impurities or degradation of product. Immunoassay and DNA hybridization are used for determination of host cell impurities. Polymerase chain reaction, which involves DNA amplification, may prove useful in detection and identification of contaminant DNA. The limulus amebocyte lysate (LAL) test is considered to be the most sensitive and specific test used to detect and measure endotoxin. A comparative study demonstrated that LAL test is more sensitive than rabbit pyrogen test. The potency of rDNA product is generally assessed by specific techniques. The choice of assay is often determined by the nature of the product and its intended therapeutic application. Animal model assay, cell culture-based assay and *in vitro* (physico-chemical) assay are used for determination of potency of rDNA product. These assays require reference standard (calibrated in international unit) and statistical support to correctly interpret the resultant data. In addition to the afore-mentioned tests for protein analysis, carbohydrate analysis for glycoprotein equally plays a major role in characterizing rDNA products. In many products, changes in carbohydrate structures are known to affect biological activity.

A few points should be considered for analysis of rDNA products. Tests for identity usually require a combination of methods. These tests should be highly specific for unique properties of the products. A combination of methods should be used to assess purity of the product; the methods should be quantitative and capable of distinguishing the desired protein from product-related impurities. Process-related impurities should be minimized. Limits for product-related impurities should be set and quantitative methods employed to assure that these limits are met. Potency assays should have wide confidence limits and may include animal-based bioassay, *in vitro* cell culture assays or biochemical assay. The FDA currently regulates certain rDNA products as drugs. All rDNA drugs undergo rigorous quality control testing in order to comply with and conform to predetermined specifications. The fundamental difference between quality control system for rDNA drugs and traditional pharmaceuticals lies in types of method used to determine drug identity, purity and potency. The use of suitable reference standard from internationally recognized sources such as WHO, NIH, etc. is important for identification and purity of rDNA-derived drugs. Potency testing is of obvious importance that ensures the drug to be efficacious when administered to the patients.

Large amounts of insert (cloned) DNA can be retrieved when required. The primary objective of recombinant DNA technology is the identification and isolation of genes. The process would not be possible without type II restriction endonucleases that cleave DNA molecules reproducibly into fragments of discrete sizes. This enzyme binds to specific sequences with a DNA molecule and symmetrically cut phosphodiester bonds of each strand at the recognition site. In addition, many other enzymes, such as T4 DNA ligase and DNA polymerase, are important for cloning genes.

Recombinant DNA (rDNA) technology has made a revolutionary impact in the area of human healthcare by enabling mass production of safe, pure and effective rDNA expression products. rDNA technology has indeed made tremendous breakthrough in the discovery of various rDNA products. Besides the products approved by FDA for human use, several products are under clinical trials. Products developed in the field of haematology, endocrinology and oncology will be most valuable for further development of rDNA products in the coming years.

SUGGESTED READING

- Anderson S, Gart MJ, Magol L, Young IG. *Nucleic Acid Res* 8, 1731 (1980).
- Backman K, Ptashne M. *Cell* 13, 65 (1978).

- Biotechnology- Potential and Limitations, Ed. Silver S, Springer, Verlag, Berlin (1985).

- Brod P. Plasmids, Freeman and Co., San Francisco (1979).

- Collins J, Bruning HJ. *Gene*, 4, 85, (1978).

- Gupta PK. Essentials of Biotechnology, Rastogi Publications, Meerut, India (1997).

- Katoh M, Ayabe F, Norikane S, *et al. Biochemical and Biophysical Research Communications* 321, 280 (2004).

- Kurpiewski MR, Engler LE, Wozniak LA, Kobylanska A, *et al. Structure* 12, 1775 (2004).

- Lipps HJ, Jenke ACW, Nehlsen K, Scinteie MF, *et al. Gene* 304, 23 (2003).

- Pezzuto JM, Johnson ME, Manesse HR Jr. Biotechnology and Pharmacy, Chappman and Hall, New York (1993).

- Pouwel PH, Enger-Valk BE, Brammar WJ. Cloning vector, Elsevier, Amsterdam (1985).

- Prokop A, Bajpai RK, Ho C. Recombinant DNA Technology and Applications, Mc Graw Hill, New York (1991).

- Watson JD et al., Recombinant DNA, 2nd ed Scientific American Book Freeman (1992).

- Wilmut I, Schnwike AE, Mc Whir J, Kind AJ, Campbell KHS. *Nature* 385, 810 (1997).

GENE AND GENE THERAPY

10.9. GENETICALLY-SELECTED MEDICINE—PHARMACOGENETICS AND SINGLE-NUCLEOTIDE POLYMORPHISMS (SNPs)

10.10. GENES, HUMAN PHYSIOLOGY, AND GENE THERAPY

10.11. DISEASES AND GENE THERAPY

10.11.1. Insulin-dependent diabetes mellitus

10.11.2. Hemophilia B

10.11.3. Cystic fibrosis (CF)

10.11.4. Cardiovascular disease

10.11.5. Nervous system disorders

10.11.6. Cancer

10.11.7. AIDS

10.12. NUCLEIC ACID DELIVERY TO MITOCHONDRIA

10.12.1. Mitochondrial genetics and gene therapy

10.12.2. Strategies for targeted DNA delivery to mitochondria

10.12.3. Mitochondrial properties, which help in the designing of carrier systems

10.12.4. Various delivery methodologies for targeted DNA delivery to mitochondria

10.12.4.1. Physical techniques

10.12.4.2. Chemical techniques

10.12.4.2.1. Conjugation with mitochondriotropics

10.12.4.2.2. Conjugation with mitochondrial leader sequence

10.12.4.2.3. DQAsomes: A mitochondriotropic vesicular system

10.1. INTRODUCTION

The ability to transfect genes into cells and effect their expression has enabled the practical emergence of human gene therapy wherein functionally active genes are putatively inserted into the (somatic) cells of a person requiring the expression of a given protein. A novel adaptation of gene therapy is the transfection of cells with non-resident genes in order to accomplish *in situ* expression of a pharmacologically beneficial protein or create a site for further therapeutic intervention. In other words, genes may act like "drugs", generating a product with a specific pharmacological effect. In simple terms, gene therapy involves insertion of genetic material into a patient's cells to make them capable of producing some therapeutic protein.

Today's gene therapy has gone beyond the original definition of gene therapy. It has created an opportunity to *fight the cause* of a disease *rather than its symptoms*. Over 45,000 human diseases related directly to genetic disorders have been identified. Until recently, treatment of genetic disorders have employed substitution therapy e.g., enzyme storage disease(s), cystic fibrosis (CF) or more rationally to replace a missing protein. In contrast, gene therapy paves the way to either replace the missing or defective gene at the origin or arrest undesired gene expression (viral and oncogene expression) at the origin.

Gene medicines are generally based on a gene expression system that contains a therapeutic gene and a delivery system. A gene delivery system controls the distribution and access of a gene expression unit to the target tissue, its recognition by cell-surface receptors and its intracellular trafficking (Tomlinson and Rolland, 1996).

With the advent of gene manipulation by biotechnological techniques it has become feasible to splice and insert a human gene into a viral or bacterial genome; the latter is referred to as vector. The technique is essentially based on recombinant DNA technology which allows isolation of genes and their subsequent utilization in the production of respective proteins; essentially it so engineers them that they act as a corrective gene system. Therapeutic protein expressions function and produce their effect in the blood stream. This is a constraint in effective delivery (cell specific gene or genome delivery and expressed protein targeting).

10.1.1. Current gene concept

No two people are the same because of difference in genotypes dependence. Genetics is the study of biologically inherited traits, including those that are influenced in part by the environment with genetic linkage. Genes are transmitted from parents to offspring at reproduction. A gene is defined as a sequence of bases that codes for an ordered amino acid assemblage in a functional product.

Bacterial genetics forms the basis of molecular genetics. In early 1900s, there was a misunderstanding of genotypic changes which arise in a single cell: they were mistaken for phenotypic adaptation (reversible changes) that occurred in all the cells of a population. It was in the 1940s and 1950s that the process of gene transfer were critically studied and in bacteria paved the way for many new developments in molecular genetics.

It is now clear that heritable changes in genes are caused by mutation. A mutation is defined as any change in the base sequence of the DNA. Some mutations are silent, i.e., without observable change in demonstrable phenotypic character (s); other mutations are wild type. The changes in various kinds of mutations can be precisely identified in terms of base sequences in DNA and amino acid sequences in the protein. The DNA changes include **nucleotide replacements, deletions, insertions** and **rearrangements**. Replacement may involve **transition**, where a purine is replaced by a purine and a pyrimidine by a pyrimidine, or transversion, where a purine is replaced by a pyrimidine or vice-versa.

Mutations affect the coding properties of the DNA. Among the replacements, **missense mutations** cause the substitution of one amino acid with another; the protein may remain functional provided there is no marked effect of substitution on its tertiary structure. In case of **nonsense** (terminator) mutations, any premature termination in the growth of the peptide chain destroys its function. Larger deletions destroy the function except when they remove small unessential parts of proteins. Deletions at the boundary between two genes, if in frame, cause the two polypeptide chains to be synthesized as a single chain (**gene fusion**), with partial retention of one or both functions. A shift of the reading frame causes the production of a jumbled distal sequence resulting in loss of function which can be corrected by another shift in the opposite direction provided the jumbled region is small and not in a critical position. Insertions are usually caused by transposons or prophages. They frequently block the function of the protein and affect the expression of distal genes. Introducing purpose-specific mutations into specific genes is called gene targeting. The specificity of gene targeting comes from the DNA sequence homology needed for homologous recombination.

While a genome means the full collection of genes encoded by a particular organism, the term gene was first defined in the early 1900s to explain the hereditary basis of traits (Morgan, 2001). At that time phenotypic traits were ascribed to hereditary factors even when the physical basis of those factors was not known. In the early 20th century, T.H. Morgan and others established and associated the heritable traits with specific chromosomal regions. In the 1930s, G.W. Beadle introduced the concept of "one gene, one enzyme", which later became "one gene, one polypeptide concept".

The advent of recombinant DNA and gene cloning made it possible to assign a gene to a specific segment of DNA leading to formation of gene product. At first it was thought that the final product of a gene was a protein but the discovery that RNA shows structural, catalytic and even regulatory properties suggested that the end product could be a nucleic acid (Eddy, 2002). Today, we define a gene in molecular terms as "a complete chromosomal segment responsible for making a functional product". This definition involves the following parts: the expression of a gene product; the requirement that it should be functional and should contain both coding and regulatory regions.

10.1.2. Open reading frames (ORFs)

An ORF is a string of triplet nucleotide codons bounded by start and stop signals. Protein-coding genes are found by identifying large ORFs in the genome, particularly in prokaryotes and other organisms having few introns (the regions spliced out of RNA) in their genes. However, some genes are short and difficult to identify in this way. Moreover, organisms with genes that undergo significant RNA splicing often contain small exons sandwiched between large introns, making ORFs difficult to identify.

10.1.3. Sequence features

After an ORF has been identified, codon bias may be used to determine whether the ORF is a gene. Genes, particularly highly expressed ones, show biased non-random use of codons. But for many genes, the bias is weak, and small ORFs (or exons) contain too few codons to show statistically significant bias. Besides overall bias, one may also look for specific patterns in the DNA sequence such as splice sites to locate genes.

10.1.4 Sequence conservation

In contrast to focusing on an individual DNA sequence, one can identify genes by comparing multiple sequences among organisms (Eddy, 2002). DNA sequence conservation among species is a good estimate of importance of the gene product. However, conserved sequences could sometimes be nontranscribed regulatory elements. Also, this method requires sequences of related organisms that are separated by appropriate evolutionary distances.

10.1.5. Transcription

A good non-sequence based approach for identifying genes is to search for RNA or protein expression commonly accomplished by using micro-array hybridization, serial analysis of gene expression (SAGE), cDNA mapping, or sequencing of expressed sequence tags (Brown and Botstein, 1999). Large scale tagging of genes with transposons has revealed several new regions in the yeast genome that can produce proteins. But the function, if any, of many of the transcribed regions is not known. Conversely, there could be some conserved ORFs that are not transcribed; their RNA or protein products have not been identified.

10.1.6. Gene activation

The function of a gene can sometime be identified by mutating or inactivating its product, accomplished by direct gene disruption or RNA interference. But there are many coding sequences which make products whose inactivation does not result in an obvious phenotype. Indeed, many genes are difficult to identify solely by inactivation. Beyond these five criteria some additional issues in gene identification include overlap, alternative splicing, and pseudogenes. Examples are known of overlapping reading frames of protein coding genes, overlapping transcriptional units (for example, where the exon of one gene is encoded within the intron of another), and even overlapping protein coding and RNA coding genes. In all cases of gene overlap, each gene has a unique functional sequence and so is distinct.

With regard to products from alternatively spliced genes, in the human genome over a half of the genes have spliced isoforms. Gene products from alternatively spliced messenger RNAs contain functionally unique and distinct sequences, and there exist no good systems for describing such variants. Furthermore, the definition of a gene is linked with the definition of a pseudogene. Pseudogenes are similar in sequence to normal genes but usually have obvious changes such as frame shifts or stop codons in the middle of coding domains-changes that prevent them from making a functional product or having a detectable effect on the organism's phenotype. Pseudogenes occur in many animals, fungi, plants, and bacteria.

The boundary between living genes and pseudogenes (dead genes) is often not sharp. A pseudogene in one individual can be a functional gene in a different isolate of the same species. Moreover, pseudogenes can be transcribed. Conversely, some pseudogenes have entire coding regions without obvious disablements but do not appear to be expressed (e.g. human ribosomal pseudogenes) presumably because they lack the regulatory elements required for transcription. Among the various organisms that have been sequenced so far, the best characterized genome in terms of functional genomics is that of the budding yeast, *Saccharomyces cerevisiae.* Its genes undergo only a small amount of splicing; that is why for this organism we have the clearest understanding of which DNA sequences are genes. When the yeast genome was first sequenced, all ORFs longer than 100 codons could be named, resulting in 6274 possible genes (Mewes *et al.,* 1997). This number has been greatly revised since then. More small genes have been identified either through new homologies found in databases or through evidence of transcription. In addition, 283 genes have been found to be "questionable ORFs" because they seem to lack transcription, function, or sequence conservation. Finally, a few pseudogenes have been found in the laboratory strain of *S. cerevisiae,* some of which may be functional in other yeast strains (Mewes *et al.*, 1997).

The yeast genome happens to be much simpler than human genome and many of the problems encountered in yeast may be greatly magnified in human. First, the human genome is expected to contain a large number of potential ORFs in view of the small size of exons and the complexity of mRNA splicing—it seems doubtful that we will find true genes among these ORFs only by analyzing their raw nucleotide sequences. In fact, initial estimates of the number of genes in the human genome ranged from 20,000 to >100, 000 (Venter *et al.*, 2001).

According to Snyder and Gerstein (2003) one solution for annotating genes in sequenced genomes could be to revert to the original definition of a gene—a sequence encoding a functional product—and use functional genomics to identify them. Ultimately, identification of genes based solely on the human genome sequence may not be practical in the near future. Only through large scale systematic functional genomics experiments together with careful sequence comparisons against related the organism will we succeed in achieving a clear annotation of the human genome.

10.1.7. "RNA" and the hidden genes

Emerging evidence contradicts conventional theories that genes make up the sole basis of heredity and the complete blueprint for all life. Some parts of the genome previously thought to be junk or redundant actually exert control over the development and the distinctive traits of all organisms. It is not the ''protein-coding genes'' alone that are important. Protein-encoding genes make up only a very small fraction of the total DNA of a cell and yet only this small fraction has attracted most of the research on DNA.

The dogma postulates that genes express themselves as proteins, which are made in four steps: first an enzyme docks to the chromosome and slides along the gene, transcribing the sequence on one strand of DNA into a single strand of RNA. Next, any introns (noncoding parts of the initial RNA transcript) are cut out, and the rest of the RNA is spliced together to generate a segment of messenger RNA. The RNA message then moves out of the nucleus to the main part (cytoplasm) of the cell, where the ribosomes translate it into chains of amino acids. Finally, each chain twists and folds into an intricate three-dimensional shape. The remarkable versatility of proteins emanates from their specific shapes. Some proteins make muscles and tissues, other functions as enzymes to catalyze, metabolize or signal; and still others regulate genes by docking to specific sections of DNA or RNA. All these properties have prompted many biologists to assume that, with very few exceptions, a DNA sequence qualifies as a gene only if it can produce a protein.

The human genome probably contains about 30, 000 genes that code for proteins; and there is no definite correspondence between the complexity of a species and the number of genes in its genome. For instance rice plants have more coding genes than humans. On the other hand interestingly, the amount of noncoding DNA does seem to scale with complexity. In higher organisms genes are broken into chunks of protein-encoding sequences separated by often-extensive tracts of non-coding sequences. The protein-coding parts account for less than 2 % of the DNA in human chromosomes. Some three billion pairs of bases that we all carry in nearly every cell must be there for some other reason – it is emerging that there is a large groups of 'genes' that do function even though they produce only RNA but no protein. In fact to call these RNA-only genes as genes is not correct – they are better termed as transcriptional units. It is also conceivable that the intervening noncoding sequences (introns as well as intergenic 'junk' DNA) probably transmit parallel information in the formation of RNA molecules (Gibbs, 2003). RNA is capable of multifarious actions. Like proteins, some RNA transcripts interact with other pieces of RNA, with DNA, with proteins and even with small chemical compounds. Proteins are more like analog molecules and bind to targets in the same way as keys fit in locks. RNA has a specific sequence, which makes it more digital, like a zip code. A segment of RNA can float around until it collides with a DNA (or RNA) having a complementary sequence; the two halves of the ladder then join rungs.

10.1.8. Pseudogenes and "RNA"

Human DNA seems to contain almost equal numbers of genes and pseudogenes – defective copies of functional genes. Pseudogenes have till recently been dismissed as molecular fossils, i.e., the remains of genes that were damaged by mutation and abandoned by evolution. But in 2003, Shinji Hirotsune and associates, Saitama Medical School, Japan discovered the first functional pseudogenes. In mice RNA made from pseudogenes regulates the expression of the true gene whose sequence it mimics, even though the two lie on different chromosomes (Gibbs, 2003). It is conceivable that many pseudogenes give rise to active RNA. Every normal protein coding gene, for instance, has a complementary or standby DNA sequence located on the other side of the ladder and which is usually not transcribed into RNA but which the cell can exploit to repair the damaged gene. In some cases, this standby has its own agenda. While the gene is producing a sensible RNA message, its backup copy can make an "antisense" RNA with a complementary sequence (Fig 10.1). Whenever matched sense and antisense RNAs meet, they interact to generate their own double-stranded ladder thereby effectively interfering with the ability of this gene to express its protein. Besides bacteria and plants even mammals are known to produce antisense. Yelin *et al.* (2003) screened human genome databases and concluded that over 1600 human genes yields antisense RNAs.

These competing RNAs probably suppress a gene by tying up or binding the gene's messenger RNA. It is also possible that they employ a built in genome censor, known as the RNA interference machinery which selectively silences individual genes. When double stranded RNA appears in a cell, enzymes dice it up, peel the two strands apart, and use one RNA fragment to seek out and destroy any other RNA messages that are attached to its sequence. This protects cells against viruses which often deliver their payloads in the form of double stranded RNA. The censor also provides an easy method for scientists to shut off any gene at will.

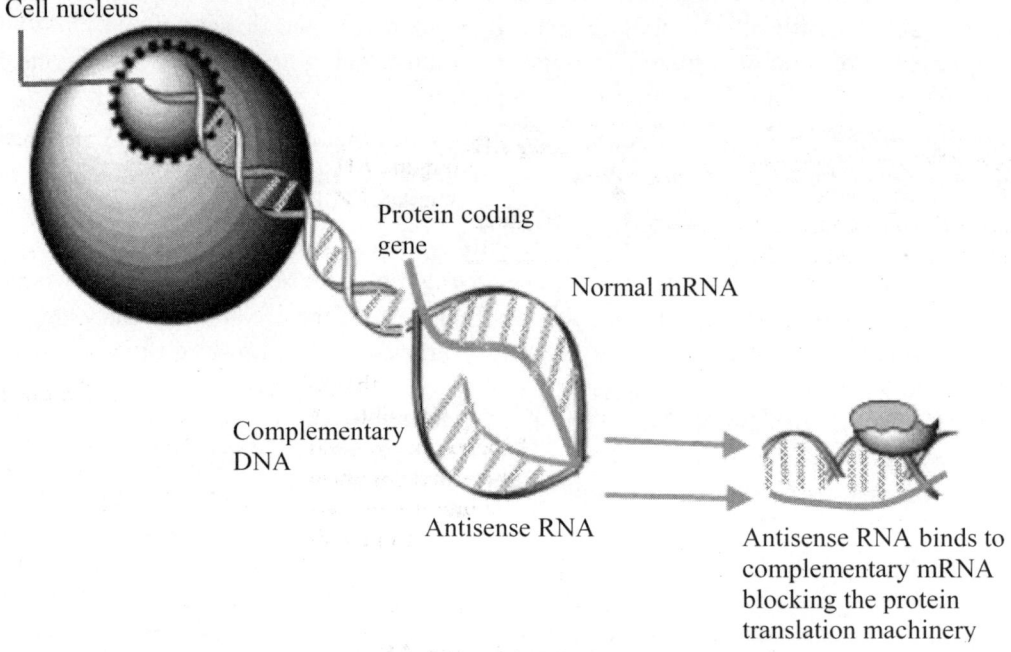

Fig. 10.1: Anticodon RNA is made from the complementary DNA strand. Antisense RNAs can intercept the messenger RNA transcribed from the gene, preventing the RNA from being translated into protein

Another novel type of active RNA is called microRNA. These are short noncoding RNAs that fold back on themselves, like hairpins (Fig. 10.2). In *Arabidopsis*, the microRNA doubles over and is then caught by the RNA interference machinery, just as if it had come out of a virus, but its sequence matches that of some different protein-making genes, members of a family that control the shape and size of the plant. The censor dutifully represses each of them by chopping up much of the messenger RNA they produce. Thus a tiny RNA-only gene serves as the main lever by which *Arabidopsis* cells adjust the volume of a bag of important protein genes. Hundreds of microRNAs have been found and seem to enable organisms to wrangle genes. Humans have over 150 microRNAs. Some of them appear to play an important role in brain development.

Another newly discovered form of RNA that acts as precision genetic switch is called riboswitch. Riboswitches are produced from noncoding DNA between known genes. A riboswitch folds into a complex shape. While one part of the folded RNA can bind to a specific target protein or chemical; yet another part carries folded RNA that can bind to a specific target protein or chemical, another part carries the RNA that codes for a protein product.

The riboswitch turns "on" and produces the protein it encodes only when its target is present (Eddy, 2001; Gibbs, 2003). Riboswitches are long RNAs having both coding and noncoding functions. When the RNA folds up, the noncoding end turns into a sensitive receptor for a particular chemical target. An encounter with the target fills up the switch, causing the other end-the protein coding end–to change shape. The riboswtich thus gives rise to a protein; much like a normal gene does– to change the shape. The riboswitch thus gives rise to a protein, much like a normal gene does – but it does so only when it senses its target.

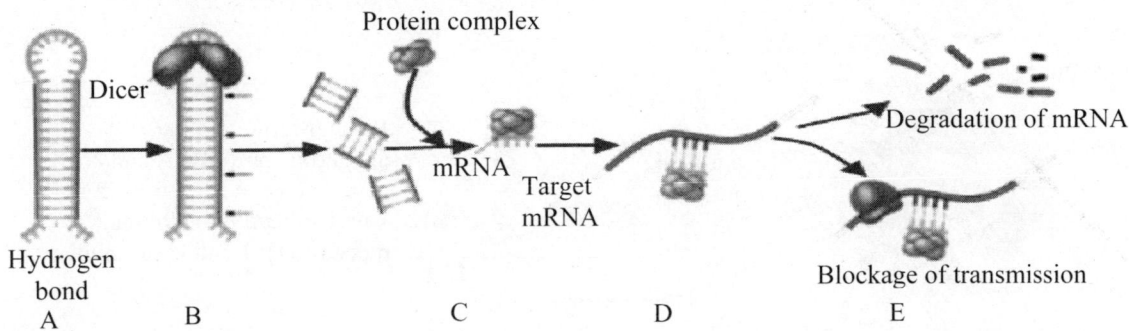

Fig 10.2: The micro RNA (miRNA) precursor folds back on itself, held together by hydrogen bonds, B. An enzyme called Dicer moves along the double stranded RNA, cutting it into shorter segments, C. One strand of each double stranded RNA is degraded; the other strand (miRNA) associates with a complex of proteins, D. The bound miRNA can base pair with any target mRNA that contains the complementary sequences, E. The miRNA protein complex prevents gene expression either by degrading the mRNA or by blocking its translation

10.1.9: Reverse genetics

Genetics has traditionally relied on mutation to provide the raw material needed for analysis. The usual procedure has been to use a mutant gene and phenotype to identify the wild type allele of the gene and its normal function. However, this approach has certain limitatioi.s. For example, it may prove difficult or impossible to isolate mutations in genes that duplicate the functions of other genes or that are essential for the viability of the organism.

Reverse genetics (Fig. 10.3) is a procedure that reverses the usual flow of study. Using recombinant DNA technology, wild type genes are cloned, intentionally mutated in specific ways, and introduced back into the organism to study the phenotypic effects of the mutations. Because the position and molecular nature of each mutation is precisely defined, a very fine level of resolution is possible in defining promoter and enhancer sequences required for transcription, RNA splicing and sequences of particular amino acids essential for protein function.

10.1.10. Vectors

Bacterial vectors are derived from plasmids or from phage genome. Both have been severely reduced in size so that they can accommodate large foreign segments while retaining the genes required for autonomous replication. The cyclic replicons of non-conjugative plasmids are excellent vectors because they can accommodate variable amounts of foreign DNA, are easy to purify, have selectable genes, and can be made to reproduce large numbers in a cell.

The host range has been extended to **eukaryotic vectors**, using plasmids or DNA from viruses. Vectors capable of replicating in both bacteria and eukaryotic cells (shuttle vectors) are created by fusing two replicons, one bacterial, and the other eukaryotic. Shuttle vectors are useful for many applications, especially those studied in animal cells but amplified in bacteria or yeast. While many vectors are designed merely to clone and amplify the foreign DNA, some are made to obtain large amounts of the protein specified by the inserted gene. These vectors are named **expression vectors**. In these, the inserted gene is under the control of a promoter and a ribosome-binding site suitable for expression in the host cells. The introduction of DNA cloning has revolutionized biology. A possible application in humans is gene therapy—introducing a cloned gene into somatic cells or into germline cells to replace or compensate for a defective gene.

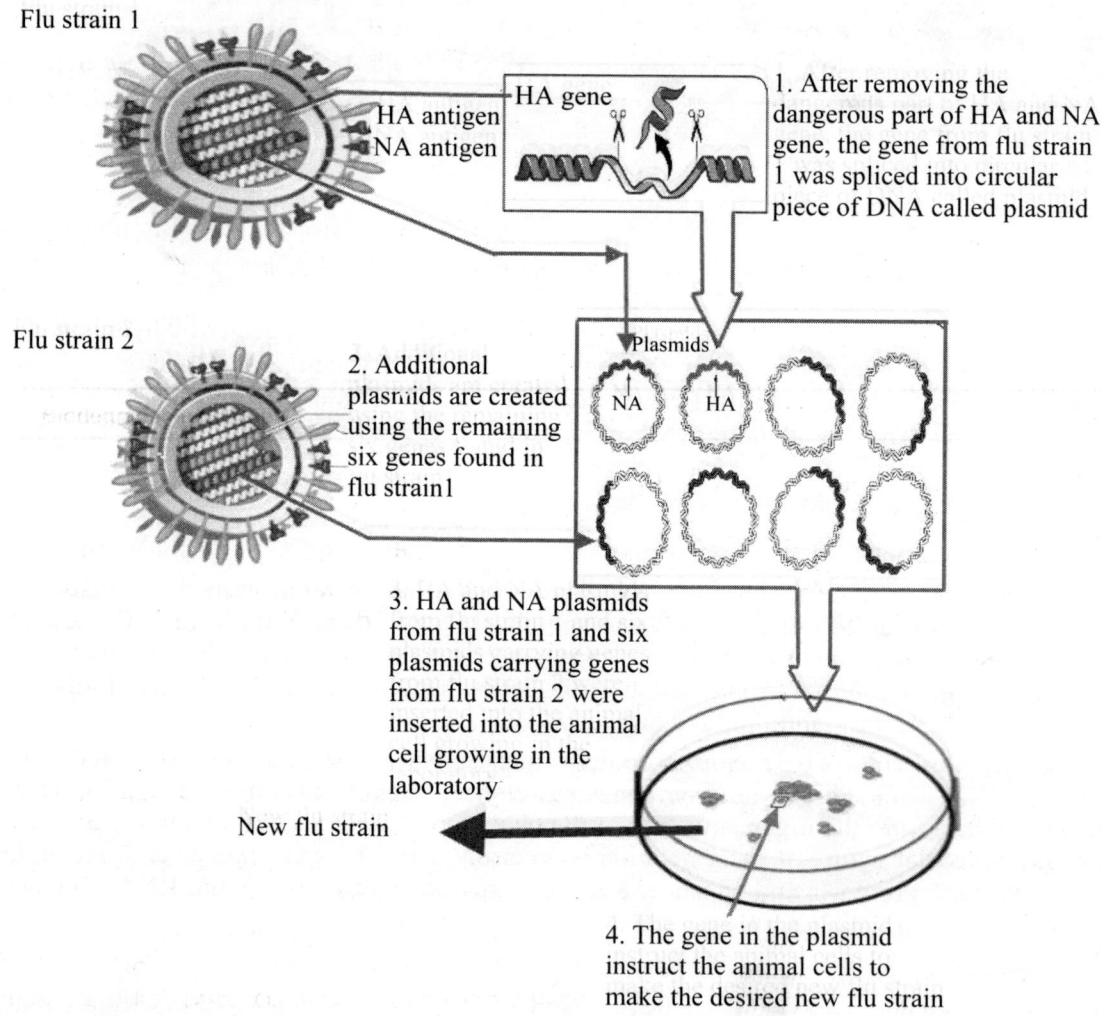

Fig. 10.3: An example of reverse genetics

10.2. APPROACHES TO GENE THERAPY

Various approaches have been tried for effective transfer of genes to appropriate target sites. These approaches broadly fall into four categories.

1. Gene modification

      a. Replacement therapy

      b. Corrective gene therapy

2. Gene transfer

      a. Physical (Microinjection, Gene gun, 'naked DNA', EPD, Electroporation, etc.)

      b. Chemical (Liposomes, cationic liposomes, oligonucleotides, etc.)

      c. Biological (Viral vectors, mammalian artificial chromosomes, etc.)

3. Gene transfer in specific cell lines

      a. Somatic gene therapy

      b. Germline gene therapy

4. Eugenic approach (gene insertion)

5. Anti sense technology

10.2.1. Gene modification

Before discussing different approaches to gene therapy, we should be clear what our ultimate goal is, replacement therapy or corrective gene therapy. In replacement therapy, a defective gene is inserted somewhere in the genome so that its product replaces that of a defective gene. This approach may be suitable especially for recessive disorders, which are marked by deficiency of an enzyme or other proteins. The gene functions in the genome by providing an appropriate regulatory sequence, however this approach may not be successful in treating dominant disorders associated with the production of an abnormal gene product which interferes with the product of a normal gene. On the other hand, corrective gene therapy requires replacement of a mutant gene or a part of it with a normal sequence. This can be achieved by using recombinant technology. Another form of corrective therapy involves the suppression of a particular mutation by a transfer RNA that is introduced into a cell.

10.2.2. Gene transfer

Gene transfer can be used for improvement of a specific disease for example, introducing a growth hormone gene to increase height. This gene transfer into cells can be brought about by physical, chemical and biological methods.

10.2.3. Gene transfer to specific cell lines

Somatic gene therapy, which has emerged as a new approach for the treatment of a variety of genetic and acquired diseases, involves the insertion of genes into specific somatic cells. If all goes well, they function during the lifetime of an individual and hence correct a genetic disease. Though it sounds well, it presents some practical problems. On the other hand, injection or insertion of genes into germ cells, i.e., into fertilized eggs is known as germ line therapy. It differs from somatic cell therapy in that the inserted genes would be passed on to future generations.

10.2.4. Eugenic approach (gene insertion)

Eugenic approach involves inserting genes to alter or improve complex traits of a person e.g. intelligence. However, it is far beyond the current technological feasibility. Two basic methods for delivery of genes are shown in Figure 10.4.

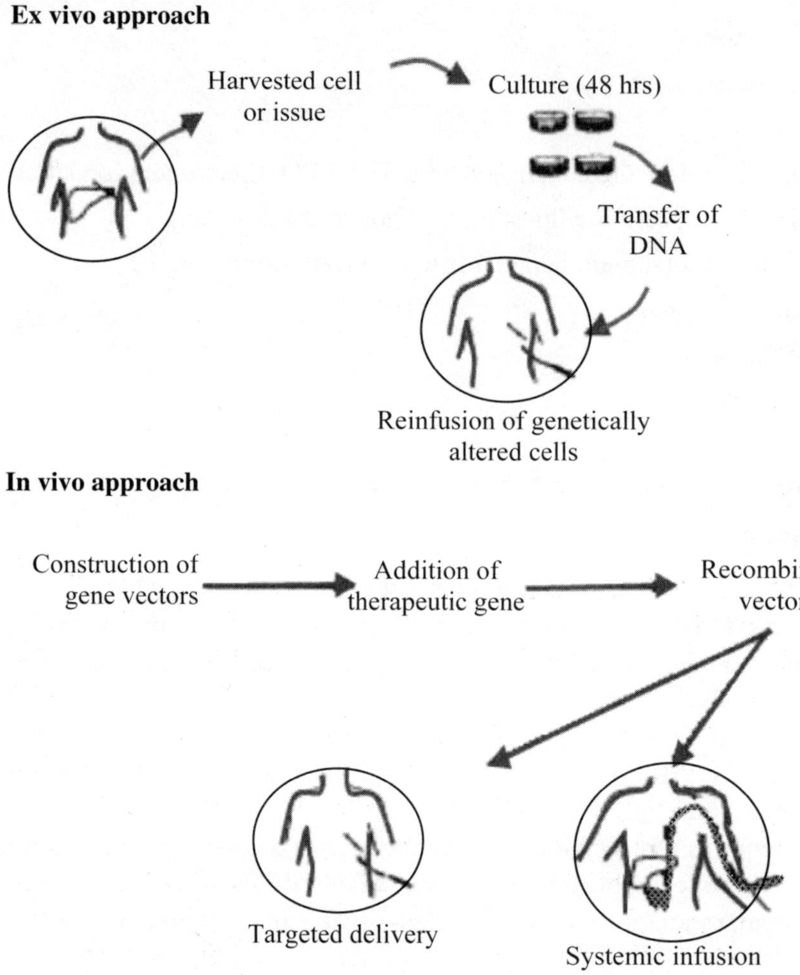

Ex vivo approach

In vivo approach

Fig. 10.4: Two basic methods for delivery of genes. The upper panel shows the ex vivo approach. It requires removal of cells or tissue, culturing of cells, and transfection. Successfully transformed cells are selected and returned to the patient where they home to the original location of removed cells or tissue. The lower panel shows the in vivo approach. A gene vector construct, suitable for the delivery of genes to the targeted cell or tissue, is generated. The therapeutic gene is incorporated into the construct and the recombinant vector is delivered to the patient by any of a number of methods. The method of choice should provide the best level of transfection with minimal side effect

10.2.5. Antisense technology

Antisense oligonucleotides (AS-ODNs) based strategies represent one of the most successful approaches to achieving suppression or elimination of a genetic message. In the past few years novel approaches to therapeutics, which involve intervention in these processes using synthetic oligonucleotides (ODNs), have been developed. These have the capability of emerging as effective pharmaceutical agents. In effect, this approach represents a novel strategy that is in some ways intermediate between the classical drug paradigm of small molecule (lock and key) inhibitors, and gene therapy that involves the introduction of whole genes into affected individuals. The antisense effect of synthetic oligonucleotide (ODN) sequence for therapeutic purpose was first proposed by Zamecnik and Stephenson in 1978. AS-ODNs are short chains of nucleic acids, usually consist of 10 to 30 nucleotides which are complementary to their target mRNA and are intermediate in size compared with smaller-size conventional drugs, such as beta-blockers, and the much larger therapeutic polypeptides, such as growth factors or monoclonal antibodies.

Hybridization of AS-ODN to the target mRNA *via* Watson-Crick base pairing can result in specific inhibition of gene expression by various mechanisms, depending on the chemical make-up of the AS-ODN and location of hybridization, resulting in reduced levels of translation of the target transcript [Zamecnik and Stephenson, 1978]. AS-ODNs therapy have many advantages such as broad applicability, direct utilization of sequence informations, selective knockout single critical target, rapid development at low costs, reduced likelihood of side effect, high probability of success and extremely high specificity (Bennet and Cowsert, 1999). In addition to antisense technology, RNA-cleaving ribozymes and small interfering RNA (siRNA) have also been established as highly effective method of suppressing gene expression in mammalian cells (Elbashir *et al.*, 2001; Paroo and Corey, 2004).

10.2.5.1. Design and development of AS-ODNs as therapeutics

AS-ODNs can be designed on the basis of nucleotide sequence of the targeted genes and on the concept of base pairing of nucleic acids, which is governed by one set of physico-chemical principles. So the selection of optimal targets is a critical step in the design of an antisense therapeutic. There are some prerequisites for AS-ODNs design (Arrigo, 2002):

1. Knowledge about the gene function;

2. Identification of highly specific targets on the sequence

3. Evaluation of the functional relevance of the selected targets;

4. Evaluation of the metabolic fate and toxicity and side effects of the AS-ODNs.

Design is critical for the clinical efficacy of ODNs and should include consideration of length, chemistry, conformation, and ability to hybridize with the target mRNA [Patil *et al.*, 2005]. The specificity and stability of an ODN also depend on its length. The suggested optimal length for ODNs with efficient antisense activity ranges from 12 to 28 bases (Engel and Uhlman, 2000). Various chemical modifications to the backbone have been used to improve ODN stability. AS-ODNs are designed primarily for their ability to hybridize with the mRNA of interest (Akhtar, 1998).

10.2.5.1.1. Chemical modification of AS-ODNs

In addition to the requirements outlined above, ASODNs must display good pharmacokinetic and pharmacodynamic properties. To address these requirements of a successful drug candidate, various structural modifications of ribo/deoxyribonucleotides are studied. Following Kurreck *et al.*, (2003) there are three possible sites on a nucleotide where protective modification could be introduced as shown in Figure 10.5. These can be broadly distinguished as:

1. Analogues with unnatural bases

2. Modified sugars (especially at the 2' position of the ribose),

3. Altered sugar-phosphate backbone

Modified AS-ODNs analogues are often employed for *in vivo* antisense applications due to their increased stability and nuclease resistance.

To make the jump from fascinating laboratory technique to clinical therapeutic agent requires overcoming several potential hurdles. It has been emerged that to act as a successful antisense drug, AS-ODNs should fulfill the following criteria:

1. Specific target recognition by Watson-Crick base pairing,
2. Good structural mimicry to the natural DNA-RNA,
3. Activation of RNase-H to promote the target mRNA cleavage,
4. Enhanced cellular uptake, and
5. Enhanced resistance to various nucleases.

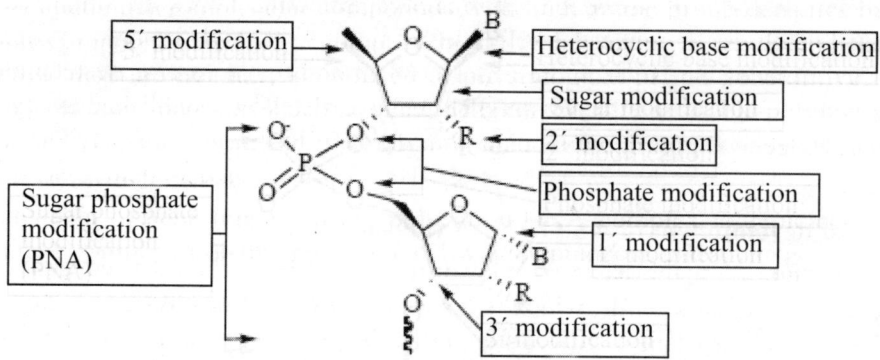

Fig. 10.5: Structurally possible DNA modification site

10.2.5.2. Ribozymes

Ribozymes are RNA molecules with catalytic activity. Naturally occurring ribozymes, with the sole exception of the ribosome, catalyze the cleavage or ligation of the RNA phosphodiester back-bone (Kruger *et al.*, 1982). In contrast to other known ribonucleases, ribozymes catalyze highly sequence-specific reactions determined by RNA-RNA interactions between the ribozyme and its substrate molecules. These behave like true enzymes: they are not modified during the reaction and one ribozyme molecule can process several substrate molecules. Substrate recognition and binding is essentially governed by Watson-Crick interactions. The capacity of ribozymes to specifically inactivate other RNAs has made ribozymes very promising molecular tools and potential gene suppressors with important applications.

10.2.5.3. RNA Interference

Only recently, research in the antisense field increased in impact by the discovery of RNA interference (RNAi). In 1998, Andrew Fire (Fire *et al.*, 1998) and coworkers described a new technology that was based on the silencing of specific genes by double stranded RNA (dsRNA); a technology they called RNA interference (RNAi). They showed that, in *C. elegans*, the presence of just a few molecules of dsRNA was sufficient to almost completely abolish the expression of a gene that was homologous to the dsRNA. The action of interfering dsRNA in mammals usually involves two enzymatic steps (Lee and Sinka, 2006) as shown in Figure 10.6.

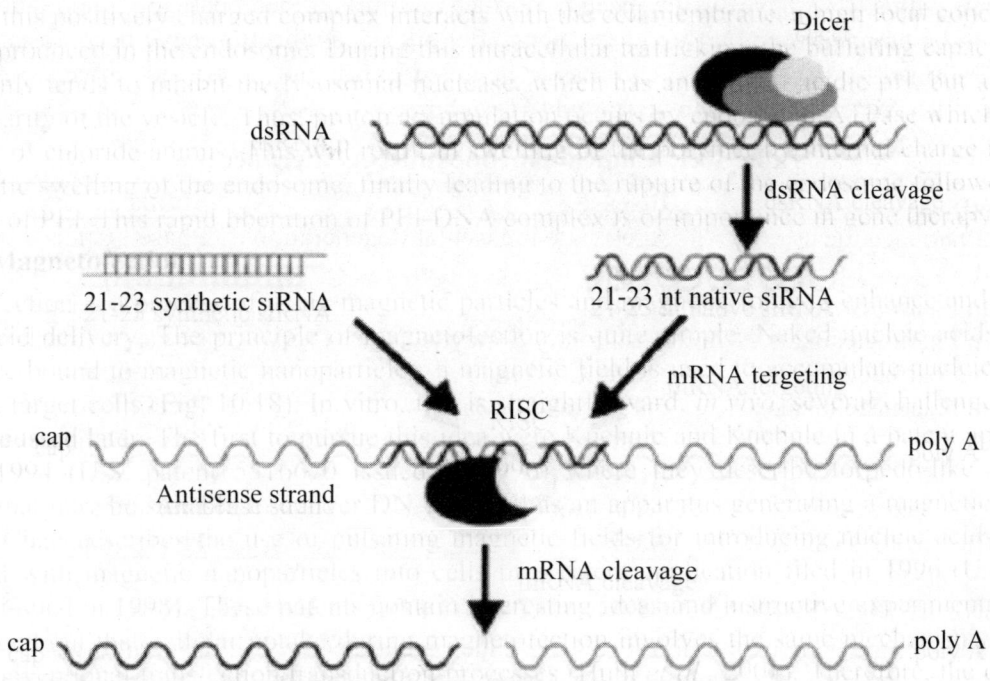

Fig. 10.6: The classical RNA interference (RNAi) pathway in mammalian cells

First, Dicer, an RNase III-type enzyme, cleaves dsRNA to 21-23-mer siRNA segments. Then, RNA-induced silencing complex (RISC) unwinds the RNA duplex, pairs one strand with a complementary region in a cognate mRNA, and initiates cleavage at a site 10 nucleotides upstream of the 5'end of the siRNA strand (Dorsett and Tuschel, 2004). This process takes place in the cytoplasm. Another common, although not universal, protein of the RNAi machinery is RNA-dependent RNA polymerase (RdRP), which synthesizes dsRNA from ssRNA templates to initiate or amplify the RNAi reaction (Martienssen, 2004). RNA interference is related to another gene-silencing mechanism that involves a group of small RNA molecules, known as microRNAs (miRNAs), which are expressed endogenously. Although genes in the host genome encode them, miRNAs are not involved in the pathway that leads to the production of a protein; instead, they regulate mRNA expression. siRNAs are tolerant of a considerable degree of chemical modification, although some alterations cause a loss of activity. In general, sense strands and 3' regions are more amenable to modification, whereas the 5' region on the antisense strand and the central region are more sensitive (Chiu and Rana, 2003). Short interference RNAs theoretically represent ideal drugs for the specific knockdown of unwanted or disease causing gene products. Intense research efforts are being aimed at developing siRNAs for therapeutic purposes (Behlke, 2006; Verma and Dey, 2004). Currently, there are a dozen or so biotechnology companies developing clinical applications of siRNA in various human diseases (Howard, 2003; Reich *et al.*, 2003) (Table 10.1).

However, it can be useful as a complement to genetic studies and as a method for investigating the function of genes identified by biochemical approaches (Maine, 2001). The use of siRNA as a therapeutic target is still in its infancy. Currently, various research groups around the world have demonstrated the clinical potential of appropriately designed siRNAs in various diseases, including cancer, viral infections and neurodegenerative disorders. Taken together, first promising *in vivo* experiments with siRNA have already been performed and further therapeutically important genes are expected to be targeted soon. No toxic reactions after siRNA application have been observed in the studies performed to date, but great care has to be taken to rule out severe side-effects of long-term induction of RNAi before trials can be started to treat human diseases.

Table 10.1: Clinical pipeline in RNAi therapeutics

Company	Disease	Status
Acuity Pharmaceuticals (Cand5)	Age-related muscular degeneration (AMD)	Phase I Clinical
Alnylam Pharmaceuticals	AMD	Phase I Clinical
Alnylam Pharmaceuticals	Respiratory Syncytial Virus (RSV)	Phase I Clinical in 2006
Alnylam Pharmaceuticals	Spinal Cord Injury	Preclinical
Alnylam Pharmaceuticals	Parkinson's disease	Preclinical
Benitec	Human immunodeficiency virus (HIV)	Phase I Clinical in 2005
Intradigm Corporation	Solid Tumour	Preclinical
Sirna Therapeutics (Sirna-027)	AMD	Phase I Clinical

10.3. GENE EXPRESSION AND GENE MAPPING FOR CLINICAL TRAITS

It appears that some gene expression levels are under genetic control in different organisms and that certain hotspot regions in the genome control the expression of many other genes. Conceivably, gene expression data might be gainfully used to localize genes that affect clinical traits (Kraft and Horvath, 2003). While traditional techniques for reverse genetics have been successful in mapping rare Mendelian diseases (caused by rare, highly penetrant alleles at a single locus), they have not been so successful in mapping complex diseases that result from the interaction of several loci and environmental factors. This seems to be partly due to the reason that genes influence diseases via their corresponding mRNA and proteins.

Gene expression data may be potentially used in conjunction with meiotic mapping techniques. Schadt *et al.* (2003) adopted two strategies involving the use of genome wide gene expression data to help map a clinical trait. One strategy; termed 'genetical genomics' by Jansen and Nap (2001) – uses the genetics of gene expression to reconstruct metabolic or regulatory pathways. The second strategy involves gene expression profiling and overcomes the problem of genetic locus heterogeneity (Kraft and Horvath, 2003). Schadt *et al.* (2003) used a mouse gene oligonucleotides microarray to monitor the gene expression levels of many genes from F2 mice. Antisense inhibition of gene expression relies on the rules of Watosn-Crick base pairing. A synthetic single strand (13-25 mer) oligonucleotide complementary to a specific gene is introduced into cells, binds with mRNA, and inhibits translation. Its hybridization with the target mRNA physically blocks the translation machinery or activates RNase H cleavage at the RNA-DNA duplex site (Crooke, 1998). Targeting of gene expression at the RNA level turns off protein production even if RNA is abundant. When the protein product of translation is important for cell growth and or viability, antisense inhibition of gene expression can produce a lethal phenotype. In principle, antisense inhibition of gene expression in humans may be exquisitely specific.

High-density cDNA microarrays enable parallel analysis of the expression of thousands of genes in a single hybridization for complex biological systems. According to Cho *et al.* (2001), antisense can modulate many genes that appear to have a tenuous or no relationship with a targeted gene. Clinical success with Geneta pharmaceuticals (Berkeley Heights, New Jersey, USA) Genasense against BCL-2 has shown the promise of antisense as an adjunct to more conventional chemotherapeutics. The work of Cho-Chung and Becker suggests that down regulating a specific protein could have unforeseen consequences in multiple cellular signaling pathways, at least with phosphorothioate oligonucleotides. This makes it important to examine the antisense effect at the genomic level rather than at the level of a single target gene. It appears that microarray studies may facilitate the study of oligonucleotide pharmacokinetics, sequence specificity, non-sequence specific effects, and toxicity. Growing adoption of this technology can facilitate development of nucleic acid medicines with high target specificity and minimal side effects (Cho–Chung *et al.,* 2003).

10.4. ARTIFICIAL CELLS

Such modern techniques as recombinant DNA, gene shuffling and knockout mutations can be used to alter the genome of a unicellular microbe or even of multicellular organisms. However, these powerful techniques do have limitations related to cost and efficiency of scale. Also, genetically modified cells require specialized nutrient media and the desired products of genetic manipulation are sometime toxic to the cell which makes combining cellular and non-biological technologies difficult. Genetic engineering also poses safety and ethical issues (Pohorille and Deamer, 2002). The above limitations can be avoided by adopting an alternative approach to make simple cell-like structures engineered for some specific application. A complex version of a hypothetical living (artificial) minimal cell should include a translation apparatus that could use sequence information in one type of polymer to direct the synthesis of a second type of polymer. In real cells, this is the ribosome, but conceivably, some simpler structures might also perform similar functions.

In principle, an idealized artificial cell should have the following properties:

- An information-carrying polymer, such as a nucleic acid, must be synthesized by a template-directed polymerization occurring in a membrane-bound structure.
- The monomers of the polymer need to be provided externally and transported across the membrane boundary to support the replication process. Other small molecules or ions needed for biosynthetic reactions also need to be delivered from the environment.
- Availability of external source of chemical energy, which can dynamically drive the biosynthetic reactions.
- Linking of a catalytic activity to the replication process, so that variations in replication affect the catalyzed reactions and so change fitness of the system, stimulating its evolution. Compartmentalization of the replicating catalytic system within a membrane-bound entity should allow selection of variations, leading to 'speciation'.
- The boundary membrane must be able to grow, whether by accumulation of membrane-forming material from the environment or by converting precursor molecules into such material.
- A mechanism that allows the assembly to separate into two or more smaller structures during the growth process—the smaller structures that possess the capabilities of the larger system.
- Effective regulation of catalysis, replication, and growth to ensure that none of the processes lags behind and one gets much ahead of other processes in the cell (Pohorille and Deamer, 2002).

Any attempt to create an idealized artificial cell having the above properties would depend first of all on making the boundary membrane itself. In fact, membranous vesicles (liposomes) made of pure lipid bilayers have been available in some laboratories for over three decades. The second component is a replicating molecular system including nucleic acid polymerases commonly used to catalyze the synthesis of DNA and RNA from template molecules, using nucleotide triphosphates as substrates. The third component—a translation system exploits the genetic information present in nucleic acids to direct the synthesis of specific proteins. Already translation systems that use ribosomes and activated amino acids to produce peptides and larger proteins are already available. Finally, there exist many natural and engineered proteins that have been optimized for certain catalytic binding and structural functions. These proteins could be used to build artificial metabolisms inside vesicles. Unfortunately, even though the individual parts of molecular machinery are available, biologists have not so far been able to integrate them effectively to produce a living cell. Pohorille and Deamer have described the various components (outlined below) and discussed the prospects for establishing an integrated system.

10.5. PROBLEMS ASSOCIATED WITH GENE THERAPY

Human gene therapy has progressed from speculation to reality within a short span. The first clinical gene transfer (albeit only a marker gene NeoR/TIL) in an approved protocol was attempted successfully on 22 May, 1989, at National Institutes of Health (NIH), Bethesda, MD for malignant melanoma. The first federally approved gene therapy protocol, for correction of adenosine deaminase (ADA) deficiency, began on 14 September 1990, at NIH, Bethesda. In spite of wide application they too have problems when brought in practice, for example those problems encountered in attempting to correct a single gene disorder like β-thalassaemia, with an objective to replace the product of a defective or missing β globulin gene with that of a normal β gene. Now the question arises what is our target cell for insertion of the normal gene? And would the 'new' genes function properly in the recipient cells? To cure a genetic blood disorder like thalassaemia, a 'good' gene must be inserted into hemopoietic stem cells, the self-sustaining cell population from which are derived all the formed elements of the blood. First, we can't identify the human stem cells, as they can only be assayed in murine systems. Secondly, till now no efficient method is available by using which successful introduction of corrective gene could be affected. Another problem is the safety in transferring genes into foreign cells. But the most worrying part is the possibility that the 'new' gene might activate an oncogene and may give rise to neoplastic change in a particular cell population.

Besides medical concerns, there are also some philosophical, ethical and theological concerns. Though there is a general consensus that somatic cell gene therapy for the purpose of treating a serious disease is an ethical therapeutic option and considerable controversy exists as to whether or not germline gene therapy would be ethical.

10.6. CANDIDATE DISEASES FOR GENE THERAPY

In general, diseases in which genetic factors play an important role can be classified as below:

Single gene disorders

Chromosomal disorders

Congenital malformation and common diseases

Multifunctional inheritance

Cytoplasmic inheritance

Somatic cell mutations

For gene therapy, it is wiser to initially focus on a genetic disease in which corrected cells might have a selective growth advantage in patients (Anderson, 1984). Alternatively, a disease wherein DNA mutation occurs during DNA replication or metabolism could be treated using appropriate gene therapy. Three diseases fall under this category: ADA deficiency, PNP (purine nucleoside phosphorylase) deficiency and HGPRT (hypoxanthine-guanine phospho-ribosyl transferase) deficiency, also known as Lesch-Nyhan disease. These diseases are caused by deficiencies of enzymes produced by housekeeping genes (genes that are expressed at a relatively low level in most cells), which are 'on' in most cells and do not require very precise regulation. In spite of various problems, i.e., the requirement of a careful regulation in terms of tissues as well as their level of expression. The first target for gene replacement therapy was globulin.

As each biological target will require a unique gene delivery and gene expression system, many of the principles and methods established in development of advanced drug delivery systems can be applied to the design and preparation of synthetic gene delivery systems. The delivery of gene(s) generally falls under two categories: ex vivo and in vivo approaches. The former involves the use of either viral or non-viral systems to insert genes into cells that have been removed from patient, followed by reimplantation of these transduced or transfected cells back into the patient (Culver and Blaese, 1994). The latter involves the administration of genes directly into the patients. Under this, two major methods have been proposed.

(a) Viral-mediated gene transfer

(b) Non-viral-mediated gene transfer

The natural ability of several viruses to infect cells efficiently leads investigators to make use of the same in *in vivo* viral-mediated gene delivery. Such viruses include retrovirus, adenovirus (A V), adeno-associated virus (AAV) and herpes simplex-I virus (HSV-I).

Besides viral mediated gene delivery, non-viral mediated gene delivery has also shown promising results and has emerged as an alternative. Cationic liposomes, polymer based gene delivery and peptide-based gene delivery exemplifies this.

10.7. VIRAL MEDIATED GENE DELIVERY

Gene delivery has become quite easy with the availability of several viral and non-viral delivery systems. Viruses used as carriers include Moloney murine leukemia virus (MoMLV) and the human immunodeficiency virus (HIV), adenoviruses (A V), adeno-associated virus (AA V), herpes simplex virus (HSV), Epstein Barr virus (EBV), Sindbis virus, bovine, human papilloma viruses (BPV and HPV), hepatitis B virus (HBV), vaccinia virus and polyoma virus. The delivery and the mechanism involved depend on the viral encoded proteins.

10.7.1. Retroviral vectors

Principally, a retroviral vector actively introduces genetic sequence into the host cell vis-a-vis proliferate in helper cell line for its own cloning. Characteristically, it offers the following advantages in effective gene delivery to the cell.

1. Facilitates entry of genetic material into a wide variety of cells.

2. Is well understood with simple molecular biology.

3. Integrates into the host genome.

4. Has a potential control over the range of cells to be infected.

5. Is capable of gene expression.

6. May carry upto 8 kb of coding information.

7. Above all, it establishes one way of non-replicative infection of target cells.

Mammalian retrovirus vectors commonly used for gene transfer are classified on the basis of their host range as they could be ecotropic, which only infect murine cells, or amphotropic, which infect murine and non- murine cells both. The main features of the genome of a typical retrovirus are as shown in Figure 10.7. Retroviruses, which are RNA viruses, pass through a DNA stage after infection and integrate into the host genome to form provirus.

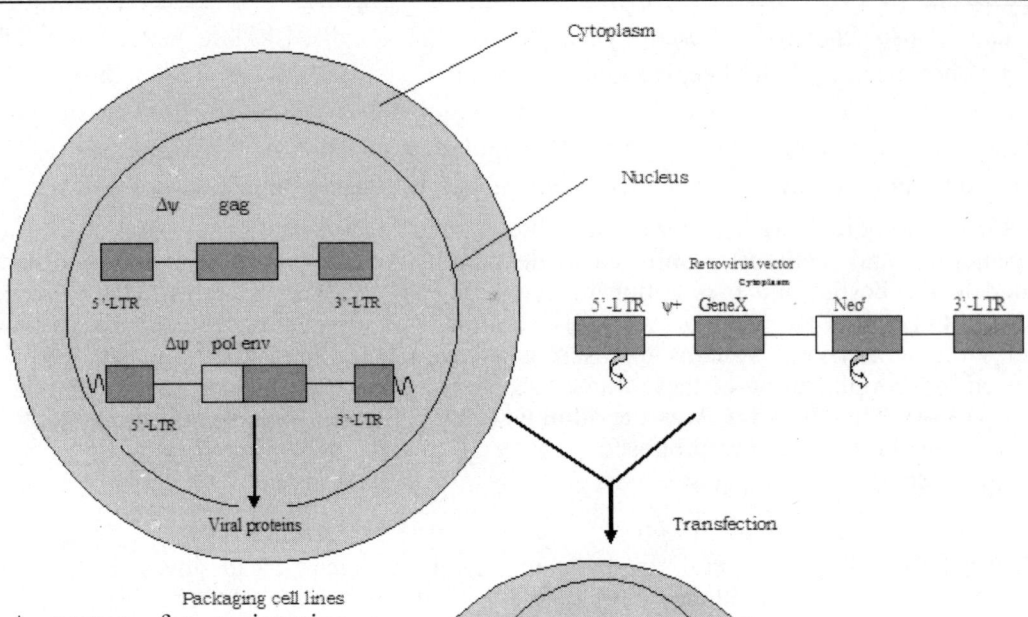

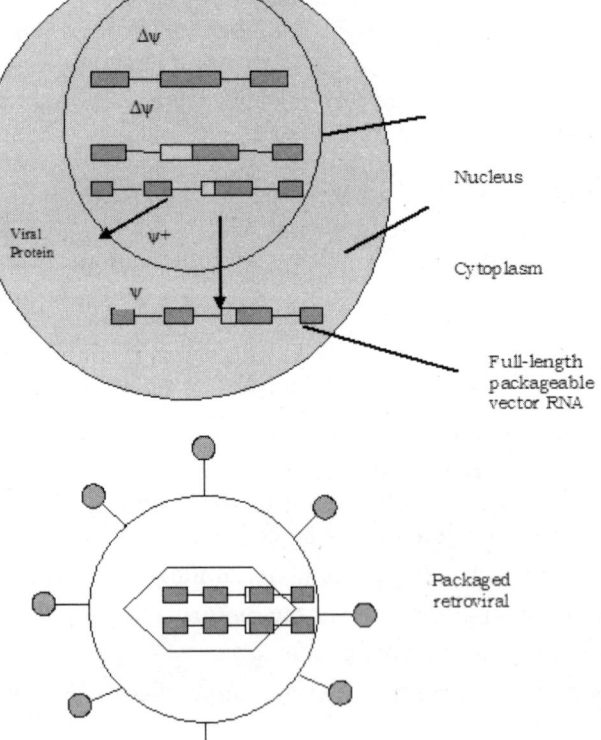

Fig. 10.7: A strategy for engineering a virus into a vector. The general genome organization of a simple retrovirus is shown. The packaging cell lines have two separate retroviral gene regions on its chromosomes; one contains the gag gene, and the other contains the *pol* and *env* genes. In each of these inserts, transcription is driven sequences within the 5' long terminal repeat (5'-LTR) region. Both virus DNA segments lack the encapsidation sequence (Δψ+) that is required fo packaging of retroviral genome into a viral capsid. The packaging cell lines synthesize vial proteins, but because there is no encapsidation sequence within either of the retroviral mRNAs, empty viral capsids are produced. The viral proteins continue to be synthesized after transfection of a packaging cell line with a full- length retroviral vector carrying a remedial (therapeutic) gene (Gene X) and a selectable marker gene (Neor). The full length RNAs from the retrovirus vector sequence is replicated, and because they have a encapsidation region (Δψ+) they are packaged into viral capsids. The released viral particles are replication defective because they do not have a *pol* gene

This provirus can be characterized for its protein coding region (*trans*-acting) and the sequences corresponding to the replication, transcription and integration signals. Cell lines which make *trans*-acting viral proteins but no functional viral particles can be constructed using the "helper gene" sequences coding for the canonical retroviral gag, pol and env proteins, linked by appropriate promoters and polyadenylation signals, but devoid of packaging sequences.

The viral genome needed for the infection, integration and transcriptional control of the genome is all contained in the long terminal repeat sequences (LTR's), which in turn are preserved together with packaging sequences (psi). At the same time, viral sequences of which the function can be supplied in *trans*, are taken out. Thus, the gag sequences which encode internal structural proteins of the virion core, *pol* genes which encode reverse transcriptase and *env* genes which encode the envelop glycoproteins are all deleted and replaced by a dominant selectable marker and the gene that we wish to transfer. Virus is continuously produced by the helper cell and can be harvested from tissue culture supernatant for infection of target cells.

The "helper cells" which provide complementing functions to retroviral vectors are then introduced into helper cells. These modified cells, called "helper cells" are replication-deficient virus, which can supply the missing viral proteins to form a new virion. They produce viral particles which are microscopically identical to genuine retroviral particles, but carry a desired foreign gene. These particles, which are capable of introducing their RNA genomes into target cells, reverse transcribing them into DNA followed by integration into the cellular genome. The new genetic information thus resides in the target cell and does not propagate further as a virus.

The first human replacement gene therapy using a retrovirus vector was approved for the replacement of a defective, missing, ADA gene in children suffering from severe combined immune deficiency (SCID) (Culver and Balese, 1994). The lymphocytes were harvested, transduced or transfected ex vivo with a retrovirus vector containing a functional ADA gene and were then reinfused into the host. Spectacular results were recorded in patients, indicating a significantly enhanced ADA level and as a result improved immune function.

Hepatic genetic deficiencies have been experimentally treated with genes introduced via retroviral vectors (Ledley *et al.*, 1991). A case of hypercholesterolemia in rabbits following ex-vivo treatment and re-implantation of hepatocytes with the LDL receptor gene has been reported by Chowdhury *et al.*, (1991). Similarly, human hepatocytes were transfected with the neomycin resistant gene in a retroviral vector followed by eventual transplantation of modified cells into the spleen of mice that suffered SCID.

A major focus of gene therapy in recent days is in the area of human immunodeficiency virus-I (HIV-I) infection. In the case of this dreaded disease, the HIV -I gp 120 binds selectively and with high affinity to the CD4 receptor, if a high concentration of circulating, soluble CD4 could compete with cellular CD4 for HIV binding, it could intercept circulating HIV -I virus before it can infect host cells (Morgan *et al.*, 1990). The other strategy involves the introduction of a mutant HIV -I envelopes which would compete with the wild-type, occupying the CD4 receptor and therefore, inhibit the spread of the wild-type virus (Buchschacher *et al.*, 1992). The third strategy (also known as "suicide" strategy) involves transfection of T -lymphocytes with a HIV regulated diphtheria toxin A chain gene (Harrison *et al.*, 1992).

The next major area of interest in gene therapy is cancer gene therapy. Studies have suggested that introducing cytokine genes directly into tumor cells, immunize the animals against the tumor (Gansbucher *et al.*, 1990; Golumbek *et al.*, 1991).

Cardiovascular diseases have also attracted possibility of gene therapy. It has been shown in the Yucatan mini pig model that both endothelial cells and vascular smooth muscle cells, when transfected ex-vivo with the galactosidase marker gene, can be inserted in predetermined arterial segments using an intravascular catheter. Two to four weeks after treatment, histo-chemical staining showed positive results (Nabel *et al.*, 1989; Plautz *et al.*, 1991). Another unique application of gene therapy is the use of transfected endothelial cells as 'coating' material for prosthetic devices (Wilson *et al.*, 1989) with the aim of continuously releasing thrombolytic agents, *e.g.,* tissue plasminogen activator (tPA) (Dichek *et al.*, 1991). The use of retrovirus is extremely efficient and results in stable insertion of the transfected gene into the host genome.

10.7.2. Adenovirus (AV) vectors

Adenovirus, a non-enveloped double-stranded DNA virus (unlike retrovirus) can be loaded with upto 36 kb DNA segments and can be used for in vivo transfection as it can also infect non-replicating cells. The A Y gene remains episomal without insertion into the host genome, after gaining cell entry via endocytosis and it subsequently releases in to the cytoplasm, which eliminates possible eventuality of insertional mutagenesis—a major obstacle with retroviral vectors (Horwitz, 1990).

Adenoviruses (AVs) can infect a wide range of cell types and live AVs have been used as vaccines in US military personnel without any major side effects. Two serotypes, Ad5 and Ad2 have been studied extensively. Of the several genes encoded by the adenoviral genome, the proteins encoded by the E I gene are crucial for virus replication and deletion of E I gene renders the virus replication defective. AVs are attractive candidates for gene therapy of lung disorders because of their natural tropism for infecting respiratory epithelium (Crystal, 1994). Unlike retroviruses, they can infect post-mitotic cells and thus their use for gene transfer to brain is of prime importance (Davidson *et al.*, 1993; Bajocchi *et al.*, 1993).

Recombinant AV vectors have been designed which are replication deficient and contain tissue-specific promoters which restrict the site of transgene expression (Berkmer, 1988). AV vectors are similarly broad in range of infectivity as retroviruses. AV infects the pulmonary epithelium avidly and has been successfully employed in in-vivo transfection of pulmonary epithelial cells with the hαlaT gene and the CFTR gene both in cotton rat (Rosenfeld *et al.,* 1991; 1992).

AV gene constructs have also been employed to correct ornithine deficiency in-vivo by transfecting the gene for ornithine transcarbamylase in a mouse model and to demonstrate *lac Z* gene expression (β-galactosidase activity) in skeletal and cardiac muscle following intravenous and intramuscular administration in mice. Two different methods of AV viral mediated gene transfer are currently under investigation. The first involves the insertion of a gene of interest into deleted A V particles similar to AV approach (Quantin *et al.*, 1992). The second method involves complexing the DNA to be inserted with transferrin-polylysine and the viral coat of AV is similar to a Sendai virus gene transfer approach (Wagner *et al.*, 1992). Using this approach, Lemarchand *et al.* (1993) successfully transferred genes into blood vessels. The major concern with A V vectors is similar to that for other viral vectors, i.e., recombination with wild-type A V, especially in the upper airways, which would lead to the generation of replicating A V with unknown pathogenicity. A significant fraction of the population has developed immunity to A V (Straus, 1984) the latter could affect the efficiency of transfection.

10.7.3. Adenovirus-associated viral (AAV) vectors

AA V is a nonpathogenic human parvovirus which has aroused a lot of interest as a vector for gene therapy. It contains a single strand of DNA of 4.7 kb (Muzyezka, 1992). Human AA V infection appears to be non-pathogenic with a majority of the population testing positive for AA V capsid protein antibodies. It is a dependovirus that requires a helper virus co-infection for viral replication. In the absence of co-infection with a helper virus such as A V, herpes virus or cytomegalovirus, the viral genome integrates into the human genome usually at a specific site, 19q 13.3qter. The biology of AA V vectors is not as well understood as of retrovirus or A V. (Berns and Linden, 1995). In terms of gene therapy, the site-specific insertion of wild-type AA V in chromosome 19 is of great interest. AA V vectors have been used to transfect a human leukemia cell line (Dixit *et al.*, 1991) and a cystic fibrosis cell line (Flotte *et al.*, 1992). They have been successfully applied in vivo to transfect a lung lobe with CAT in Sprague-Dawley rats.

10.7.4. Herpes simplex virus-1 (HSV-1) vectors

Among viral vectors, HSV-1 has potentially the largest DNA carrying capacity. It can establish long term, non-cytopathic relationships with the neurons that it infects. Like A V, HSV -I, infects non-dividing cells (Geller and Breakefield, 1988). In addition, HSV does not generally integrate into the host genome. This provides an element of safety, as there is little opportunity for insertional mutagenesis of infected cells. However, these viruses contain a genome of much greater complexity (152 kb) than the more familiar retroviral gene transfer vector (10 kb). This makes development of these vectors, quite difficult.

Three general strategies are available to develop HSV for use as gene transfer vector (Breakefield and DeLuca, 1991). A replication-competent virus with a transgene introduced into a non-essential part of the viral genome (Palella *et al.*, 1989). However, whose limitation is their ability to retain and propagate the cytotoxic properties which are not clinically useful. HSV vectors are promising vehicles for gene transfer in neural disorders especially of brain cells. Initial studies of the effectiveness of the HSV vector were carried out using a marker gene encoding β galactosidase. The expression of the transgene can be assessed both quantitatively and with a simple histochemical strain.

10.7.5. Alpha viruses as vectors

Alpha viruses are a group of arthropod-borne Toga viruses that infect many types of host ranging from mosquito to avian and mammalian species (Strauss and Strauss, 1994). The genome of alpha viruses consists of a single stranded RNA molecule of positive polarity; a productive infection can be initiated either by infection or by transfection of a cell by the isolated RNA. This strategy of self-replication with its highly efficient production of new RNA molecules and protein products provides the basis for recently developed alpha virus expression vectors (Lijestrom, 1994; Schlesinger, 1993). The genome is divided in such a way that the replicase is encoded by one ORF on the genomic RNA while the structural proteins are encoded by a second ORF on separate subgenomic species. Alpha viruses are manipulated by means of subgenomic sequences which do not affect the replication capacity of the system.

Alpha virus vectors have established themselves as a basic tool in research and show remarkable versatility for gene delivery. These vectors can be applied in-vivo for the development of recombinant vaccines. Viral replicase will initiate RNA synthesis from any subgenomic promoter on a minus-strand molecule, thus making possible the expression of a foreign sequence packed in infectious viral RNA simply by adding a second transcription unit either upstream or downstream from the structural gene.

Delivery of recombinant RNA (rRNA) into the cell can be negotiated in several ways; the simplest and efficient method to transfect RNA is to transcribe *in vitro* using electroporation or lipofection (Lijestrom and Garoff, 1994). Transfection efficiencies of up to 100% can be achieved under *in vitro* cell culture conditions. However, it is a cumbersome process when different cell types are used especially in *in vivo* application. Therefore, a preferable mode of delivery is to make use of the very broad host-range of these viruses for infecting cells. Helper vectors that allow rRNA to be packed into infectious virus particles have been developed with high titer values (10^9–10^{16} /ml).

Although several alpha viruses are pathogenic, the two viruses SFV and SIN commonly used as vectors are avirulent in humans (Strauss and Strauss, 1994). For safety and economic reasons a novel strategy involving a layered DNA'-RNA vector system has been developed (Fig. 10.8). This system is independent of helper vectors. Recombinant alpha virus expression-cassette cDNA is controlled by a eukaryotic promoter, such as the cytomegalovirus early promoter (pCMV). This plasmid-DNA construct can be delivered directly into the cell by DNA transfection method. Here, in the cell nucleus, RNA polymerase transcribes the complete unit into RNA which is transported to the cytoplasm. This provides a positive polarity. The RNA is translated to form the viral replicase, which takes over the replica of the whole molecule in the same manner as during normal replication of alpha virus RNA molecule.

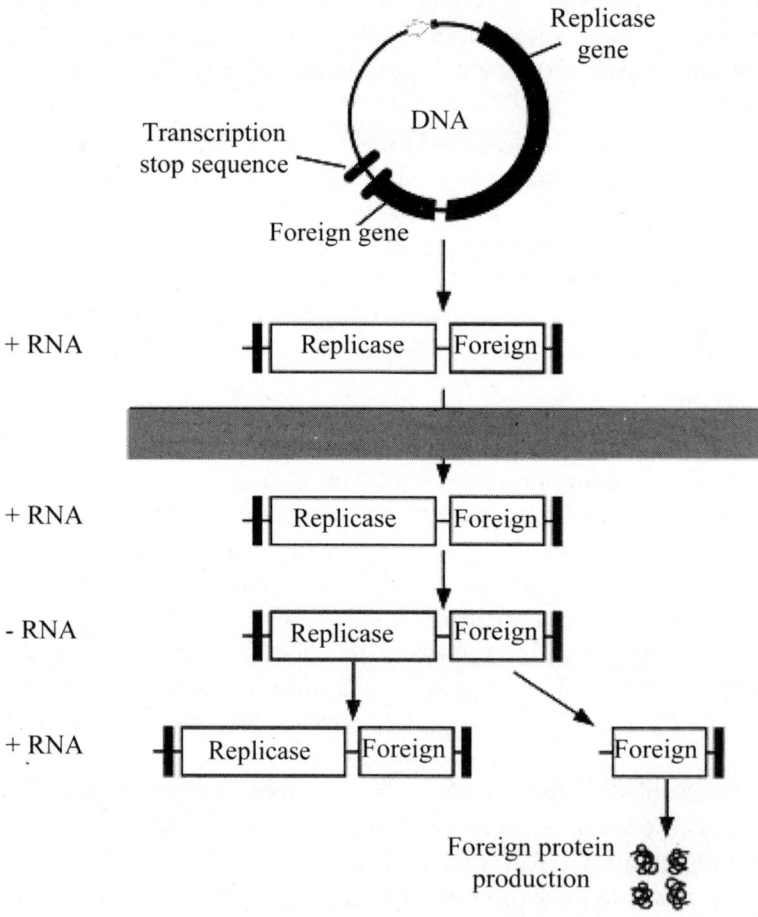

Fig. 10.8: Layered DNA-RNA vector system

Alpha virus vectors have been successfully used to study the structure and function of protein and for protein production. It is a useful tool in targeting of transient, high level protein expression to desired areas. They have also proved useful found in development of recombinant vaccines (Berglund *et al.,* 1996).

10.7.6. Epstein Barr Virus (EBV)

Long term gene expressions are required for certain applications that do not involve the integration of transferred DNA. For this, persistent gene expression and episomal maintenance are required. An ideal-long term expression system bears the following features:

- Nuclear retention by attachment of DNA to the nuclear matrix.
- Autonomous replication
- Enhanced gene expression
- Prevention of plasmid degradation
- Efficient delivery into the nucleus

These goals can be achieved by using parts of viral systems. One such system is the Epstein Barr Virus (EBV), which provides autonomous replication and nuclear retention. EBNA 1 protein that interacts with the EBV origin of replication (*ori*P) provides such a function. Mammalian artificial chromosomes also provide such features.

10.7.7. Suicide genes

In the present scenario none of the existing DNA delivery systems can mediate a transfection in all cells *in-vivo*—a major drawback in cases like cancer where the treatment requires 100% selective delivery of therapeutic genes to tumor cells. Toxin or suicide gene delivery represents a potentially powerful approach in cancer gene therapy. The therapeutic index is largely dependent on the specificity of gene delivery and efficiency of gene transfer in vivo to target tumor cells.

10.7.7.1. Toxin gene therapy

Cell suicide by expression of the diphtheria toxin A chain coding sequence has been demonstrated in cell culture and in animals. Diphtheria toxin is an extremely potent inhibitor of protein synthesis in eukaryotic cells. It has been estimated that one molecule of diphtheria toxin A per cell is sufficient to kill murine L cells. The toxin is composed of two subunits. The B chain (342 amino acids) is adsorbed to the cell surface for internalization and the A chain (193 amino acids) specifically modifies histidine residues of elongation factor 2 by ADP-ribosylation, which prevents protein synthesis and kills the cell. Expression of the toxin may be induced by linking the diphtheria toxin A coding sequence with tissue-specific transcription regulatory elements (promoters and enhancers). This approach has been tested in B-lymphoid cells, in which a plasmid was transfected that carried the diphtheria toxin A chain coding sequence under control of the engineered immunoglobulin K light chain gene regulatory sequences. This construct specifically expressed diphtheria toxin A in mature B cells but not in pre-B cells, suggesting that the construct may be further developed to allow therapeutic ablation of malignant B cells of mature stages while sparing normal progenitor cells.

Another similar approach used Pseudomonas exotoxin, which was conjugated with IL-4 to treat murine sarcoma and colon adenocarcinorna cells that express high-affinity IL-4 receptors. The chimeric IL-4 Pseudornonas exotoxin protein is cytotoxic to the tumor cells by inhibiting cellular protein synthesis in a dose-dependent manner. A non chimeric Pseudomonas exotoxin protein that could not bind to the IL-4 receptor did not inhibit protein synthesis in tumor cells. A chimeric mutant protein that could bind to the IL-4 receptor but did not have the capacity to inhibit protein synthesis was not cytotoxic to tumor cells. The protein synthesis-inhibitory activity of the IL-4/Pseudornonus exotoxin fusion protein could be completely abolished by a neutralizing antibody against IL-4. These data suggest that a receptor-mediated toxin therapy might be effective.

10.7.7.2. Suicide gene therapy

Suicide gene therapy is based on introducing a drug sensitivity gene into target cells, which are then killed by the drug at doses that are not detrimental to normal cells. One such "suicide" gene that has been successfully used to confer drug sensitivity in an animal model system is the herpes simplex virus thymidine kinase gene (HSV-tk). The HSV-tk enzyme can specifically catalyze the phosphorlyation of a number of nucleoside analogs, such as acyclovir or ganciclovir, which are poor substrates for the tk enzymes of mammalian cells. The phosphorylated acyclic nucleoside becomes active when incorporated into newly synthesized DNA, resulting in a cytocidal effect by induction of DNA strand breaks and inhibition of DNA polymerase activity.

In a syngeneic mouse model, subcutaneous tumors developed from the HSV-tk-transduced tumor cells went into complete regression following intraperitoneal administration of ganciclovir, while tumors derived from the nontransduced tumor cells were not affected. An analogous approach has been taken for treatment of brain tumors in a rat model. In these experiments, the HSV-tk retrovirus producing cells were stereotactically injected into rat cerebral gliomas in vivo. The HSV-tk retroviruses generated from the producer cells were expected to preferentially infect the proliferating tumor cells, which would be selectively killed by ganciclovir administered intraperitoneally. Indeed, complete regression of the glioma was observed in 11 of 14 rats. Since it was unlikely that all of the tumor cells became infected with the HSV-tk retroviruses, it was suggested that this regression may have been due to a "bystander effect." This effect was demonstrated by a coculture experiment in vitro, in which HSV-tk-transduced human fibrosarcoma cells induced the ganciclovir killing effect on non-transduced coculture cells through a gap junction-mediated metabolic cooperation.

Although the mechanism of the bystander effect in vivo was not well understood, the remarkable success of this technique in the treatment of a very aggressive tumor that has an extremely poor prognosis when treated with conventional therapy has led to human clinical trials.

Gene-directed enzyme prodrug therapy (GDEPT) is an emerging strategy used to improve the selectivity of cancer chemotherapy. This is accomplished through tumor-specific activation of non cytotoxic prodrugs to active drugs by drug-metabolizing enzymes. The general scheme consists of transfection of tumor cells with an enzyme responsible for the bioactivation of a non cytotoxic prodrug and treatment with the prodrug: only cells expressing the transfected drug-metabolizing enzyme can metabolize the prodrug into cytotoxic metabolites, leading to cell death (Fig. 10.9). The use of viral vectors for transgene introduction is more specifically referred to as virus directed enzyme prodrug therapy (VDEPT).

The therapeutic approach called "virus-directed enzyme/prodrug therapy" (VDEPT) is another example of suicide gene therapy. In treatment of hepatocellular carcinoma with VDEPT, the varicella zoster virus thymidine kinase (VZV-tk) gene that was transcriptionally regulated by either the hepatoma-associated α-fetoprotein or liver-associated albumin promoters was constructed into a retroviral vector. After infecting the cancer cells with this vector, nontoxic prodrug 6-methoxypurine arabinonucleoside (araM) activated by VZV-tk expressed preferentially in hepatoma cells. The final product, adenine arabinonucleoside triphosphate (araATP), selectively induced cytotoxicity in the hepatoma cells that expressed the gene.

The gene encoding cytosine deaminase can also be used to prime cell death upon administration of a drug that is not normally toxic to eukaryotic cells. Cytosine deaminase converts the nontoxic substance 5-fluorocytosine to a toxic derivative, 5-fluorouracil. Thus, only genetically modified cells carrying and expressing the cytosine deaminase gene are able to synthesize 5-fluorouracil and induce the cytocidal effect. Retrovirus-mediated cytosine deaminase gene transfer in various cell types has demonstrated this specific cell killing effect after treatment of the transduced cells with 5-fluorocytosine.

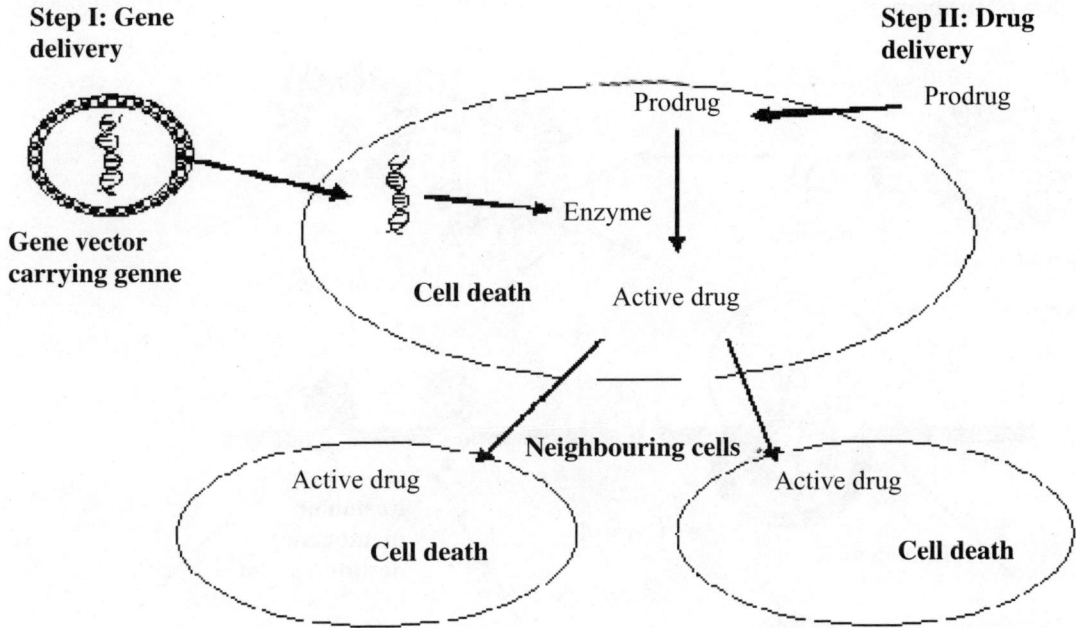

Fig. 10.9: Mechanism of gene-directed enzyme prodrug therapy (GDEPT)

10.8. NON-VIRAL MEDIATED-GENE THERAPY

At present, majority of the approved clinical trials on gene therapy in human subjects have involved viral transfection using viral vector mediated transfer. Non-viral gene medicines (Fig. 10.10) have emerged as potentially safe and effective gene therapy options for a wide variety of acquired arid genetic diseases.

10. 8.1. Barriers to non-viral gene delivery

The current understanding of the various biological barriers that face efficient gene delivery include the ability to

        I.   Package therapeutic genes

        II.   Gain entry into cells

        III. Escape the endo-lysosomal pathway

        IV. Effect DNA/vector release

        V.   Traffic through the cytoplasm and into the nucleus

        VI. Enable gene expression

        VII.   Remain biocompatible. These points are diagrammatically represented in Figure below (Fig. 10.11).

10.8.2. Disadvantages of viral mediated gene therapy

1. Retroviral vectors are not capable of replication although they infect and introduce the provirus into the target.

2. These vectors function as single hit gene transfer systems.

3. Retroviral vectors can only infect dividing cells.

4. The transgenes inserted by retroviral vector do not remain transcriptionally active, thus posing a "viral shut down" problem.

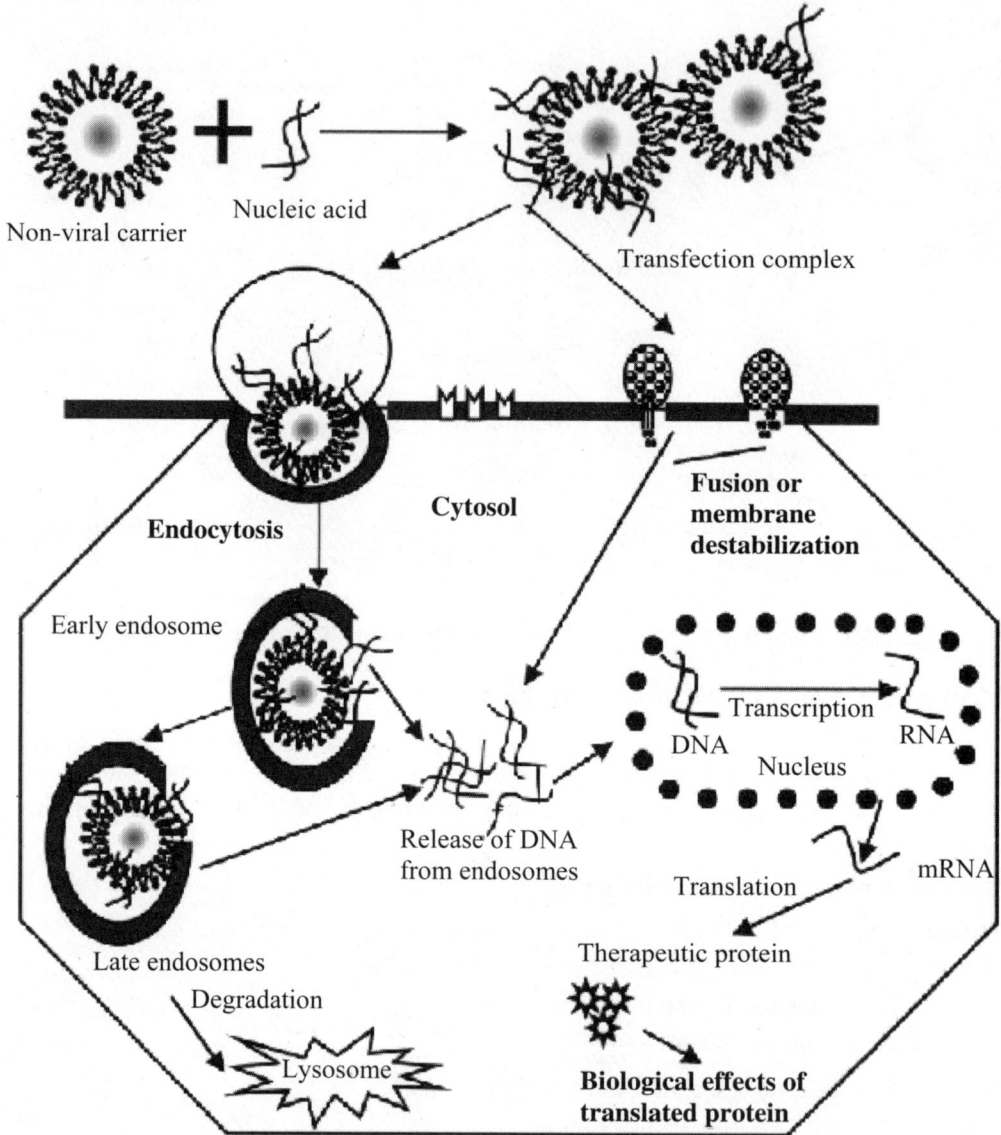

Fig. 10.10: Mode of action of non-viral gene delivery system

5. Difficulty in targeting certain cells.

6. Requirement for a packaging cell line.

7. They show a low DNA transfer.

8. Size limitation of DNA constructs.

9. Production of high titer viral vectors is difficult.

10. No assurance for completely free replication-competent virus.

11. Severe immunogenic reactions and safety concerns.

12. Toxic side effects.

13. Possibility of insertional mutation.

14. Possible triggering of oncogene(s) or desirable tumor suppresser gene(s).

15. Above all, the possibility to revert back or to retain an infectious form.

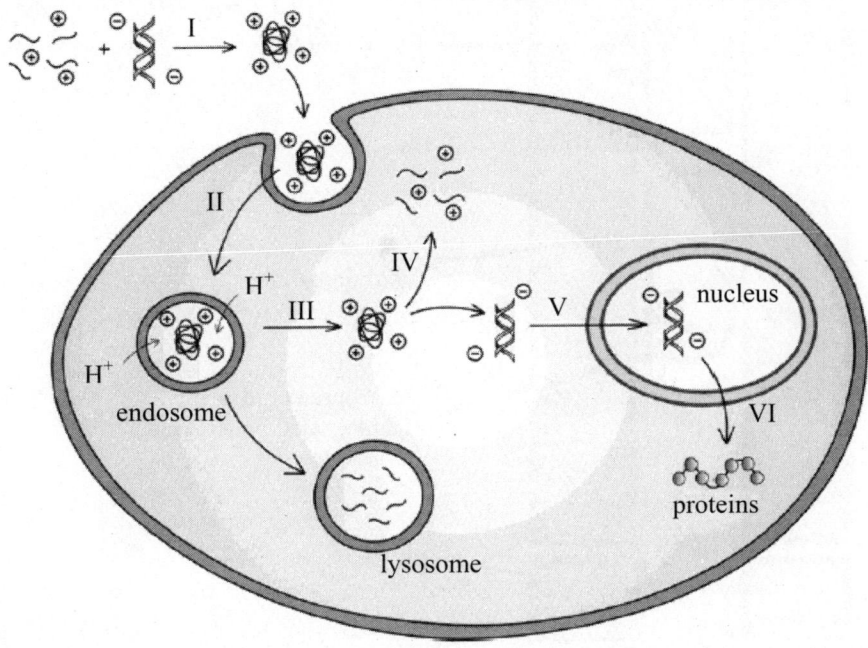

Fig. 10.11: Barriers to gene delivery

10.8.3. Biolistic and needle free delivery

Interstitial administration of plasmid-gene expression systems using needle-free jet injection devices, e.g. 'gene guns' or 'golden guns' and 'hypospray' or direct injection have been reported and suggested that these genes are taken by a variety of cells *in vivo* (Hickman *et al.*, 1994; Sikes *et al.*, 1994; Raz *et al.*, 1994). These gene guns (Fig.10.12) use tissue bombardment with gold or tungsten microparticles coated with a DNA plasmid-based gene expression system. Ballistic methods that use particle-mediated or 'gene gun' technology have shown up to 100 fold greater gene expression levels both in ex vivo and *in vivo* in comparison to cationic lipid delivery or other non viral gene delivery systems. This method has been successfully used to deliver DNA *in vivo* into liver, skin, pancreas, muscle, spleen, and tumors. Expression of reporter genes (e.g. firefly luciferase and β-galactosidase) or therapeutic genes (human growth hormone) has also been reported (Cheng *et al.*, 1993; Andree *et al.*, 1994). 'Hypospray' devices which do not require non-biodegradable microparticles have been used for the in-vivo administration to mouse skin either as a skin-specific gene expression system (driven by human keratin K6 promoter) or as a non-tissue-specific construct (driven by a viral CMY promoter); both the systems contained a β-galactosidase reporter gene (β -gal) (Selheyer *et al.*, 1993; Furth *et al.*,

1992; Ledley *et al.,* 1994). These studies concluded that there was a significantly increased level of gene expression as compared to the administration of the same in the form of saline suspensions.

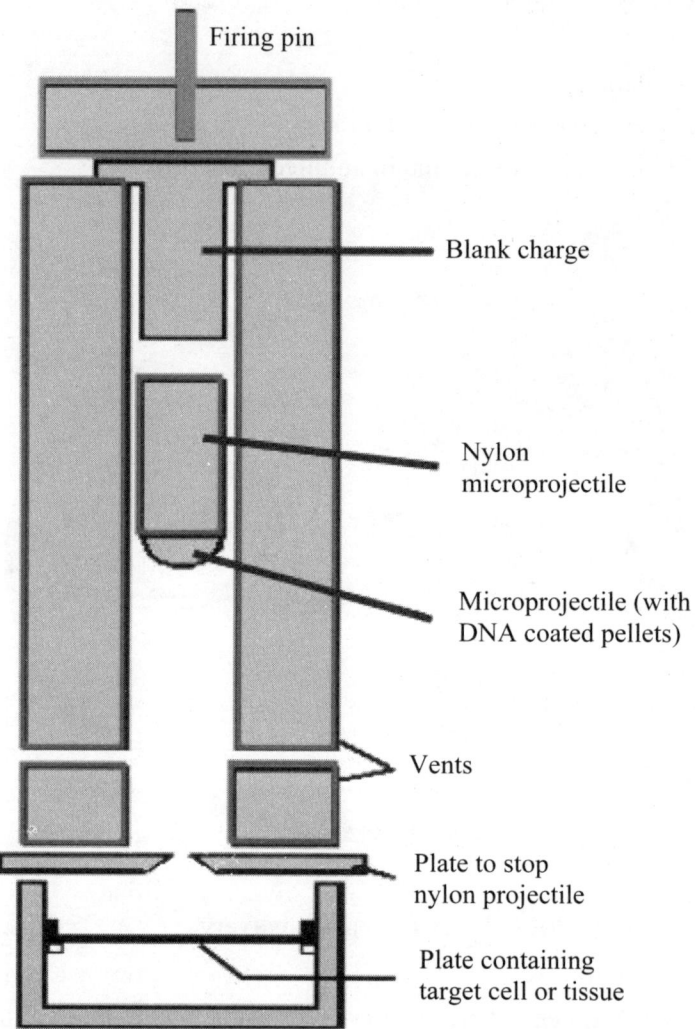

Fig. 10.12: Diagrammatic presentation of a gene gun

Interstitial administration of plasmid-based gene expression has shown low levels of gene expression with the exception of such systems for vaccination purposes (Ulmer *et al.,* 1993; Davis *et al.,* 1993). Such results have led to designing novel approaches for enhancing the location and amount of genes to the nuclei of target cells. These approaches include (Feigner and Ringold, 1989; Feigner *et al.,* 1987; Wu *et al.,* 1991):

1. Cationic lipids.

2. Charged synthetic polymers.

3. Peptides that act in a non-specific manner.

4. Peptide and carbohydrate-based targeting ligands.

10.8.4. Liposome-mediated delivery

Liposomes have been well studied for the controllable delivery of drugs to specific sites. Nicolau and co-workers in 1983 demonstrated the delivery of prepro-insulin gene to the liver of rats. The DNA plasmids were encapsulated in lactosylceramide based liposomes which were then administered intravenously. Intracellular trafficking of DNA following endocytosis by cells has also been demonstrated using pH-sensitive liposomes and proteoliposomes (Wang and Huang, 1987; Nicolau and Cudd 1989; Kato *et al.,* 1991).

Liposomes are being used by the pharmaceutical industry as drug delivery agents. Lipid vesicles were first prepared in the mid 1960s and are referred to as multi-lamellar vesicles (MLVs). These have certain limitations which prompted the production of more homogeneous preparations consisting of small unilamellar vesicles (SUVs), prepared by sonication of MLV, having dimensions in the range of 25 nm to 100 nm. Large unilamellar vesicles (LUVs) (100 nm to 1 μm diameter), first reported in 1976 are standard preparations today (Fig. 10.13). They are commonly prepared by extrusion through polycarbonate filters.

Table 10.2: Compositional lipids of liposomes

Name of lipid	Carbon: unsaturation	Transition temperature (°C)	Net charge
DLPC	12:0	-1	0
DMPC	14:0	23	0
DPPC	16:0	41	0
DSPC	18:0	55	0
DOPC	18:1	-20	0
DMPE	14:0	50	0
DPPE	16:0	63	0
DOPE	18:0	-16	0
DMPA.Na	14:0	50	-1.3
DPPA.Na	16:0	67	-1.3
DOPA.Na	18:1	-8	-1.3
DMPG.Na	14:0	23	-1
DPPG.Na	16:0	41	-1
DOPG.Na	18:1	-18	-1
DMPS.Na	14:0	35	-1
DPPS.Na	16:0	54	-1
DOPS.Na	18:1	-11	-1
DPPE-mPEG-2000.Na	16:0	N/A	-1
DPPE-mPEG-5000.Na	16:0	N/A	-1
DPPE-Carboxy PEG-2000.Na	16:0	N/A	-2
DOTAP	18:1	-0	+1

Liposomes are concentric bilayered vesicles in which an aqueous core is entirely enclosed by a membranous lipid bilayer mainly composed of natural ad synthetic phospholipids. The lipid molecules are usually phospholipids- amphipathic moieties with a hydrophilic head group and two hydrophilic lipidic tails. On the addition of excess water, such lipidic moieties spontaneously originate to give the most thermodynamically stable conformation, in which polar head groups face outwards into the aqueous medium, and the lipidic chains turn inwards to avoid the water phase, giving rise to double layered or bilayer lamellar structures. Both water and lipid soluble drugs can be entrapped into the liposomes. Hydrophilic drugs can entrap in the aqueous environment and lipophilic drugs remain within the bilayer region. Liposomes may also contain glycerol, glycolipids, organic acids, membrane proteins, hydrophilic polymers and other agents depending upon the type of vesicle required.

Table 10.3: Properties of various vesicular systems

Properties	Large Unilamellar Vesicles (LUVs)	Small Unilamellar Vesicles (SUVs)	Multilamellar vesicles (MLVs)
Entrapped volume	High	Low	Medium (<LUVs)
Thermodynamic stability	Less stable	Unstable	Stable
Energy requirement	Low	High	Low
RES uptake	Rapid clearance	Long circulating higher $T_{1/2}$	Rapid clearance (less $T_{1/2}$)
Preparation methods	Reverse phase evaporation, Ether injection, Double emulsion, Detergent dialysis	Solvent injection French pressure Cell method Probe sonication	Thin film hydration method

As the smallest living cells are 0.2–0.5 μm in diameter, in principle LUVs could contain a sufficient number of macromolecules to form artificial cellular systems. These are convenient in that they are readily prepared and reasonably stable. The pH-sensitive liposomes can fuse with lipid membranes in the acidic environment of the endosomes, facilitating endosomal release of encapsulated gene expression systems into the cytoplasm of transfected cells. The limiting step, however, is the transfer of the encapsulated plasmid DNA from the endosomal compartment to the nucleus of the target cell. Legendre and Szoka (1992) attempted unsuccessfully to facilitate the translocation of encapsulated gene expression systems to the nucleus by incorporating a nuclear localization (specific) peptide into the expression system. It was found that addition of a lysosomotrophic agent like chloroquine, which raises the acidic pH of the endosomes, lowers the fusing efficiency of the liposome with endosomal membrane and consequently reduces the probability of gene transfer to the nucleus. Proteoliposomes (chimerasomes) have been shown to transfer genes effectively. But some problems in their action and characterization have limited their use. Proteoliposomes containing sendai virus glycoproteins can, however, mediate the cellular entry and fusion of the liposomes with the endosomal membrane (Gould-Fogerite *et al.*, 1989).

10.8.4.1. Transport across cell walls

Being just an envelope for an artificial cellular system, a vesicle has to be turned into a functional unit by mechanisms for exchange of nutrients, waste products, regulatory molecules and ions between the vesicle and their environment. The internal volume of a typical liposome with a diameter of 0.2 μm is only 4×10^{-18} liters, implying that in a 0.1 mM substrate concentration only 2400 substrate molecules for a given enzymatic reaction might be captured. All these would be fully consumed in less than a second at typical enzymatic reaction rates, making transmembrane transport is essential.

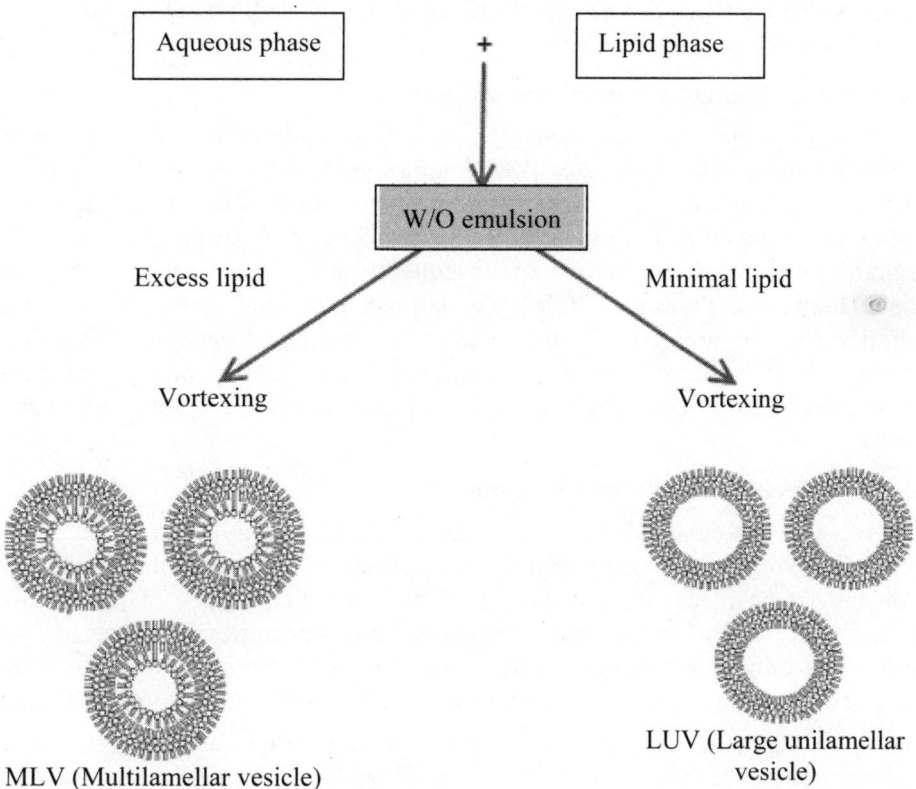

Fig. 10.13: Formation of different liposomes using reverse phase evaporation. MLV-REVs are formed in presence of excess phospholipid whereas LUV-REVs are formed in absence of extra lipid

Many small, neutral molecules readily diffuse through vesicle walls but lipid bilayers create permeability barriers to charged, zwitterionic and macromolecular species. Therefore, to achieve efficient, controlled and selective transport, an assisted mechanism is necessary. It can be provided by carrier molecules or transmembrane proteins, channels and pumps. Channels and carriers mediate passive transport (along the concentration gradient) whereas pumps actively use energy to transport species against the gradient.

It is possible to design synthetic channels or re-engineer natural ones so that they have the desired transport properties, by manipulations of the amino acid sequence along the pore, helix orientation and the diameter of the transmembrane cavity. The commonest design may be based on four to six helices arranged about a central axis. Another category of transmembrane channels is based on cyclic peptides that adopt flat ring structures and stack up to make hollow cylindrical nanotubes stabilized by backbone-backbone hydrogen bonding interactions. In these channels, rings are formed either by alternating D – α-amino acid and L–α –amino acid or by homochiral β-amino acids. As no sidechains project into the lumen of the channel, their specificity is altered by changing the diameter of the cavity rather than the identity of residues forming the ring. Tubular channels are stable, well oriented in the bilayer and can transport solutes ranging in size from protons to glucose (Hartgerink *et al.*, 1998). The hemolysin channel can transport even such large linear polymers as single stranded nucleic acids (Kasianowicz *et al.*, 1996). Channel activity may be regulated by including either triggers that turn the channel on or off once, or switches that modulate channel activity in response to a signal. Triggers and switches can be either chemical or physical, where the stimulus is provided by light, pH or voltage (Nir and Nieve, 2000).

10.8.4.2. Energy requirement for liposome uptake

Chemical energy is required to drive metabolic reactions inside an artificial cell. Energy may come from the environment as ATP molecules if the membrane bilayer is made fairly permeable to ATP, but this is usually difficult and very slow. An alternative option is to mimic the energy transduction process used by all living cells. In this, light or chemical energy from the environment is converted to a transmembrane proton gradient, which is subsequently used in the production of ATP from ADP and phosphate (Lanyi and Pohorille, 2001). The simplest artificial system for the continuous, light-driven generation of ATP consists of two membrane proteins viz., bacteriorhodopsin that works as a proton pump, and ATP synthase (ATPase), which couples the flow of protons through the enzyme to the phosphorylation of ADP. Use of thermophilic ATPase makes the system stable and functional for several months.

10.8.4.3. Macromolecules within the liposome

Any artificial cell-like system needs to encapsulate metabolic functions catalyzed by macromolecules, but it is a challenging task to assemble an encapsulated system containing catalysts: first, the encapsulation must take place without damaging the catalytic activity of the macromolecule. One approach is to inject the molecules into sufficiently large liposomes (Wick *et al.*, 1996). But these latter are limited to only a few vesicles and cannot be used for industrial scale preparation. Chang (1985) reviewed other techniques for encapsulating multienzyme systems in non-lipid membranes.

Some complex enzyme systems have been successfully demonstrated to function after encapsulation in liposomes (Oberholzer *et al.*, 1995, 1999). Attempts to encapsulate ribosomes in liposomes have yielded modest amounts of a translation product directed by mRNA (Oberholzer *et al.*, 1999). Indeed, Griffiths and Tawfik (2000) even captured the entire *in vitro* transcription/translation system and a library of genes linked to a substrate for the desired reaction in the compartmentalized system of a water-in-oil emulsion. However, it may be better to encapsulate a similar system inside liposomes as compared with the water-in-oil emulsions, as this would continuously supply substrates to the reaction compartments.

Keefe and Szostak (2001) described a novel multiple-turnover strategy for selecting novel proteins–this could make possible creating proteins that catalyze technologically interesting chemical reactions having no equivalents in biological systems (Pohorille and Deamer, 2002). Should the transcription-translation system in liposomes be captured it could be easily extended to encapsulate 'mini-genomes' yielding products that cannot be obtained from a single enzymatic reaction but instead require a metabolic pathway. This could then be coupled to the energy supply, thereby enhancing the system. In a hypothetical cell-like structure, DNA is transcribed to RNA and translated to the protein with the aid of the encapsulated transcription and translation system. The amino acids needed for translation are delivered from the environment through the transmembrane channel and activated by ATP. ATP is synthesized from ADP and phosphate by a light-driven bioenergetics system composed of bacteriorhodopsin and ATP synthase (ATPase). Expression in such a system could be regulated exogenously by including, for example, the Lac promoter in the mini-genome. However, accumulation of reaction products at high concentrations would result in product inhibition causing reactions to be markedly slowed down.

10.8.5. Cationic liposomes

The use of cationic liposomes to deliver antisense constructs has attracted recent attention. Cationic lipids are used to reduce the net negative surface charge on DNA plasmid-based gene expression systems in order to reduce charge-charge repulsion at the surface of biological membranes. Such lipids form a stable complex with the gene expression system (Felgner and Rigold 1989; Gao and Huang 1991; Felgner *et al.*, McLachlan *et al.*, 1994; Staedel *et al.*, 1994; Rojanasakul, 1996).

Cationic liposomes consist mainly of a positively charged lipid. "Lipofection", a novel highly efficient DNA transfection system based on lipofectins, was introduced in 1987 (Felgner *et al.*, 1987). The lipofection system consisted of the positively charged quaternary amino lipid N- [1-(2,3-di-oleyloxy) propyl] -N, N, N-trimethylammonium chloride (DOTMA) in a 1:1 weight mixture with dioleylphosphatidyl ethanolamine (DOPE). As DOPE can fuse with endosomal membrane, it is generally included to effect the endosomal release of a gene expression system. DNA on mixing with cationic liposomes produces a condensed DNA along with tubular structure and liposome aggregate. The mechanism by which DNA-cationic liposome complex delivers the DNA is understood to be as follows. The complex first interacts with the cell membrane, followed by endocytosis and finally disruption of endosomes. These lipid-based transfective agents have been employed successfully for genetic loading of a variety of cell lines *in vitro* and *in vivo*. Luciferase mRNA was transfected into NIH 3T3 cells using the DOTMA-DOPE liposome complex. Lipophilic polylysines, i.e., lipopolylysine (LPLL) mediated gene delivery has been reported (Zhao and Huang 1991). LPLL when mixed with DOPE and followed by sonication readily forms unilamellar liposomes, which effectively promote the transfer of gene into cell line(s). D-Chol, nothing but 313-(N-(N',N'-dimethylaminoethane)carbamoyl] cholesterol along with DOPE, is a cationic liposome that can accomplish efficient delivery of nucleic acids (Li *et al.*, 1996).

The use of cationic liposomes as synthetic viral vectors for gene delivery has the following therapeutic, toxicological and technological attributes.

1. Complexation of cationic lipid and DNA is quantitative and needs separation of unencapsulated DNA.
2. Production of such complexes is rapid, highly reproducible, and involves only one step.
3. DNA vectors directly complex with cationic lipid. There is no need for virus production or screening.
4. Due to the net negative charge, transfection is spontaneous.
5. The DOPE component of cationic liposomes is responsible for the escape of the complex from the endosomal compartment into the cytosol.
6. Cationic liposomes are non immunogenic.

10.8.6. Reconstituted sendai virus envelopes (RSVE)

This is a unilamellar proteoliposome, which incorporates the fusogenic protein(s) of the sendai virus (an enveloped virus of the paramyxovirus family) (Fig. 10.13). The vesicles are reconstituted sendai virus envelopes (RSVE). The potential of RSVE to deliver encapsulated materials intravascularly has been reported (Ardizzoni *et al.,* 1988; Gitman *et al.,* 1985; Bartzatt 1987; 1988; Bagai and Sarkar, 1993; 1994).

In general, the encapsulation of the genetic material into the sendai virus is accomplished as follows:

Two types of proteins (Haemagglutinin (HN) and fusion (F) protein) are inserted into the sendai virus in which the nucleocapsid is encapsulated within the lipid membrane or envelope (Fig.10.14).

HN mediates viral attachment to cell surfaces, while its neuraminidase activity prevents unproductive binding to cell receptors. The other protein is the F protein, which as the name suggests is a fusion protein involved in fusion of the virus envelope to the plasma membrane of the cell. Fusion of the RSVE results in microinjection of the viral genome into the cell cytoplasm (Fig. 10.15), where it is replicated in a productive infective manner or phase.

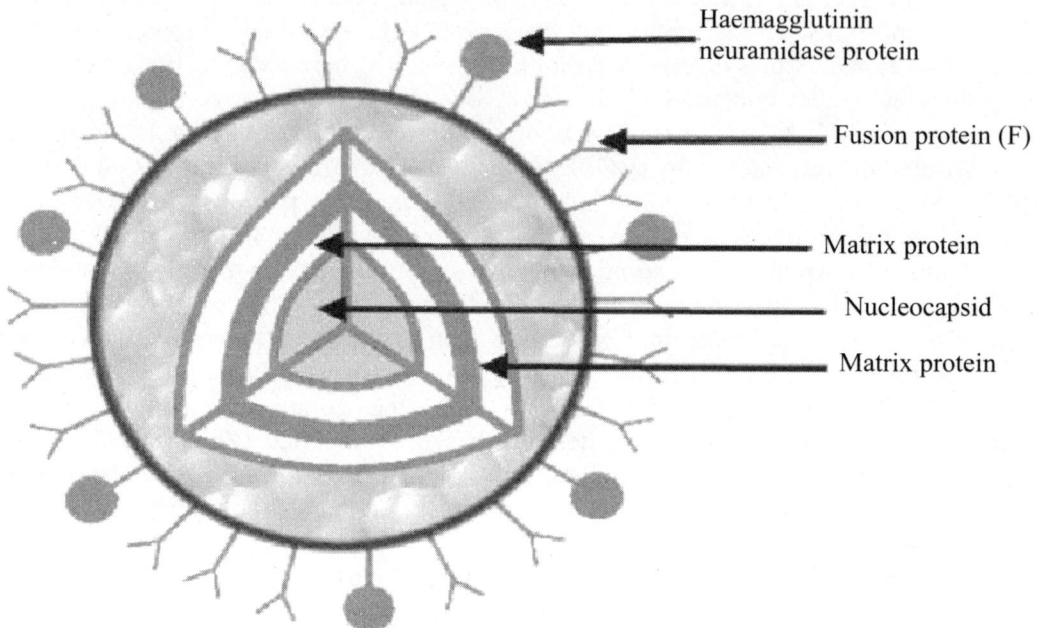

Fig. 10.14: Structure of a sendai virus particle

10.8.7. Synthetic retrotransposon vectors

10.8.7.1. Transposable elements

Cells contain a variety of transposable elements that can be inserted at many places in the bacterial chromosome, and can be excised by site-specific recombination. The important feature is that after transposing with high frequency at a given set of conditions, they become quite stable under others. Transposable elements are of importance especially in transfer of drug resistant genes to other bacteria.

Transposable elements are not replicons. They are usually duplicated, leaving the original element intact while inserting a copy elsewhere, thereby increasing the total number in the cell. In this transfer, **transposase**, an enzyme specified by a gene of the element itself, interacts with ends of transposon and with target sequences in the recipient DNA. The enzymes of different transposable elements recognize different targets, which differ in abundance. **Insertion sequences** (ISs), the simplest transposable elements, were discovered as mutagens, whose trans-position into a gene usually inactivates it. The ISs are short (150–1500 base pairs), with inverted repeats of 15 to 40 base pairs at the ends. Large ISs contain the gene for the transposase. Transposons are larger and contain additional genes, often for antibiotic resistance.

The prokaryotic transposons can be categorized under three classes. Class I are bounded by two ISs (e.g., TnIO, a gene for tetracycline resistance), while class II are bounded by two short repeats, 30 to 40 base pairs long instead of terminal ISs (e.g., Tn3, with a gene for ampicillin resistance). Class III transposons are phages.

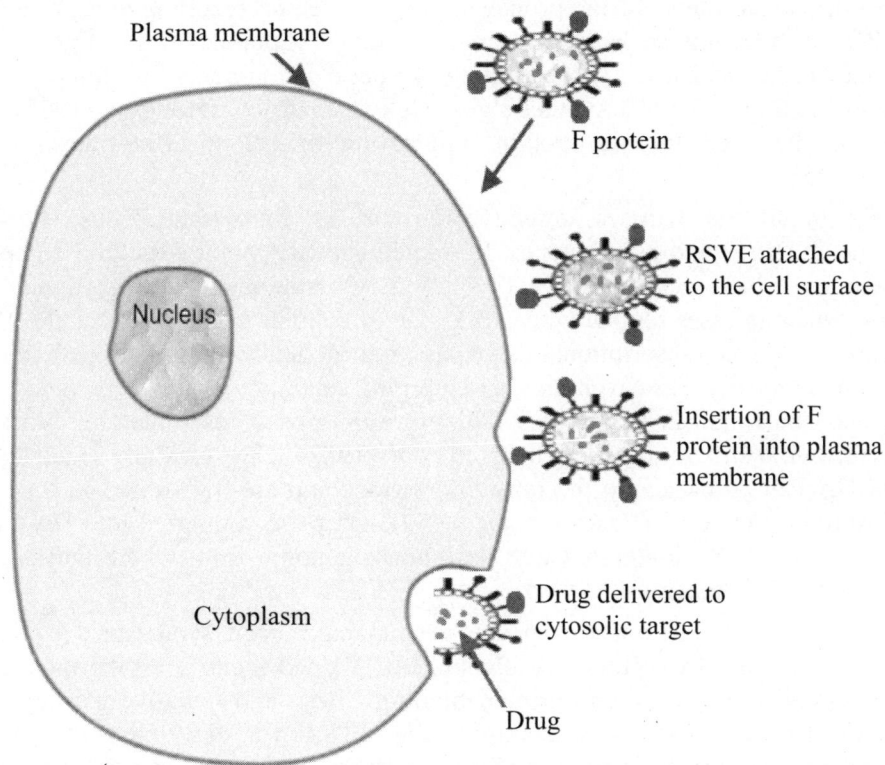

Plasma membrane

F protein

RSVE attached to the cell surface

Insertion of F protein into plasma membrane

Nucleus

Cytoplasm

Drug delivered to cytosolic target

Drug

Fig. 10.15: RSVE - mediated drug delivery

10.8.7.2. Mechanisms of transposition

Some transposons (e.g., Tn7) can integrate essentially at a single site, causing the appearance of hot spots for transposition. Some others (e.g., Tn10) integrate at many sites which are related in sequence. Still others (e.g., ISI) integrate almost anywhere, although they prefer certain sequences.

Transposition can give rise to **simple insertions** or just **co-integrate**. In simple insertion, a conservative transposition displaces the transposon from its location to a new location without replication. In cointegrate formation, each strand of the transposon is copied, resulting in two complete copies separated by a lost chromosome segment and integrated in direct orientation.

10.8.7.3. Consequences of transposition

Transposons may benefit the host cells by introducing new genes. They may inactivate a host gene by interrupting a coding sequence or by terminating transcription or translation upstream. However, the gene can be reactivated by precise excision of the transposon. Finally, transposons can activate neighboring genes by initiating transcription. In this function some transposons act as switches for adjacent genes (**gene switches**) by reversible recombination between inverted repeats. In one direction, they initiate transcription whereas in the other they either fail to initiate it, or terminate it.

Today's gene therapy vectors are either viral or nonviral. Among the viral vectors, retroviral vectors have been studied widely for their ability to integrate that a single copy of the gene precisely and permanently into an active region of host chromatin. In retroviral vectoring systems, the viral genome is split into its *cis*-acting sequences (the vector), and its *trans*-acting viral structural genes (latter inserted into vector produced cells). The shortcoming in this approach is that the cis and trans-acting sequences often recombine during propagation of the vector, resulting in replication-competent retrovirus (RCR). To overcome such shortcomings of this most popular form of gene therapy, some improvements have been suggested: (i) substituting synthetic components for viral ones, starting with the vector and proceeding towards a synthetic gene delivery particle (Hodgson, 1995) and (ii) some retro elements can be used for site-specific integration or cell-specific transcription targeting (Krichner *et al.,* 1995).

Retroelements include retroviruses, defective retroviruses, retro transposons, short interspersed repetitive elements (SINES) and pseudogenes. Retroelements are major structural components of the genome, wherein they have both positive (evolutionary) and negative (insertional mutagenesis) effects. They also in some cases regulate the expression of cellular genes (Mc Donald, 1993). Among the retro elements studied as transcriptional promoters, murine leukemia viruses (ML Vs) are the only retrovectors studied clinically. However, another emerging candidate of this class is the virus-like 30s (VL30) retrotransposon found in vertebrates. This retrotransposon resembles retrovirus in structure but contains no retroviral structural gene (Hodgson *et al.,* 1983). They lack any sequence similarity to retrovirals. But they can co-pack into the retroviral virions and are transferred to the recipient cells along with the retroviral genome (Besmer *et al.,* 1979). They are converted into DNA via retroviral reverse transcriptase and then integrated into the human genome from where they are transcribed. Thus, VL30 can be used to transmit DNA efficiently.

Minimal *cis* acting synthetic retrotransposon vectors have been synthesized by comparing the sequences of two types of retrovectors (VL30s and ML V) and identifying the most essential ones such as L TR boundaries, adjoining primer binding sites, and putative packaging. Synthetic oligonucleotide primers were used to gene-amplify the L TRs of a VL30 element (NVL-3) together with essential and non-essential *cis*-acting sequences with convenient linking and gene insertion sites. They are then synthesized using the polymerase chain reaction (PCR), the LTR blocks are isolated from agarose gels (to eliminate primers and spurious products), digested with the appropriate restriction endonucleases at the joining region, re-purified on agarose gels, ligated at common restriction sites to create cohesive termini, digested at the distal termini and finally ligated to a compatible plasmid (pGEM3) (Chakraborty *et al.,* 1993). The so formed synthetic retrotransposon vectors were biologically active in the sense that they transmit via retrovirus particles, integrate properly, and express their gene(s) as RNA and protein.

10.8.8. Oligonucleotide carrier systems

Introduction of a potent gene inhibitor is just as important as introducing a missing gene or correcting a mutant gene. These are especially required in cases like neoplastic infections and some inherited diseases (Cohen, 1991). Various "antisense" strategies have been developed.

"Antisense" compounds/oligonucleotides are short synthetic strands of nucleic acid which bind to DNA, mRNA or extracellular proteins in a complementary fashion and arrest protein synthesis by inhibiting transcription or translation (Inouye, 1988; Miller and Ts'O, 1988; Stein and Cohen, 1988).

Three basic approaches have been explored in this area.

1. Antisense oligonucleotides bind to mRNA and block translation. This approach was used to inhibit translation of HIV tat RNA (Stevenson and Iversen 1989).

2. Triple-helix-forming oligonucleotides which bind in a sequence-specific manner in the major groove of duplex DNA (Shaw *et al.,* 1991).

3. Oligonucleotides which bind to extracellular proteins and inhibit their enzymatic activity (Wang *et al.*, 1993).

The rapid degradation *in vivo* by 3'-exonuclease digestion (Tidd and Warenius 1989) limits the use of natural oligodeoxynucleotides. Therefore, nuclease resistant oligonucleotides were synthesized by modifying the phospho-diester backbone. Among them, the widely investigated ones are phosphorothioates (anionic) and methyl-phosphonate analogs (nonionic) (Goodchild 1990).

The major problem of oligonucleotide delivery is their limited access to the intracellular (and intranuclear) space. Chemical means to overcome cell exclusion, e.g. the design of more lipophilic compounds are limited as they may compromise the selectivity and binding affinity for the intended target DNA or RNA. Such problems can be addressed by employing intracellular carrier systems. Both cellular as well as intranuclear delivery of an antisense oligonucleotide hybridized to ICAM- I was found to be increased in the presence of a cationic liposome carrier (Lipofectin®).

10.8.9. Self-organized DNA-photonic nanostructures

Some techniques developed for the synthesis and modification of nucleic acids for their potential use in clinical diagnostics are "DNA probes" and, as therapeutic agents, "antisense DNA". Synthetic nucleic acids are generally referred to as "oligonucleotides". These synthetic nucleic acids have inherent recognition properties and can be easily functionalized. They are ideal candidates for creating molecular photonic and electronic devices. Oligonucleotides incorporated with simple electronic/photonic devices, which self-assemble into organized structures have been studied and are exemplified by fluorophore labelled oligonucleotides; these carry out an efficient Forster non-radiative energy transfer process (Heller *et al.*, 1983; Heller and Morrison 1985; Heller and Jablonski 1987).

Forster non-radiative energy transfer is the process by which a fluorescent donor (D) group excited at one wavelength transfers its absorbed energy via resonant dipole coupling process to a suitable fluorescent acceptor (A), which emits it at a second wavelength (Lakowicz, 1983). When two fluorophore labelled oligonulceotides are designed to bind (hybridize) to adjacent positions of a complementary target nucleic acid strand, they transfer fluorescent energy efficiently. Since these functional molecular components can be programmed, via their nucleotide sequence, they can be designed to self-assemble and organize into large and more complex but defined nano structures.

10.8.10. Polymer-based gene delivery systems

Like cationic lipids, cationic polymers such as polybrene and DEAE-dextran have been studied for transfecting cells *in vitro*. However, their *in-vitro* use has been was limited *by* low efficiency, cytotoxicity and non-biodegradability (Ishikawa and Homey 1992; Kawai and Nishizawa 1984). Recently, non-linear polycationic polymers have been synthesized and proposed for non-viral gene delivery (Haensler and Szoka 1993).

Intramuscular administration of plasmid-based gene expression systems results in lower uptake of plasmids from an isotonic saline formulation leading to varying levels of therapeutic protein expression *in vivo* (Manthotp *et al.*, 1993; Levy *et al.*, 1994). To overcome such problems, an interactive polymeric gene delivery system that enhances the delivery of genes to muscle cells has been reported (Mumper *et al.*, 1995). This system offers opportunities for the treatment of both muscle and peripheral nerve disorders.

The polymeric gene delivery system using interactive polymers like polyvinylpyrrolidone (PVP) and polyvinyl alcohol (PVA) and other polyvinyl derivatives has been reported to interact with a DNA plasmid via hydrogen bonding and hydrophobic interactions. Among this class of polymers,

PVP and PVA interact with plasmids through hydrogen bonding (Mumper *et al.*, 1995). This type of interaction protects the plasmids from the action of nucleases probably via hydrophobic coating of the plasmid. Being hypo-osmotic, PVP based gene formulations elicit improved dispersion of plasmids through the extracellular matrix of the muscle tissue, probably due to osmotically increased intracellular space.

The function of administered genes within muscle cells can be controlled by using muscle-specific gene expression systems. An *in vivo* pulsatile production of proteins may be beneficial for certain therapeutic applications. This type of *in vitro* and *in vivo* pulsatile production of proteins can be achieved by using 'gene switches' that are activated by low molecular weight drugs (Wang *et al.*, 1994). 'Gene switches' are modified receptors which do not bind to their respective hormone or other endogenous hormones, but selectively bind with antagonistic drugs that act as agonists at low doses (Wang *et al.*, 1994). These gene switches are constitutively expressed within the target cells and are designed to be part of a gene expression system. This gene expression system contains both the gene switch and a therapeutic gene.

Starburst ^{TM} polyamidoamine (PAMAM) dendrimers are a new type of synthetic polymer characterized by a branched spherical shape and a high density surface charge. These charges help bind various forms of nucleic acid by electrostatic interactions. This ability has been explored for effective delivery of 'antisense oligonucleotides' and 'antisense expression plasmids' (Bielinska *et al.*, 1996). PAMAM dendrimers are a new class of highly branched spherical polymers that are highly soluble in aqueous solution and have a unique surface of primary amino groups (Latallo *et al.*, 1996). They can be precisely synthesized and produced in large quantities like proteins. These molecules fall in the size range of 10 to 100 °A. The well defined structures of these molecules with their large number of surface primary amino groups interact on an electrostatic charge basis with biologically relevant polyions, such as nucleic acids, antibodies, or contrast agents.

Gene expression systems encoding reporter genes have been complexed with different generations of dendrimers (e.g. PAMAM; Tomalia *et al.*, 1990; Service, 1991). These dendrimers appear to condense DNA through electrostatic interaction of their terminal amines with the phosphate groups of DNA molecules. Such complexes seem to control the efficiency of delivery. The ability of PAMAM as carriers to enhance transfer of DNA into mammalian cell lines has been confirmed by using well defined analytical techniques based on such reporter gene systems as firefly luciferase and bacterial β-galactosidase. Structures of some widely used gene-packaging polymers are shown in Table 10.4.

10.8.11. Peptide-based gene delivery system

Site-specific delivery of gene expression system to target cells has involved the use of ligands that recognize cell-surface receptors and use them for receptor-mediated cell entry. A current limitation for efficient gene delivery via both non-specific and receptor mediated gene transfer is the effective elimination of a gene expression system by endocytic vesicles. Poly-L-lysine, a cationic carrier, has been studied by many workers (Wilson *et al.*, 1992; Wagner *et al.*, 1991) for delivery of DNA via the endocytic pathway. In order to impart tissue selectivity, the carrier was covalently coupled to a receptor selective targeting molecule such as asialoorosomucoid, a galactose-terminal asialoglycoprotein targeted to the hepatocyte asialoglycoprotein receptor, to human transferrin or antithrombomoulin antibody 34°A. The release of viral genome from endosomes by either disruption or fusion with endosomal membranes was reported by Curiel *et al.*(1991) and Cotton *et al.* (1992), wherein replication-defective adenoviral particles were added to DNA/ transferrin-poly-L-lysine complexes. To reduce the risk of immunogenicity associated with polypeptides, in particular polylysine, a novel synthetic condensing peptide with a shorter amino acid sequence was reported.

Table 10.4: Structures of some widely used gene-packaging polymers

Polycations

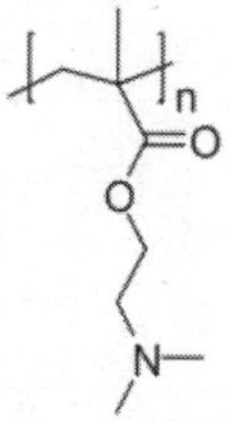

poly(2-(dimethylamino)ethyl
methacrylate)
(PDMAEMA)

branched
poly(ethylenimine)
(b-PEI)

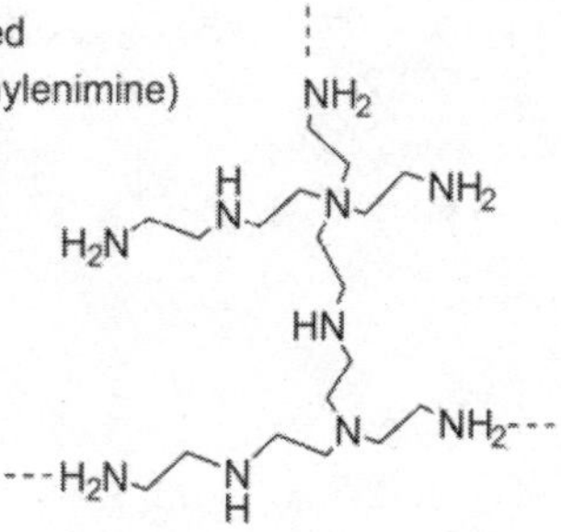

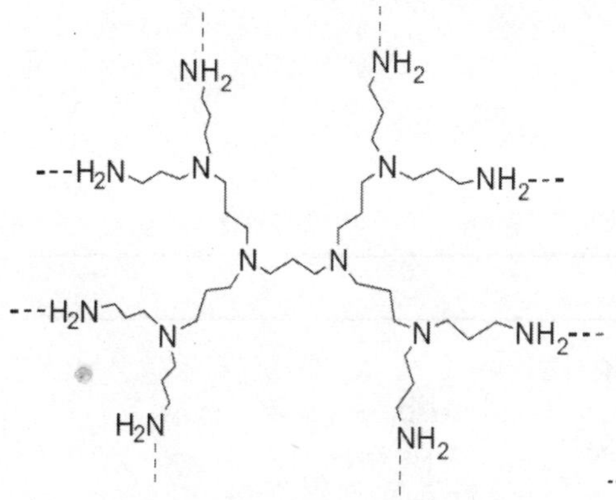

poly(propylenimine)
(PPI)

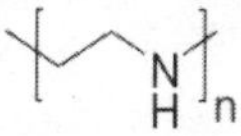

linear poly(ethylenimine)
(L-PEI)

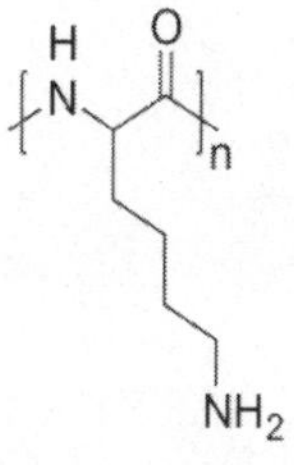

poly(lysine)
(PLL)

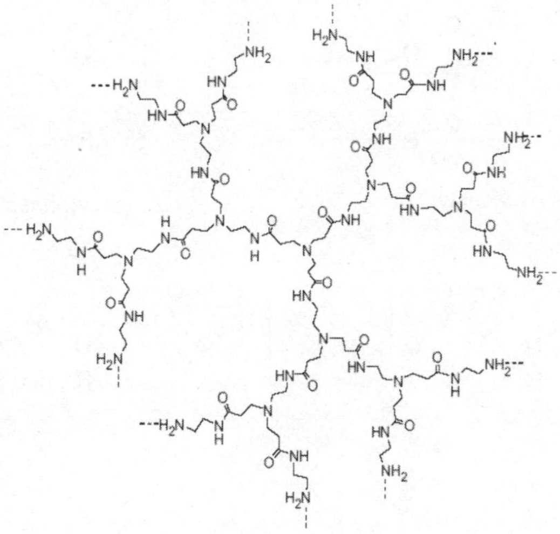

poly(amidoamine)
(PAMAM)

Polycations *(continued)*

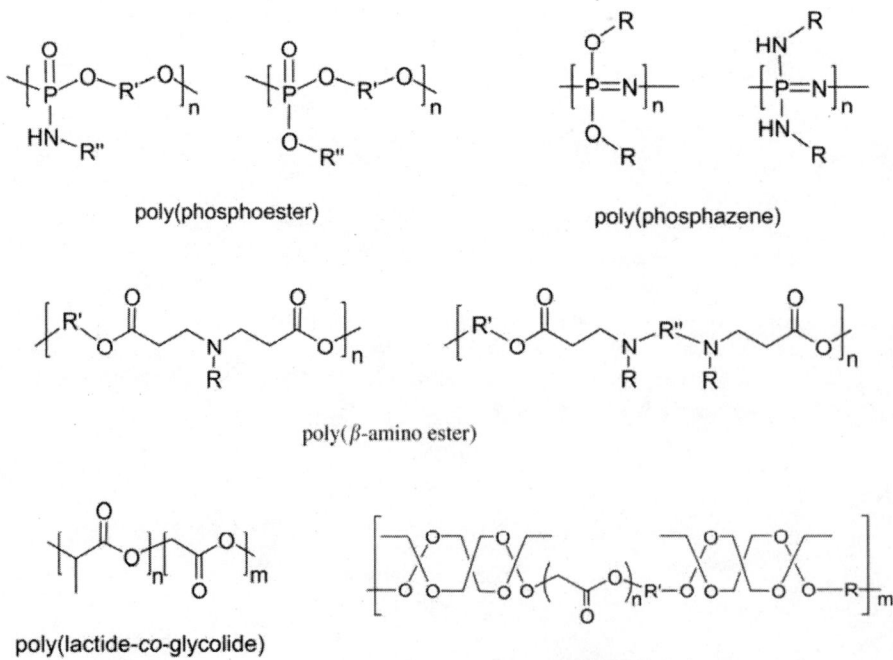

cyclodextrin-containing polycations

spermine

chitosan

Biodegradable polymers

poly(phosphoester)

poly(phosphazene)

poly(β-amino ester)

poly(lactide-*co*-glycolide)
(PLGA)

poly(orthoester)

Biodegradable polymers *(continued)*

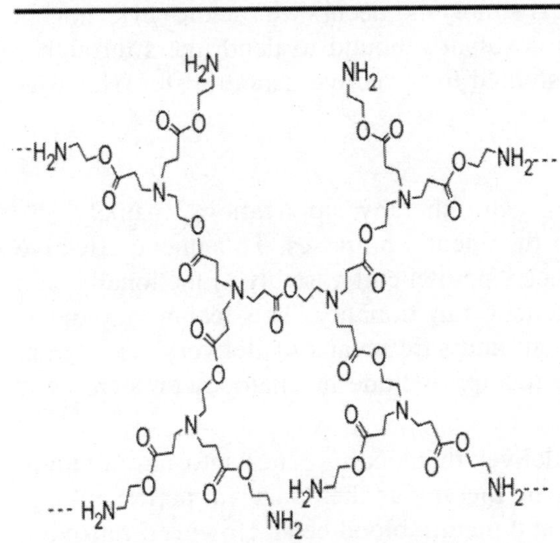

hyperbranched poly(amino ester)
(h-PAE)

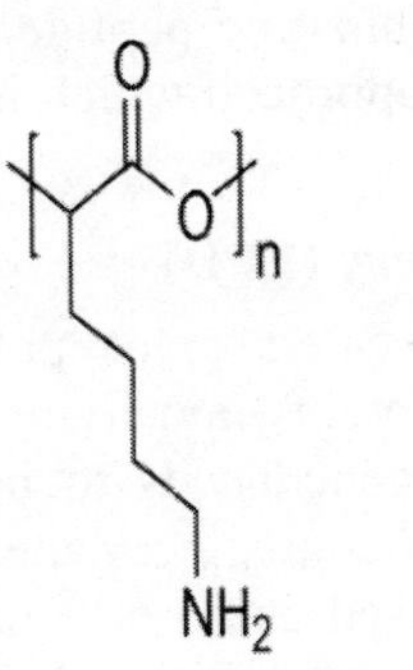

poly(α-[4-aminobutyl]-1-glycolic acid)
(PAGA)

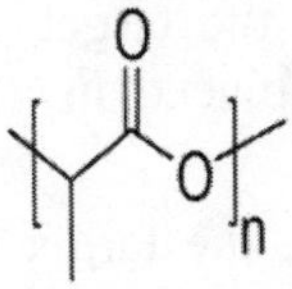

poly(lactic acid)

(PLA)

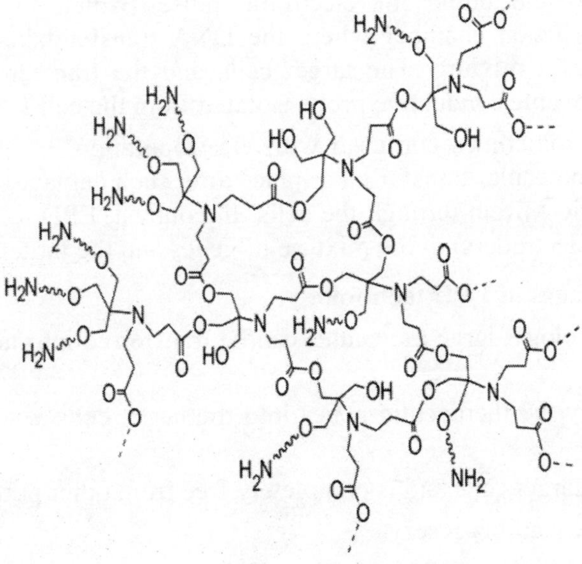

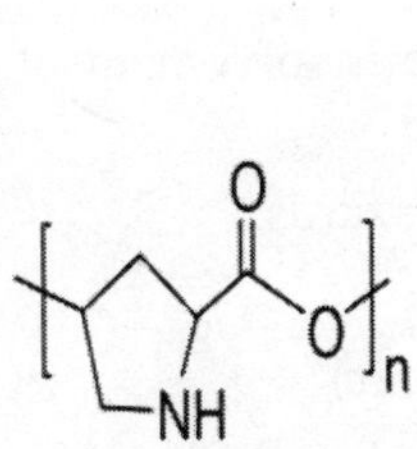

poly(4-hydroxy-1-proline ester)

(PHP-ester)

networked poly(amino ester)

(n-PAE)

These peptides form α-helices with a hydrophobic face with strong apolar amino acids; their hydrophilic face is dominated by negatively charged glutamic acid residues. The haemolytic activity of these novel fusogenic peptides is pH dependent. Haemolysis occurs in acidic pH, not in physiologic pH. Synthetic amphipathic peptide (GALA) covalently bound to dendrimers through a disulfide bond exemplifies the approach which has been studied for effective gene transfer (Haensler and Szoka 1993).

10.8.12. Electronic pulse delivery (EPD)

The EPD technology has revealed great potential in gene therapy applications, namely, by transferring DNA, RNA and proteins into living cells for therapeutic purposes. To achieve effective gene therapy, the therapeutic gene needs to be introduced permanently, stably, functionally and heritably into the target cells to confer permanent new genetic functionality. This technology meets the above criteria and can be used as an effective, efficient and safe means of delivery. The target cells suitable for EPD delivery and for protein and gene therapy include haematopoietic stem cells (HSCs), hepatocytes, fibroblasts and myoblasts.

The major challenge facing gene therapy is how to deliver therapeutic genes into non-dividing cells such as the HSCs. These cells are ideal targets for gene therapy as their survival period is long. They can renew themselves and produce new progenitors and mature blood cells. However, retroviral vector mediated delivery to these cells is problematic as the cells are quiescent. This problem can be overcome by using EPD technology.

EPD is a sophisticated method which subjects the targeted cells to precisely controlled pulses of electric field in a computer controlled molecular transfer system (Zhao 1995). The EPD system consists of a controller and a reaction chamber. The controller, driven by an EPD computer, accurately controls the output of electronic pulses which in turn are controlled by different parameters. The reaction chamber where the DNA transfer takes place holds the target cells and therapeutic gene as a mixture. The target cells and the transfer material are placed in a reaction chamber with a movable conductive probe isolated from the cell/DNA solution.

EPD has been sometimes confused with electroporation. In electroporation, the target cells are damaged and the molecular transfer takes place after such damage. Also, electroporation often applies a significant electric current through the cells. In contrast, EPD technology limits the electric current and no contact of electrode(s) to the mixture of genes and the target cells is needed.

10.8.12.1. Advantages of EPD technology

1. Using this technology, large molecules can be transferred into target cells (e.g. DNA construct, 15 kb).

2. EPD inserts only the therapeutic genes into the target cells without the involvement of any other molecules.

3. It is toxic to the target cells and is completely free from other potential hazards.

4. It has a good cell viability reserve.

5. EPD technology has remarkable transfer efficiency (about 80–90% transfer)

6, It offers a wide spectrum from which to select device parameters for different transferring applications.

7. It can be operated as a batch or continuous process.

8. The time taken by this method for transfer is very short (from a few seconds to a minute). (Zhao *et al.,* 1990; 1993; Hoeben *et al.,* 1992; Palemer *et al.,* 1989; 1991; Lu *et al.,* 1993).

10.8.13. Electroporation

Electroporation is a physical method which involves the use of non-viral delivery system. In this process, gene is transferred into cells in suspension by applying pulses of high-voltage electricity that creates pores in cell membranes.

Electroporation is one of the several physical methods used for gene transfer (Grierson, 1991). It involves the use of short electrical impulses of high field strength. The generated impulses increase permeability of the protoplast membrane, thereby facilitating the entry of DNA molecules into the cells. The pulse required for an efficient transfer of the DNA by electroporation is generated by discharging a capacitor across the electrodes from a specially generated electroporation chamber. The generated pulse may be either a high voltage (1.5 kV) rectangular wave pulse for a short duration or a low voltage (350 V) pulse for a longer duration. DNA transfer takes place by suspending the protoplast-containing vector DNA in an ionic solution between the electrodes. Using electroporation successful transfer of genes has been achieved into protoplasts of tobacco, petunia, maize and rice.

10.8.14. Aquasomes as gene carriers

Self-assembled molecular carriers ("aquasomes") (Kossovsky *et al.,* 1996) have been formed from preformed carbon ceramic nanoparticles and self-assembled calcium phosphate dihydrate particles with a glassy carbohydrate coating. They have been studied for the delivery of genes (Kossovsky *et al.,* 1995). *In vitro* studies have been carried out by immobilizing DNase (a therapeutic enzyme used in the treatment of cystic fibrosis) onto a ceramic carbon nanocrystalline particulate core coated with pyridoxal-5-pyrophosphate (Hnatyszyn, 1995). A marked retention of biological activity was observed with surface immobilized DNase on colloidal calcium- phosphate nanoparticles coated with polyhydroxyl oligomeric films. Kossovsky (1996) suggested a model to explain how the synthetic product of self-assembling chemistry using non-covalent forces comprising lithium ceramic nanocrystalline core with a polyhydroxyoligomeric film coating appears (Fig. 10.16)

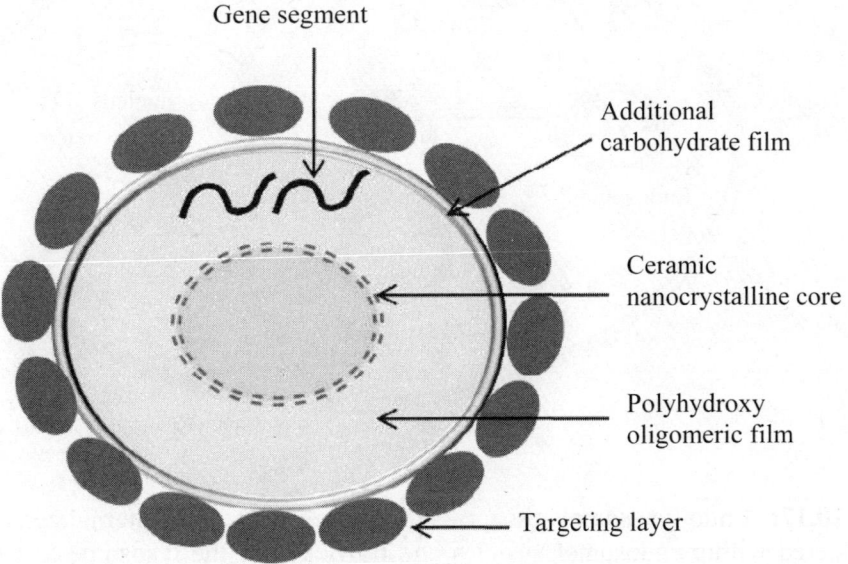

Fig. 10.16: Aquasomes for gene therapy

10.8.15. Proton sponge

Any vector used to deliver a DNA to the nucleus functions either by cell membrane rupture or by nuclear targeting. This membrane rupture occurs either directly at the cell surface or after endocytosis. In both cases, the viral fusogenic protein undergoes a major conformational change induced either by binding to a cell surface receptor or by the acidic nature of the endosomal compartment. Use of different cationic vectors, i.e., cationic lipids and cationic polymers raises the question of the buffering capacity of a vector under physiological conditions and its transfection potentials. To understand this issue, several polycations like lipopolyamines and polyethylenimines with substantial buffering capacity below physiological pH have been studied as efficient transfection agents. These agents can transfect without any addition of lysosomotropic bases, cell transfecting agents, or membrane disrupting agents. These agents/vectors deliver genes as well as oligonucleotides (Demenix and Behr 1996).

Several synthetic macromolecular compounds with high amine group densities have been studied. These cationic compounds are able to compact the DNA, but owing to repulsion between like charges near each other they are not fully protonated at physiological pH. A constitutive candidate for the development of proton sponge system has been the commercially available polymer polyethylenimine (PEl): as one in every three atoms of this polymer is an amine group, the system shows variability in protonation level, which increases between pH 7 to 5.

The mechanism of gene transfer using polycation/DNA complex is depicted in Fig. 10.17. The polycation/DNA complex probably enters the cell via spontaneous endocytosis.

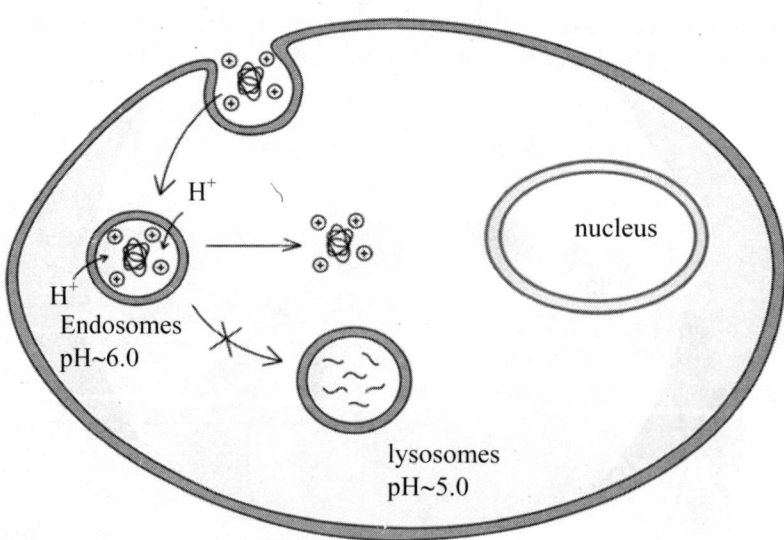

Fig. 10.17: Endo-lysosomal escape—Polyplexes that are internalized via endocytosis can be sequestered within endosomal vesicles and trafficked to the lysosome to be enzymatically degraded. Vesicles acidify (pH reduces from ~6 to ~5), through the action of vesicle-bound proton pumps, as they mature along the endo-lysosomal pathway. Strategies to escape lysosomal degradation have exploited the influx of protons by incorporating 1pH-sensitive moieties into vector designs

When this positively charged complex interacts with the cell membrane, a high local concentration of PEl is produced in the endosome. During this intracellular trafficking, the buffering capacity of the PEl not only tends to inhibit the lysosomal nuclease, which has an optimal acidic pH, but also alters the osmolarity of the vesicle. Thus, proton accumulation occurs by endosomal ATPase which leads to the influx of chloride anions. This will result in swelling of the polymer by internal charge repulsion and osmotic swelling of the endosome, finally leading to the rupture of the endosome followed by the liberation of PEl. This rapid liberation of PEl-DNA complex is of importance in gene therapy.

10.8.16. Magnetofection

Magnetofection is a process of using magnetic particles and magnetic force to enhance and to target nucleic acid delivery. The principle of magnetofection is quite simple. Naked nucleic acids or gene vectors are bound to magnetic nanoparticles, a magnetic field is used to accumulate nucleic acids or vectors at target cells (Fig. 10.18). In vitro, this is straightforward, *in vivo*, several challenges remain as are discussed later. The first to pursue this idea were Kuehnle and Kuehnle in a patent application filed in 1994 (U.S. patent 5516670 issued in 1996) where they describe torpedo-like magnetic particles that may be suitable to deliver DNA as well as an apparatus generating a magnetic field for delivery. Chan describes the use of pulsating magnetic fields for introducing nucleic acids that are associated with magnetic nanoparticles into cells in a patent application filed in 1996 (U.S. patent 5753477 issued in 1998). These patents contain interesting ideas and instructive experimental setups. It has turned out that cellular uptake during magnetofection involves the same mechanisms that also govern conventional transfection/transduction processes (Huth *et al.*, 2004). Therefore, the chemical, physical, and biological characteristics of nucleic acids and vectors are as essential in magnetofection as they are in conventional nucleic acid delivery. Important characteristics of vectors and their components to be assembled with magnetic nanoparticles are predominantly charge, size, and the possibility of chemical coupling reactions. Accordingly, strategies of assembling vectors with magnetic particles can be developed and magnetic particle synthesis can be adjusted to the needs of the assembly process.

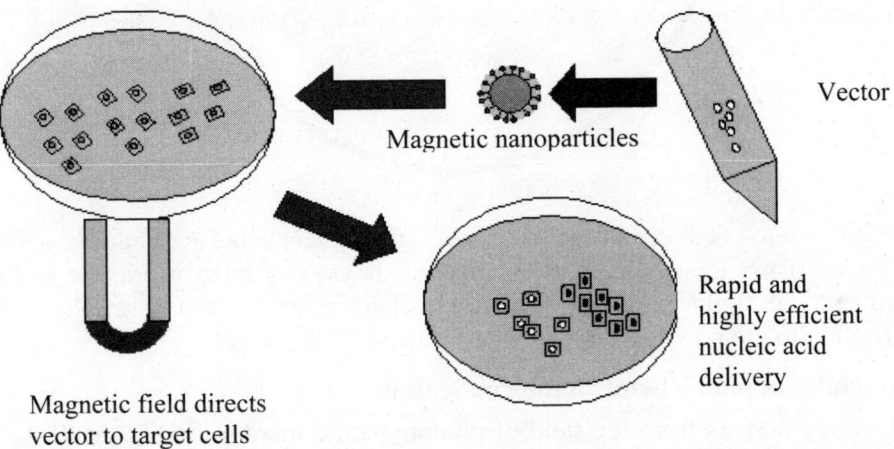

Fig. 10.18: Magnetofection in cell culture. Nonviral or viral vectors associated with magnetic nanoparticles (magnetofectins) are accelerated onto a cell layer in a culture dish through magnetic force. The result is rapid and efficient transfection, even at lower vector doses

10.8.17. Photochemical internalization

Photochemical internalization (PCI) is a technology for efficient and site-specific gene delivery. This technology enables light-directed delivery of a variety of therapeutic molecules into the cell cytosol. The technique can be used in vitro and in vivo for site-specific delivery of proteins, DNA carried by non-viral and viral vectors, peptide nucleic acids (PNA), and small interfering RNA (siRNA). PCI is based on light activation of amphiphilic photosensitizers that localize in the membranes of the endocytic vesicles. When photosensitizer containing cells or tissues are exposed to light at wavelengths absorbed by the photosensitizers, photochemical reactions are induced that rupture the membranes of the endocytic vesicles. Hence, the constituents of these vesicles (e.g., drugs or nucleic acids) can be released into the cytosol where they may act on their target or further translocate to the nucleus. As the effect of the photochemical treatment is dependent on light exposure, the enhancement of drug- or gene delivery is achieved only at illuminated regions (Fig. 10.19).

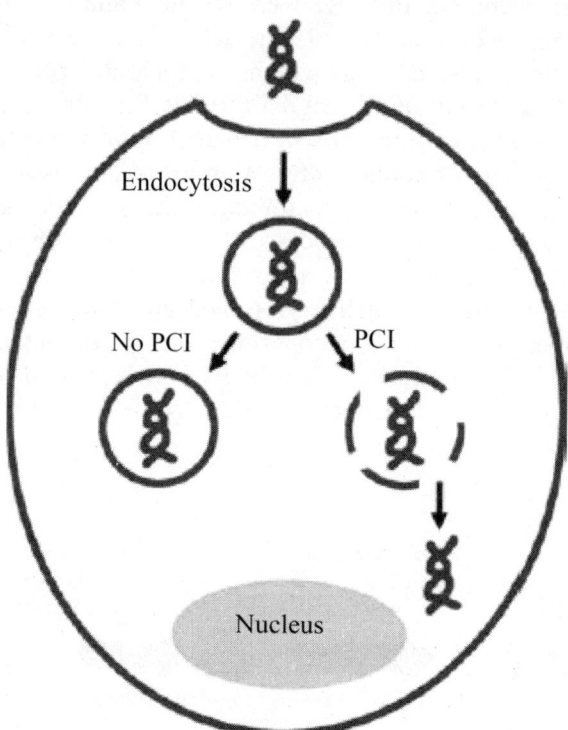

Fig. 10.19: PCI-mediated delivery of nucleic acids. The nucleic acids are endocytosed and localize in endocytic vesicles. If not translocated, the nucleic acids are degraded inside the endocytic vesicles. The PCI treatment (i.e., light exposure of photosensitizer treated cells) permeabilizes the endocytic membranes, leading to the release of the nucleic acids into the cytosol

10.8.17.1. Principles of photochemical internalization

The PCI technology derives from the field of photodynamic therapy (PDT). In PDT, the phototoxic effects induced by a photosensitizer, light, and oxygen are used therapeutically (Brown *et al.*, 2004). It is a minimally invasive treatment with great potential in malignant disease and pre-malignant conditions. PDT involves the application of a photosensitizer in combination with the targeted delivery of light, at a wavelength specific for the activation of the photosensitizer. Usually, wavelengths in the 600–800 nm range are used for optimal therapeutic effects. Upon light-dependent activation, the photosensitizers undergo photophysical reactions that lead to generation of reactive oxygen species (ROS) under aerobic conditions, most predominantly $^1O_2$. In PDT, the photochemical generation of ROS results in apoptosis or necrosis, harnessed therapeutically for the purpose of eliminating malignant tissue. However, as $^1O_2$ has a short lifetime (<0.04 µs) and a short range of action (10–20 nm) in cells (Moan *et al.*, 1991), only structures very close to the photosensitizer will be affected after light exposure. The phenyl rings are the most efficient photosensitizers for enhancing gene delivery. Photosensitizers that localize to other cellular structures than the endocytic vesicles are not efficient for inducing the PCI effect (Prasmickaite *et al.*, 2001; Berg *et al.*, 1999; Engesaeter *et al.*, 2006). The light source used to induce the photochemical reactions may be any source emitting light of wavelengths absorbed by the photosensitizer.

10.8.18. Miscellaneous approaches

A synthetic lipophilic polylysine-phosphatidylethanolamine conjugate ("lipopolylysine") has been used successfully as transfecting agent. A non-viral delivery system involving a chemical method of calcium- phosphate or DEAE-dextran conjugate formation that mediated gene transfer has been reported.

Other approaches include insulin as a receptor-specific carrier, linked to positively charged N-acylurea, albumin, plasmid packed with a polylysine-asialoorosomucoid conjugate. An albuminemia in nonobese rats by hepatic transfection of the structural human gene which resulted in albumin secretion has been demonstrated.

The ambiguous transferrin receptor may serve as a target for more generalized gene delivery of polylysine-transferrin conjugate. This concept is generally utilized in achieving high level of iron by rapidly dividing neoplastic cells. In place of "forced" cell entry by cationic liposomes, a method involving physiologic pathway of endocytosis may be utilized in effective targeting. This method also has the disadvantage that it is enzymatically degraded during endolysosomal pathway. Accordingly, augmentation of gene expression was accomplished using chloroquine to suppress lysosomal degradation. An escape mechanism from endolysosomal compartment has been designed by hybridizing polylysine-DNA complex and A V. Here, A V enables the complex to escape endolysosomal degradation.

10.8.18.1. Targeted modification of human genes

Targeted modification of genes by exogenous DNA has gained wide attention in recent years especially in the alteration of the human genome. It involves a site directed approach to the replacement of defective genes. The rationale behind this is the "Nature's" way of mixing the gene, i.e., the exogenous DNA should contain a region with the same nucleotide sequence as of the target gene, so that homologous recombination can occur. Depending on the arrangement of the incoming sequences relative to the target, the recombination may either introduce new sequences into the recipient chromosome by a single crossover, or substitute sequences by gene conversion or double crossover events. One recent advance in this field includes linearized plasmids with restriction enzymes to produce a double strand break within the region homologous to the gene target.

10.8.18.2. Transgenic approaches

Transgenic animals have been developed as models for studying gene regulation. The DNA is introduced into fertilized eggs and subsequently integrated into both somatic cells and germ cells. For example, the introduction of metallothionine/growth hormone fusion genes into mice stimulates the production of growth hormone in tissues that normally synthesize metallothionine. Induction of metallothionine promoters with metals causes treated mice to grow to about twice their normal size. Several genetic diseases in mice, including thalassaemia, have been treated by using tissue-specific expression from a variety of human genes.

10.8.18.3. Gene therapy with engineered stem cells

Treatment of disorders involving blood cells can be cured by gene therapy. Hematopoietic stem cells are removed from an affected individual and transfected with functional genes. The engineered stem cells are then reinjected into the individual. This method has been studied with individuals suffering from severe combined immunodeficiency disease (SCID) resulting from a defective gene encoding adenosine deaminase (ADA).

10.9. GENETICALLY-SELECTED MEDICINE—PHARMACOGENETICS AND SINGLE-NUCLEOTIDE POLYMORPHISMS (SNPs)

Identifying the genetic factors associated with common ailments is like trying to find a needle in a haystack. Efforts are underway to speed up the search by packaging human genetic variations into more manageable bundles, under the International HapMap Project. While the human genome sequencing project, completed in April 2003, gave us the "Book of Life', the HapMap will help gene–hunters to zoom in quickly on informative chapters or pages. It is expected to "provide the missing link between the DNA sequence of the genome and the way in which the genome influences the risk of disease (Dennis, 2003).

Geneticists who wish to know why some of us are more susceptible than others to succumb to a particular disease, proceed by sampling populations that are affected by the disease, and study single nucleotide polymorphisms (SNPs). These SNPs are points in the genome at which one base can differ between individuals. If a particular SNP is inherited with the disease, it strongly indicates that a gene that confers susceptibility lies somewhere nearby.

Clinical pharmacogenetics deals with the study of individual responses of people to different drugs. Countless deaths worldwide probably result from the side effects of drugs: on the other hand, thousands of patients happen to take drugs that for them have no effect at all. These diverse responses to drugs usually arise from SNPs.

Regulatory agencies are greatly interested in pharmacogenetics in the context of drug-regulatory decision-making, and to frame guidelines to encourage those who wish to market new drugs to submit relevant genomic data. Biomedical researchers have started thinking about how to use genomic data to avoid prescribing drugs that may either kill, have serious side effects, or just won't work. Adverse reactions to prescription drugs annually extract a heavy toll of human life. Millions of patients are treated with drugs that, for them, never do much good. Beta-blockers, prescribed to reduce blood pressure, are ineffective in one-third of patients; some antidepressants are ineffective in half of the people who take them (Abbott, 2003). In the past, most pharmaceutical companies have been afraid of being forced to abandon their traditional blockbuster approach to drug development in favour of the potentially less lucrative method of targeting therapy to restricted groups of patients most likely to benefit. But now they are attracted by the possibility of greatly reduced costs for clinical trials (Anonymous, 2003).

It is our genes that determine the way we react to drugs. Small genetic variations between people–or polymorphisms–can change the activity of proteins that carry a drug to its target cells or tissues, inactivate the enzymes that activate a drug or aid its removal from the body, or modify the structure of the receptor to which a drug binds. Variation in immune system genes can influence how particular drugs are tolerated. All these small genetic variations mean that the dose at which a drug will be effective may vary greatly from person to person–contrary to the current general practice of 'one-size-fits-all' prescribing.

The genomics revolution has created the tools to identify people who don't fit the standard prescribing mould. SNPs are single-letter changes in the genetic code that are found scattered throughout the genome. They can be used to highlight polymorphic genes that influence our response to individual drugs. Regulatory agencies are considering whether or not some drugs should be labeled as being suitable only for individuals with a defined genetic profile.

Studies on SNPs and their predictive value are also enhancing understanding of the working of approved drugs. As the price of identifying SNPs falls, physician may expect to receive more pharmacogenetic data from drug companies, along with appropriate genetic tests, to help them select the best therapy for an individual patient. While pharmacogenetics will undoubtedly improve therapeutics, their arrival and adoption will be gradual. The rationale of the HapMap project is to exploit our understanding of the genetic shuffling that occurs during the production of sex cells to increase the efficiency of gene searches. When the cells divide to give rise to eggs or sperm, pairs of chromosomes line up and exchange portions of genetic material in a process that is not entirely random: the breaking, exchange and rejoining occur at particular points. So block of sequences have been inherited down the generations from our common ancestors without being split up. Although the blocks vary widely in size, most are about 10,000 bases or more in length (Gabriel *et al.*, 2002).

The DNA sequence of a block is termed a haplotype. Common haplotypes can be identified by sampling only a few key SNPs. For each block, only a few common haplotypes in the population seem to exist. The HapMap should therefore enable geneticists to examine the entire genome rapidly for disease genes, perhaps by analysing as few as 300,000 SNPs (Gabriel *et al.*, 2002). The map may also prove useful to study how people respond differently to prescription drugs, according to their particular genetic make-up. The HapMap project consortium intends to produce a haplotype map based on the similarities in block structure and common haplotypes for the European, African and Asian populations. Although the block architecture will be similar, the common haplotypes may vary between different populations in terms of composition and frequency. The aim is to provide useful tools for gene discovery.

The project does face some technical challenges: the first being to determine which of the millions of SNPs identified so far will be most useful in making the maps. Some SNP variants, for instance, occur at such low frequencies that they cannot be studied in the sampled populations. Another challenge is to ensure that the researchers have a good, even coverage of SNPs across the entire genome. The plans are to construct the initial map by studying 600,000 SNPs scattered across the genome al intervals of around 5,000 bases. Further SNPs are then to be identified where needed to define haplotype blocks. A parallel study is going on to scrutinize every known SNP in ten selected regions of the genome, each some 500,000 bases long, to reveal whether the map can be produced using fewer SNPs or whether more will be required. A third issue relates to patenting problems. It is feared that some people could combine the consortium's data (which is open and accessible) with their own, and then patent the findings in a manner that restricts other's ability lo work freely with the HapMap data. Haplotypes, unlike SNPs, come closer to patentability.

In fact, one company, Perlegen (Mountain View. California) claims already to have made its own haplotype map. In 2001, the company unveiled its data for human chromosome 21 (Patil *et al.*, 2001). Some leading pharmaceutical firms have enlisted Perlegen to sift through their clinical DNA samples to track down genetic markers that might explain why individual patients respond differently to drugs (Dennis, 2003). Pharmacogenetics involves the study of the influence of genetic variation on drug responses. An early example was in the 1950s with a muscle relaxant succinylcholine. Some patients who were given this drug suffered serious respiratory arrest on the operating table. Succinylcholine is normally metabolized very efficiently by an enzyme called cholinesterase. But 1 in 2,500 people carry two defective copies of the gene for this enzyme, and suffer severe paralysis of muscles, including those needed for breathing, when given the drug.

Being rare, such reactions are often missed in clinical trials which typically involve a few thousand patients. They are revealed when a drug is widely prescribed. If such reactions occur in an identifiable group of patients, the drug label can specifically exclude them. In the case of succinylcholine bad responders may be detailed by measuring cholinesterase activity in the blood. The Food and Drug Administration (FDA) is now on the verge of deciding to re-label an approved drug to exclude bad responders identified by SNP analysis alone. Mercaptopurine, approved in the 1950s, is used to treat childhood leukaemias and other cancers. Like all anticancer agents, it is intrinsically toxic, and there is only a narrow dose range within which the therapeutic benefit exceeds its toxicity. But some patients suffer life-threatening bone-marrow damage at doses that are tolerated well by others.

In the mid-1990s researchers began to compare the sequences of the gene for the enzyme thiopurine methyltransferase, which metabolizes the drug in patients with and without the toxic reaction. Three SNPs have since been identified, either of which results in an enzyme that allows mercaptopurine to linger in the body at dangerous levels. Thus SNP testing enables clinicians to estimate the risk of mutations rather than measuring activity of the enzyme. In fact, some hospitals have already started subjecting patients to genetic tests before prescribing mercaptopurine (Abbott, 2003).

10.10. GENES, HUMAN PHYSIOLOGY, AND GENE THERAPY

Our genes code for all the proteins of the body. If an enzyme, hormone, or other protein needed by the body is not made, or is made incorrectly, severe diseases can result. Recent developments in recombinant DNA technology, molecular genetics, and gene therapy have provided diagnostic and therapeutic tools for several neurological disorders. Great achievements have been made in neurogenetics and have led to the chromosomal localization of many diseases. The chromosomal loci of disease genes that cause Mendelian-inherited neurologic disorders may be identified by the use of restriction fragment length polymorphisms (RFLPs). Linkage strategy makes use of the way genes are inherited. An ordinary human cell contains 23 pairs of homologous or matching chromosomes. Somewhere among thousands of genes on the 23 pairs, there may be a single defective gene that may be responsible for the disease. The symptoms and progression of various diseases have been known for centuries, but their biochemical defects are still in most cases not understood. This is true for most of the known genetic diseases.

It has become possible to localize and identify the defective gene itself. In most diseases tremendous effort is required as a vast territory of 23 pairs of human chromosomes consisting of linear molecules of double-stranded DNA with a total length of almost 3 billion base pairs has to be searched. A "gene" is a tiny but complete unit of genetic information consisting of about 10,000 base pairs. The task of finding the gene itself involves correlating the inheritance of a distinctive segment of DNA – a "marker"– with the inheritance of disease. This strategy can help localize the mutant gene within about 2 million base pairs, i.e., to less than a thousand of the human genome. The identification of a genetic marker closely linked with a disease means that the gene's inheritance pattern can be followed. This approach enables one to design tests for diagnosing carriers and future disease victims. Modern biotechnology has made practicable prenatal detection of disease and production of therapeutic agents for the treatment of disease. Recombinant DNA technology permits human disease to be defined at the molecular level. It provides an opportunity to map and clone receptors and design drugs to fit them, making it possible to develop specific therapy for many a disease. Missing enzymes can be replaced in people suffering from such metabolic neurological disorders as Gaucher's disease or Tay-Sachs disease.

The identity of a DNA marker linked to the Huntington's disease locus has brought within reach locating an autosomal gene, permitting the development of pre-symptomatic testing in families afflicted with the disorder. Use of "positional cloning" (earlier termed "reverse genetics") has led to the identification of the gene products for many diseases. Some 500 genetic diseases are known to affect the brain and the nerves. Some common diseases for which the gene product has already been identified include retinitis pigmentosa, retinoblastoma, chronic granulomatous disease, cystic fibrosis, neurofibromatosis-1, Duchenne-Becker muscular dystrophy, and Huntington's disease.

Ever since the invention of recombinant DNA technology, which made genetic engineering feasible, most research in genetics, has been run in "reverse". Reverse genetics begins with a particular gene of interest. The scientist fiddles with that gene in a cell culture or a living organism, watches what happens, and then tries to deduce the gene's function. It is a classic, powerful, reductionist approach. But the finding that the genome includes hidden genes –functional sequences that were misclassified as junk–highlights a major problem with reverse genetics: it can lead to tunnel vision. So recently several geneticists have reverted back to the older practice of "forward" genetics as a way to identify both conventional and unconventional genes that they don't know about.

Phenomix, a biotechnology company in LaJolla, California, has set up a production line for making mutant mice. In each group of mice, mutations to random points in the genome disable not just standard protein-coding genes but also hidden genes that make only active forms of RNA (Gibbs, 2003). The company starts with both healthy mice and mice that have diseases analogous to common human illnesses, such as diabetes, asthma, arthritis and Parkinson's disease. Some mutations induce or alleviate symptoms of these disorders in the mice. Genetic screening then determines which mutations accounted for the effects. Whether the approach will inspire better drug designs remains to be seen. But forward genetics has already unearthed genetic phenomena such as functional pseudogenes that no one knew were possible (Gibbs, 2003).

In principle, gene therapy is based on the simple and appealing idea that if one has the wrong version of a given gene; one just exchanges it for the correct version and gets cured. In practice, it is not so simple because no suitable and efficient vector exists that can carry the desired genes into human cells in a fully controllable manner. Gene therapy is aimed at efficient, specific and safe delivery of therapeutic DNA molecules to the inside of cell nuclei. Even though over 12 years have elapsed since the first gene therapy trial (Anderson, 1990) and even after intense research and more than 600 clinical trials, no gene therapy has yet been approved (Luo, 2004) because of difficulties relating to delivery. The major hurdle is the lack of efficient, specific and safe DNA delivery system, and particular cancer gene-therapy for solid tumors because the therapeutic agent is a large sized macromolecule (DNA) and because the solid tumor represents unique difficulties in DNA drug distribution, interstitial penetration and cellular targeting (Luo, 2004). Identifying barriers along the DNA delivery route is extremely important for the efficient delivery of DNA drugs to solid tumors.

The most serious barriers appear to be interstitial penetration, transportation, and cellular targeting. The idea is to provide adequate amounts of drugs that are close to targeted cells because the actual destination for all gene delivery is the cell nucleus. One important but challenging task for cancer-gene therapy is how to increase the expression level of the therapeutic gene (usually toxic) in targeted tumor cells while at the same time avoiding its expression in normal tissue. Some approaches have been suggested to cross the above barriers (Luo and Saltzman, 2000; Lundstrom, 2003; Wiethoff and Middaugh, 2003). One involves intratumoral injection, which boosts drug convection, enlarges tissue pore sizes and increases interstitial connectedness, but a problem with intratumoral injection of viral vectors is systemic toxicity – expression of therapeutic genes in normal tissues, particularly in the liver. Also, some leakage during the injection can contribute to viral dissemination to healthy tissue (Wang *et al.*, 2003). It is likely that some more hitherto undetected barriers may be identified in the coming years. It is however clear that no single delivery method or vector can meet all the requirements in cancer gene-therapy (Luo and Saltzman, 2003). Viruses show higher efficiency in DNA delivery *in vivo*, but non-viral approaches have better safety profiles, tighter controls in composition and more flexibility in design. A viral and non-viral hybrid system (e.g., virus combined with polymers, polymers modified with viral properties, or both) may possibly be a better option for drug delivery in general and DNA delivery in particular (Luo, 2004). Various viral vectors for the gene delivery are shown in Figure 10.20.

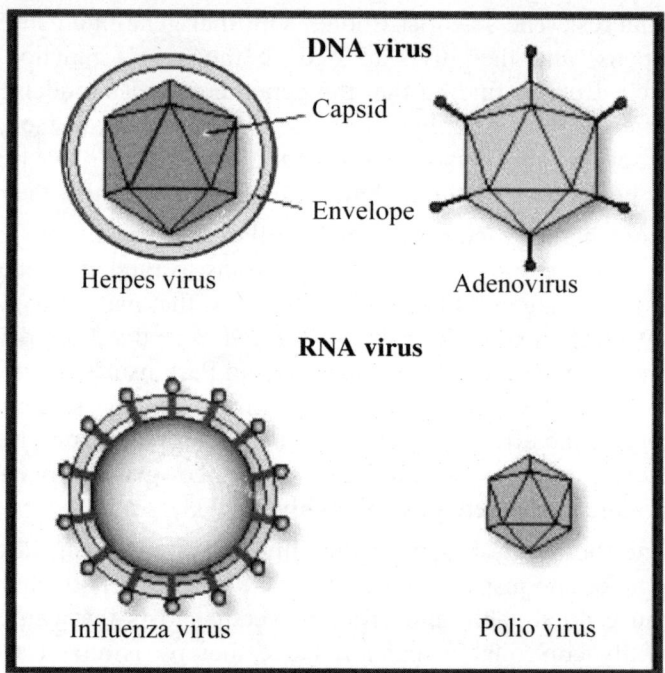

Fig. 10.20: Viral morphology. Herpesvirus, adenovirus and polioviruses all have icosahedral capsids or protein coats that surround and protect the viral genome, which may be DNA or RNA. Herpes and influenza viruses are also surrounded by a lipid bilayer that may be studded with proteins

The history of gene therapy has witnessed both high and low points. One particularly low point was the death of 18-year-old Jesse Gelsinger in 1999, whose immune system overreacted to the invasion of a retroviral vector. The high point occurred when the Necker Hospital in Paris successfully cured the X-linked severe combined immune deficiency (X-SCID) of several so called bubble babies, using a retrovirus coaxed into delivering the missing gene into the children's bone marrow cells (Gross, 2003). This was in fact the first example showing that gene therapy could actually cure a human disease. Unfortunately, however, after some time, in early 2003, there was severe set back when the second of the 10 children treated was diagnosed with leukemia- it emerged that there was a small risk that the gene transfer might activate an oncogene, but the observed frequency of cases points to the susceptibility that the vector prefers inserting the gene I a place where it can cause cancer. There is need to determine why the inserted gene tends to land in the wrong place. Various approaches for gene therapy and their merits and demerits are shown in Table 10.5

Table 10.5: General characteristics of gene therapy vectors for gene transfer

Gene transfer	Advantage	Disadvantage	Clinical application
Retrovirus	Efficient entry into cells	Need high titer Limited payload	Suitable for permanent correction
Adenoassociated Herpes poxvirus HIV-1	Stable integration Biology known	Immunogenetic Difficult to control and stabilize expression Can induce adverse events Random insertion	Extensive use in marking studies Specific virus for specific disease, e.g., herpes-neurology
Liposomes	Commercially available Easy to use Targetable Large payload	Entry into cells Integration rate	
Naked DNA	Ease in preparation; Safe no size limitation;	Inefficient entry into cells; not stable	Topical application
Complexed DNA	More efficient uptake than naked DNA; protected from degradation; targetable Unlimited construct size	Not stable Inefficient cell entry Limited tragetability	Limited clinical use; Vaccination
Artificial chromosomes	Autonomous vectors No insertion required	Unpredictable chromosome and centromere formation	Experimental: only in human transformed cells
Artificial cells	Designer potential	Complexity	Conceptual

The above setback has affected work on gene therapy around the world. In Germany, there is cautious support and around 250 patients are undergoing experimental treatment involving gene transfer, but a few have been halted. In the United States, a new gene therapy trial targeting age dependant macula degeneration was allowed to proceed in February 2003. In Britain, a smaller scale trial of X-SCID gene therapy, similar to the one at Paris, has now been allowed to continue. Meanwhile, the UK government released an official report on genetics, entitled *'Our inheritance our future'*: Realizing the potential of genetics in the NHS with plans of incorporating recent advances in genetics into the mainstream health care offered by the National Health Service (NHS). This document lists the attempts to find new treatments, including gene therapy, alongside enhanced antenatal screening, genetics-related counseling, and legislation against DNA theft. According to this document, gene therapy might become available within 5 to 10 years. It pledges substantial government funding for gene therapy research targeting disorders caused by mutations of a single gene, and to develop a gene transfer therapy against cystic fibrosis, the commonest of such diseases in Britain. It is also intended to provide ready access to facilities where suitable vectors for gene therapy can be produced by geneticists (Gross, 2003).

10.11. DISEASES AND GENE THERAPY

Diseases wherein gene therapy has been focused upon include -

- Cystic fibrosis
- Thalassaemia
- Malignant melanoma
- Pediatric AML
- Neuroblastoma
- Adenosine deaminase deficiency SCID
- Hemophilia B
- Chronic myleogenous leukemia
- Hepatitis B
- Hypercholesterolemia
- Diabetes
- Cardiovascular diseases
- Phenylketonuria
- Acquired immunodeficiency syndrome (AIDS)

The basis of gene therapy of a few of the above diseases is discussed below in brief.

10.11.1. Insulin-dependent diabetes mellitus

Diabetes can be classified into Type-1 or insulin dependent diabetes mellitus (IDDM) and Type-2 or non-insulin dependent diabetes mellitus (NIDDM). Among the two, IDDM is an autoimmune disease, produced as a result of destruction of insulin-producing β-cells of the pancreas. At present, careful monitoring of blood glucose levels, multiple injections of insulin, diet control and exercise regimens are the treatments prescribed for IDDM.

As the β-cells are destroyed in IDDM, any attempt to restore and reconstitute the insulin gene expression must be directed to an ectopic organ. The liver fits in as the right target, as it is the principal effector organ in maintaining blood glucose homeostasis and ketogenesis. A somatic gene therapy has been attempted. The results observed were encouraging (Kolodka *et al.*, 1995). A recombinant retroviral vector, LX/rINS, encoding the complete sequence for rat pre-proinsulin lcDNA under the transcriptional, control of the viral LTR promoter was constructed and used to transduce rat hepatocytes *in vivo* (Ullrich *et al.*, 1977).

10.11.2. Hemophilia B

Hemophilia B is a X-linked blood coagulation disorder resulting from a deficiency of factor IX production, which ultimately leads to severe bleeding. Normally, the treatment for this is protein replacement therapy. Due to the short half-life of factor IX in the circulation, the goal is not achieved. To overcome this problem and to provide an effective therapy, recombinant retroviral and adenoviral vectors encoding canine factor IX to transduce the hepatocytes to hemophilia B in dogs have been studied (Kay *et al.*, 1993; 1994). An infusion of amphotropic retroviral vector encoding the canine factor IXcDNA under the transcriptional control of the viral L TR (LX-CFIX) was administered into the portal vasculature of hemophilia B dogs. An increase in plasma factor IX concentration was recorded (Evan *et al.*, 1989).

10.11.3. Cystic fibrosis (CF)

Cystic fibrosis is a complex, multi-system disease which is inherited in an autosomal recessive pattern. The goal of gene therapy in young children is to prevent the generation of infectious lung disease, whereas the realistic goal in CF patients with established lung disease is to prevent a further loss of lung function. CF is due to a mutation in the CFTR gene, which perturbs the salt and water composition of secretions, slows the mucocilliary clearance of airways and promotes infection. However, this does not explain the predilection for infection in CF with Staphylococcus aureus and Pseudomonas aeruginosa. CF is dominated by the respiratory tract involvement which characterizes airway obstruction caused by accumulation of thick purulent secretions and progressive deterioration of lung functions. Majority of the patients acquire broncho pulmonary infections due to *Pseudomonas aeruginosa*. The current therapy involves the use of antibiotics and approaches to improve, mucous clearance. A large number of studies have established that many gene transfer vectors are highly efficient *in vitro*. It has been found that transformed and primary cultures of human airway epithelia in non-polarized and polarized culture conditions have been relatively easy to transduce with the help of adenoviral vectors containing CFTR, with correction of the CF CI- transport defect (Zabner *et al.* 1994). Fig.10.21 depicts the cystic fibrosis gene and it protein product.

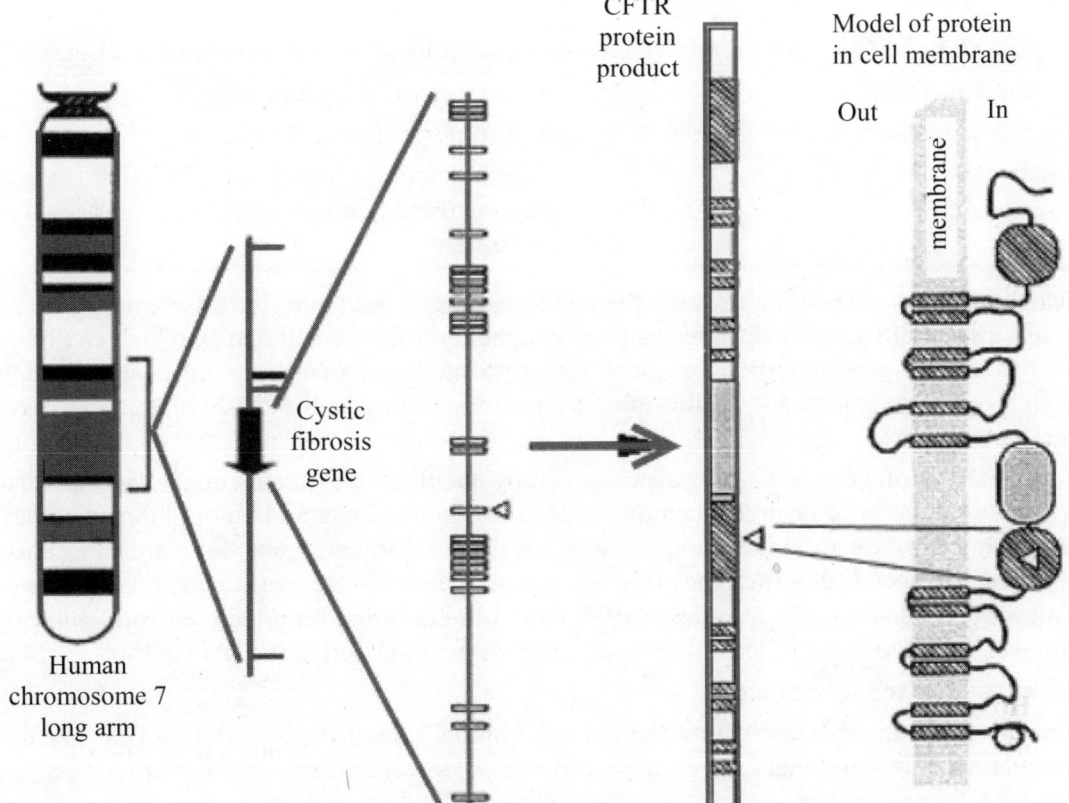

Fig. 10.21: Cystic fibrosis gene and it protein product

The efficiency of adenoviral vectors has shown substantial variation in-vivo. However, adenoviral gene transfer efficiency to the uninjured airway of primates and man appears to be very low. New generation modalities in the treatment of CF utilize recombinant human deoxyribonuclease I (rhDNase) which reduces the viscoelasticity of respiratory tract (Shak *et al.*, 1990). A plasmid encoding for chloramphenicol acetyl transferase (pRSY2-CAT) complexed with Lipofectin liposomes has demonstrated for its in vivo functioning by Brigham *et al.*, in 1989. Similarly, cationic liposomes have also been reported for the delivery of CFTR to the respiratory tract (Logan *et al.*, 1995). For a detailed review refer Schreier and Swayer 1996. Inspite of the wide advantages there are certain problems posed for CF gene therapy. The preeminent problem for CF gene therapy is the functional efficiency of the system in vivo. The second problem is the safety profiles of the various vectors that continue to be uncovered both in *in vitro* studies and in clinical trials. Certain vectors like adenoviral vectors can slow the cell cycle and induce apoptosis. Novel cationic lipid formulations appear to be more inflammatory in lungs. In addition the amount of liposomal lipid delivered to the lung and surfactant metabolism in pulmonary surface liquids will have to be evaluated.

10.11.4. Cardiovascular disease

Cardiovascular disease is currently the commonest cause of mortality. Over 7 million individuals suffer from cardiovascular ailments every year around the globe. Although significant progress has been made in the areas of treatment and prevention of various cardiac diseases, these diseases remain the leading public-health problem. In spite of many recent advances there are still diseases which are not having an effective therapy; familial hypercholesterolemia (FH) and retenosis after angioplasty are just two example.

Table 10.6: Various gene transfer techniques applicable to cardiovascular diseases

Viral mediated methods	Retrovirus, sendai virus, adenovirus
Lipid-mediated methods	Liposomes, cationic liposomes
Other methods	Microinjection, mechanical (high energy microparticle bombardment), implantation (myoblast)

Research has been diversified towards the use of gene as a medicine for different ailments. Gene therapy towards cardiovascular diseases can be brought about by gene transfer, which can be carried by three methods of gene modification, gene replacement, gene correction and gene augmentation. Among them gene augmentation is the most promising technique for modifying targeted cells in cardiovascular therapy.

The application of gene in cardiovascular therapy includes the treatment of vascular diseases, cardiac diseases, metabolic disorder, hereditary coagulation disorders and autoimmune diseases. The vascular wall: heart, liver, kidney and muscle have been target organs for cardiovascular gene therapy. There has been little experience of in vivo gene transfer to the heart. Direct injection of DNA is the only way of gene transfer into the heart to date. Lin et al, first reported the expression of β-Gal in cardiomyocytes in vivo for at least four weeks after direct injection in the left ventricle.

10.11.5 Nervous system disorders

Gene therapy has attracted focus as a therapeutic approach to diseases such as CF, cancer, HIV infection and various hormonal and enzyme disorders. However, disorders of the central nervous system (CNS), though of prime importance, have not gained much attention possibly in view of that structurally and functionally complicated CNS which also involves differentiated cells having different functions and different anatomical connections. Similarly the neurons are also highly complicated both functionally and anatomically. In case of other candidate diseases, gene therapy was possible because these diseases are relatively easy for *in vitro* gene manipulation.

Despite these difficulties, some neurological disorders are promising gene therapy models. Indeed that for certain disorders gene therapy may not require the brain cells: "surrogate" cells, such as autologous fibroblasts, may be useful for delivery of the therapeutic gene products after gene manipulation and transplantation to the brain (Gage *et al.*, 1987). A second factor which has helped in achieving effective gene transfer is the availability of the novel gene transfer vectors capable of transferring the gene directly into neurons and glia *in vivo*. Cultured cells can be genetically modified with retroviral vectors, followed by grafting the cells into living animals.

Table 10.7: Cardiovascular and other diseases and suitable target genes for treatment

Indication	Target gene
Systemic gene therapy	
Familial hypercholesterolemia	Low density lipoprotein receptor
Atherosclerosis	High density lipoprotein
Hypercoagulable states	Tissue-plaminogen
Refractory diabetes mellitus	Insulin
Local gene therapy	
Restenosis after angioplasty	Cell-cycle regulatory gene
Transplant rejection	Leukocyte adhesion molecule
Transplant vasculopathy	Cytokine
Myocardial infarction	Fibroblast growth factor
Cardiac remodeling; Angiogenesis	Transforming growth factor β
Myocarditis	Cytokine
Congenital heart disease	Myocyte differentiation factors
Glomerular diseases	Cytokine, cell-cycle regulatory gene
Aortic aneurisms	Protease

Alzheimer's disease is a neurodegenerative disorder in which there is a progressive loss of cholinergic neurons in the basal forebrain, with associated profound cognitive impairment. Its treatment involves the delivery of nerve growth factor (NGF) which prevents the neuronal loss in addition to ameliorating deficits in learning and memory associated cells. Intracerebral transplantation of genetically modified fibroblasts has been applied to an animal model wherein a sparingly small amount of cholinergic neurons has been observed to produce NGF (Rosenberg *et al.*, 1988).

Parkinson's disease is a disorder in which degeneration of dopaminergic neurons of the nigrostriatal pathways is associated with a severe impairment of voluntary movement. Studies involving grafts of fetal substantia nigra dopamine neurons into dopamine-depleted brain indicated that delivery of dopamine from grafted cells lessens movement disturbances. These studies led to the suggestion that non-neural cells that have been genetically modified to produce dopamine or the dopamine precursor L-DOPA, might also be effective.

While intracerebral transplantation of genetically modified cells may be suitable for some disorders, other disorders will almost certainly require the delivery of genetic material directly into resident brain cells. For this purpose, considerable effort has been devoted to the development of viral mutants to serve as vectors for introducing genetic material into the brain. The first candidate for such a function has been a derivative of neurotropic viruses such as herpes simplex viruses (Breakefield and DeLuca, 1991). Initial studies have shown that herpes virus vectors can be used to infect neurons and glia both *in vitro* and *in vivo*. Lesch-Nyhan disease is one of the first neurogenic disorders chosen as a model for gene therapy (Wills *et al.*, 1984); it was the first disease model to be tackled with a herpes-virus vector. Lesch-Nyhan disease is an inborn error of metabolism resulting from deficiency of the purine-salvage-pathway enzyme by Poxanthine-guanine phosphoribosyl-transferases (HPRT). It involves several prominent neurological abnormalities, including involuntary movements, retardation and self-mutilation. Herpes-virus vectors are promising vehicles for direct gene transfer into brain cells but there are a number of problems which remain to be circumvented.

Adenovirus vectors are also potentially useful vehicles for gene transfer into the brain. Transgenes introduced into the genomes of adenoviral mutants by recombination can be expressed in a wide variety of recipient cell types, including neurons, glia and ependymal cells lining the centricles (Le Gal La Salle *et al.*, 1993).

Gene transfer into peripheral organs for correction of CNS diseases is also in focus. One such example is the inborn error of amino acid metabolism involving phenylketonuria, which is mainly due to a defect in hepatic phenylalanine hydroxylase. Despite this enzyme being expressed predominantly in the liver, the major clinical manifestations of the disease are attributable to the accumulation of toxins, which impair neural function. Similarly, some of the Iysosomal storage disorders which organize in neurophathological changes might respond to genetic modification of bone-marrow stem cells, since these cells are thought to give rise to migratory macrophages that can populate the brain (Hoogerbrugge *et al.*, 1988). Several different approaches, including intracerebral transplantation of genetically modified cells, direct intracerebral introduction of gene transfer vectors, and genetic alterations targeted to peripheral organs, are being actively pursued in animal studies as models for gene therapy of neurological disease (Table 10.8).

Table 10.8: Gene therapy models for neurological disorders

Disorder	Transgene	Method
Neurodegenerative disorders		
Alzheimer's disease	NGF or other tropic factors	Surrogate cells grafted to basal forebrain or cortex
Parkinson's disease		Direct delivery of vector to basal forebrain or cortex
Genetic disorders	Tyrosine hydroxylase	Surrogate cells grafted to the basal ganglia
Phenylketonuria	Phenyalanine hydroxylase	Direct delivery of vector to basal ganglia or midbrain
Lesch-Nyhan disease	HRPT	Transplants of genetically modified hepatocytes
		Direct delivery of vector to liver
Lysosomal storage disease	Lysosomal enzymes	Surrogate cells grafted to brain
		Direct delivery of vector to brain
		Transplants of genetically modified bone marrow cells

Each of these approaches has its own merits and demerits, which render it useful under different circumstances. Further studies will be necessary to characterize the long-term viability of the transplanted cells or vectors and the stability of gene expression. Immunological responses are potentially promising for inducing direct or indirect neuro-pathological changes.

10.11.6. Cancer

Cancer is a disorder of the genetic make-up of somatic cells, which results as clone cells with abnormal pattern of growth control. Human genome contains both normal genes and oncogenes. When a favorable condition is created (for growth) inside the body it converts pro-oncogenes into oncogenes which then multiply and ultimately lead to tumor formation due to uncontrolled growth of such genetically modified cells.

Conventional cancer treatment with chemotherapy, radiotherapy, and surgery aims at destroying the tumor while leaving the normal host tissues intact. In fact, in chemotherapy, a curative dose ultimately turns out to be a toxic dose which destroys normal body tissue(s) while the same in low doses develops resistant tumors. The problem with both surgery and radiotherapy is, however, one of tumor invasion and spread outside areas that are directly accessible to these treatments. In addition, the growth of tumor is observed in adjacent areas other than the main region. Nucleic acid-based gene therapies for cancer are summarized in Table 10.9.

Table 10.9: Nucleic acid-based gene therapy strategies for cancer treatment

Approach	Structure	Mechanism	Target
Antisense	DNA or RNA	Translation arrest RNase activation	mRNA-oncogenes
Antigene	DNA or RNA	Triplex formation Transcription blockage	DNA-oncogenes Transcription factors
Aptamer	DNA or RNA	Binding and inhibition of protein function transcription factors	Protein transcription factors
Ribozyme	RNA	mRNA cleavage	mRNA of growth factors; drug resistance gene; oncogenes

Biological approaches to the treatment of cancer have been realized under certain circumstances where not only the tumor cells are recognized by the host immune responses but also by the effective destructive mechanism (Mestrangelo *et al.*, 1988). Genes encoding cytokines involved in the control of immune system have been produced in sufficient quantities. These cytokines (interferons and interleukins) have shown sufficient biological action against certain types of tumors but their mechanism of action is not clear.

Current research is focused upon human genome mapping by which a comparison between the genetic constitutions of cells exhibiting abnormal growth pattern against their normal growth pattern can be appreciated; Analysis of oncogenes and tumor suppresser genes will, almost certainly, reveal targets for therapy at the molecular level. Gene manipulation has become easier with the help of homologous recombination, retroviral and other gene transferring vectors and antisense technology along with powerful analytical tools such as the polymerase chain reaction (PCR). It will be helpful in manipulating and monitoring cell cultures.

A major difference between normal and cancer cells is the decrease or functional impairment of major histocompatibility complex (MHC) on the surface of tumor cells. The importance of this observation is attested by the fact that tumor cells transfected with MHC class I can not only prevent tumor spread when administered as a prophylactic vaccine, but also induce metastatic remission in established disease in a number of murine models including lymphoma, carcinomas and melanomas.

10.11.7. AIDS

Acquired immunodeficiency syndrome (AIDS), a fatal retroviral-disease is caused by the human immunodeficiency virus (HIV). Its cure is attracting highest priority (Fig. 10.22). The disease is caused by an RNA virus. Researchers wish to seek an agent that can inhibit the *in vitro* multiplication of the virus. Of two different approaches, one aims at finding a nucleoside candidate and the other aims to target reverse transcriptase (RT) present in RNA viruses.

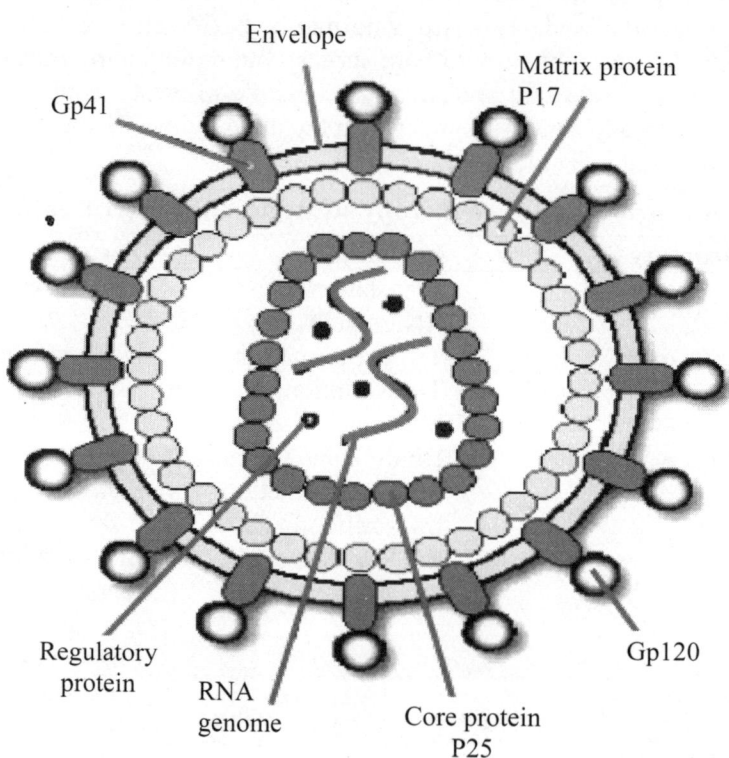

Fig. 10.22: Structure of HIV (an enveloped retrovirus that has a double-stranded RNA genome containing nine genes the capsid consists of a spherical matrix and an inner, cone-shaped protein core. Glycoproteins (Gp) 41 and 120, embedded in the envelope, are crucial for cell entry. Several regulatory proteins, including reverse transcriptase, are stored in the core)

Human immunodeficiency Virus type-l (HIV -I) has circumvented most conventional anti-viral strategies at large through its rapid rate of replication and resultant genetic heterogeneity. However, ribozyme engineering coupled with gene therapy applications may have some potential as a strategy for countering HIV-I infection *in vivo*. "Hairpin ribozyme", an enzymatic RNA molecule, was first isolated from the negative strand satellite RNA (viroid) from a plant pathogen, Tobacco Ringspot

Virus {TRSV} (Hampel and Tritz, 1989). The ribozyme complex consists of a 50 nucleotide (nt) catalytic domain with a 14 nt substrate binding region (Hampel *et al.*, 1990). These two domains fold and anneal into a loop resembling a hairpin. The loop is utilized during rolling circle replication of the small RNA genome. The 14nt tail region of the hairpin binds through complementary base pairing with the substrate and results in the formation of two adjacent helical structures. This helix acts as a handlebar to form a bulge in the center of the substrate strand which is cleaved by the 50nt catalytic domain of the ribozyme. Mutagenesis studies have identified N*GUC sequence as the cleavage site (*-cleavage site) on the substrate. These minimal requirements for ribozyme binding and cleavage made possible the synthesis or genetically engineered base pairing with any other heterologous RNA region surrounding the N*GUC sequence. As this reaction was found to occur at near physiological conditions *in vitro*, it may have potential use in fighting infectious agents.

10.12. NUCLEIC ACID DELIVERY TO MITOCHONDRIA

Mitochondria are composed of a double membrane with an intermembrane space. The innermost mitochondrial space is the matrix. Like all membranes, mitochondrial membranes are composed of a phospholipid bilayer with embedded proteins. The outer membrane, like the plasma membrane, has a lipid to protein ratio of 1:1. It does not offer a barrier to small molecules (<5 kDa), which can simply diffuse through pores in the membrane formed by a membrane spanning protein called porin. The composition of the inner membrane differs from that of the outer membrane in that it is more proteinacious and contains an unusual phospholipids cardiolipin. The mitochondrial matrix is the innermost space enclosed by the cristae membrane and contains a soup of metabolic enzymes, mitochondrial ribosomes and specialized transfer RNAs as well as several copies of circular non-chromosomal mitochondrial DNA (mtDNA). mtDNA is the only extrachromosomal DNA in humans. It is a circular 16.5 kbp DNA which encodes 13 polypeptides, 22 tRNA and 2 rRNA (Fig. 10.23). All 13 polypeptides are the components of mitochondrial enzymes (Vaidya *et al.*, 2009b).

The majority of diseases are originated from mitochondria. They are largely due to incorporation of damaged or mutated proteins into complexes of the electron transport chain. Because complexes are composed of subunits encoded by both mitochondrial and nuclear genes, mutation in any of gene may cause diseases. Since mtDNA is free of exons, it possesses a much higher information density compared to nuclear DNA. Therefore, mtDNA is more susceptible to mutation than nuclear DNA (>20 fold), resulting in a high frequency of mitochondrial diseases.

10.12.1. Mitochondrial genetics and gene therapy

The polyploid nature of the mitochondrial genome (up to several thousand copies per cell) gives rise to an important feature of mitochondrial genetics, i.e., homoplasmy and heteroplasmy. When all copies of the mitochondrial genome are identical it is referred as homoplasmy whereas in case of heteroplasmy there is a mixture of two or more mitochondrial genotypes. The importance of these homoplasmy and heteroplasmy is apparent in reference to mtDNA mutations that lead to mitochondrial diseases. The majority of patients who harbour pathogenic mtDNA defects have a mixture of mutated and wild-type mtDNA (heteroplasmy). The clinical features of mtDNA disease are intimately dependent upon the ratio of mutated and wild-type mtDNA *in vivo*.

The phenotypic defect is only expressed when the percentage of mutated mtDNA exceeds a critical threshold. Gross *et al.*, (1969) demonstrated that mtDNA, unlike nuclear DNA, is continuously being copied and degraded with an estimated half-life between 0.7 and 30 days. By specifically inhibiting the turnover of mutated mtDNA, it is theoretically possible to correct the biochemical defect, prevent clinical progression and potentially reverse some of the pathological features of mtDNA disease.

As described earlier that mammalian mtDNA encodes 13 polypeptides for oxidative phosphorylation complexes, along with the rRNA and tRNA required for their translation, mtDNA defects often lead to dysfunctional ATP synthesis and a range of progressive neuromuscular disorders in patients. First time it was reported in 1988 that mutations of mitochondrial genome can cause human diseases. Genetic mutations that are responsible for mtDNA associated diseases can be categorized into four types: missense, point mutation, deletion, and copy number (Fig. 10.23). A first step towards developing mitochondrial gene therapies is to deliver DNA or RNA molecules to the mitochondria within target cells. Possible approaches are based on delivery of complete genes encoding expressing polypeptides to mitochondria to replace or complement defective genes, or to deliver mRNA molecules to mitochondria to complement defects in mitochondrial tRNA or rRNA genes. Progress towards these goals requires the effective and targeted delivery of nucleic acids to mitochondria.

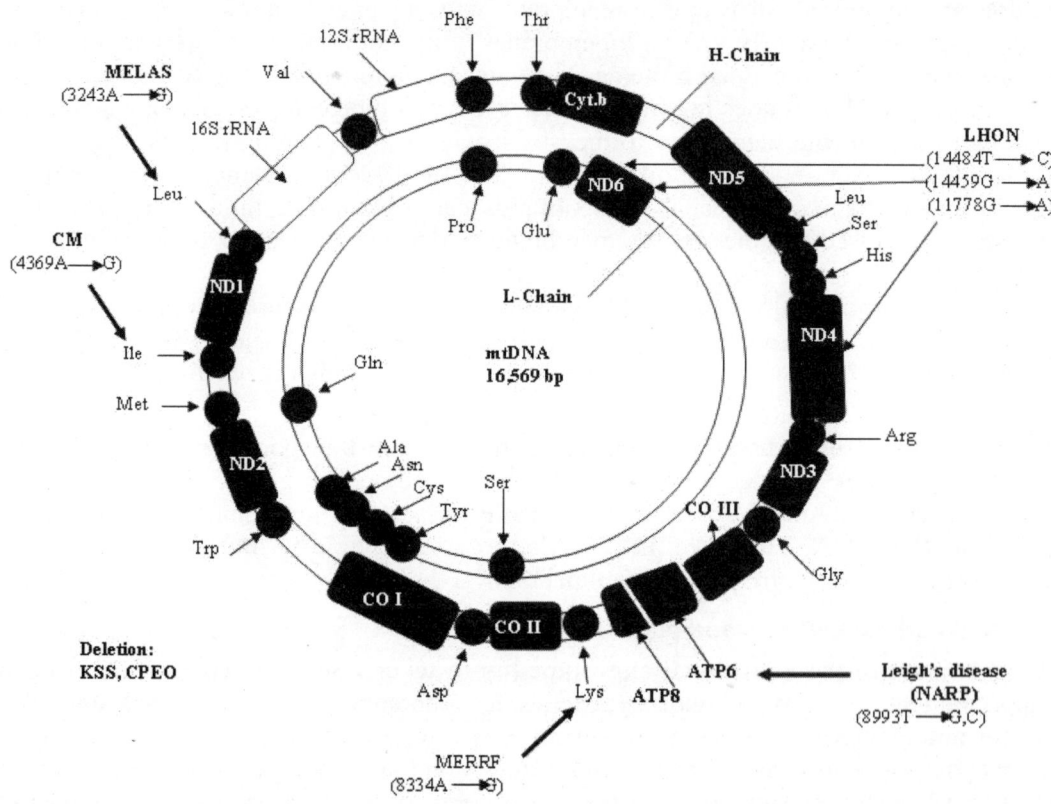

Fig. 10.23: Map of human mitochondrial DNA. It is 16,569 bp long and contains 13 polypeptide-encoding genes, 2 rDNA and 22 tRNA. ND: NADH dehydrogenase coding subunits; CO: cytochrome oxidase coding subunits; ATP: F1F0-ATP synthase coding subunits

10.12.2. Strategies for targeted DNA delivery to mitochondria

There are therapeutic agents including antioxidants, DNA alkylating agent, diazoxide, plasmid DNA, peptide nucleic acids, and fusion proteins which have been tried for their selective targeting to mitochondria. A large number of experiments have been concluded for delivery of these bioactives to selectively alter functioning of one of the mitochondrial membranes, matrix or mtDNA. These bioactives were delivered to the mitochondria either by conjugating them to mitochondriotropic molecules or by selectively complexing them with mitochondria selective vesicular systems like DQAsome or mitochondriotropic liposome.

For efficient and selective targeted delivery of DNA, the therapeutic DNA has to cross the plasma membrane as well as the outer and the inner mitochondrial membrane in order to reach the matrix space. To overcome these barriers, a mitochondria specific delivery system needs to be designed. Such a delivery system must possess the following properties.

- It should bind and condense pDNA.
- It should neutralize the charge of DNA.
- It should protect DNA from nuclease digestion.
- It should be helpful in cellular uptake.
- It should transport the DNA selectively to mitochondria.
- Finally, it should become destabilized upon contact with mitochondrial membranes leading to the release of DNA.

10.12.3. Mitochondrial properties, which help in the designing of carrier systems

Any delivery system can be localized into the mitochondria by using one of the two specific mitochondrial properties- high inner membrane potential of mitochondrial membrane and protein import machinery of mitochondria. These properties can be used for selective transport of the bioactives into the mitochondria from cell cytoplasm after selective localization of the molecule in to the correct cell type and for *in vivo* study into isolated mitochondria. Mitochondrial membrane potential is useful for higher accumulation of positively charged lipophilic cationic molecule in to the mitochondria as compared to other organelles of the cell whereas protein import machinery is useful to deliver therapeutic protein molecules to the mitochondria because mitochondria itself import some necessary peptides from cytoplasm, which are synthesized by nuclear genome of the cell.

10.12.4. Various delivery methodologies for targeted DNA delivery to mitochondria

After years of research it has been known that gene transfer mechanism is a complex process during which the vector has to surpass a plenty of biological and cellular barriers. As a consequence, non-viral gene therapy has captured the attention of biomedical scientist. Nonviral approaches are further classified into two categories: physical and chemical technique.

10.12.4.1. Physical techniques

Several strategies have been developed with an aim to enhance the efficiency of gene transfection using pDNA *in vitro* and *in vivo*. The following physical methods for gene delivery are explored: microinjection and particle bombardment (gene gun); electroporation, sonoporation, laser irradiation; and magnetofection. Electroporation is a process in which controlled electric fields is applied to facilitate the cell permeabilization. It is routinely employed to introduce DNA up to several kilo base pairs in size into isolated yeast mitochondria and has been used to transform mammalian mitochondria as well. Biolistic bombardment with DNAcoated tungsten particles has achieved significant success in isolated yeast mitochondria and living yeast cells. However, this technique has failed so far in mammalian cells. Similar to electroporation, the major advantage of gene gun method is that it does not require the use of complex (and sometimes toxic) delivery systems. In mammalian systems, physical methods like electroporation and biolistic bombardment are restricted to the use of isolated mitochondria. Therefore the use in clinical treatment is dependent on some novel intracellular mitochondrial delivery strategies.

10.12.4.2. Chemical techniques

Chemical carriers are straightforward modules for gene delivery. These may be constructed either by direct conjugation, i.e., homing device conjugated with therapeutic molecules or by carrier based methods, i.e., the carrier systems contain genetic molecules for *in vivo* site specific delivery.

10.12.4.2.1. Conjugation with mitochondriotropics

Mitochondriotropics are molecules which possess high affinity for mitochondria. These molecules have tendency to accumulate inside the mitochondrial membrane because of mitochondrial membrane potential. These molecules have common structural features. Firstly, they are all amphiphilic, i.e., they combine a hydrophilic charged center with a hydrophobic core. Secondly, in the structures of these molecules the π-electron charge density extends over at least three atoms or more instead of being limited to the internuclear region between the heteroatom and the adjacent carbon atom. This tends to the distribution of the positive charge density amongst two or more atoms i.e., delocalization of the positive charge therefore these are also known as delocalized cations (DLCs). There are so many examples of these agents which have been described earlier by various reviewers. Some examples of these agents include rhodamine 123, dequalinium chloride, triphenyl phosphonium ions, cyanine dyes such as N,N,-bis (2-ethyl-1,3-dioxolane) kryptocyanine, Victoria Blue BO. Linking neutral molecules as large as 500 Da to these molecules facilitates their lipid bilayer transport and delivers them to the mitochondria within cells. These agents have been used for selective targeting of antioxidants to mitochondria in intact cells. For mitochondria selective delivery vitamin E was covalently coupled to lipophilic triphenylphosphonium cations (TPP). It was reported that such positively charged compounds could accumulate within the mitochondria up to a thousand-fold higher content in fully energized mitochondria because of negative transmembrane electric potential of approximately 200 mV. Skulachev *et al.* also synthesized new type of compounds (SkQs) comprising plastoquinone (an antioxidant), penetrating cation, and a linker for mitochondrial targeting. The penetrating cations used were triphenylphosphonium and rhodamine 19. Studies concluded that SkQs might be potential tools for treatment of senesence and age-related diseases. Muratovska *et al.*, (2001) also used mitochondriotropics for targeted delivery of peptide nucleic acid (PNA) to the mitochondria. The PNA oligomers used were: H2N-Cys- GTTGGCTCTCT-CO2H and Biotin-OO-GTTGGCTCTCTO-Cys-CO2H, the spacer O was 8-amino-3,6-dioxanoic acid. The oligomers were conjugated with lipophilic phosphonium cation. The developed system reportedly acquires the properties of both lipophilic cation as well as intrinsic properties of mitochondria for the delivery of nucleic acid to the mitochondria in cells. Such as (1) the lipophilic cation facilitates transport of nucleic acid through the lipid bilayers of the plasma membrane and the mitochondrial inner membrane; (2) the plasma membrane potential drives accumulation of phosphonium–PNA conjugates into the cytoplasm; and (3) higher negative inner potential of the energised mitochondria helps in the accumulation of phosphonium–PNA conjugates selectively to the mitochondria.

10.12.4.2.2. Conjugation with mitochondrial leader sequence

An alternative mitochondrial targeting strategy for the delivery of bioactives to mitochondria is based on the mitochondrial protein import machinery. The signal peptide that directs the transport of proteins to the mitochondrial matrix has a sequence consisting of an alternating pattern with a few hydrophobic amino acids and a few positive-charged amino acids. These are short (3–60 amino acids long) peptides. These are also called the mitochondrial targeting signal (MTS) or mitochondrial leader sequences (MLS). The MTS can be linked to other non-mitochondrial proteins to create a chimeric protein that is taken up in to the mitochondrial matrix via the protein import pathway. For example, a MTS has been linked to green fluorescent protein and cytosolic enzymes such as dihydrofolate reductase and cytochrome C oxidase for the targeted delivery of these molecules to the mitochondria. The mitochondrial protein import pathway has also been used for mitochondrial gene replacement. Therefore the pathway could potentially be implied to selectively deliver the nucleic acid (target) and to correct a mutant mitochondrial genome just in a similar way to classical gene replacement therapies that is used to replace a defective nuclear gene by its corrected copy/version. A number of studies have been performed in which DNA was introduced into isolated mitochondria by covalently linking the mitochondria targeting signal peptide (MTS) to ODN, double-stranded DNA, or PNA. It was reported by Seibel *et al.* that these conjugates are transported to the mitochondria through the outer and inner membranes through the protein import machinery. It was also reported that DNA of 17-322 bp in length can be used in this strategy. Thus, the targeting of covalently linked MTS-DNA molecules to mitochondria via the protein import pathway may open up new avenues for the development of mtDNA delivery strategies. As described earlier in the text that CPP or protein transduction domain (PTD) may deliver bioactives and carriers directly to the cytosol, Shokolenko *et al.* developed a combination system consisting of PTD and MTS for the targeted delivery of exonuclease III protein (Exo III) to the mitochondrial matrix. A MTS–Exo III–TAT-fusion protein was constructed by the fusion of MTS and TAT with Exo III at the N- and C-terminus, respectively. In the strategy, PTD functions as a cytoplasmic delivery device whereas MTS performs mitochondrial targeting activity (Fig. 10.24). Choi *et al.*, (2006) also developed a combination carrier system for the targeted delivery of DNA to mitochondria by conjugating mitochondrial leader peptide (LP) to polyethyleneimine (PEI). Mitochondrial LP conjugated PEI (PEI-LP) was synthesized with low molecular weight PEI (2,000 Da, PEI2K). Cell-free DNA delivery assay showed that PEI2K-LP delivered more DNA to mitochondria at a 1.8/1 weight ratio as compared to naked DNA or PEI. This result suggested that PEI2K-LP might be useful for the development of mitochondrial gene therapy system with lower cytotoxicity.

10.12.4.2.3. DQAsomes: A mitochondriotropic vesicular system

As described earlier that mitochondria-specific vectors must possess two properties. First, they should be able to transport DNA to the site of mitochondria. Second, they must not release DNA during endocytosis. Various studies showed that viral and non-viral vectors hardly meet these requirements. Viral vectors are nucleus-bound by virtue of their nature whereas cationic liposomes deliver DNA to the nucleus. It was suggested by Xu and Szoka, 1996 that cationic lipid/DNA complexes destabilize the endosomal membrane and induce flip-flop of anionic lipids from the cytoplasm facing monolayer. The resulting formation of charge neutral ion pairs with the cationic lipid causes the release of the DNA from its vector/carrier into cytoplasm. All these studies showed that cationic liposomes and various viral vectors/carrier are not appropriate vectors for mitochondria specific DNA delivery.

DQAsomes, a mitochondriotropic vesicular system, was investigated by Weissig *et al.* in 1998. Dequalinium chloride is a bolaamphiphile which aggregates in to vesicular system upon sonication. Initially, it was investigated that this system might be used for intracellular delivery of bioactives. In sequential studies it was observed that DQAsomes may be useful for mitochondrial targeting (Weissig *et al.*, 2000, 2001, Vaidya *et al.*, 2009a). For pDNA delivery DQAsomes was mixed with requisite quantity of DNA. DQAsomes form complex with DNA and protect it from deoxyribonuclease-I (DNAse-I) digestion. It was assumed on the basis of various studies that DQAsomes have endosomolytic activity, i.e., it ruptures endosomes when comes in contact with the

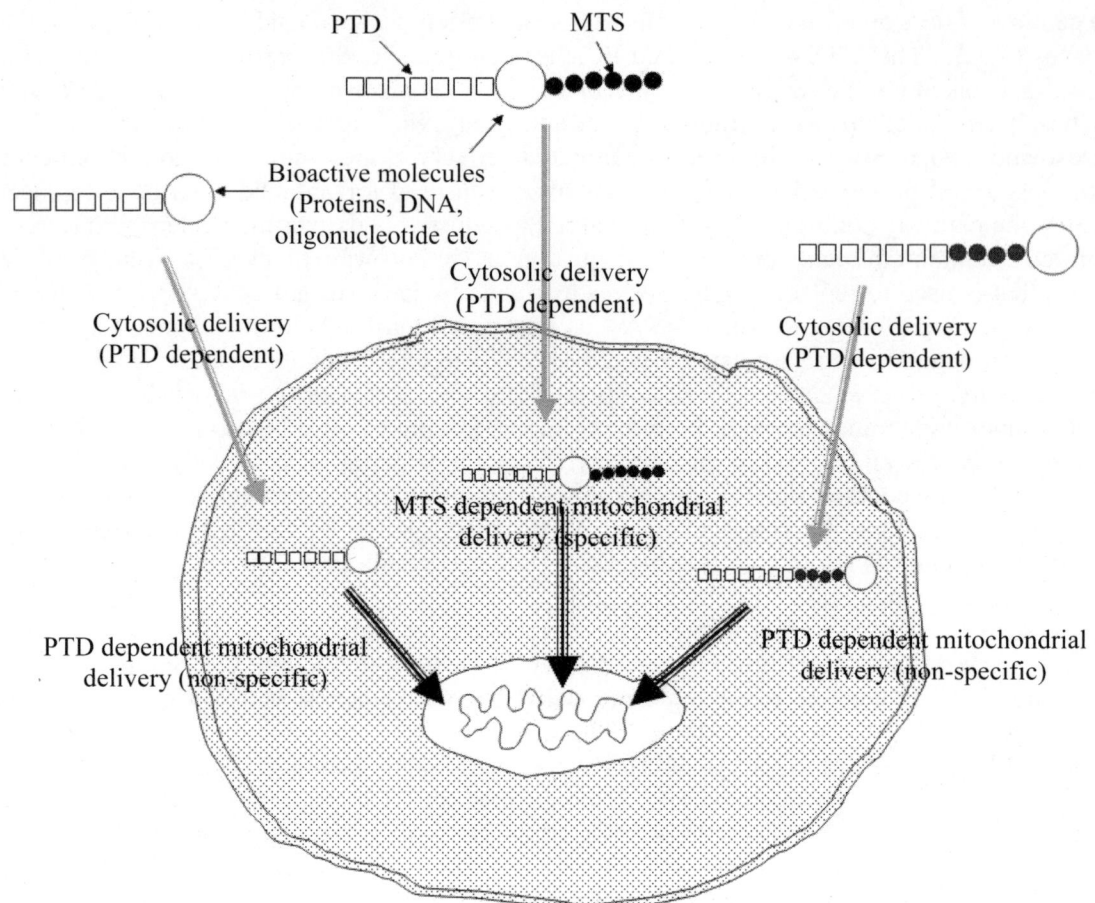

Fig. 10.24: Schematic diagram showing direct entry to mitochondria: cell penetrating peptide (CPP) or protein transduction domain (PTD) dependent cellular internalization. PTD dependent mitochondrial targeting is non-specific delivery however when MTS is conjugated to the PTD conjugated molecules it transverse in to the mitochondria via mitochondrial protein import machinery dependent pathways

endosomal membrane and release its DNA content in the proximity/vicinity of mitochondrial membrane. It was suggested by D'Souza *et al.*, (2003) that after endocytotic uptake DQAsome/DNA complexes release the DNA to a much lesser extent on contact with anionic lipids of the inner cytosolic membrane. However, when these systems come in contact with Cardiolipin-rich mitochondrial membranes the DNA is released. It was suggested that DQAsome–DNA complexes become destabilized upon contact with intact mitochondria resulting in the release of DNA from DQAsomes. Based on the intrinsic property of dequalinium to accumulate in mitochondria and the selective release of DNA from DQAsome/DNA complexes at mitochondria-like membranes, DQAsomes can be considered as the first described potential mitochondria-specific transfection vector. However, the problem remains unresolved as to how DNA could be internalized in mitochondrial matrix? To solve this problem D'Souza *et al.*, demonstrated that oligonucleotides as well as plasmid DNA conjugated to a mitochondrial leader sequence (MLS) co-localize with mitochondria when delivered into mammalian cells by DQAsomes. The MLS-oligonucleotide (mOTC-oligo) consisted of a 5' fluorescein labelled oligonucleotide (5'-CTCCCTCACCATTGGCAGCCTA-3') coupled at the 3' end to the Nterminal end of the mouse ornithine transcarbamylase (mOTC) mitochondrial leader sequence (H2N–FNLRILLNNAAFRNGHNFMVRNFRCGQPLQN–COOH). In case ofplasmid DNA human mitochondrial matrix protein malate dehydrogenase (hMDH) (H2N–MLSALARPAG AALRRSFSTS AQNNAKVAVLGASC–COOH) with a C-terminal cysteine was used as leader sequence. This study was based on DQAsomes mediated transport of the DNA into the close proximity of mitochondria followed by the MLS mediated uptake into the mitochondrial matrix.

SUGGESTED READING

- Akhtar S. *J Drug Target* 5, 225 (1998).
- Akhtar S, James H, Gibscn I. *Nature Medicine* 1, 300 (1995).
- Akli S, Caillaud C, Vigne E, *et al. Nature Genet* 3, 224 (1993).
- Anderson WF. *Science* 226, 401 (1984).
- Andree C, Swain WF, Page CP, *et al. Proc Natl Acad Sci* USA 91, 12188 (1994).
- Anonymous. Eat up your vaccines. *Seedling* Newsletter (GRAIN, Barcelona) 17, 2-12 (2000).
- Ardizzoni SC, Michaels A, Arendas GW. *Science* 239,183 (1988).
- Arrigo P, Scartezzini P, Romano P. *IEEE* 1(4), 167 (2002).
- Bagai S, Sarkar DP. *J Biol Chem* 268, 1966 (1994).
- Bagai S, Sarkar DP. *Biochim Biophys Acta* 1152, 15 (1993).
- Bajocchi G, Feldman SH, Crystal RG, *et al. Nature Genet*, 3, 229 (1993).
- Bartzatt R. *Biotechnol Appl Biochem* 11, 133 (1988).
- Bartzatt R. *Med Sci Res Biochem* 15, 791 (1987).
- Bass B, Weintrab H. *Cell* 55, 1089 (1988).
- Bayley H. *Curr Opin Biotechnol* 10, 94 (1999).
- Behlke MA. *Molecular Therapy* 13(4), 644 (2006).
- Bennet CF, Chiang MY, Chan H, *et al. J Liposome Res* 3, 85 (1993).
- Bennet CF, Chiang MY, Chan H, *et al. Mol Pharmacol* 41, 1023 (1992).
- Bennett CF, Cowsert LM. *Biochim Biophys Acta* 1489, 19 (1999).
- Berg K. *et al. Cancer Res* 59, 1180, (1999).
- Berglund P, Tublekas I, Liljestrom P. *Trends Biotechnol* 14, 130 (1996).
- Berkner KL. *Biotechniques* 6, 616 (1988).
- Berns KI, Linden RM. *Bioessays* 17, 237 (1995).
- Besmer P, Olshevsky U, Baltimore D, *et al. J Virol* 29, 1168 (1979).
- Bielinska A, Kukowska-Latallo JF, Johnson J, *et al. Nucleic Acids Res* 24, 2176 (1996).
- Brazhnik P, de la Fuente A, Mendes P. *Trends in Biotech* 20, 467 (2002).
- Breakefield XO, De Luca NA. *N Biol* 3, 203 (1991).
- Breaker RR, Joyce GF. *Trends Biotechnol* 12, 268 (1994).
- Bringham KL, Meyrick BO, Christman BW, *et al. Am J Med Sci* 298, 278 (1989).
- Brown PO, Botstein D. *Nat Genet* 21, 33 (1999).

- Brown SB, Brown EA, Walker I. *Lancet Oncol* 5, 497, (2004).
- Buchschacher GL, Free EO, Panganiban AT. *Hum Gene Ther* 3, 391 (1992).
- Chakraborty AK, Link MA, Hodgson CP. *FASEB J* 7, 971 (1993).
- Chang TMS. *Methods Enzymol 112,* 195 (1985).
- Chang TMS. *Trends in Biotech* 17, 61 (1999).
- Cheng L, Zielhoffer PR, Yang NS. *Proc Natl Acad Sci* USA 90, 4455 (1993).
- Chiu YL, Rana TM. *RNA*, 9, 1034 (2003).
- Cho YS, Kim M, Cheadle C, *et al. PNAS* (USA) 98, 9819 (2001).
- Cho-Chung YS, Becker KG. *Nat Biotechnol* 21, 492 (2003).
- Choi JS, Choi MJ, Ko KS, *et al. Bull Korean Chem Soc* 27, 1335 (2006).
- Chowdhury JR, Grossman M, Gupta S, *et al. Science* 254, 1802 (1991).
- Cohen JS. *Pharmacol Ther* 52, 211 (1991).
- Consortium TGO. *Genome Res* 2, 1425 (2001).
- Cotton M, Wagner E, Zatloukai K, *et al. Proc Natl Acad Sci* USA 89, 6094 (1992).
- Crooke S. (ed.). *Antisense Research and Application.* Springer, New York (1998).
- Crystal RG. *Nature Genet* 8, 42 (1994).
- Culver, K.M., Blaese, R.M., Gene therapy for adenosine deaminase deficiency and malignant solid tumor, In: *Gene Therapeutics: Methods and Applications of Direct Gene Transfer*, J.A. Wolff (Ed.), Birkhauser, Boston, pp. 263-280 (1994).
- Curiel DT, Agarwal S, Wagner E, *et al.* Proto Natl Acad Sci USA 88, 8850 (1991).
- Curiel KM, Agarwal S, Romer MU, *et al. Am J Respir Cell Mol Biol* 6, 247 (1992).
- D'Souza GG, Rammohan R, Cheng SM, Torchilin VP, Weissig V. *J Control Rel* 92,189 (2003).
- Davidson BL, Allen ED, Kozarsky KF, *et al. Nature Genet* 3, 219 (1993).
- Davis HL, Micher ML, Whaien RG. *Hum Mol Genet* 2, 1847 (1993).
- Demenix, B.A., Behr, J.P., In: *Artificial Self-Assembling Systems for Gene Delivery*, P.L. FeIgner, M.J. Heller, P.Lehn, J.P. Behr, F.C. Szoka, Jr. (Eds.), Proceedings, American Chemical Society, Washington, DC, p146-151 (1996).
- Dennis C. *Nature 424,* 711 (2003).
- Dichek DA, Nussbaum O, Degen SJF, *et al. Blood* 77, 533 (1991).
- Dixit M, Webb MS, Smart WC, *et al. Gene* 104, 253 (1991).
- Dorsett Y, Tuschl T. *Nat Rev Drug Discov* 3, 318 (2004).
- Earl, R.T., Drug Delivery and Targeting Systems Latest Advances, Conference documentation, Organized by IBC Technical Services Ltd (1989).
- Eddy S. *Cell* 109, 137 (2002).
- Eddy SR. *Nat Rev Genet* 2, 919 (2001).
- Eisenbraun MD, Fullwer DH, Haynes JR. *DNA Cell Biol* 12, 791 (1993).
- Elbashir SM, Harborth J, Lendeckel W, Yalcin A, Weber K, Tuschl T. *Nature* 411, 494 (2001).
- Engesaeter BO. *et al. J Gene Med* 8, 707 (2006).

- Evans JP, Brinkhous KM, Brager GD, *et al. Proc Nat Acad Sci* USA 86,10095 (1989).

- Fahn S. *New Engl J Med* 327, 1589 (1992).

- Feigner OL, Gadek TR, Holm M, *et al. Proc Nat Acad Sci* USA 84, 7413 (1987).

- FeIgner PL, Ringold GM. *Nature* 337, 387 (1989).

- Fielding RM, Lasic DD. *Expert Opin Therapeut Patent* 9, 1679 (1999).

- Fire A, Xu SQ, Montgomery MK, Kostas SA, Driver SE, Mello C. *Nature* 391, 806 (1998).

- Flotte TR, Solow R, Owens RA, *et al. Am J Respir Cell Mol Biol* 7, 349 (1992).

- Freed CR, Reeze RE, Rosenberg NL, *et al. New Engl J Med* 327, 1549 (1992).

- Friedmann T. *HPRT Gene Transfer as a Model for Gene Therapy*, Plenum Press (1985).

- Furth PA, Shamy A, Wall RJ, *et al. Anal Biochem* 20, 365 (1992).

- Gabriel SB, Schaffner SF, Nguyen H, *et al. Science* 296, 2225 (2002).

- Gage FH, Wolff JA, Rosenberg MB, *et al. Neurosciences* 23, 795 (1987).

- Gansbacjer B, Zier K, Baniels B, *et al. J Exp Med*, 172, 1217 (1990).

- Gao XA, Huang L, *Biochim Biophys Res Commun* 179, 280 (1991).

- Geller AI, Breakefield XO. *Science* 241, 1667 (1988).

- Geller AI, Keyomarsi K, Bryan J, *et al. Proc Natl Acad Sci* USA 87, 8590 (1990).

- Gibbs WW. *Sci Amer* 47 (2003).

- Gitaman AG, Graessmann A, Loyter A. *Proc Nalt Acad Sci* USA 82, 7309 (1985).

- Golumbek PT, Lazenby AJ, Levitsky HI, *et al. Science* 254, 713 (1991).

- Goodchild J. *Bioconjugate Chem* 1, 165 (1990).

- Gould-Forgeite S, Mazurkiewicz JE, Raska K, *et al. Gene* 84, 429 (1989).

- Grierson D. Plant Genetic Engineering, In: *Plant Biotechnology*, Vo.l, Blackie, Glasgow (1991).

- Griffiths AD, Tawfik DS. *Curr Opin Biotechnol* 11, 338 (2000).

- Gross NJ, Getz GS, Rabinowitz M. *J Biol Chem* 244, 1552 (1969).

- Gross M. *Current Biology* 13, R577 (2003).

- Gygi SP, Aebersold R. *Curr Opin Chem BioI* 4, 489 (2000).

- Hampel A, Tritz R. *Biochemistry* 28, 4919 (1989).

- Hampel A, Tritz R, Cruz P. *Nucleic Acid Res* 18, 299 (1990).

- Hanensler J, Sroka FC Jr, *Bioconjugate Chem* 4, 372 (1993).

- Hanison GS, Long CJ, Curiel TJ, *et al. Hum Gene Ther* 3,461 (1992).

- Hartgerink JD, Clark TD, Ghadiri MR. *Chem Eur J* 4, 1367 (1998).

- Heller MJ, Jablonski EJ. European Patent Application No. 0229 943 (1987).

- Heller MJ, Morrison L. In: *Rapid Detection and Identification of Infectious Agents*, D.Kingsbury and S. Falkow (Eds.), Academic Press, New York, p345-356 (1985).

- Heller MJ, Morrison LE, Prevatt WD, *et al.* European Patent Application No. 070685, (1983).

- Hetherington S, Hughes AR, Mosteller M, *et al. Lancet* 359, 1121 (2002).

- Hickman MA, Malone RW, Lehmann K, *et al. Hum Gene Ther* 5, 1477 (1994).

- Hnatyszyn HJ, Ph.D. Thesis, University of California, Los Angeles (1995).
- Hodgson CP. *Biotechnology* 11, 222 (1995).
- Hodgson CP, Elder PK, Ono T, *et al. Mol Cell Biol* 3, 2221 (1983).
- Hoeben RC, Valerio D, Van der EB, *et al. Clin Rev Oncol Hematol* 13, 33 (1992).
- Hoogerbrugge PM, Suzuki K, Poorthuis BJHM, *et al. Science* 239, 1035 (1988).
- Horwitz MS. *Adenovirus and their replication.* In: *Virology,* Fields, B.N. Knipe, D.M. (Eds.), Vol. 2, Raven Press, New York, pp. 1679-1721 (1990).
- Howard K. *Nat Biotechnol* 21(12), 1441 (2003).
- Huckett B, Ariatti M, Hawtrey AO. *Biochem Pharmacol* 40, 253 (1990).
- Huth S, *et al. J Gene Med* 6, 923 (2004).
- Inouye M. *Gene* 72, 25 (1988).
- Johnston WK, Unrau PJ, Lawrence MSJ, *et al. Science* 292, 1319 (2001).
- Kasianowicz JJ, Brandin E, Branton D, *et al. PNAS* (USA) 93, 13770 (1996).
- Kato K, Kaneda Y, Sakurari M, *et al. J Biol Chem* 266, 22071 (1991).
- Kauffman SA. *The Origins of Order: Self-Organization and Selection in Evolution.* Oxford Univ. Press, New York (1993).
- Kay MA, Landen CN, Rottenberg SR, *et al. Proc Natl Acad Sci* USA 91, 2353 (1974).
- Kay MA, Rothenberg S, Landen CN, *et al. Science* 262, 117 (1993).
- Keefe AD, Szostak JW. *Nature* 410, 715 (2001).
- Kell DE, King RD. *Trends in Biotech* 18, 93 (2000).
- Kolodka TM, Finegold M, Moss L, *et al. Proc Natl Acad Sci* USA 92, 3293 (1995).
- Kossovsky N, Gelman A, Rajguru S, *et al. J Control Rel* 39, 383 (1996).
- Kossovsky N. In: *Artificial Self-Assembling Systems for Gene Delivery*, P.L. Feigner, M.J. Heller, P.Lehn, J.P. Behr, F.C. Szoka, Jr. (Eds.), American Chemical Society, Washington, DC. p 152-168 (1996).
- Kossovsky N. Presented at the Cambridge Healthtech Institute Conference on *Artificial Self-Assembling System for Gene Transfer*, Boston, M.A., September (1995).
- Kraft P, Horvath S. *Trends in Biotech* 21, 377 (2003).
- Krichner J, Connolly CM, Sandmeyer SB. *Science* 267, 1488 (1995).
- Kruger K, Grabowski PJ, Zaug AJ, Sands J, Gottschling DE, Cech TR. *Cell* 31, 147 (1982).
- Krynetski EY, Evans WE. *Oncogene* 22, 7403 (2003).
- Kuile BH, Westerhoff HV. *FEBS Lett* 500, 169 (2001).
- Kukowska-Latallo JF, Billinska AU, Johnson J, Spindler R, Tomalia DA, Baker JR Jr. *Proc Natl Acad Sci* USA 93, 4897 (1996).
- Kurreck J. *Eur J Biochem* 270, 1628 (2003).
- Lakowicz JR. In: *Principles of Fluorescent Spectroscopy*, Plenum Press, New York, p305-337 (1983).
- Lanyi JK, Pohorille A. *Trends in Biotech* 19, 140 (2001).

- Le Gal La Salle G, Berrard JJR, Ridoux V, Stratford-Perricaudet LD, Perricaudet M, Mallet J. *Science* 259, 988 (1993).
- Ledley FD, O'Malley BWJr, Borchardt J, *et al. J Cell Biochem* 18A, 226 (1994).
- Ledley FD, Woo SL, Ferry GD, *et al. Hum Gene Ther* 2, 331 (1991).
- Lee SH, Sinko PJ. *Eur J Pharm Sci* 27, 401 (2006).
- Lee Y, Jeon K, Lee JT, Kim S, Kim VN. *EMBO J* 21, 4663 (2002).
- Legendre JY, Szako FC Jr. *Pharm Res* 9, 1235 (1992).
- Lemarchand P, Jones M, Yamada I, *et al Circ Res* 72, 1132 (1993).
- Levy MY, Meyer KB, Barron L, *et al. Pharm Res* 11, 317 (1994).
- Li S, Gao X, Son K, *et al. J Control Rel* 39, 373 (1996).
- Liljestrom P. *Curr Opin Biotechnol* 5, 495 (1994).
- Liljestrom P, Garoff H. In: *Current Protocols in Molecular Biology* (Ausubel, F.M. *et al.,* Eds.), pp. 16.20.1-16.20.16., Greene Publishing Associates and Wiley Interscience (1994).
- Lindvall O, Brundin P, Widner H, *et al. Science* 247, 574 (1989).
- Logan JJ, Bebok Z, Walker LC, *et al. Gene Ther* 2, 38 (1995).
- Loomis WF, Sternberg PW. *Science* 269, 649 (1995).
- Lu DR, Zhou JM, Zheng B, *et al. Sci China* 36, 1342 (1993).
- Lundstrom K. *Trends in Biotech* 21,117 (2003).
- Luo D, Saltzman WM. *Nat Biotechnol* 18, 33 (2000).
- Luo D, Saltzman WM. *Synthetic DNA Delivery Systems* Kluwer, Dordrecht (2003).
- Luo D. *Trends in Biotech* 22, 101 (2004).
- Maine EM. *Dev Biol* 239, 177 (2001).
- Manthorpe M, Comefert-Jensen F, Hartikka J, *et al. Hum Gen Ther* 4, 419 (1993).
- Markowitz D, Goff S, Bank A. *Virology* 167, 400 (1988).
- Martienssen R. *Nature Genet* 35, 213 (2004).
- Mastrangelo MJ, Schultz S, Kane M, *et al. Semi Oncol* 15, 589 (1988).
- Mc Lachlan G, Davidson H, Davison D, *et al. Biochemic* 11,19 (1994).
- McDonald JF, *Curr Opin Genet Dev* 3, 855 (1993).
- McKusick VA. *Mendelian Inheritance in Man*, 8th Ed, Johns Hopkins University Press, Baltimore,MD (1988).
- Mendes P. Modeling large scale biological systems from functional genomic data: parameter estimation. In *Foundations of Systems Biology* (Kitano, H., ed.). pp. 163-186, MIT Press (2001).
- Mewes HW, Albermann K, Bähr M, *et al. Nature* 387, 7 (1997).
- Miller AD, Buttimore C. *Mol Cell Biol* 6, 2895 (1986).
- Miller AD, Eckner RJ, Jolly DJ, *et al. Science* 225, 630 (1984).
- Miller AD, Jolly DJ, Friedmann T, *et al. Proc Natl Acad Sci* USA 80, 4709 (1983).
- Miller PS, Ts'O POP. *Annu Rep Med Chem* 23, 295 (1988).
- Moan J, Berg K. *Photochem Photobiol* 53, 549 (1991).

- Morgan M. *The Misunderstood Gene.* Harvard Univ. Press, Cambridge, MA (2001).
- Morgan R, Looney DJ, Muenchau DD, *et al. Res Hum Retrovir* 6, 183 (1990).
- Moseley MA. *Trends in Biotech* 19, S10 (2001).
- Mumper RJ, Barron MK, Anwer K, *et al. Pharm Res* 12, 80 (1995).
- Muzyezker N. *Curr Top Microbiol Immunol* 158, 97 (1992).
- Nabel EG, Plautz G, Boyce FM, *et al. Science* 244, 1342 (1989).
- Nicolau C, Cudd A. *Crit Rev Ther Drug Carrier Syst* 6, 239 (1989).
- Nicolau C, Le Pape A, Soirano P, *et al. Proc Natl Acad Sci* USA 80, 1068 (1983).
- Nir S, Nieve JL. *Prog Lipid Res* 39, 181 (2000).
- Noordewier MA, Warren PV. *Trends Biotechnol* 19, 412 (2001).
- Nurse P. *Nature* 424, 883 (2003).
- Oberholzer T, Nierhaus KH, Luisi PL. *Biochem Biophys Res Comm* 261, 238 (1999).
- Palella TD, Hidaka Y, Silverman T J, *et al. Gene* 80, 137 (1989).
- Palmer TD, Rosman GJ, Obsborne WRA, *et al. Proc Natl Acad Sci* USA 88, 1330 (1991).
- Palmer TD, Thompson AR, Miller AD. *Blood* 73, 438 (1989).
- Paroo Z, Corey DR. *Trends Biotechnol* 22(8), 390 (2004).
- Patil N, Berno AJ, Hinds DA, *et al. Science* 294, 1719 (2001).
- Patil SD, Rhodes DG, Burgess DJ. *AAPS Journal* 7(01), E61 (2005).
- Pirmohamed M, Park BK. *Toxicology* 192, 23 (2003).
- Plautz G, Nabel EG, Nabel GJ. *Circulation* 83, 578 (1991).
- Pohorille A, Deamer D. *Trends in Biotech,* 20, 23 (2002).
- Prasmickaite L, Høgset A, Berg K. *Photochem Photobiol* 73, 388, (2001).
- Pushparaj PN, Melendez AJ. *Clin Exp Pharmacol Physiol* 33, 504 (2006).
- Quantin B, Perricaudet LD, Tajbakhsh S, *et al. Proc Natl Acad Sci* USA 89, 2581 (1992).
- Raz E, Carson DA, Parker SE, *et al. Proc Natl Acad Sci* USA 91, 9519 (1994).
- Reich SJ, Fosnot J, Kuroki A, Tang W, Yang X, Maguire AM, Bennett J, Tolentino MJ, *Mol Vis* 9, 210 (2003).
- Rojanasakul Y. *Adv Drug Deliv Rev* 18, 115 (1996).
- Romer K, Friedmann T. *Eur J Biochem* 208, 211 (1992).
- Rosenberg MB, Friedmann T, Robertson RC, *et al. Science* 242, 1575 (1988).
- Rosenfeld MA, Siegfried W, Yoshimura K, *et al. Science* 252, 431 (1991).
- Rosenfeld MA, Yoshimura K, Trapnell BC, *et al. Cell* 668, 143 (1992).
- Schadt EE, Monks SA, Drake TA, *et al. Nature* 422, 297 (2003).
- Schlesinger S. *Trends Biotechnol* 11,18 (1993).
- Scjreoer J, Sawuyer S. *Adv Drug Del Rev* 19, 73 (1996).
- Seegmiller JE, Rosenbloom FM, Kelly WN. *Science* 155, 1682 (1967).
- Selheyer K, Bickenbach JR, Rothnagel JA, *et al. Proc Nat Acad Sci* USA 90, 5237 (1993).

- Service RF. *Science* 267, 458 (1995).
- Shak S, Caponm DJ, Hellniss R, *et al. Proc Natl Acad Sci* USA 87, 9188 (1990).
- Shaw JP, Milligan JF, Krawczyk SH, *et al. J Am Chem Soc* 113, 7765 (1991).
- Sikes M, O'Malley BW Jr., Finegold M, *et al. Hum Gene Ther* 5, 837 (1994).
- Snyder M, Gerstein M. *Science* 300, 258 (2003).
- Somogyi R, Greller LD. *Drug Discov Today* 6, 1267 (2001).
- Staedel C, Remy JS, Hua Z, *et al. J Invest Derrnatol* 102, 768 (1994).
- Starford-Perricaudet LD, Makeh L, Perricaudet M, *et al. J Clin Invest* 90 , 626 (1992).
- Stein CA, Cohen JS. *Cancer Res* 48, 2659 (1988).
- Stevenson M, Iversen PL, *J Gen Virol* 70, 2673 (1989).
- Strarford-Perricaudet LD, Levrero M, Chasse JF, *et al. Hum Gene Ther* 1, 241 (1990).
- Straus SE. Adenovirus infections in humans. In: *The Adenovirus*, H.S. Ginsberg (Ed.), Plenum Press, New York, pp. 451-496 (1984).
- Strauss JH, Strauss EG. *Microbiol Rev* 58,491 (1994).
- Szostak JW, Bartel DP, Luisi PL. *Nature* 409, 387 (2001).
- Tidd DM, Warenius HM. *Br J Cancer* 60, 343 (1989).
- Tomalia DA, Naylor AM, Goddard WA. *Angew Chem Int Ed Engl* 29,138 (1990).
- Tomlinson E, Rolland AP. *J Control Rel* 39, 357 (1996).
- Ullrich A, Shine KL, Chirgwin J, *et al. Science* 196,1313 (1977).
- Ulmer JB, Donnelly JL, Parker SE, *et al. Science* 149, 1745 (1993).
- Vaidya B, Mishra N, Dube D, Tiwari S, Vyas SP. *Curr Gene Ther* 9(6), 475 (2009a).
- Vaidya B, Paliwal R, Rai S, *et al. Cancer Therapy* 7, 141 (2009b).
- Varmus H. *Science* 240, 1427 (1988).
- Venter JC, Adams MD, Myers EW, *et al. Science* 291, 1304 (2001).
- Verma NK, Dey CS. *J Clini Pharm Therap* 29, 395 (2004).
- Wagner E, Cotton M, Foisner R, *et al. Proc Natl Acad Sci* USA 88, 42545 (1991).
- Wagner E, Zatloukal K, Cotton M, *et al. Proc Natl Acad Sci* USA 89, 6099 (1992).
- Wang CY, Huang L. *Proc Natl Acad Sci* USA 84, 7851 (1987).
- Wang KY, McCurdy S, Shea RG, *et al. Biochemistry* 32, 1899 (1993).
- Wang Y, Hu JK, Krol A, *et al. Mol Cancer Ther* 2, 1233 (2003).
- Wang Y, O'Malley BW Jr., Tsai SY, *et al. Proc Natl Acad Sci* USA 91, 8180 (1994).
- Weissig V, D'Souza GG, Torchilin VP. *J Control Rel* 75, 401 (2001).
- Weissig V, Lasch J, Erdos G, *et al. Pharm Res* 15, 334 (1998).
- Weissig V, Lizano C, Torchilin VP. *Drug Deliv* 7, 1 (2000).
- Wick R, Luisi PL. *Chem Biol* 3, 105 (1996).
- Widner H, Tetrud J, Rehncrone S, *et al. N Engl J Med* 327, 1556 (1992).
- Wiethoff CM, Middaugh CR. *J Pharm Sci* 92, 203 (2003).

- Willis RCW, Jolly DJ, Miller AD, *et al. J Biol Chem* 259, 7842 (1984).
- Wilson C, Szostak JW. *Nature* 374, 777 (1994).
- Wilson JM, Bimiyi LK, Salomon RN, *et al. Science* 244, 1344 (1989).
- Wilson JM, Grossman M, Wu CH, *et al. J Biochem* 167, 963 (1992).
- Xu Y, Szoka FC. *Biochemistry* 35, 56163 (1996).
- Yelin R, Dahary D, Sorek R, *et al. Nat Biotechnol* 21, 379 (2003).
- Zamecnik PC, Stephenson ML. *Proc Natl Acad Sci* 75, 280 (1978).
- Zhao X. *Adv Drug Del Rev* 17, 257 (1995).
- Zhao X, Batten B, Singh B. *Oncogene* 1727 (1990).
- Zhao X, Klibanov AL, Huang L. *Biochim Biophys Acta* 1065, 8 (1991).
- Zignani M, Drummond DC, Meyer O, *et al. Biochim Biophys Acta* 1463, 383 (2000).

11

IMMUNOLOGY AND VACCINES

11.1. INTRODUCTION

11.2. NATURAL IMMUNITY

11.3. ACQUIRED IMMUNITY

    11.3.1. Naturally acquired active immunity

    11.3.2. Artificially acquired active immunity

    11.3.3. Naturally acquired passive immunity

    11.3.4. Artificially acquired passive immunity

11.4. THE IMMUNE SYSTEM

    11.4.1. The innate immune system

        11.4.1.1. Endocytes and phagocytes

        11.4.1.2. Inflammatory response

        11.4.1.3. Natural killer (NK) cells and soluble factors

    11.4.2. Adaptive/Acquired/Specific immunity

        11.4.2.1. Antigen presentation

        11.4.2.2. Humoral immunity

        11.4.2.3. Cell mediated immunity

11.5. CYTOKINES

11.6. CELL AND ORGANS OF THE IMMUNE SYSTEM

    11.6.1. Hematopoiesis

    11.6.2. Cells of immune system

    11.6.3. Organs of immune system

    11.6.4. Complement system

11.7. IMMUNOLOGICAL PROPERTIES OF ANTIGEN

11.8. MAJOR HISTOCOMPATIBILITY COMPLEX (MHC)

11.9. ANTIBODIES OR IMMUNOGLOBULINS

    11.9.1. Immunoglobulin structure

    11.9.2. Immunoglobulin sequences

    11.9.3. Antigenic determinants on immunoglobulins

11.1. INTRODUCTION

Our environment contains a large variety of invading, pathogenic microbes/microorganisms against which an effective, protective cover is given by the immune system. The immune system is a remarkably adaptive defense system. It can generate a variety of cells and molecules capable of specifically recognizing and eliminating a variety of foreign invaders from the system. The immunity can be broadly classified into two types natural and acquired. It is further classified into active and passive, each category again sub-classified into natural and acquired (Fig. 11.1).

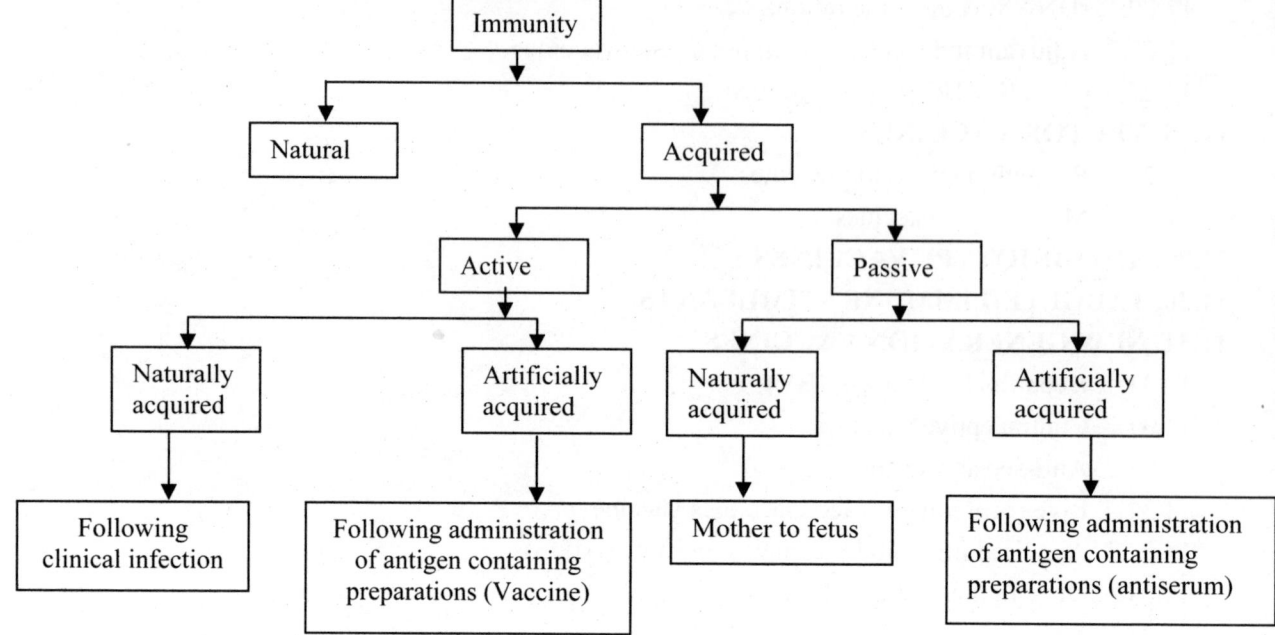

Fig. 11.1: Classification of immunity

11.2. NATURAL IMMUNITY

Natural immunity is resistance to a disease possessed by an individual. Nature has given advantage to certain individuals, species and races by providing them immunity against some diseases. For example, some individuals are more resistant to certain infections than others. Similarly the dreaded disease, plague, which attacks humans, does not harm fowls. Again, among races there are differences; Negroes are highly resistant to yellow fever while the whites are highly susceptible.

11.3. ACQUIRED IMMUNITY

It is difficult to survive only under cover of natural immunity. Hence, immunity is provided by either stimulating an individual's antibody production or by introducing antibodies acquired from a person or an animal. Acquired immunity is developed during a person's lifetime; it is not inherited. Immunity can be acquired actively or passively. This actively or passively acquired immunity may be either natural or acquired.

11.3.1. Naturally acquired active immunity

Naturally acquired immunity develops when a person is exposed to natural infection by pathogens or to some antigens in day-to-day life. Following exposure, the immune system responds by producing specialized lymphocytes and special proteins called antibodies. Immunity of this kind lasts long in most cases as it results in development of memory cells. Immunity developed following clinical and sub-clinical infections also falls under this category.

11.3.2. Artificially acquired active immunity

Artificially acquired active immunity arises from the stimulation of antibody production following the administration of specially prepared antigens called vaccines into the body by safe means. This is also termed as vaccination or active immunization. Vaccines are composed of inactivated bacterial toxins (toxoids), killed micro-organisms or living but attenuated (weakened) micro-organisms that are subjected to treatment wherein they lose their toxicity or the ability to cause a disease but are still capable of stimulating the immune system.

Table 11.1: Comparison between active and passive immunity

Active	Passive
Developed immunity	Produced immunity
Develops slowly and last long	Relatively fast and short lived
If required, a booster dose can be given to provide lifelong immunity	A booster dose also doesn't help in maintaining it for long
It is mainly to prevent a disease and is administered before infection	Generally develops after the subject has been exposed to an infection.
Given in long term prophylaxis	Given in short term prophylaxis and therapeutically
Antigens are administered	Antibodies are administered

11.3.3. Naturally acquired passive immunity

It involves the natural transfer of antibodies from a mother to fetus *via* placenta and so provides immunity to the newborn for a few days to few months. Here, the fetus is immune to those diseases to which the mother is immune, but only for a short period. For example, if the mother is immune to diphtheria, chicken pox, and polio, the newborn is also immune to the same diseases but only for a period not exceeding six months. Similarly, certain amount of immunity is provided through breast-feeding. Certain antibodies can pass from the mother to the infant *via* the breast milk. A comparison between active and passive immunity is given in Table 11.1.

11.3.4. Artificially acquired passive immunity

Since a long lasting immunity can be generated by administering antigens, consequently an artificial-active lasting immunity can also be generated administering antibodies. These antibodies are produced either in animals or humans and then administered to the subject. The antibodies appear in the serum of the immune animal or human and hence the term serum or sera or antisera is frequently used.

11.4. THE IMMUNE SYSTEM

The immune system is basically involved in protection against pathogens and opportunistic organisms. It involves different components; the diversity allows defense against different types of attack from microbes (Fig.11.2).

On the basis of the characteristics of immune system, it can be divided into two types, namely innate and adaptive. The first line of defense is provided by innate immune system. If this first line defense fails, then the adaptive system is activated. While the innate system checks out potential pathogens even before they establish an infection, the adaptive system produces a specific reaction to each infectious agent, which normally eradicates that agent. In addition, the latter remembers that particular infectious agent and recalls whenever they come across next time, thus preventing the agent from causing disease. Adaptive arm is the immune response which is comparatively delayed and generates a specific response towards a particular antigen, the specificity being conferred by antigen specific receptors on B-cells and T-cells. There has been considerable progress in understanding of the molecular basis of adaptive responses *via* elucidation of genes and structures of the B-cell receptor (BCR) and T-cell receptor (TCR). Less is known about the innate arm of the immune system which recognizes microbial components. For instance lipopolysaccharide (LPS), a component of gram-negative bacteria, activate B cells and macrophages. LPS is also responsible for endotoxic shock, resulting in hypotension and multi organ failure.

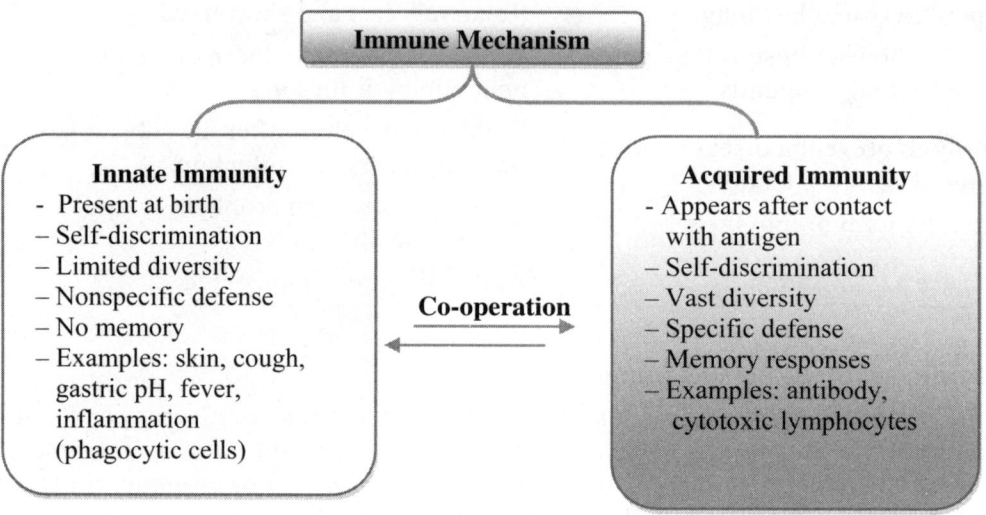

Fig. 11.2: Simplified view of immune mechanism

Immune responses are mediated by leukocytes, which derive from precursors in the bone marrow. A pluripotent hematopoietic stem cell gives rise to the lymphocytes responsible for adaptive immunity, and also macrophages and dendritic cells that participate in both innate and adaptive immunity. Neutrophils, eosinophils, and basophils are collectively known as granulocytes these are the other cells of immune system; they circulate in the blood unless recruited to act as effector cells at sites of infection and inflammation. Macrophages and mast cells complete their differentiation in the tissues where they act as effector cells in the front line of host defense and initiate inflammation. Macrophages phagocytose bacteria and recruit other phagocytic cells such as the neutrophils, from the blood. Mast cells are exocytic and thought to orchestrate the defense against parasites as well as trigger allergic inflammation; they recruit eosinophils and basophils, which are also exocytic. Dendritic cells enter the tissues as immature phagocytes where they specialize in ingesting antigens. These antigen-presenting cells subsequently migrate into lymphoid tissue. There are two major types of lymphocyte: B lymphocytes, which mature in the bone marrow; and T lymphocytes, which mature in the thymus. The bone marrow and thymus are thus known as the central or primary lymphoid organs. Mature lymphocytes recirculate continually from the bloodstream through peripheral or secondary lymphoid organs, returning to the bloodstream through lymphatic vessels. Most adaptive immune responses are triggered when a recirculating T cells recognizes its specific antigen on the surface of a dendritic cell. The three major types of peripheral lymphoid tissue are spleen, which collects antigens from blood; the lymph nodes, which collect antigen from sites of infection in tissues; and the mucosal-associated lymphoid tissues (MALT), which collect antigens from the epithelial surfaces of the body. Adaptive immune responses are initiated in these peripheral lymphoid tissues: T cells that encounter antigen proliferate and differentiate into antigen-specific effector cells, while B cells proliferate and differentiate into antibody-secreting cells.

11.4.1. The innate immune system

Innate immune system comprise of the cells and functional mechanism of immune system that act in nonspecific manner. The innate system is thought to constitute an evolutionarily older defense strategy, and is the dominant immune system found in plant, fungi, insects and primitive multicellular organisms. Intact skin acts as an effective barrier to most of the organisms. This is very clear from patients suffering from burns. Here, the prime entry of infection is *via* the damaged skin. Most infections enter the body *via* the epithelial surface of the nasopharynx, gut, lungs and genito-urinary tract. A variety of physical and biochemical defense mechanisms exist in these areas and protect them from most infections (Table 11.2). For example, lysozyme an enzyme widely distributed in different secretions and capable of splitting a bond found in the cell wall of many bacteria.

Table 11.2: Physical and biochemical defense mechanisms

Intrinsic Epithelial Barrier to Infection	
Mechanical	Epithelial cells joined by tight junction
	Longitudinal flow of air or fluid across epithelium
	Movement of mucous by cilia
Chemical	Fatty acid(Skin)
	Enzymes: Lysozyme (Saliva, sweat, tears), pepsin (gut)
	Low pH : Stomach
	Antimicrobial Peptides: defensins (skin, gut), Cryptidins (intestine)
Microbiological	Normal flora compete for nutrients and attachment to epithelium and can produce antimicrobial substances

11.4.1.1. Endocytes and phagocytes

If an organism penetrates an epithelial surface, a special type of innate defense mechanism also comes into play that involves the influx of extracellular macromolecules. This is brought in either by endocytosis or phagocytosis. Endocytosis is a mechanism wherein the macromolecules contained within the extracellular tissue fluids are internalized by either of the two processes: pinocytosis or receptor-mediated endocytosis (Fig.11.3). Internalization of macromolecules through non-specific membrane is known as pinocytosis. This process depends upon the concentration of macromolecules. In receptor-mediated endocytosis, macromolecules are selectively internalized after binding to specific membrane receptors.

The organism which penetrates an epithelial surface is encountered by phagocytic cells of the reticulo-endothelial system. The specialized phagocytic cells are derived from bone marrow of stem cells and include neutrophils, monocytes and tissue macrophages. The function of phagocytes is to engulf particles, internalize them and destroy them. They act as the soldiers of immunity, guarding us against microbes. Phagocytes occur everywhere within us, in lungs, liver, and in blood. Some of them can move through liquids and tissues, penetrating through vascular walls, whereas others remain fixed. Phagocytes devour foreign particles including bacteria. The free (mobile) phagocytes include white blood cells, leucocytes, and certain connective tissue cells. The immobile or fixed phagocytes are present in all organs, especially spleen, liver, lymph nodes, bone marrow, and vascular cells.

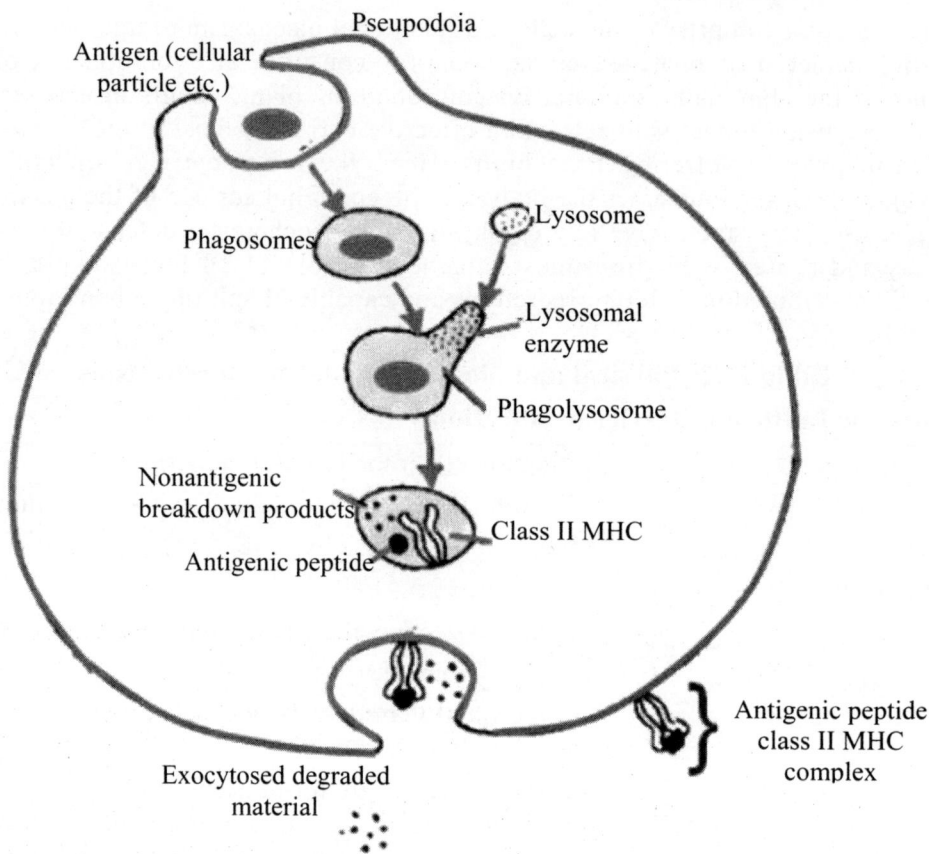

Fig. 11.3: Phagocytosis and processing of endogenous antigen by macrophages

11.4.1.2. Inflammatory response

Inflammation is the body's reaction to an injury or to an invasion by an infectious agent and defined as local accumulation of fluid, plasma proteins and WBC that is initiated by physical injury, infection, or a local immune response. Inflammation is manifested by:

1. An increase in blood supply to the infected area.

2. Increase in capillary permeability caused by retraction of endothelial cells.

3. Influx of phagocytic cells.

The increase in capillary permeability permits larger molecules to traverse across the endothelium and thus allows soluble mediators to reach at site of infection. Similarly, the migration of leukocytes out of capillaries into the surrounding tissues makes them move towards site of infection by process of chemotaxis (the process by which phagocytes are attracted to site of inflammation also known as extravasation). This extravasation into tissues occurs by initial attachment of lymphocytes to endothelium in the vascular lumen, followed by migration between endothelial cells and through the basement membrane (Fig.11.4). The process is reversed as lymphocytes leave tissue *via* lymphatics.

Lymphocytes interact with certain components found in both the basement membrane, interstitial matrix and potentially also on the endothelium. Major events that occur at the time of tissue injury during an infection are summarizes in figure 11.5.

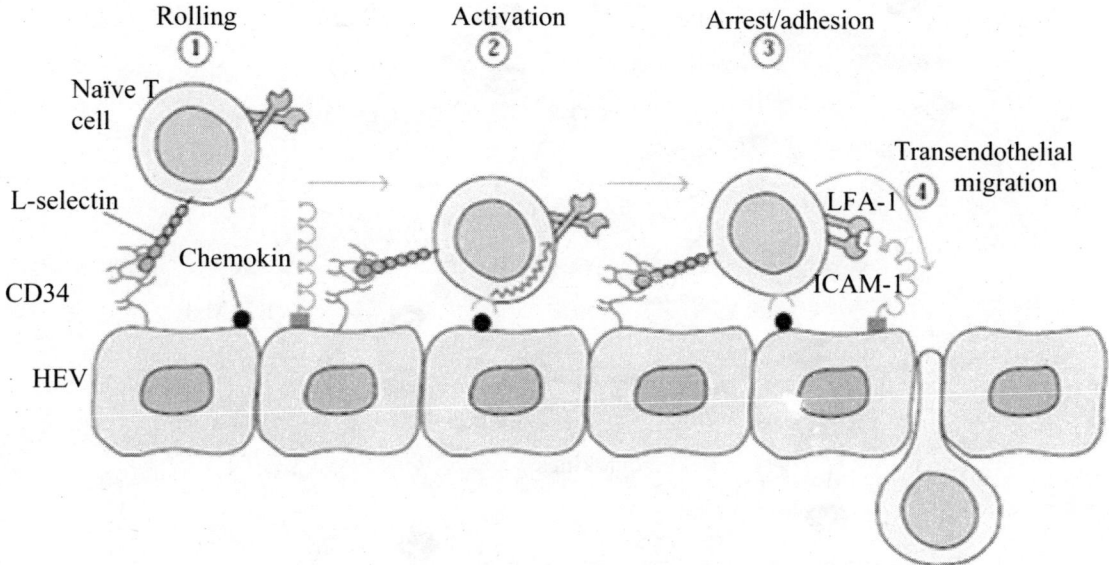

Fig. 11.4: Migration of lymphocytes through tissue

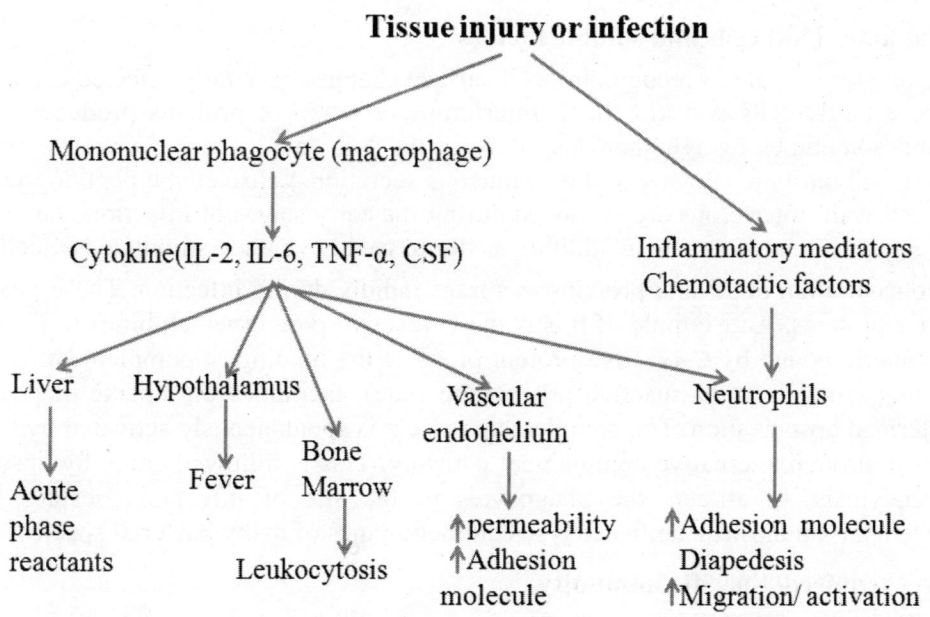

Fig. 11.5: Innate immune response following tissue injury or infection

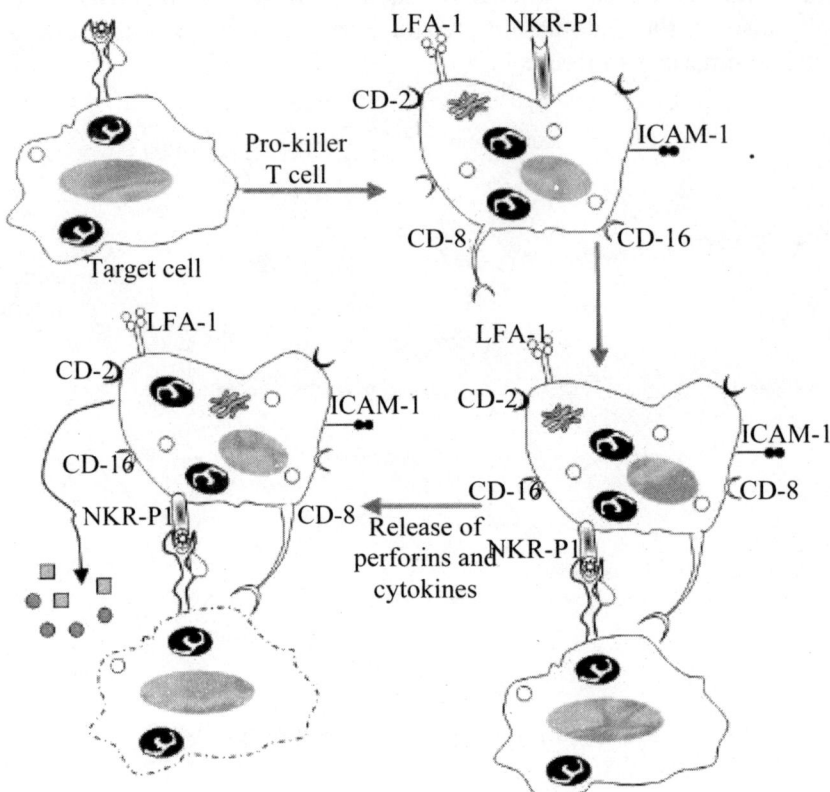

Fig. 11.6: Mode of action of killer and helper T cells

11.4.1.3. Natural killer (Nk) cells and soluble factors

NK cells are leukocytes capable of recognizing cell surface changes on virally infected cells. The NK cells bind to these target cells and kill them. Interferons, a group of proteins produced by virus-infected cells and sometimes by lymphocytes, activate the NK cells. Among a variety of soluble factors, lysozyme (a hydrolytic enzyme found in mucous secretions) cleaves the peptidoglycan layer of the bacterial cell wall. Interferons are produced during the early stages of infection and act as first line of resistance against many viruses. In addition as discussed above, they stimulate NK cells.

The serum concentration of several proteins increases rapidly during infection. These proteins are called acute phase proteins. An example of this is the C reactive protein which binds to C protein of *pneumococci*. Bacteria bound by C-reactive protein promote the binding of complement (a group of serum proteins that circulate in an inactive proenzyme state), facilitates the uptake of phagocytes. This process is termed opsonization. The complement system is spontaneously activated by surface of the microorganism through alternative complement pathway. This is followed either by opsonization leading to phagocytosis, or attracts the phagocytes to the site of infection. Besides this, the complement system has an intrinsic ability to lyse cell membranes of many bacterial species.

11.4.2. Adaptive/Acquired/ Specific immunity

The **adaptive immune system** is composed of highly specialized, systemic cells and processes that eliminate or prevent pathogenic challenges. The adaptive immune response provides vertebrate immune system with ability to recognize and remember specific pathogens (to generate immunity), and to mount stronger attacks each time pathogen is encountered. It is adaptive immunity because the body's immune system prepares itself for future challenges. The adaptive immunity displays four characteristic attributes

- Antigen specificity
- Diversity
- Immunological memory
- Self/nonself recognition

The system is highly adaptable because of somatic hypermutation (a process of accelerated somatic mutations), and V(D)J recombination (an irreversible genetic recombination of antigen receptor gene segments). This mechanism allows a small number of genes to generate a vast number of different antigen receptors, which are then uniquely expressed on each individual lymphocyte. Because the gene rearrangement leads to an irreversible change in DNA of each cell, all of the progeny (offspring) of that cell will then inherit genes encoding the same receptor specificity, including the Memory B cells and Memory T cells that are the keys to long-lived specific immunity. Immune network theory is a theory of how the adaptive immune system works, that is based on interactions between variable regions of receptors of T cells, B cells and of molecules made by T cells and B cells that have variable regions. Any of Pathogen entered in the body will be first recognized and then are ingested by antigen presenting cell. Following processing the antigens will be presented on to the surface of MHC molecule (either MHC-I or MHC-II). These cells then migrate to lymph node and present the antigen to naïve T cell and finally lead to generation of adaptive immunity against the antigen.

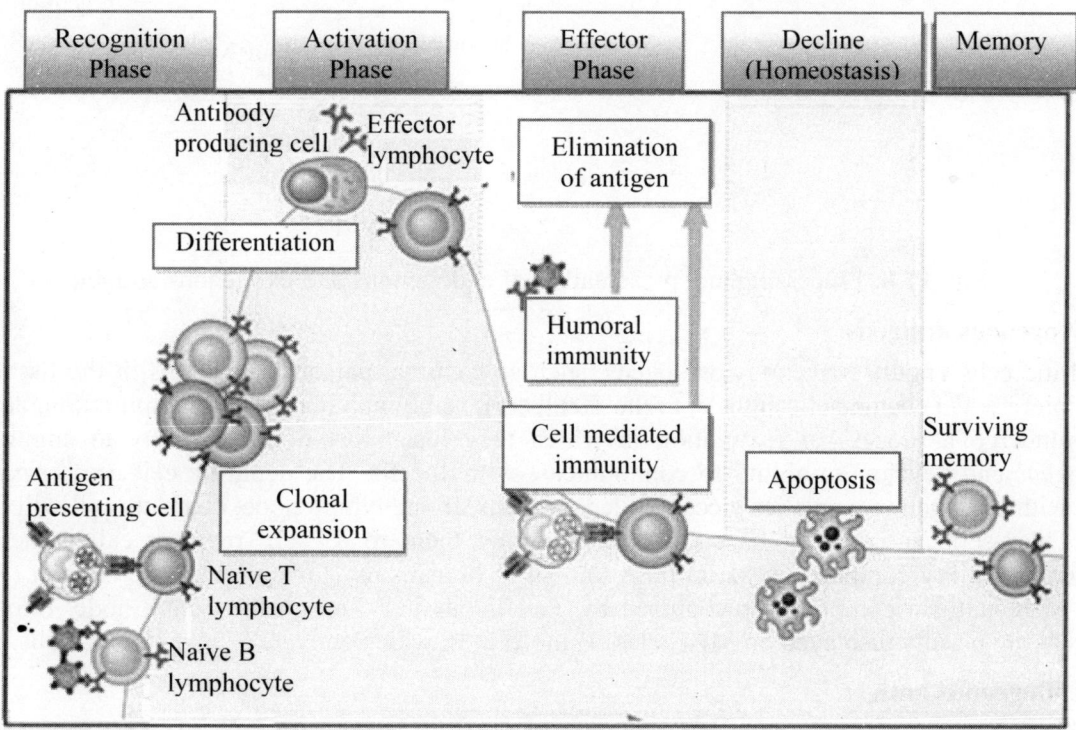

Fig. 11.7: Phases of adaptive immunity

11.4.2.1. Antigen presentation

Adaptive immunity relies on the capacity of immune cells to distinguish between the body's own cells and unwanted invaders. With the exception of non-nucleated cells (including erythrocytes), all cells are capable of presenting antigen and of activating the adaptive response. Some cells are specially equipped to present antigen, and to prime naive T cells. Dendritic cells and B-cells (and to a lesser extent macrophages) are equipped with special immunostimulatory receptors that allow for enhanced activation of T cells, and are termed professional antigen presenting cells (APC). Several T cells subgroups can be activated by professional APCs, and each type of T cell is specially equipped to deal with each unique toxin or bacterial and viral pathogen. The type of T cell activated and the type of response generated depends in part on the context in which APC first encountered with antigen.

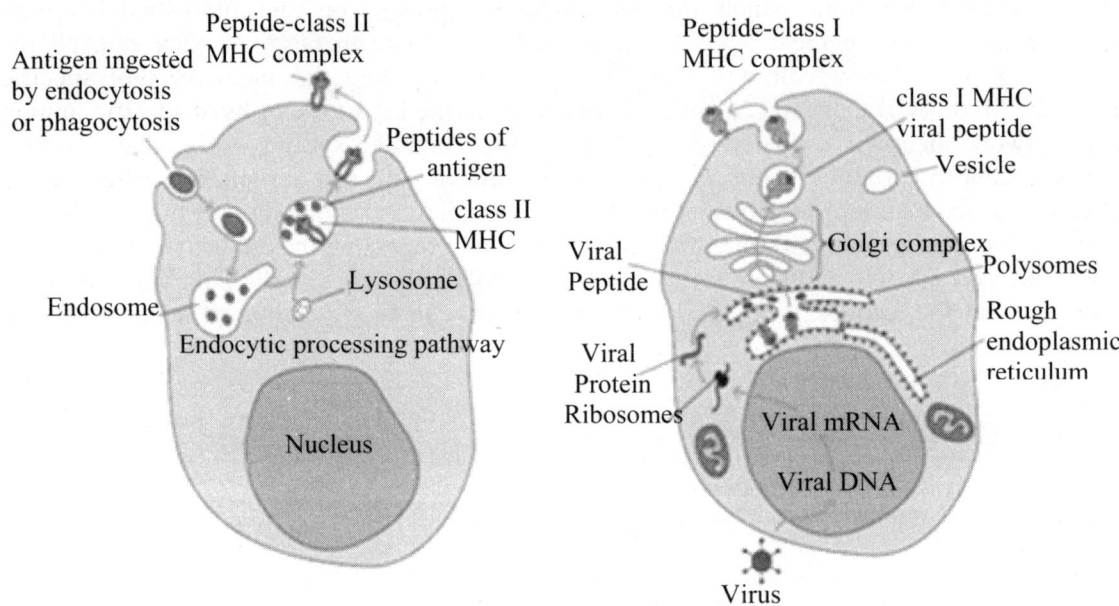

Fig. 11.8: Processing and presentation of endogenous and exogenous antigen

(a) Exogenous antigens

Dendritic cells engulf exogenous pathogens, such as bacteria, parasites or toxins in the tissues and then migrate, *via* chemotactic signals, to the T cell enriched lymph nodes. During migration, dendritic cells undergo a process of maturation in which they lose most of their ability to engulf other pathogens and develop an ability to communicate with T-cells. The dendritic cell uses enzymes to chop with pathogen into smaller pieces, called antigens. In the lymph node, dendritic cell will display these "non-self" antigens on its surface by coupling them to a "self"-receptor called the Major histocompatibility complex, or MHC [also known in humans as Human leukocyte antigen (HLA)]. This MHC-antigen complex is recognized by T-cells passing through the lymph node. Exogenous antigens are usually displayed on MHC class II molecules, which activate CD4^{+} helper T-cells.

(b) Endogenous antigen

Endogenous antigens are produced by viruses replicating within a host cell. The host cell uses enzymes to digest virally associated proteins and displays these pieces on its surface to T-cells by coupling them to MHC. Endogenous antigens are typically displayed on MHC class I molecules, and activate CD8$^+$ cytotoxic T-cells. With the exception of non-nucleated cells (including erythrocytes), MHC class I is expressed by all host cells.

11.4.2.2. Humoral immune response

Humoral Response (HI) is the aspect of immunity that is mediated by secreted antibodies (as opposed to cell-mediated immunity, which involves T lymphocytes) produced in the B lymphocyte lineage (B cell). B Cells (with co-stimulation) transform into plasma cells which secrete antibodies. Humoral immunity is so named because it involves substances found in the humours, or body fluids. The study of the molecular and cellular components that comprise the immune system, including their function and interaction, is the central science of immunology. Induction of the humoral immune response begins with the recognition of antigen. Through a process of clonal selection, specific B-cells are stimulated to proliferate and differentiate.

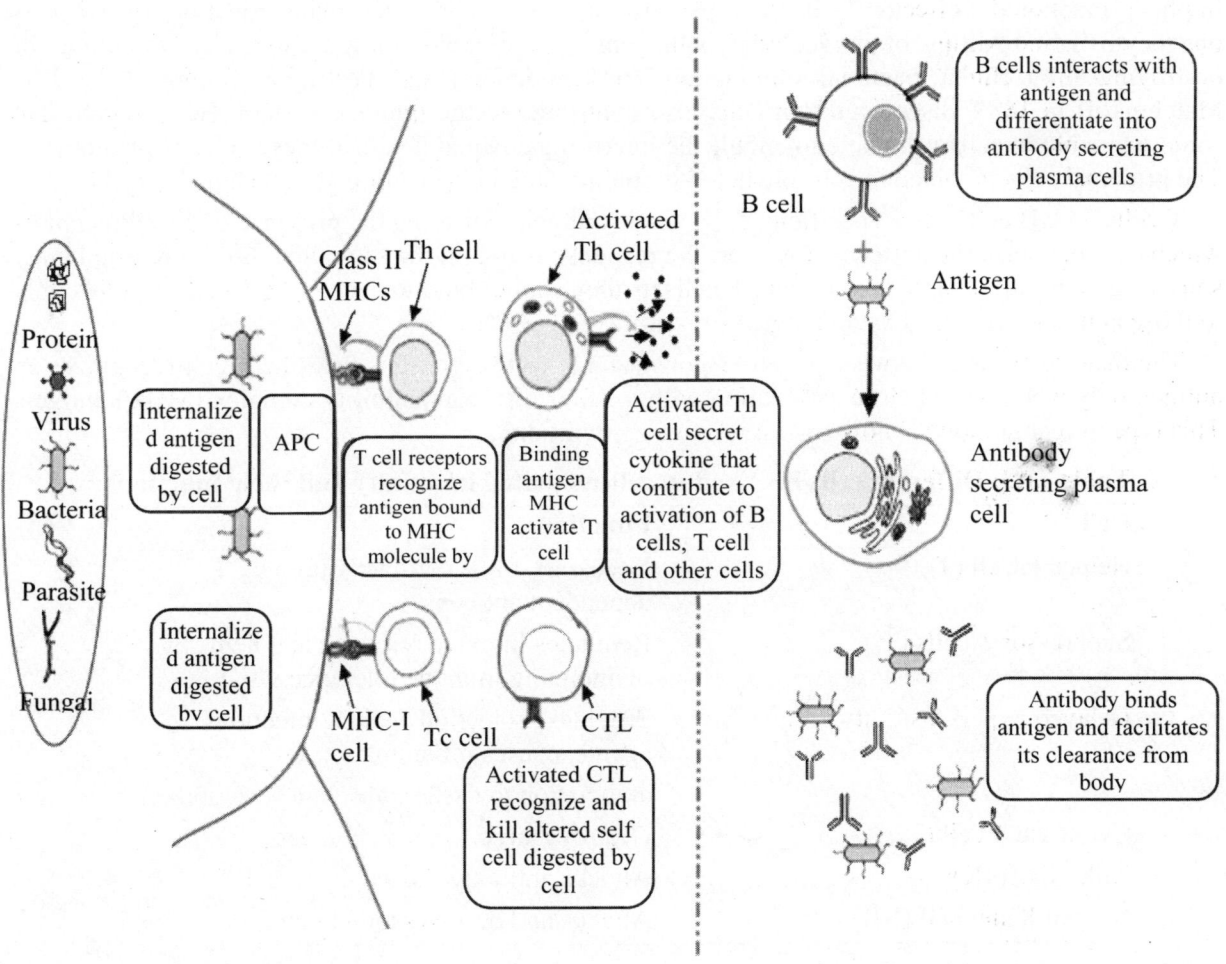

Fig. 11.9: Overview of generation of cell mediated and humoral immune response

However, this process requires the intervention of specific $CD4^+$ T-helper-2 cells that are themselves stimulated to produce lymphokines and are responsible for activation of the antigen-induced B-cells (plasma cell) and memory cell. In other words, B cells recognize antigen *via* immunoglobulin receptors on their surface but are unable to proliferate and differentiate unless prompted by the action of T-cell lymphokines. Plasma cell secrete antibodies that bind to antigens on the surfaces of invading microbes (such as viruses or bacteria), which flags them for destruction. Memory cell preserve experience and are ready in future to react with same antigen again. These memory cells are the basis of vaccination. As the humoral immunity is mediated by antibody and immune response is transferred from mother to fetus in the form of antibody as they remain functional in serum for prolonged period of time.

11.4.2.3. Cell-mediated immunity

The second arm of immune response is referred to as Cell Mediated Immunity (CMI). Cell mediated immunity is mediate by T lymphocytes (cytotoxic T lymphocytes and T Helper cells). As name implies, functional "effectors" of this response are the cells. The main function of CMI is phagocytosis and killing of intracellular pathogens. These responses are especially important for destroying intracellular bacteria, eliminating viral infections and destroying tumor cells. Elie Metchnikoff in 1883, discovered that cells also contribute to the immune system. He observed that some white blood cells were able to engulf the micro-organism and named these cells as phagocytes. The principal cells involved in cell- mediated immunity and their function are given in Table 11.3.

T cells, like B cells, have specificity for a single antigen indicating the presence of T cell receptors which can recognize the antigen. However, the response is not on the same line, for the reason being, soluble antigens are unable to stimulate T cells as they cannot bind to T cells. A T cell responds only to those antigens processed by an antigen-presenting cell (APC).

The major difference between T cell response and B cell response is that, the T cell recognizes an antigen only when it is in close association with a major histocompatibility complex (MHC) antigen. This type of recognition is known as associative recognition.

Table 11.3: Different cells involved in cell-mediated immunity and their functions

Cell	Function
Helper T Cell (T_H)	Necessary for B cells activation by T - dependent antigens
Suppressor T cells (T_s)	Regulates immune response and helps In maintaining immune tolerance
Delayed hypersensitivity T cell (T_D)	Provides protection against infectious agents; causes inflammation in association to tissue transplant rejection
Cytotoxic T cell (T_c)	Destroys target cells on contact
Killer CI:II (K)	Attacks antibody-coated target cells
Natural Killer cell (NK)	Attacks and destroys target cells

Once the APC are stimulated by an antigen, the cell starts secreting a substance called interleukin-l (IL-1), a monokine (secreted by macrophages and biologically active). This biologically active substance in turn activates the T cell, which in turn begins to synthesize interleukin-2 (IL-2). The T cell also synthesizes surface receptors for IL-2. When the receptors bind to IL-2, T cells begin to proliferate and differentiate into different effector cells; IL-2 receptors on T cells are present only if the T cell has been stimulated by an antigen (Fig. 11.10). A list of some diseases based on phagocytic, humoral, cell-mediated and combined humoral and cell-mediated deficiencies is given in Table 11.4.

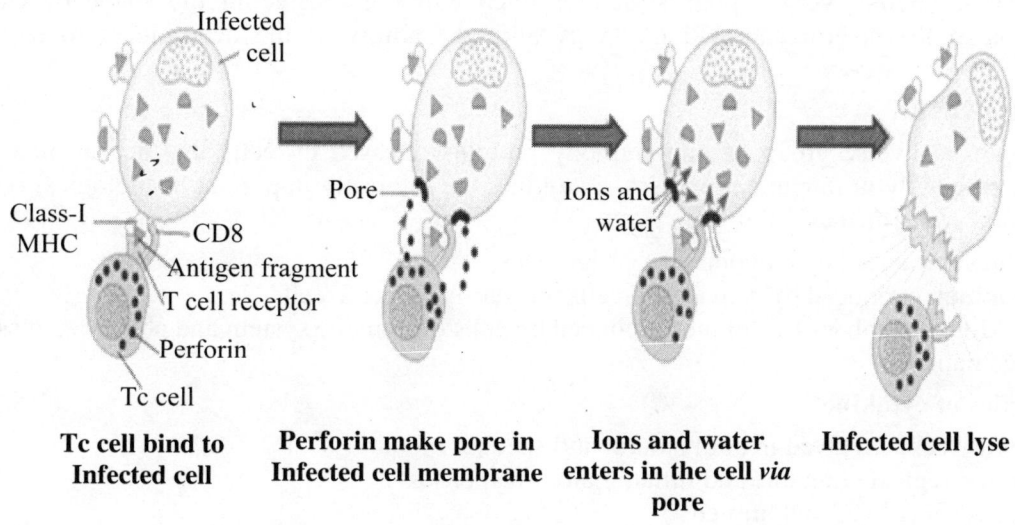

Tc cell bind to Infected cell | Perforin make pore in Infected cell membrane | Ions and water enters in the cell *via* pore | Infected cell lyse

Fig. 11.10: Cytotoxic T cell lyse the bacteria

Table 11.4: Immunodeficiency related diseases based on cells involved in immune response

Phagocytic deficiencies	Humoral deficiencies	Cell-mediated Deficiencies	Combined Humoral and Cell mediated deficiencies
Congenital agranulocytosis	X-linked agammaglobuli-nemia (XLA)	Di-George Syndrome	Reticular dysgenesis
Leukocyte-adhesion deficiency (LAD) syndrome	X-linked hyper Ig M (XHM)	Nude mice	Bare-lymphocyte syndrome
lazy-leukocyte syndrome	Common variable hypogammaglobulinem a (CVH)		X-linked SCID
Chronic granulomatus disease (CGD)	Selective immunoglobulin Deficiencies		Autosomal recessive SCID
			ADA deficiency SCID
			PNP deficiency SCID
			CB-17 scid mouse
			Wiskott-Aldrich syndrome (WAS)

Antigens are substances of various chemical natures capable of stimulating the immune system to produce a response specifically directed at the inducing substance and not towards unrelated substance. The molecular properties of antigens and specificity of immune response to chemical structures (antigenic determinants), plays a central role in understanding the immune system. An antibody directed towards an antigenic determinant of a particular molecule will react only with this determinant or another very similar structure. Even a minor change in the shape or chemical modification in the determinant will markedly alter the ability of the determinant to react with antibody.

11.5. CYTOKINES

Cytokines are a diverse group of non-antibody proteins released by cells that act as intercellular mediators, especially in immune processes. Cytokines are clinically important as biological response modifiers and are termed as following:

1. Monokines: produced by mononuclear phagocytes.
2. Lymphokines: produced by activated T cells, primarily helper T cells.
3. Interleukins: a number of cytokines produced by cells of immune system and abbreviated as IL with a given number.

A. **Properties of cytokine**

1. Produced by cells involved in both natural and specific immunity
2. Mediate and regulate immune and inflammatory responses
3. Secretion is short-lived and limited

      a. Cytokines are not stored as pre-formed molecules
      b. Synthesis is initiated by new short-lived gene transcription
      c. mRNA is short-lived and results in production of cytokines as needed

4. A number of individual cytokines are produced by many cell types and act on various cell types (they are pleiotropic).
5. In many cases cytokines have similar actions (they are redundant). This redundancy is due to the heterodimeric (sometimes heterotrimers) receptors of cytokines as they can be grouped into families in which one subunit is common to all members of a given family.

Since the subunit is common to all members of the family functions in binding cytokine and in signal transduction, a receptor for one cytokine can often respond to another cytokine in the same family. Thus, an individual lacking IL-2, for example, is not adversely affected because other cytokines (IL-15, IL-7, IL-9, etc.) assume its function. Similarly, a mutation in a cytokine receptor subunit other than the one in common often has little effect. On the other hand, a mutation in the common subunit has profound effects. Again, as an example, mutation in the gene for the IL-2 gamma subunit causes human X-linked severe combined immunodeficiency (XSCID) characterized by a complete or nearly complete T cell defect.

6. Often influence the synthesis of other cytokines:

      a. They can produce cascades, or enhance or suppress production of other cytokines.
      b. They exert positive or negative regulatory mechanisms for immune and inflammatory responses.

7. Often influence the action of other cytokines. Effects can be:

      a. antagonistic
      b. additive
      c. greater than additive (synergistic).

8. Bind to specific receptors on target cells with much higher affinity as compared with antigen binding to antibody or peptide binding to MHC molecules.

9. Cells that can respond to a cytokine are:

      a. same cell that secreted cytokine: autocrine
      b. a nearby cell: paracrine
      c. a distant cell reached through the circulation: endocrine

10. Cellular responses to cytokines are generally slow (hours), and require new mRNA and protein synthesis

Table 11.5: Classification of cytokines according to their functions

Functions	Examples
Mediators and regulators of Natural immunity	Tumor Necrosis Factor (TNF) Interleukin-1 (IL-1) Chemokines Interleukin-10 Interferon-gamma (IFN-gamma)
Mediators and regulators of specific immunity	Interleukin-2 (IL-2) Interleukin-4 (IL-4) Interleukin-5 (IL-5) Interleukin-10 (IL-10) Interferon-gamma (IFN-gamma)
Stimulators of hematopoeisis	Interleukin-3 (IL-3) Colony-Stimulating Factors (CSFs)

B. Functions of selected cytokines: I. Mediators and regulators of natural immunity

1. Tumor Necrosis Factor (TNF) also called TNF-gamma

(a) It is produced by activated macrophages.

(b) It is the most important mediator of acute inflammation in response to Gram-negative bacteria and other infectious microbes.

(c) Mediates the recruitment of polymorphonuclear leukocytes (PMNs) and monocytes to the site of infection:

      (i) Stimulates endothelial cells to express new adhesion molecules that make the cell surface "sticky" for PMN and monocytes.

      (ii) Stimulates endothelial cells and macrophages to produce chemokines that induce leukocyte chemotaxis and recruitment.

(d) Acts on the hypothalamus to produce fever.

(e) Promotes the production of acute phase proteins by the liver.

2. Interleukin-1

(a) Produced by activated macrophages.

(b) Effects are similar to those of TNF.

3. Chemokines

The name chemokine is a contraction of chemotactic cytokines

(a) These are large family of substances (more than 50) produced by many different leukocytes and tissue cells.

(b) They recruit leukocytes to sites of infection.

(c) They play a role in lymphocyte trafficking.

4. Interleukin-10

(a) Is produced by activated macrophages.

(b) Acts as an inhibitor of activated macrophages by blocking production of TNF.

II. Mediators and regulators of specific immunity

1. Interleukin-2

(a) It is produced mainly by helper T cells (CD4$^+$); less by cytoxic T cells (CD8$^+$).

(b) Mainly functions to promote T cell division and to increase production of other cytokines.

(c) It has autocrine functions on T cell proliferation as depicted in Figure 11.11.

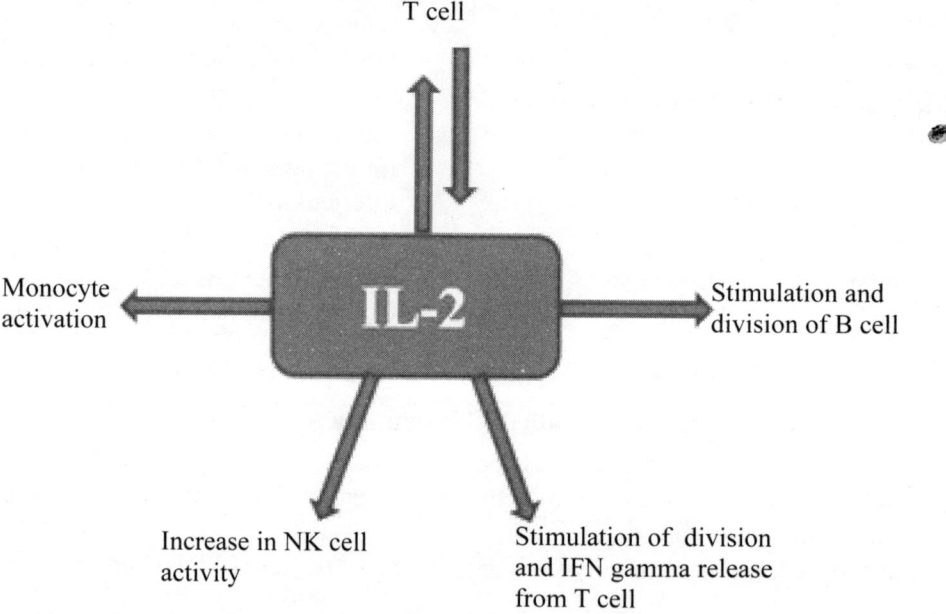

Fig. 11.11: Autocrine function of T cell proliferation mediated by IL-2

2. Interleukin-4

(a) Is produced mainly by Th2 subpopulation of helper T cells (CD4$^+$). Recall that Th2 cells are required for antibody production by B cells.

(b) Stimulates immunoglobulin class switching to the IgE isotype (IgE is involved in eosinophil-mediated elimination of helminths and arthropods).

(c) Stimulates development of Th2 cells from naive CD4$^+$ T cells.

(d) Promotes growth of differentiated Th2 cells.

3. Interleukin-5

(a) Is produced mainly by the Th2 subpopulation of helper T cells (CD4$^+$).

(b) Promotes growth and differentiation of eosinophils.

(c) Activates mature eosinophils.

IL-4 and IL-5 function together with IgE opsonizes helminths that then bind to eosinophils which upon activation kills the helminth.

Interferons (IFN)

There are three groups of interferons: IFN-alpha, IFN-beta , IFN-gamma

(a) IFN-alpha: Twenty variants are produced by leukocytes in response to viruses.

(b) IFN-beta: This is a single protein produced by fibroblasts and other cells in response to viruses. Both, IFN-alpha and IFN-beta inhibit viral replication and increase expression of class I MHC on cells.

(c) IFN-gamma:

(i) This protein is produced by the Th1 subpopulation of helper T cells (CD4$^+$), cytotoxic T cells (CD8$^+$), and NK cells. Since the Th1 cells are involved in the elimination of pathogens residing intracellularly in vesicular compartments.

(ii) IFN-gamma functions in both natural and specific immunity.

Natural Immunity:

- IFN-gamma enhances the microbicidal function of macrophages through formation of nitric oxide and reactive oxygen intermediates (ROI).

Specific Immunity:

- IFN-gamma stimulates the expression of class I and class II MHC molecules and co-stimulatory molecules on antigen presenting cells.
- IFN-gamma promotes the differentiation of naive helper T cells into Th1 cells.
- IFN-gamma activates polymorphonuclear leukocytes (PMN) and cytotoxic T cells and increases the cytotoxicity of NK cells.

Its functions are shown in Figure 11.12.

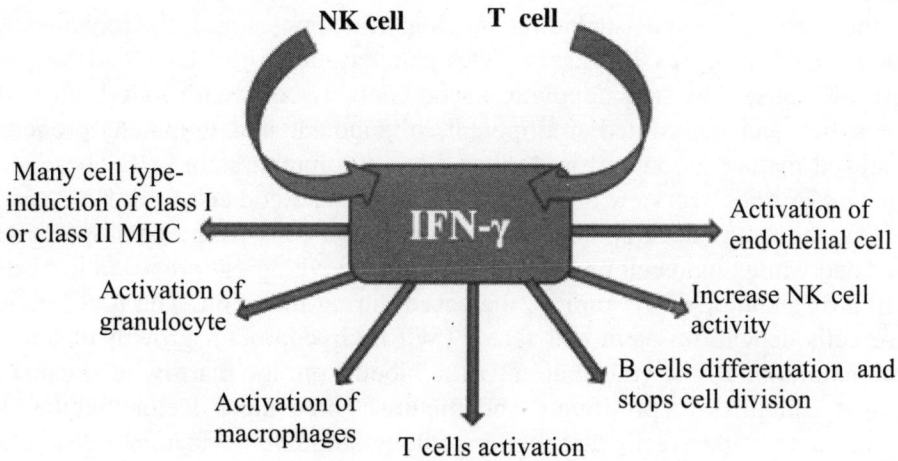

Fig. 11.12: Function of IFN-γ

5. Transforming growth factor (TGF-beta)

(a) It is an inhibitory cytokine produced by T cells, macrophages, and many other cell types.

(b) Inhibits proliferation and differentiation of T cells.

(c) Inhibits activation of macrophages.

(d) Acts on PMN and endothelial cells to block the effects of pro-inflammatory cytokines.

III. Stimulators of hematopoiesis

1. Interleukin-3

(a) Produced by helper T cells.

(b) Promotes growth and differentiation of bone marrow progenitors.

2. Colony-stimulating factors (CSFs)

(a) Produced by T cells, macrophages, endothelial cells, fibroblasts.

(b) Granulocyte-macrophage colony-stimulating factor (GM-CSF) promotes growth and differentiation of bone marrow progenitors.

(c) Macrophage colony-stimulating factor (M-CSF) is involved in the development and function of monocytes/macrophages.

(d) Granulocyte colony-stimulatory factor (G-CSF) stimulates the production of PMN.

11.6. THE CELLS AND ORGANS OF THE IMMUNE SYSTEM

11.6.1. Hematopoiesis

Haematopoiesis (from Ancient Greek: haima blood; poiesis to make) is the formation of blood cellular components. All cellular blood components are derived from haematopoietic stem cells. In humans, this process begins in the yolk sac in the first weeks of embryonic development. By the third month of gestation, stem cells migrate to the fetal liver and then to the spleen (between 3-7 months gestation these two organs play a major hempatopoietic role). Next, the bone marrow becomes the major hematopoietic organ and hematopoiesis ceases in the liver and spleen. In a healthy adult person, approximately 10^{11}–10^{12} new blood cells are produced daily in order to maintain steady state levels in the peripheral circulation. Hematopoietic stem cells (HSCs) are multipotent stem cells that give rise to all the blood cell types including myeloid (monocytes and macrophages, neutrophils, basophils, eosinophils, erythrocytes, megakaryocytes/platelets, dendritic cells), and lymphoid lineages (T-cells, B-cells, NK-cells). The hematopoietic tissue contains cells with long-term and short-term regeneration capacities and committed multipotent, oligopotent and unipotent progenitors. Every functional specialized mature blood cell is derived from a common stem cell. These stem cells are therefore, pluripotent. A brief overview of generation of various blood cell form HSC is summarize in Figure 11.13A that shows the development of different blood cells from hematopoietic stem cell to mature cells. Red and white blood cell production is regulated with great precision in healthy humans, and the production of granulocytes is rapidly increased during infection. The proliferation and self-renewal of these cells depend on stem cell factor (SCF). Glycoprotein growth factors regulate the proliferation and maturation of the cells that enter the blood from the marrow, and cause cells in one or more committed cell lines to proliferate and mature. Three more factors which stimulate the production of committed stem cells are called colony-stimulating factors (CSFs) and include granulocyte-macrophage CSF (GM-CSF), granulocyte CSF (G-CSF) and macrophage CSF (M-CSF). These stimulate a lot of granulocyte formation. They are active on either progenitor cells or end product cells. Erythropoietin is required for a myeloid progenitor cell to become an erythrocyte. On the other hand, thrombopoietin makes myeloid progenitor cells differentiate to megakaryocytes (thrombocyte-forming cells).

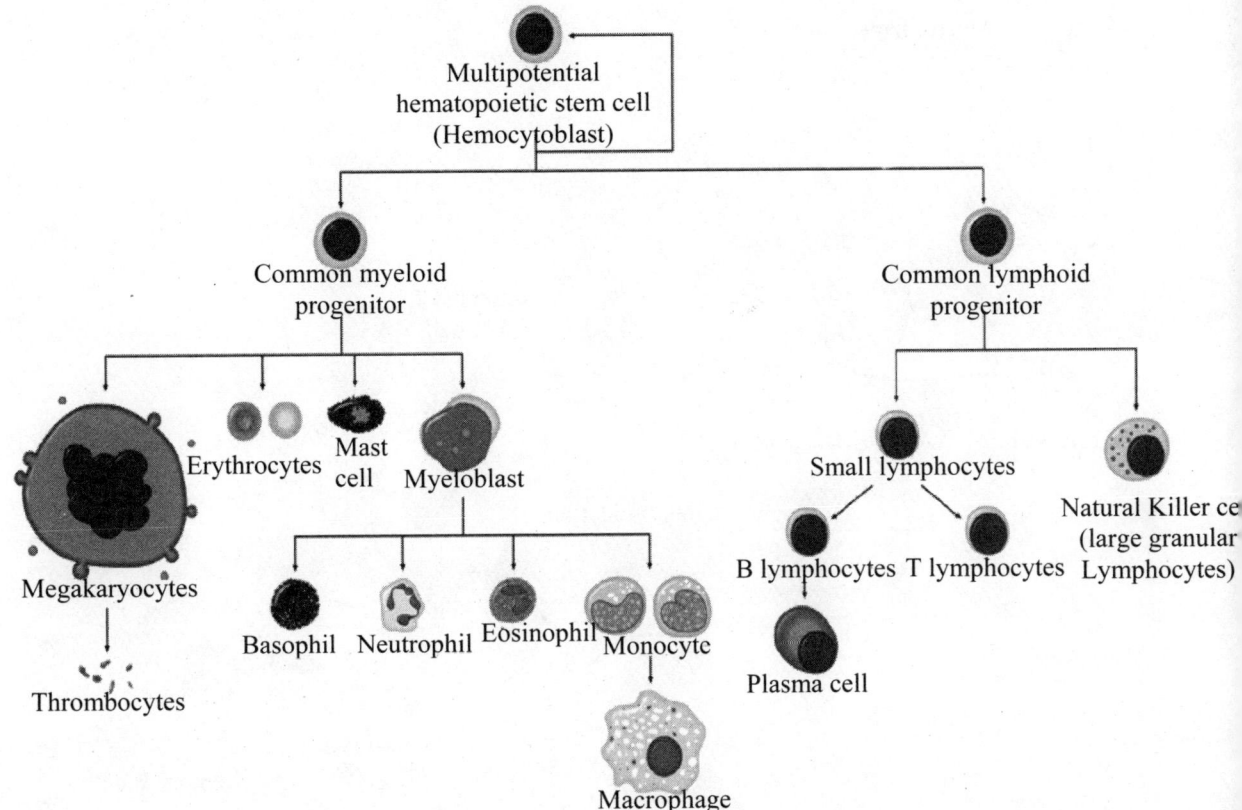

Fig. 11.13A: Diagram that shows the development of different blood cells from hematopoietic stem cell to mature cells

11.6.2. The cells of immune system

Generation of an effective immune response involves a number of organs and several; different cell types which can accurately and specificaliy recognize non-self antigens on micro-organism and to eliminate those organism. Two major groups of cells fall under this category:

1. Lymphocytes
2. Antigen presenting cells (APC)

Among the two different kinds of lymphocytes, T cells differentiate initially in the thymus whilst B cells differentiate in fetal liver, spleen and in bone marrow. In addition to these cells, non-B or non-T cells or third population cells/null T cells are also present. Further, a number of auxiliary cells are involved in generating immunity against invading organism.

11.6.2.1. Lymphoidal cells

1. B lymphocytes or B cells

Classically, the B lymphocytes are defined by the presence of endogenously produced immunoglobulins (antibody). That is the B cell receptor is an antibody molecule, a membrane-bound glycoprotein. They mature in the bone marrow and leave the marrow with a unique antigen-binding receptor on the membrane (Fig. 11.13B).

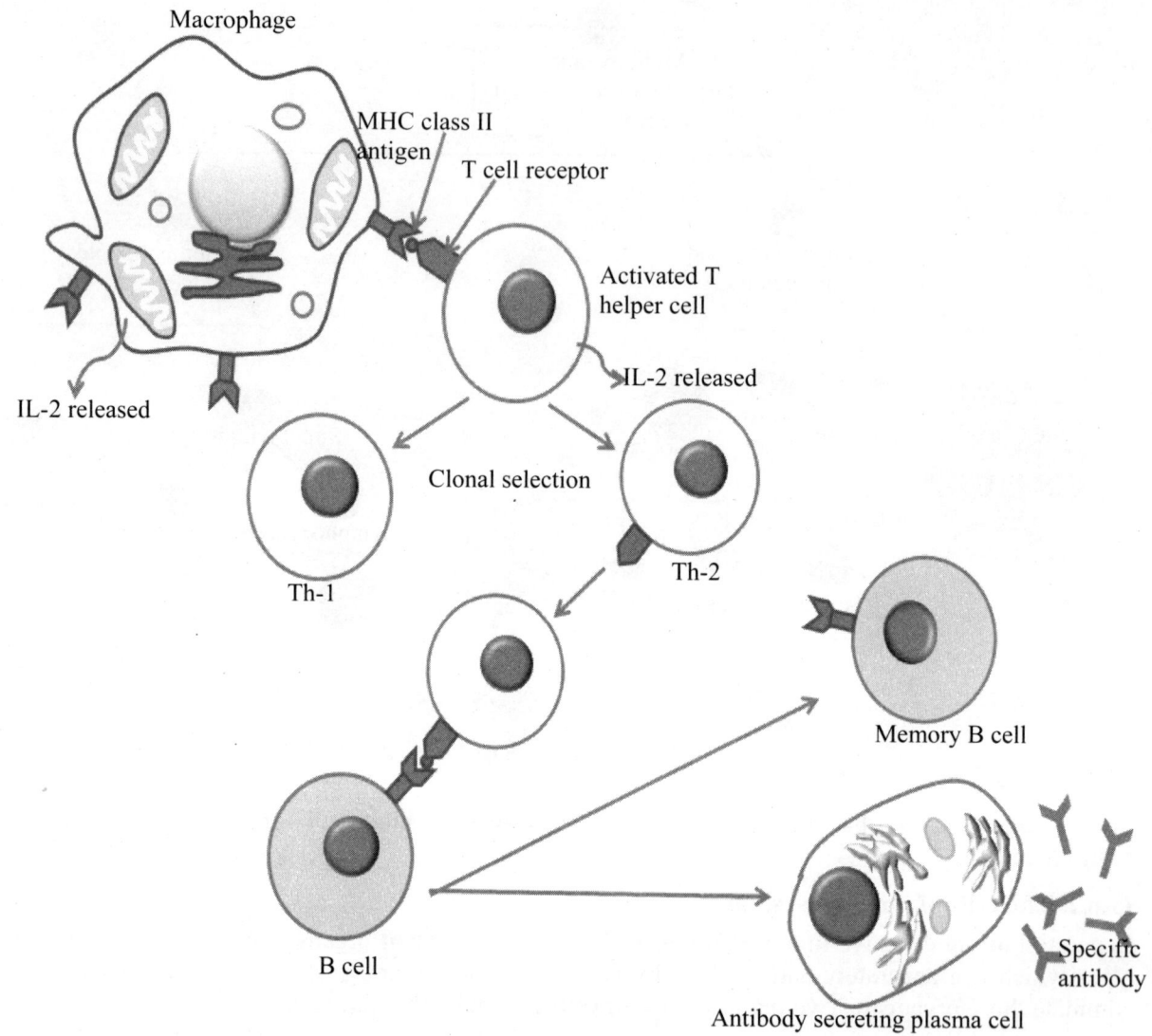

Fig. 11.13B: T cell dependent antigen triggering of a B cell

They constitute about 5–15% of the circulating lymphoidal pool. They are detected on the surface of mature cells by staining cell suspension with fluorescent labeled, specific antibodies. When a virgin B cell first encounters the antigen, the cell begins to divide rapidly. They differentiate themselves into memory B cells and plasma cells or effector cells. The memory B cells have a longer life span and resemble their parent in their function. Plasma cells do not produce membrane-bound antibody instead they produce the antibody in a form that can be secreted. They are short living cells, secreting enormous amount of one of the five classes of antibody within their life span. These secreted antibodies are the major effector molecules of humoral immunity. The human peripheral blood B lymphocytes express both surface IgM and IgD antibodies. Very few cells express surface IgG, IgA or IgE in the circulation.

2. T-Lymphocytes or T cells

The name originated from their site of maturation namely the thymus (Fig.11.14). Like B cells, they have structurally distinct antigen binding receptor site. T cells can be distinguished from B cells, as the former has different surface proteins which can bind to sheep erythrocytes. T cell receptors can recognize antigens only when they are associated with self-molecule encoded by genes within the major histocompatibility complex (MHC). This is the basic difference between humoral and cell-mediated immunity.

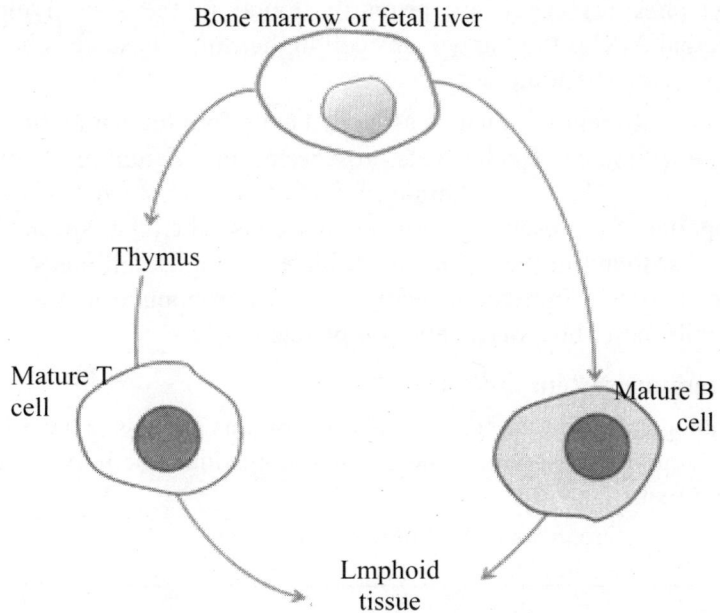

Fig. 11.14: Difference between B and T cell production

The T cells have two major sub-population namely T helper cells (T_H) and T cytotoxic cells (T_c) while a third, namely the T suppressor cells (T_s) is also said to be in existence.

3. Null cells

The null cells are a group (small) of peripheral-blood lymphocytes which do not bear the necessary membrane proteins to differentiate themselves between B and T lymphocytes. These cells also fail to display antigen-binding receptors as either of the lymphocyte cells. A population, of null cells namely the natural killer (NK) cells first described in 1976, constitutes 5–10% of the peripheral-blood lymphocytes. The NK cells produce cytotoxic activity against a wide range of tumor cells in spite of any previous immunization against that particular tumor. These NK cells play an important role in displaying host defense against tumor cells. The defense is said to be created in two different ways; by creating a direct membrane contact with the tumor cells in a non-specific way, i.e. antibody-independent process, secondly by antibody dependent cell-mediated cytotoxicity wherein NK cells bind to antitumor antibodies present on the surface of tumor cells.

4. Mononuclear cells

The prime cells of mononuclear phagocytic system are the circulating monocytes and macrophages in the tissues. Macrophages which are dispersed throughout the body can be classified into fixed macrophages and wandering or free macrophage. The fixed macrophages serve different functions in different tissues and their names reflect their location. These cells in the liver are called Kupffer cells, histocytes in the connective tissue; alveolar macro phages in the lungs; mesangial cells in the kidney and microglial cells in brain. Generally, the macrophages are in resting stage, but in the course of an immune response, a variety of stimuli activate macrophages.

11.6.2.2. Antigen-presenting cells (APC)

APCs are one among the two types of mononuclear cells. Their role is to present antigen to specific antigen-sensitive lymphocytes. They are primarily found in the skin, lymph nodes, spleen and thymus. The--archetypal APC is the Langerhans cell in the skin. These cells have characteristic tennis racket granules termed Briback granules.

They migrate via the afferent lymphatics as 'veiled cells' into the paracortex of the draining lymph node and interdigitate with many T cells. This provides as an efficient mechanism to present antigen, carried from the skin, to T cells in the draining lymph nodes. These APCs are rich in class II MHC antigens and are important for presenting antigens to T cells. The other specialized APCs include, the follicular dentritic cells, found in the secondary follicles of the B cell areas of the lymph nodes and spleen. The other cells of the immune system are polymorphonuclear granulocytes which include neutrophils, eosinophils, basophils, mast cells and platelets.

11.6.3. Organs of immune system

A number of morphologically and functionally diverse organs and tissue have various functions in the development of an immune response. These can be distinguished by function as primary and secondary lymphoid organs.

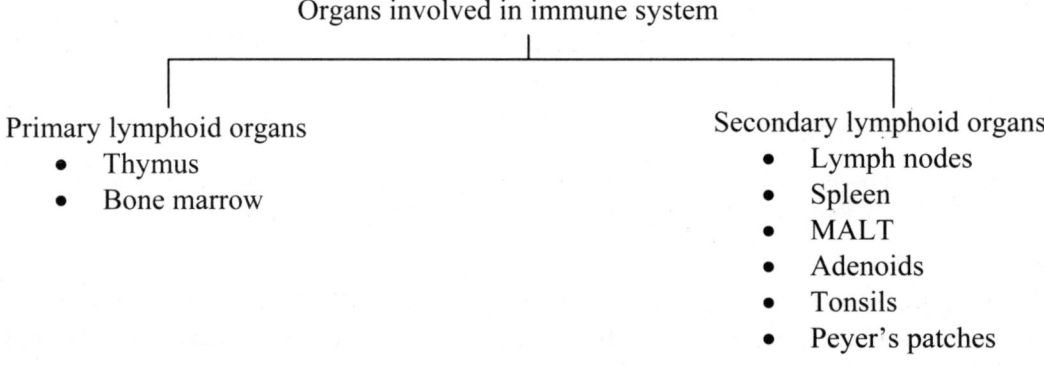

Organs involved in immune system

Primary lymphoid organs
- Thymus
- Bone marrow

Secondary lymphoid organs
- Lymph nodes
- Spleen
- MALT
- Adenoids
- Tonsils
- Peyer's patches

A. *Primary lymphoid organs*

Immature lymphocytes generated in hematopoiesis mature and become committed to a particular antigenic specificity within the primary lymphoid organs. Only after a lymphocyte has matured within a primary lymphoid organ is the cell immunocompetent (capable of mounting an immune response). T cells arise in the thymus, and in many mammals, humans and mice for example-B cells originate in bone marrow.

I. Bone marrow

It is the site of hematopoiesis and B lymphocyte development. Bone marrow is a loosely-organized grouping of cells located in central soft tissue portion of bones (surrounded by the calcified matrix) throughout the body. Reticular cells form a matrix within which the other bone marrow cells interact. The other cells found here include hematopoietic stem cells and progenitor cells, as well as immature and mature forms of all blood cells. Hematopoietic stem cells (HSC) present in the bone marrow are responsible for development of all blood cells after about the seventh month of gestation in humans. B lymphocytes, granulocytes, monocytes and erythrocytes all develop to maturity in the bone marrow before they are released into the bloodstream for transport to other locations in the body.

Pro T lymphocytes (immature T cells) are released into the bloodstream before final maturation as a matter of course in contrast to granulocytes and erythrocytes, which may be released into the bloodstream in immature forms in times of great need.

II. Thymus-site of T lymphocyte development

The thymus is the site of T-cell development and maturation. It is a flat, bilobed organ situated above the heart. Each lobe is surrounded by a capsule and is divided into lobules, which are separated from each other by strands of connective tissue called trabeculae. Each lobule is organized into two compartments: the outer compartment, or cortex, is densely packed with immature T cells, called thymocytes, whereas the inner compartment, or medulla, is sparsely populated with thymocytes. Both the cortex and medulla of the thymus are crisscrossed by a three-dimensional stromal-cell network composed of epithelial cells, dendritic cells, and macrophages, which make up the framework of the organ and contribute to the growth and maturation of thymocytes.

The function of the thymus is to generate and select a repertoire of T cells that will protect the body from infection. As thymocytes develop, an enormous diversity of T-cell receptors is generated by a random process that produces some T cells with receptors capable of recognizing antigen-MHC complexes. However, most of the T cell receptors produced by this random process are incapable of recognizing antigen-MHC complexes and a small portion react with combinations of self antigen-MHC complexes. MHC and pose a danger of causing autoimmune disease. More than 95% of all thymocytes die by apoptosis in the thymus without ever reaching maturity.

B. Secondary lymphoid organs

I. Lymph nodes

They are bean-shaped, encapsulated nodules located at junctions of lymphatics at strategic areas of the body. It filters particulate and soluble molecules out of lymph (interstitial tissue fluid picked up by the lymphatics for transport to the lymph ducts that empty into the subclavian veins) thus capturing immunogens for immune system stimulation. Three types of tissue (in addition to the ubiquitous reticular cells that form the tissue matrix along with trabecular connective tissue) are found in lymph nodes:

(a) Cortical (cortex) tissue: Located in the outer region of lymph nodes, just inside the subcapsular sinus (into which lymph drains from afferent lymphatics) B cells are the primary lymphoid cells found here (but there are some T cells and follicular dendritic cells present as well). Lymphoid follicles (loosely-organized clusters of lymphoid cells) characterize the cortical region of lymph nodes germinal centers develop within lymphoid follicles as a result of antibody responses that occur here.

(b) Paracortical (paracortex) tissue: Located in the intermediate region of lymph nodes and partially surrounding lymphoid follicles (on the medullary side of the cortex). T cells are the primary lymphoid cells here (but there are some macrophages and dendritic cells present as well) but they migrate into lymphoid follicles following antigenic stimulation by APCs to "deliver" cytokines to B cells responding to immunogens present migrate from lymph into blood and from blood into lymph *via* high endothelial venule cells in lymph nodes.

(c) Medullary (medulla) tissue: Located in the central region of lymph nodes as a loosely-organized aggregate of predominantly phagocytic cells Macrophages and dendritic cells (both are APCs) are the primary lymphoid cells here (but there are variable numbers of plasma cells, especially during active immune responses) APCs migrate into the paracortical region of lymph nodes when they have processed antigen and are presenting immunogen fragments on their APCs so they can stimulate T cells to initiate immune responses.

II. Spleen

It is a lumpy, rather amorphous encapsulated lymphoid organ (much larger than a normal lymph node) located ventral to the stomach in the abdominal cavity and filters particulate and soluble molecules out of blood thus capturing immunogens for immune system stimulation. Trabecular connective tissue forms the splenic matrix, which contains two major types of tissue:

(a) Red pulp consists of a network of sinusoids containing reticular macrophages and erythrocytes plus the other elements of blood being filtered at the time of organ examination.

(b) White pulp consists of splenic lymphoid cells and is organized into two major regions that form concentric sheaths around each of the arterioles that deliver the blood into the sinusoids:

Periarteriolar lymphatic sheath (PALS) areas surround each of the arterioles and contain many T cells admixed with interdigitating dendritic cells. Marginal zone surrounds the PALS and contains numerous B cells, some of which are loosely organized to form primary lymphoid follicles these primary follicles develop into secondary lymphoid follicles with germinal centers as antibody responses occur in the spleen.

III. Mucosal-associated lymphoid tissue (MALT)

The mucous membranes lining the digestive, respiratory, and urogenital systems have a combined surface area of about 400 m^2 (nearly the size of a basketball court) and are the major sites of entry for most pathogens. These vulnerable membrane surfaces are defended by a group of organized lymphoid tissues mentioned earlier and known collectively as mucosal-associated lymphoid tissue (MALT). Structurally, these tissues range from loose, barely organized clusters of lymphoid cells in the lamina propria of intestinal villi to well-organized structures such as the familiar tonsils and appendix, as well as Peyer's patches, which are found within the submucosal layer of the intestinal lining. The functional importance of MALT in the body's defense is attested to by its large population of antibody-producing plasma cells, whose number far exceeds that of plasma cells in the spleen, lymph nodes, and bone marrow combined.

The tonsils are found in three locations: lingual at the base of the tongue; palatine at the sides of the back of the mouth; and pharyngeal (adenoids) in the roof of the nasopharynx. All three tonsil groups are nodular structures consisting of a meshwork of reticular cells and fibers interspersed with lymphocytes, macrophages, granulocytes, and mast cells. The B cells are organized into follicles and germinal centers; the latter are surrounded by regions showing T-cell activity. The tonsils defend against antigens entering through the nasal and oral epithelial routes.

IV. Cutaneous-associated lymphoid tissue

The skin is an important anatomic barrier to the external environment, and its large surface area makes this tissue important in nonspecific (innate) defenses. The epidermal (outer) layer of the skin is composed largely of specialized epithelial cells called keratinocytes. These cells secrete a number of cytokines that may function to induce a local inflammatory reaction. In addition, keratinocytes can be induced to express class II MHC molecules and may function as antigen-presenting cells. Scattered among the epithelial-cell matrix of the epidermis are Langerhans cells, a type of dendritic cell, which internalize antigen by phagocytosis or endocytosis. The Langerhans cells then migrate from the epidermis to regional lymph nodes, where they differentiate into interdigitating dendritic cells. These cells express high levels of class II MHC molecules and function as potent activators of naive TH cells. The epidermis also contains so-called intraepidermal lymphocytes. These are similar to the intraepithelial lymphocytes of MALT in that most of them are CD8$^+$ T cells, many of which express T-cell receptors, which have limited diversity for antigen. These intraepidermal T cells are well situated to encounter antigens that enter through the skin and some immunologists believe that they may play a role in combating antigens that enter through the skin. The underlying dermal layer of the skin contains scattered CD4$^+$ and CD8$^+$T cells and macrophages. Most of these dermal T cells were either previously activated cells or are memory cells.

11.6.4. Complement system

The complement system is a biochemical cascade that helps the ability of antibodies to clear pathogen from an organism. It is the part of innate immune system and consists of more than 30 proteins. Many complement proteins occur in serum as inactive enzyme precursors (zymogens); others reside on cell surfaces. These proteins can recognize some pathogen surface intrinsically, or can recognize Ab molecules bound to pathogen infected cells. The recognition and activation of the complement system results in activation cascade and massive amplification of the response finally activation of cell killing membrane attack complex on infected cells which results in lysis of infected cells. The complement system bridges innate and acquired immunity and serve following functions (Fig.11.15):

(a) **Lysis of cell bacteria and virus-** polymerization of Polymerization of specific activated complement components on a foreign cell or enveloped virus leads to the formation of pores. The lipid bilayer of the cell or virus is disrupted.

(b) **Opsonization-**Certain complement proteins can bind to virions. Phagocytic cells with receptors for these complement proteins can then engulf the virus particles and destroy them. This process is called opsonization.

(c) **Activation of inflammation-**Several peptides produced by proteolytic cleavage of complement proteins bind to vascular endothelial cells and lymphocytes. These cells then produce cytokines which stimulate inflammation and enhances responses to foreign antigens.

(d) **Solubilization of immune complexes**–Some virus infections that are not cytopathic, the virus does not kill cells and lead to the accumulation of antibody-virus complexes. When these immune complexes lodge in blood vessels they can cause damage. An example is glomerulonephritis caused by deposition of antibody-antigen complexes in the kidney. Some complement proteins can disrupt these complexes and facilitate their clearance from the circulatory system.

11.6.4.1. Complement activation: There are 3 pathways of complement activation

- Classical
- Lectin
- Alternative

A. Classical pathway: The classical pathway activation is Ab dependent and is triggered by activation of the C1-complex (C1q, two molecules of C1r, and two molecules of C1s thus forming $C1qr^2s^2$), which occurs when C1q binds to IgM or IgG complexed with antigens (a single IgM can initiate the pathway, while multiple IgGs are needed), or when C1q binds directly to the surface of the pathogen. The binding leads to conformational changes in the C1q molecule and leads to the activation of two C1r (a serine protease) molecules. They then cleave C1s (another serine protease). The $C1r^2s^2$ component now splits C4 and then C2, producing C4a,C4b,C2a,and C2b. C4b and C2a bind to form the classical pathway C3-convertase (C4b2a complex), which promotes cleavage of C3 into C3a and C3b; C3b later joins with C4b2a (the C3 convertase) to make C5 convertase (C4b2a3b complex). The inhibition of C1r and C1s is controlled by C1 inhibitor. C3-convertase can be inhibited

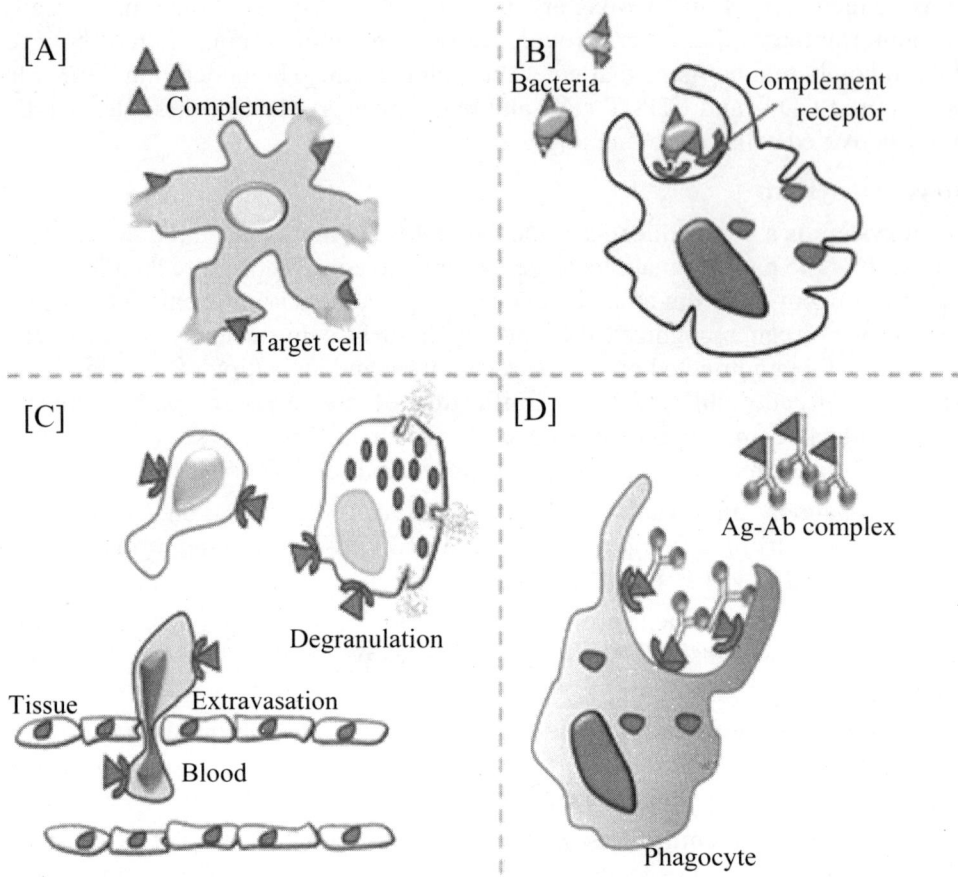

Fig. 11.15: Functioning of complement system [A] lysis [B] opsonization [C] activation of inflammatory response [D] clearance of immune complexes

by Decay accelerating factor (DAF), which is bound to erythrocyte plasma membranes *via* a GPI anchor.

B. Lectin pathway: The lectin pathway is homologous to the classical pathway, but with the opsonin, mannose-binding lectin (MBL), and ficolins, instead of C1q. This pathway is activated by binding mannose-binding lectin to mannose residues on the pathogen surface, which activates the MBL-associated serine proteases, MASP-1, and MASP-2 (very similar to C1r and C1s, respectively), which can then split C4 into C4a and C4b and C2 into C2a and C2b. C4b and C2a then bind together to form the C3-convertase, as in the classical pathway. Ficolins are homologous to MBL and function *via* MASP in a similar way. In invertebrates without an adaptive immune system, ficolins are expanded and their binding specificities diversified to compensate for the lack of pathogen-specific recognition molecules.

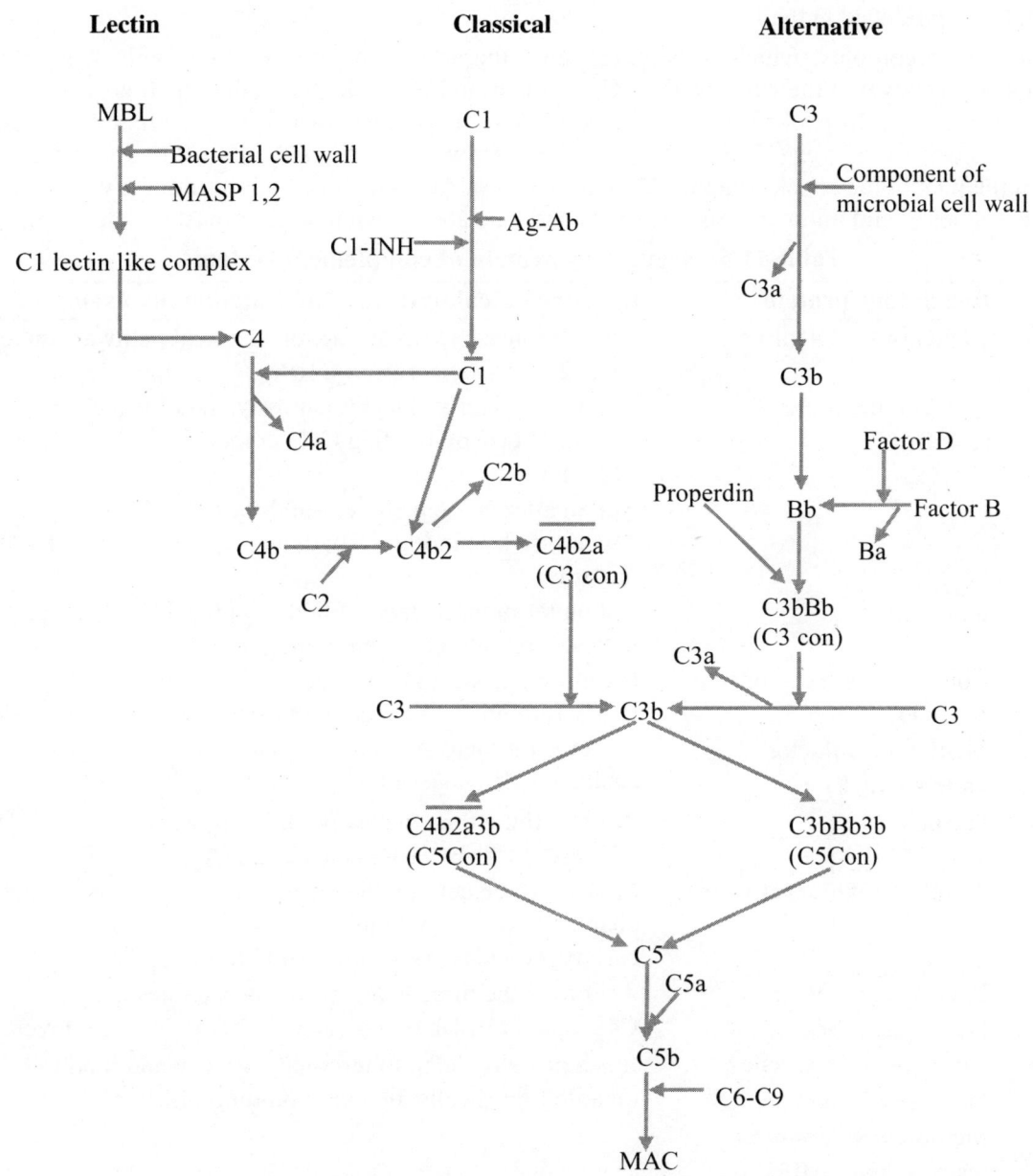

Fig. 11.16: Pathway of complement activation

C. Alternative pathway: The alternative pathway is triggered by spontaneous C3 hydrolysis directly due to the breakdown of the thioester bond *via* condensation reaction (C3 is mildly unstable in aqueous environment) to form C3a and C3b. It does not rely on pathogen-binding antibodies like the other pathways. C3b is then capable of covalently binding to a pathogenic membrane surface if it is near enough. If there is no pathogen in the blood, the C3a and C3b protein fragments will be deactivated by rejoining with each other. Upon binding with a cellular membrane C3b is bound by factor B to form C3bB. This complex in presence of factor D will be cleaved into Ba and Bb. Bb will remain covalently bonded to C3b to form C3bBb which is the alternative pathway C3-convertase. The protein C3 is produced in the liver.

The C3bBb complex, which is "hooked" onto the surface of the pathogen, will then act like a "chain saw," catalyzing the hydrolysis of C3 in the blood into C3a and C3b, which positively affects the number of C3bBb hooked onto a pathogen. After hydrolysis of C3, C3b complexes to become C3bBbC3b, which cleaves C5 into C5a and C5b. C5b with C6, C7, C8, and C9 (C5b6789) complex to form the membrane attack complex, also known as MAC, which is inserted into the cell membrane, "punches a hole," and initiates cells lysis. C5a and C3a are known to trigger mast cell degranulation.

Table 11.6: Regulatory protein of complement system

S. No.	Regulatory protein	Immunological pathway and function involved
1.	C1 inhibitor (C1Inh)	Serine protease inhibitor: act on classical pathway and causes C1r2s2 to dissociate from C1q
2.	C4b-binding protein (C4bBP)	Act on classical and lectin pathway and blocks formation of C3 convertase by binding C4b; cofactor for cleavage of C4b by factor I
3.	Factor H	Act on alternative pathway and blocks formation of C3 convertase by binding C3b; cofactor for cleavage of C3b by factor I
4.	S protein	Act on terminal pathway. Binds soluble C5b67 and prevents its insertion into cell membrane
5.	Complement-receptor type 1 (CR1) Membrane-cofactor protein (MCP)	It acts on classical alternative and lectin all the three pathway. Block formation of C3 convertase by binding C4b or C3b; cofactor for factor I-catalyzed cleavage of C4b factor I-catalyzed cleavage of C4b
6.	Factor-I	Act on all the three pathway Serine protease: cleaves C4b or C3b using C4bBP, CR1, factor H, DAE, or MCP as cofactor
7.	Anaphylatoxin inactivator	Protein which act on effector pathway which inactivates anaphylatoxin activity of C3a, C4a, and C5a by carboxypeptidase N removal of C-terminal Arg
8.	Decay-accelerating factor (DAE or CD55)	Act on all the three pathway and accelerates dissociation of C4b2a and C3bBb (classical and alternative C3 convertases)
9.	Homologous restriction factor (HRF) and Membrane inhibitor of reactive lysis (MIRL or CD59)	It is a protein bound to terminal pathway and bind to C5b678 on autologous cells, blocking binding of C9

11.6.4.2. Biologic activities of complement: Complement components have other immune functions that are mediated by complement receptors (CR) on various cells.

- CR1 (CD35) promotes phagocytosis and helps clear immune complexes.
- CR2 (CD21) regulates Ab production by B cells and is the Epstein-Barr virus receptor.
-

(a) CR3 (CD11b/CD18), CR4 (CD11c/CD18), and C1q receptors play a role in phagocytosis.

(b) C3a, C5a, and C4a (weakly) have anaphylatoxin activity: They cause mast cell degranulation, leading to increased vascular permeability and smooth muscle contraction.

(c) C3b acts as an opsonin by coating microorganisms and thereby enhancing their phagocytosis.

(d) C3d enhances Ab production by B cells.

(e) C5a is a neutrophil chemoattractant; it regulates neutrophil and monocyte activities and may cause augmented adherence of cells, degranulation and release of intracellular enzymes from granulocytes, production of toxic oxygen metabolites, and initiation of other cellular metabolic events.

11.6.4.3. Regulation of complement system

Since many component of complement system are capable of attacking host cell as well as foreign cell a regulatory mechanism has evolved to restrict its activity to designed target. The regulation in all complement pathways occur by two main mechanisms. One the inclusion of highly labile components in regulation of complement, which undergo spontaneous inactivation if are not stabilized by reaction with other components. In addition, the second mechanism involve a series of regulatory proteins can inactivate various complement components. For example, the glycoprotein C1 inhibitor (C1Inh) can form a complex with C1r2s2, causing it to dissociate from C1q and preventing further activation of C4 or C2. The regulatory protein of complement system and there function are summarized in Table 11.6.

11.7. IMMUNOLOGIC PROPERTIES OF ANTIGENS

Based on the immunological properties, antigens can be categorized as immunogenic, antigenic, allergenic and tolerogenic.

Immunogenic substances are those which can induce a humoral or cell-mediated immune response.

B cells + antigen → plasma cells + memory cells

T cells + antigen → T effector cells + memory cells

All immunogenic substances are antigenic. Antigenic substances have the ability to combine specifically with the final products of an immunogenic response (i.e., antibodies/or cell-surface receptors). In contrast, some small molecules referred to as haptens are not capable by themselves of inducing a specific immune response. In simple terms, they lack immunogenicity. In order to induce immune response, the hapten requires to be attached to a carrier molecule (usually a serum protein such as albumin). The hapten molecule then acts as a determinant of antigenic specificity and is referred to as an antigenic determinant.

Allergenic substances are those which have the ability to induce various types of allergic responses. Allergens are immunogens that tend to activate specific types of humoral or cell-mediated responses. Tolerogenic substances are those which can induce specific immunologic non-responsiveness in either the humoral or cell-mediated branch.

11.7.1. Factors influencing immunogenicity

The following factors are influential in providing an effective protection against infectious agents.

1. The immune system must be able to recognize bacteria, bacterial products, fungal parasites and viruses as immunogens.

2. Immune system usually recognizes some particular macromolecules of an infectious disease, generally proteins or polysaccharides.

3. Lipids and nucleic acids do not serve as immunogens.

4. When complexed to proteins or polysaccharides, lipids and nucleic acids can serve as immunogens.

5. Soluble proteins or polysaccharides are used as immunogens for study of humoral immunity [e.g., Bovine serum albumin (BSA)].

6. Only proteins serve as immunogens for cell mediated immunity, but they are not recognized directly; instead, they are processed into small peptides and then presented alongwith and in association with major histocompatibility complex (MHC).

7. Immunogenicity is not an intrinsic property of a macromolecule.

8. To elicit an immune response, a molecule must be recognized as non-self by the biological system. This is termed as foreignness.

9. Generally, a substance to be immunogenic should have a molecular weight of not less than 5,000 Da.

10. Copolymers of sufficient size, containing two or more different amino acids are immunogenic while polymers composed of a single amino acid or sugar lack immunogenicity.

11. Macromolecules that cannot be degraded and processed by antigen-presenting cells are poor immunogens.

12. Large, insoluble macromolecules are generally more immunogenic as they are readily phagocytosed and processed.

13. Intermolecular chemical cross-linking, heat aggregation and attachment to insoluble matrices are used to increase the insolubility of macromolecules and hence the immunogenicity.

14. Genetic constitution of an immunized animal also influences the type of immune response manifested.

15. Genes encoding B-cell and T-cell receptors and various proteins involved in immune regulation also play a key role in immune response.

16. The dose of an immunogen is important in eliciting immune response; the dose should be neither too high nor too low.

17. The route by which the immunogens are administered is also critical. Generally, they are administered by routes other than oral, e.g. intradermal, subcutaneous, intravenous or intramuscular.

18. Immunogenicity of an antigen may be increased by using adjuvants (substances which when mixed with an antigen, serve to enhance immunogenicity of that antigen).

19. Low molecular weight substances (e.g., aspirin, penicillin and sulfonamides) are antigenic as they form a covalent bond complex with tissue proteins.

20. Particle size also plays an important role in determining antigenicity. Example, aggregated BSA is more effective as compared to non-aggregated BSA.

11.7.2. Haptens

In the 1920s, Landsteiner chemically defined a system for studying the binding of an individual antibody to a unique epitope on a complex protein antigen. In his approach he coupled small organic molecules called haptens to larger protein molecules called carriers. The resulting hapten-carrier conjugate was used to immunize animals. Haptens are small molecules that can bind to antibodies but cannot by themselves function as immunogens. The system developed by Landsteiner does not stimulate a clonal selection alone. However, if multiple copies of a hapten are coupled to a large non-immunogenic homopolymer, the molecule does sometime behave as an immunogen. Here, the homopolymer provides the requisite size, and the hapten provides the complexity and multivalency.

The chief advantage of the hapten carrier system is that it provides immunologists with a chemically defined determinant that can be chemically modified to determine the effect of various chemical structures on immune specificity. The specific reaction of the anti-hapten antibodies in the immune serum and that of antibodies to the original carrier epitopes has also been studied. Landsteiner further tested that an antihapten antibody could bind to other haptens having a slightly different chemical structure. Many biologically important substances, including drugs, peptide hormones and steroid hormones can function as haptens. The home pregnancy test kit, which determines the presence or absence of human chorionic gonadotropin (HCG) in a woman's urine, is a classical hapten-inhibition assay.

11.7.3. Mitogens

Mitogens are agents that can induce cell division in a high percentage of T or B cells. Unlike immunogens, which activate only lymphocytes bearing specific receptors, mitogens activate many clones of T or B cells regardless of their antigen specificity. Because of this ability, mitogens are known as polyclonal activators. Various diverse agents function as mitogens. Many common mitogens are proteins (called lectins) that are derived from plants and bind sugars. However all lectins are not mitogenic in nature. Lectins recognize different glycoproteins on the surface of various cells, including lymphocytes. Their binding often leads to agglutination, or clustering of the cells, followed by cellular activation. Some mitogens preferentially activate B cells, others activate T cells, and some activate both. Three commonly used lectins with mitogenic activity are concanavalin A (Con A), phyto-hemagglutinin (PHA) and pokeweed mitogen. Each of these binds to carbohydrate residues in glycoproteins and is able to crosslink glycoproteins on the surface of cells. The lipopolysaccharide (LPS) component of the gram-negative bacteria cell wall functions as a B-cell mitogen, Con A and PHA are T-cell mitogens, while pokeweed mitogen acts as both. Among the group of T cell mitogens, an unusual group of substances, known as superantigens, is found to be most potent. These superantigens can bind to residues in the Vf3 domain of the T cell receptor and residues in class II MHC molecules outside of the antigen binding cleft. In this way the superantigen cross-links a T cell to a class II MHC molecule in an antigen-independent manner, and activates distinct set of $V\beta$ expressing T cells. Staphylococcal enterotoxins (Ses) and toxic-shock syndrome toxin I (TSSTI) exemplify superantigens. These toxins activate many TH cells by crosslinking the T cell receptors with any class II MHC molecule expressed on an antigen-presenting cell.

11.8. MAJOR HISTOCOMPATIBILITY COMPLEX (MHC)

The major histocompatibility complex (MHC) is a large genomic region or gene family found in most vertebrates. It is the most gene-dense region of the mammalian genome and plays an important role in the immune system, autoimmunity, and reproductive success. The proteins encoded by the MHC are expressed on the surface of cells in all jawed vertebrates, and display both self antigens (peptide fragments from the cell itself) and nonself antigens (e.g., fragments of invading microorganisms) to a type of white blood cell called a T cell that has the capacity to kill or co-ordinate the killing of pathogens and infected or malfunctioning cells.

MHC complex is group of genes on a single chromosome that codes the MHC antigens. Major as well as minor histocompatibility antigens (also called transplantation antigens) mediate rejection of grafts between two genetically different individuals. However, the role played by the major histocompatibility antigens supersedes the minor histocompatibility antigens. HLA (human leukocyte antigens) are the MHC antigens of humans, and called so because they were first detected on leukocytes. H-2 antigens are their equivalent MHC antigens of mouse. A set of MHC alleles present on each chromosome is called an MHC haplotype. Monozygotic human twins have the same histocompatibility molecules on their cells, and they can accept transplants of tissue from each other. Histocompatibility molecules of one individual act as antigens when introduced into a different individual. George Snell, Jean Dausset and Baruj Benacerraf received the Nobel Prize in 1980 for their contributions to the discovery and understanding of the MHC in mice and humans MHC gene products were identified as responsible for graft rejection. MHC gene products that control immune responses are called the immune response (Ir) genes. Immune response genes influence responses to infections. The essential role of the HLA antigens lies in the induction and regulation of the immune response and defence against microorganisms. The physiologic function of MHC molecules is the presentation of peptide antigen to T lymphocytes. These antigens and their genes can be divided into three major classes: class I, class II and class III.

Table 11.7: The MHC region is divided into three subgroups, class I, class II, and class III

Name	Function	Expression
MHC Class-I	Encodes heterodimeric peptide binding proteins, as well as antigen processing molecules such as TAP and Tapasin	Found in all nucleated cells. MHC class I proteins contain α chain and β_2 micro-globulin. They present antigen fragment to cytotoxic T cells *via* CD8 molecule and also bind on inhibitory receptor on NK cell.
MHC Class-II	Encodes heterodimeric peptide binding protein and proteins that modulate antigen loading n to MHC class II protein in the lysosomal compartment such as MHC II DM, MHC II DQ, MHC II DR, and MHC II DP.	On most immune system cells, specifically on antigen-presenting cells. MHC class II proteins contain α & β chains and they present antigen fragments to T-helper cells by binding to the CD4 receptor on the T-helper cells.
MHC class III region	Encodes for other immune components, such as complement components (e.g., C2, C4, factor B) and some that encode cytokines (e.g., TNF-α) and also hsp.	Variable

11.8.1. Structure

The MHC complex resides in the short arm of chromosome 6 and overall size of the MHC is approximately 3.5 million base pairs. The complete three-dimensional structure for both class I and class II MHC molecules has been determined by x-ray crystallography. The class I gene complex contains three loci A, B and C, each of which codes of α chain polypeptides. The class II gene complex also contains at least three loci, DP, DQ and DR; each of these loci codes for one α and a variable number of β chain polypeptides. Class III region is not actually a part of the HLA complex, but is located within the HLA region, because its components are either related to the functions of HLA antigens or are under similar control mechanisms to the HLA genes. Class III antigens are associated with proteins in serum and other body fluids (e.g.C4, C2, factor B, TNF) and have no role in graft rejection.

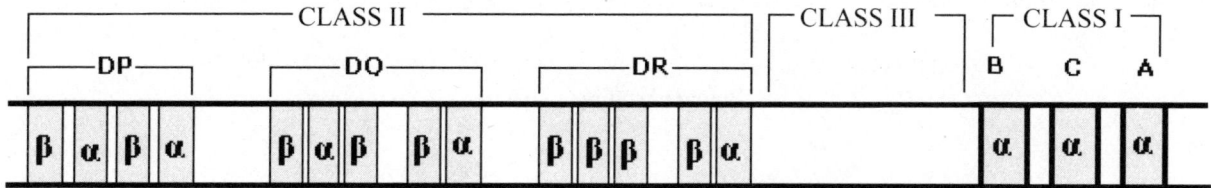

Fig. 11.17: Composition of MHC molecule

11.8.2. Expression

Class I antigens are expressed on all nucleated cells (except those of the central nervous system) and platelets. The class II antigens are expressed on antigen presenting cells such as B lymphocytes, dendritic cells, macrophages, monocytes, Langerhans cells, endothelial cells and thymic epithelial cells. Cytokines, especially interferon gamma (IFN-γ), increase the level of expression of class I and class II MHC molecules.

11.8.3. MHC class I molecule

Class I MHC molecules contain two separate polypeptide chains, the heavier (44-47 KDa) alpha chain and the lighter (12 KDa) beta chain. The carboxyl end of α chain resides inside the cell while the amino end projects on the surface of cell with a short intervening hydrophobic segment traverses the membrane. The α chain is coded by the MHC genes and has three globular domains α1, α2 and α3. B2-microglobulin is encoded by a gene on another chromosome. The α3 domain is non-covalently associated with the β2 microglobulin. Both α chain and β2-microglobulin are members of the Ig superfamily. Without the β2 microglobulin, the class I antigen will not be expressed on the cells surface. Individuals with defective β2 microglobulin gene do not express any class I antigen and hence they have a deficiency of cytotoxic T cells. A peptide-binding groove is formed between α1 and α2 helices with beta-pleated sheet as its floor. A peptide of 8–10 amino acids long can be presented in this groove. The alloantigenic sites that carry determinants specific to each individual are found in the α1 and α2 domains. The greatest variability in amino acids (or polymorphism) occurs in the α1 and α2 sequences that line the wall and floor of the groove that binds the peptides. The polymorphism among class I MHC gene products creates variation in the chemical surface of the peptide-binding groove so that various peptide molecules can be accommodated. The specific binding of a peptide molecule in the peptide-binding groove of MHC requires the peptide to have one or more specific amino acid at a fixed position. Such sites are termed anchor sites. The other amino acids can be variable so that each MHC molecule can bind many different peptides. The α1 and α2 domains also bind T cell receptor (TCR) of CD8+ T lymphocytes. The parts of these domains that are in contact with TCR also show polymorphism. The immunoglobulin-like region of α3 domain is constant (shows no variation) and is non-covalently bound β2 microglobulin. The importance of the highly conserved region of α3 is that CD8 molecules present on CD8+T lymphocytes binds to this region.

CD8+ T lymphocytes recognizes peptide antigen only when it is presented by the antigen presenting cell in the peptide binding groove of MHC I molecules. Class I molecules present peptide fragments in the cytosol (endogenous antigen, which could be fragments of viral or tumour proteins) to the $CD8^+$ lymphocytes.

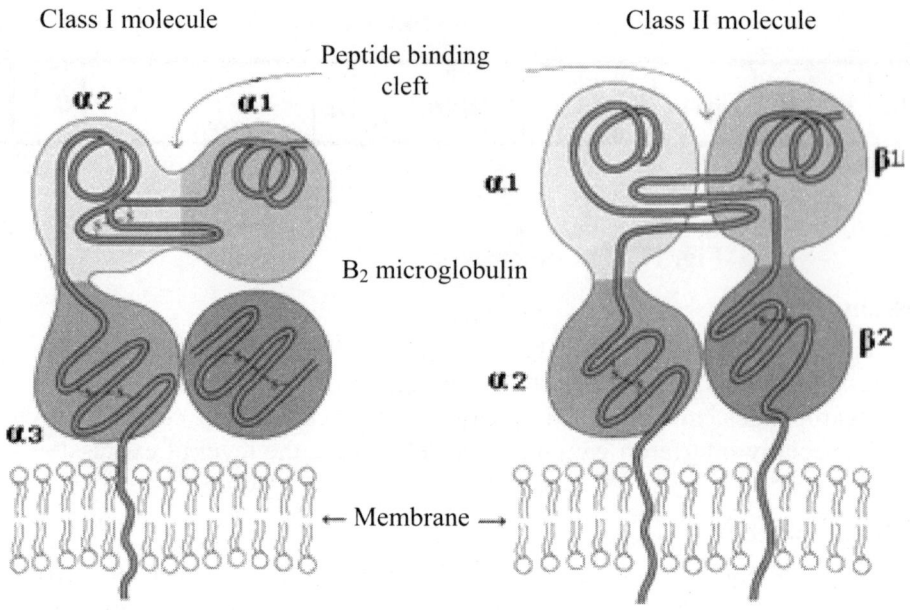

Fig. 11.18: Structure of MHC class-I and MHC class-II molecule

11.8.4. MHC class II molecule

MHC class II molecules comprise two non-identical and non-covalently associated polypeptide chains (α and β). These two chains have amino ends on the surface, a short transmembrane stretch and intracytoplasmic carboxyl ends. Both α chain (34 kDa) and β chain (28 kDa) are MHC-encoded and polymorphic. The domains closest to the membrane in each chain are structurally related to immunoglobulins. With the exception of the $\alpha 1$ domain, all domains are stabilized by disulfide bridges. The β chain is shorter than α chain and contains the alloantigenic sites. A peptide binding groove is formed in between $\alpha 1$ and $\beta 1$ domains with a beta pleated floor. As in the case for class I MHC, the greatest polymorphic variability in the amino acids is in those facing the groove. This in turn determines the chemical structure of the groove and influences the specificity and affinity of peptide binding. Peptides associated with class II MHC are 13–25 amino acids long. As with class I MHC, anchor sites for one or more amino acids also exist in the groove of the class II MHC molecule, $\alpha 2$ and $\beta 2$ are largely non-polymorphic. During antigen presentation, CD4 molecule of helper T lymphocyte binds to $\beta 2$ domain of the class II MHC molecules. Exogenous antigens (fragments of bacterial cells or viruses that are engulfed and processed by antigen presenting cell) are presented to helper T-cells along with MHC II molecules.

11.9. ANTIBODIES OR IMMUNOGLOBULINS

Immunoglobulins or antibodies are a group of glycoproteins present in the serum and tissue fluids of all animals. Immunoglobulins function as antibodies, the antigen binding proteins present on the B cell membrane and are secreted by plasma cells. Secreted antibodies serve as the effector molecules of humoral immunity. They circulate in the blood, seeking out and neutralizing or eliminating antigens. Their production is induced when the host's lymphoid system comes in contact with immunogenic foreign molecules (antigens); they bind specifically to the antigen which induces their formation. All immunoglobulins share certain structural features and thus to a significant extent govern the specificity and effective functions of immunoglobulins. Here, the main focus will be on the structure and function of immunoglobulins. In 1939 Tiselius and Kabat subjected the serum of ovalbumin immunized rabbits to electrophoresis and obtained four fractions; albumin, alpha (α), beta (β) and gamma (γ) globulins. The same serum when reacted with an antigen formed a precipitate. The serum left over after separating the precipitate, when subjected to electrophoresis showed a significant drop in the amount of γ globulin fraction; thus it was inferred that the γ globulin fraction; contained serum antibodies, which they named as immunoglobulins (Ig).

11.9.1. Immunoglobulin structure

Porter and Edelman in 1960s first separated the γ globulin fraction of serum into a high molecular weight fraction with a sedimentation constant of 19S and a low molecular weight fraction with a sedimentation constant of 7S with a molecular weight of 1,50000. They designated this 7S fraction of γ globulins as immunoglobulin (IgG).

The chain structure of IgG was first suggested by Edelman and was later confirmed by Porter. The IgG (1,50,000 MW) is composed of two 50,000 MW polypeptide chains designated as heavy (H) chain and two 25,000 MW chains, designated as light (L) chains. Porter in 1962 proposed a prototype structure of IgG (Fig.11.19). He found that on brief digestion with papain, IgG fragmented. Among the fragments, two were identical (each with 45,000 MW) called Fab fragments due to their 'antigen-binding' activity and one fragment, the Fc fragment, so named because they crystallized during cold storage. However, Alford Nisonoff found that on digestion with pepsin, IgG produced only a single fragment with molecular weight 1,00,000, He named this as F(ab')2 fragment which, like Fab, could precipitate antigens.

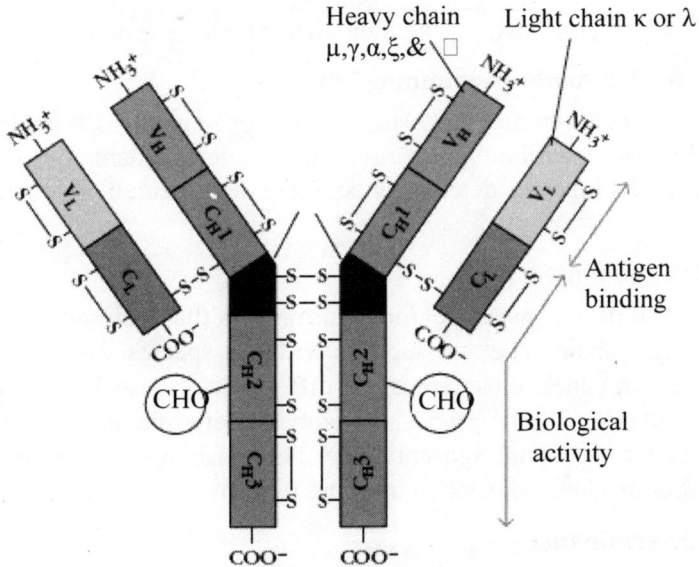

Fig. 11.19: Prototype structure of IgG

A single antibody has two identical heavy chains and two identical light chains. Immunoglobulins have similar basic structure and similar chemical properties. However, their antigen binding specificity and exact amino acid sequences differ. Light chain sequencing: Studies carried out on various amino acid sequences revealed that the amino-terminal half of the amino acid chain varied among different proteins. This region is called Variable (V) region. The carboxyl terminal half of the molecule is called Constant (C) region. The constant region was found to have two basic amino acid sequences named Kappa (K) and Lambda (λ). In human beings, 60% of the light chains are Kappa and 40% Lambda, whereas in mice 95% of the light chains are Kappa and only 5% are Lambda. A noteworthy point is that a single antibody molecule expresses either K light chains or light chains but never both.

Heavy chain sequencing: The heavy chains of antibodies like their counter parts (light chain) showed a variation in their amino terminal which was again designated as variable (V) region. However, the remaining part of the protein revealed five basic amino acid sequence patterns (μ,γ,α,δ and E) corresponding to five different heavy chain constant (C) regions (Fig.11.20). It is these chains (heavy) which determine the class on antibody, i.e. IgG, IgA, IgM, IgE and IgD. A single antibody molecule has two identical light and heavy chains. However, the light chain may be K or λ (Table 11.7).

Table 11.7: Composition of immunoglobulin chain among the five different classes in human (*)

Class	Heavy chain	Subclasses
IgG	γ	$\gamma1,\gamma2,\gamma3,\gamma4,$
IgA	α	$\alpha1,\alpha2$
IgM	μ	----
IgD	δ	----
IgE	ε	----

* Note: The light chain in all cases is k/λ

11.9.3. Antigenic determinants on immunoglobulins

As we know by now that antibodies are made of glycoproteins, which is alone can function as potent immunogens and induce an antibody response. Antigen determinants fall into three major categories; isotypic, allotypic and idiotypic determinants; these are located in characteristic portions of the molecule.

11.9.4. Isotypic determinants

Isotypic determinants define constant region determinants that distinguish each heavy chain class and subclass and each light chain type and subtype within a species. However, different species inherit different constant region genes, thus expressing different isotypes. Therefore, when an antibody from one species is injected into another species, the isotypic determinants are recognized as foreign and so elicit antibody response to the foreign antibody. This enables researchers to determine the class or subclass of antibodies produced during an immune response.

11.9.5. Allotypic determinants

These refer to genetic variations within species. Although all members of a species inherit the same set of isotypic genes, multiple alleles exist for some genes. These alleles introduce a difference in amino acid sequence. In humans, allotypes have been characterized for all four IgG subclasses, for one 19A subclass and for the k light chain. Antibodies to allotypic determinant can be produced following a blood transfusion or transferred from mother to fetus, or by injecting antibodies from one species to another.

11.9.6. Idiotypic determinants

Variation in the variable domain (in particular in the highly variable segments) produces idiotypes. Idiotypes are usually specific for individual antibody clone, but are sometimes shared between different clones. Each individual antigenic determinant of the variable region is referred to as an idiotope. Many vertebrate animals are capable of rejecting foreign particles, skin, or soluble substances by specific antibodies. These immune reactions are mediated by lymphoid cells, which are endowed with immunological memory and hence can mount a rapid and strong immune response when repeatedly challenged by an antigen. The immune system consists of leukocytes (i.e., lymphocytes. macrophages, granulocytes), dendritic cells, epidermal Langerhans cells, and specialized epithelial cells. They are present in such tissues and organs as bone marrow, lymph nodes, spleen, patches of intestine, tonsils, and thymus. A major fraction of the leukocytes constitutes a recirculating pool of cells found in the blood and lymph vessels.

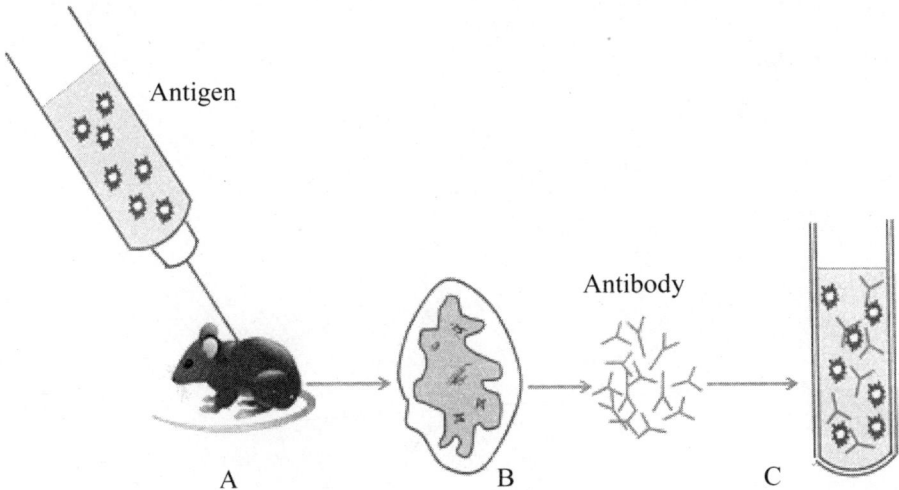

Fig. 11.20: Production of antibodies by injecting antigens in rabbit A, injection of rabbit with an antigen (foreign protein), B, production of distinct Y-shaped antibodies by the rabbit's white blood cells as a response to injection; C, precipitation occurs, when some of the rabbit's blood serum containing antibodies are mixed with the antigen

An antigen is a material (generally a protein) that is foreign to some animal. When the antigen is injected into the animal, it initiates a series of reactions resulting in the synthesis of antibodies. These distinctive proteins made by the animal have sites that are paratactic to the features of the antigen. We can detect antibodies because they bind so strongly to antigens. For instance, when antigens are combined with blood serum containing antibodies (immune serum) there is no reaction with a non-immune serum. The antigen-antibody reaction is thus very specific.

The immunologic system is anatomically and histologically very similar in all vertebrates. At least two directing mechanisms are involved. The first causes acute rejection of foreign skin within two weeks. The second facilitates chronic rejections of transplants within the span of a month or more. In those vertebrates, which are able to reject within a fortnight, a short chromosomal region has been identified in which many genes controlling immune reaction appear to be located close together. This region is called the major histocompatibility region or complex or system, and abbreviated as MHR, MHC or MHS. Examples of these vertebrates (acute rejections) include mammals and birds. In contrast, reptiles and several amphibians can reject foreign skin chronically; in these cases the genes are scattered over the entire genome. Interestingly, even in mammals and birds, which have a compact histocompatibility system, there is another, much weaker, system of genes which is distributed over the entire genome as in the case of reptiles.

In man, the MHR is called the HLA system, HLA being derived from Human Lymphocyte System A. An organism is able to respond to antigens because of the presence of the lymphocytes. An adult human being has over 10^6 different lymphocyte clones, each having receptors for distinctive antigens (Figs 11.21 and 11.22).

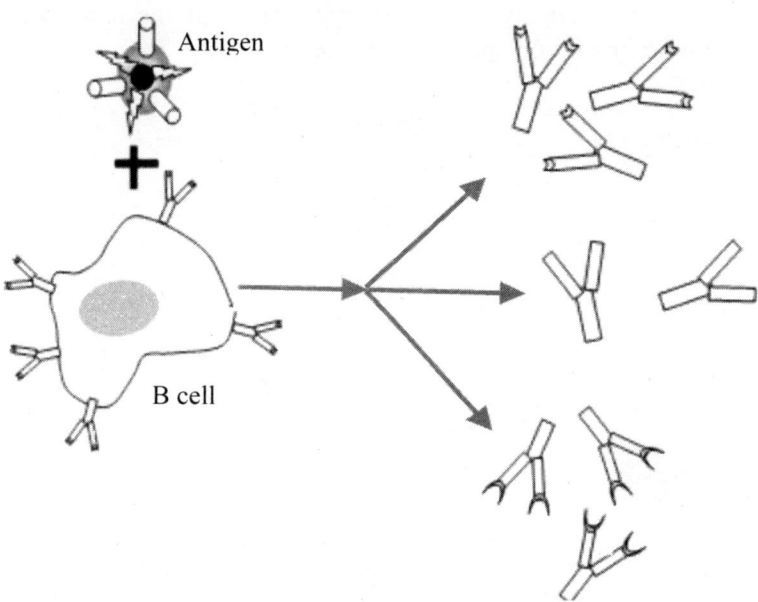

Fig. 11.21: Production of polyclonal antibodies by B-lymphocytes. A polyclonal antibody pool contains antibodies from many different clones of plasma cells. Here, only three antibodies are shown. The antigen stimulates the B-lymphocytes, which produce the antibodies. The antibody in the polyclonal pool binds to different epitopes on the antigen

The immune system generates an enormous diversity of proteins that act as deadly weapons against the myriads of microorganisms that attack us. The immune system remembers throughout life the pathogenic microbes or other harmful agents that we have encountered. So it can deploy the weapons instantaneously on subsequent infection.

11.10. ANTIBODY GENES

Researches on mammalian immune system have shown that shuffling of a few hundred genes in pre-lymphocyte cells generates the enormous diversity of antibody molecules produced by the mature lymphocytes. An antibody molecule results from the assembly of some protein chains. Since a mammal produces an enormous number of antibody molecules, there exist millions of genes corresponding to the antibodies. But we know that a mammalian genome does not exceed about 35,000 genes, and only a fraction of these can direct the synthesis of antibodies. The explanation of this paradox is that the germ cells or embryonic cells do not contain a complete set of all the antibody genes but rather have a basic kit of genetic elements which are shuffled during the course of development, differentiation, and maturation of the cells of the immune system (i.e., the B-lymphocytes). This is how different combinations result in each of the millions of cell lines.

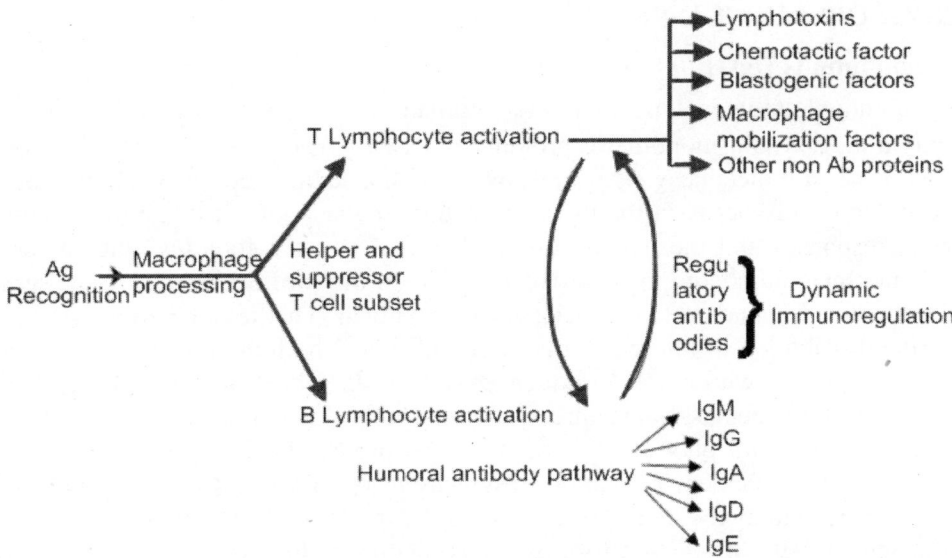

Fig. 11.22: Major pathways of mammalian immune response

11.11. Antibody diversity and hypermutation

Upon encountering foreign molecules, our antibodies can mutate. This allows them to bind to the intruders more strongly. The immune system fights off intruders by producing protective antibody proteins which recognize and neutralize foreign molecules. Antibodies are secreted by B-cells and are unique among our proteins in having unlimited potential for diversity (Gearhart, 2002). Half of each antibody molecule is encoded by the so-called variable genes. When a B-cell recognizes and responds to a foreign molecule, these variable genes mutate at very high frequency. DiNoia and Nauberger (2002) discovered the elusive mechanism behind this 'hypermutation'. They showed that the activation-induced cytosine deaminase (AID) protein, which is needed for hypermutation, leads to DNA mutations when expressed in bacteria. More mutations of the cytosines in DNA occur in bacteria that lack the enzyme uracil glycosylase, suggesting that AID converts cytosines to uracils. Normally, these erroneous uracils would be removed by the glycosylase before they caused a problem. It has now been proved that the generation of uracil from cytosine in B-cell DNA triggers hypermutation when the cells try to fix the errors (Gearhart, 2002). DiNoia and Neuberger (2002) confirmed the conversion of cytosine to uracil in DNA in eukaryotic cells.

Hypermutation creates new protein sequences that can bind the antigen more strongly and specifically than their precursors. This allows people to respond quickly and effectively to pathogens that they have encountered previously. Individuals who fail to mutate their antibodies suffer recurring bacterial and viral infections, and do not respond to vaccination (Gearhart, 2002).

Hypermutation occurs only in B-cells that have been stimulated with antigen during hypermutation. Many single mutations and, rarely, small insertions and deletions, are introduced into the variable regions of antibody encoding genes, The identification of AID generated uracil as the likely starting point constitutes a major breakthrough in understanding hypermutation. But one unresolved question is how AID targets the rearranged variable genes. One possibility is that AID is delivered to these genes by interacting with transcription factors, also before the model is fully accepted it needs to be shown that AID actually does deaminate cytosine in DNA, and that uracil are present in the variable genes.

11.12. IMMUNOGLOBULIN CLASSES

11.12.1. Immunoglobulin G (IgG)

IgG, the major immunoglobulin isotype in normal human serum constitutes 70-75% of the total serum immunoglobulin. IgG is a monomeric protein with two γ heavy chains and two k or λ light chains (Fig.11.23). It has a molecular weight of 1,46000 with a sedimentation coefficient of 7S. The IgG class is distributed evenly between the intra and extravascular pools. It is the major antibody of secondary immune responses and the exclusive-toxin class. There are four IgG subclasses namely IgG1, IgG2, IgG3 and IgG4 numbered in accordance with their order of occurrence in the serum. One important thing to be noted is that no two subclasses are identical. This may be either with reference to the number or the distribution of interchain disulfide linkages. The four subclasses are encoded by different germ-line CH genes whose DNA sequences are 90-95% homologous. The differences in amino acid sequence in IgG subclasses are directly related to biological activity. While IgG1, IgG3 and IgG4 cross the placenta and play an important role in protecting the fetus, IgG2 crosses only partially in some cases. Complement activation efficiency also differs; IgG3 is the most effective, followed by IgG1, IgG2 and IgG4 and said to be totally ineffective in activating a complement sequence. The opsonin activity of IgG is attributed to its binding to Fc receptors on phagocytic cells. Again, the different subclasses have different affinity. IgG1 and IgG3 have a higher affinity to Fc receptors while IgG4 has an intermediate affinity; IgG2 shows an extremely low affinity.

11.12.2. Immunoglobulin A (lgA)

Immunoglobulin A (lgA), the predominant immunoglobulin in mucous secretions, constitutes 15-20% of the normal human serum immunoglobulin pool. It is protected from proteolysis by combination with another protein; the secretory component IgA is predominantly seen in external secretions such as breast milk, saliva, tears and mucus of the bronchial, genitourinary and digestive tracts. Hence, they are frequently known as secretory IgA (slgA). In serum, IgA exists as a monomer; however, in most cases it is polymeric, i.e. dimers, trimers, etc. The slgA consists of a dimer or tetramer, a J chain polypeptide and a polypeptide chain called secretory component. The secretory component is a polypeptide with 70,000 MW and is produced by epithelial cells of mucous membranes. It consists of, five immunoglobulin like domains that bind to the Fc region of IgA dimer.

11.12.3. Immunoglobulin M (lgM)

IgM accounts for about 10% of the total serum immunoglobulin with an average serum concentration of 1.5% mg/ml. Unlike IgG or IgA, IgM has a pentameric structure in which individual heavy chains have a molecular weight of approximately 65,000 while the total molecular weight amounts to 9,70,000. The monomeric units consist of two μ heavy chains and two light chains. The subunits are held together by disulfide bonds between their carboxyl terminal (Cμ 4/Cμ4) domains and Cμ3/Cμ3. The subunits are so arranged that their Fc region lies in the center of the pentamer. It is believed that IgM has 10 antigen binding sites but they are unable to combine with the antigen with similar efficiency; this makes it difficult to demonstrate the presence of 10 sites. In addition to the above, Fc linked polypeptide called J (joining) chain, is disulfide bonded to the carboxyl terminal cysteine residue of two of the 10μ chains.

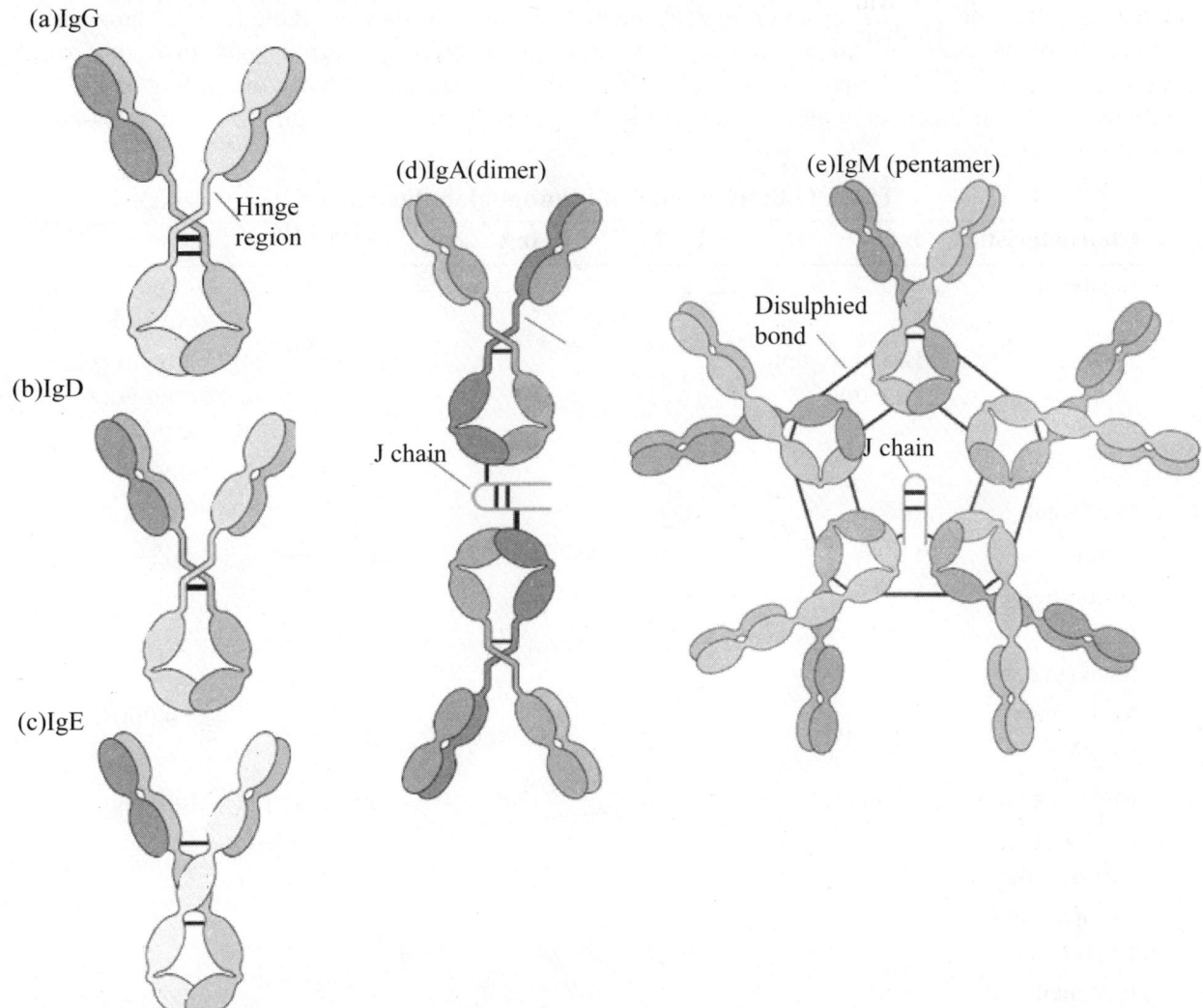

Fig. 11.23: General structure of five major classes of secreted antibody

The J chain appears to be required for polymerization of the monomer. The presence of the J chain allows IgM to bind to receptors on secretory cells, which helps them in transporting across the epithelial linings to external secretions that bathe mucosal surfaces. IgM is largely confined to the intravascular pool and is the predominant 'early' antibody frequently directed against antigenic complexes after a primary response. It is also the first to be synthesized by the neonate. Monomeric IgM is expressed as membrane bound antibody on B cells. Because of its pentameric structure, serum IgM has higher valance than others. For example, it takes 100–1000 times as many molecules of IgG as of IgM to achieve the same level of agglutination. Due to its large size, diffusion to the intracellular tissue fluids is very low.

11.12.4. Immunoglobulin D (IgD)

IgD constitutes less than 1 % of the total plasma immunoglobulin with a serum concentration of 30μg/ml. IgD, together with IgM, is the major membrane bound immunoglobulin expressed by mature B cells. Though their exact biological function is not clear they are thought to function in the activation of B cells by an antigen. IgD is more susceptible to proteolysis than any other immunoglobulin class. IgD has a simple disulfide bond between the δ chains and a high content of carbohydrate distributed in multiple oligosaccharide units. One of these units is rich in N-acetyl galactosamine.

Table 11.8: Summary of immunoglobulin classes

Characteristics	IgG	IgM	IgA	IgD	IgE
Location	Blood, lymph, intestine	Blood. Lymph. B-cell surface			Bound to mast and basophil cells throughout the body, blood
% of total serum antibodies	80-85	5-10	15	0.2	0.002
Normal serum level (mg/ml)	3	1.5	2	0.03	0.0003
Molecular weight	1,50,000	9.00,000	3,20,000	1,85,000	2,00,000
Molecular form	Monomer	Pentamer	Dimer	Monomer	Monomer
In vivo serum half life (days)	23	5	6	3	2
Complement fixation	+	+	-	-	-
Placental transfer	+	-	-	-	-
Functions	Enhances Phagocytosis	First Ab produced	Localized	Unclear, but presence of B cells may indicate function in initiation of immune response	Allergic reactions

11.13. IMMUNOMODULATING SUBSTANCES

A variety of substances are used as adjuvants, in combination with specific vaccines enhance immunity levels above those which the vaccine elicits by itself, Agar, tapioca, lecithin, and some other substances show this potentiating effect. Certain peptides of animal origin are potent stimulants (or adjuvants) of the immune system whereas others act as inhibitors and in some cases the same peptide stimulates under certain conditions and on the contrary inhibits under other conditions the immune response. These peptides with dual function are called immunomodulators. Good examples of immunomodulator peptides include interferon, interleukin, muramyl peptides of microbial origin (e.g., murabutide and lipopeptides which attack phagocytic cells and T-lymphocytes), several peptides of animal origin, including thymic hormones (e.g., thymulin promotes many T-cell functions and inhibits the generation of cytotoxic T-lymphocytes), tuftsin (stimulates phagocytic cells, pinocytosis, phagocytosis, motility, and antigen processing), peptides derived from fibrinogen, and certain peptides from colostrums and from milk. Furthermore, some neuropeptides (neuroendocrine hormones) are thought to play an essential role as signals from the central nervous system to the immune system. Somatostatin is a tetradecapeptide, isolated from the hypothalamus that inhibits the secretion of growth hormone. It is present in neural and gastrointestinal tissues and can also inhibit secretion from several endocrine and exocrine glands. Specific functional receptors for a variety of neuropeptides have been demonstrated in diverse cell populations of the immune system.

11.14. MONOCLONAL ANTIBODIES

Antibodies are routinely obtained by injecting an animal (or man) with the antigen against which an immune response is sought. The immune system then reacts by generating a variety of antibodies, each specific to a different part of the injected antigen molecule. Blood serum taken from such an animal contains this antibody mixture. Most immunogens tend to be rather weak because of the heterogeneity of the immune response which results in each antiserum being a mixture of antibodies with varying affinity, cross reactivity and effector functions. They react with the immunizing antigen that was being originally generated by the spleen cells. These hybrids can grow continuously in culture, recover after freezing and induces tumours when injected into animals. The hybrids produce a homogeneous antibody having a constant, specific amino acid sequence. The formation of the tumour in the recipient animal (following injection of the hybrid) confers upon it the capacity to accumulate large amounts of the particular antibody in its serum or ascites fluid.

However, it is fairly easy to produce rodent MAbs, but problems is the production of human MAbs. Indeed, it is possible to produce genetically-altered immunoglobulin molecules and thus improve existing MAbs. Organization of the antibody genes is such that they can be easily manipulated as each domain of the protein is found on a separate exon. This makes it possible to produce antibodies with novel combinations of domains by assembling the appropriate exons. Further, the introns become spliced from the primary transcript and do not appear in mature mRNA. Therefore any change within introns does not alter the protein product.

The foregoing approach has been exploited for making chimeric antibodies that combine exons from different species. By joining the variable domains from mouse hybridomas to human constant region domains, one can make mostly human antibodies possessing the wide spectrum of specificities available in mouse MAbs. It has been found that a chimeric antibody may be some 100 times as effective as the mouse antibody, from which the variable region was derived, in interacting with human immune cells to mediate antibody-dependent cellular cytotoxicity. The production of monoclonal antibody has been given in following section:

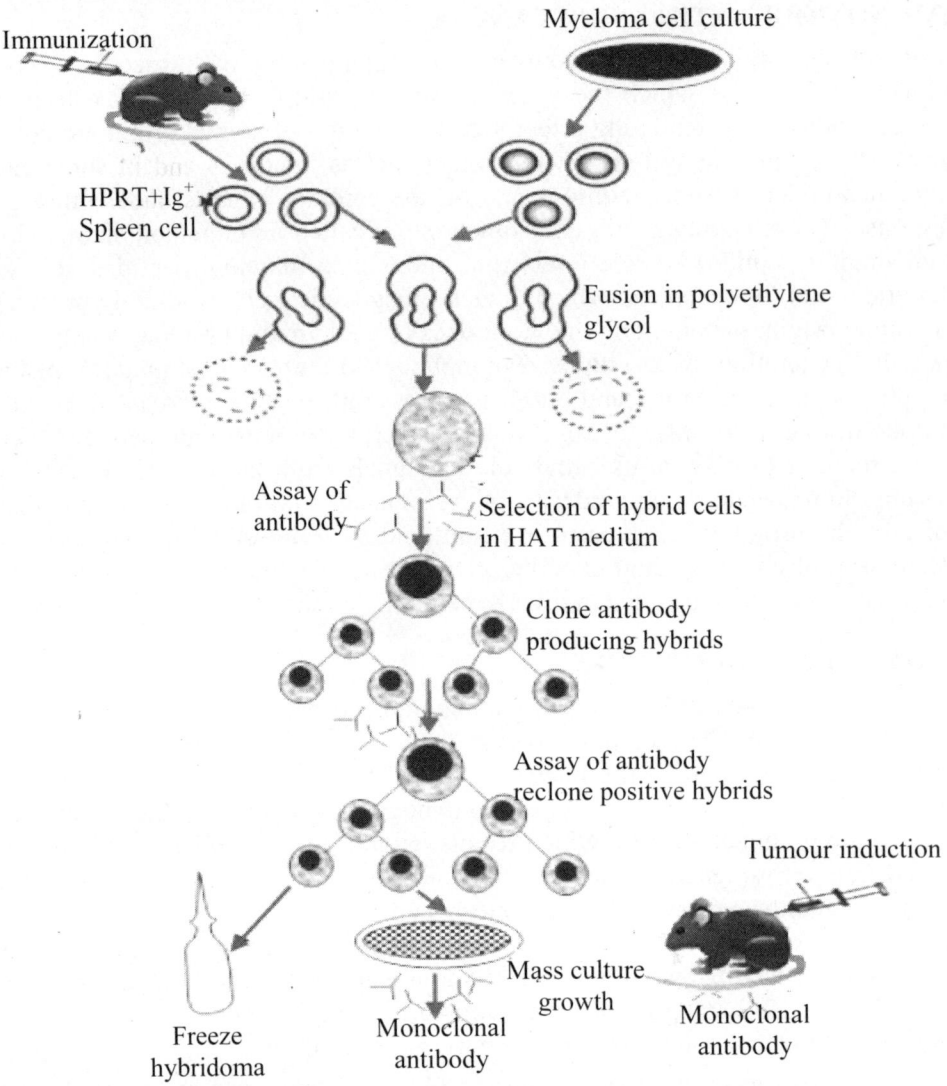

Immunization

Myeloma cell culture

HPRT+Ig⁺ Spleen cell

Fusion in polyethylene glycol

Assay of antibody

Selection of hybrid cells in HAT medium

Clone antibody producing hybrids

Assay of antibody reclone positive hybrids

Tumour induction

Mass culture growth

Monoclonal antibody

Freeze hybridoma

Monoclonal antibody

Monoclonal antibody

Fig. 11.24: Procedure for production of monoclonal antibodies

11.14.1. Production of monoclonal antibodies

Four basic steps are involved in the production of a given monoclonal antibody:

1. Immunization
2. Generation of B cell hybridomas by fusing primed B cells and myeloma cells
3. Selection and the screening of the resulting clones for those that secrete antibody with the desired specificity.
4. Cloning by propagating the desired hybridomas.

Immunization

Immunization of animals with immunogens is performed by injecting microgram or milligram quantities of immunogen mixed with an adjuvant (aluminum salts, Freund's complete or incomplete adjuvant), intradermlly or subcutaneously at multiple sites repeatedly at different times. The serum of animal is assayed for the relative concentration of antibodies of desired specificity at various time intervals. When the concentration of antibodies is found to be nearly optimal, the animal is sacrificed and the spleen, which contains a large number of plasma cells, is dissociated into single splenocytes by mechanical and/or enzymatic method.

Cell fusion

Splenocytes are then mixed with plasmocytoma cells in an appropriate medium. This mixture is exposed to a high concentration (e.g. 50%) of PEG for short period of time and fusion is allowed to proceed over a period of time Mouse has been used in the production of monoclonal antibody secreting hybridoma with splenocytes,because these animals are inexpensive and several billion cells can be obtained from a mouse spleen. In contrast, mice are rarely used for the production of poly clonal antisera, because of their very low blood volume (= 2ml). The use of HGPRT cells (that cannot grow in HAT medium) assured that only hybridomas (hybrid myeloma-spleen cells) are selected. After 7-10 days of culture in the HAT medium most of the wells contain dead cells, but a few wells contain small clusters of viable cells. Each cluster represents clonal expansion of a hybridoma. After HAT selection, single cells are transferred and cultured in separate wells to ensure the monoclonality of the secreted antibody. Wells containing viable clusters are then screened for antibody production and antibody positive clones are subcultured at low cell densities, again to ensure clonal purity in each microwell.

The first hybridoma obtained by Kohler and Milstein secreted not only antibody from the spleen B cell but also unwanted antibody from the myeloma cell as well as' one hybrid antibody containing heavy or light chains from both original parent cells. To avoid this difficulty a HGRPT, Ab-myeloma cell was chosen as ideal fusion partner. This fusion partner has the immortal properties of a cancer cell but does not secrete its own antibody or gene product. Hybridomas generated with this fusion partner thus secrete only the antibody from the B cell partner. These hybridomas can be propagated in tissue culture to give rise to large clones secreting homogenious monoclonal antibody.

Selection and screening of the clones for monoclonal antibody specificity

Once pure clones of antibody-secreting hybridomas are obtained, they must be screened for the desired antibody specificity. Selection of hybridoma cells in HAT medium is usually followed by screening of hybridomas for secretion of antibodies of the desired specificity. After fusion, the cells may be transferred to HAT medium in tissue culture flasks. After an appropriate incubation time, all viable cells will be hybridomas. They are removed from the flasks, transferred to regular culture medium and aliquots are distributed among the well of 96-well plastic culture plates. The supernatant of each hybridoma culture can be assayed for a particular antigen specificity in various ways. Two methods are frequently used (a) ELISA and (b) RIA. Both are easily adapted to mass screening with 96-well plastic culture plates. In both assays, antigen that reacts with the desired antibody is bound to the bottom of 96-well plates, and washed to remove unbound antigen. Supernatant from each hybridoma well is added to separate well and incubated for an appropriate period of time. If a sample of supernatant contains the desired antibody it will bind to the antigen and will remain associated with the well as unbound material is washed off.

In ELISA, this antibody is then -detected by an immunoconjugate consisting of two components covalently linked to each other One component is' an antibody specific for an epitope in the constant domain of the first antibody (e.g., mouse Fc or mouse Y chain). The second component is an enzyme such as alkaline phosphates or horse radish peroxidase. After another washing step, a colorless substrate that is converted to a colored product by the enzyme of immunoconjugate is added. After an appropriate incubation, the enzymatic reaction is stopped and the optical density of each well is determined at the respective λ max. with a specialized colorimeter known as a 'plate reader'. In RIA the anti-isotype antibody is radio labelled; bound label can be detected by counting the wells individually in a gamma counter or the entire plate can be exposed to X-ray film. If the desired monoclonal antibody is specific for a cell membrane molecule, immunofluorescent techniques can be used for screening. In this case, target cells with the particular cell membrane antigen are stained with monoclonal antibody in micrometer wells and visualized by the addition of fluorochrome-conjugated anti-isotype antibody.

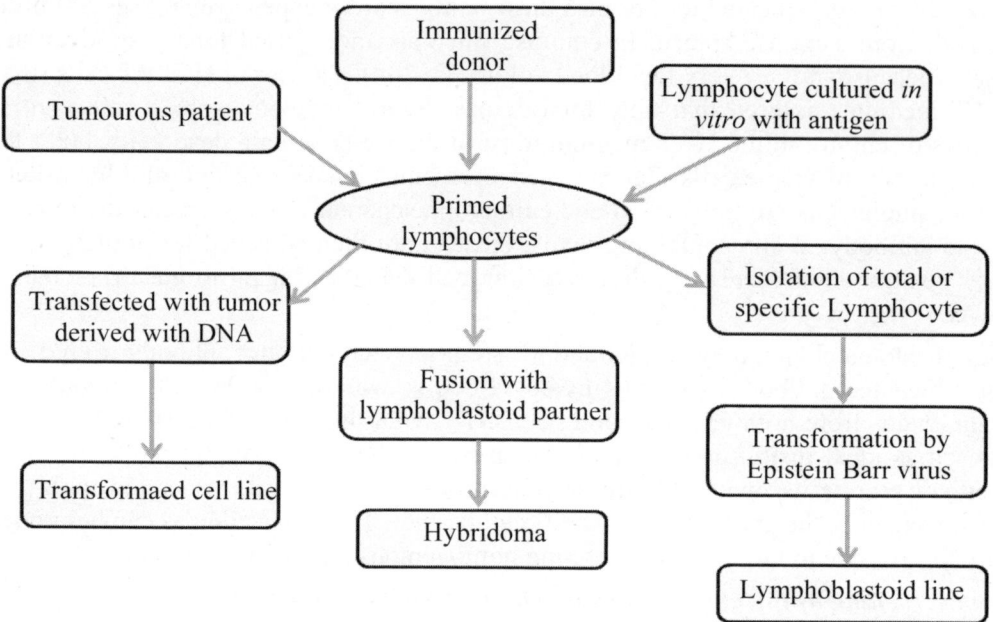

Fig. 11.25: Protocol for producing specific antibody-secreting lines of human origin

Cloning of hybridomas secreting specific monoclonal antibody

Single cells secreting the desired antibody are isolated from positive cultures and propagated into cell lines). There are two cloning techniques which are most widely used:

1. Limiting dilution

2. Soft agar

In limiting dilution, the cells in the culture are enumerated, diluted and aliquoted into new wells so that only one cell found in any well. Cells are allowed to regrow and the procedure is repeated several times to increase the probability that all the cells in a given well are monoclonal. The second method is based on the fact that many malignant cells will proliferate, forming spherical colonies, in a semisolid medium containing low amounts of agar. If the culture can be reliably dispersed into single cells and the cell concentration, is such that the colonies will be well spaced, then visible colonies picked out of the agar are likely to be monoclonal..

When a hybridoma is grown in tissue culture flasks, the antibody is secreted into the medium at fairly low concentration (10-100μg/ml). An increase in the yield of monoclonal antibody secreting hybridoma can also be propagated in the peritonea] cavity of histocomplatible mice, where it secretes the monoclonal antibody into the ascites fluid at concentrations of 1-25mg/ml. The antibodies can be purified from the mouse ascites fluid by chromatography. To meet the increased demand of monoclonal antibodies, biotechnology companies have been developing various techniques to increase yield. Damon Biotech Company encapsulates hybridomas in alginate gels, which allow nutrients to flow in and waste products and antibodies to flow out. In these capsules, a much higher concentration of hybridoma cells can be achieved than in tissue culture, as a result 100 fold greater yield of antibody production has been obtained. Another approach has been used by Cell Tech in UK. In this method hybridomas are grown in 100 liter fermenters, which yield 100gm of monoclonal antibodies in a 2 week period.

11.14.2. Human monoclonal antibody

The homogeneity and specificity of monoclonal antibodies make them particularly suitable for in vivo administration in humans for diagnostic or therapeutic purposes. However, a major problem to the clinical use of monoclonal antibodies in human is that they are usually mouse antibodies and therefore are recognized as foreign, including an anti-isotype response, for human clinical trials, the use of human monoclonal antibodies is preferable, thus avoiding any anti-isotype response

The production of human monoclonal antibody has been hampered by a number of technical difficulties which are as follows:
1. Difficulty in obtaining antigen prone B cell in humans (equivalent to mouse spleen);
2. One cannot immunize a human volunteer with the range of antigens that can be given to mice or other animals;
3. Another major difficulty in producing human monoclonal antibodies has been finding partner for the B cell. To overcome these difficulties normal human B lymphocytes can be transformed with Epstein Barr Virus (EBV). When lymphocytes are cultured with antigen in the presence of EBV, some of the B cells acquire the immortal-growth properties of the transformed cell while continuing to secrete the desired antibody. Cloning of such primed, transformed cells has permitted production of human monoclonal antibodies.EBV is a lymphotrophic DNA herpes virus which is capable of converting normal human and mouse B-lymphocytes into cancer cell lines that proliferate indefinitely in vitro. The major difficulty with the method is the danger of the presence of the virus and the loss of antibody production with time.

EBV transformation can be brought about by many ways e.g., (i) isolate the peripheral blood lymphocytes and culture them in vitro with antigen and EBV or (ii) first select the isolated peripheral blood lymphocytes for a specific antigen and these selected cells are then used for EBV transformation. Human myeloma cell fusion is another method by which human hybridomascan be produced. The technique proposed by Kohler and Milstein involves the availability of a suitable HAT (a selective biochemical killer) for sensitive myeloma cell line. However, the success in fusing mouse x human cells using this technique is limited. Olsson and Kaplan in the year 1980 produced the first human-human myeloma (SKO-007), against the hapten 2,4-dinitrophenyl(DNP). Similarly, 19G secreting myeloma have been studied. The major drawback in producing human hybridomas is the limitation for its production only at in vitro conditions. This is because of the need of human volunteers for in vivo cultivation.

11.14.3 Advantages of monoclonal antibodies

Monoclonal antibodies are of exceptionally high quality; represents only one molecular species and which may be obtained virtually in a homogeneous state. Conventional antiserums possess certain disadvantages, for e.g., they consist of a mixture of antibodies and a major portion of the sample contain irrelevant immunoglobulin. These properties of conventional antiserum lead to cross reactions with other antigens. A summary of the advantages of MAbs over conventional antisera is listed below:

1. Pure one molecular species only.
2. Specificity for one antigenic determinant.
3. Cross reaction means shared determinants.
4. Antiserum titer values obtained are very high.
5. Antibodies with high avidity can be produced.
6. Immure immunogen can be used.
7. *In vitro* or *in vivo* production is possible with high production rate.
8. Maintenance of farm/animals is not required for immunization and bleeding.
9. Immortal cell lines.
10. Antiserum having identical antibody with an identical specificity and constant property can be obtained worldwide.
11. High reproducibility with respect to specificity and avidity.
12. Production of cell lines to individual components of a mixture is possible.
13. Radiolabelling and fluorescent conjugation or enzyme marking of MAbs are easy.

11.14.4. Limitations of monoclonal antibodies

The first and foremost limitation is the initial cost involved in the technique. However, on continues production, the cost is less as compared to conventional antiserum production. The method is time consuming and has its own drawbacks.

Precipitate formation

In general, MAbs do not form a precipitate in a standard double-immuno diffusion method. This leads to the necessity to produce a lattice framework for precipitation in tests like ouchterlony assays (refer chapter 16).

Complement fixation

Conventional antiserum possesses better complement fixing capabilities than 40 MAbs. For an efficient complement fixation, binding of Clq component to two antibody, the molecules (Fc regions) are required either adjacent to them or nearby to the determinants. IgM and IgG are the classes of antibody which fix complement easily. Among them IgM is the best. MAbs produced via cell fusion contain mainly IgG class. Yet, they show complement fixing capabilities. The reason given is related to the population density of antigenic determinants present. Henceforth, a blend of MAbs required to produce the necessary synergism.

Antibody specificity

Production of MAbs is against a single antigenic determinant .principally incorporates high. level of selective specificity In to the MAbs thus rendering them Incapable to distinguish between a groups of different molecules, cells bearing the chemical structure or determinants except one against which they are raised. A conventional antiserum contains antibodies to all the determinants on an antigen and can be precisely used-as 'fingerprint' identification for that antigen(However, complete cross reactions can occur for MAbs and may pose problems in assays where one molecular species amongst several very similar molecular entities is to be detected. The well identified problem of crossreactivity could effectively be addressed by production of determinants specific antibody clone. The approached adds to the precision and efficiency of MAbs based analytical techniques.

Antibody avidity

The energy of binding to an antigen is 'precise' in case of MAb whereas it is 'average' in case of conventional antiserum. The high antibody avidity of a MAb has advantages as well as disadvantages. It is advantageous in case of immunoassay methods and undesirable for purification process (affinity chromatography).

11.15. REGULATION OF IMMUNE RESPONSE

Specific T and B-lymphocytes respond against infection on the basis of parameters of receptor specificity and antigen that determines whether an immune response can be accurately measured against model antigens and how this relates to protection against a given pathogen. Some balance is attained between host and infectious agents that promotes their mutual survival. For the pathogen, this balance depends on level of direct cell and tissue damage caused by infectious agent and on kinetics of infection. For the host, survival depends on mechanisms of innate resistance and on the repertoire of T-and B-lymphocytes that confer adaptive immunity (Mims, 1987).

Producing an immune response in general costs a host significantly because some collateral damage to the host's own cells and tissues is an inevitable side effect and outcome of immunity. Therefore, evolution of beneficial immune protection has developed in equilibrium with potentially lethal damage that immune responses can cause, namely, immunopathology. Further, the immune system needs to control foreign infections without reacting specifically against the host's own antigens and cells. The balance of host and infectious agent might therefore be seen to reflect the strengths and weaknesses of a system that is exploited by infectious agents to promote the coexistence of both.

Whether the immune system reacts to antigen depends on relative frequencies of responding T and B-cells and on the thresholds of binding avidity of their receptors display on their surface (Zinkernagel and Hengartner, 2001). Further, it depends upon levels of antigen present and the period during which antigen remains in secondary organized lymphatic tissues, where primary immune responses are initiated. T and B-cells respond to antigens that become transiently localized within organized lymphatic tissues for at least 3 to 5 days. In contrast, T-cells do not generally react against antigens such as self-proteins that are continuously present at some level in blood, thymus, spleen, lymph nodes and bone marrow. This is because such T-cells have been functionally and physically eliminated by exhaustive induction or clonal deletion. Some noncytopathic persistent systemic infections that are transmitted from mother to offspring, as well as chronic noncytopathic infections or lymphatic tumors in immunocompetent hosts, can also delete T-cells. Persistence of antigen in the lymphohemopoietic system eventually activates and deletes all T-cells specific for that antigen. A low precursor T-cell frequency, together with persistent self-antigen is also characteristic of the thymus. In the thymus, therefore, optimal conditions exist for early induction of self-reactive T-cells, leading to deletion in the absence of immunopathology. In contrast, adult hosts with adequate numbers of reactive precursor T-cells often induce immune responses that cause severe immunopathology when a noncytopathic virus becomes widely disseminated within a particular organ. Antigens that do not reach organized lymphatic tissue not only fail to induce an immune response but are also unable to delete T-cells.

The B-cell (antibody) responses differ from those of T-cells. B-cells are induced efficiently when an antigen is presented in a repetitive rigid form, such as that found on the surface of infectious agents or when linked to polyclonal B-cell activators such as lipopolysaccharides (LPS). Such antigens can induce immunoglobulin M(IgM) B-cell responses independent of T-cell help. Other antigen configurations, e.g. some multimeric antigens present on flexible backbones as well as monomeric or oligomeric protein antigens induce B-cells only if helped by specific $CD4^+$ T-cells; antigen concentration also determines the extent of help required from T-cells. The smaller the concentrations of antigen the more directly dependent the B-cell response is on T-cell help. Further, efficient switching from short-lived IgM production (IgM half life is about 24 hours) to other classes, in particular long-lived immunoglobulin G (IgG) responses (IgG half life is about 20 days), requires conventional T-helper cell activity (Zinkernagel and Hengartner, 2001).

11.16. TUNING OF IMMUNE RESPONSES

The immune system can make qualitatively distinct responses against different microbial infections. An integral component of the immune system is a network of cells known as dendritic cells (DCs), which sense different microbial stimuli and transport this information to lymphocytes. A better understanding of DC biology has allowed a model to be constructed in which the type of immune response to an infection is considered as a function of several determinants, including the subpopulation of DCs, nature of microbe, microbe recognition receptors, and the cytokine microenvironment (Pulendran *et al.*, 2001). In response to intracellular microbes such as viruses and certain bacteria, $CD4^+$ T-helper (T_H) cells differentiate into T_H1 cells, which secrete interferon-γ (IFN-γ) and possess a specific range of functions. In contrast, extracellular pathogens such as helminths induce the development of T_H2 cells, whose cytokines [interleukin 4 (IL-4), IL-5, and IL-10] direct immunoglobulin E- and eosinophil-mediated destruction of the pathogens. Although, B and T-lymphocytes respond to antigens with high specificity, they alone cannot make these complex decisions. These choices are made jointly by the nature of the microbe and by DCs. DCs are scattered throughout the body, including the various portals of microbe entry where they reside in an immature form. Immature DCs act as "immunological sensors' alert to potentially dangerous microbes, and can decode and integrate such signals. They then convey this information to naive T-cells in the T-cell areas of secondary lymphoid organs, undergoing a maturation process. Here, the mature DCs present this information to T-cells, thus launching an immune response and immune memory through which the antigenic encounter can be remembered even for a lifetime.

11.17. DEFENSINS

Defensins constitute a family of versatile antimicrobial peptides abundant in such immune cells as white blood cells (specifically neutrophils), intestinal paneth cells, and barrier epithelial cells. In these settings, defensins directly contribute to the killing of microbes. Zhang *et al.* (2002) and Biragyn *et al.* (2002) implicated defensins in novel specific activities: defensins seem to be important for the anti-HIV activity of human $CD8^+T$ lymphocytes and for the induction of cell-mediated antitumor immunity in mice (Ganz, 2002). $CD8^+T$ lymphocytes from some HIV-infected patients secrete a substance (CD8 antiviral factor or CAF) that interferes with the ability of HIV to infect cells. This factor is abundant in AIDS patients who are doing well clinically and in those HIV-infected patients (nonprogressors) who do not develop the symptoms of the disease for many years after the initial infection. According to Zhang *et al,* $CD8^+T$ cells from long-term nonprogressor HIV patients secrete α-defensins-1, 2, and 3 when stimulated. These α-defensins account for much of the antiviral activity of CAF. The activity of defensins as a component of CAF has important implications, α-defensins and β-chemokines appear to be causally involved in slowing down the progression of HIV infection in patients favored by specific environmental or genetic factors. Better understanding of the regulation of defensins production in CD8$^+$T lymphocytes may conceivably extend these benefits to other HIV patients, and eventually a pharmacological substitute for these natural defensins could be developed. Alternatively, defensins may serve as markers of nonprogression.

Biragyn *et al.* studied the ability of defensins to signal the cells involved in adaptive immunity. In response to infection defensins are produced within a few hours by neutrophils or specialized epithelial cells. Some defensins act as chemoattractants for immature dedritic cells (Yang *et al,* 1999) that present antigen to T-cells when stimulated. Murine β-defensin-2, are being a chemoattractant binds to and signals through a chemokine receptor and also induces dendritic cells to mature by binding to Toll-like receptor-4; this receptor is essential for the host response to bacterial lipopolysaccharide. Further, murine β-defensin-2 when linked to nonimmunogenic tumour antigen augment a potent cell-mediated immune response and antitumor activity in mice (Ganz, 2002). Thus it appears that defensins act as a potent immunological adjuvant and they may be useful in the designing of therapeutic antitumour vaccines for use in human cancer patients. However, defensin sequences vary considerably between humans, mice, and other animals and it is not clear if a human defensin with similar properties will be found, or that the mouse defensin will retain its activity in humans.

11.18. IMMUNITY ENGINEERING

The idea of eliminating certain immunodeficiency diseases by replacing the defective parts of the immune system with healthy parts has gained momentum in recent years and has catalyzed the rise of the new discipline of immunoengineering. Transplantations of bone marrow cells (producers of B-lymphocytes), lymph nodes, spleen, or thymus (producer of T-lymphocytes) are already being increasingly brought into clinical practice. Some techniques for minimizing tissue incompatibility problems in organ transplantation are also available; an example is the use of immunosupressive preparations weakening the rejection of grafted tissues or organs.

A defective B-cell system is somewhat easier to replace as compared to a defective T-cell system. The latter can only be compensated by transplanting T-lymphocytes or the thymus. Whereas the B-system defects can often be alleviated by giving injections of immunoglobulins, the T-system deficiencies can only be treated by transplantation operations. Seven types of transplantation can be used for healing various immuno deficiencies. These are:

(1) Transplantation of bone marrow, spleen and lymph node cells, and blood lymphocytes from healthy adult donors.

(2) Transplantation of thymus from a healthy adult donor, or from an incompatible embryo.

(3) Combined liver and thymus transplantations from the same incompatible embryo donor.

(4) Transplantation of bone marrow from a donor compatible with recipient in tissue compatibility antigens.

(5) Transplantation of stem cells (isolated from the bone marrow) of an immunologically-mature compatible donor.

(6) Transplantation of isolated stem cells or the whole bone marrow from the parents preceded by the introduction of antibodies against the tissue compatibility antigens of the patient.

(7) Transplantation of stem cell fractions isolated from the bone marrow of the parent, in conjunction with immunodepressive therapy.

11.19. SOME GENERAL AREAS OF RESEARCH IN BASIC IMMUNOLOGY

- Study of the components and mechanisms involved in the innate immune response, and understanding the mechanisms by which this response modulates the adaptive immune response.
- Activation, proliferation, death and homeostasis in lymphocytes (T cells, B cells and NK cells).
- Mediators and mechanisms involved in the interaction of lymphoid and non-lymphoid cells under normal, pathogenic and aberrant (e.g. autoimmune, allergic) conditions.
- Characterization of cells and mechanisms involved in immunological memory.
- Genes involved in immune defects/modulation of immune responses and the role of genetic polymorphism in the immune response, disease resistance and susceptibility.

The adaptive immune response is subdivided into two types of humoral response, mediated by the secretion of immunoglobulins by B-cells and cellular response governed by T-cells. Cytotoxic T cells kill infected cells whereas T-helper cells produce interleukins (IL), the 'hormones' of immune system, and modulate B cell responses. Unlike B cells which recognize epitopes on native antigen, T-cells recognize peptides presented on major histocompatibility complex (MHC) encoded proteins. There are two broad classes of MHC molecules, namely MHC class I and class II and are highly polymorphic. These molecules play a dominant role in the T cell-mediated adaptive immune response, scan cells for the lack of expression of MHC class I, and are aided by NK receptors which scan cells for MHC class I expression; cells which do not express MHC class I proteins are targeted for lysis. Usually, recognition of MHC molecules by NK receptors prevents lysis of target cells; but occasionally NK receptors activate target cell lysis. Many of the peptides bound to MHC molecules are generated from cellular proteins. Indeed, in the absence of a peptide, cell-surface expression of MHC molecules is quite weak. During infection, a small proportion of peptides derived from the pathogen bind to MHC molecules and become expressed on the surface of antigen presenting cells (APCs). On recognition of this peptide/MHC complex *via* TCRs, specific T-cells are activated and proliferate.

On activation, T cells produce high levels of interleukins IL-2 and IL-4 to modulate the immune response. The ratio of various different interleukins results in dominance of T-helper, Th1 or Th2 type of immune responses, which influences development of autoimmune diseases and allergic responses. Normally, there exists about one antigen-specific T-cell among some ten thousand T-cells. But upon infection, these specific T-cells proliferate ($\sim 10^4 - 10^5$ times) and constitute the bulk of the immune response. It is dangerous to have such a large number of activated T-cells because the large amounts of interleukins or other factors produced by these cells can damage other cells of the body, creating problem of immunopathology. As the antigen is cleared, most such activated T-cells suffer apoptosis, but a few memory T-cells remain to fight future battles. The immune system has somehow devised mechanisms to down modulate an acute immune reaction.

Lymphocytes die in both thymic and peripheral tissues. This death ensures tolerance and maintenance of immune homeostasis. Lymphocyte deletion may be triggered *via* signals through antigen receptors, which recruit death receptor-ligand interactions and tumour necrosis factor (TNF) receptors into this process. These receptors interact with cellular proteins to cause death of cells. However, the regulation of these events (the decision of the lymphocyte to trigger apoptotic death as opposed to proliferation or survival in response to antigen receptor cross-linking) is not known. Caspases are a family of cysteine proteases and appear to be the key effectors of apoptotic pathways. Two major apoptotic pathways involving these death proteases have been identified in lymphocytes

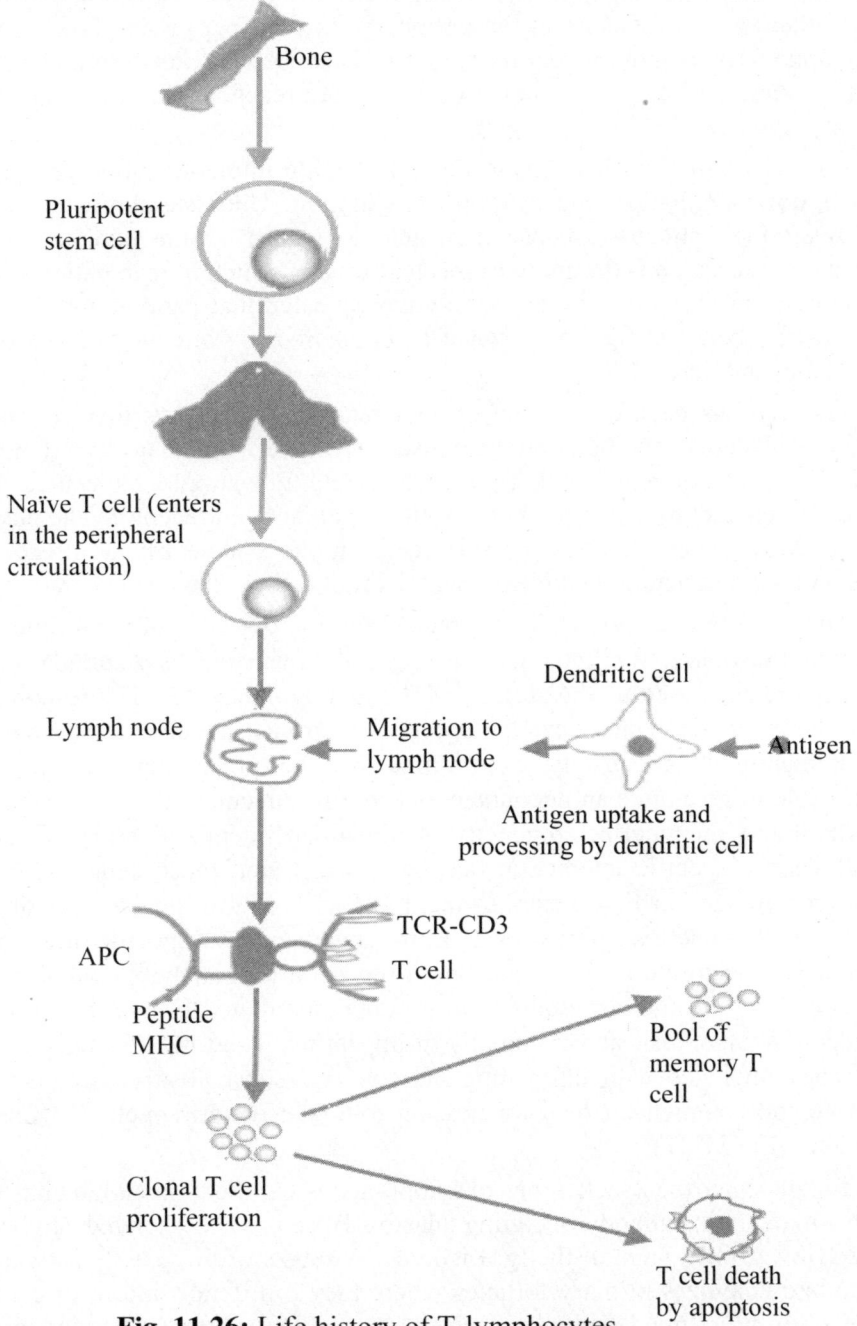

Fig. 11.26: Life history of T-lymphocytes

and in other cells. The first is triggered *via* the death receptors listed above whereas the second involves mitochondria. The mitochondria is a key checkpoint in the death pathway and molecules like cytochrome c, apoptosis activating factor-1 (Apaf-1) and a novel flavoprotein, the apoptosis inducing factor (AIF) are some of the apoptogenic molecules associated with this organelle. Most of these molecules are located in the intermembrane space (IMS) of the mitochondria.

MHC class I and class II molecules are important not only in selecting T-cells in the thymus, but also in maintaining naive T-cells in the periphery. In fact, peripheral T-cells transferred into hosts lacking lymphocytes result in proliferation of these newly transferred T-cells in a self-MHC-dependent manner, until a certain number of T-cells are reached. However, uncontrolled proliferation is somehow prevented.

Viruses show various mechanisms to down-modulate immune responses, including MHC class I and class II down-regulation and cytokine modulation. Understanding the mechanisms by which viruses subvert the immune response may help to identify some potential drug targets. Another promising area of research is the study of mechanisms by which human patients resist viral infections. Work on human survivors of HIV and Ebola has revealed that patients who secrete higher levels of cytokines stand a better chance of survival as compared to patients with a slow and low cytokine response (Nandi and Sarin, 2001).

Much research has been carried out on understanding processes that govern both initiation and progression of T-dependent humoral responses. However, the majority, if not all, of these have employed as model antigens-small, rigid and structurally simple molecules providing a minimal surface area for contact by either antibody or the B-cell antigen receptor. The physiologically relevant antigens normally experienced by B-cells (e.g., in the course of an infection) are much larger molecules with high structural complexity and diversity (Rao, 2001).

The adaptive immune system is characterized by two distinct but interrelated activities of recognition and response. While the overall recognition capacity is a cumulative property of diverse antigen receptors expressed on the surface of B and T-lymphocytes. The response is clonally derived from those lymphocytes which bear the appropriate antigen receptors. The recognition potential of adaptive immunity is adequately exemplified by the pre-immune B-cell repertoire which is collectively able to recognize an uncountable array of molecular species encompassing wide ranging size, structural and chemical heterogeneity. Antigen-dependent activation of 'naïve', resting B cells occurs following a specific interaction between antigen and those cells which express appropriate receptors. This interaction first occurs in the T-cell-rich extrafollicular sites of secondary lymphoid organs. This, with some exceptions, leads to the appearance of specific antibody producing B cells (AFCs), which concentrate in the periphery of the periarteriolar lymphoid sheath (PALS). Antigen-activated B cells in the foci differentiate to produce unmutated Ig over the next ten to twelve days, before undergoing apoptosis and eventually disappearing. The low affinity Ig that is produced in this period forms complexes with circulating antigen and subsequently, becomes sequestered on the surface of Fc and complement receptor-bearing follicular dendritic cells (FDCs) residing in primary B-cell follicles (Fig.11.27).

Naïve B-cells enter the T-cell zones of lymph nodes *via* the high endothelial venule (HEV) where they differentiate into antibody secreting plasma B cells. The secreted antibodies are genetically unmodified (low affinity) and of the IgM isotype. A subset of these early activated B-cells, however, migrates to and colonizes primary follicles where they proliferate and form germinal centers (GCs). Within GCs, proliferating B-cells are subject to a mutation and selection process that increases affinity and functional efficiency of the memory immunoglobulins repertoire. These latter processes are governed by the antigen present as immune complexes on the surface of follicular dendritic cells (FDCs). This secondary phase eventually gives rise to relatively long lived plasma cells that produce high affinity (genetically modified) and high titer, predominantly non-IgM (Usually IgG with some IgE) antibodies and memory B-cells capable of differentiating into similar plasma cells upon subsequent exposure to antigen. One dramatic event in the functioning of the immune system is the steady enhancement of the binding efficiency of antibodies being generated in the course of an immune response. Whereas early in the immune response to a vaccine antigen, the efficiency of antibody-antigen binding is quite low, this efficiency can undergo huge exponential increments in late phase of the response.

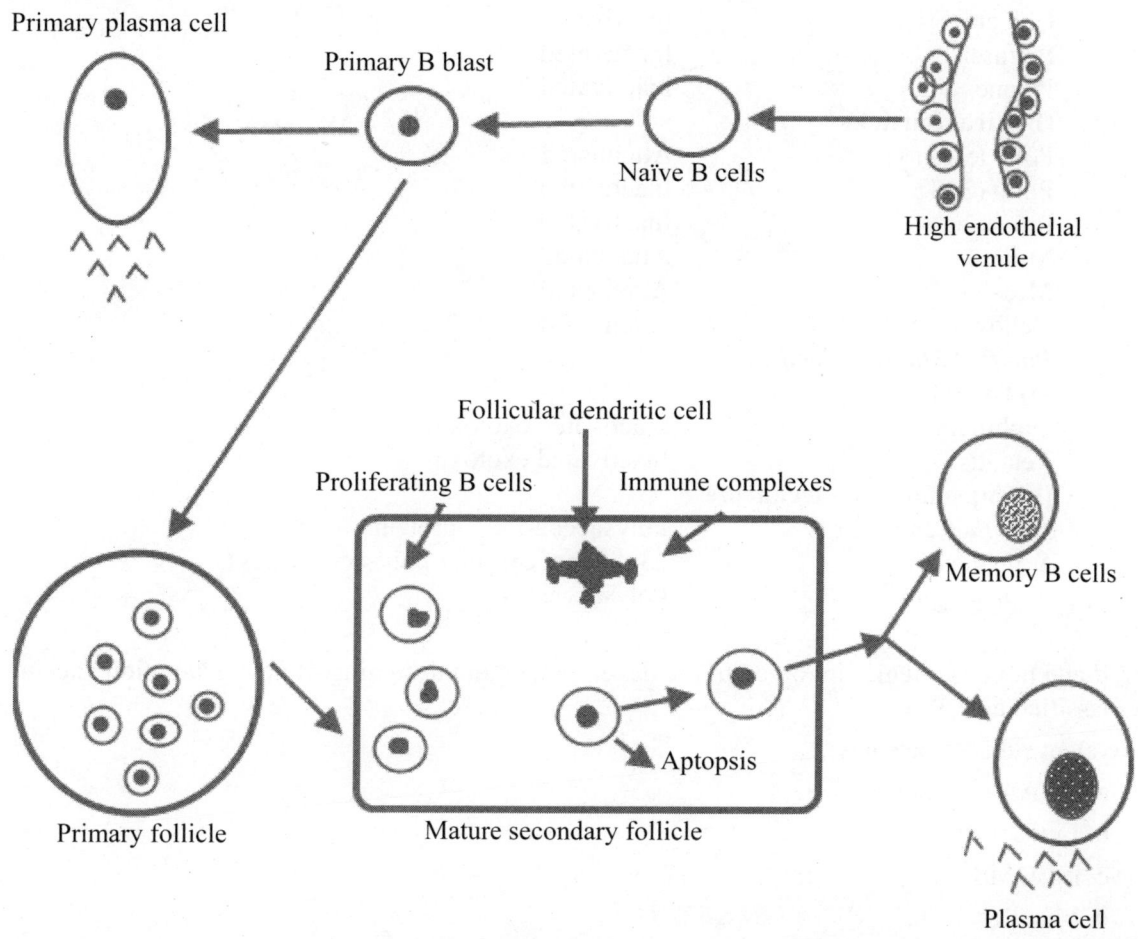

Fig. 11.27: B cell maturation in secondary lymphoid tissue

11.20. VACCINES

Recent advances in immunology have led to the development of new and promising vaccine strategies. Knowledge of differences in epitopes recognized by T cells and B cells has enabled immunologists to design vaccines to maximize activation of the humoral or cell mediated branch of the immune system. Genetic engineering techniques facilitate development of vaccines which maximize the immune response to selected epitopes. This chapter focuses on some existing vaccination strategies and some experimental designs that may become the vaccines of the future. Table 11.9 indicates some currently used vaccines.

Table 11.9: Classification of commonly used vaccines

Disease	Type of vaccine
Whole organism	
(a) Bacterial cells	
Tuberculosis	Attenuated
Cholera	Inactivated
Pertussis	Inactivated
Plague	Inactivated
(B)Viral particles	
Polio (Sabin)	Attenuated
Polio (Salk)	Inactivated
Influenza	Inactivated
Mumps	Attenuated
Measles	Attenuated
Yellow fever	Attenuated
Purified Macromolecules	
(a)Toxoids	
Diphtheria	Inactivated exotoxin
Tetanus	Inactivated exotoxin
(b)Capsular polysaccharide	
H. influenza type b	Polysaccharide + protein
S. pneumonia	23 distinct capsular polysaccharides
N. meningitis	Polysaccharide

Improved and novel strategies involved in the development and designing of new generation vaccines can be classified as

1. Multivalent subunit vaccines

    a. SMAA complexes

    b. Liposomes

    c. ISCOMS

    d. Micelles

2. Purified macromolecules

3. Synthetic peptides as vaccines

4. Immunoadhesin(s)

5. Antigen vaccines

    a. Recombinant antigen vaccines

    b. Adjuvant independent immunotargeted vaccines

    c. Class II MHC target antigen

6. Vector vaccines

    a. Recombinant vector vaccines

    b. Minicells as vaccines

7. Anti-idiotype vaccines

8. Targeted immune stimulants

9. Miscellaneous

    a. Antisense oligonucleotides

    b. Competitive inhibition of ribosome binding to 5' unsaturated region (5'-VTR)

11.21. HOW VACCINES WORK

Vaccines work by priming the immune system to swiftly destroy the disease causing agents before they can multiply enough to cause symptoms. To date, this priming has been achieved by presenting the immune system with whole viruses or bacteria that have been killed or attenuated (made too weak to proliferate much). The immune system responds to this vaccine as if it was under attack by a fully potent antagonist and mobilizes its forces to destroy the foreign body. Memory cells are then left behind on alert, ready to unleash whole armies of defenders if real pathogen ever finds its way into the body.

Classic vaccines create a small risk in that the killed or attenuated microorganism may sometimes spring back to life, causing the disease for which vaccine was meant to prevent. For this reason, 'subunit' vaccines (which contain no genes, just proteins derived from them) are now favored since they reduce this risk. They are however, often not as effective as live vaccines. Subunit vaccines are also expensive, because they are produced in cultures of bacteria or protozoan cells and have to be purified and refrigerated.

Many researchers hope to develop edible vaccines which are similar to subunit preparations, containing only the genes coding for certain antigens, not the whole virus or bacterium. One main hurdle to be overcome here is that the antigens could be degraded in stomach before having time to act. Typical subunit vaccines have to be delivered by injection precisely because of this. Researchers working on an edible hepatitis B vaccine suggest that oral doses may need to be 10-100 times higher than an injectable dose to elicit a comparable immune response.

11.22. THE IDEAL VACCINE

An ideal vaccine should be safe, efficacious, cheap, easily administered (e.g., orally), and thermally stable. It should confer long-term immunity. A single vaccine should preferably protect against several locally important infectious diseases, i.e. should be multivalent. Some of the currently available viral vaccines meet many of these requirements. The efficacy of a vaccine depends primarily upon the nature and persistence of the induced immune response. Some understanding has come from the study of model viral-host systems, such as the murine influenza model. Four stages are readily identified and include: (1) prevention of infection, (2) limitation of viral replication, (3) recovery from infection, and (4) generation of memory cells. Vaccines function by stimulating adaptive immune response. They are usually administered before exposure to the wild-type agent has occurred. The time interval may be weeks, months or years. The vaccine should stimulate B-cells, T-helper (Th) cells and Tc cells. In the case of an antigenically stable infectious agent, neutralizing antibody is the most important immune parameter.

The four requirements of an ideal vaccine are: (1) activation of antigen-presenting cells to initiate antigen processing and production of interleukins; (2) activation of both T- and B-cells to give a high yield of memory cells; (3) due generation of antibody to two or three B-cell epitopes and of Th and Tc cells to several epitopes; and (4) persistence of antigen, probably mainly on follicular dendritic cells in lymphoid tissue resulting in the continuing presence of antibody. A scores of efforts have been made by researchers with the objective to develop an ideal vaccines are discussed in following sections.

11.23. MULTIVALENT SUBUNIT VACCINES

Synthetic peptide vaccines and recombinant protein based vaccines are poorly immunogenic. Additionally, they also tend to induce humoral antibody production but are less able to induce a cell-mediated immune response. These limitations call for a method of structuring vaccine to contain immunodominant B-cell and T-cell epitopes. Also, if a CTL response is required, the vaccine should be delivered intracellularly so that the peptides can be processed and presented on MHC-I together with class II MHC molecules. Some techniques for developing multivalent subunit vaccines are discussed below:

      1. Solid matrix antigen antibody (SMAA) complexes

      2. Liposomes

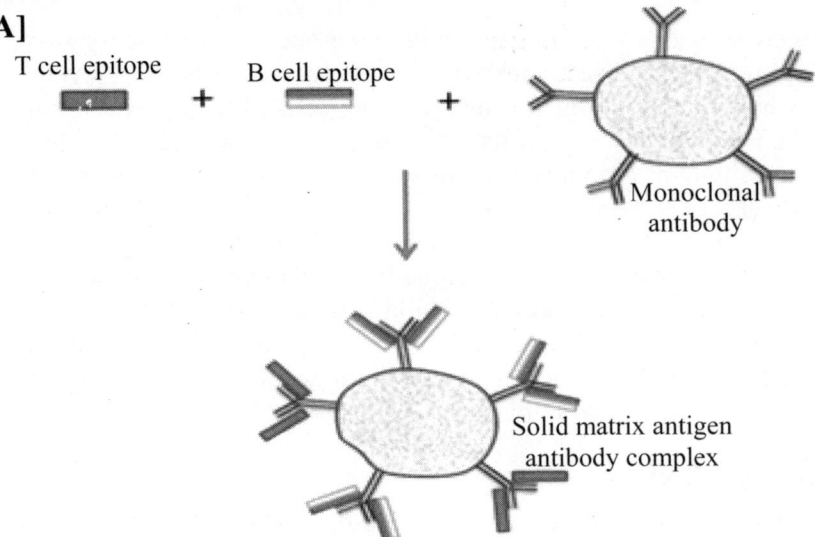

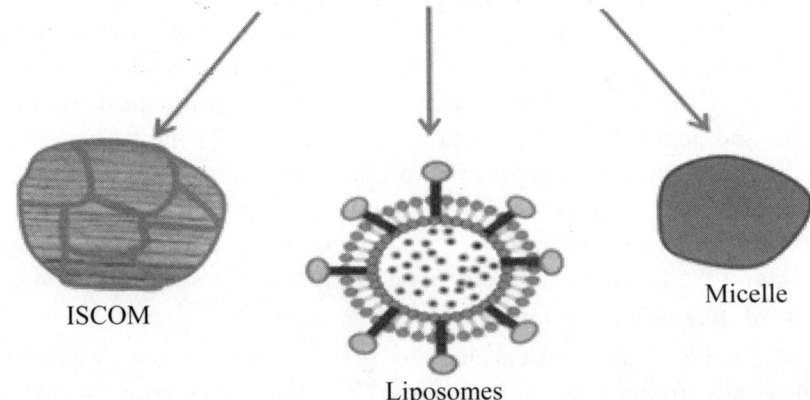

Fig. 11.28: Multivalent subunit vaccines (A) solid matrix antigen-antibody complexes; (B) ISCOM, liposomes and protein micelles prepared with extracted antigens or antigenic peptides

3. Immunostimulating complexes (ISCOMS)
4. Micelles

11.23.1. SMAA Complexes

SMAA complexes are prepared by coupling monoclonal antibodies to solid particulate matrices followed by saturating the antibodies with the desired antigen. These complexes are then utilized as vaccines. A variety of monoclonal antibodies can be attached to the solid matrix (Fig.11.28). This property can be exploited to bind a mixture of peptides/proteins to the solid matrix so that immunodominant epitopes for both T cells and B cells can be composed. These multivalent complex vaccines may induce vigorous humoral and cell-mediated responses. Their particulate disposition facilitates phagocytosis by phagocytic cells which play an important role in augmenting their immunogenicity.

11.23.2. Liposomes

Another approach of obtaining a multivalent vaccine is utilization of detergent to incorporate peptide/protein antigens into lipid vesicles called liposomes. Pharmaceutical research in the field of drug delivery systems has advanced greatly with the help of medical research. Novel drug delivery systems have attracted great attention in delivering the drug to the target site in a targeted or controlled manner. They have also been tried as vaccines and vaccine adjuvants. This has made possible the development of vaccines against newly emerging pathogens that cause infectious diseases.

Liposome-based vaccines are an attractive choice as they are biocompatible, biodegradable and composed of natural products that are non-toxic and immunologically inert. Besides, they can be frozen and freeze-dried without any deleterious effects. The classical dehydration-rehydration vesicles (DRVs) and emulsion reverse phase evaporation technique(s) have been used for successful incorporation or encapsulation of antigen(s), microbes, etc. Protein antigens associated with or encapsulated within liposomes are converted from soluble antigens to particulate antigens. Thus, by association of small soluble antigens with liposomes they can be targeted to macrophages. The toxicity of some antigens may be reduced by their incorporation in liposomes and at the same time their immunogenicity is increased several fold by this procedure.

Immunopotentiation has been established both for antigens encapsulated within the liposomes and for antigens exposed on to the liposomal surfaces. Liposome encapsulated antigens are masked and prevented from recognition by surface receptors present on lymphoid cells so that the liposomes are phagocytosed by macrophages. Thus, phagocytosis of liposomes followed by unmasking of the encapsulated antigens appears to be a logical first step in the induction of an immune response. It has been reported that macrophages are necessary and sufficient for presentation of antigens encapsulated in liposomes to T-cells; B-cells by themselves are incapable of presenting the same. Like B cells, dendritic cells show only limited phagocytosis and may not take up any appreciable amount of liposomes. Also, the macrophages that had been fed liposome encapsulated antigen in culture seem to enhance the immune response.

Liposomes have a unique structural versatility. It is possible to manipulate their membrane fluidity, size, surface charge and phospholipid to antigen mass ratio so that optimal adjuvanticity can be achieved for a number of antigens. Amplification in adjuvanticity has been observed by receptor mediated targeting to antigen presenting cells and the co-entrapment of adjuvants such as IL-2 with the antigen.

11.23.2.1. Cloned gp120 liposomal vaccines

This strategy is based on cloning gp120 soluble HIV virus envelope protein. The recombinant gp120 protein is non virulent and induces significant $CD8^+CTL$ response. However, to evoke significant $CD8^+CTL$ response it is desirable that the gp120 antigen(s) must be processed and presented by MHC class I molecules. Liposomal immobilization of gp120 antigen presents them to MHC class I molecules, thus enabling contained gp120 to be processed by class I MHC *via* endogenous pathway. Further, the system i.e. recombinant gp120 antigen (envelope protein) could be administered in the form of ISCOMS (particles with mean diameter 35-40nm) carrying antigen in adjuvant based micelles. Moreover, concerns regarding gp120 originated syncytia formation leading to $CD4^+T$ cell depletion is yet to be evaluated.

11.23.3. Immunostimulating complexes (ISCOMS)

ISCOMS comprise of a carrier structure and antigens which are incorporated into this matrix through hydrophobic interactions. The building blocks of ISCOMS are triterpenoids. On association with cholesterol and phosphatidylcholine some of these triterpenoids form a typical 40nm size cage-like structure. Other terpenoids in the Quil A mixture show adjuvant activity. Some cause side effects in higher doses whereas others produce none or negligible side effects. Recently, structure forming triterpenoids giving rise to ISCOM-like particles that are virtually non-toxic for mice have been isolated.

For an adjuvant like aluminum hydroxide or oil, the important immunopotentiating factor is depot effect at the site of injection. On the contrary, antigens in ISCOMS are rapidly transported from site of injection to draining lymphatic organ. Therefore, in comparison to aluminum hydroxide and oil adjuvants negligible local inflammatory reaction and no granulomas are observed with ISCOMS. Following subcutaneous injection of high doses of ISCOMS only transient redness is observed. After intraperitoneal immunization with radiolabelled antigens contained in ISCOMS, many of the antigens associate with cells and are transported to spleen when they localize for a longer period of time as compared to the same antigen when administered in micellar form.

Macrophages internalize ISCOM borne antigen more efficiently than do native B cells or monocytes. Splenic dendritic cells are less efficient than macrophages but more active than monocytes or native B cells in taking up ISCOM borne antigen. Cytokine studies have indicated that ISCOMS and their matrix may induce macrophages to produce IL-1 and IL-6. ISCOMS have a unique ability to induce immune response *via* both MHC class I and class II pathways. The prospects for future development of ISCOMs as immunological carrier system are bright: they are useful for defined antigens produced by any means e.g., by chemical synthesis, gene technology techniques or in conventional microorganisms. ISCOMS can be formulated for parenteral or mucosal administration. Formulation with purified components from Quil A has proved innocuous in toxicological studies.

11.23.4. Micelles

Micelles are formed by mixing proteins in detergent and then removing the detergent by dialysis. The individual proteins orient themselves with the hydrophobic residues packed towards center, thereby largely avoiding their interaction with the outer aqueous environment towards which the hydrophilic residues are oriented. An antigen may be incorporated in micelles and used as an adjuvant for improved immunogenicity.

11.24. PURIFIED MACROMOLECULES

The risk involved in vaccines based on attenuated or killed microorganisms can be avoided with vaccines that comprise of specific purified molecules. For instance, vaccines for Meningococcal meningitis and Pneumococcal pneumonia consist of a mixture of purified capsular polysaccharides as the immunogen. Polysaccharide vaccines cannot activate the cells; this is a serious limitation in their utility. They activate B cells in a thymus-independent manner, producing only IgM and not IgG. There is also hardly any development of memory cells. Several options have been explored to circumvent this limitation. One such technique is conjugation of the polysaccharide antigen to some sort of protein carrier. The vaccine for Haemophilus influenza type b (Hib), major cause of bacterial meningitis in childrens less than 5 years of age. It consists of type b capsular polysaccharide covalently linked to tetanus toxoid, a protein carrier. As compared to polysaccharide alone, the polysaccharide-protein conjugate is relatively more immunogenic and as it activates Th cells, it enables class switching from IgM to IgG. This type of vaccine can only induce memory B cells but not memory T cells specific for the pathogen. For the Hib vaccine, it appears that memory B cells can be activated to some extent in absence of a memory Th-cell population and in all probabilities this accounts for the efficacy of this vaccine.

One problem associated with vaccines containing purified surface macromolecules is the difficulty of obtaining the purified component. This limitation can be overcome with recombinant DNA techniques whereby a gene encoding an immunogenic protein is expressed in bacterial, yeast or insect cells. For example, diphtheria and tetanus vaccines can be made by purifying the recombinant bacterial exotoxin and then inactivating the toxin with formaldehyde to form a toxoid. Vaccination with the toxoid induces antitoxoid antibodies, which can also bind to the toxin and neutralize its toxicity. Production of toxoid vaccines requires rigorous control so that detoxification can be achieved without excessive modification of the epitope structure.

11.25. SYNTHETIC PEPTIDE VACCINES

Recent developments in identifying and synthesizing specific B and T-cell epitopes offer the potential to induce disease neutralizing immune response with completely synthetic structures. As short chain peptides can be used to mimic antigenic sites of viruses, they provide a basis for vaccine development. This has inspired attempts to synthesize peptides that act as surrogate immunogens, as an alternative to the existing conventional vaccines such as chemically modified toxins, attenuated strains of microbes and killed but antigenic microbes. The following reasons motivate researchers to develop synthetic peptides:

- Relatively easy and cheap to produce;
- Prolonged stability without the need for refrigeration; and
- Scaling up of production and purification is easier than for conventional vaccines.

Synthesizing a peptide which can induce production of antibodies reacting with the coat proteins of viruses requires, identification of the critical epitopes involved in providing protective immunity and determining the sequence of amino acids that constitute an epitope.

11.25.1. B and T-cell epitopes: A prerequisite for antigenicity of peptides

Several predictive and experimental approaches can be used to identify potential immunogenic determinants. In the past it was believed that owing to relatively smaller molecular size, synthetic peptides behave like haptens and are necessarily poor immunogens that require some means of enhancing their immunogenicity (e.g., coupling to carrier proteins). Synthetic peptides, like any other antigen, must contain appropriate B-cell epitopes (antibody recognition sites) and Th-cell epitopes (site capable of eliciting help for antibody production), in order to evoke antibody responses. These Th-cell epitopes must be capable of binding class-II MHC molecules on the surface of host APC and B-cells and should subsequently interact with the T-cell receptor in the form of a trimolecular complex so that the differentiation and proliferation by B-cells can be induced.

Potential B-cell epitopes of a protein antigen are identified by examining its structure for peptide sequences representing sites that are accessible, hydrophilic and mobile. Generally, B-cell epitopes are chosen by identifying strongly hydrophilic sequences. This is based on the assumption that strongly hydrophilic sequences are most likely to represent accessible surface regions that constitute B-cell epitopes. For induction of humoral immunity, a vaccine should include peptides composing immunodominant B-cell epitopes. Such epitopes are identified by determining the dominant antibody in the sera of individuals recovering from a disease. This has to be followed by testing peptides for their ability to react with that antibody with a high affinity.

A vaccine must also include immunodominant T-cell epitopes, since an effective memory response for both humoral and cell-mediated immunity requires generation of a population of memory Th cells. Owing to the unpredictable role played by MHC in influencing immunodominance for the T-cell system, it is very difficult to identify those epitopes with synthetic peptide vaccines. In most cases T cells recognize processed peptides that appear to represent internal amphipathic peptides. These peptides should possess a site (the agretope) that enables them to interact with MHC molecules and a site (the epitope) that enables them to interact with the T-cell receptor. MHC molecules differ in their ability for peptide presentation. Thus, MHC polymorphism within a species influences the level of T cell responsiveness by different individuals to different peptides. Also, different sub-populations of T cells recognize different epitopes. Studies have identified some peptides that induce immunologic suppression and other peptides that induce a strong helper response. Generally, these helper and suppressor peptides represent different, non-overlapping amino acid sequences. For instance, immunization with the amino terminal residues (1-17) of hen egg-white lysozyme suppresses the response to native lysozyme. Immunity can be enhanced by the identification (and thereby elimination) of the suppressing peptides. These suppressing peptides can also be exploited in cases where the immune response is to be decreased, as in the treatment of autoimmune diseases.

The current approach in designing synthetic peptide vaccines against viruses involves location of invariant regions whose amino acid sequence is highly conserved. For example, some regions of the hemagglutinin (HA) molecule of influenza virus display high levels of amino acid variation. This generates the type and subtype differences that enable the virus to escape the immune system. But invariant regions mediating essential biological functions are also present in the HA molecule. For instance, the sialic acid-binding site on HA allows the virus to bind to sialic acid residues on cell surfaces. Normally, this region on the intact viral particle does not induce antibody formation and yet synthetic peptide vaccines of this conserved region have been found to neutralize viral infectivity against several different influenza types and sub-types. However, if a peptide is a poor immunogen or is non-immunogenic, as in the case of peptides which contain only a B-cell epitope, they can be rendered immunogenic by:

(a) Coupling to a large carrier protein (that contains many TH-cell epitopes);

(b) Polymeric presentation of such peptides;

(c) Incorporating an identified TH-cell epitope into the peptide.

11.25.2. Synthetic peptides and T-helper cell determinants

Cell determinants play a crucial role in designing synthetic immunogens. Synthetic peptides can be highly immunogenic in their soluble form (free form) provided that they carry appropriate antibody recognition sites, i.e. B cell epitopes should also carry sites capable of eliciting help for antibody production *via* the cell epitopes. The latter in turn must bind to class II MHC molecules on the surface of host antigen presenting cells and B cells and subsequently should interact with T cell receptor *via* trimolecular complex orientation which could induce B cell to differentiate and proliferate. If however, a free peptide turns to be a poor immunogen or produces an immune response that is genetically restricted, then in such cases appropriate cell epitopes may be added. This widespread concept of combination of B cell and T cell epitopes introduces an important class of vaccines of interest.

The combination could be accomplished by chemical co-polymerizing of epitopes of B and T cells. In a typical case Chedid and his colleagues used glutaraldehyde to polymerize four peptides from two bacterial antigens, i.e. *S. pyrogen,* M protein, diphtheria toxoid or HBsAg and proteinoid *Plasmodium knowlensii.* The approach exhibited enhanced immunogenetics as compared to their homopolymers.

11.25.3. Carrier coupling

A low molecular weight foreign substance (hapten) is usually not antigenic unless made larger by attachment to a carrier molecule. Once an antibody against the hapten is formed, however, the hapten alone reacts with antibodies (Fig.11.29) an example: penicillin is not antigenic by itself, but it combines with serum proteins of some persons and the resulting molecule initiates an immune response. In fact coupling to large carrier proteins is the most convenient and straightforward approach to enhance the immunogenicity of a poor/non-immunogenic synthetic peptide. The carrier proteins provide T-cell help for B-cell antibody production to poor/non-immunogenic peptides. Several studies have indicated that protective immunity can be induced in experimental animals with synthetic peptides coupled to carrier proteins. Full protection of animals against foot and mouth disease virus (FMDV) and hepatitis-B virus (HBV) has been demonstrated.

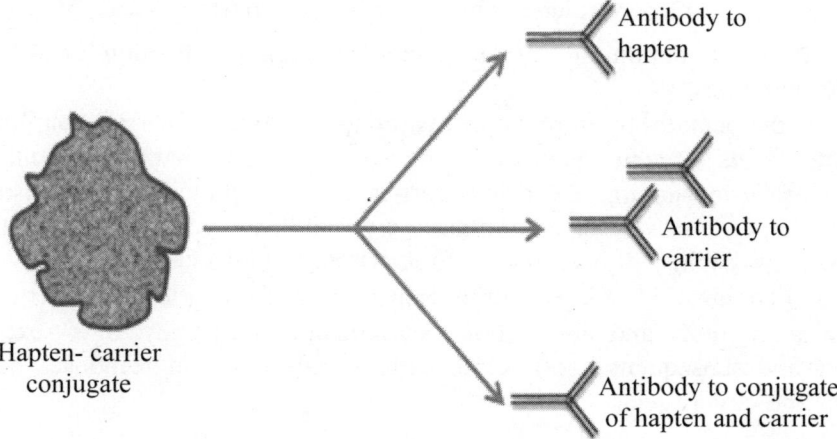

Fig. 11.29: Formation of antigenic molecules by attachment of hapten to carrier molecules

11.25.3.1. Mechanism of immunogenicity

More than one different mechanism may be involved in the immunogenicity enhancement effect of carrier peptides. Some possibilities are:

- The coupling of small synthetic peptides to carrier proteins increases the molecular mass of peptide thereby improving uptake by APC.
- Biological half life of small peptides is increased *via* their linkage to carrier proteins.
- The synthetic peptide itself is immunogenic (as in case of peptides having B and T-cell epitopes).

11.25.3.2. Commonly used carriers and selection of suitable carrier

Carrier proteins which are commonly used for synthetic peptides include:
(a) Keyhole limpethemocyanin (KLH) and sperm whale myoglobin (SWM).
(b) Albumins (bovine serum albumin, ovalbumin).
(c) Bacterial toxoids (tetanus toxoid, diphtheria toxoid) and other bacterial proteins used in vaccines such as PPD from BCG.
KLH and SWM are the traditional carrier proteins and offer a number of distinctive advantages such as-

- likely to be highly foreign to species to be immunized;
- unlikely to elicit cross-reactive or interfering antibodies;
- well established model immunogens;
- SWM is extensively characterized;
- When used in man, KLH does not produce any obvious side effects.

While albumins offer the advantage of free availability, the generation of anti-carrier antibodies with these carriers is a drawback. Bacterial toxoids and bacterial proteins have also been used as carriers believing that a pre-primed human population exists which may produce an enhanced response to the peptide linked to these carriers. However, some researchers observed that no pre-priming occurs or even active suppression takes place.

Following factors must be considered while selecting a carrier:

- Is the purpose of coupling to immunize an animal against infection, or to elicit high titer anti peptide antibodies?
- Nature of the peptide- hydrophilic or hydrophobic, effect of carrier coupling on the residues important for its antigenicity; presence of cysteine residues that may form disulfide bridges.
- Choice. of carrier -natural or artificial carrier, common protein; or an unusual protein, risk of eliciting hypersensitivity or autoimmunity; possibility to elicit cross-reactive or interfering antibodies; possibility of occurrence of pre priming against carrier.
- Method of conjugation-effect on antigenicity of peptide; peptide to carrier ratio.
- Immunization route and dose; choice of adjuvant; frequency; age; sex; interval between primary and subsequent booster inoculations; difference in responses between laboratory animals and target species.

11.25.3.3. Coupling methods

Carrier proteins require some form of chemical coupling to the synthetic peptide molecules to enhance their immunogenicity. Various methods and reagents can be used for this purpose. Some important chemical agents employed for coupling are listed in Table 11.10 of which glutaraldehyde is the commonest. However, the reaction is relatively uncontrolled and may deleteriously affect antigenic sites on the peptide. The problem can be overcome by use of hetero-bifunctional crosslinking agents which, unlike glutaraldehyde, facilitate specific linkages.

Table 11.10: Chemical agents employed and the functional groups involved in coupling reaction

Reagents	Functional groups involved in the coupling reaction
Glutaraldehyde	Amino, imidazole, phenolic hydroxyl, sulfhydryl
Carbodiimides	Amino, carboxyl, phenolic hydroxyl, sulfhydryl
Bis-imido esters	Amino
Heterobifunctional cross-linkers	Amino, sulfhydryl
Homobifunctional NHS esters	Amino

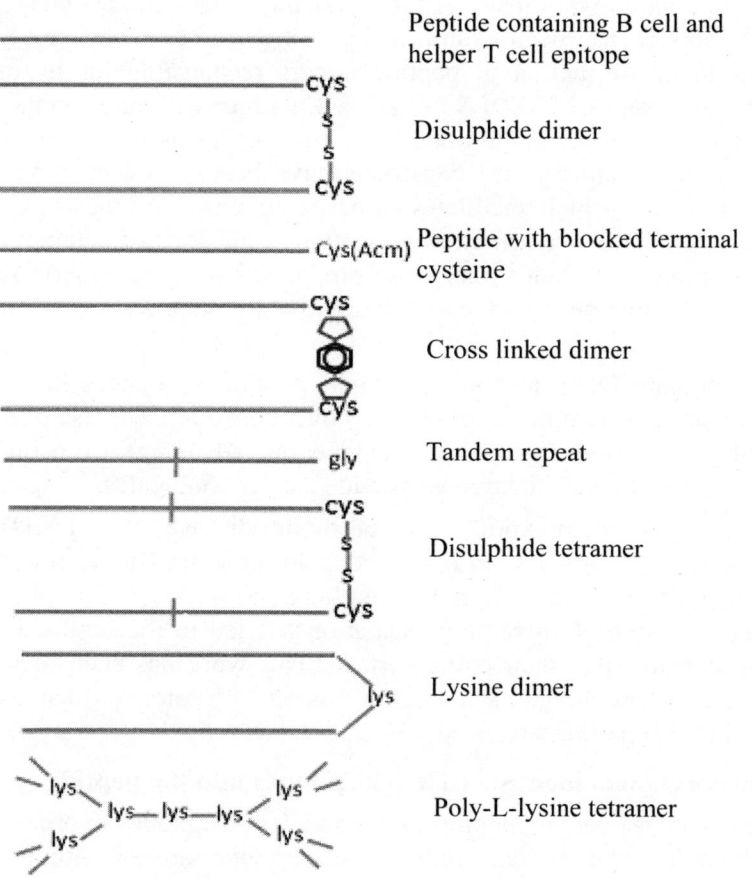

Fig. 11.30: Various forms of uncoupled synthetic peptides used for comparative immunogenicity studies

11.25.3.4. Potential drawbacks

While the method of chemical coupling of carrier proteins to synthetic peptides offer advantage of being a quick simple and convenient method, it inherits certain drawbacks which include -

- Poor batch-to-batch reproducibility as the coupling reaction is poorly defined and difficult to control.

- Carrier induced suppression and hypersensitivity to the carrier.

- Adverse effect on antigenicity of the peptide, i.e. masking or modification of important antigenic sites on the peptide.

11.25.4. Polymeric presentation of peptides

Polymeric presentation of peptides is a *via*ble approach that improves the immunogenicity of synthetic peptides significantly. Various researchers have conducted different studies to establish such presentation systems as commercially *via*ble wholly synthetic vaccines. A number of synthetic forms of 141-160 peptides from VPI of FMDV have been prepared and subsequently tested for their immunogenicity. Various forms that were prepared are presented in figure 11.30.

The role of non natural terminal free thiol cysteine residue in the enhancement of immunogenicity of free FMPV peptide has been examined by many workers. The presence of free thiol cysteine residue results in the formation of peptide dimers responsible for its increased immunogenicity. Similarly, tandem repeats of FMPV VPI 137-162, with or without terminal cysteine residue, produce higher titer value of neutralizing antibodies in guinea pigs as compared to single copy peptides. In addition, polylysine octamer based constructs have been produced by utilizing multiple antigenic peptide (MAP) system which facilitates direct solid phase synthesis of a peptide antigen onto a branching lysine backbone. Presentation of peptide in the form of octamer or tetramer induces higher neutralizing antibody titer values than those produced by lysine dimeric forms. Therefore, it is now established that effective quantitative and qualitative immune response can be induced by polymeric forms of synthetic peptides.

Using recombinant DNA technology, small peptide sequences have been fused to the genes encoding larger proteins in order to produce a novel construct. The use of peptidal sequences fused to bacterial proteins as immunogens has the potential advantage of being uniform with a defined structure as compared to uncharacterized peptide/carrier conjugates.

In an interesting work, to express foot and mouth disease virus (FMDV), peptides were fused to the N-terminus of β-galactosidase in *E. coli* cells. Preliminary studies revealed that multiple copies of the inserted peptide sequence might be beneficial. Similarly, in another development, the fusion protein concept for multiple peptide presentation has led to the production of particulate structures with epitopes repeated over their entire surface. This work has been focused on hepatitis B surface antigen, hepatitis B core antigen (HBsAg) and yeast Ty protein, which spontaneously self assemble into 22, 27 and 60 nm particles respectively.

11.25.5. Incorporation of identified Th-cell epitopes into the peptide

Synthetic peptides must contain appropriate B and T-cell epitopes in order to be immunogenic in their free form. Peptides that contain only B-cell epitope are non-immunogenic. Incorporation of appropriate Th-cell epitopes into such peptides is another approach to render them immunogenic. Different methods of generating such combinations of B and Th-cell epitopes are:

(1) Polymerization of B and T-cell peptides

(2) Chemical linkage

(3) Co-linear synthesis

11.25.5.1. Polymerization of B and T-cell peptides

This is the simplest method of combining B and T-cell epitopes. Co-polymers of a number of individual peptides can be produced by chemical means.

Some limitations of this approach are:

- Uncontrolled nature of polymerization reaction.
- Risk of affecting antigenic properties of peptides.

Table 11.11: Production of combination of B-cell and T-cell epitopes

Work done	Significant findings
Francis 1990	Demonstrated the importance of location of the T-cell epitope in relation to B-cell epitope using FMDV system.
Borras-Cuesta *et al.* 1987	Synthesized two peptides from major coat protein VPG of bovine rotavirus (which contained non-immunogenic B-cell epitopes) and a peptide from influenza virus (which contained T-cell epitope). Both the peptides induced anti-rotavirus responses in mice greater than those produced by the same rotavirus sequences conjugated to bovine serum albumin.
Good *et al.* 1987	Linked the malaria-encoded sequence (NANP)n from circumsporozoite (CS) protein to another peptide from the CS protein. The resultant conjugate raised anti (NANP)n antibodies in mice which were non-responders to (NANP)n Antibodies sequence alone.
Francis *et al.* 1987	140-160 peptide from VPI of FMDV (which contained B-cell epitope and H-k T-cell epitope) was co-synthesized with three different sequences containing $H-2^d$ and T-cell epitopes. one from ovalbumin and two from sperm whale myoglobin. The resultant three peptides produced anti-FMDV peptide antibodies in both $H-2^k$ and $H-2^d$ haplotype mice.
Chedid *et al.* 1984	Polymerized four peptides from two bacterial antigens, one viral antigen and one parasitic antigen using glutaraldehyde. Association of peptides enhanced their respective immunogenicities.
Leclerc *et al.* 1987	Co-polymerized a streptococcal protein peptide (which contained B-&T-cell epitopes) with a hepatitis-B virus surface antigen peptide (containing B-cell epitope)
Francis *et al.* 1989	Five predicted ten amino acid cell epitopes (TI to T5) from HRV (human rhinovirus) were used to improve the performance of a non-immunogenic B-cell epitope peptide from the same virus.
Jolivet *et al.* 1990	Showed the importance of T-cell epitopes in the polymers.
Ho *et al.* 1990, Pollur *et al.* 1988, Rusche *et al.* 1988, Goudssmit *et al.* 1988	Raised virus neutralizing antibodies with synthetic peptides for a linear B-cell epitope of human immunodeficiency virus (HIV). These antibodies neutralized HIV *in-vitro*.

11.25.5.2. Chemical linkage

This is a more controlled method as it utilizes a heterobifunctional cross-linking reagent, such as M-maleimidobenzoyl-N-hydroxysuccinimide ester (MBS). This compound has an amino-reactive NHS-ester as one functional group and a sulfhydryl reactive group as the other. Amino groups on one peptide (e.g. B-cell epitope) are acylated with the NHS-ester *via* the hydroxysuccinimide group. This is followed by the introduction of a second peptide (e.g. Th-cell epitope) having a free sulfhydryl group that can react with the maleimide group of the coupling reagent. Good *et.al*, (1987) have used this method to link the malaria-encoded sequence (NANP)n from the circumsporozoite (CS) protein to another peptide from the CS protein. However, this technique may require the synthesis of a specific peptide with a non-natural cysteine residue added to its carboxyl terminal. Also, the presence of essential natural cysteine or lysine residues within either peptide may ultimately affect the nature and final antigenicity of the conjugate produced.

11.25.5.3. Co-linear synthesis

This technique overcomes the limitations associated with the first two methods. A peptide with known immunological properties can be synthesized by adopting this approach. The method offers the flexibility to alter position of one epitope in relation to another and to synthesize.

11.26. IMMUNOADHESIN(S)

The major problem with CD4 clone prophylaxis is fast clearance of these molecules. In the case of CD4 vaccines biological half-life is reported to be 30-120 minutes in serum necessitating frequent injections. Immunoadhesin gene strategy reported by Capon and colleagues is principally based on recombinant technology where CD4 gene is linked with constant region gene of IgG1. The immunoglobulin-CD4 gene hybrid formed is immunoadhesive and exhibits high affinity for gp120 (typical characteristics of CD4) as well as longer biological half-life that corresponds to IgG1. The biological half-life of CD-IgG1 has been reported to be 200 fold longer than of soluble CD4 whose expected half-life in humans is about 21 days. This opens up vistas for diverse immunoadhesive expressions, and for various associated factors and functions like opsonization or complement activation.

11.27. RECOMBINANT ANTIGEN VACCINES

11.27.1. r-DNA vaccines -The rationale

In the last two decades, recombinant DNA (rDNA) technology has revolutionized basic and applied biomedical research. A wide range of new impressive products have been developed by using recombinant techniques and are available in the market. These products include biologicals such as insulin and tissue plasminogen activator (TPA); genetically engineered organisms protect valuable fruit crops; enzymes utilized in the manufacture of foods; and new generation vaccines. Diagnostic kits have been developed that helps in detection of infections at early stage. In forensic laboratories, "finger printing" tests can be made on blood and semen samples. Our focus here in on the use of recombinant technology in development of new generation vaccines. Certain vaccines currently available in market are efficacious and cost effective but are being produced by using older techniques. The rDNA technique effectively and successfully could be used to make the products safer and cost effective provided that certain problems relating to handling infectious agents and the safety concerns of personnel handling the same are addressed. Since vaccines are developed to prevent infectious diseases, traditional approaches to vaccine development are arousing concerns about safety. rDNA vaccines have clear advantages over those where the organisms are used to produce the vaccine. The disadvantages associated with traditional micro-organism based vaccine systems are mentioned below:

(a). It is dangerous to handle;

(b). It could produce disease in vaccinated hosts;

(c). It needs to be attenuated, and/or

(d). It could-produce toxic end products.

Use of highly virulent organisms poses an obvious problem in developing, producing and using any vaccine made from them. This is one of the reasons for failure of the conventional technique in developing a vaccine for hepatitis B. Application of rDNA technique has facilitated successful development of hepatitis B vaccine (HBV) which has now flooded the market. Cloning the genes required to produce HBV-soluble antigen (the protective antigen) in a bacterial host made possible to create a nonvirulent, recombinant organism capable of synthesizing large amount of the protective antigens of HBV. The rDNA technology can help in increasing the amount of antigen produced by an organism. Isolation and cloning of DNA encoding antigenic determinants can be carried out in yeast, bacteria or mammalian cells. A number of genes from viral, bacterial, and protozoan pathogens have been successfully cloned and attempts are being made to develop them as vaccines. The first recombinant vaccine was developed successfully for the major antigen (VPI) of the foot and mouth disease viruses. The viral RNA encoding the VPI surface antigen was transcribed into cDNA using reverse transcriptase. The VPI cDNA was then inserted into an *Escherichia coli* plasmid and cloned in *E. coli*. With this procedure, large quantities of the VPI antigen can be produced, which are then purified and used as a vaccine in animals.

Hepatitis B vaccine was the first recombinant antigen vaccine approved for human use. It was developed by cloning gene for the major surface antigen of hepatitis B virus (HBsAg) in yeast cells. The recombinant yeast cells are grown in fermenters and accumulation of HBsAg occurs intracellularly in the cells. The yeast cells are harvested and disrupted by high pressure thereby releasing the recombinant HBsAg which is then purified by conventional biochemical techniques. The recombinant hepatitis B vaccine has been tested successfully and has immense potential for exploitation.

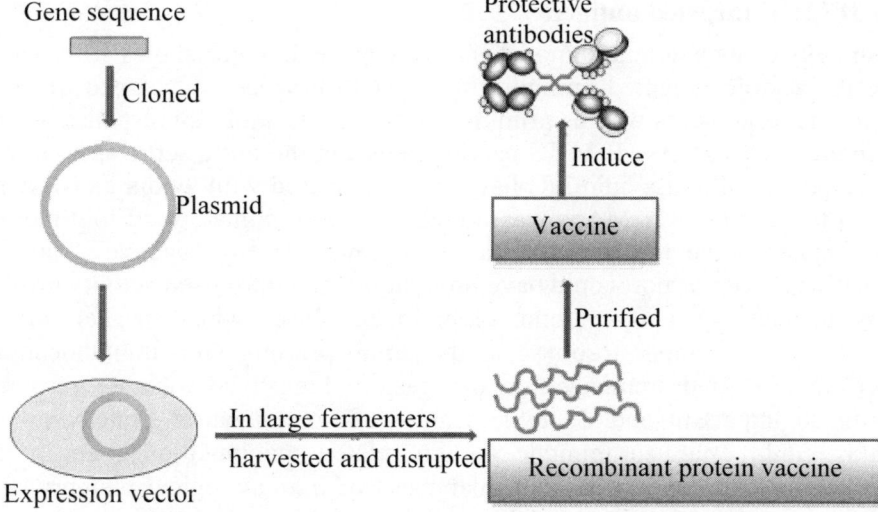

Fig. 11.31: Production of recombinant antigen vaccine

Studies are presently being carried out for development of recombinant vaccines for human immuno-deficiency virus. Other recombinant vaccines are being developed in animal models and include the circumsporozoite protein of the malaria parasite, the B subunit of cholera toxin, a glycoprotein membrane antigen from Epstein-Barr virus and the enterotoxin of *E. coli*. In some cases promising results have been obtained with a protective immune response to a subsequent challenge. The chief limitation of recombinant protein or glycoprotein vaccines is that they are processed as exogenous antigens and therefore fail to induce much activation of class I MHC-restricted Tc cells.

For weakly immunogenic recombinant proteins some safe and powerful adjuvants have been designed so that their immune response can be augmented. One approach utilizes genetic grafting of immuno-stimulatory lymphokines, such as IL-1 or TNFα into a recombinant protein. However, their practical application is strongly limited in humans due to their toxic, proinflammatory and pleiotropic effects. For example, IL-1 is an important modulatory molecule of the immune system which also induces *in vivo* after administration of several adjuvant molecules, such as bacterial products. But IL-1 cannot be used as such because it is also a potent pyrogen and proinflammatory agent. To alleviate this problem, 163-171 sequence of human IL-1β has been proposed as adjuvant for poorly immunogenic vaccines. This non peptide was found to be the minimal structure responsible for immunostimulatory properties of the entire molecule. It lacked many undesired *in vivo* and *in vitro* pro-inflammatory activities of IL-1. In addition, it can stimulate the immune response to both T-dependent and T-independent antigens. Use of recombinant antigens with 'built-in' adjuvanticity opens up new vistas in designing vaccines in which poorly immunogenic proteins are coupled to domains endowed with immunostimulatory properties.

11.27.2. Adjuvant independent immuno targeted vaccines

This approach involves antigen-antibody conjugation. The complex is presented to determinant expressed *in vivo* on surface of cells of immune system. The immunization as such a parenteral preparation administered intravenously with saline has referred as antigen independent. Thus, physical properties and passivasion for disposition of conjugate itself presumably dominated the event *via* antibody specific binding affinity of conjugate. Thus antigen is presented and in turn localized at the surface of specific preidentified target cells.

11.27.3. Class II MHC targeted antigen

In a classical strategy using avidin as a model antigenic protein, which shows affinity to MAb specific for class II MHC, a target oriented immunization system has been developed. In order to have an appreciable immune response as well as priming for secondary antibody response, both B-cell and T-cell recognition are needed. Class II MHC bearing cells can therefore serve as a target cell line. The immunogenic responses of anti avidin IgG have been compared with avidin anti-IgA MAbs in mice. Avidin bound to the anti-class II MAbs was found to be approximately 40 fold more immunogenic than avidin conjugated to the anti-NP MAb (a control antibody, non reactive). Thus, it was inferred that ligand specific to receptor port could have brought by the improvised activity profile.

The results indicate an early immunoglobulin response, which peaked after 10 days of immunization. A strong memory response to the initial priming with immunoconjugate could be induced by avidin. Targeted immunization can restore long-lived memory response. This is in accordance with an important and desirable feature of immunization strategy to vaccine design. Immunotargeting could establish immune system related manipulation even in the absence of adjuvants. Furthermore, in context of molecular basis of immunological memory, the anti-class II MHC immunoconjugates seem able to deliver antigen to the cellular level selectively where the maintenance of long term memory is desirable.

Cells bearing class II MHC have potential for antigen presentation, employing that beginning with an uptake followed by proteolytic processing and in turn the association of released T-cell epitopes (peptides) together with class II MHC can result in the activation of T-cells. It is likely that following subcutaneous immunization anti-classII MHC immunoconjugates encounter classII specific determinants present on specialized antigen presenting cells such as dendritics, and interact with class II MHC on B cells. The antigen specific T cells determinants are presented following their processing by the cascade of events described above; as a result it leads to activation of class II MHC restricted T helper (TH) cells capable of signaling through cytokine(s) regulation necessary for B cell differentiation and proliferation. However, only B cells which have already received traditional signal can respond to this "help". The traditional signals originate and/or induced by engagement of antigen specific receptors with B cell epitopes on the antigen. Thus the process favors enhanced uptake of class II MHC specific antigens by APC and could possibly augment the immunogenicity of antigens *via* their targeted presentation.

11.28. VECTOR VACCINES

11.28.1. Recombinant vector vaccines

Genes encoding major antigens of virulent pathogens can be introduced into attenuated viruses or bacteria. The attenuated organism serves as a vector, which replicates within the host and expresses the gene product of the pathogen. Various organisms have been utilized for vector vaccines and include adenoviruses, attenuated poliovirus, and vaccinia virus, BCG strain of *Mycobacterium bovis* and attenuated strains of *Salmonella*.

Vaccinia virus, used to eradicate smallpox is widely employed as a vector vaccine. This large and complex virus containing a genome of about 200 genes can be manipulated to carry scores of foreign genes without any impairment in its capacity to infect and replicate in host. The gene encoding desired antigen is inserted into a plasmid vector adjacent to a vaccinia promoter and is flanked on the two sides by vaccinia thymidine kinase sequences. Simultaneously, tissue culture cells are infected with vaccinia virus and transfected with the recombinant plasmid. The desired gene and promoter are inserted into the vaccinia virus genome by homologous recombination at the site of the non-essential vaccinia thymidine kinase gene. This results in a thymidine kinase-negative recombinant virus. Selection of tissue culture cells infected with recombinant (thymidine kinase-negative) vaccinia viruses are then carried out by adding bromodeoxyuridine (Budr), a thymidine analog which kills all thymidine kinase-positive cells (Fig.11.32).

The genetically engineered vaccinia expresses high levels of the inserted gene product which can later serve as a potent immunogen in an inoculated host. Attempts have been made to insert genes from hepatitis B virus, influenza and herpes simplex viruses into vaccinia virus. This engineered vaccinia induces antibodies to all three engineered gene products. As with smallpox vaccine, genetically engineered vaccinia can be administered simply by dermal scratching so that a limited, localized infection is caused in host cells. If the foreign gene product expressed by the vaccinia is a viral envelope protein, it is inserted into the membrane of the infected host cell, inducing development of both T-cell-mediated immunity and antibody-mediated immunity.

Vaccinia virus engineered with the glycoprotein envelope of the human immunodeficiency virus (HIV) is being examined as a potential vaccine for AIDS. However, the vaccinia vector vaccine may not be suitable for individuals with AIDS, because 'in immunity deficient individuals even an attenuated vaccine can be fatal. Various other attenuated vector vaccines safer than the vaccinia virus have been tried. An attenuated strain of *Salmonella typhimurium* has been engineered with genes from the bacterium that causes cholera. This vector vaccine is advantageous in that *Salmonella* infects cells of the mucosal lining of the gut and thereby inducing secretory IgA production. For various diseases like cholera and gonorrhoea, an increased level of secretory IgA at mucous membrane surfaces is required for immunity. Another potential candidate for a safe and effective vector vaccine is the Sabin vaccine strain of poliovirus. Here the poliovirus vector is genetically engineered to replace a portion of the gene encoding the outer capsid protein of poliovirus by DNA encoding the epitope of choice. The resulting poliovirus chimera expresses the desired epitope(s) in a highly accessible presentation protruding from the poliovirus nucleocapsid. In animal models a chimeric poliovirus vector vaccine expressing epitopes from the envelope glycoproteins of HIV has been shown to induce high levels of neutralizing antibodies specific for HIV.

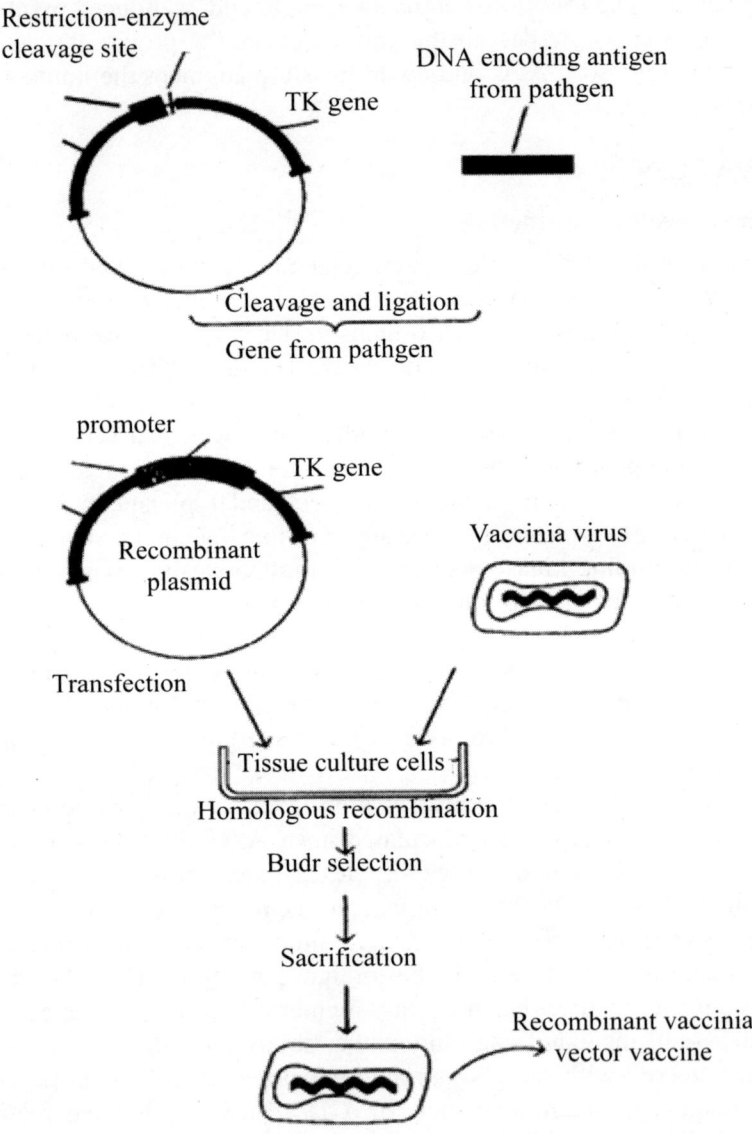

Fig. 11.32: Production of vaccinia vector vaccine containing a gene encoding an antigen from a pathogen

11.28.2. Minicells as vaccines

The use of whole cell organisms has the disadvantage that once they enter the Gut-associated lymphoid tissue (GALT) they produce antibodies. However, they create their own environmental challenges and problems. To overcome such regeneration problem, a non-regenerating vaccine carrier such as minicells can be used. Strains of *E. coli* (minicell-producing) and *S. typhimurium* have been reported. Minicells are non-regenerating vaccine carriers containing somatic and surface antigens. They do not express any pathogenic activity and can elicit both humoral and cellular immune responses.

11.28.2.1. The concept

When a rod-shaped bacterium undergoes cell division at the midcellular axis, it generates two daughter cells, each containing not only the cellular constituents of the mother cell but also a full complement of the genetic material. Chromosomal genes responsible for the replication of the chromosome (genophore) and its partitioning between the two daughter cells ensure the preservation of the cell size and the inheritance of a genophore. Under most normal growth conditions, some variations in the distribution of daughter cell sizes are observed. On the other hand, under some special physiological conditions, such as aged culture or in cells treated with antibiotics, anomalous cell division leads to asymmetrical cells, that is the formation of daughter cells of unequal sizes.

The daughter cells resulting from cell division in rod shaped bacteria perpetuate the cell cycle and formation of progeny cells. The formation of daughter cells is controlled both physiologically and genetically. Once there is an intervention with the normal process of cell division in rod-shaped bacteria through antibiotics, mutation or metabolic disorders, it yields daughter cells of unequal size called anucleated minicells (AMCs).

The term minicells refers to small daughter cell of an unequally divided rod-shaped bacterial cell. These minicells can be produced after subjecting the growing cultures to a number of physiological treatments. The principal chromosomal lesion responsible for the production of a minicell in *E. coli* is in the *min B* gene. Some other taxa of minicell producing rod-shaped bacteria include *Salmonella, Haemophilus, Bacillus, Shigella, Pseudomonas,* and *Erwinia*. The genetic event takes place due to multiple mutations. The size of minicell obtained from *E. coli* is 1/5 to 1/10 the size of the parent cell. They contain most of the cellular contents, which help them in carrying out the physiological activity. Minicells can be produced by means of continuous or batch fermentation. The so produced minicells are stored at low temperature (+4 to -70°C) until used.

Tankersly and Woodward in the 1974 were the first to demonstrate the potential use of minicells as vaccines. They used a strain of *S. typhimurium* obtained from a clinical specimen and treated it with triethylene melamine. They recovered the minicell-producing derivative and cultured it. The minicells were purified and then injected into adult rabbits. After completion of the immunization regimen, the rabbits were bled and the sera collected; the latter contained antibodies against group *B. Salmonella*.

11.28.3. Nucleic acid vaccines

Immunization using nucleic acid is becoming a promising new field. It is achieved by administering plasmid DNA containing genes encoding antigen. The plasmid DNA enters cells and the antigen is expressed *via* normal cellular mechanisms. These nucleic acid vaccines act by delivering the antigen for presentation *via* MHC class I and class II mechanisms. Similar to live-attenuated vaccines, nucleic acid based immunization can induce both antibody and MHC class I restricted CD8$^+$ cytotoxic T lymphocyte (CTL) responses. Clinical trials of DNA vaccines against HIV-I are underway.

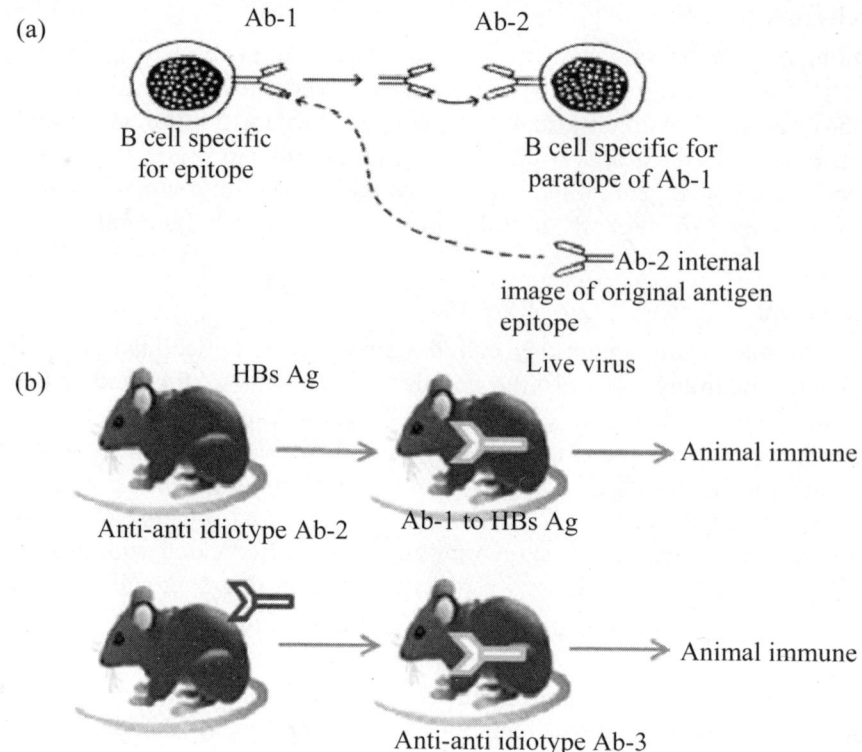

Fig. 11.33: The use of anti-idiotype antibody as vaccine (a) The binding site on the same anti-idiotype antibodies (b) Immunization with anti-idiotype antibody

11.29. ANTI-IDIOTYPE VACCINES

Anti-idiotype antibody specific for the antigen-binding site (the paratope) on anti-pathogen antibody can potentially serve as a vaccine. This approach holds promise since effective immune response to pathogenic antigen is generated without exposure of the vaccinated individual to any form of pathogen, i.e. attenuated or killed whole-pathogen vaccine. This avoids any undesirable or uncontrollable side effects. When anti-idiotype antibody specific for the paratope is administered, an animal makes antibody to the binding site on the anti-idiotype antibody, and this antibody (called anti-anti-idiotype antibody) will also bind to the original antigen (Fig11.33). In this manner an animal can become immune to an antigen without having come across the antigen itself; instead, it is exposed to anti-idiotype antibody. For example, if animals are immunized with anti-idiotype antibody specific for the binding site of TEPC-15, they will be immune if these are later challenged with live *pneumococci*.

Anti-idiotype antibodies to HIV antigens have been produced and injected into animals to produce anti-anti-idiotype antibody that binds to HIV antigens as well. Immunizing with the virus or viral components can be precisely avoided. Following the same principle, vaccines have been designed to bind to a conserved region on the gp 120 envelope glycoprotein that is required for binding to the CD4 membrane molecule on host cells. Anti-idiotype vaccines have been reported to induce protective immunity in mice against hepatitis B virus, Sendai virus, rabies virus, *Listeria monocytogenes*, *Schistosoma mansoni*, *Streptococcus pneumoniae* and *Trypanosoma rhodesiense*. An anti-idiotype vaccine for humans may materialize in the near future and holds much promise in avoiding the unacceptable risks associated with a killed or attenuated virus.

11.30. TARGETED IMMUNE STIMULANTS

Bacillus Calmette Guerin (BCG) has recently been recognized as general immunostimulant and has been introduced into clinical practice as a mode of treatment for superficial blood tumors. The mode of action of BCG particularly against tumors can be broadly divided into three phases: (1), organ targeting to superficial tumor cells; (2), stimulation of immune response; and (3) phagocytosis of tumor cells.

Targeting: Fibronectin receptor and fibronectin interaction have been explored for targeted delivery of BCG cells to the super bladder tumor by Ratllief and co-workers in 1987. It appears that fibronectin is excreted in very close proximity of tumor cell surface. When BCG is administered to normal intact urothelium, virtually no BCG is found to be associated, suggesting that direct contact occurred between BCG and urothelial cells. However, it was shown that human T24 carcinoma cell line is capable of capturing, adhering and ingesting BCG. BCG fibronectin receptor is virtually a member of the group of antigens (85 protein complexes) which are the major components of protein excreted by BCG in culture and have molecular weights of around 30-32 kDa. However, even larger proteins may be responsible for actual attachments to the cell wall. Thus, tumor site is approached *via* receptor ligand mediation, whereas necrotin receptor is approached by BCG surface associated antigen protein complexes.

Immunological response: BCG-evoked immune response is local in nature and interesting a delayed hypersensitivity, or undoubtedly the phagocytes stimulation involving partially a phagocytic response followed by a granulomatous reaction generated and localized in bladder wall. T-lymphocytes, monocytes, macro and leukocytes are the prime infiltrating cells that respond to intravesicle BCG treatment. The expression of class II MHC has also been observed on urothelial tumor cell wall and leads to alteration of the phenotype with implications for at least one of the possibilities of BCG showing antitumor activity. Thus, local response is crucial in overall antitumor activity.

Phagocytosis: It was reported that BCG cells are internalized and digested by both human bladder tumor and murine bladder tumor cell lines. After getting internalized, BCG cells kill murine sarcoma cells. The possibility persists that BCG may contain a stable cytotoxic component such as lipopolysaccharide which has chemical affinity to lipoarabinomannan (LAMP) identified as toxic composed from M. tuberculosis. Hopefully, defining that mode and mechanism of new generation of targeted drug delivery in immunization, could yield a vaccination system of choice with potential to prevent or effectively treat diseases.

11.31. NEW GENERATION VACCINES

11.31.1. Hepatitis B vaccine (HBV)

Several hepatitis B vaccines (HBV) are available in the market. They are broadly classified as hepatitis B surface antigen (HBsAg) and recombinant HBV. The drawbacks of HBsAg particles are their low efficacy, low response and low stability during freezing as well as at high temperature. This problem may be addressed by incorporating the particles into liposomes and produce a liposomal vaccine.

11.31.1.1. Liposomal vaccine

An HBsAg particle contains three peptides: small (S), middle (M) and long (L) peptides. On encapsulation into liposomes the particle serves as an adjuvant-carrier. The three peptides are coded by ORF Pre-S/S genes. The S-peptide corresponds to the 3' region of the ORF. The M peptide includes the pre-S2 region and the S peptide. The L peptide contains amino acid sequences of Pre-S I, Pre-S2 and S peptides. The Pre-S 1 and Pre-S2 amino acid sequences have antigenic determinants independent of the S proteins. The presence of the Pre-S I region induces specific T cell response which can bypass non-responsiveness to the Pre-S2 and S regions of HBsAg.

Liposomal vaccines are prepared by using dimyristoyl phosphatidylcholine (DMPC) and dimyristoyl phosphatidylglycerol (DMPG). The negative charge of DMPG results in the enlargement of the aqueous volume entrapped in the liposomes by electrostatic repulsion between the bilayer leaflets. HBsAg particles are obtained by isolating HBV DNA and transfecting them into Chinese hamster ovary (CHO) cells. Following selection and cloning, these cells secrete 22nm HBsAg particles. The efficiency of the vaccine is examined by vaccination of BALB/c mice with different doses of HBsAg entrapped in liposomes.

11.31.1.2. Adenovirus vectored hepatitis B vaccines

Immunization against one of the major infectious liver diseases, hepatitis, caused by hepatitis B virus is done by either using an HBsAg or recombinant hepatitis vaccine derived from yeast. This preparation is too expensive to be brought under the World Health Organization's (WHO) immunization scheme. Live recombinant hepatitis vaccines using adenovirus vectors provide an alternative that offers the advantage of low cost and ease of administration. Considerable progress in making recombinant adenoviruses that express large amounts of HBsAg *in vitro* has occured. *In vivo* studies in cotton rat hamster, dog and chimpanzee have been encouraging.

11.31.2. Contraceptive vaccines

Fertility control by immunological approach has become a reality today. Birth control vaccines for human use have reached the stage of clinical trials both in India and abroad. A strong need for birth control vaccine was identified in the 1970s. Today, vaccines against three hormones (leuteinizing hormone releasing hormone LHRH, follicle stimulating hormone (FSH) and human chorionic gonadotropin hormone, HCG) are undergoing clinical trials.

11.31.2.1. Human chorionic gonadotropin vaccine

HCG is an early signal of pregnancy as it essential for establishment and maintenance of pregnancy during the first seven-week period. This hormone is normally responsible for missing of the menstrual period, which by its action on corpus luteum continuously produces progesterone. This hormone can be a good target for devising a birth control vaccine. HCG neutralizes the hormonal signal by neutralizing circulating antibodies and so blocking the HCG support to corpus luteum, which leads to continual menstrual cycle.

The strategy behind targeting HCG hormone can be well documented by its need by corpus luteum which brings in continual synthesis of progesterone by ovaries which in turn prepares the endometrium which will receive the embryo. Blocking HCG by anti-HCG antibodies abolishes support by corpus luteum and intervenes at post-ovulatory phase but prior to -the onset of pregnancy. However, the immunological sequence does not interfere with normal physiological functions such as ovulation and secretion of normal steroidal sex hormones. The vaccine approach has an edge over contraceptives which normally act by blocking ovulating and stops secretion of normal steroidal sex hormones.

Above all, HCG comes from a natural source. Its primary subunit structure and composition are well known. HCG is composed of two subunits, α and β. As the α-subunit is common to three other pituitary hormones, the β-subunit or a part of it is chosen. Based on the selection, two types of vaccines have been made: first, the 37 amino acid carboxy terminal peptide (CTP) of β-HCG and secondly, entire β-HCG was employed. CTP was chosen as it does not exist in β-HLH, thus preventing the antibodies from cross-reacting with HLH. However, it was found that CTP-induced antibodies react with somatostatin-producing cells of the pancreas. Use of entire β-subunit of HCG has the advantage that they are more immunogenic than CTP and the antibodies have better capacity. However, cross reactivity with HLH was observed and did not deplete the monthly LH surge below the amount necessary for ovulation.

β-HCG and CTP are 'self molecules' and thus cannot elicit an antibody response on themselves. Therefore they are either hapten-modified or linked to a carrier. The first prototype vaccine, linked p-HCG with tetanus toxoid (TT). This vaccine evoked antibodies against both HCG and TT. Linking HCG with TT has the added advantage that immunoprophylaxis against tetanus infection is achieved. HCG did not act as a booster on itself. Steps have been taken to improve the immunogenicity of p-HCG- TT vaccine and are listed below:
1. Sodium phthalyl derivative of lipopolysaccharide (SPLPS) from *Salmonella enteritidis* is included as an adjuvant in the first injection.
2. Diphtherial toxoid (DT) is selected as a carrier in addition to TT.
3. The intrinsic immunogenicity of p-HCG was augmented by associating it with a heterospecies a-subunit of bovine origin.

11.31.2.2. Recombinant products

The genes for β-HCG and α-HLH have been cloned and expressed in vaccinia virus and baculovirus. The vaccinia-expressed products are fully glycosylated and identical to the native hormonal subunits. However, baculovirus expression system showed better yield but the products were partially glycosylated. In both cases, the p-HCG is immunoreactive. The β-subunit could bind with the a-subunit to generate bioactive hormone. p-HCG has also been expressed in *E. coli* which produced higher yield; the amino acid composition was the same as that of the human β-HCG; and the product was not glycosylated. A live recombinant vaccine has been developed by inserting β-HCG in vaccinia virus along with a transmembrane 48 amino acid fragment. When tested in rodents, this vaccine was highly immunogenic.

11.31.2.3. LHRH vaccine

Luteinizing hormone releasing hormone (LHRH) or gonadotropin releasing hormone (GRH) (a decapeptide), controls the secretion of luteinizing hormone (LH) and follicle stimulating hormone (FSH) from the pituitary. These in turn act on the male or female gonads to generate sperms or egg and also steroidal sex hormones. Activation of LHRH impairs fertility and fails to produce steroidal sex hormones. Besides fertility control in human, they are also useful in animal fertility control. This is possible because of the conserved sequence of the hormone in mammals. Immunization against LHRH is also useful in animals grown for the purpose of meat. Here, the suppression of the androgen hormone will have an impact on the quality of the meat. Immunization can be both active and passive. Passive immunization is achieved by parenteral administration of monoclonal antibodies.

LHRH of natural origin has neither an amino terminal nor carboxy terminal end for carrier-linkage but molecules can be chemically synthesized to have one or the other group. TT linked at the N-terminal amino position generates higher immunogenicity than the one produced with a carboxyl end linked TT. The vaccine was designed by substituting a D-lysine at position 6 for glycine, thereby producing an analogue that is resistant to metabolic degradation, with an additional spacer group for linkage. The so obtained vaccine showed higher immunogenicity.

11.31.2.4. Paraneem vaccine

Research on fertility control has led to a natural source for vaccination. A single instillation of purified neem (*Azadirachta indica*) seed extract (paraneem) into the uterus prevents pregnancy without impairing ovulation. Paraneem vaccine induces local cell-mediated immunity, leading to immunosuppression at the genital tract which reacts against the sperm, which is foreign to the women's immune system. Following the immunological response, activated by the sperm, it locally produces cytokines such as γ-interferon, IL2 and TNF that reject implantation.

11.31.2.5. Male fertility control

Male fertility control is brought about by using FSH vaccine. An alternate approach is to exploit the in-built developmental potential of selective immunosuppression of spermatogenesis by cell-mediated immune response. At puberty, many proteins are 'foreign' to the body's immune system. Leydig cells producing testosterone are recognized as 'self' as they are present in, and function from, the fetal stage. Injecting a suspension of BCG vaccine induced spermatogenesis without decline of testosterone. This effect was observed in every mammal that was studied. However, the effect was reversible and spermatogenesis was regained with time. By injecting purified neem seed extract into the vas deferens, spermatogenesis can be induced without any significant reduction in testosterone level.

11.31.3. Anti-sepsis vaccine

Septic shock occurs as a consequence of the introduction of a pathogen into a sterile tissue; this leads to a battle between the pathogen and the host. To design a vaccine against septic shock, one should be well versed with the strategy of the disease at each stage. The entire act begins with the replication of pathogenic bacteria or fungus in the tissue. The shock is usually caused by gram negative bacteria. A vaccine has been developed against sepsis resulting from gram-negative bacteria. Lipopolysaccharide (LPS), a complex molecule, is shed by gram negative bacteria when they replicate. The vaccine targets the important component (lipid A portion) of this LPS. LPS is a potent stimulant of immune reaction and is the major contributor to the lethal consequences of septic shock. The anti-sepsis vaccine comprises of lipid A in lipid vesicle (liposomes), whereby the inherent toxicity of lipid A is masked, while retaining the adjuvanticity property through which an immunologic reaction is stimulated. The liposome-bearing lipid A acts as the antigen stimulating an immune response.

11.31.4. Live recombinant vaccinia–Rabies vaccine

Rabies is a viral disease, which affects all-warm-blooded animals and is widespread throughout the world. Dogs represent the major vector in our country. The disease is transmitted through the bite of an infected animal whose saliva contains large amount of virus. As rabies is nearly always fatal, immune populations do not exist. Rabies virus (RV), a rhabdovirus, is an enveloped negative single-stranded RNA virus related to vesicular stomatitis virus. The glycoprotein (G), present on the exterior surface of the virion is the only protein capable of inducing or reacting with virus-neutralizing antibody (VNA) and appears to be the main viral protein capable of eliciting protection. Oral route administration is the only appropriate route for vaccination of a large number of animals. Live attenuated rabies virus is used for vaccination. However, attenuated viruses remain pathogenic and may revert to virulence. Inactivated rabies virus is ineffective when administered orally. Vaccinia virus (VV), a large (180 kb) double-stranded DNA virus, has been used extensively to control and eradicate smallpox in man. They are being studied as live vector for viral antigens and derivatives thereof.

A recombinant vaccinia virus (VVTGgRAB) bearing the rabies G coding sequence and expressing the rabies surface antigen was developed by Kidney and co-workers. They inserted the rabies G cDNA into a plasmid vector downstream of the vaccinia virus p7.5K promoter into the non-essential vaccinia TK gene. Double reciprocal recombination *in vivo* between this plasmid the vaccinia virus genome allows integration of the DNA inset into the viral genome. Infection of cell cultures with VVTGgRAB elicited the production of a correctly processed rabies G which was found to react strongly with rabies neutralizing antibodies.

11.31.5. Acquired immunodeficiency syndrome (AIDS)

AIDS was first reported in the year 1981 in the *New England Journal of Medicine*. The report indicated that the victims had decreased counts of $CD4^+$ T cells, confirming their suspected linkage to a compromised immune system. In 1982, the Centers for Disease Control (CDC), an agency of the U.S. Public Health Services, suggested that this distinct new disorder be called acquired immunodeficiency syndrome, now commonly known as AIDS. Although the disease was first reported and identified in homosexual men in the United States, it was soon observed in other groups including hemophiliacs, blood-transfusion recipients, intravenous drug users, sexual partners of AIDS patients, and eventually in infants of mothers with the disease. In 1983 Luc Montaginer's group at the Pasteur Institute isolated a retrovirus from a lymph node biopsy of an AIDS patient. The retrovirus was named human immunodeficiency virus or HIV in 1986. It was also observed that there existed an antigenic variation in the virus. Thus, the original virus was designated HIV-I and the variant HIV-2. Both were found to be genetically related to the simian immunodeficiency virus (SIVs), found in African primates. Another variant, designated HIV-O, has been identified in Cameroon. Development of a vaccine for disease of this nature requires a thorough knowledge about the infectious agent, characterization of the immune response to the agent, and determination of what type of immune response is protective.

11.31.5.1. Structure of HIV

All members of the lentivirus family of retroviruses, including the three types of HIV and various SIVs, share numerous structural and molecular similarities. The viruses have an RNA genome and two associated molecules of reverse transcriptase which catalyze "reverse transcription" of viral RNA into DNA. Other nucleoid proteins include the p10 protease and p32 integrase. Surrounding the viral genome and nucleoid proteins are two layers of core proteins; in HIV these core proteins are designated as p17 and p24. The viral core, or nucleocapsid, is surrounded by an envelope derived from the host-cell membrane, which is modified by the insertion of two HIV glycoproteins, gp120 and gp41. The gp41 glycoprotein spans the membrane; gp120 is noncovalently associated with gp41 but extends beyond the membrane. Both gp 120 and gp41 have important roles in the binding of HIV to cells in the process of infection. The HIV envelope is studded with human proteins (including class I and class II MHC molecules) acquired by the virus as it buds from the human cell membrane.

Entry of the HIV into the target cells involves two steps: binding of virions to receptors on target cells is followed by fusion of the viral envelope with the plasma membrane of the cells. The glycoproteins gp 120 and gp41 play vital roles in these steps: gp 120 in binding and gp41 in fusion. Upon entering the target cell, the viral RNA is copied into DNA which then integrates into the host cells' DNA, forming a provirus which may remain in a latent state or may be activated and transcribed into viral proteins.

11.31.6. Development of an AIDS vaccine

Since the identification of HIV as the causative agent of AIDS, serious efforts have been made to develop a safe and effective vaccine. Some vaccines that have been designed are inactivated whole virus, live recombinant viruses, attenuated virus, synthetic peptides, anti-idiotype antibodies and recombinant DNA products.

11.31.6.1. Inactivated whole viruses

The procedure involved is similar to the one used in developing the Salk polio vaccine. Here, preparations of HIV-l and SIV have been produced by irradiating the virus followed by formaldehyde treatment. This inactivates the retroviral genome and releases much of the gp120 from the envelope. The resultant, noninfectious SIV or HIV preparations are used as vaccine. Initial trials in animals look promising. However, the results have been challenged as the SIV vaccine was prepared by growing SIV in human T-cell cultures.

11.31.6.2. Attenuated viruses

This method of vaccine development is also similar to that of Sabin polio vaccine, wherein live poliovirus is grown in monkey kidney. When a live virus is grown under unusual culture conditions, the viruses are forced to mutate to survive in the new growing conditions. Most viral vaccines used today are attenuated vaccines. As the vaccine is live, it is able to infect cells and grow for a limited period of time before the immune response eliminates the virus. However, during this period, the attenuated virus is able to induce a potent immune response, often including generation of cell-mediated cytotoxic T-lymphocytes specific for the endogenously produced viral antigens. In addition, they have an added advantage that the attenuated viral vaccines induce a good memory cell response that accounts for the life-long immunity developed by these vaccines.

HIV being a highly mutant virus, using attenuated strains was considered to be too dangerous. In 1992, Desrosiers and co-workers developed an attenuated strain of SIV by eliminating the regulatory gene 'nef' from a highly virulent strain of SIV. When this nef-deleted strain was injected into six macaques, the animals did not develop any symptoms of simian AIDS (SAIDS). When the animals were challenged with huge doses of infectious SIV, they remained healthy. However, the blow came when it was found that the attenuated strain caused SAIDS in the newborn macques.

11.31.6.3. Cloned envelope glycoproteins

The first cloned gp 160 vaccines were produced by MicroGeneSys, Inc. in the year 1987. Several groups have applied gene-engineering techniques to clone either the gp120 gene or the entire gp160 gene in order to produce large quantities of gp120 or gp160 for immunization. The cloned gp160 vaccine when administered induced humoral immunity. Antibodies elicited in the volunteers inhibited viral replication *in vitro*, and the inhibition was always strain specific.

11.31.6.4. Recombinant viruses carrying HIV genes

Another strategy for effective AIDS vaccine development depends on the use of recombinant vectors. Vaccinia virus and the Sabin polio virus are both live attenuated vaccines used effectively as vaccines. These viruses can be engineered to carry genes from HIV -1, and the recombinant virus can then be used as a vaccine. As the recombinant virus is attenuated but not inactivated, it is capable of infecting host cells and is therefore expected to induce CTL activity. Vaccinia virus, a large virus, can be engineered to carry several dozen foreign genes without impairing its capacity to infect host cells and to replicate in them. The engineered vaccinia virus can be administered easily and simply by dermal scratching. It causes a limited localized infection in the host cells. The foreign genes are expressed by the vaccinia, and if the foreign gene product is a viral envelope protein, it is inserted into the membrane of the infected host cell where it stimulates the development of T-cell mediated immunity. Vaccinia virus carrying gp160 infects host cells at the site of scarification. The gp 160 is glycosylated, cleaved into gp 120 and gp41, and inserted into the plasma membrane of the infected host cells. Some HIV genes that have been engineered into vaccinia virus are *enve, tat, pol* and *gag*.

11.31.6.4. Synthetic crown-sequence peptides

Synthetic peptides of different HIV crown sequences, including MN sequence, have been prepared and tested for ability to activate T-cell proliferation and cytotoxicity in vitro. The principal neutralizing epitope of HIV overlaps with V3100p of gp120. Antibodies to the V3 loop protect chimpanzees from HIV infection. Because of the high level of variation in the V3 loop, antibody neutralization is always strain specific. However, the so-called crown sequence in the V3 loop is conserved to a considerable degree. These synthetic peptides appear to activate a population of the cells and to induce some cytotoxic activity; however, because these peptides are processed as exogenous antigens, the cytotoxic cells induced were all $CD4^+$, class II restricted. These studies suggest that cocktails of synthetic peptides, representing the crown sequences of the predominant HIV isolates, might induce protective antibody or $CD4^+$ T cytotoxic cells.

11.31.7. Malaria vaccine

Malaria, a protozoan disease, is responsible for 1-2 million deaths every year and infecting about 600 million people around the world. Malaria is caused by various species of the genus *Plasmodium* of which *P. falciparum* is the most virulent and prevalent. The alarming rise in resistance developed by *Plasmodium* to multiple drug therapy has led to the development of new strategies to control the spread of malaria. One such development is the designing of a vaccine. Keeping in view the present situation in developing countries, an effective malaria vaccine is of utmost importance. It should be designed to maximize the most effective immune defense mechanisms, unfortunately, little is known of the roles that humoral and cell-mediated responses play in the development of protective immunity to this disease.

Current vaccination strategies are aimed at producing synthetic subunit vaccines consisting of epitopes that can be recognized by T cells and B cells. One such vaccine, designated SPf66, consists of three merozoite-derived proteins together with a conserved domain from the circumsporozoite protein. Approaches to design a malaria vaccine largely focus on the sporozoite stage. However, the results are not encouraging as the life span of this stage in blood is only 30 minutes, too short a period for a vaccine to be effective.

11.32. NOVEL VACCINE DELIVERY SYSTEMS

Vaccination is probably the most efficient, cost-effective means for the prevention of a wide variety of infectious diseases. Concerted immunization programs have resulted in the eradication of smallpox. With few exceptions, most vaccines are administered as part of routine childhood immunization programs. Perhaps the greatest problem faced in effective delivery of such vaccines is that multiple dose primary immunization regimens are essential. In addition, periodic boosters are required throughout life to maintain immunity. New vaccine delivery technologies are clearly needed both to remedy the limitations of existing immunization regimens and to allow for the development of new or improved vaccines. Novel vaccine delivery systems, distinct from classical adjuvants, are being investigated as means to modulate the immune response following vaccination. Several such systems have undergone clinical evaluation with promising results. These systems have been widely acclaimed for their ability to present antigens in a better way.

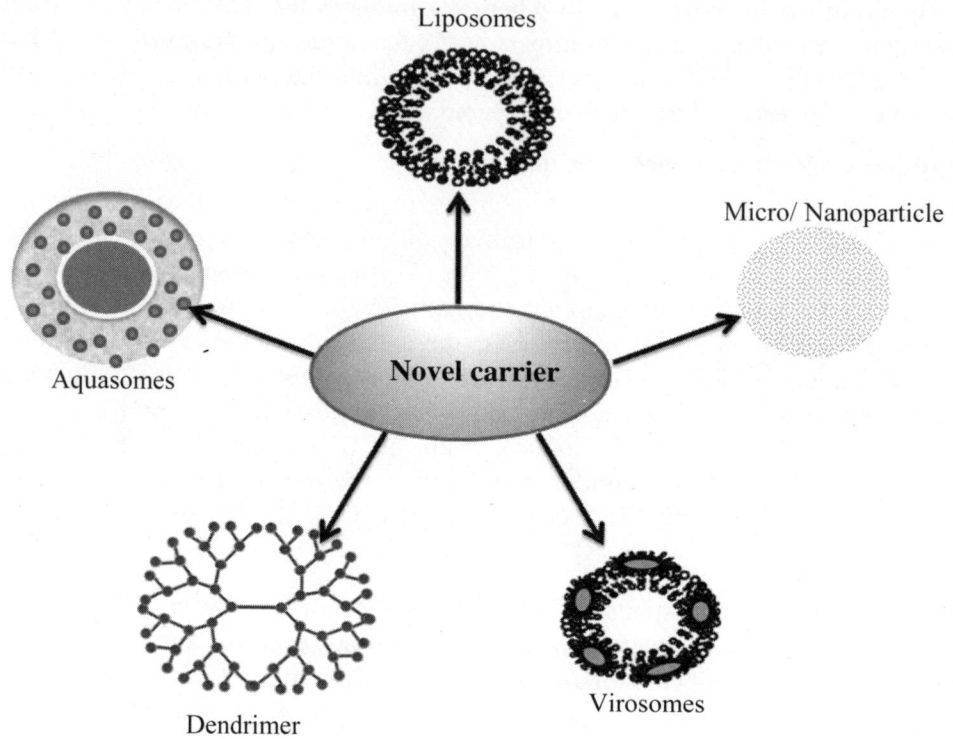

Fig. 11.34: Novel carriers for vaccine delivery

Processing and presentation of antigens by antigen presenting cells (APCs) is critical to the recruitment and activation of T cells. Uptake of exogenous antigens generally leads to presentation in association with class II MHC molecules. Cytolytic T lymphocytes (CTLs) are normally CD8$^+$, and recognize peptides in association with class I MHC molecules. Presentation of antigen by class I or class II MHC proteins is thus dependent upon its route of introduction into the cell and its susceptibility to degradation. These factors can be influenced by the use of specific delivery systems, which are therefore important determinants of the immune response; vaccination should endeavor to direct the immune response into activation of cells and processes appropriate for each pathogen.

11.32.1. Liposomes

Liposomes are microscopic phospholipids bubbles with bilayer membrane structure in which an aqueous volume is enclosed in lipid bilayer. The ability of liposomes to act as a potent and non-toxic immunological adjuvant was first observed in 1974 by Allison and Gregoriadis using diphtheria toxoid as a model antigen. Approximately three decade after discovery of immunoadjuvant property of liposomes presently they are the major delivery adjuvant for scores of candidate vaccines, with a liposome-based vaccine licensed for use in humans Epaxal Berna$^®$ against hepatitis A for use in Switzerland. The reason of such extensive use is their ability to encapsulate almost every molecule, protection from enzymatic and pH dependent degradation, antigen presentation to cells of immune system, biocompatibility and biodegradability. Both humoral and cell-mediated immunity were observed to be induced with the use of liposomes. Liposomes are versatile in terms of structural characteristics, mode of antigen localization within the vesicles, and options in the route of administration. Liposomes can also induce immunity against the associated antigen *via* noninvasive route including mucosal (oral, nasal, vaginal) and transdermal route.

Liposomes containing antigens can also induce systemic and mucosal immune responses following intranasal administration. The effectiveness of rectal administration of liposomes has also been reported. Furthermore, liposomes also offer advantage of co-encapsulation of antigen along with immunostimulatory adjuvant. This is of particular advantageous for the adjuvant is required to be present in close milieu to act on same cluster of antigen presenting cell.

11.32.2. Aquasomes

Aquasomes are three layered self assembled molecular carriers with diameter between 30-300nm. Aquasome comprise of central ceramic carbon nanocrystalline core coated with glassy cellobiose or alternatively degradable calcium phosphate nanoparticulate core coated glassy pyridoxal-5 phosphate or by sugar molecules such as cellobiose, trehalose, maltose, sorbitol and lactose. Subsequently drug or antigen is adsorbed to the outer coating. The solid core provides the structural stability to the structure. The carbohydrate covering on the central core creates a quasi- aqueous film, which act as dehydroprotectant and offer freedom of bulk movement, prevent denaturation or degradation of protein and also allocate freedom of internal molecular rearrangement induced by intermolecular rearrangement. Aquasome (also known as water like body) are biocompatible, economical, simple to manufacture, reduce the side effects and enhance the duration of the immune response. Furthermore they have the potential to selectively trigger a defined class of immune response such as the CD4$^+$ T-cells response and CD8$^+$ T cell (cell mediated immune) response.

11.32.3. Archaeosomes

Archaeosomes are liposomes made from the polar ether lipids of Archaea. These lipids are unique and distinct in structure from the ester lipids found in eukaryotes and bacteria. It has been shown that total polar lipids of archaeobacteria and purified lipid fractions can form liposomes. These lipid structures provide formulary advantages and contribute to the excellent physicochemical stability of the archaeosomes and their efficacy as self-adjuvanting vaccine delivery vesicles. In addition, archaeosomes enhance the recruitment and activation of professional antigen-presenting cells *in vivo*, and deliver the antigen to both MHC class I and II pathways for antigen presentation, without eliciting overt inflammatory responses. In general archaesomes demonstrate to possess relatively higher stability to oxidative stress, high temperature, alkaline pH, action of phospholipase, bile salt and serum protein furthermore they induces superior humoral response conventional liposomes.

11.32.4. Virosomes

Virosomes are lipidic envelope devoid of genetic information, which retain the antigenic profile and fusogenic properties from their viral origin. Reconstituted lipid vesicles equipped with viral glycoproteins seems to possess many ideal properties for mucosal delivery of immunogens such as no limitation of size of encapsulated immunogens, high efficiency for cytosolic delivery, simplicity in handling and brevity of incubation time. Human parainfluenza viruses are extensively investigated for preparation of vesicles hemagglutinin-neuraminidase (HN) and fusion (F) glycoproteins of human parainfluenza virus type-3 (PI3) was solubilized with octylglucoside and reconstituted into lipid vesicles following removal of the detergent by dialysis. The binding of the filamentous hemagglutinin (FHA) with the liposome surface is advantageous for targeting towards the mucosal tissue for administration of the heterologous protein. The FHA imparted two actions: first increasing the mucoadhesivity and targeting property with respect to mucosal issue, and second increasing the immune response against antigen of the heterologous protein.

11.32.5. Polymeric nano/microspheres

Nano/Microparticles based on polylactide-co-glycolide have gained much attention as carriers for antigens in view of the fact, that they are more stable than any other carrier and can protect encapsulated drug from harse environment (pH, temperature, enzymatic degradation etc.). Adding up they allow manipulation of physiochemical parameters (i.e. size, zeta potential, *in vitro* release) by the choice of polymer and its composition and also could be designed to provide pulse of antigen similar mimic boosting. Impressive results have been attained for both humoral and cell mediated effects. PLGA has the advantage that it has already been approved for human use and is biodegradable and biocompatible. Such polymers have the advantage that they can be freeze dried and hence avoid the need for cold storage. The incorporation of antigens into biodegradable microspheres has several advantages including the protection of antigen from proteolysis and possible co-incorporation of immunological adjuvants that may further enhance the immune response.

Most of the evaluation for vaccination involving microspheres has focused on oral route. Induction of mucosal and systemic responses by this route is influenced by the size of the microspheres: < 5μm in diameter are not retained in the Peyer's patches but are found in the spleen and in lymph nodes where they induce systemic immunity. Those in the size range 5-10 μm remain in Peyer's patches and induce mucosal immunity. Microspheres other than PLGA have also been studied for immunization. These include alginate, albumin, chitosan, Hyaluronic acid, carbopol etc. and gelatin microspheres.

11.32.6. Dendrimer

Dendrimer are highly branched three dimensional macromolecule with vastly controlled structure consisting of all bands emanating from a central core. During dendrimer formation molecule stem out from a core, like a tree and they more and more ramify with each subsequent branching unit referred as generation. The unique molecular architectures and interesting characteristics such as defined structures, inner cavities able to encapsulate guest molecules, and controllable multivalent functionalities in their inner or outer part make these materials attractive for the gene and drug delivery applications. The surface of dendrimer have functional group that offer multiple attachment sites e.g. for conjugation of drugs and/or targeting moieties, and therapeutic molecules can also be incorporated within the core. This multiple binding of dendrimer mimics the structure of a bacteria or virus, i.e. membrane protein binding with a solid core that is of further advantage to enhance immune recognition of protein. Advances in the understanding of the role of molecular weight and architecture on the *in vivo* behavior of dendrimers, together with recent progress in the design of biodegradable constitution, has enabled the application dendrimer for vaccine antigens delivery.

11.32.7. Cochleates

Fusogenic proteoliposomes, prepared by the protein cochleate method have been developed and tested for immunogenicity after oral or parenteral administration. Cochleates consist of stable protein-phospholipid-calcium precipitates. Antigens like glycoproteins from influenza or parainfluenza virus or a 12 amino acid peptide from SIV gag protein that contains an epitope for cytotoxic T lymphocytes have been incorporated in such structures. A strong and prolonged immune response was observed after oral administration, or as parenteral injection. It manifests as mucosal and systemic antibodies and cytotoxic T cells.

11.32.8. Mucoadhesive polymers

Mucoadhesive and other bioadhesive polymers are used for drug delivery, particularly in transdermal and buccal devices. Mucoadhesive polymers also have many pharmaceutical applications. Some (e.g. sodium alginate) have adjuvant properties when injected, and others such as carboxymethyl cellulose are used as depot forming agents. Mucoadhesives have been tested for nasal immunization and are being studied as adjuvant vehicle/carrier for oral drug delivery. Influenza vaccine administered orally in mucoadhesive polymers elicited a high antibody titer value and appears to be promising.

11.33. EDIBLE VACCINES

Vaccines are designed to elicit an immune response without causing disease. Vaccines that one can eat, called edible vaccines, are among the most unusual approaches for administering new vaccines. The idea of plant derived edible vaccines is continuing to be developed, with the help of emerging innovations in medical sciences and plant biology, for the creation of efficacious and affordable pharmaceuticals. Edible vaccines are like subunit preparation, in that they are engineered to contain antigen, but bear no genes that would enable whole pathogen to form. Edible vaccines are currently being developed for a number of human and animal diseases, including measles, cholera, foot and mouse disease, and hepatitis B and C. Many of these diseases require booster vaccination or multiple antigens to induce and maintain protective immunity. Plants have capacity to express more than one transgene, allowing delivery of multiple antigens for repeated inoculations. A concern with oral vaccines is the degradation of protein components in stomach (due to low pH and gastric enzymes) and gut before they can elicit immune responses, but the rigid plant cell wall could provide protection from intestinal degradation. It was, therefore, not surprising when Hiatt and co-workers attempted to produce antibodies in plants, which could serve the purpose of passive immunization. The first report of edible vaccine (a surface protein from *Streptococcus*) in tobacco, at 0.02% of total leaf protein

Table 11.12: Examples of edible vaccines

S. No.	Vaccine	Vector used	Diseases/Condition it is used for
1.	Hepatitis B virus	Tobacco Potato Lettuce	Hepatitis B
2.	Norwalk virus	Tobacco Potato	Diarrhoea Nausea Stomach cramps
3.	Rabies virus	Tobacco	Rabies
4.	Transmissible gastroenteritis Corona virus	Tobacco Maize	Gastroenteritis
5.	Rabbit hemorrhagic diseases virus	Potato	Hemorrhage
6.	HIV virus	Tomato	AIDS
7.	*Vibrio cholera*	Potato	Cholera

level, appeared in 1990 in the form of a patent application published under the international patent cooperation. The concept of edible vaccine got impetus after Arntzen and co-workers expressed hepatitis B surface antigen in tobacco plants. Today's development of novel vaccines stresses the need for edible vaccines that are inexpensive, easily administered and capable of being stored and transported without refrigeration. Without these characteristics, developing countries find it difficult to adopt vaccination as the central strategy for preventing their most devastating diseases. Some examples of edible vaccines are shown in Table 11.12.

11.33.1. Transgenic plants and edible immunogen concept

Introduction of genes encoding microbial antigens in plants represents a novel and potentially important approach in vaccine administration. Manson and co-workers developed a recombinant bacterial vector *Agrobacterium tumefaciens* with a gene for the surface antigen of hepatitis B virus and infected tobacco plants which subsequently expressed this antigen. An alternative approach to deliver the gene is by infecting the plant with *Clavibacter*, tobacco mosaic virus, or by using gene gun. Antigens of hepatitis B virus, rotavirus, Norwalk virus and B subunit of *E. coli* heat-labile enterotoxin (LT-B) have been expressed in such plants. Haq and co-workers have immunized mice with purified LT-B produced in tobacco and potato plants, or with raw transgenic potatoes and observed that both systemic and mucosal anti-LT-B neutralizing antibodies were secreted. 'Using this technique inexpensive edible immunogens suitable for immunization of large populations particularly in developing countries can be produced.

11.33.2. Genes going wild

Genetic engineering is inherently hazardous because it depends on developing gene transfer vectors (carriers) specifically designed to cross wide species barriers. It promotes the transfer of genes horizontally across species, Instead of vertically within species by inheritance. It is also increasingly designed to overcome the species defense mechanisms, which degrade or inactivate foreign genes. It is still a very crude science, with genes being inserted at random points in the host's genetic material (genome), rather than being carefully pinpointed as happens in traditional breeding. For these and other reasons, genetic engineering destabilizes the genomes of its plant and animal hosts, and the effects ricochet through the neighboring ecosystem. There is growing evidence that by facilitating horizontal gene transfer and recombination, genetic engineering may be contributing to the emergence and re-emergence of infectious, drug-resistant diseases. Edible vaccines (even subunit vaccines) will always entail the ingestion of recombinant viral genetic material, and hence pose considerable risks to the environment and health.

Edible subunit vaccines are likely to be less dangerous than those that may be produced by using genetically modified viruses and viruses used as vectors (carriers) for the vaccine. But they still involve the insertion of foreign genes into plants and the implications thereof. Genetically tweaking the pathogen to reduce its potency is even more risky. Minor genetic changes in, or differences between, viruses can result in dramatic changes in host spectrum and disease-causing potential. According to Terje Traavik of the Norwegian Institute of Gene Ecology, "For all these vaccines, important questions concerning effects on species other than the targeted one are left unanswered so far." There are also considerable risks related to the possibility of a genetically engineered vaccine virus engaging in recombination with naturally occurring relatives. New viruses resulting from such events may have totally unpredictable characteristics with regard to host preferences and disease-causing potential."

Table 11.13: Selected patents on edible vaccine technologies

Patent Holder	Claim
Ribozyme-Pharm	Nucleic acid vaccine to treat or prevent viral infections in plants, animals or bacteria
Found. Advan. Mil. Med (USA)	Antibacterial vaccine expressed in plant cells, particularly useful against shigellosis
Loma Linda University	Gene constructs used to produce edible vaccines to treat autoimmune diseases, including diabetes and multiple sclerosis
Rubicon-Lab	Retrovirus expressed in animal or plant cells useful as virus and cancer vaccine
Biosource (now Large Scale Biology)	Plant viral vector with potential as anti-AIDS vaccine; recombinant proteins for use in vaccines to protect against parasitic infection, e.g. malaria
Applied Phytologics	Gene constructs for disease resistance, vaccine production in rice, barley, wheat, corn
University of Texas	Hepatitis B virus core antigen recombinant vaccine
University of Yale	Vaccine against invertebrates (insects, arachnids. helminths, etc.)
Biocem; Rhone-Merieux Institute Pasteur	Rabies vaccine in transgenic plants Attenuated *E. coil* vaccine for use in gene therapy
University of Texas A&M/ Tulane University	Transgenic plants containing *E. coli* enterotoxin B for edible vaccine application in animals
USDA/ Univ. Philadelphia	Rabies vaccine expressed in tomato plant
Cornell University	Increasing foreign protein expression
Scripps Research Institute	Recombinant antigen production in lettuce, spinach, tobacco, kidney bean, or *Chenopodium amaranticolor*
Prodigene	Recombinant antigen production and transfer to plant cells using plasmid vector system; Transmissible Gastroenteritis Virus in tomato and potato; broad patent for edible vaccine technology in all plants
Mycogen/Washington Uni.	Series of broad patents covering plant-based edible vaccine technology,
Agr. Genet/Purdue Research Foundation	Modified viruses used for vaccine production in plants, esp. against foot and mouth disease, HIV and human rhino virus

11.34. GENETICALLY MODIFIED YEAST FOR VACCINES

Genetically engineered proteins can be produced in yeasts (Wiseman, 1993). As vaccine production with genetically modified (GM) yeasts will discharge human proteins, these proteins must be subjected to rigorous and stringent criteria of clean production. Vectors for expressing desired gene sequences in the appropriate yeast systems could in principle be based on either the yeast episomal plasmid (YEP) or the yeast artificial chromosome (YAC) for large protein assemblies. Yeast cell-surface display enables attachment of the presenting-antigen epitope to a carrier protein on the yeast protoplast; some applications include vaccine production, for instance, by using hepatitis A, HIV and SARS surface-antigen displayed on novel-surface GM yeasts grown aerobically in deep culture fermentation vessels at high glucose concentration (Wiseman, 1993).

The yeast *Saccharomyces cerevisiae* is known to 'surface-display' such enzymes as invertase and acid phosphatase in its periplasmic space (between the cytoplasmic membrane and the cell wall). The latter is made of mannan-glucan-glycopeptide complexes. This means, for example, that sucrose is accessible to the invertase; so when sucrose is added in brewing biotechnology processes, it becomes converted into glucose and fructose. Some GM yeasts display cytochromes P450. These yeasts can prove valuable for food bioprocessing industries (Wiseman, 2003 a,b) which use redox enzymes, such as many isoforms of cytochromes P450 including numerous human isoforms (Lewis, 2001; Wiseman and Woods, 2003).

11.34.1. *Lactobacilli* for vaccine delivery

Since long people have known that eating such fermented products as yoghurt has a positive effect on gastrointestinal health. These probiotic effects are attributed to the presence of *lactobacilli*; evidence has accumulated that different strains of *Lactobacillus* have different effects on the immune system. This immunomodulatory capacity is important for the development of the immune response, and also identifies *Lactobacillus* as a potent oral vaccine carrier. This has aroused interest in the use of these bacteria for vaccination purposes, and *lactobacilli* are now being investigated for use in active vaccination, passive vaccination and tolerance induction.

Passive vaccination depends on the delivery of pathogen or toxin-neutralizing agents, most commonly immunoglobulins. Intact immunoglobulins are large complex molecules that cannot be easily produced in bacteria; therefore strategies are being developed for secretion and cell wall anchoring of single-chain polypeptides, which comprise only the binding domain of the immunoglobulins (Kruger *et al.*, 2002). Parenteral vaccination usually proves effective in eliciting some protective immune response. Pathogens that enter an organism at first elicit a mucosal or a systemic response, depending on the route of entry; each of these responses has a humoral and a cellular component (Medzhitov and Janeway, 1997; Janeway and Medzhitov, 2002). Whereas humoral response at the mucosa is mediated predominantly by secretory immunoglobulin A (sIgA) antibodies, systemic humoral response occurs in secondary lymphoid organs and is mediated chiefly by IgG antibodies. For pathogens that enter the organism *via* the systemic route, e.g., in wounds, parenteral vaccination is quite effective. But for most pathogens, before it becomes systemic infection occurs at the mucosa of the lungs and intestines. Therefore, parenteral vaccination reduces but does not prevent the spread of infectious agents to nonimmune individuals. Ideally, initial infection and replication of the pathogen should be prevented; therefore through mucosal immunity, much research is focused on the development of adequate mucosal vaccines, and various vaccine delivery systems are being tried for oral application (Ryan *et al.*, 2001). One popular delivery system is the use of live bacterial vaccine vectors such as *lactobacilli*.

Lactic acid bacteria (LAB) are widely used for making cheese, yoghurt and dried sausages and so are consumed in large amounts by humans. This makes them suitable materials for developing safe oral vaccines. Their potential as vaccine vectors has been shown in prototype vaccines against *Brucella abortis, Helicobacter pylori,* HIV and measles. With *Lactobacillus,* prototype vaccines against anthrax and rotavirus are being developed, and have already been developed against tetanus (Seegers, 2002). Some merits of LAB as candidates for oral vaccination are their intrinsic immunogenicity, their resistance to bile acid, and their persistence in the gastrointestinal tract. Some beneficial effects for health, attributed to LAB in general, and to *lactobacilli* in particular, range from relieving gastrointestinal disorders to protecting against colon cancer (Marteau, 2002). Repetitive feeding of live *lactobacilli* results in a three to five-fold increase in virus-neutralizing antibodies elicited after a normal (parenteral) immunization with influenza haemagglutinin subunit vaccine (Marteau, 2002).

Live *lactobacilli* exert two effects on the immune response: (i) an activation of the immune response and (ii) a suppression of the (undesired) immune response, for example in autoimmunity and allergy. Immune responses may notably be enhanced in immunocompromised populations such as the elderly, by increased (live) yoghurt consumption (Meydani and Ha, 2000). Satisfactory cloning systems have been developed for the genetic transformation of *lactobacilli*. Important features of cloning vectors for the delivery of antigens include promoter sequences that allow either constitutive or inducible expression. Some inducible expression systems are the nisin-inducible expression system especially adapted for use in *Lactobacillus,* and systems based on sugar metabolism with promoters regulated by catabolite repression such as the xylose promoter (Lokman *et al.,* 1997). These vectors have secretion and anchor signals, which allow expression of proteins in different cellular compartments. However, in using similar expression systems in different *Lactobacillus* strains it should be realized that promoters differ in their activity levels, depending on the strain in which they are used (McCracken and Timms, 1999) and that replication efficiencies and plasmid copy numbers can differ. Also, codon usage of heterologous genes tends to differ from the expression host, which can lower expression levels in *Escherichia coli* (Kane, 1995). As *Lactobacillus* strains show different preferences for codon usage, this could influence the efficiency of translation of a specific antigen (Seegers, 2002).

While some immunization experiments have pointed to the feasibility of using *lactobacilli* for mucosal immunization, only limited success has been obtained with several antigens. It is a challenging task to elicit the desired immune response (tolerance or protection) with any antigen. *Lactobacillus* strains have different adjuvant characteristics with a differential influence on the immune system, thereby advantageously combining delivery and adjuvant in one system. For most studies, *L. casei* and *L. plantarum* strains have been used as delivery vectors for antigens and many more strains need to be tested.

SUGGESTED READING

- Allison AC and Gregoriadis G, *Nature*, 252:252 (1974).
- Anderson WF, *Hum. Gene. Ther.* 1: 371-372 (1990).
- Andrianov AK, Payne LG, *Adv. Drug Deliv. Rev.* 34: 155-170(1998).
- Beck G and Habicht GS, *Scientific Am.*, 275(5), 60 (1996).
- Bellanti JA, *Immunology* III, 3 rd ed., W.B. Saunder, Philadelphia (1985).
- Bhatt AD, Bhatt, *N.S. Indian J. Gastroenterol.* 15: 63-67 (1996).
- Bier DG, DaSliva WD, Gotze D, et al., *Fundamentals of Immunology*, Springer-Verlag, New York (1981).
- Biragyn A, Ruffini PA, Leifer CA *et al., Science* 298: 1025 (2002).
- Braciale TJ and Trowsdale J, *Current Opin Immunol.*, 5, I-55 (1993).
- Coleman RM, Lombard M and Sicard R, *Fundamental Immunology*, 2 ed, Wm. C. Brown Publishers, USA (1992).
- Davis GL*: Br. Med. J.* 323: 1141-1142 (2001).
- Desowitz RS, *The thorn in the starfish: How the human immune system works*, Norton, New York (1987).

- DiNoia J, Neuberger MS, *Nature* 419: 43-48 (2002).
- Fearon DT, Manders P, Wagner, S.D. *Science* 293: 248 (2001).
- Ganz T, Versatile defensins. *Science* 298: 977-979 (2002).
- Gearhart PJ, *Nature* 419: 29-30 (2002).
- Green M, Loewenstein PM, *Cell 55:* 1179-1188 (1988).
- Gref R. *Science.* 263: 1600-1603 (1994).
- Gregoriadis G, Allison AC and Poste G (Eds.), *Vaccines: Recent Trends and Progress*, Plenum Publishing Corp., NY (1991).
- Gregoriadis G, *Immunology Today*, 11,89 (1990).
- Gregoriadis G, Allison AC and Poste G (Eds.), *Immunological Adjuvants and Vaccines*, Plenum Publishing Corp., NY (1989).
- Gregoriadis, G, McCormack B, Allison AC and Poste G (Eds.). *New Generation Vaccines: the Role of Basic Imrnunology*, Plenum Publishing Corp., NY (1987).
- Hoglund S, Dalsgaard K, Lovgren K *et al.*, *Subcell Biochem.* 15:39-68 (1989)
- Hood LE, Weissman IL, Wood WB et al., *Immunology*, Benjamin/Cumming Publishing Company Inc. California (1984).
- Hudson L and Hay FC, *Practical Immunology*, Blackwell Scientific Publications, London (1980).
- Hughson PM *Curr. Biol.* 5: 265-274 (1995).
- Janeway CA and Travers P, *Immunology: The Immune System in Health and Disease*, Blackwell Scientific Publishers, Oxford, (1996).
- Janeway CAJ, Medzhitov R, *Annu. Rev.immunol. 20:* 197-216 (2002).
- Kane JF, *Curr. Opin, Biotechnol.* 6: 494-500 (1995).
- Khaja MN, Munpally SK, Hussain MM *et al.*, *Curr. Sci.* 83: 219-224 (2002).
- Kohler G, Milstein C, *Nature* 256: 495-497 (1975).
- Kruger C, Hu Y, Pan Q *et al. Nat. Biotechnol.* 20: 702-706 (2002).
- Kuby J, Immunology W.H. Freeman and Company, New York (1994).
- Langel U. (Ed.). *Cell-penetrating Peptides: Processes and Applications* CRC Press, Boca Raton (2002).
- Langer R, Cleland JL, Hanes J. *Adv. Drug Deliv. Rev.* 8: 97-119 (1997).
- Litman GW, *Scientific Am.*, 275(5), 67 (1996).
- Lokman BC, Heerikhuisen M, Leer RJ *et al.*, *J. Bacteriol.* 179: 5391-5397 (1997).
- Marteau, P.R. *Clin. Rev. Allergy* 22: 255-273 (2002).
- McCracken A, Timms P, *J. Bacteriol.* 181: 6569-6572 (1999).
- Medicine Series, Vol.12, Kluwer Academic Publishers.
- Medzhitov R, Janeway CA, *J. Cell* 91: 295-298 (1997).
- Meydani SN, Ha WK, *Am. J. Clin. Nutr.* 71: 861-872 (2000).

- Mims CA, *Pathogenesis of Infectious Disease.* Academic Press, London (1987).
- Murthy N, Campbell J., Fausto N. *et al., Bioconjugate Chem.* 14: 412-419 (2003b).
- Murthy N, Campbell J, Fausto N *et al., J. Control Release* 89: 395-374 (2003a).
- Murthy N, Xu M, Schuck S *et al., PNAS* (USA) 100: 4995-5000 (2003).
- Nandi D, Sarin A, *Current Science* 80: 647-652 (2001).
- Nori A, Jensen KD, Tijerina M. *et al., Bioconugate. Chem.* 14: 44-50 (2003).
- Pal SK, *Current Science* 83J 1058-1059 (2002).
- Paul WE, *Fundamental Immunology*, 2nd ed., Raven Press, New York (1990).
- Poynard T, Leroy V, Cohard M *et al. Hepatology,* 32: 1131-1137 (2000).
- Prescott LM, Harly JP and Klein DA, *Microbiology*, 2 nd ed., Wm. C. Brown Publishers, USA. (1993).
- Pulendran B, Palucka K, Banchereau J, *Science* 293: 253-254 (2001).
- Rao JVRP, HIV/AIDS: *Challenges in the new era.* Abstracts (p. 12), 67th Meeting of Ind. Acad. Sci., Tirupati (9-11 Nov., 2001).
- Rath S and Bal V, *Resonance*, 2, 90-93 (1997).
- Roitt IM, Brostoff J and Male DK, *Immunology*, 2 nd ed., C.V. Mosby, St. Louis (1989).
- Roitt I, *Essential Immunology*, Blackwell Scientific Publications, London (1986).
- Ryan EJ, *Trends Biotechnol.* 19: 293-304 (200I).
- Schwarze SR, Hruska KA, Dowdy SF, *Trends Cell Biol.* 10: 290-295 (2000).
- Seegers JFML, *Trends Biotechnol.* 20: 508-515 (2002).
- Simecka JW, *Adv.Drug. Deliv. Rev.* 34: 235-259 (1998).
- Sprent J, Tough DF, *Science* 293: 245-248 (2001).
- Stayton PS, *Trends Biotechnol.* 21: 465-467 (2003).
- Stites DP, Stobo JD, Fudenberg HH, and Wells JV, *Basic and Clinical Immunology*, 5 th edition, Lange Medical Publications Los Altos (1984).
- Tizard IR, *Immunology: An introduction*, 2 nd ed., W.B. Saunders, Philadelphia (1988).
- Vives E, Brodin P, Lebleu B, *J. Biol. Chem. 272:* 16010-16017 (1997).
- Weir DM, *Handbook of Experimental Immunology*, Blackwell Scientific Publications, London (1979).
- Wiseman A. (Ed). *Production and Control of Genetically-engineered Proteins in Yeasts* Ellis Horwood, Chichester (1993).
- Wiseman A, Woods LFJ, *Trends Biotechnol.* 21: 7 (2003).
- Yang D, *et al. Science* 286: 525 (1999).
- Zanetti M, Sercarz E and Salk J, *Immunology Today*, 8, 18 (1987).
- Zhan H, Oh KJ, Shin YK *et al., Biochemisty* 34: 4856-4863 (1995).
- Zhang J, Campbell RE, Ting AY *et al. Nat. Rev. Mol. Cell Biol.* 3: 906-918 (2002).
- Zinkernagel RM, Hengartner H, *Science* 293: 251-253 (2001).

DNA VACCINES: THIRD GENERATION GENETIC VACCINES

12.1. INTRODUCTION

Over the past 100 years, the development and widespread use of vaccines against infectious agents has been one of the triumphs of medical science. One reason for the success of these vaccines is that they excel at inducing antibodies, the principal agents of immune protection against most viruses and bacteria. There are, however, exceptions, including medically important intracellular organisms like *Mycobacterium tuberculosis*, malarial parasite *Plasmodium, Leishmania major* and possibly the human immunodeficiency virus (HIV), in which protection depends more on cell mediated immunity than on the induction of antibodies (humoral immunity). Conventional active vaccines are made of a killed or attenuated form of the infectious agents, a modified product of infectious agents (toxoid) or a constituent of an infectious agent (such as capsule). Viable attenuated vaccines are usually more effective as compared to non-viable vaccines. Relatively high and repeated doses are administered when a non-viable (killed organism, toxoid, capsule) vaccine is used and protective immunity obtained does not last long. Moreover, only humoral immune response is induced. On the other hand, low doses are administered when a viable attenuated vaccine is used, both humoral and cell mediated immune responses are generated and immunity is usually long lasting (Weiner *et al.* 1999). However more efforts are needed to seek safer antigens that can be processed by the endogenous pathway and eventually activate cytotoxic T-lymphocytes (CTL). The activated CTLs generated in this way can destroy the parasite-infected cells.

In 1965, Youmans and Youmans first reported the immunogenicity of mycobacterial ribosomal and ribonucleic acid preparations, Berry and Vernneman (1972) reported immunogenicity of pure RNA extracted from *Salmonella typhimurium*. Both reports suggested the ability of RNA preparations to induce a cell-mediated immune response. The idea of using nucleic acids as vaccines was later abandoned because it was thought that RNA was behaving as an adjuvant for the antigen contaminants in the ribosome / RNA vaccines (Eisenstein *et al.*, 1975). In 1990, direct gene transfer of plasmid DNA into mouse muscle *in-vivo* without any need for a special delivery system was demonstrated and led to induction of protein expression in muscle cells. Later, Tang *et al.,* 1992 demonstrated the production of anti-human growth hormone (hGH) antibodies in mice injected with plasmid DNA encoding hGH, and Ulmer *et al.,* 1994 showed that both antibody and CTL responses were elicited in mice injected with a plasmid DNA encoding an influenza virus protein. Moreover, the mice were protected against influenza infection. DNA vaccines are new types of sub-unit vaccines whose delivery into living cells leads both to expression of the protein of interest *in vivo* as well as effective induction of both humoral and cellular immunity to the expressed protein.

Various attempts have been made to prepare vaccines that mimic the effectiveness of an attenuated vaccine for those intracellular parasites for which no effective vaccines are available. These novel vaccines also provide safety against the possibility of attenuated vaccines reverting to their virulent form, and inability to use them in immunodeficiency diseases. These possibilities highlighted the need to develop alternative of attenuated vaccines that would be effective and also safer to use. DNA vaccines induce both humoral and cell mediated immune responses. The immunity conferred by them has been demonstrated in many animal models of various diseases including HIV, tuberculosis, and cancer (Lee *et al.,* 2004).

12.2. DNA VACCINES

A DNA vaccine is based on a circular double stranded DNA molecule, referred to as a plasmid, containing genes encoding one or more proteins of a pathogen. Plasmids are extra-chromosomal circular DNA molecules that are often present in multiple copies in bacterial cells. A plasmid contains a bacterial origin of replication (Fig. 12.1) by virtue of which it can replicate autonomously inside bacterial cells but not in eukaryotic cells. Such plasmids can be isolated from bacteria by using simple, inexpensive protocols. Recombinant DNA technique allows inserting a foreign gene into the plasmid molecule to generate a recombinant plasmid. When the gene is inserted downstream of DNA sequences referred to as promoter and enhancer elements to which eukaryotic RNA polymerase II and a host of proteins known as transcription factors bind, then the resultant plasmid is referred to as an expression plasmid

When such plasmids are introduced into eukaryotic cells, the gene of interest is transcribed by the RNA polymerase II and other accessory proteins resulting in the synthesis of messenger RNA (mRNA) that is translated into the corresponding protein in the cytoplasm of host cells. In brief, the basic requirements for the backbone of a plasmid DNA vector are a eukaryotic promoter, a cloning site, a polyadenylation sequence, a selectable marker, and a bacterial origin of replication. The principle of DNA vaccination has been successfully utilized for a variety of infectious diseases and in shown in Table 12.1.

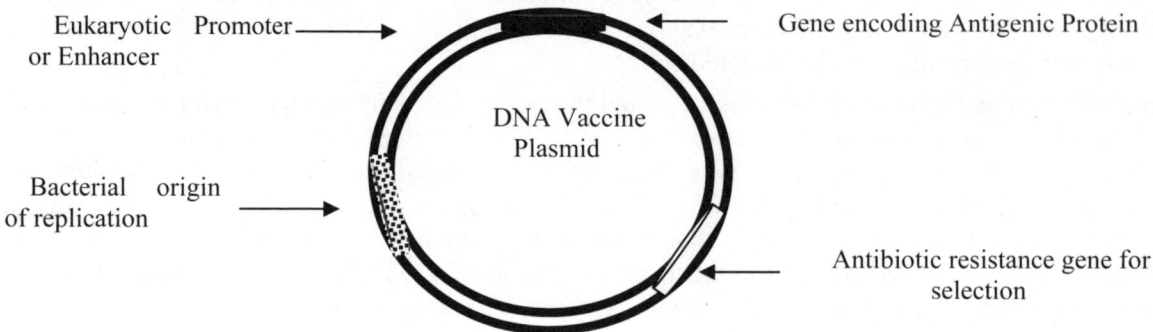

Fig. 12.1: DNA vaccine plasmid

Table 12.1: Effectiveness of DNA vaccines against diseases by induction of protective immune response in animal models

Causative Agents	Diseases
Bacteria	*Borrelia burgdorfer*, cholera, Enterotoxic *E. coli, Moroxella bovis, Mycobacterium tuberculosis, Mycoplasma, Salmonella,* tetanus toxin.
Viruses	*Avian influenza, Bovine herpes*, dengue fever, encephalitis, hepatitis B, hepatitis C, herpes, human cytomegalovirus, herpes simplex virus, human immunodeficiency virus, Ebola, influenza, measles, papilloma, rabies, pseudorabies, rotavirus, simian virus.
Parasites	*Cryptosporidium parvum, Leishmania, Plasmodium falciparum* (Malaria), *Schistosoma.*
Cancer-associated antigens	Carcinoembryonic antigen (CEA), Melanoma associated antigen, MHC molecule HLA-B7

12.2.1. Mechanism of uptake of DNA vaccines and induction of immune response

General steps of DNA vaccination are shown schematically in Figure 12.2.

Step I

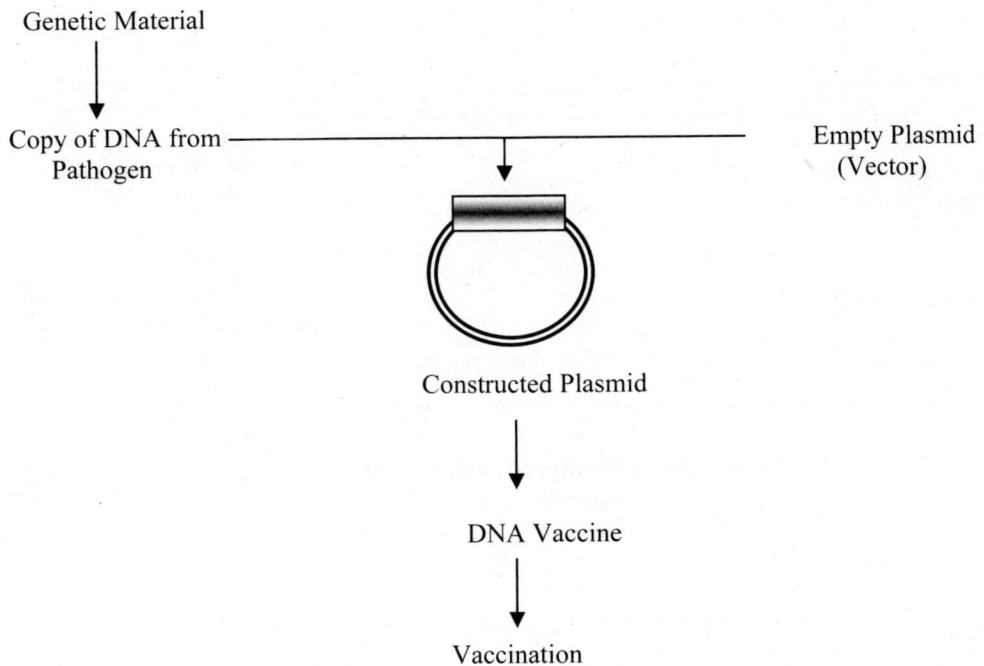

Step II

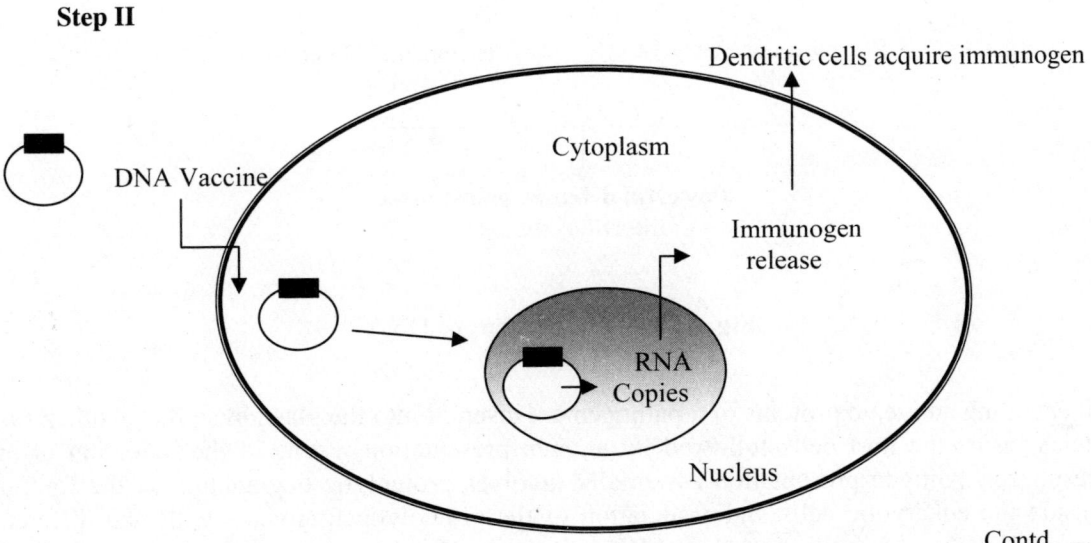

Contd….

Step III

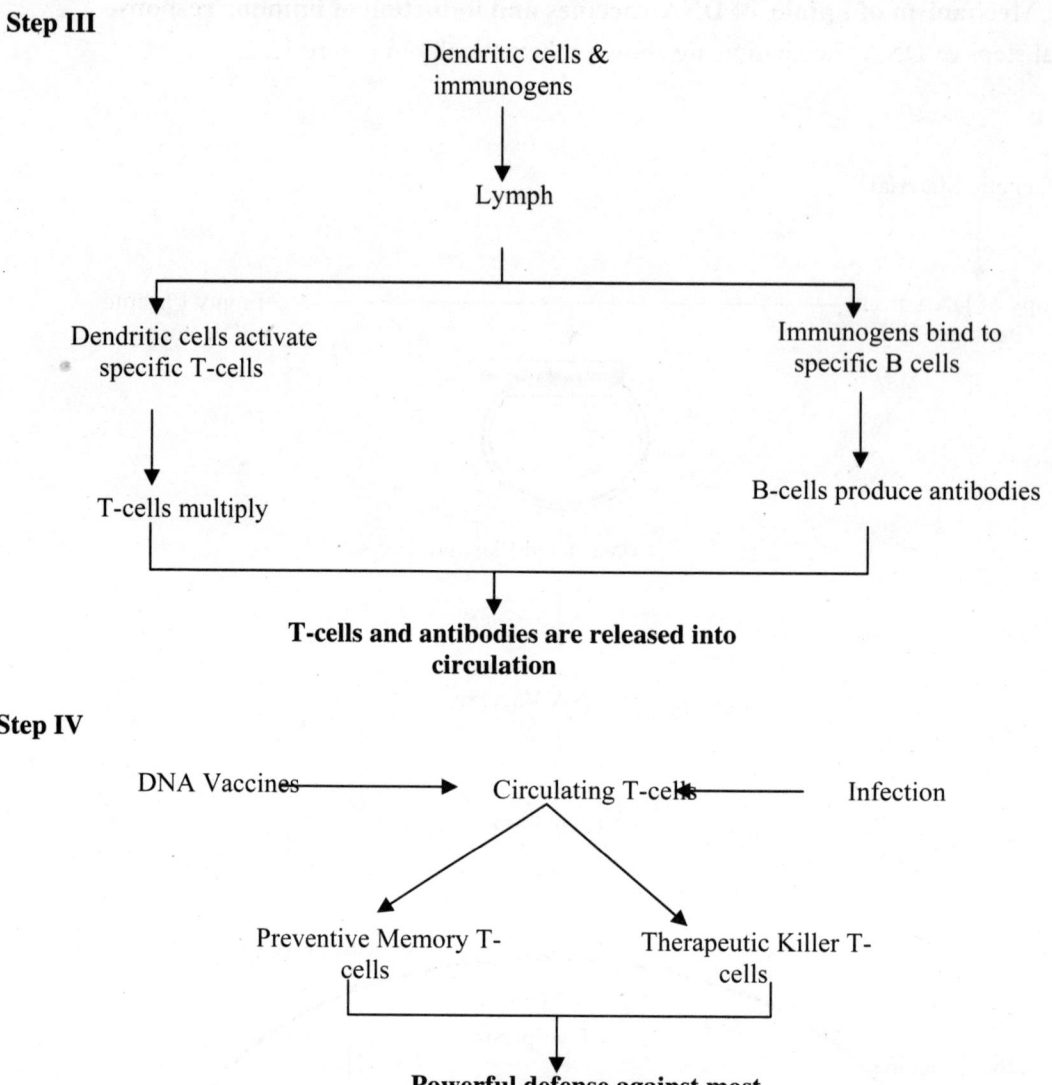

Fig. 12.2: General steps of DNA

Gene (s) encoding antigenic proteins of a pathogen are inserted into the plasmid so that synthesis of these proteins inside the host cells followed by antigen presentation results in the induction of an immune response. Antigen presentation essentially involves proteolytic degradation of the foreign proteins inside the eukaryotic cells and association of the proteolytic fragments with two different types of major Histocompatibility complex (MHC) proteins referred to as class I and class II MHC proteins. Class I molecules present protein fragments to cytotoxic T-cells. Class II molecules present the fragments to T-helper cells (Fig. 12.3). In case of DNA vaccination, since the pathogenic proteins are synthesized inside the host cells, both humoral and cell-mediated immune responses are induced.

(A) CYTOSOLIC PATHWAY

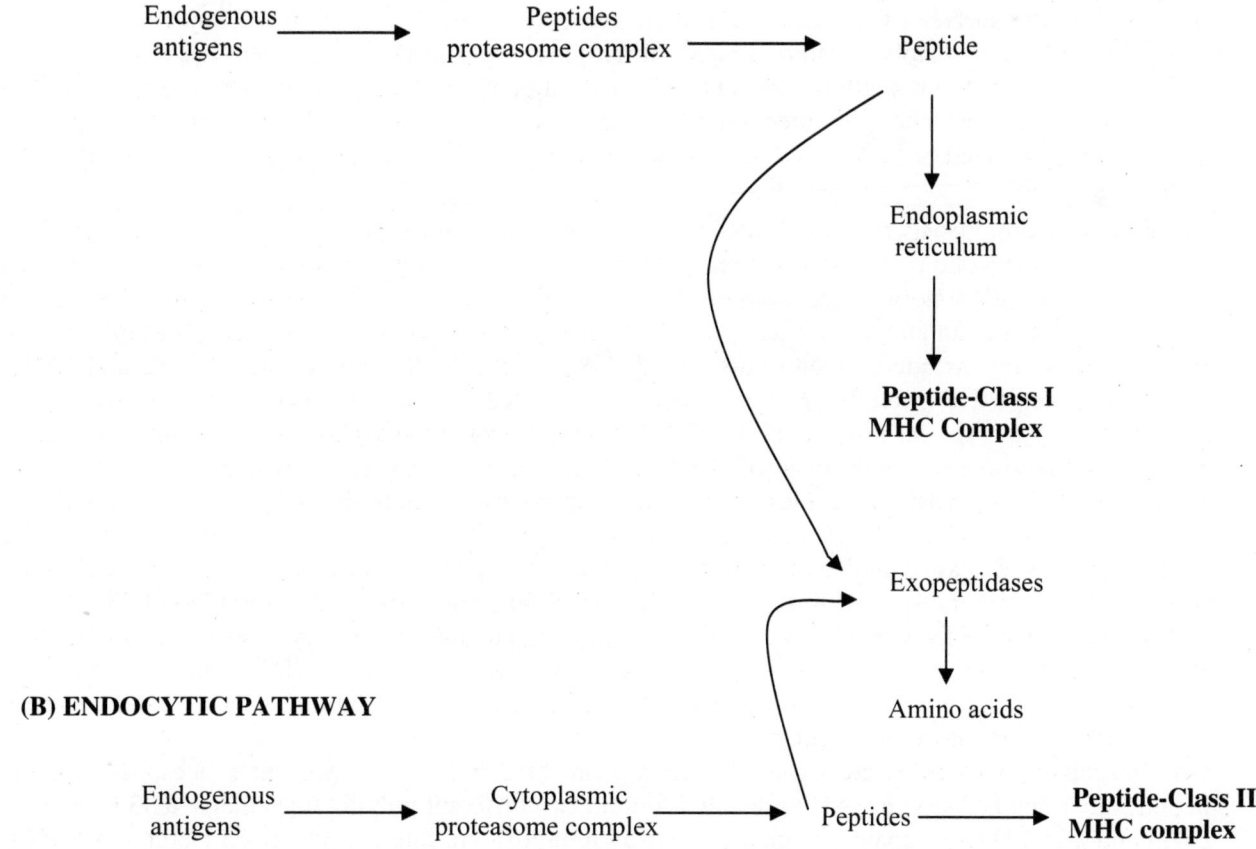

Fig. 12.3: Cytosolic and endocytic pathways for antigen processing

12.2.2. Mechanism of antigen processing/presentation

Activation of both humoral and cell mediated branches of the immune system requires cytokines produced by T_H cells. To ensure carefully regulated activation of T_H cells, they recognize only antigen that is displayed together with MHC class II molecules on the surface of antigen presenting cells (APCs). Antigen Processing/Presenting cells (APC) degrade a protein antigen into smaller peptides and present the peptide to T-lymphocytes which eventually are activated. A variety of cells can function as APC. Their distinguishing feature is the ability to express class II MHC molecules and to deliver a co-stimulatory signal. Three cell types are classified as professional APCs : dendritic cells, macrophages and B-lymphocytes. Several other cell types, classified as non-professional APCs, can be induced to express class II MHC molecules or a co-stimulatory signal (Table 12.2).

Table 12.2: List of professional and non-professional APCs

Professional	Non-professional
Dendritic cells	Fibroblasts, Thyroid epithelial cells
Macrophages	Glial cells, Thymic epithelial cells
B-cells	Pancreatic β-cells, Vascular endothelial cells

Major Histocompatibility Complex (MHC) class I and class II molecules have a major role in presenting a processed antigen to T-lymphocytes and B lymphocytes. MHC class I molecules are expressed on the surface of practically all nucleated cells (York *et al.,* 1996). They consist of two polypeptide chains: an alpha chain and beta-2 microglobulin. The immune system uses two different pathways to eliminate intracellular and extracellular antigens. Endogenous antigens are processed in the cytosolic pathway and presented on the membrane with class I MHC molecules; exogenous antigens are processed in the endocytic pathway and presented on the membrane with class II MHC molecules.

Intracellular proteins such as viral, protozoal, bacterial and tumor proteins are degraded into short peptides by a cytosolic proteolytic system present in all cells. The proteins targeted for proteolysis often have a small protein called ubiquitin attached to them. Ubiquitin-protein conjugates can be degraded by a multi-functional protease complex called a "proteasome". The proteasomes involved in antigen processing include two sub-units encoded within the MHC gene cluster, LMP2 and LMP7 and a third non-MHC protein LMP10. Peptides generated in the cytosol by the proteasome are translocated by transporter proteins (TAP1/TAP2) into the rough endoplasmic reticulum (RER) by a process that requires the hydrolysis of ATP. TAP is optimized to transport peptides to RER and eventually to class I MHC molecules. Molecular chaperones facilitate the folding of polypeptides in order to form stable class I MHC molecular complex that exit the RER along with the peptide in the binding groove of class I molecule. The tri-molecular complex (alpha chain, beta-2-microglobulin and peptide) is then transported to the cells outer membrane and presented to the $CD8^+$ CTL. These lymphocytes become fully activated following second signals that include cytokine-receptor (such as IL-2 and IL2R) and co-stimulatory molecule-receptor (such as B7 and CD28) interactions. The activated $CD8^+$ CTL produce perforins that polymerize in the cell membrane of the target cell (e.g. virus infected cell) causing its death.

MHC class II molecules are expressed mainly on APC where they present processed antigenic peptides to T_H cells. MHC class II molecules contain two different polypeptide chains, a 33 kDa alpha chain and a 28 kDa beta chain, which associate by non-covalent interactions. Each chain in a class II molecule contains two external domains-α_1 and α_2 domains in one chain and β_1 and β_2 domains in the other, a transmembrane region and an intracytoplasmic region.

APC internalizes exogenous antigens by phagocytosis, endocytosis or both (Mach *et al.* 1996). Once an antigen is internalized it is degraded into peptides within compartments of the endocytic-processing pathway. Internalized antigen moves from early to late endosomes and finally to lysosomes, encountering hydrolytic enzymes and a lower pH in each environment. When class II molecules are synthesized within the RER, three pairs of class II α, β chains associate with the pre-assembled trimer of a protein called invariant chain. This trimeric protein interacts with the peptide binding cleft of the class II molecules, preventing any endogenously derived protein from binding to the cleft while the class II molecule is within the RER. As the proteolytic activity increases in each successive compartment, the invariant chain is gradually degraded. However, a short fragment of the invariant chain termed CLIP (for class II associated invariant chain peptide) remains bound to the class II molecule after the invariant chain has been cleaved within the endosomal compartment. A non-classical class II MHC molecule called HLA-DM is required to catalyze the exchange of CLIP with antigenic peptides. The complex formed is than transported to the plasma membrane and is presented to $CD4^+$ T-lymphocytes (T-helpers). These lymphocytes become activated following second signals that include cytokine-receptor and co-stimulatory molecule-receptor interactions. There are at least 2 sub-populations of T-helpers (Th) i.e. Th1 and Th2. Activation of either of the two sub-populations predominates, depending on the cytokines produced; interleukin-12 (IL-12) favors the Th1 response and IL-4 favors a Th2 response, the co-stimulatory molecules involved also decide the type of response(B7.1-CD28 interaction favors a Th1 response; B7.2-CD28 interaction favors a Th2 response). Activated Th1 mailny produces IL-2 and gamma-interferon whereas activated Th2 mailny produces IL-4, IL-5, IL-6, IL-10 and IL-13. Cytokines produced in a Th1 response mediate Delayed Type Hypersensitivity and are involved in the activation of CTL, macrophages and NK-cells, also help B-lymphocytes to eventually produce IgG2a and IgG3 class antibodies. On the other hand, cytokines produced in a Th2 response promote eosinophil proliferation, also production of IgG1 and IgE class antibodies by B-lymphocytes. Maximized Th1 and CTL responses are both needed for protection against intracellular parasites and tumors.

These are indications that exogenous proteins may be processed, complexed to MHC class I molecules and presented to CTL. By a yet not well-defined mechanism called cross priming, the antigen may be either shuttled directly into the cytosol of the APC, or it may be engulfed by phagocytosis and may leak out from the endosome/lysozome compartment into the cytosol.

12.2.3. Generation of an immune response to the protein encoded by the gene of interest

Administration of plasmid DNA vaccine containing a gene of interest induces immune response against the expressed protein or antigen. The plasmid DNA enters the cell and then the nucleus where it undergoes transcription and translation to express encoded the gene product in the cytoplasm, which leads to generation of both humoral and cell-mediated immune response.

12.3. ANTIGEN PROCESSING/PRESENTING CELLS (APCs)

APCs are specialized cells that share two properties 1. They express class II MHC molecules on their membranes; 2. They are able to deliver a co-stimulatory signal that is necessary for T_H cell activation. A number of studies have been performed to determine the ability of APC to take up plasmid DNA, process it, and activate both humoral and cell-mediated branches of immune system. Studies performed by Wolff *et al.,* (1990) and Ulmer *et al.,* (1993) suggested that myocytes behaved as APCs on administration of plasmid DNA by intramuscular route but lacks the co-stimulatory signals. Agadjanyan *et al* showed that antigen-specific CTL responses could be induced by muscle cells only when the mice were vaccinated with plasmid DNA possessing an antigen and a B7 (co-stimulatory molecule) reporter genes. Klinman *et al.,* (1997) suggested that keratinocytes and/or Langerhans cells might be the APCs that are transfected.

12.4. ROLE OF PLASMID DNA AS AN ADJUVANT

An immunologic adjuvant is an agent that can increase the rate, level and duration of an immune response to an antigen. An adjuvant that is added to some vaccines for human use is alum (aluminium hydroxide and/or aluminium phosphate), which creates a biased Th2 response. The immunostimulatory effect of bacterial DNA was reported by Tokunaga *et al.,* (1984). They showed that a DNA-rich fraction extracted from *Mycobacterium bovis* exhibited strong anti-tumor activity, stimulated mouse NK activity and induced the production of interferon and macrophage activating factor. Bacterial DNA contains immunostimulatory sequences (ISS) or motifs that trigger innate immunity in the host. ISS consists of unmethylated CpG dinucleotides flanked by two 5' purines and two 3' pyrimidines. Sequence analysis of the ampicillin resistant gene of plasmid DNA vaccines indicated that it contains two repeats of a palindromic CpG hexamer 5'AACpGTT3'. This 6 base motif proved to be a potent adjuvant in mice. They stimulate the production of cytokines, in particular gamma interferon and IL-12, which favor a Th1 response. CpG motifs are about 20 times more common in bacterial than in mammalian genome. Moreover, less than 5% of the cytosine residues in the CpG dinucleotides of bacterial DNA are methylated as compared to 70-90% of cytosine residues in eukaryotic DNA. Methylation of cytosine residues in the plasmid DNA abolishes immunostimulatory effect.

12.5. Th1 AND Th2 LYMPHOCYTE RESPONSES

When injected intramuscularly or intradermally, plasmid DNA vaccines induce a Th1 response because the CpG motifs stimulate the production of IL-12 that favors the activation of Th1 lymphocytes. On the other hand, if the plasmid DNA is administered with a gene gun, a Th2 response is generated.

In a number of animal models of infection, dominant Th1 responses have been correlated with protection. BALB/c mice are susceptible to *Leishmania major* because they are unable to generate a Th1 response unless they are given IL-12. Injection of BALB/c mice with a plasmid DNA vaccine containing gp63 reporter gene from *L. major,* induced a dominant Th1 response that was protective. In the case of Influenza virus, intra-muscular injection of mice with a plasmid DNA vaccine encoding influenza NP induced a protective Th1 response. An enhanced pulmonary inflammatory response with a predominant Th2 pattern and an unfavorable outcome was observed in mice immunized with an inactivated vaccine and infected with Respiratory Syncytial Virus (RSV). However, a predominant Th1 protective response against RSV was induced in mice injected with a plasmid DNA vaccine.

Moreover, a Th1 response rather than a Th2 response to a potential allergen appeared to abrogate an allergic reaction. Plasmid DNA encoding the house dust mite allergen (Der p 5) injected intradermally to rats inhibited specific IgE synthesis, histamine release and airway hyper-responsiveness upon aerosolized allergen challenge. In another report, mice were first sensitized to the latex allergen (Hev b 5) with alum that is an adjuvant that favors a Th2 response. Injection of these mice with plasmid DNA encoding the Hev b 5 antigens significantly decreased antigen-specific IgE levels. In yet another recent work, an oral DNA vaccine containing the gene for the main peanut allergen (Aruh-2) was shown to protect mice against peanut induced anaphylaxis. This effect was accompanied by a reduction in IgE levels. Thus it appears that plasmid DNA vaccines can both prevent allergic responses and downregulate an ongoing Th2 response.

On the other hand, in autoimmune diseases, a Th1 response appears to correlate with progression of the disease. Waisman *et al.,* (1996) used a DNA vaccine coding for a T cell receptor to protect mice against experimental autoimmune encephalitis. Protection was associated with a decrease in the Th1, and an increase in the Th2 response.

12.6. CYTOLYTIC T-CELL (CTL) RESPONSES

The initial interest in DNA vaccines arose from their ability to induce potent cellular response mediated by MHC class I restricted $CD8^+$ cytolytic T-cell in animal models. Effector cytolytic T-cells that recognize epitope peptides appropriate to the MHC restriction element have been demonstrated in mice immunized with DNA encoding the nucleoprotein from influenza virus, Hepatitis B surface antigen and core antigen, rabies, rota virus and ebola virus. In addition, cytolytic T-cells that recognize and kill virus-infected targets have been demonstrated in models of influenza virus, Lymphocytic chorio meningitis virus and herpes simplex virus.

Experiments using mouse models of infection revealed that CTL contributed to immunity against a number of protozoan parasites. Malaria remains an overwhelming problem in tropical developing countries, with 200-300 million cases and 1-2 million deaths per year. DNA vaccines against malaria tested in mice induced a specific CTL response and protection. Tuberculosis is another world health problem. Tascon *et al.,* (1996) reported a high degree of protection in mice immunized with a plasmid DNA vaccine containing the gene that codes for the 65 kDa heat shock protein of *M.*

tuberculosis. Tumor cells may behave as professional APC, if they express a tumor peptide MHC class I complex and co-stimulatory molecules. It has been reported that a vaccine containing the gene that codes for the carcino-embryonic antigen effectively generates a CTL response in mice and Graham *et al.,* (1996) reported that a plasmid vaccine containing the polymorphic epithelial mucin (PEM) gene protects mice against PEM – expressing tumor cells.

12.7. HUMORAL RESPONSES

Conventional vaccines in current use induce protective antibody responses. Plasmid DNA vaccines also induce the production of antibodies. Peak antibody levels are reached 4-12 weeks post immunization. DNA vaccines elicit antibodies against various viral, bacterial, parasitic tumor and eukaryotic proteins, including proteins from influenza, HIV, hepatitis B surface antigen, rabies virus glycoprotein, herpes simplex glycoproteins B and D, papilloma virus L1, hepatitis C nucleocapsid protein, hepatitis B core protein, *Mycoplasma pulmonis, Mycobacterium tuberculosis* antigen 85 and heat shock proteins, plasmodial antigens and Leishmania and Schistosoma antigens. However, comparison of humoral immune responses obtained in animals immunized with a DNA vaccine and a conventional vaccine or a sublethal dose of an infectious agent revealed that antibody levels achieved using the latter immunizing agents were higher.

Boyle *et al.,* (1996), and Deck *et al.,* (1997) reported that influenza virus antibody titers in mice immunized with a DNA vaccine were lower than that in mice immunized with live influenza virus. Similar results were obtained when mice immunized with DNA encoding a malaria surface protein and those immunized with the malaria protein alone were compared. Many infectious diseases enter the host through mucosal surfaces. Thus, it would be advantageous to generate mucosal antibody responses in addition to systemic responses. To date, intra-muscular injection and gene gun delivery of naked plasmid DNA have had limited ability to induce secretory mucosal IgA responses. However, formulation of plasmid DNA with cationic lipids, monophosphoryl lipid A, or Q5-21, encapsulated in poly-(lactide-co-glycolide) microparticles, macro-aggregated polyethyleneimine-albumin conjugates or biodegradable alginate microspheres that are delivered intramuscularly, orally or intranasally, induce significant secretory IgA responses at mucosal sites.

Wang *et al.,* (2004) reported induction of strong mucosal immunity against the similar immunodeficiency virus in primates by using DNA encoding intact noninfectious virions. The levels of secretory IgA in the rectal secretions of the immunized primates were higher than the levels achieved through natural infection. In recent development, Hattori *et al.,* (2004) have induced immune responses by DNA vaccination through targeted gene delivery using mannosylated cationic liposomes (mann-liposomes) formulations following intravenous administration in mice. In cultured mouse peritoneal macrophages, MHC class-I restricted antigen presentation of man-liposome-antigen complex was significantly higher than that of naked antigen and that complexed with plain liposomes. As regards antibody classes and sub-classes produced in an immune response to a DNA vaccine, it appears to depend on the method of vaccine administration. Using a gene gun, a biased TH_2 response would be obtained and the production of IgG1 and IgE antibodies would predominate. On the other hand, if the DNA vaccine were administered by injection, a biased Th1 response and the production of IgG2a would predominate.

12.8. DNA IMMUNIZATION ROUTE AND EFFECTIVE DOSE

Several routes of plasmid DNA inoculation have been explored in animal models: intramuscular, subcutaneous intra-periotoneal, intra-dermal, sub-cutaneous, intra-venous, oral, rectal, intra-bursal, intra orbital, intra-tracheal, intra-nasal and vaginal routes.

A plasmid DNA vaccine for a tumor can be directly injected into the tumor site. The commonest routes of administration are injecting the plasmid DNA dissolved in saline intra-muscularly or intra-dermally by using a hypodermic needle, or bombarding plasmid DNA coated onto colloidal gold microparticles in the dermis or muscle by means of a gene gun. The dose used in mice depends on the method of administration. Usually an immune response is generated when 10-100 μg of plasmid DNA is injected; it is 0.1-1 μg when administered with a gene gun. The immune response increases when 1 or 2 boosters are given. However, the time intervals between boosters appear to be critical. Two studies showed that increase in the time interval between immunizing doses elicits an enhanced immune response.

12.9. DURATION AND STRENGTH OF IMMUNE RESPONSE

Long lasting immunity is attained when a DNA vaccine is used. Akbari *et al.,* (1999*)* reported that antigen-specific $CD4^+$ T-lymphocytes remained elevated for up to about 10 months following immunization with a DNA vaccine, and Gurunathan *et al.,* (1998) reported long term antigen- specific Th1 activity in mice immunized with a DNA vaccine containing a gene encoding a *Leishmania* antigen. CTL responses and antibody levels were observed for up to about 17 months in mice immunized with a DNA vaccine containing a reporter gene coding for an influenza virus protein and a DNA vaccine containing a reporter gene coding for hepatitis B protein, respectively.

The prolonged immune response in the above-mentioned studies was probably due to persistence of the antigen produced in the host. Wolff *et al.,* (1992*)* detected antigen in muscle for longer than a year, and influenza virus nucleoprotein was detected in the dermis at one month post plasmid DNA inoculation. An immunization regimen that may result in an optimal immune response involves priming the host by using the DNA vaccine and subsequently boosting it with the antigen. Letvin *et al.,* (1997) primed rhesus monkeys with plasmid DNA containing HIV *env* gene. Subsequent boosters were given by using a combination of the plasmid DNA and HIV *env* protein. Strong CTL and neutralizing antibody activity were obtained.

12.10. ANIMAL MODELS OF DNA VACCINES

Table 12.3 shows the various experimental models of DNA vaccination. Most pathogens studied have been viruses-consistent with the method used; since the genes transferred by the plasmids require the host cellular machinery to be expressed, DNA based immunization strongly resembles a viral infection. However, genes from other microorganisms have also been used with success. The types of polypeptides expressed are often the envelope proteins of virus, but various other proteins have also been used. In the case of immunization for HBV surface antigen, the fine specificity of the humoral response in mice mimics, to a certain extent, that observed during infection in humans. T-cell proliferation and cytokine secretion have been studied in several models, and the cytokine profile indicates a Th1 type response characterized by the secretion of interleukin-2 and α-interferon.

The immune response can be remarkably long-lasting; however, its duration or persistence does not appear to have any deleterious effects on the animals because they remain protected against challenge long after immunization. One human trial used plasmid vector expressing HIV-1 genes delivered to HIV-seropositive individuals by intra-muscular injection. This protocol used Marcaine (Bupivacaine hydrochloride, a local Anesthetic) to facilitate DNA uptake, although the mechanism of this effect has not been clearly delineated. More clinical trials are also being initiated (Table 12.4) since plasmid DNA is now considered an innocuous substance compared with other genetic vectors used in therapy.

12.11. CLINICAL TRIALS

The traditional focus for vaccines is on infectious diseases. This is also true for DNA vaccines. Most data available are on vaccines against HIV, Hepatitis B and malaria. Immune responses induced by

Table 12.3: Animal models of DNA vaccines

Pathogens	Antigen	Animals
Bovine herpesvirus	Glycoprotein	Cattle, mouse
Hepatitis B virus	Capsid (core antigen)	Mouse
Hepatitis B virus	Envelope protein (surface antigen)	Mouse, Rabbit, Rat, Chimpanzee
Hepatitis C virus	Core/nucleocapsid	Mouse
Herpes simplex virus	Glycoproteins B, D.ICP27	Mouse
Human immuno-deficiency virus-1	Envelope glycoprotein gp160	Mouse
	Noninfectious particles	Nonhuman primates
House dust mite	Allergen	
Influenza virus	Hemagglutinin	Chicken
	Matrix protein	Ferrets
	Nucleoprotein	Nonhuman-primates
Leishmania major	Major surface glycoprotein	Mouse
Lymphocytic chorio-meningitis virus	Glycoprotein Nucleoprotein	Mouse
Mycobacterium tuberculosis	*M. leprae* hsp65	Mouse
Mycoplasma pulmonis	*M. pulmonis* DNA	Mouse
	M. pulmonis DNA expression library	
Papillomavirus	Major capsid protein L1	Rabbit
Plasmodium yoelli	Circumsporozoite protein	Mouse
Rabies virus	Glycoprotein	Mouse
Simian immunodeficiency virus	Env, gag	Monkeys
Schistosoma japonicum	Paramyosin (Sj97)	Mouse

plasmid DNA vaccines can be modulated or oriented by using different means of administration and / or co-administering an immunomodulator gene established in animal studies. Clinical trials of DNA vaccines have been performed or are underway for various diseases including cancer, influenza, Hepatitis B, HIV and malaria. It remains to be established if DNA plasmid vaccines operate in the same manner in humans. Some differences between mice and humans have been observed. Higher doses of plasmid DNA are needed to induce an immune response in humans. Whereas in mice immune responses are usually elicited using 0.1-1μg of plasmid DNA administered by a gene gun, or 10-100μg administered by injection.

Phase I clinical trials were initiated to evaluate the safety and immunogenicity of HIV-1 env/rev DNA constructs in infected and uninfected persons. The uninfected persons who received the highest dose of DNA vaccine had antigen specific lympho-proliferative responses and antigen specific production of interferon γ and β-chemokines, but these responses were weak and short lived. In the infected persons, an HIV-1 env/rev DNA vaccine construct boosted the env- specific antibodies; however no consistent effect was observed on cellular responses to HIV. Another phase I clinical trial evaluated HIV regulatory genes, such as *rev*, *nef* and *tat*. Immunization of infected persons with these genes enhanced cellular responses but produced no consistent changes in lymphocyte subsets or viral load .The DNA vaccines were well tolerated in doses from 20µg upto 2500µg; no significant local or systemic reactions were observed, and no participant dropped out of the study.

In the study by Wang *et al.*, (1998) involving phase I clinical trial of malaria DNA vaccines, 20 subjects were vaccinated with plasmid DNA encoding *P. falciparum* circumsporozoite protein. Each subject received a total of three intramuscular injections of 20, 100, 500 or 2500µg of plasmid DNA, given at four week intervals. After immunization 11 of the 20 subjects were shown to have malaria specific, classic cytotoxic T-cells (cytolytic activity restricted by HLA class I antigens) in their blood. There was some indication that immunization with either a 500µg dose or a 2500µg dose of DNA induced a better cellular response than that immunization with a 20µg or 100µg dose of DNA. These results point to the ability of DNA vaccines to induce specific cellular immunity in humans. But, the protective effects of the vaccine against malaria are still not confirmed. A phase I trial of an experimental HIV vaccine that includes an HIV A subtype *gag* gene and more than 40 bits of DNA encoding regions of HIV proteins is in progress in Kenya. This is the first component of a prime boost vaccination strategy, and will be followed by a second vaccine using modified vaccinia virus as a vector. Another phase I clinical trial was recently started in infected and uninfected person to directly compare vaccines in which the gene is delivered as naked DNA or by attenuated adenovirus. A DNA vaccine against Hepatitis B virus has been evaluated for safety and immunogenicity in a phase I clinical trial involving naïve healthy volunteers. A gene gun was used to propel the DNA into the skin. The hepatitis B DNA vaccine was found to be safe, well tolerated, and immunogenic. Current phase I and phase II trials are studying DNA vaccines as potential immunotherapy for various cancers including colon cancer, human follicular lymphoma and cutaneous T-cell lymphoma.

12.12. COMPARISON OF DNA VACCINES AND TRADITIONAL VACCINES

Upon *de novo* synthesis of antigen in transfected cells, DNA vaccines induce a full spectrum of immune responses including antibodies, T helper cells and cytolytic T cells. This is also achieved by live attenuated vaccines or viral recombinant vaccines but DNA vaccines lack inherent risks associated with the use of attenuated vaccines. Unlike recombinant vaccines, immune responses to the vaccine carrier are not an issue upon vaccination with plasmid DNA.

Unlike viral recombinant vaccines, DNA vaccines can be used repeatedly for different immunogens. Inactivated vaccines and protein vaccines produce only minor side effects and induce antibodies and T helper cells - two immune mechanisms that fully suffice for protection against many pathogens. Nevertheless, most inactivated vaccines or protein vaccines require addition of adjuvants which induce a local inflammatory reaction that acts as the danger signal to the immune system. The severity of the inflammatory reaction, which commonly correlates with the efficacy of the adjuvant, limits the use of many adjuvants in humans. DNA vaccines provide their own adjuvant through unmethylated cytosine linked to guanine (CpG) sequences present in the bacterial part of the vector. Inactivated vaccines and proteins commonly induce Th2 responses which, in the case of some infections such as those with respiratory syncitial virus, might actually exacerbate disease upon infection. Upon intramuscular immunization, DNA vaccines induce Th1 responses. Peptide vaccines induce monospecific B or T cell responses. This might be particularly useful for treatment of cancer where known point mutation of a self protein, such as p53 creates a T-cell epitope. Peptides require the addition of adjuvants, especially if the induction of CD8$^+$ T cells is sought. Furthermore, peptides are in general poorly immunogenic, which in part reflects their short half-life in serum. DNA

Table 12.4: Selected list of DNA vaccines currently under development

Target species	Product type	Development stage	Company
Cytomegalovirus	DNA vaccine	Research/ preclinical	Vical (San Diego, CA)
Hantavirus	Naked DNA vaccine	Lead preclinical research	Powderject Vaccines (Madison, WI)
Hepatitis B virus	Therapeutic DNA vaccine	Clinical I	Powderject Vaccines
Hepatitis B virus	Prophylactic DNA vaccine	Clinical I	PowderjectVaccines
Hepatitis B virus	Therapeutic naked DNA	Research/ preclinical	Vical
Herpes simplex virus	Naked DNA vaccine	Preclinical	Merck & Co.
Herpes simplex virus	Naked DNA vaccine	Lead preclinical research	Powderject Vaccines
HIV	Naked DNA vaccine	Phase I	Merck & Co.
HIV	Therapeutic DNA vaccine	Research/ preclinical	Vical
HIV	Therapeutic DNA vaccine	Lead preclinical research	Powderject Vaccines
HIV	Prophylactic DNA vaccine	Lead preclinical research	Powderject Vaccines
Human papillomavirus	Naked DNA vaccine	Phase II	Merck & Co.
Influenza virus	Preventive DNA vaccine	Phase I	Vical
Influenza virus	Naked DNA vaccine	Phase I	Merck & Co.
Influenza virus	Naked DNA vaccine	Lead preclinical research	Powderject Vaccines
Tuberculosis	Naked DNA vaccine	Preclinical	
Cancer (melanoma/ sarcoma)	Granulocyte Macrophage Colony Stimulating Factor (GMCSF) –DNA vaccine	Phase I	Powderject Vaccines
Cancer	DNA vaccines	Lead preclinical	Powderject Vaccines
Various cancers	Therapeutic DNA vaccines	Research/ Preclinical	Vical

vaccines carrying minigenes for expression of single epitopes can readily be made to replace peptide vaccines. Many of the traditional vaccines fail to induce immune responses in neonates, whereas DNA vaccines readily stimulate T and B cell responses to most traditional vaccines which is impaired in the presence of maternally transferred antibodies.

Compared with many traditional vaccines, DNA vaccines induce comparatively low immune responses (see Table 12.5). This might limit their usefulness for pathogens that invade their host at high numbers or that replicate very efficiently. For reasons, the potency of DNA vaccines in priming the immune response is still not very clear. Experimental animals inoculated with a DNA vaccine develop very high immune responses upon booster immunization with a low dose of traditional vaccine expressing the same antigen. This might be linked to the adjuvant effect of CpG sequences that by creating a unique cytokine might favour activation of memory T-helper cells. For that reason, even if DNA vaccines on their own are eventually shown to lack efficacy for many of the human pathogens, they might still secure their place in vaccinology as prime agents.

12.13. SECOND GENERATION VACCINES

As simple plasmids, DNA vaccines effectively induce immune responses and protection in various animal models of disease, but they have induced only modest immune responses in clinical trials. Various strategies have been employed to improve the expression of antigens: incorporation of immunostimulatory sequences in the backbone of the plasmids, co-expression of stimulatory molecules, utilization of localization/secretory signals and utilization of the appropriate delivery system. Another important consideration is the utilization of methods designed to optimize transgene expression.

12.14. REGULATORY ELEMENTS

Various reports have described the strength of promoters/enhancers or other transcriptional elements in DNA vaccines. In general, virally-derived promoters have provided greater gene expression *in vivo* than other eukaryotic promoters. In particular, the cytomegalovirus immediate early enhancer/promoter (CMVp) directs the highest level of transgene expression in eukaryotic tissues as compared to other promoters. For example in one study a plasmid expressing human immunodeficiency virus type 1 (HIV-1) Gag/Env under the regulation of CMV promoter/enhancer was compared to a comparable plasmid utilizing the endogenous AKV murine leukemia long terminal repeat. Analysis of the immune responses in macaques injected with the plasmids showed that the CMV-containing plasmid elicited higher Gag-and Env-specific humoral and T-cell proliferative responses, reflecting the greater transcriptional activity of the CMV promoter. Inclusion of the CMV intron A improved the level of expression of transgenes expressed by the CMV promoter or other promoter/enhancers. It is thought that the beneficial effect of introns on expression is primarily due to an enhanced rate of polyadenylation and/or nuclear transport associated with RNA splicing. However, some widely used virally derived promoters, such as the CMV promoter, may not be suitable for some gene therapy applications since treatment with interferon-γ or tumour necrosis factor-α may inhibit transgene expression from DNA vaccines containing these promoters. Thus, alternatives to the CMV promoters/enhancers, which control expression of the muscle-specific cytoskeletal protein desmin, was used effectively to drive expression of the hepatitis B surface antigen. These responses were shown to be of a comparable magnitude to those in mice immunized with comparable DNA vaccines containing the CMV promoter. Other tissue-specific promoters that have been studied include the creatine kinase promoter, also specific to muscle cells, and the metallothionein and 1,24-vitamin D(3) (OH) (2) dehydroxylase promoters, both of which are specific to keratinocytes. Since the rate of transcriptional initiation is generally increased by the use of strong promoter/enhancers, the rate of transcriptional termination may become rate limiting. The polyadenylation sequence used within a DNA vaccine may also have significant effects of transgene expression. For example, it was demonstrated that the commonly used SV40 polyadenylation sequence was less efficient than the minimal rabbit β-globin and bovine growth hormone polyadenylation sequences in mouse liver, although addition of a second SV40 enhancer downstream of the SV40 polyadenylation signal did increase expression to a level comparable to the other signals. Therefore, it is possible that the strategy of inserting a second SV40 enhancer downstream of a SV40 polyadenylation sequence may be utilized in the construction of more efficient vectors.

Table 12.5: Comparison of DNA vaccines with other traditional vaccines

Properties	Attenuated pathogen	Inactivated pathogen	Live recombinant vector	Protein vaccine	Peptide vaccine	DNA vaccine
Antibody response	Yes	Yes	Yes	Yes	Yes	Yes
Antibody rise	Fast	Fast	Fast	Fast	Fast	Slow
CTL induction	Yes	No	Yes	No	Variable	Yes
T-helper induction	Yes	Yes	Yes	Yes	Yes	Yes
Complete antigen repertoire	Yes	Yes	No	No	No	Possible
Immune response to the vaccine carrier	No	No	Possibly	No	No	No
Duration of response	Long	Short	Long	Short	Short	Long
Vaccine doses required	One	Multiple	Multiple	Multiple	Multiple	One or more
Safety (especially for pregnant & immuno-suppressed individuals)	No	Yes	No	Yes	Yes	Probably
Risk of reversion	Yes	No	Yes	No	No	No
Impaired efficacy in the presence of maternal antibodies	Yes	Yes	Yes	Yes	Yes	No
Ease of production	Variable	Difficult	Difficult	Difficult	Difficult	Easy
Cost	Variable	Expensive	Expensive	Expensive	Expensive	Inexpensive

12.15. KOZAK SEQUENCES

Sequences flanking the AUG initiator codon within mRNA influence its recognition by eukaryotic ribosomes. As a result of studying the conditions required for optimal translational efficiency of expressed mammalian genes, the' Kozak' consensus sequence has been shown to be important. It has been proposed that this defined translational initiating sequence ($^{-6}$GCCA/GCCAUGG $^{+4}$) should be included in vertebrate mRNAs located around the initiator codon. It has also been suggested that efficient translation is obtained when the −3 position contains a purine base or, in the absence of a purine base, a guanine is positioned at +4 (134). Prokaryotic genes and some eukaryotic genes do not possess Kozak sequences. Therefore, the expression level of these genes might be increased by the insertion of a Kozak sequence.

12.16. CODON USAGE

Codon bias is observed in all species, and the use of selective codons in genes often correlates with gene expression efficiency. In general, taxonomically close organisms, such as *E. coli* and *Salmonella enterica* subspecies 1 *serovar Typhimurium* use similar codons for their protein synthesis whereas taxonomically distant organisms, such as *E.coli* and *Saccharomyces cerevisiae*, utilise very different codons. Mammalian codon usage is also different from that of microorganisms. Nagata *et al*, (1999), studied the effect of codon optimization for mammalian cells of cytotoxic T-lymphocyte (CTL) epitopes derived from the intracellular bacterium *Listeria monocytogenes* and the parasite *Plasmodium yoelii*. They found that the codon optimisation level of genes correlated well with translational efficiency in mammalian cells.

The greatest deviation from random codon usage in an organism occurs in the most highly expressed genes as a result of selection for codons that maximize translational efficiency. Minor tRNA species are avoided in highly expressed genes. Thus, differences between codon usage in a heterologous gene and the host organism may affect expression. A DNA vaccine vector encoding a synthetic epitope of listeriolysin O with mammalian codon usage showed higher translation efficiency than a vector containing the wild-type sequence in murine cells. Furthermore, the first DNA vaccine was capable of inducing specific CD8^{+} T cells able to confer partial protection against challenge with *L. monocytogenes* whereas the second DNA vaccine could not. Several other studies revealed that increased immune responses may be obtained by DNA vaccination with a transgene sequence with optimised codon usage.

In some circumstances it may be desirable to optimise DNA vaccines to produce reduced transgene expression. For example, the weaker SV40 promoter has been used instead of CMV promoter to drive expression of antigens that induce cell death upon overexpression. Tissue-specificity is also important: Tissue-specific expression systems may promote stable expression by reducing the probability of inducing an immune response to the transgene. Restricting the site of expression of genes should minimise risks related to aberrant expression of a gene product. Finally, enhanced knowledge of the regulation of expression of antigens has facilitated production of it is now possible to produce multivalent systems whereby multiple antigens are expressed from a single DNA vaccine vector.

The backbone of a DNA vaccine vector may be further modified to enhance immunogenicity *via* the manipulation of the DNA to include certain sequences, so that the DNA itself will have an adjuvant effect. DNA vaccine vectors contain many CpG motifs (consisting of unmethylated CpG dinucleotides flanked by two 5' purines and two 3' pyrimidines) that, overall, induce a Th1-like pattern of cytokine production, and are thought to account for strong CTL responses often seen following DNA vaccination. It is possible to augment responses to DNA vaccine vectors by incorporating CpG motifs into the DNA backbone of the plasmid. Alternatively, immune responses may be modulated or enhanced by the co-expression of stimulatory molecules or cytokines or through the use of localisation or secretory signals or ligand fusions to direct antigens to sites appropriate for immune modulation.

12.17. ADVANTAGES AND LIMITATIONS OF DNA VACCINES

12.17.1. Advantages

As compared to live attenuated vaccines or viral carrier systems, plasmid DNA is non-infectious and non-replicating; it encodes only the antigen of interest. It induces both cell-mediated (Th1 and CTL) and humoral immunity. Activations of both these immunity pathways account for the improved performance of the vaccine. First, cell-mediated immunity imparts longer-lasting memory, so lifelong immunity after just one application of the vaccine may be feasible. Second, the cell based immune system has rather broad spectrum and provides protection against one serotype as well as against heterologous strains of a pathogen. Third, by combination of both immunity pathways, it is possible to target not only free viruses but also virus-infected cells.

Many microbial proteins have folded structures that are altered during purification. If the shape of the recombinant protein differs from that of the native proteins of the pathogen, the antibodies induced by the recombinant protein will not recognize the native protein of the pathogen and lead to vaccine failure. DNA vaccines induce *in-vivo* expression of immunogens, thus conserving the native conformation of epitopes. An appropriate tertiary conformation should be conserved for the induction of conformational specific antibodies and cellular responses. They may be constructed to include more than one immunogen gene, potentially decreasing the number of vaccinations required in children.

DNA vaccine plasmids can be constructed using simple recombinant DNA techniques, enabling co-inoculaion of multiple plasmids encoding different antigens of the same pathogen or of different pathogens. Such a multivalent approach is especially important for diseases such as malaria, AIDS and tuberculosis where a single antigen alone may not offer complete protection. DNA vaccines therefore offer the possibility of generating effective immune responses against diseases where other types of vaccines have failed. Moreover, they may be safer to use than live attenuated vaccines especially in immuno-compromised hosts.

Another major advantage of DNA vaccines is that they do not require a cold-chain storage that refers to the series of refrigerators required to maintain the viability of a vaccine during its distribution. Currently, maintaining the cold-chain represents nearly 80% of the cost of vaccinating individuals in developing nations. Since DNA vaccines can be stored dry or in an aqueous solution at room temperature there is no need for the cold chain. Thus, DNA vaccines are stable, easy to freeze dry and reconstitute, and can be manufactured inexpensively in large quantities in pure form.

12.17.2. Limitations of DNA vaccines

While DNA vaccination offers several advantages over conventional vaccines, plasmid DNA vaccines have some limitations and potential dangers. DNA vaccination approach induces immune responses only against the protein components of the pathogen and cannot substitute for polysaccharide based subunit vaccines, for diseases caused by pathogens such as *Pneumococcus*. Although induction of protective immune responses following DNA vaccination has been demonstrated for a variety of diseases, the mechanism of DNA vaccine action is still not completely understood.

The potential risks of using plasmid DNA encoding cytokines or co-stimulatory molecules in the host are not known. A major concern about DNA vaccines is whether the plasmid DNA integrates into the genome randomly, potentially leading to insertional mutagenesis. If plasmid DNA integrates into the host genome it may either activate oncogenes or suppress tumor suppressor genes, which may lead to a malignant transformation. Efforts to integrate DNA vaccine plasmids into mouse genomic DNA have failed to detect insertions of the injected plasmid. Thus, the level of integration, if it does occur, may not pose a significant safety concern. If the vaccine is administered intradermally, the transfected epidermal cells are lost within 10-14 days because of the normal sloughing of keratinized skin tissue. If administered intramuscularly, the transfected muscle cells are non-dividing and random insertion is more likely to occur in replicating cells in which DNA is being actively synthesized. Moreover, Nicholas *et al.,* (1995) did not detect integration of plasmid DNA into the host cell genome at 3,6,12 and 18 weeks after intramuscular administration.

Another major concern is the induction of anti-DNA antibodies by plasmid DNA. Antibodies to DNA can cause disease and are associated with systemic lupus erythematosus (SLE). SLE is an autoimmune disease characterized by the presence of anti-double stranded DNA antibodies in patient's serum. The injection of plasmid DNA may induce the production of anti-DNA antibodies and SLE.

On the other hand, one way by which immunological tolerance may be induced in adults is by administration of minute amounts of antigen. The minute amount produced by transfected cells may induce a state of tolerance of plasmid –encoded antigen that appears to persist for long periods of time but, unresponsiveness, rather than protective immunity might result. Potential harmful effects of bacterial ISS (CpG motifs) must also be considered. Schwartz *et al.,* (1997) reported that CpG motifs in bacterial DNA cause inflammation in lower respiratory tract.

12.18. RECENT PROGRESS ON DNA VACCINES

➢ DNA vaccines induce broad immune responses in animals. Several adjuvants have been tried to increase the intrinsic capacity of DNA, such as cytokine genes, granulocyte macrophage-colony stimulatory factor, or a recombinant protein. A new adjuvant imidazo quinoline compound imiquimod has been studied. Imiquimod was topically delivered to a mouse model as an adjuvant to DNA immunization so as to induce cellular and humoral immune responses against the p37 [gag] gene of HIV-I.

➢ The responses obtained represented broader antigenic stimulus and mediated total protection against HIV-I/MuLV challenge. MuLV (Murine Leukemia Virus) is a pseudo-virus.

➢ DNA vaccines are being used as an effective mucosal priming agent to stimulate a protective immune response for AIDS prevention and HIV infection occurring at an alarming rate.

➢ Immune responses have been enhanced by DNA vaccination through targeted gene delivery by using mannosylated cationic liposome (man-liposomes) formulations following intravenous administration in mice. Ovalbumin (OVA) was selected as a model antigen for vaccination. OVA-encoding pDNA (pCMV-OVA) was constructed to evaluate DNA vaccination. The potency of the man-Liposome/pCMV-OVA complex was compared with that of naked pCMV-OVA and that complexed with 3-β-[n-[(N',N'-dimethylamino)ethane]carbamoyl]cholesterol (DC-Chol) liposome.

➢ Targeted delivery of DNA vaccine by Man-Liposomes is a potent vaccination method for DNA vaccine therapy.

> BALB/c mice have been vaccinated with plasmid DNA encoding ESAT 6 protein of *Mycobacterium tuberculosis* and with Esat 6 protein in IFA adjuvant or a combined DNA prime-protein boost regimen. While DNA immunization induced Th1 polarized immune responses, protein-in-adjuvant vaccination elicited a Th2 dominant response.

> In a recent study, it was found that activity of BAT antibody enables DNA vaccination to inhibit the progression of established autochthonous Her-2/ neu carcinomas in BALB/C mice and thus provide protection against incipient carcinomas.

> Immunization with naked DNA requires considerable amounts of DNA in order to be effective. Therefore, a strategy has been evaluated to reduce the amount of DNA by using Ag85 DNA adsorbed onto cationic PLG microparticles.

> DNA vaccine constructs expressing Pvs 25 and Pvs 28 (*Plasmodium vivax*), prevent further development within the mosquito vector halting the transmission of parasite.

> DNA vaccine might provide an alternative to the live smallpox vaccine in providing protective efficacy in an orthopox virus (OPV) lethal respiratory challenge model.

12.19. FUTURE PROSPECTS

DNA vaccines have successfully generated protective immunity not only against viral infections but also against bacterial infections and cancer. But the area of concern is the risk-benefit ratio of the treatment for a given disease. It is important to carefully evaluate the safety of DNA vaccines in pre-clinical and clinical trials, while at the same time considering the benefit of a protective vaccination. Unlike other recombinant protein pharmaceuticals, in DNA vaccines the plasmid DNA itself, rather than the protein produced by it, is the final product. For some applications the potential benefits clearly outweigh the risks, and expeditious approval of DNA vaccine clinical trials will provide important safety information for applications where the potential risks initially appear of greater importance.

While DNA vaccine research has taken off in a big way, some researchers are already toying with the idea of using the genome sequence data of several pathogenic microbes to develop genomic vaccines. This approach, also known as expression library immunization, envisages immunization of animals with groups of plasmids encoding 100:1000 genes of a pathogen. The group that confers protection against the pathogen is split into a smaller group of 10-100 genes and re-tested. Using such a reductionist approach, a single gene in each group responsible for protection can be identified.

Barry *et al.,* (1995) took advantage of the very small amounts of DNA required with the particle bombardment method. Since a single nanogram of DNA coated on the gold particles can induce an immune response, 1µg can potentially introduce 1000 different genes. On this basis a library of gene fragments was prepared from *Mycoplasma pulmonis* by cloning the genomic DNA into a plasmid expression vector. So, protection against *M. pulmonis* has been achieved after immunization with different expression libraries. The manner of administration of the DNA vaccines, amount of plasmid DNA to be administered, delivery of plasmid DNA to appropriate antigen presenting cells, antigen expression by DNA vaccines, number of boosters to be given and time interval between boosters need to be optimized. Still, more efforts are needed to improve and optimize antigen expression. The major challenge is to establish the clinical utility of DNA vaccines.

SUGGESTED READING

- Abdelnoor AM. *Critical Reviews in Oncogenesis* 3, 81 (1997).
- Agadjanyan MG, Kim JJ, Trivedi N, *et al. J Immunol* 162, 3417 (1999).

- Akbari O, Panjwani N, Garcia S, *et al. J Exp Med* 189,169 (1999).
- Allen TM, Vogel TV, Fuller DH, *et al. J Immunol* 164, 4968 (2000).
- Amara RR, Villinger F, Altman JD *et al. Science* 92, 69 (2001).
- Aris A, Feliu JX, Knight A, *et al. Biotechnol Bioeng* 68, 688 (2000).
- Barnett SW, Lu S, Srivastava I, *et al. J Virol* 75, 5526 (2001).
- Barouch DH, *et al., Proc Natl Acad Sci* USA 97, 4192 (2000).
- Barouch DH, Craiu A, Santra S, *et al. J Virol* 75, 2462 (2001).
- Barouch DH, Santra S, Tenner-Racz K, *et al., J Immunol* 168, 562 (2002).
- Barry MA, Lai WC, Johnston SA. *Nature* 377, 632 (1995).
- Bartlott RJ, Secore SL, Singer JT, *et al. Cell Transplant* 5, 411 (1996).
- Berry LJ, Vennman MR. In *Cellular Antigens*, Nowotny, A, Ed. Springer-Verlag New York, pp. 3-13 (1972).
- Bevan MJ. *Nature* 325, 192 (1987).
- Bourne N, Stanberry LR, Bernstein DI, *et al. Infect Dis* 173, 800 (1996).
- Boyer JD, Chattrgoon M, Shah A, *et al. Dev Biol Stand* 95, 147 (1998).
- Boyer JD, Cohen AD, Ugen KE, *et al., AIDS* 14, 1515 (2000).
- Boyer JD, Cohen AD, Vogt S, *et al. J Infect Dis* 181, 476 (2000).
- Boyle CM, Morin M, Webster RG, *et al. J Virol* 70, 9074 (1996).
- Boyle JS, Koniarasm C, Lew AM. *Int Immunol* 9, 1897 (1997).
- Breman JG, Campbell CC. *Bull WHO* 66, 611 (1988).
- Butts C, Zubkoff I, Robbins DS. *Vaccine* 16, 1444 (1998).
- Calarota S, Bratt G, Nordlund S, *et al. Lancet* 351, 1320 (1998).
- Calarota SA, Kjerrstrom A, Islam KB, *et al. Hum Gene Ther* 12, 1623 (2001).
- Carbone FR, Bevan MJ. *J Exp Med* 171, 377 (1990).
- Casares S, Inaba K, Brumeanu TD, *et al. J Exp Med* 186, 1481 (1997).
- Caselli E, Boni M, Luca D, *et al. Comp Immunol Microbiol Infec Dis* 28, 155 (2005).
- Castellino FG, Zhong G, Germain N. *Human Immunol* 54, 159 (1997).
- Chapman BS, Thayer RM, Vincent KA, *et al. Nucleic Acids Res* 19, 3979 (1991).
- Cherpelis S, Shrivastava I, Gettie A, *et al. J Virol* 75, 1547 (2001).
- Cohen J, *Science* 292, 24 (2001).
- Conry RM, Widera G, Lo Buglio AF, *et al. Gen Ther* 3, 67 (1996).
- Cox GJ, Zamb TJ, Babuik LA. *J Virol* 67, 5664 (1993).
- Davis HL, *Curr Opin Biotechnol* 8, 635 (1997).
- Davis HL, Mancini M, Michel ML, *et al. Vaccine* 14, 910 (1996).
- Davis HL, Michel ML, Mancini M. *et al. Vaccine* 12, 1503 (1994).
- Davis HL, Michel ML, Whalen RG. *Hum Mol Genet* 2, 1847 (1993).
- Davis HL, Schirmbeck R, Reimann J, *et al. Hum Gene Ther* 6, 1447 (1995).
- Deck RR, Dewitt CM, Donnelly JJ, *et al. Vaccine* 15, 71 (1997).

- Deliyannis G, Boyle JS, Brady JL, *et al.*, *Proc Natl Acad Sci* USA 97, 6676 (2000).
- Demil L, Bojak A, Steck S, *et al*. *J Virol* 75, 10991 (2001).
- Denkers EY, Yap G, Scharton-Kersten T, *et al.*, *J Immunol* 159, 1903 (1997).
- Donnelly JJ, Martinez D, Jansen KU, *et al.*, *J Infect Dis* 24, 1375 (1996).
- Donnelly JJ, Ulmer JB, Liu MA. *Ann NY Acad Sci* 772, 40 (1995).
- Donnelly JJ, Ulmer JB, Liu MA. *Life Sci* 60, 163 (1997).
- Doolan DLo, Hoffman SL, *Parasit Today* 13, 171 (1997).
- Eisenbraun MD, Fuller DH, Haynes JR, *DNA Cell Biol* 12, 791 (1993).
- Eisenstein TK. *Infect Immun* 12, 364 (1975).
- Fuller DH, Corb MM, Barnett S, *et al*. *Vaccine* 15, 924 (1997).
- Fuller DH, Haynes JR, *AIDS Res Hum Retrover* 10, 1433 (1994).
- Fuller DH, Murphey-Corb M, Clements J, *et al.*, *J Med Primatol* 25, 236 (1996).
- Fynan EF, Webster RG, Fuller DH, *et al.*, *Proc Natl Acad Sci* USA 90, 11478 (1993).
- Galvin TA, Muller J, Khan AS, *Vaccine* 18, 2566-2583 (2000).
- Gebhard JR, Ahu J, Cao X, *et al*. *Vaccine* 18, 1837 (2000).
- Ghiasi H, Cai S, Slanina S, *et al*. *Antiviral Res* 28, 147 (1995).
- Graham RA, Burchel JM, Beverely P, *et al.*, *Int J Cancer* 65, 664 (1996).
- Grosjean H, Fliers W, *Gene* 18, 299 (1982).
- Gurunathan S, Klinman DM, Seder RA. *Ann Rev Immunol* 18, 927 (2000).
- Gurunathan S, Prussin C, Sacks DL, *et al.*, *Nat Med* 41, 409 (1998).
- Haddad D, Ramprakash J, Sedegah M, *et al.*, *J Immunol* 165, 3772 (2000).
- Harms JS, Oliveira SC, Splitter GA. *Braz J Med Biol Res* 32, 155 (1999).
- Hattori Y, Kawakami S, Suzuki S, *et al.*, *Biochem Biophys Res Comm* 317, 992 (2004).
- Herrmann JE, Chen SC, Fynan EF, *et al.*, *J Infect Dis* 174, S93 (1996).
- Hoffman SL, Sedegah M, Hedstrom RC. *Vaccine* 12, 1529 (1994).
- Hsu CH, Chua KY, Tao MH, *et al.*, *Nat Med* 2, 540 (1996).
- Huang MT, Gorman CM, *Nucleic Acids Res* 18, 937 (1990).
- Hung CF, Cheng WF, Chai CY *et al.*, *J Immunol* 166, 5733(2001).
- Huygen K, Content J, Denis O, *et al.*, *Nat Med* 2, 893 (1996).
- Ikemura T, *J Mol Biol* 158, 573(1982).
- Ikemura T, *Mol Biol Evo* 2, 13(1985).
- Itali K, Sawamura D, Meng X, *et al.*, *Clin Exp Dermatol* 26, 531 (2001).
- Jones DH, Corris S, McDonald S, *et al.*, *Vaccine* 15, 814 (1997).
- Kang Y, Calvo PA, Daly TM, *et al.*, *J Immunol* 161, 4211 (1998).
- Kevissa M, Von Kampen J, Zurbriggen R, *et al.*, *Vaccine* 18, 2337 (2000).
- Klinman DM, Yamshchikov G, Ishigatsubo Y, *J Immunol* 158, 3635 (1997).
- Klinman DM, Barnhart KM, Conover J. *Vaccine* 17, 19 (1999).
- Klinman DM, Sechler JM, Conover J, *et al.*, *J Immunol* 160, 2388 (1998).

- Kongkasuriyachai D. *Vaccine* 22, 3205(2004).
- Kovacsovics – Bankowski M, Clark K, Banacerraf B, *et al.*, *Proc Natl Acad Sci* USA 90, 4942 (1993).
- Kovacsovics–Bankowski M, Rock KL. *Science* 267, 243 (1995).
- Kozak M, *EMBO J.* 16, 2482 (1997).
- Kozak M. *J Mol Biol* 196, 947 (1987).
- Kreig AM, Yi AK, Matson S. *Nature* 374, 546 (1995).
- Krieg AM, Yi AK, Schorr J, Davis HL. *Trends Microbiol* 6, 23 (1998).
- Kuhober A, Pudorlek HP, Reifenberg K, *et al.*, *J Immunol* 156, 3687 (1996).
- Kuhrober A, Wild J, Pudollek HP, *et al.*, *Int Immunol* 9, 1203 (1997).
- Kumar S, Tarleto RL, *Parasite Immunol* 20, 207 (1998).
- Lagging LM, Meyer K, Hoft D, *et al.*, *J Virol* 69, 5859 (1995).
- Lai WC, Bennett M, Johnston SA, *et al.*, *DNA Cell Biol* 14, 643 (1995).
- Le TP, Hedstrom KM, Charoenvit Y, *et al.*, *Vaccine* 18, 1893 (2000).
- Lee D, Graham BS, Chiu YL, *et al.*, *J Infect Dis* 190, 903 (2004).
- Lee SW, Sung YC. *Immunology* 94, 285 (1998).
- Leitner WW, Seguin MC, Ballou WR, *et al.*, *J Immunol* 159, 6112 (1997).
- Letvin NL, Montefiori DC, Yasutomi Y, *et al.*, *Proc Natl Acad Sci* USA 94, 9378 (1997).
- Lewis PJ, Cox GJM, Hurk S, *et al.*, *Vaccine* 15, 861 (1997).
- Li X, Sambhara S, Li CX, *et al.*, *Exp Med* 188, 681 (1998).
- Liu MA, Yasutomi Y, Davies ME, *et al.*, *Antibiot Chemother* 48, 100 (1996).
- Ljungberg K, Rollman E, Eriksson L, *et al.*, *Virology* 302, 44 (2002).
- Lodmell DL, Ray NB, Ewalt LC. *Vaccine* 16, 115 (1998).
- Lodmell DL, Ray NB, Parnell MJ, *et al.*, *Nat Med* 4, 949 (1998).
- Lopez-Macias C, Lopez-Hernandez MA, Gonzalez CR. *Ann NY Acad Sci* 772, 285 (1995).
- Lowrie DB, Tascon RE, Clston MJ, *et al.*, *Vaccine* 12, 1537 (1994).
- Lu S, Manson K, Wyand M, Robinson HL. *Vaccine* 15, 920 (1997).
- Lu S, Santoro JC, Fuller DH, *et al.*, *Virology* 209, 147 (1995).
- Lu S, Wyatt R, Richmond JF, *et al.*, *J Virol* 72, 9092 (1998).
- MacGreger RR, Boyer JD, Ugen KE, *et al.*, *J Infect Dis* 178, 92 (1998).
- MacGreger RR, Boyer JD, Ciccarelli RB, *et al.*, *J Infect Dis* 181, 406 (2000).
- Mach B, Steimle V, Martinez – Soria E, *et al.*, *Immunol* 14, 301 (1996).
- Major ME, Vitvitski L, Mink MA, *et al.*, *J Virol* 69, 5859 (1995).
- Makoff AJ, Oxer MD, Romanos MA, *et al.*, *Nucleic Acids Res* 17, 10191 (1989).
- Manickan E, Rouse RJ, Yu Z, *et al.*, *J Immunol* 155, 259 (1995).
- Manickan E, Yu Z, Rouse RJ, *Wire* 8, 53 (1995).
- Martins LP, Lau LL, Asano MS, *et al.*, *J Virol* 69, 2574 (1995).
- Mc Clements WL, Armstrong ME, Keys RD, *et al.*, *Proc Natl Acad Sci* USA 93, 11414 (1996).

- McDonnel WM, Askari FK. *N Engl J Med* 334, 42 (1996).

- Michel ML, Davis HL, Schleef M, *et al.*, *Proc Natl Acad Sci* USA 92, 5307 (1995).

- Mitchell WM, Rosenbloom ST, *J Immunotechnology* 1, 2119 (1995).

- Mittal SK, Aggarwal N, Sailaja G, *et al.*, *Vaccine* 19, 253 (2000).

- Mollenkipf HJ, Dietrich G, Fensterle J, *et al.*, *Vaccine* 22, 2690 (2004).

- Moore AC, Kong WP, Chakrabarti BK, *et al.*, *J Virol* 76, 243 (2002).

- Mor G. *Biochem Pharmacol* 55, 1151 (1998).

- Mor G, Klinman DM, Shapiro S, *et al.*, *J Immunol* 155, 2039 (1995).

- Mumper RJ, Ledebur HC, Rolland AP, *et al.*, DNA Vaccines-Methods and Protocols: Humana Press, 267 (2000).

- Mustafa F, Richmond JF, Fernandez-Lorsson R, *et al.*, *Virology* 229, 269 (1997).

- Nagata T, Uchijima M, Yoshida A, *et al.*, *Biochem Biophys Res Comm* 261, 445 (1999).

- Narum DL, Kumar S, Rogers WO, *et al.*, *Infect Immun* 69, 7250 (2001).

- Nichols WW, Ledwith BJ, Manam SV, *Ann NY Acad Sci* 772, 30 (1995).

- Norbury CC, Hewlett LJ, Prescott AR, *et al.*, *Immunity* 3, 783 (1995).

- Orson FM, Kinsey BM, Hua PJ, *et al.*, *J Immunol* 164, 6313 (2000).

- Ourmanov I, Bilska M, Hirsch VM, *et al.*, *J Virol* 74, 2960 (2000).

- Pavlenko M, Roos AK, Lundquist A, *et al.*, *Br J Cancer* 91, 686 (2004).

- Pisetsky DS, *Nat Med* 3, 829 (1997).

- Prince AM, Whalen RG, Brotman B. *Vaccine* (1996).

- Proudfoot NJ. *Trends Biochem Sci* 14, 105 (1989).

- Pulford DJ. *Vaccine* 22, 3358 (2004).

- Qin L, Ding Y, Pahud DR, *et al.*, *Hum Gen Ther* 8, 2019 (1997).

- Quaglino E, Mastin C, Iezzi M, *et al.*, *Vaccine* 23, 3280 (2005).

- Raz E, Carson DA, Parker SE, *et al.*, *Proc Natl Acad Sci* USA 91, 9519 (1994).

- Reis C, Sousa E, Germain RN. *J Exp Med* 182, 841 (1995).

- Reynolds FH, Todaro GJ, Fryling C, *et al.*, *Nature* 292, 259 (1981).

- Rice J, King CA, Spellerberg MB, *et al.*, *Vaccine* 17, 3030 (1999).

- Richmond JF, Lu S, Santoro JC, *et al.*, *J Virol* 72, 9092 (1998).

- Richmond JF, Mustafa F, Lu S, *et al.*, *Virology* 230, 265 (1997).

- Robertson JS. *Vaccine* 12, 1526 (1994).

- Robinson HL, Boyle CA, Feltquate DM, *et al.*, *J Infect Dis* 176, S50 (1997).

- Romagnani S. *Immunol Today* 18, 263 (1997).

- Romero P, Maryanski JL, Corrandin G, *et al.*, *Nature* 341, 323 (1989).

- Rouse RJ, Nair SK, Lydy SL, *et al.*, *J Virol* 68, 5685 (1994).

- Roy K, Mao HQ, Huang SK, *et al.*, *Nat Med* 5, 387 (1999).

- Roy MJ, Wu MS, Barr LJ, *et al.*, *Vaccine* 19, 1764 (2000).
- Sasaki S, Tsuji T, Asakura Y, *et al.*, *Anticancer Res* 18, 3907 (1998).
- Sato Y, Roman M, Tighe H. *Science* 273, 352 (1996).
- Schodel F, Aguado MT, Lambert PH. *Vaccine* 12, 1491 (1994).
- Schwartz DA, Quinn TJ, Thorne PS, *et al.*, *J Clin Invest* 100, 68 (1997).
- Sedegah M, Hedstrom R, Hobartm P, *et al.*, *Proc Natl Acad Sci* USA 91, 9866 (1994).
- Sedegahm M, Jones TR, Kaur M, *et al.*, *Proc Natl Acad Sci* USA 95, 7648 (1998).
- Segal BM, Klinman DM, Shevach EM. *J Immunol* 158, 5087 (1997).
- Shen Z, Reznikoff G, Dranoff G, Rock KL. *J Immunol* 158, 2723 (1997).
- Shirmbeck R, Bohn W, Ando K, *et al.*, *J Virol* 69, 5929 (1995).
- Shiver JW, Davies ME, Yasutomi Y, *et al.*, *Vaccine* 15, 887 (1997).
- Shiver JW, Perry HC, Davies ME, *et al.*, *Ann NY Acad Sci* 772, 198 (1995).
- Simmonds RS, Shearer MH, Kennedy RC. *Parasitol Today* 13, 328 (1997).
- Slater JE, Zhang YL, Arthur-Smith A, *et al.*, *J Allergy Clin Immunol* 99, S504 (1997).
- Spier RE, *Vaccine* 14, 1285 (1996).
- Stratford R, Douce G, Zhang-Barber L, *et al.*, *Vaccine* 19, 810 (2001).
- Sundaram P, Xiao W, Brandsma JL. *Nucleic Acids Res* 24, 1375 (1996).
- Suzuki Y, Remington JS, *J Immunol* 140, 3943 (1988).
- Tang DC, De Vit M, Johnston SA. *Nature* 356, 152 (1992).
- Taracha EL, Bishop R, Musoke AJ, *et al.*, *Infect Immu* 7, 6906 (2003).
- Tarleton RL, *J Immunol* 144, 717 (1990).
- Tarleton RL, Koller BH, Latourm A, *et al.*, *Nature* 356, 338 (1992).
- Tascon RE, Colston MJ, Ragno S, *et al.*, *Nat Med* 2, 888 (1996).
- Taubes G. *Science* 278, 1711 (1997).
- Thomson SA, Sherritt MA, Medveczky J, *et al.*, *J Immunol* 160, 1717 (1998).
- Tokunaga T, Yamamoto H, Shimada S, *J Natl Cancer Inst* 72, 955 (1984).
- Trinchieri G. *Annu Rev Immunol* 13, 251 (1995).
- Uchijima M, Yoshida A, Nagata T, *et al.*, *J Immunol* 161, 5594 (1998).
- Ulmer JB, Deck RR, Dewitt CM, *et al.*, *Immunology* 89, 59 (1996).
- Ulmer JB, Deck RR, Dewitt CM, *et al.*, *Vaccine* 12, 1541 (1994).
- Ulmer JB, Donnelly JJ, Parker SE, *et al.*, *Science*, 259, 1745 (1993).
- Ulmer JB, Liu MA, Momtogomery CM, *et al.*, *Vaccine* 15, 792 (1997).
- Vinner L, Nielson HV, Bryder K, *et al.*, *Vaccine* 17, 2166 (1999).
- Waisman A, Ruiz PI, Hirschberg DL, *et al.*, *Nat Med* 2, 899 (1996).
- Wang B, Boyer J, Srikantan V, *et al.*, *DNA Cell Biol* 12, 799 (1993).
- Wang B, Boyer J, Srikantan V, *et al.*, *Virology* 211, 102 (1995).

- Wang B, Ugen KE, Srikantan V, *et al.*, *Proc Natl Acad Sci* USA 90, 4156 (1993).
- Wang QM, Sun SH, Hu Z, *et al.*, *Vaccine* 22, 3622 (2004).
- Wang R, Doolan DL, Le TP, *et al.*, *Science*, 282, 476 (1998).
- Wang S, Bertley FMN, Kozlowski PA, *et al.*, *Vaccine* 22, 846 (2004).
- Wang S, Heilman D, Liu F, Lus A. *Vaccine* 22, 3348 (2004).
- Wang SW, Kozlowski PA, Schmelz G, *et al.*, *J Virol* 74, 10514 (2000).
- Waris ME, Tsou C, Erdman DD, *et al.*, *J Vinol* 720, 2852 (1996).
- Watts C, *Annu Rev Immunol* 15, 821 (1997).
- Weerathna R, Millan CLB, Krieg AM, *et al. Nucleic Acid Drug Devel* 8, 351(1998).
- Weiner DB, Kennedy RC, Genetic Vaccines, *Sci Amer* July (1999).
- Weiss WR, Berzofsky JA, Houghten RA, *et al.*, *J Immunol* 149, 2103 (1992).
- Weiss WR, Sedegah M, Beaudoin RL, *et al.*, *Proc Natl Acad Sci* USA 85, 573 (1988).
- Whalern RG, Davis HL. *Clin Immunol Immunopathol* 75, 1 (1995).
- Wolff JA, Mallone RW, Williams P, *et al.*, *Science* 247, 1465 (1990).
- Wolff JA, Ludtke JJ, Acsadi G, *et al.*, *Hum Mol Genet,* 1, 363 (1992).
- Wu Y, Wang X, Csencsits KL, *et al.*, *Proc Natl Acad Sci* USA 98, 9318 (2001).
- Xeang ZQ, Spitalnik SL, Cheng J, *et al.*, *Virology* 209, 569 (1995).
- Xiang Z, Ertl HCJ. *Immunity* 2, 129 (1995).
- Xiang ZQ, Spitalnik S, Tran M, *et al.*, *Virology* 199, 132 (1994).
- Xiang ZQ, Spitalnik SL, Cheng J, *et al.*, *Virology* 209, 569 (1995).
- Xu D, Liew FY. *Immunology* 84, 173 (1995).
- Xu L, Sanchez A, Yang ZY, *et al.*, *Nat Med* 4, 37 (1998).
- Xu ZL, Mizuguchi H, Ishii-Watabe A, *et al.*, *Gene* 272, 149-156 (2001).
- Yamamoto S, Yamamoto T, Kataoka T. *J Immunol* 148, 4072 (1992).
- Yang W, Waine GJ, McManus DP. *Biochem Biophys Res Commun* 212, 1029 (1995).
- Yankauckas MA, Morrow JE, Parker SE, *et al.*, *DNA Cell Biol*, 12, 771 (1993).
- Yasutomi Y, Robinson HL, Lu S, *et al.*, *J Virol* 70, 678 (1996).
- Yokoyama M, Zhang J, Whitton JL. *J Virol* 69, 2684 (1995).
- York IA, Rock KL. *Annu Rev Immunol* 14, 369 (1996).
- You Z, Huang X, Hester J, *et al.*, *Cancer Res* 61, 3704 (2001).
- Youmans GP, Youmans ASJ. *Bacteriol* 89, 1291 (1965).
- Zarozinski CC, Fynan EF, Selin LK, *et al.*, *J Immunol* 154, 4010 (1995).
- Zuber AK, Brave A, Engstrom G, *et al.*, *Vaccine* 22, 1791 (2004).

PROTEINS, PROTEOMICS AND THERAPEUTICS

13.1. INTRODUCTION

The terms *proteomics* and *proteome* were coined by Wilkins *et al.* in 1997 to describe the entire collection of proteins encoded by genomes in the human organism. Proteomics differs from protein chemistry at this point since it focuses on multiprotein systems rather than individual proteins and uses partial sequence analysis with the aid of databases. Proteins are the bricks and mortar of the cells, carrying out most of the cellular functions essential for survival of the organism. The definition of proteomics can be summarized in four parts as given in Table 13.1. Each part represents a different aspect of proteomic research and some have even acquired names for all or part of what they encompass.

Table 13.1: Proteomics - a universal definition

- Determination of the structure and function of the complete set of proteins produced by the genome of an organism, including co- and posttranslational modifications
- Determination of the all of the interactions of these proteins with small and large molecules of all types
- Determination of the expression of these proteins as a function of time and physiological condition
- The coordination of this information into a unified and consistent description of the organism at the cellular, organ and whole animal levels

The first part deals primarily with the identification of all the protein components that make up the proteome and can be viewed in some respects as a giant catalog. The simplest form of this list would be the one to one match up of proteins with genes. This can be most easily accomplished in prokaryotes where mRNA splicing does not occur, but still is a realizable, if much larger and more elusive, goal in eukaryotes. It is this aspect of proteomics that most closely parallels genomics and transcriptomics and what undoubtedly gives workers from those fields the highly questionable sense that the proteome is a finite and therefore determinable entity. The final component of this part of the definition is the determination of function for each protein and it is here that one must begin to seriously depart from the cataloging concept. While one can usually connect one or more functions (catalytic, recognitive, structural, etc.) to most proteins, ascribing single functions to proteins is at best a gross simplification of the situation. As taken up in part three, protein-protein interactions, with their resultant effects on activity, are enormously widespread and since the presence or absence of these interactions, along with many co- /posttranslational modifications are time (expression) dependent, simple listings are at best a draconian description of a proteome and are really inadequate to describe function in the cellular context.

While the concept of a 'protein catalog' undoubtedly existed, at least in the minds of some people, prior to the coining of the term proteome, the realization that protein-protein interactions were a dominant feature of proteome function was certainly considerably less clear. However, such is the case and the second part of the definition requires a detailed knowledge of all of these recognitive events, both stable and transient. The elucidation of these interactions and the underlying networks has been termed cell-mapping proteomics (Blackstock & Weir, 1999). This in fact has been a quite productive area of proteomic research, as described below. The third part of the definition clearly represents the greatest challenge in terms of data collection. If the first two parts can be said to loosely represent the 'who, what and how' of proteomics, then the third part is the 'when and where', and is by far the most dynamic of the three. Obtaining this information requires perturbation almost by definition and in essence represents what has been described as 'systems biology'. It is commonly known as 'expression proteomics' (Blackstock & Weir, 1999) and forms the heart of signal transduction studies, a field that has thrived independently and has been one of the major areas of molecular and cellular biology research for the past ten years or more. Major Proteomics directions are shown in Fig. 13.1.

The final part of the definition can, to complete the analogy, is considered the 'why' of proteomics. This part also encompasses the bioinformatics component of proteomics, another vaguely defined discipline that arose from the realization, as genomics moved into full swing, that the amount of information being obtained was increasing, and would continue to do so in an exponential manner and that 'managing' this inundation was a serious challenge in its own right. Proteomics, far more than genomics and transcriptomics, will accelerate this trend and hence data management must be an integral part of the definition.

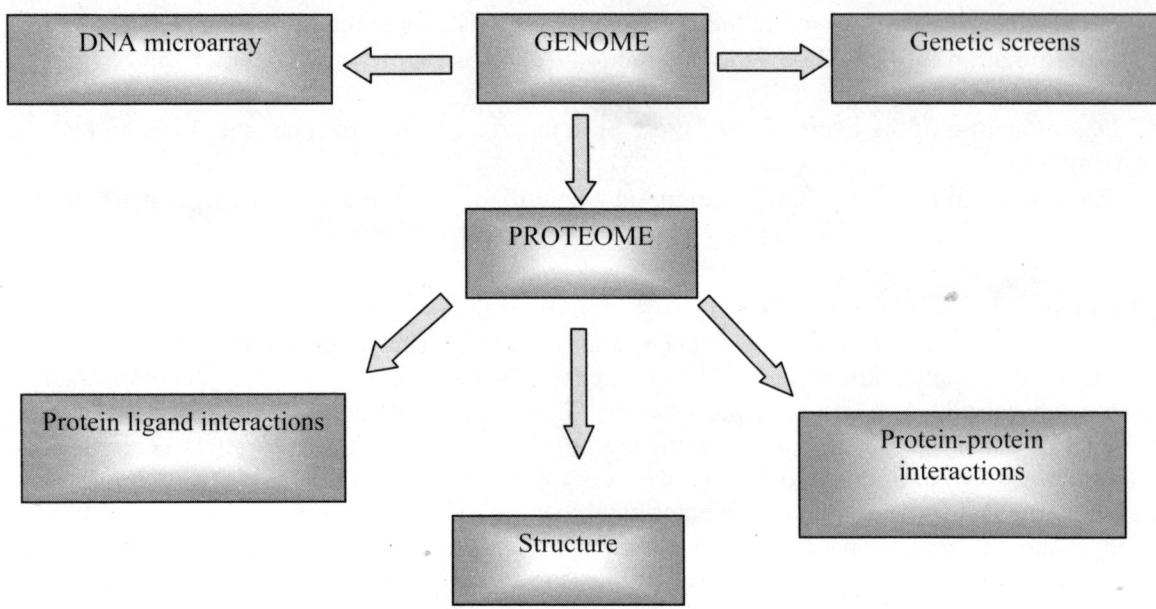

Fig. 13.1: Major proteomics directions

13.2. WHAT IS A PROTEOME?

The term proteome defines a complete protein entity encoded by a specific gene of an organism or cell. Proteome is susceptible to any change in environment unlike the genome. Proteome plays a key role in intracellular signaling pathways of the immune system and intercellular metabolism as being the interface between the cell and the environment. A specific gene produces a protein molecule following a complex pathway (Fig. 13.2).

The amino acid sequence of the molecule can easily be predicted from the nucleotide sequence of the gene. Subsequently, the protein molecule undergoes further modifications at the post-translational stage, resulting in the formation of a protein with different biological activities at the cellular level. Approximately 200 different types of post-translational modifications (folding, oxidation of cysteine, thiols, carboxylation of glutamate) have been described. Modified proteins are then delivered to specific locations in cells to function. Posttranslational modifications significantly influence the process of degradation. For example, some proteins undergo degradation following conjugation with ubiquitin. Proteins have a modular structure comprised of motifs and domains.

Short peptide sequences bring specificity for certain modifications while in most cases longer ones form domains reflecting bulk physical properties as a result of formation of helices in the secondary structure. The translation of the peptide sequence to functions in a protein molecule can be expressed as modular units (motifs and domains) that confer similar properties or functions in a variety of proteins.

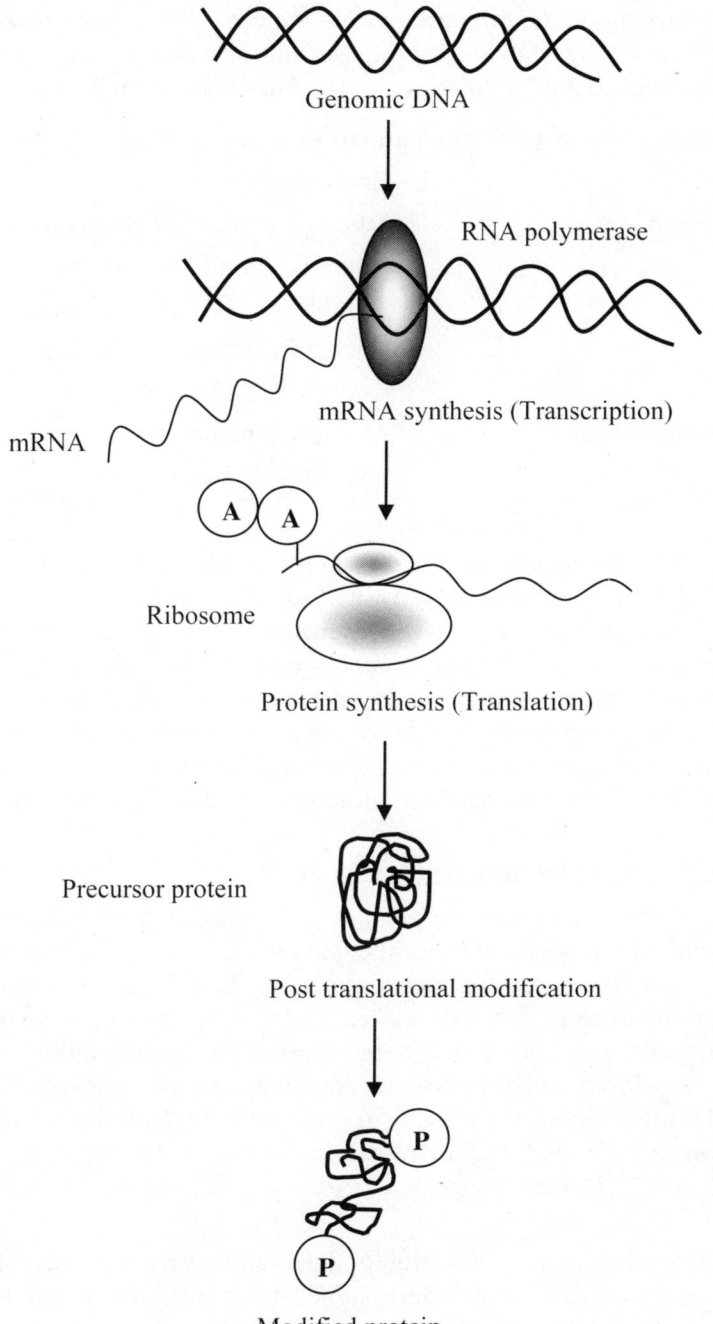

Fig. 13.2: Protein synthesis

Based on characteristics of modular units, proteomes can be classified into families of proteins possessing related functions. For instance, some proteins play a key role in intercellular signaling pathways and some are structural, while others participate in metabolism. Up to 40% of proteins are encoded by the genome and carry out unknown functions, which still need to be discovered. The classification of proteomes revealed the occurrence of "core proteome," indicating the complexity of an organism or a genome and varying number of paralogs among organisms. What makes the human organism complex is not the size of the human genome, but the diversity of human proteomes. A general comparison of protein chemical and proteomic experiments is shown in Table. 13.2

Table 13.2: A comparison of protein chemical vs. proteomic experiments

Protein Chemistry	Proteomics
Function/identity generally known	Function/identity often unknown (Identification from sequences)
Single entity	Complexes of multiple entities (including protein machines)
Single function	Coordinated functions
Free standing (studied as an isolated entity)	Multiple interactions
Focused studies	High throughput

Another important issue is what can be used to predict change in protein levels. In a review of the literature, it is apparent from the measurements in yeast and mouse liver that there is yet no strong correlation between mRNA level and that of proteins, especially in the case of poorly expressed genes. Therefore, conducting gene expression measurements may not be sufficient to infer protein expression. Thus, the analytical methods used in proteomics must provide detection of proteomes present in multiple-modified forms at relatively low levels. Sequences of proteome can be predicted by analytical methods and these will be covered in later parts of this chapter and can be used to define biological activity of proteins. The connection between proteomics and Bioinformatic is given in Fig. 13.3.

13.3. SYSTEMS BIOLOGY – PROTEIN MODIFICATIONS

Systems biology can help us to understand how the genome and proteome respond to environmental changes through the signal-transaction mechanisms of the cell (Kitano, 2002). Suitable mathematical and computational tools have been developed for such approaches. Lee *et al.* (2002) have shown the feasibility of a computational approach to correctly assign all the regulators of a complex network, such as the cell cycle. An algorithm to automatically reconstruct the corresponding transcriptional regularity architecture could be devised without previous knowledge of the molecules involved. This work materialized because the transcriptional mechanism governing the cell cycle follows the same type of patterns off interconnections that are involved in a wide range of complex networks encompassing ecological systems, neuronal synapses, electric circuits, and the Internet (Milo *et al.*, 2002).

Although experimentally-derived genome-wide protein interaction networks have helped in the elucidation of functional information that cannot be obtained from examining individual proteins, analysis of these networks is complicated and time consuming. To tackle this difficulty some computational methods for predicting protein networks in novel genomes have been developed (McDermott and Smudrala, 2004). Phylogenetic profiling can be employed for elucidating novel pathways in proteomes that have not been experimentally characterized. This method, together with other computational methods for generating protein interaction networks, might help identify novel functional pathways and enhance functional annotation of individual proteins (McDermott and Smudrala, 2004).

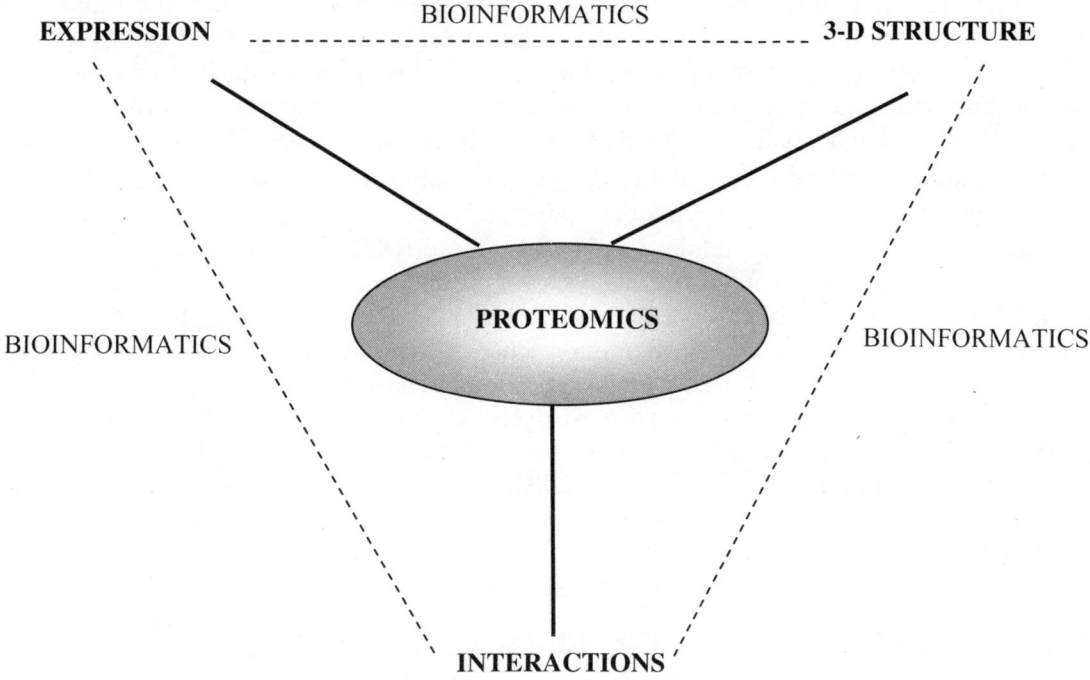

Fig. 13.3: The connection between proteomics and bioinformatics

For instance, experimental techniques have been developed to derive protein interaction networks for yeast and *Helicobacter pylori* (Ito *et al.*, 2001; Rain *et al.*, 2001; Uetz *et al.,* 2000). These networks have a specific topology and functional modularity. The interactions between complexes in specific metabolic pathways are highlighted and many hitherto uncharacterized proteins can be associated with known pathways. Highly connected proteins in the yeast networks have been found to correlate well with essential proteins (Jeong *et al.,* 2001). Besides the transcriptional network, the genome, protenome, metabolome and physiome all follow a power-law distribution in which very few nodes become hubs dominating the entire network by attaching themselves to other, already well interconnected networks (Rangel-Aldao, 2003). A meaningful synthesis of genomics, protenomics, signal transduction, network theory, computing science, non-linear dynamics, and clinical practice, can help in designing appropriate algorithms to visualize dynamic maps of the molecular networks that underlie clinical manifestations of disease (Hasty *et al.,* 2002). These, in turn, can facilitate early diagnosis, prognosis, and risk management (Rangel-Aldao, 2003).

Mass spectrometry has long been a method of choice for characterizing biomolecules such as proteins. But its major limitation has been the inability to quantitative protein levels. Recently developed new methods have overcome this limitation, making possible the study of protein dynamics in cells (Raghothama and Pandey, 2003). To achieve quantitation, certain proteomic methods involving the 'tagging' of proteins or peptides to distinguish different states have been developed. In particular the use of tagged peptides as internal standards has enhanced the utility of mass spectrometers to facilitate absolute quantitation of proteins and post-translational modifications (PTMs). However, while absolute quantitation is sometimes required, in most biological systems it is sufficient to determine relative levels of protein abundance and PTMs. For this purpose, several labelling methods are available that involve chemical modifications *in vitro* by heavy-isotope-containing tags, or labelling *in vivo* by heavy-isotope-containing nutrients (Cagney and Emili, 2002). Examples of *in vitro* methods are biotinylared isotope coded affinity tags (ICATs) for labelling cysteine residues, labelling of N-termini of peptides and labelling of C-terminal lysine residues by guanidination. Likewise, examples of *in vivo* labelling approaches include the use of heavy isotope-labelled media (e.g., ^{15}N) and labelled amino acids (Raghothama and Pandey, 2003).

Two of the commonest PTMs in vertebrate systems that enable absolute or relative quantitation of PTMs are phosphorylation and glycosylation. These regulate, for instance, enzymatic activities, protein- protein interactions and subcellular localization (Wold, 1981; Steen and Pandey, 2002). Use of differentially labelled tags can facilitate analysis of phosphopeptides by mass spectrometry by replacement of the phosphate moiety by a different chemical group during the purification process that provides both enrichment and quantitative information. Quantitation without enrichment may be achieved by employing methods that do not involve introduction of a chemical group. No single available method can allow a comprehensive analysis of the proteome. But recourse to mass spectrometry and refined techniques for quantitation can tackle the huge task of unraveling its dynamic nature. According to Navarro *et al.* (2003), protein databases containing quantitative information are crucial for a systems biology approach. No such databases exist today, but the increasing emphasis being placed on data storage and retrieval, makes it virtually certain that such databases will become available to fulfill the growing needs of the proteomic community.

13.4. PROTEIN FOLDING: NANOENGINEERING OF ALLOSTERY

Several pressing questions of protein folding face scientists today. While the ultimate goal is to be able to predict *de novo* protein folding and unfolding pathways (structure, stability, function and activity from primary structure), some success in moving towards this goal may be achieved by focusing on those aspects of the problem that have some chance of near-term solution. Important areas in this context can be *de novo* design and evolution, protein misfolding, and protein dynamics and allostery (Sagermann *et al.,* 2003). Sagermann *et al.* (2003) described a phage T4 lysozyme mutant that incorporates a tandem duplication of a α- helix. Although only one repeat can occupy the equivalent wild-type location, structure can be induced to switch to the alternative repeat by modifications to an adjacent turn. This finding highlights the interactions between the stabilizing forces of adjacent secondary structures and suggests a novel mechanism for allostery over long distances (Blaber, 2003). The work identifies a design principle by which a defined conformational change may conceivably be engineered and regulated to generate allostery. The structural changes associated with allostery have always interested protein researchers because the dynamic motions of proteins in relation to their overall 3D structure are crucial to their function. The structural change reported in the tandem-repeat T4 lysozyme mutant exemplified a type of helical shift that was observed in the allostery of aspartate receptors by Yu and Koshland (2001); it constitutes a mechanism by which structural changes are transmitted over long distances.

13.5. THE EVOLUTION OF ALLOSTERY

Some of the many known fundamental protein superfolds (e.g., triose phosphate isomerase (TIM) barrel, β-trefoil, 'jelly roll', IG-like and 'up-down' superfolds) show a marked structural symmetry and many proteins probably evolved through gene duplication or fusion events (Mukhopadhyaya, 2000; Ponting and Russel, 2000; Lang *et al.,* 2000; Blaber, 2003). From this it follows that the manner in which a protein responds to a duplicated region results from protein evolution – although the symmetry of protein superfolds can be quite high at the level of the tertiary structure, it is often lacking at the level of the primary structure. It is conceivable that the constraints that primary structure symmetry could impose on protein folding and stability may well be a critical factor in the *de novo* protein synthesis (Blaber, 2003). A common connection between structural duplication, turn stability, allostery, symmetry, evolution and *de novo* protein design may exits. Enhancing our understanding of the nature of the energetics of turn secondary structure should be a high priority goal for advancing our understanding of the protein-folding problem.

One of the dogmas in molecular biology has been that the biological function of a protein is strictly related to its three-dimensional structure in the folded state. This dogma now needs to be slightly modified: recent evidence points to the existence of soluble proteins that either lack a well-defined folded structure, or contain disordered segments (Wright and Dyson, 1999; Dyson and Wright, 2002). A computer analysis of known proteins with intrinsic disorders has indicated unstructured regions of 40 or more consecutive residues in up to about 60 % of the genome of five eukaryotes (Dunker and Obradovic, 2001). Some proteins are partially unstructured under physiological conditions and assume a well-defined three-dimensional structure only upon binding to another protein or macromolecular complex. Several such examples have been found among proteins involved in regulatory functions in eukaryotic cells (Caflisch, 2003). Verkhivker *et al.* (2003) investigated the coupled folding and binding of p27 to the cyclin A-cyclin dependent kinase 2 (CDK2) complexes, which is involved in cell cycle regulation. They derived an atomic picture of the transition state assemble (TSE) and the sequence of events for folding and binding. By carrying out computer simulations of protein unfolding and unbinding, Verkhivker *et al.* (2003) have proposed a sequence of structural events for p27, with to the cyclin A-cyclin dependent kinase 2 (CDK2) complexes, which is involved in cell cycle regulation. The derived an atomic picture of the transition state ensemble (TSE) and the sequence of events for p27, with β-hairpin and β-strand folding preceding α-helix formation. It is intended to validate such simulations experimentally by site-directed mutagenesis and rate measurements.

According to Caflisch (2003), it might prove rewarding to study the behavior of p27 with (partial) flexibility in the cyclin A-CDK2 complex, so as to eventually compare this with high temperature molecular dynamics simulations (Frenkel and Smit, 2002; Karplus and McCamman, 2002). The sugar coatings that are used to decorate proteins are actually more than ornamental frosting – the specific sugars and their manner of attachment ensure that proteins undergo correct folding and remain stable. GlycoFi is now producing   sugar-coated human proteins in yeast – a feat that could provide much higher yields than the current standard method of manufacturing proteins in Chinese hamster ovary cells, which takes over a fortnight to produce even small amounts. Yeast is expected to do the same in three days. But yeast does not normally have chemical pathways to put the right sugars on proteins; therefore, GlycoFi is engineered assembly lines of enzymes from variety of species, with a view to obtain better yields, lower production costs and longer-lasting, more potent drugs.

13.6. PROTEIN TRANSDUCTION TECHNOLOGY

The human cell membrane happens to be impermeable to most peptides, proteins, DNA and oligonucleotides. This property limits the therapeutic potential of these biological agents. But some short cationic peptides can cross the plasma membrane efficiently. This has generated new possibilities for the intracellular delivery of these peptides, commonly referred to as protein transduction domains (PTDs). PTDs have been successfully used to transport heterogeneous, proteins, peptides and other types of cargo into cells (Kabouridis, 2003). As PTDs can transducer the cell membrane, they can be employed *in vivo* to deliver biologically active cargo into various tissues.

Determining and controlling the function of a protein in a living cell requires either expression of mutant forms of the proteins or silencing of its concerned gene. This has been achieved by transgene expression, either using recombinant vectors or directly introducing proteins into cells by such cumbersome techniques as microinjection, electroporation or red-dell ghost fusion (Gomperts and Fernandez, 1985; Chang *et al.,* 1991). A novel technology for the direct delivery of biological material has recently emerged with the finding that certain proteins can enter cells in an unconventional way. The TAT protein, which transactivation factor from the human immunodeficiency virus 1 (HIV-1) has been the first reported polypeptide that can enter into cells when supplied in the culture medium (Green and Loewenstein, 1988; Mann and Franke, 1991). Some other proteins also can cross the plasma membrane. The identification of short membrane-permeable cationic peptides derived from these proteins, and synthesis of certain other amphipathic peptides prompted the development of a new technology for delivering biological agents into cells (Wadia and Dowdy, 2002). These peptides are generally termed protein transduction domains (PTDs).

Several proteins, both wild type and mutated, have been transduced into cells after their fusion to PTDs (Fawell *et al.*, 1994; Kabouridis, 2003). PTDs have also been used to deliver drug carriers such as liposomes, DNA-DNA or liposome DNA complexes, peptide nucleic acids, and phage particles (Torchilin *et al.,* 2001, 2003). Several recent reports have appeared on using this technology to deliver bioactive agents *in vivo*. This points therapeutic potential of protein transduction technology. In most work so far, transduction tissues *in vivo* have been achieved by injection of purified PTD-protein. It appears that membrane transducing peptides may aid the absorption of those drugs that penetrate poorly in tissues, such as the cyclosporine A (CsA), which is only weakly absorbed by the skin.

Protein transduction technology has become a useful tool in biology and medicine. It could have considerable potential application not only in the clinic but also in the regulation of signal transduction pathways that underlie some pathological disorders. Although viral vectors are being used to introduce genes into cells, they suffer from simultaneous entry of unwanted and/or harmful genetic material and also because expression levels of the transgene cannot be controlled. By contrast, PTD-mediated delivery makes possible temporal and reversible regulation of a biological process by directly controlling intracellular levels of inhibitors (Kabouridis, 2003). Inhibitors can be administered, stopped and administered again to minimize detrimental side effects. Unfortunately, two major limitations of PTD technology are its inadequacy for *in vivo* applications, and lack of targeting specificity. At the least it would be essential to establish that PTD-chimera benefits diseased cells while producing no adverse effects on healthy tissue (Kabouridis, 2003).

13.7. PROTEINS FOR PROTEOMICS – UNDERSTANDING PROTEIN FUNCTION FOR HUMAN HEALTH

Proteins being the engines of biological systems, not only most pharmaceuticals act on them but proteins themselves are being increasingly used therapeutically. Many assays are based on the use of highly purified proteins. Biology having already entered the post-genomic era, the exciting opportunity has arisen of studying proteins in high throughput (HT) experiments, by means of a great variety of techniques that range from enzyme catalysis assays to interaction and structural studies (Braun and LaBaer, 2003). Countless novel protein-coding sequences have been discovered. The increasing availability of large cDNA sequences has made it possible to study protein function critically at an unprecedented scale. There is an urgent need for developing HT methods for protein isolation and proteome scale protein expression systems. There are two broad classes of applications of high-throughput protein expression and purification. In one class HT protein expression is used as a first step to screen for optimal conditions or gene constructs before scaling up for high yield protein production. Most protein crystallization and the production of protein affinity reagents require at least milligram quantities of protein. It is often quite difficult to obtain such large quantities because proteins sometimes express poorly or fold improperly when produced in heterologous systems (Braun and LaBaer, 2003). The trial-and error attempts to express different versions of the target protein are often highly time consuming and usually fail unless and until a well-expressing, soluble, correctly folded construct is identified. Many constructs have to be screened simultaneously in a multi-well format so as to speed up this screening process.

In the category of applications, the HT expression of proteins is used directly. Several methods for HT biochemical experiments have been reported. Applications such as protein microarrays (MacBeath and Schreiber, 2000; Zhu *et al.*, 2001), multi-well solution biochemistry (King *et al.*, 1997), and isolation of protein complexes for mass spectrometric analysis (Gavin *et al.*, 2000; Ho *et al.*, 2002) can gain much from better methods for HT protein isolation, and HT protein expression systems may soon become an important common application in the post genomic era. *Escherichia coli* happen to be the simplest and the most widely used organism for protein expression. Its advantages include its speed, ease of use and low cost, but these advantages are sometimes offset by the lack of eukaryotic post-translational modifications (PTMs) and the low solubility of some proteins (Braun *et al.*, 2002; Hammarstrom *et al.*, 2002; Waldo, 2003). One crucial aspect of recombinant protein production is the functional integrity of the produced proteins. The estimates made by Christendat *et al.* (2000) showed that more than one-half of 100 soluble proteins from *E. coli* might be in a state of aggregation and hence potentially nonfunctional. Yee *et al.* (2002) also found that the NMR spectra of 27% to 55% of proteins (depending on the organism) that were soluble in *E. coli* suffered aggregation or conformational instability of the protein. However, although these reports have generated some skepticism, the fact remains that thousands of functional proteins have been successfully produced in bacteria and also that *E. coli* remains the most widely used protein expression system (Braun and LaBaer, 2003).

Cell-free expression systems are especially useful for HT applications because the absence of a cell membrane obviates the need for any harsh steps associated with introducing DNA into cells, lysing cells and clearing lysate. Expression systems from eukaryotic cell lysates have the additional benefit that most PTMs take place properly. Some widely used open expression systems are bacterial, wheat germ and reticulocyte lysates. Protein yields from such systems can give high yields of up to 6 mg ml^{-1} for individual proteins (Kigawa *et al.*, 1999). Indeed, the exclusively in bacterial cell-free expression systems. In recent years, the yeast (*Saccharomyces cerevisiae*) has attracted considerable interest as a protein expression system. It has the advantages of an inexpensive, fast growing unicellular organism as well as the properties of a eukaryotic cell.

13.8. PROTEOMICS FOR BIOMAKERS AND DRUG TARGETS

Although protenomics5 technologies (i.e., a basket of technologies and tools for studying the proteome) have greatly aided the discovery of potential biomarkers and drug targets, this success has also created a bottleneck. While throughput and high-output technologies are used to discover potential biomarkers and drug targets, the preliminary validation methods are low-throughput and low-output (Bodovitz and Joos, 2003). This constraint can however be addressed by adopting several strategies. The first is to reduce the number of potential biomarkers and drug targets by dividing the proteome into smaller segments. Another possibility is to widen the bottleneck with higher-output and higher-throughput screening technologies. Also, a more preliminary validation may be incorporated into the discovery process.

Today, the rate of discovering potential biomarkers and drug targets exceeds the rate of preliminary validation, and the gap is expected to increase (Bodovitz and Joos, 2003). It appears that our ability to collect large datasets also exceeds the ability to validate, interpret and integrate these data for generating biological knowledge (Patterson and Aebersold, 2003). Several recent technological advances are enabling more and more protein features to be studied rapidly. These modern technologies can reveal many of the underlying differences between the proteomes of healthy and diseased tissues (Bodovitz and Joos, 2003). But, differences alone do not necessarily always make potential biomarkers and drug targets valuable. Preliminary validation is no less important. The best way to fully validate potential biomarkers is to test them across a large number of subjects. Potential drug targets can be fully validated only by testing the corresponding potential therapeutics in clinical trials. Since full validation is extremely costly, recourse is had to preliminary triage. Here the problem is that such high-output technologies for discovery as 2D-gel electrophoresis, chromatography and mass spectrometry give way to low throughput, low-output technologies for preliminary validation. Researchers depend on such basic methods as western blots, immuno-histochemistry, and enzyme and pathway activation assays. The limitation of these methods is that they cannot even deal with a few dozens of potential leads in parallel, *let al*one the thousands that emerge regularly from dedicated proteomics program (Page *et al.,* 1999).

One way to address this constraint is to improve fractionation to reduce sample complexity. The simplest methods for sampling the proteome are based on the general physical properties of proteins. 2D-gel electrophoresis, the commonest method for dividing the proteome, fractionates based on solubilization, isoelectric point and size, and proves highly suitable for the separation of intricate patterns of differentially modified and processed proteins, but its low sensitivity and low resolution limit the number of proteins that can be identified. Chromatography can be an attractive gel-free alternative. Proteins from complex mixtures may be divided effectively by using two or three orthogonal separation methods in sequence, such as cation exchange and capillary reverse-phase chromatography. Exciting breakthroughs in fractionation methods to widen the bottleneck are likely to come from those that are based on function and/or functional associations. One biologically significant fractionation method involves the isolation of protein complexes. Hartwell *et al.* (1999) put forward the interesting idea that a cell is not merely a collection of isolated proteins, but rather a collection of interconnected modules. The study of protein complexes can lead to an initial assessment of the feasibility of further development by linking a potential biomarker or target with a protein of known function. Indeed Gavin *et al.* (2002) and von Mering *et al.* (2002) have used affinity-tagged bait proteins expressed in yeast cells to isolate protein complexes. Thousands of protein interactions could be identified in these studies many of which were hitherto unknown.

13.9. BETTER SCREENING

Another option to broadening the bottleneck is to use parallel screening methods such as bead-based and protein-biochip technologies. These new technologies enable researchers to take thousands of leads from discovery and examine them in parallel. Specific proteins and/or post-translational modifications can be captured and quantitated by using beads or biochips with immobilized antibodies or antibody fragments and interactions as well as post-translational modifications are studied by using beads or biochips with immobilized peptides, proteins or carbohydrates. Unfortunately, growth of the capture segment is limited by the lack of high-quality capture agents having high affinity and selectivity suitable to be used in combination on the surface of a bead or biochip, and that can be generated in a time-scale compatible with that of the rate of discovery (Bodovitz, 2003).

13.10. VALIDATION FOLLOWING DISCOVERY

The bottleneck can also be reduced by constraining the discovery process in such a way that the potential biomarkers and drug targets arise with some preliminary validation. For this, proteomics has to be combined with, for instance, chemistry or cell biology. The integration of proteomics and chemistry exploits compounds and/or structure-activity relationships to identify druggable targets. Also, small molecule modulators may be used as tools to either inhibit or strengthen the activity of a protein target and observe the physiological results, enabling even better validation. Likewise, an integration of proteomics and cell biology facilitates the discovery of protein targets connected to specific phenotypic changes, showing that the targets play dominant roles in physiologically significant pathways. It is now emerging that success in discovery cannot accrue for long without concomitant advances in preliminary validation.

The polymerase chain reaction (PCR) and other forms of target amplification have catalyzed many advances in the development of effective tools for detecting and quantifying DNA targets for clinical applications (Nam *et al.,* 2003). The development of comparable target amplification methods for proteins could substantially improve medical diagnostics and the developing field of proteomics. Although one cannot yet chemically duplicate protein targets, it is possible to tag such targets with oligonucleotide markers that can be subsequently amplified with PCR and then use DNA detection to identify the target of interest (Schweitzer *et al.,* 2002). This so called immuno-PCR approach makes possible the detection of proteins with DNA markers in a variety of different formats. Nam *et al.* (2003) designed a sensitive method for detecting protein analytes. It relies on magnetic microparticle probes with antibodies that specifically bind a target of interest e.g., prostate-specific antigen (PSA), and nanoparticle probes that are encoded with DNA that is unique to the protein target of interest and antibodies that can sandwich the target captured by the microparticle probes. Magnetic separation of the complexed probes and target followed by dehybridization of the oligonucleotides on the nanoparticle probe surface allows the finding of the target protein by identifying the oligonucleotide sequence released from the nanoparticle probe. Because this probe carries with it a large number of oligonucleotides per protein binding event, there is substantial amplification and PSA can be detected at 30 attomolar concentration. Alternatively, a polymerase chain reaction on the oligonucleotide bar codes can boost the sensitivity to 3 attomolar. Comparable clinically accepted conventional assays for detecting the same target have sensitivity limits of - 3 picomolar six orders of magnitude less sensitive than what is observed with this method (Nam *et al.,* 2003).

13.11. QUANTITATIVE PROTEOMICS

Two possible proteomics approaches for determining the function of proteins (i) the identification of components of protein complexes, or (ii) study of protein-protein interactions. Identification of proteins cannot provide all the required information for assessing protein pathways. Monitoring of protein levels is indispensable for understanding various biological processes. The abundance of proteins within cells is regulated at three different levels, viz., transcriptional, translational, and post-translational. This generates discrepancies between mRNA and protein levels (Griffin *et al.,* 2002; Steen and Pandey, 2002). The relative abundance of proteins can be compared in two related states and quantitated by comparing staining intensities of proteins separated by using gel electrophoresis. Fluorescent dyes with high sensitivity and a large linear dynamic range have been developed (Berggren *et al.,* 2000). Mass spectrometry, *per se,* does not provide quantitative information, but some labeling approaches in combination with mass spectrometry do facilitate quantitatation of relative protein levels. Schematic representation of high-resolution mass spectrometry is shown in Fig. 13.4.

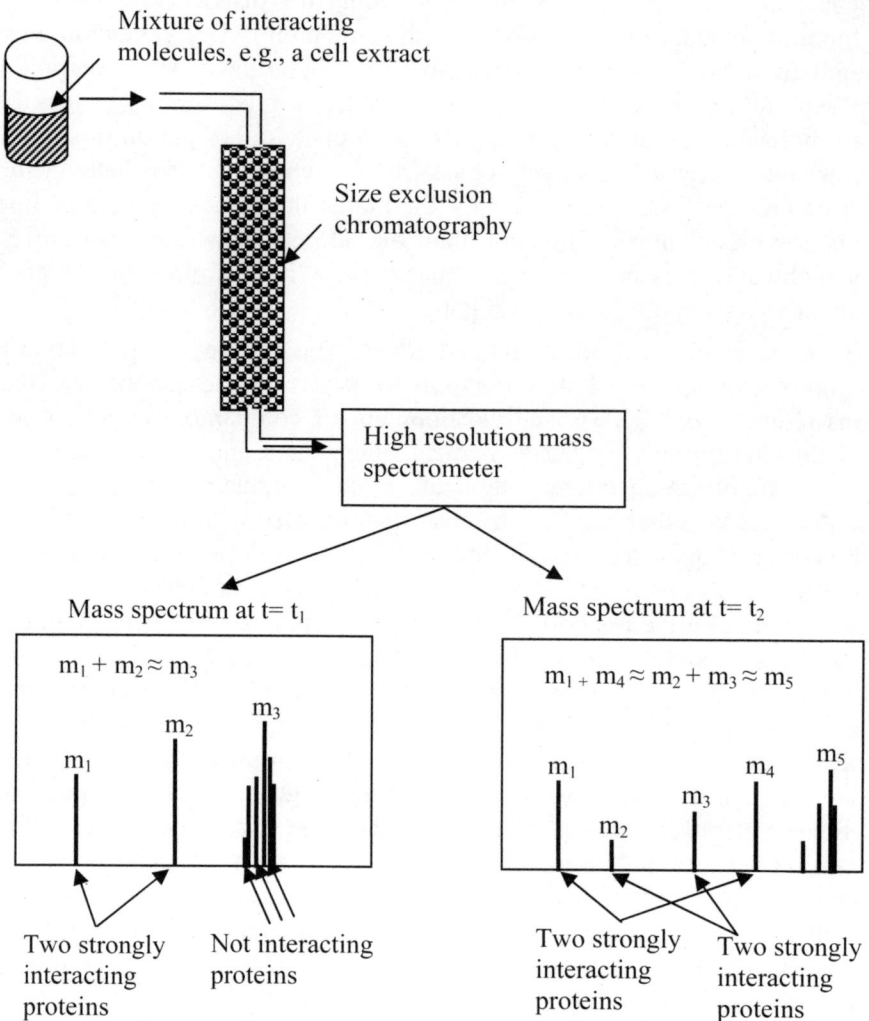

Mixture of interacting molecules, e.g., a cell extract

Size exclusion chromatography

High resolution mass spectrometer

Mass spectrum at t= t_1

$m_1 + m_2 \approx m_3$

m_1 m_2 m_3

Two strongly interacting proteins

Not interacting proteins

Mass spectrum at t= t_2

$m_1 + m_4 \approx m_2 + m_3 \approx m_5$

m_1 m_2 m_3 m_4 m_5

Two strongly interacting proteins

Two strongly interacting proteins

Fig. 13.4: High-resolution mass spectrometry allows the simultaneous mapping-out of a large number of protein-protein and protein-drug interactions without needing microarrays: A fast size exclusion chromatography separates the complicated mixture of interacting molecules into fractions. The parameters for chromatography were chosen such that strongly interacting molecule complexes remain together. Chromatographic fractions are then mass-spectrometrically analyzed. Strongly interacting dimers of molecules appear in the spectrogram as pairs with a total mass of about that of the monomers in the fraction

In fact, protein-based methodologies are rapidly catching up with established DNA-based methods. Recent developments in mass spectrometry enable high throughput automated identification of proteins, as is already the case with DNA sequencing methods. Furthermore, methods for the quantitation of relative protein abundance at the protein level are getting more advanced and these can complement gene expression monitoring at the mRNA level (Zhang and Regnier, 2002; Oda *et al.,*

2002; Cagney and Emili, 2002; Steen and Pandey, 2002). Schematic representation of MALDI-TOFF analyzer is shown in Fig. 13.5.

Some notable mass spectrometry-based methods for relative quantitation of proteins are the following:

- ICAT (Isotope-coded affinity tags).
- MCAT (Mass-coded affinity tags).
- Modification of the N-termini
- Methyl esterification.
- ^{18}O labelling of C-termini.
- Growth in media having stable isotope containing amino acids.

Most of the labeling approaches can only be used for relative quantitation of protein abundance because one sample set is used as internal standard without further knowledge of the absolute amounts. Another limitation is the quantitation of dynamic protein modifications such as phosphorylation where the abundance of the protein remains virtually unchanged. Future research should be directed to the development of a series of isotope labels that could allow the relative quantitation of more than two cell states or more than one modification at a time (Steen and Pandey, 2002). Common proteomic methods are shown in Fig.13.6 Researchers on molecular biology can easily detect very minute quantities of genetic material in a molecular sea by means of the polymerase chain reaction (PCR). Very soon biochemists may also have access to an equally revolutionary technique that can enable them to spot minuscule amounts of particular proteins in a biochemical soup (Service, 2003).

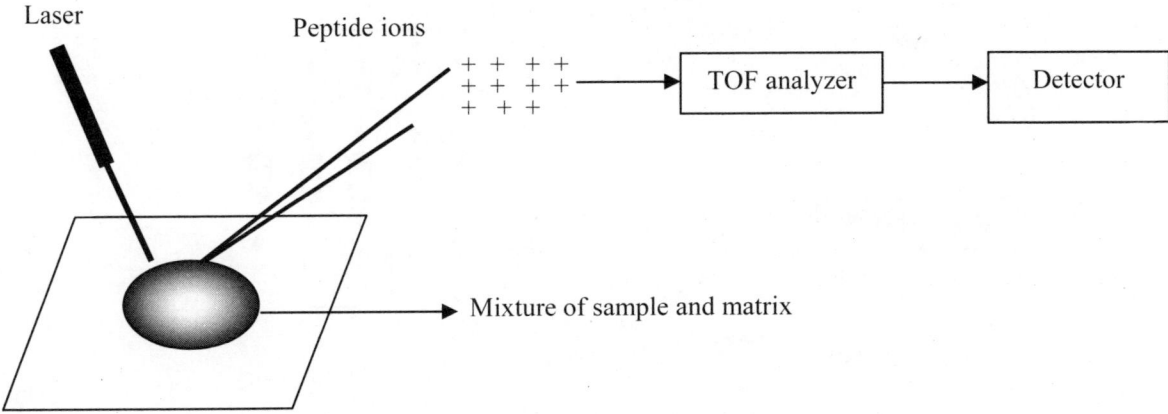

Fig. 13.5: Schematic representation of MALDI-TOFF analyzer

13.12. TINY PARTICLES FOR LOCATING SCARCE PROTEINS

Nam *et al.* (2003) have described a new technique that can turn specks of iron and gold into biochemical bloodhounds that detect target proteins with a million fold higher sensitivity than in the conventional approach. This revolutionary technique may help researchers on proteomics to spot proteins present in only small traces and link their changing concentrations to a variety of diseases.

This can potentially help doctors in diagnosing ailments before they overwhelm the body. Nam *et al.* (2003) have been using tiny metal particles to detect DNA sequences that can point to the presence of anything from cancer cells to the anthrax bacteria. But this approach could not compete with PCR. So Mirkin and associates experimented on something that PCR cannot detect-proteins. They focused on prostate-specific antigen (PSA), a protein that can indicate prostate cancer in men. To detect PSA, the researchers started with two types of particles; 1-μm plastic spheres with magnetic iron cores, and even smaller nonmagnetic gold nanoparticles. The iron particles were linked to genetically engineered proteins called monoclonal antibodies, designed to bind to PSA using the same molecular handle. The gold nanoparticles were linked to "polyclonal" antibodies designed to bind to PSA at different sites, and the researchers also tagged them with numerous pieces of single stranded DNA bound to even shorter complementary strands. These short strands served as "bio-bar codes" for identifying the PSA protein to which the nanoparticles bound (Serivce, 2003; Nam *et al.*, 2003).

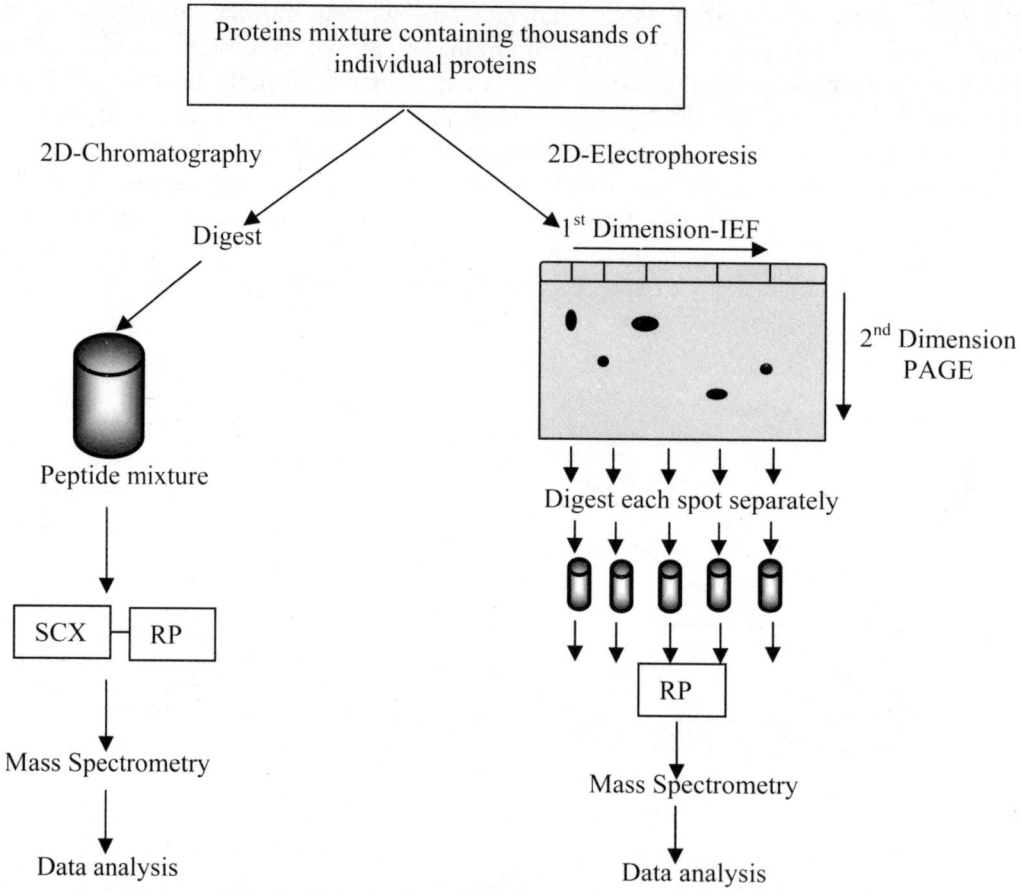

Fig. 13.6: Proteomics methods

Both sets of nanoparticles were added to solutions containing PSA proteins. Both the monoclonal and polyclonal antibodies bound to the PSA, sandwiching the target proteins between the particles. A magnetic field was then applied so as to attract the magnetic particles to the side of the test tube. When PSA was present, both it and any attached DNA-toting nanoparticles were dragged along as well. Another standard solution was then used to make the DNA fragment release the "bar code" strands; the bar codes were tested using standard DNA detection schemes (Service, 2003). The approach was successful. The bar codes on each gold nanoparticle amplified the signal, thus making it possible to detect extremely small quantities of their target protein. The team (Nam *et al., 2003*) claims to be able to detect proteins at concentrations of just 3 attomolar, or about 18 to 20 copies of a protein in 10 microliters of a solution. By contrast, the conventional antibody-based PSA detection scheme can spot only PSA present at 3 picomolars, a million fold higher concentrations.

13.13. APPLICATIONS OF FUNCTIONAL 'RNAs' IN PROTEOMICS AND GENOMICS

Short interfering (si) RNAs and other non-natural, functional RNA molecules modulate gene function at the mRNA or protein level. Famulok and Verma (2002) discussed some recent advances reported in the expression and application of these functional RNAs and explained how engineered, intracellularly active RNAs can serve as potential therapeutic agents.

Table 13.3: Biotechnology companies using NMR and X-ray for proteomic studies

Company	Technologies Used for Proteomics
Vertex Pharmaceuticals	NMR, x-ray, computational chemistry, chemogenomics
RiboTargets	NMR, x-ray, RiboDock software
Gene Formatics	NMR, x-ray, Fuzzy Functional Form Technology, bioassay development
Integrative Proteomics	NMR, x-ray, high throughput protein production
Metabometrix	NMR metabonomics
Novaspin Biotech	NMR, software development, biochemistry

Rapidly accumulating data through numerous genome-wide sequencing projects has created an urgent need to not only develop novel tools for the discovery and validation of drug targets, but also to generate novel concepts in drug therapy. Functional, synthetic RNA molecules, such as siRNAs, protein-binding RNA motifs (aptamers) and catalytic RNAs (ribozymes, maxizymes and aptazymes, (Kuwabara, 2000), are effective, specific tools in functional genomics and proteomics, possibly leading to newer approaches in gene therapy. Such genetic knockdown technologies as antisense, ribozymes and RNA interference (RNAi) permit inactivation of genes without directly manipulating the gene of interest (Rossi, 1995, 1999; Branch, 1998). Alternatively, intracellularly expressed RNA aptamers (intramers) may be used to modulate gene function at the protein level.

13.14. INTRACELLULARLY EXPRESSED CATALYTIC NUCLEIC ACIDS

Ribozymes and deoxyribozymes can be used to suppress the expression of therapeutically relevant genes in cells, tissues and organisms, to analyze the function of genes in eukaryotic cells', and in gene repair. Sometimes, a target site on a mRNA becomes inaccessible to ribozymes owing to complex secondary and tertiary nucleic acid structures. This limitation has been overcome by Warashina *et al.* (2001) who engineered RNA-protein hybrid ribozymes that can access sites on target RNA, independently of its folding. Hybrid ribozyme libraries, containing randomized substrate-binding arms, have been introduced into a breast carcinoma cultured cells (MCF-7) using a retroviral expression system (Kawasaki and Taira, 2002). Surviving clones can be collected after 72 h and genomic DNAs containing ribozymes isolated, PCR amplified with ribozyme-specific primers, and the resulting ribozyme sequences are determined. Cognate target gene sequences of various ribozymes have been located and identified by database searches. Poly (A)-linked ribozyme pools are more effective for gene function studies than are non poly (A) linked ribozymes. The poly (A)-connected ribozymes can potentially increase the efficiency of their own co-localization with the target mRNA (Famulok and Verma, 2002).

13.15. EXPRESSION OF "siRNAs"

siRNAs are RNA duplexes containing "21-23 nucleotides" that can inhibit expression of mammalian genes with complementary sequences by RNAi (Tuschl, 2001). Vector systems have been constructed that allow stable intracellular expression of siRNAs, facilitating development of a powerful method for rapid analysis of loss-of-function phenotypes in mammalian cells; this may have potential application in the generation of transgenic animals. Several recent studies (Tuschl, 2002; Lee *et al.,* 2002; Miyagishi and Taira, 2002) have shown that intracellular siRNA expression reliably inhibits expression of targeted genes. Stable expression of si RNAs should enable functional analysis of cellular genes that are difficult to treat with exogenous siRNAs (e.g., human T-cells); also serve as a starting point for novel gene-based therapeutic applications to treat persistent viral infections (Tuschl, 2002).

13.16. TARGETING OF INTRACELLULAR PROTEINS BY "RNA" INTRAMERS

Although the above approaches are extremely useful for assessing gene function, they do not usually indicate whether a target qualifies for inhibition by antagonistic mechanisms (Famulok and Verma, 2002). This limits the utility of genetic knockdown approaches for comprehensive validation of a protein target direct recognition and inhibition of a protein target by an inhibitory molecule is required. This has focused attention to approaches yielding additional information about the function of a protein by inactivating it directly in its natural compartment. Rapid identification of specific inhibitors for such targets is badly needed to meet increasing demand for validation of many potential targets in the post-genomics era. The more important requirements include: routine applicability; performance independent of the target; ready automation; compatibility with molecules that cover nearly unlimited shape-space and which can be unambiguously identified within complex mixtures; and finally, applicability in an intracellular context (Famulok and Verma, 20(2). All these requirements are satisfied by *in vitro* selection of functional nucleic acids, so that they allow rapid selection of aptamers, specific binders and potential protein inhibitors, which are easily isolated from randomized nucleic acid libraries containing up to 10^{15} different molecules. Aptamers are readily expressed inside cells and can change cell phenotypes by modulating the biological function of the targeted protein. These intracellularly expressed functional aptamers are termed 'intramers'. Intramers permit precise investigation of specific molecules, for example specific discrimination of homologous proteins; indeed, they are just as effective as monoclonal antibodies in studying some functional characteristics. Intramers have been successfully applied for inhibiting HIV-I Rev protein function (Good *et al.*, 1997; Konokpa *et al.,* 2000). These functional probes also inhibit endogenous proteins in the nucleus and in the cytoplasm. Blind *et al.* (1999) has reported intramer-mediated modulation of cytoplasmic membrane-protein domain function leading to highly specific cellular effects.

In fact, intramers have emerged as powerful tools for modulating cytoplasmic membrane-protein domain function, leading to highly specific cellular effects (Kolanus and ZeitImann, 1998). Efficient combinatorial selection of an inhibitor, combined with an active intracellular expression in an appropriate cellular compartment, may probably be successfully applied for studying individual protein function. The availability of several other intracellular RNA expression systems has generated the possibility to express intramers in the same ways as to siRNAs or ribozymes. According to Famulok and Verma, aptamers can be obtained more easily by automated selection techniques but they still need to be characterized biochemically to determine whether or not they act as inhibitors. In this context, siRNA and helicase-recruiting technologies provide a more simple and viable rationale for the design of the targeting agent than does aptamer (intramer) technology. But since intramer technology does provide some valuable information about the proteome, it effectively complements siRNA and helicase-recruiting technologies for target validation and drug discovery processes. What has not so far been demonstrated is whether intramers can target a wide variety of proteins inside cells. Moreover, it would be desirable to design generally applicable systems that allow expression of intramers under the control of inducible endogenous promoters to ascertain that the intramer is reliably co-localized with the target.

13.17. INTEGRATING ANTIBODY PHAGE DISPLAY WITH PROTEOMICS

The current challenge in 'post genomic' research is to understand gene function by analyzing the proteome. This challenge can be addressed by means of antibodies. Analysis of over 90,000 human gene products requires high throughput methods for antibody generation. In contrast to animal-based methods, *in vitro* selection systems using recombinant antibodies offer this capability (Hust and Dubel, 2004). Antibody phage display is the most commonly used contemporary system, which has provided a large number of antibodies for therapy and diagnostics. Numerous cloning and mutagenesis strategies have been developed to create, preserve and exploit maximal antibody diversity, and libraries of different antibody formats have been created from different genetic sources (Hoogenboom, 1997). Studies of various phage-display libraries indicate that the present focus on generating human therapeutic antibodies has yielded methods that are not readily applicable to postgenomic research. A streamlined process needs to be defined by closely integrating antigen logistics with library and antibody formats, panning procedures and robotic handling (Hust and Dubel, 2004). Only by optimizing the interplay of biology, bioinformatics and technology can an affordable high-throughput process be generated to meet the demands of proteome analysis and microarray technology (Hust and Dubel, 2004).

After the sequencing of the genome of any organism, the research focus shifts to the analysis of gene products and their functions. The human genome codes for about 31,000 genes but as a result of alternative mRNA splicing and posttranslational modifications such as glycosylation and phosphorylation the number of different proteins of the human proteome is more than about 90,000 (Harrison *et al.,* 2002). This means that for each gene, we need tools to determine the amount, location and function of its products-while the genotype defines the species of an organism, the proteome defines the phenotype (Hust and Dubel, 2004).

Biologists use protein arrays (or chips) as tools to study protein expression on a global scale. These arrays are made by spotting hundreds of capture molecules onto a solid surface, which is then used to analyze a particular sample for protein content. Many of the first protein arrays used antibodies as capture molecules (Macbeath and Schreiber, 2000; Haab *et al.,* 2001), because antibodies display a very high specificity of action (even distinguishing between functional groups on a molecule) as a result of the elegant structure of their binding sites. However, recent studies have generated doubts about the usefulness of antibodies in such formats in view of concerns as to whether antibodies really are sufficiently specific (Service, 2001; Mitchell, 2002). This may be because the investigators do not select antibodies for the properties that they are expected to display in a particular application. For instance, if the application is antibody microarrays, then the antibodies must be stable and functional in the microarray format. This problem may be addressed by designing a recombinant antibody library on the basis of a single framework, such as that based on single-chain Fv (scFv) fragments. As all scFvs in such a library share the same molecular scaffold, the most stable framework can be adopted, resulting in very similar on-the-chip behavior by scFvs with different specificities (Wingren *et al.,* 2003). Indeed Wingren *et al.* could construct a cFv array with specificities against nine different cytokines. Upon being allowed to interact with crude extracts of human dendritic cells containing >10,000 different proteins, scFvs directed against interleukin (lL)- 1a-IL-8, IL-16, IL- 18, and monocyte chemotactic protein (MCP)-4 did not cross-react with any other proteins from the crude cell lysate. The differential intensity of spots showed a specific upregulation of four of the cytokines derived from the activated cells. Hence, recombinant antibody fragments were found to be well suited for the array format, but only if selected for that application and not simply taken off the shelf (Wingren *et al.,* 2003).

The next formidable challenge for antibody arrays will be how to scale up so that global analysis of up to 10,000 proteins may be achieved. Conceivably, nanoengineering approaches coupled with new formats may facilitate analysis on a large scale. Applications of two-dimensional electrophoresis and mass spectroscopy have given us an insight into proteome variations either for different phenotypes, tissues and cells, or in response *to* external stimuli or differentiation processes. However, the throughput of these two techniques is limited. In genomics, microarrays can enable the parallel analysis of whole genomes (Lockhart and Winzeler, 2000). But a bottleneck hinders development of microarrays for proteome analysis-generating a molecule that binds specifically to a given protein is much more laborious than designing an oligomer to identify its encoding mRNA. Fortunately, we can choose antibodies as suitable protein binding agents since the antibody pool in vertebrates has evolved admirably well to strongly bind to any possible protein specifically.

There are many methods to obtain antibodies, as recently reviewed by Bradbury *et al.* (2003, 2003a). But only the *in vitro* methods can potentially meet the requirements of the highly parallel processes needed for proteomics (Wingren *et al.* 2003). Unlike in animal-based methods, the biochemical conditions during the selection step are fully controllable and allow the *in vitro* selection of "conformation specific antibodies". Another great advantage of this approach is that no immune system is involved, so antibodies to toxic compounds, lethal pathogens and highly conserved antigens can be obtained by *in vitro* methods (Nizak *et al.,* 2003).

Table 13.4: Phage-display antibody selection systems for developing therapeutic antibodies and research applications in proteomics

Applications	Therapeutics	Proteomics
Target proteins	Few	Many
	Known, available	Usually not known, not available
	Well characterized	Not well characterized
Selection process	Number of steps not an issue	Number of steps minimal
	Selection cost not crucial	Optimized for low selection cost
	Failure rate should be lowest	Failure rate may be somewhat higher
Optimization of product (antibody) for	Low immunogenicity	Robustness
	Good pharmacokinetics	Compatibility to established assays
	Binding its antigen	No individual optimization possible

For the *in vitro* selection of antibodies, phage display happens to be a powerful technology that has yielded most of the recombinant antibodies generated so far. So far, the technology for development of antibody phage display has been driven chiefly towards methods to obtain therapeutic products, and the process has been optimized for factors that are not really relevant to generating research agents (Table 13.4). Hust and Dubel have reviewed the available technologies from the angle of their applicability as tools for proteome research. According to them we need a new model for both antibody library formats and the selection process so as to meet the requirements of proteomics.

The pioneer work of Smith (1985) on peptides spurred the development of antibody phage display (Hoogenboom *et al.* 1991). The genotype and phenotype of a polypeptide were linked by fusing antibody gene fragments to a gene coding for the minor coat protein of the filamentous bacteriophage M13. The work led to the expression of an antibody, fusion protein on the surface of phage, thereby allowing the affinity purification of antibody-coding genes by antigen binding. Antibody libraries with diversities of up to 10^{11} independent clones have so far been assembled as molecular repertoires for phage-display selections (Sblattero and Bradbury, 2000), and several methods have been developed for 'panning' the desired specificity from vast repertoires (Hust and Dubel, 2004). The size of the repertoire is correlated with the affinities of the antibodies isolated from it. Also various types of phage-display library have been successfully constructed. Methods have been designed to clone the genetic diversity of antibody repertoires. While immune libraries are usually built by a two-step cloning or assembly PCR method after mRNA isolation and cDNA preparation from the desired cell type, native libraries can be made by two or three cloning steps (Hoogenboom and Winter, 1992). It has now emerged that, antibodies with nanomolar affinities can be selected from both native libraries and synthetic libraries (which can be assembled by either cloning or PCR) provided that the molecular complexity is carefully preserved during library construction and if library sizes of at least 10^{10} are reached.

A robust molecular format compatible with current assay is a pre-requisite for applications of antibodies to proteome research. A reagent needs to be fully interchangeable with commercially available IgG used for western blotting, immunoprecipitation, immunohistochemistry, enzyme-linked immunosorbent assay (ELISA) and antibody microarrays. This issue not only concerns stability and affinity, but also concerns compatibility with detection systems, which usually are secondary antisera labelled with an enzyme or a fluorescent dye. Throughput being crucial, the optimal format should be produced directly by the library selection process without any need for subsequent cloning setups (Hust and Dubel, 2004).

13.18. ANTIGEN CHOICE

Many antibodies have been derived by immunization or by panning on purified or recombinantly expressed antigen. For large-scale proteomic research, the large number of antigens each of which requires individual characterization and purification methods creates problems of handling and costs. This means that despite high antigen quality (e.g. folding and post-translational modifications), the use of antigens purified from native material is limited to special niche applications only. There are two other possibilities for producing antigens, viz., synthesis from cDNA libraries, and the use of synthetic peptides. Both these methods have been validated by the production of numerous monoclonal and polyclonal antibodies in animals. For creating recombinant antigen, large cDNA collections and rapid *in vitro* translation and transcription systems that yield milligrams of protein within 2 days have become available (Sawasaki *et al.*, 2002). Conceivably, one may use many different peptides per antigen in high-throughput screening (HTS) approach. It is also possible that by using, for instance, phosphorylated variants, peptides may aid the search for post-translational modifications. Some recently developed methods of synthesizing peptides in array formats on solid phase for phage panning can greatly reduce the number of experimental steps and so improve throughput greatly (Frank, 2002; Hallborn and Carlsson, 2002). Another emerging possibility is that antibody fragments might be replaced by an alternative scaffold (Skerra, 2000).

13.19. PREDICTIVE MEDICINE AND PROTEIN THERAPEUTICS

Our ability to design drugs that exploit disease phenotype is limited and the ability to customize drugs specific for human subpopulations is beyond reach. The drug production pipeline is too long and very expensive. Happily, however, biology is becoming a predictive, quantitative science with a rational basis for rapid design and discovery-the coming, few decades are likely to see a sharp increase in the number of available drugs and targets and in their clinical efficacy and safety, along with a reduction in their cost of production and time to market. Advanced experimental and computational technologies have recently generated new approaches to the early phases of the drug production pipeline. The revolution in DNA microarray technologies and the imminent emergence of its analogue for proteins, along with machine learning algorithms, can potentially speed up the identification of potential drug targets and facilitate development of high-throughput screens for subpopulation-specific toxicity. Likewise, advances in structural genomics in conjunction with *in vitro* and in silico evolutionary methods can greatly accelerate the number of lead drug candidates and substantially augment their target specificity. All such advances can usher in an era of predictive medicine, which could move medical practice from reactive therapy after disease onset, to proactive prevention (Weng and DeLisi, 2002).

This emerging era is defined and symbolized by the genomic revolution–a revolution that encompasses high-throughput sequencing, and the technologies that exploit and add to the information it generates. Such technologies are exemplified by a variety of DNA microarray methods that monitor genomic change, emerging array methods for monitoring protein profiles, (MacBeath and Schreiber, 2000; Figeys and Pinto, 2001; Kruglyak and Nickerson, 2001; Roos, 2001), high-throughput methods for genetic characterization of disease diathesis and resistance, high-performance computing for biological discovery and real-time data analysis and data integration. All these technologies can catalyze and hasten the discovery and molecular characterization of disease-specific genetic pathways and of ligand specific toxicity and metabolic pathways. They will not only speed up the discovery of protein therapeutics and the identification of candidate drug targets but will propel us toward individualized medicine (therapy that takes into account genetic markers for predisposition to drug side effects and/of efficacy) (Debouck and Goodfellow, 1999; Bodor and Buchwald, 2000; Archer, 1999).

Suitable DNA microarrays are being developed to monitor the expression of some or many of the expressed genes of a cell as well as for characterizing the change in genomic expression that accompanies normal development and disease progression. These arrays will help in identifying highly specific disease targets and in customizing drugs (Garrett and Workman, 1999; Freeman, 2000). The microarray technology has already been applied to disease biology and diagnosis, especially to cancer (Golub *et al.*, 1999; AIon *et al.*, 1999). Alon *et al.* (1999) studied gene expression in samples of tumor colon tissue and could distinguish them from normal colon tissue samples on the basis of gene expression. Besides revealing that expression patterns cluster to form diagnostic fingerprints, several recent results have yielded clues to identifying genes and pathways that are potential therapeutic targets (Golub *et al.*, 1999). The chief merit of microarrays is high-throughput screening, which can be for target validation as well as for identification. Thus if a gene deletion or mutation produces a genomic expression pattern similar to that of a disease, the gene and its product are potential drug targets (Weng and DeLisi. 2002). Likewise, microarrays are used to test the efficacy and toxicity of drug candidates by selecting those that can best recover the normal pattern of gene expression. Conducting these experiments on cells with different genotypes helps in predicting functional variation in the response of individuals to different drugs. In due course, such studies, when coupled with advances in protein technologies, should provide not only the extensive and diverse data-structures but also a deeper understanding of cell biology-prerequisites for predictive medicine.

Although analogous technologies for monitoring changes in protein abundance are not yet available, the field of proteomics is growing rapidly (Zhu and Snyder, 2001; Kumar, 2004). The importance of proteome technologies stems from the fact that most current drug targets are proteins; also in view of the variable and unreliable correlation between gene and protein expression, and in the posttranslational protein modifications (Parekh and Rohlff, 1997); it is these factors that are responsible for realizing the signaling and information processing that regulate cell behavior (Weng and DeLisi, 2002; Garrett and Workman, 1999). Once a protein is considered to be a drug target, its biological ligand logically becomes a drug candidate. The availability of all full-length cDNAs in the human genome has made it possible for three proteomic methods (viz. mass spectrometry, yeast two-hybrid system. and display technologies) to be developed to identify binding partners (Pandey and Mann, 2000). Display technologies make possible combinatorial generation of diversity followed by selection and amplification of molecules with the desired property; for example, tight binding to a receptor. These technologies are able to associate every protein with its genetic material (RNA or DNA). The 'displayed entity' is the protein whose function can be screened for. Linking every protein molecule to its respective oligonucleotide facilitates the rapid 'decoding' of desirable proteins once they have been selected from the library.

The interplay between proteins and their genes can assume many forms; this leads to different kinds of display technologies. Bacteriophage-based methods were the first to be developed and are being widely used (Sidhu, 2000). The oligonucleotide coding for the target protein is fused with the gene of a phage coat protein. By fusing oligonucleotides containing random mutations with the phage gene, a library of phages, each carrying a distinct peptide sequence as part of its coat protein is produced. This links the target protein to its DNA through a phage particle. The phage library is placed on a dish coated with the receptor molecule and unbound phages are washed away. Binding phages are harvested, amplified and sequenced to show the mutations that cause the improved binding. Ribosomal display is based on the direct attachment of the target protein to its mRNA molecule through ribosome. The RNA-peptide fusion technique involves a covalent bonding of a protein to its mRNA. Other examples are flagellum display, yeast display and mammalian cell-based display (Sidhu, 2000; Boder and Wittrup, 2000; Li, 2000; Williams, 2000; Colas, 2000). Stemmer (1994) invented an elegant technique termed gene shuffling for generating sequence diversity. Related DNA sequences (e.g. all 20 copies of interferon in the human genome) are amplified and randomly fragmented. The fragments are reassembled using DNA polymerase in a self-priming fashion. The resulting chimeric molecules are selected by means of a display technology. Desirable progeny molecules are selected and may be bred again, thereby concentrating multiple beneficial mutations. Shuffling allows highly efficient exploration of the genetic diversity of natural sequences.

Exploring natural mutations is analogous to searching through an infinitesimal sequence subspace that is largely free of deleterious mutations in the mean time; beneficial mutations become enriched (Weng and DiLisi, 2002). Computational approaches to small-molecule drug discovery are based on geometric recognition algorithms to search small-molecule databases for structures complementary to target molecules (Zeng, 2000; Gane and Dean, 2000), in the hope that they will bind to the target, and so modulate its activity. This is a good starting point for both high-throughput screening and rational drug design. Small molecules have proven suitable for targeting enzymes and ion channels but are not as effective as proteins in blocking interactions between large macromolecules. Further, non-biological small molecules are usually much more toxic than human proteins. Proteins thus represent a growing class of therapeutic agents, despite difficulties related to their pharmacokinetic properties (Cho and Juliano, 1996).

13.20. PROTEIN DESIGN *IN SILICO*

One important goal of protein design is to achieve improved stability for a monomeric protein (Hellinga, 1998). The same design principles (Dahiyat and Mayo, 1997; Malakauskas and Mayo, 1998; Marshall and Mayo, 2001) that are used to increase the stability of a monomer are applicable to increase the stability and specificity of complexes; the goal here is to achieve improved stability to meet some design specification and not necessarily to achieve most stable complex (Looger and Hellinga, 2001; Weng and DeLisi, 1998, 2002).

13.21. THERAPEUTIC PEPTIDES

Some recent advances have generated new strategies for the administration of peptide drugs and improvements of clearance half-lives in vivo. Despite some potential obstacles that remain, peptide therapeutics is poised to play a significant role in the treatment of diseases ranging from Alzheimer's disease to cancer. The clinical trend of using some peptides as therapeutic drugs has been gaining popularity in recent years. A therapeutic peptide results when several (<100) amino acids are linked by amides (Wieland, 1995). A few good examples are oxytocin, vasopressin and insulin. Such long peptides can be chemically synthesized easily by using solid-phase synthesis (Merrifield, 1995). Some naturally derived peptides have also proven to be good drugs. With the advent of large biological and synthetic peptide libraries and high-throughput screening, many promising candidates will soon be added to the growing list of peptides under development. Peptides can also be produced through natural or recombinant microbial fermentations. However, chemical synthesis allows the conjugation of other small molecules or incorporation of non-natural amino acids and peptides. Combining small molecules to peptides enhances their potential application as targeted cytotoxic agents for anti-tumor therapy. Likewise, inserting non-natural amino acids into the peptide generates not only greater chemical diversity but also high-affinity, high-specificity molecular recognition. Non-natural amino acids tend to prevent rapid degradation of the peptide, as the latter cannot be recognized by proteases. Not all peptides are proteolytically labile. The fairly small size of many peptides is conducive to their removal from the circulation by rapid filtration of the kidney. But this can sometime limit the therapeutic use of a peptide. The use of cytotoxic reagents for cancer therapy and their rapid clearance is often beneficial provided the dose is appropriate (Boerman *et al.*, 2000). For treating cancer, another advantage of peptides over larger proteins (e.g., antibodies) is that peptides penetrate better in tumors (Shockley *et al.*, 1991).

In cancer treatment, which often suffers from lack of specificity, and causes significant side effects, use of therapeutic peptides can enhance cellular uptake, drug targeting and vaccination (Luhrs *et al.*, 2002; Curnis *et al.*, 2000; Zwaveling *et al.*, 2002). Synthetic peptide vaccines have been developed on the rationale that whereas cancerous cells display epitopes on their surface, normal cells do not (Sahin *et al.*, 1997). Clinical trials on using synthetic peptide vaccines to various tumor antigens have not shown any major toxicity (Sundaram *et al.*, 2002). However, these trials have also revealed fairly low efficacy (Lien and Lowman, 2003). The low immunogenicity of peptides leads to inefficient priming of the immune system. A possible strategy to address this problem may be to incorporate several peptide epitopes in the vaccine as discrete peptides. Drug targeting is another good role for peptides in cancer therapy. In mice, proliferating endothelial cells have been targeted by peptides that were isolated by in vivo panning of combinatorial phage libraries in mice (Arap *et al.*, 1998, 2002). Some of these peptides can target angiogenic (tumor) tissue while blocking integrins from binding to their ligands, or can inhibit matrix metalloproteases (Lien and Lowman, 2003). Either of these actions results in apoptosis of the endothelial cells in the newly formed blood vessels-this stop or reverses tumor progression in mouse models. For tumor targeting in humans, peptides must have specifically to tumor epitopes rather than to normal human tissue.

Table 13.5: Some representative peptide therapeutics already approved or undergoing clinical trials (after Lien and Lowman, 2003)

Drug	Company(s)	Natural source	Indications
Plenaxis™	Praecis Pharma	GnRH	Prostate cancer. Endometriosis
Apan™	Praecis Pharma	amyloid	Alzheimer's disease
Exubra^R	Inhale, Pfizer, Aventis Pharma	Insulin	Diabetes
Oral insulin	NOBEX, Glaxo, SmithKline	Insulin	Diabetes
Oratonin TM	NOBEX,	Calcitonin	Osteoporosis
Oral calcitonin	Emisphere, Novartis	Calcitonin	Osteoporosis
Oralin™	Generex	Insulin	Diabetes
HER-2/neu vaccine	Corixa	HER-2/neu	Breast and ovarian cancer
Fuzeon™, T-1249	Trimeris	gp41, HIV2, SIV, gp41	AIDS
Lupron depot^R	Abbott Pharma	GnRH, LH-RH	Prostate cancer, Endometriosis

In the light of the fact that higher organisms naturally produce a large number of antimicrobial peptides (e.g. defensins and cathelicidins), it appears that peptides could potentially be used as antimicrobial therapeutics. Many of these peptides are short, cationically charged, and capable of forming amphipathic structures in non-polar solvents. They probably disrupt negatively charged bacterial cell membranes to which they are electrostatically attracted, rather than mammalian cell membranes, which are usually neutral. Upon binding, the hydrophobic side of the amphipathic structure breaks the lipid bilayer by some unknown mechanisms (Lien and Lowman, 2003). Antimicrobial peptides have also been used for inducing apoptosis in cancer cells. When these peptides were linked to sequences isolated from in vivo phage panning, they targeted to angiogenic vasculature in mice suffering from breast and prostate carcinomas (Ellerby *et al.,* 1999; Arap *et al.,* 2002). Internalization of the peptides by the proliferating endothelium disrupts the mitochondrial membrane (resembling that of bacteria) and, hence, kills the cell. The high selectivity of antimicrobial peptides and the lack of resistance to them enhance the value of these peptides as potential therapeutics. Most of these peptides have been derived from natural products. But now combinatorial peptides library screening is playing an important role in the lead discovery process. Combinatorial chemistry has identified several potential novel peptides therapeutics (Aina *et al.,* 2002). Although many of the peptides found by combinatorial library screening have turned out to be highly specific, potent and structured, they need to be pharmacologically characterized.

13.22. MINIMIZING CLEARANCE OF PEPTIDES

A therapeutic peptide can be modified and enhanced by glycosylation, conjugation with polyethylene glycol or substituting D-amino acids for L-amino acids so as to reduce its susceptibility to certain proteases. Another option is engineer the peptide's association with serum albumin so as to limit proteolysis and filtration clearance from the body (Stiles, 2002; Hinds and Kim, 2002). Albumin happens to be the most abundant protein in serum. Its circulating half-life is 19 days in humans (Peters, 1985). Peptides that fuse directly to serum albumin by the incorporation of chemical groups or linkers that bind albumin, or through the addition of a peptide sequence that binds albumin in vivo have been designed (Koehler *et al.*, 2002; Dennis *et al.*, 2002).

Being smaller than antibodies and other proteins, therapeutic peptides can be injected intravenously. Other potential benefits are patient compliance and reduction of overall treatment costs. Some other novel delivery methods for novel peptides include transdermal patches, transdermal electrophoresis sonication, inhalation, and oral formulations (Henry *et al.*, 1998; Kanikkannan, 2002; Mitragotri *et al.*, 1995). Some hurdles still remain in the widespread development of peptides as therapeutics. Results from *in vitro* models have been quite promising, but their *in vivo* efficacy is not established. Interactions with proteases and the immune system cause particular concern. Peptides made entirely of L-amino acids are potential immunogens. Immunogenicity can sometimes produce dramatic effects including loss of drug activity, rapid drug clearance or hypersensitivity reactions. It may be advisable to go in for peptide agonists that act as single-administration, low-dose therapeutics, but it is quite difficult to identify the high-affinity, mechanism-specific molecules of this class in typical screens of chemical and biological diversity libraries (Lien and Lowman, 2003). There seems little doubt that, despite some remaining obstacles, peptides are destined to comprise a large part of future therapeutics, owing to the ease with which combinatorial peptide libraries can be produced and screened, their (potentially) low immunogenicity, their potential for delivery by less-invasive methods than intravenous injection, and the ability to manipulate them chemically.

13.23. PROTEINS FOR THERAPY

Since the advent of monoclonal antibodies (Kohler and Milstein, 1975) some 12 therapeutic antibodies have been approved for such disease indications as rheumatoid arthritis, non-Hodgkin's lymphoma and respiratory syncytial virus infection. Indeed antibodies have become well established as highly potent and well tolerated therapeutics. However, some formatting and manufacturing issues with conventional antibodies (e.g., the reliance on mammalian cell expression) have led to a clear preference for smaller fragments of antibodies that can be manufactured by high-volume bacterial or yeast cell culture in liquid media. Domain antibodies (dAbs) are the smallest known antigen-binding fragments of antibodies; they range from 11 kDa to 15 kDa (Holt *et al.*, 2003). They occur naturally in 'heavy chain' immunoglobulins from camels, and are now being produced in fully human form. dAbs are the robust variable regions of the heavy and light chains of immunoglobulins (V_H and V_L respectively). They can be highly expressed in microbial cell culture; they show good solubility and temperature stability, and are well suited to selection and affinity maturation by *in vitro* selection systems such as phage display (Davies and Reichmann, 1995). dAbs are bioactive as monomers and, owing to their small size and inherent stability can be formatted into larger molecules to create drugs with prolonged serum half-lives or other pharmacological activities (Holt *et al.*, 2003). Both recombinant Fabs (~ 57 kDa) and single chain Fv fragments (scFvs–27 kDa, each a V_H domain fused to a V_L domain via a polypeptide linker) are undergoing clinical trials.

In vitro technologies have been developed for selecting binders from large libraries of polypeptides. As Fabs, scFvs and dAbs can readily express in bacteria, they can be isolated using phage display;

this means that antibody fragments specific for a chosen target may be isolated without any need for animal immunization (Davies and Reichmann, 1995). Because of their smaller size, scFvs and dAbs can be produced in bacterial culture at higher yields than Fabs and are better suited to phage display because a single polypeptide chain is expressed. Many companies are using phage display of human scFvs and/or dAbs as an important part of their discovery programs.

Holt *et al.* (2003) summarized the current options for isolating fully human dAbs that bind therapeutic targets, and discussed how their small size relates to their pharmacological properties. The likelihood of creating fully human dAbs with high affinity and specificity for several targets raises the hope for producing a novel class of therapeutic drug with all the advantages of conventional antibodies but without the drawbacks encountered in manufacturing and formatting. For commercially useful dAbs must be extremely soluble and resistant to proteolysis, aggregation, denaturation and chemical degradation. These properties can be introduced by replacing specific residues at specific positions in human V_H domains with those frequently found in camel V_H domains (Davies and Riechmann, 1994). Such a "camelisation" can at least partially eliminate the tendency to aggregate but the modified V_H domains may still be poorly expressed and less thermodynamically stable than their wind-type counterparts owing to β-sheet deformation (Davies and Riechmann, 1995, 1996; Riechmann, 1996). Several camelid V_H domains regain antigen-binding specificity after prolonged incubation at temperatures of ~ 80-92°C (Dumoulin *et al.,* 2002); this has been attributed to a reversible unfolding behavior. In contrast, antibodies and their fragments derived from other species including human V_H dAbs usually aggregate irreversibly on thermal denaturation. With regard to thermostability, such approaches as site-directed mutagenesis, molecular evolution and in silico molecular design have been attempted with a view to optimizing antibody fragments including dAbs (Worn and Pluckthun, 2001).

Phage display has proven useful for selecting human, murine and camelid dAbs with high specificity and affinity to several antigens and antigen types, including binders against haptens, enzyme active sites and proteins as diverse as transcription factors and cytokines (Davies and Riechmann, 1995). For commercial-scale production of a dAb to be used as drug, a good expression system needs to be chosen so as to maximise the quality of purified product and to minimise the drug cost. The commonest system for expressing dAbs is periplasmic expression in *Escherichia coli.* Some other systems include yeasts such as *Saccharomyces* and *Pichia.* Recombinant proteins, including antibodies and antibody fragments, have also been expressed in the milk of cows or rabbits, or in bird eggs (Houdebine. 2002; Ivarie, 2003).

The small size of highly specific high affinity dAbs appears to make them suitable for targeting antigens in such obstructed locations as tumours where penetration into poorly vascularised tissue is crucial to the success of the drug. The delivery of toxins or radioisotopes to diseased tissues (Carter, 2001; Holt *et al.*, 2003) could also be greatly facilitated through a dAb – it would deliver the toxin to the tumour and minimize the length of time over which the toxin could cause damage to healthy cells in the blood. The short half-life of dAbs also enhances their other applications requiring rapid clearance.

13.24. HEAT-SHOCK PROTEINS FOR CANCER THERAPY

In the salivary gland chromosomes of the fruitfly Drosophila, the gene products encoded on chromosome puffs have been isolated and termed heat-shock proteins, or Hsps whose production accelerates in response to temperature stress; these proteins are also abundant in unstressed cells. Hsps are more accurately called 'molecular chaperones', because they protect other cellular proteins from becoming disorted as a result of high temperature or other environmental insults, and certain

Hsps also enable newly synthesized proteins to attain the correct conformation (Neckers and Lee, 2003).

One promising anticancer strategy seems to be to target a specific protein or a single signaling pathway that is required for the survival of tumour cells but not normal cells. But few such unique targets exist, and inhibiting a single pathway might not suffice to treat cancers that result from several genetic abnormalities. Therefore, focus is shifting to heat-shock proteins such as (Hsp90) that regulate many signaling pathways in cancer cells. One important trait of Hsp90 is that although cancer cells can produce high levels of the protein it is also abundant in normal cells (Neckers and Lee, 2003). This makes drugs targeting Hsp90 potentially toxic. Surprisingly, however, the first Hsp90 inhibitor to be tested in clinical trials (the drug 17-AAG) is well tolerated by patients. Kamal *et al.* (2003) reported that Hsp90 found in tumour cells has a much higher affinity for 17-AAG than does Hsp90 from normal cells. The chaperone Hsp90 regulates the function and stability of many key-signaling proteins that enable cancer cells to escape the inherent toxicity of their environment and to evade the effects of chemotherapy. This raises the possibility that inhibitors of Hsp90 could attack cancer cells and either kill them or at least weaken them so much that they could be controlled by chemotherapy or radiotherapy.

Despite this rationale for Hsp90-directed anticancer therapy, the high abundance of the protein in normal cells has generated concerns that Hsp90 inhibitors (e.g.17-AAG) may prove toxic to patients. But actual pre-clinical data and clinical trial revealed that this drug targets tumour cells in preference to normal cells. Kamal *et al.* (2003) found that Hsp90 derived from tumour cells binds to 17-AAG up to 100 times more tightly than does Hsp90 isolated from normal cells. Intriguingly, Hsp90 from normal cells binds the drug with nearly the same low affinity as does purify Hsp90 (Neckers and Lee, 2003). According to Kamal *et al.*, (2003) the chaperone seems to interact with other proteins inside tumour cells and normal cells-Hsp90 assembles with other chaperones and associated proteins forming a 'super-chaperone' machine. In tumour cells, the bulk of Hsp90 exists in such an assembly, whereas most of the Hsp90 in normal cells exist in a free form. This means that the affinity of 17-AAG for Hsp90 probably depends on the incorporation of the chaperone into a multi-protein machine. The drug 17-AAG, which is related to geldanamycin, binds more tightly to Hsp90 when the protein is part of a 'super-chaperone machine' that actively modulates the shape of 'client' proteins. Conceivably, Hsp90 itself catalyses the conversion of drugs like 17-AAG-the super-chaperone machine might be a more efficient catalyst of this process than uncomplexed Hsp90.

13.25. IMPROVING THERAPEUTIC PROTEINS

Negative design principles have recently been used to improve the pharmacokinetic properties of important therapeutic proteins (Sarkar *et al.,* 2002; Berg *et al.,* 2003). Rather than enhancing specific activity, the central strategy consisted of the removal of states that compromise efficacy through the use of rational engineering and better understanding of the in vivo clearance biology of a biotherapeutic (Desjarlais and Lazar, 2003). The concept of negative design has been frequently applied in the protein design process to bias against undesired states (e.g., DeGrado *et al.,* 1989). A major challenge of negative design problem is that the protein positions, which contribute to the favored state(s) also directly, contribute to the unwanted state(s).

A common goal for protein therapeutics is enhanced pharmacokinetics (PK). Lowering the *in vivo* turnover rate of proteins often leads to enhance therapeutic potency and the possibility of less frequent dosing. Several effective methods for improving the pharmacokinetics of protein therapeutics are available including attachment of polyethylene glycol (PEG) or fusion to a long-lived carrier protein (such as human serum albumin or the antibody Fc region) they effectively lower *in vivo* clearance rates that are dominated by a small set of mechanisms. More recently, some new approaches have offered intringuing alternatives suited to the clearance biology of each protein and are potentially applicable to several systems (Desjarlais and Lazar, 2003). One such recent approach is directed at reducing the receptor-mediated clearance of G-CSF– the therapeutic protein granulocyte colony-stimulating factor (Sarkar *et al.*, 2002). G-CSF is a leukocyte-stimulating cytokine currently used to treat chemotherapy-induced neutrophil depletion (neutropenia).

Sarkar *et al.*, (2002) redesigned G-CSF to lose affinity for its receptor in a pH dependent manner. The pH stability of G-CSF (and interleukin-2) variants was found to be correlated with ligand trafficking and depletion, suggesting that engineering aimed at balancing lysosomal degradation and recycling might be a general strategy for enhancing the efficacy of biotherapeutics with primarily "cell based clearance" mechanisms (Ricci *et al.*, 2003). Another recent strategy, adopted by Berg *et al.* (2003), involved decreasing inhibition of activated protein C. Berg *et al.*, (2003) re-engineered activated protein C (APC) for improved pharmacokinetics. APC (drotrecogin alpha) is an anticoagulant and anti-inflammatory agent currently used to treat sepsis. The therapeutic use of APC derives partly from its ability to attenuate the clotting cascade that can result from infection, specifically through its cleavage and inactivation of its clotting factor substrates Factors Va and VIIla. Unfortunately, for use as a drug, APC is rapidly inactivated by certain serine protease inhibitors (SERPINS) which first act as substrates and then as irreversible inhibitors after cleavage by the protease via formation of a covalent complex (Desjarlais and Lazar. 2003). As in the G-CSF case, for APC design there are desired states that need to be maintained (specifically, the APC-clotting factor complexes) and undesired states that must be removed (specifically the APC-SERPIN complexes). Further, negative design is equally challenging because the same set of amino acids in APC interact directly with both clotting factors and SERPINs. Some molecular modeling work done by Berg *et al.* (2003) has yielded valuable clues to pinpoint APC substitution sites that can impact substrate recognition. This would prove rewarding in efforts at negative designing.

13.26. STRUCTURE-BASED ENGINEERING OF BIOTHERAPEUTICS

The above new approaches bring out the utility of structural- and computational based protein engineering for improving biotherapeutics efficacy. Rational, structure guided approaches have enabled researchers to keep the number of mutations to a minimum, thereby weakening the impact of engineering on the immunogenicity of the protein (Desjarlais and Lazar, 2003). The above works also demonstrate the power of negative design for creating improved protein therapeutics.

13.27. PRODUCTION OF RECOMBINANT PROTEINS IN TRANSGENIC ANIMALS

As pointed out by Dove (2002), our current manufacturing capacity for recombinant therapeutic proteins is extremely short. This has prompted evaluation of several different biological systems for the production of these proteins. Factors such as scale up, total annual production, speed of production set-up, post-translational modifications and regulatory issues are critical in choosing the most suitable system (Table 13.6)

While bacteria are useful as bioreactors because of the ease of cultivation, they have only limited ability to perform the post-translational protein modifications essential for many targets (Balbas, 2001; Swartz, 2001). Certain eukaryotic systems, e.g., yeast, filamentous fungi and unicellular algae can be scaled-up fairly easily and do carry out post-translational modifications but suffer from the limitation of duplicating human patterns of protein processing and so can yield recombinant products with such undesirable properties as immunogenicity or lack of activity. Insect cell systems work well when used at the laboratory scale but they have unique glyeosylation patterns, and the baculovirus system is more appropriate for laboratory scale production (Dyck *et al.*, 2003). Bioreactors based on metazoan cell culture systems are quite expensive to maintain and difficult to scale up. While mammalian cells do carry out complex post-translational modifications, their scaling up costs for mass-production is extremely high (Andersen and Krummen, 2002). Transgenic plants animals and insects have the merit of large production capacity at lower costs than mammalian cell culture but suffer from fairly slow production set-up and have still to cross many regulatory hurdles (Dyck *et al.*, 2003). According to Dyck *et al.*, transgenic animal bioreactors meet the growing need for therapeutic recombinant proteins. Their ability to produce complex, biologically active recombinant proteins efficiently and economically has aroused much interest; genetically modified animals of several species expressing foreign proteins in various tissues are being developed. However, the production of transgenic animals is a cumbersome process and there are problems in the application of this technology.

Table 13.6: Relative merits of different systems for producing proteins*

Parameters

	Worst		Suitability		Best
Speed	An	P	Mc	F	Bac
Cost/g	Mc	F	Bac	An	P
Post-translation modifications	Bac	F	P	An	Mc
Scale-up	Mc	F	Bac	An	P
Regulatory	An	P	F	Bac	Mc

*Speed, gene to production time, Cost/g, total cost of goods, scal up, ease and speed regulatory, accumulated products approval history.

Key: Bac (Bacteria), F (Fungi), Mc (Mammal cells), P (Plants), An (Animals).

The mammary gland is the tissue of choice to express valuable recombinant proteins in transgenic animal bioreactors in view of the fact that milk can be easily collected in large volumes. As a result, transgenic bioreactors are usually based on sheep, goats and cows (Eyestone, 1999). Foreign proteins usually express into transgenic milk at rates of several grams per litre. However, the production of proteins in milk suffers from the fairly long interval from birth to first lactation that occurs in domestic livestock the discontinuous nature of the lactation cycle and the substantial time and material investments required to produce transgenic dairy animals (Houdebine, 1995; Wall *et al.*, 1997). This problem may be addressed by producing transgenic rabbits and pigs, expressing foreign proteins in their mammary glands, but milk production rates and the number of animals needed to produce sufficient amounts of protein are some limitations.

Another possible method for large-scale production of recombinant proteins is the use of transgenic eggs. A single hen can produce up to 330 eggs per year and egg white naturally contains ~ 4 g of protein. Unfortunately this method suffers from the absence of a good system of transgenesis in poultry. There is considerable potential for producing valuable proteins with transgenic animals but the purification of these proteins from their source, whether milk or eggs, is a hurdle yet to be overcome. Although no doubt transgenic animal bioreactors are a welcome means of producing recombinant proteins, the generation of transgenic domestic animals by the commonly employed method of DNA microinjection is quite difficult and highly inefficient (usual success rate only about 1%) and so limits their application. Such high inefficiency, together with the long oestation and high maintenance costs of domestic farm animals, makes the production of transgenic livestock fairly time-consuming and expensive.

Retroviruses (Varmus, 1988) represent a natural means of efficiently introducing foreign DNA into animal cells and may be better than DNA microinjection. Viral gene sequences are deleted from the organism and replaced with a transgene. The retroviruses so modified are introduced into developing embryos to affect the transfer of the foreign DNA into an animal. The merit of retroviral vectors for transgenesis is that only a single copy of the transgene is integrated in the host genome and the virus can be introduced into oocytes or embryos at different stages. But retroviral vectors are limited in the size of constructs that they can carry (Friedrich and Soriano, 1993; Cepko *et al.*, 2000). Actively motile sperm have been used as vectors to introduce foreign DNA into oocytes. This process involves the incubation of washed spermatozoa in the presence of DNA fragments; it led to the production of transgenic mice when these (mouse) spermatozoa were used for *in vitro* fertilization (Lavitrano *et al.*, 1989). Transgenic pigs can also be produced with this technique (Lavitrano *et al.*, 2002). Brinster (2002) further extended the use of sperm as DNA carriers by manipulating the cells responsible for spermatogenesis (viz., spermatogonia) rather than the sperm themselves. One may recover spermatogonial stem cells, genetically manipulate them *in vitro* and transplant the cells into a recipient testis (Dym, 1994). The recipient animals produce male gametes originating from the genetically modified spermatogonia. Resulting transgenic offspring can contain the gene introduced into the male stem cells *in vitro*. Brinster and Nagano (1998) extended the processes for transplanting testis cells from one male to another, as well as culturing spermatogonial cells to the mouse. For livestock, this interesting technology has so far been limited to the manipulation of the pig male stem cells in vivo (Honaramooz *et al.*, 2003).

Embryonic stem (ES) cells and primordial germ (PG) cells make up a suitable medium for the production of transgenic animals particularly poultry. Genetically modified pluripotent ES or PG cells are injected into developing embryos to produce chimeric animals. In case the modified cell line does contribute to the production of sperm and oocytes, the resulting offspring incorporates some transgenic progeny. The advantages of ES cells as a mode of gene transfer include: (1) transformation *in vitro* with foreign DNA and screening before being used to produce chimerics; (2) controlling the site of transgene integration in the genome by homologous recombination to replace existing genes. Chimeric animals have already been produced with ES or PG cell technology in mice, rabbits, pigs, cattle and poultry. But transmission of the ES or PG genome into the gametes to produce transgenic offspring from a chimeric animal has only been achieved in mice (Anderson, 1999).

The uses of transgenic animals for commercial protein production are subject to patenting constraints for agricultural or biomedical applications. For expressing a particular protein in the mammary gland, the required functional promoter and its regulatory sequences are covered by patent limitations. Also, if the desired product to be produced in milk contains a known DNA sequence, the protein and its use as a therapeutic may also have been patented. If nuclear transfer or cloning constitutes a part of the process, diverse patents may have already been granted for certain aspects of this procedure. All the regulatory processes involved in the commercialization of a given product require the description of detailed procedures and help in the enforcement of intellectual property rights (Dyck *et al.*, 2003).

Some other concerns associated with these technologies are the ethical and environmental aspects of transgenesis. Integration of a transgene into the genome can potentially disturb endogenous gene expression in the resulting animals. Any genetic manipulation that causes animal suffering is not acceptable to researchers, the public or regulatory agencies. In general, many current methods for producing transgenic animal founders are fairly inefficient and time-consuming. The inefficiency of transgenesis in the reproductively less prolific cattle species, coupled with some inherent disadvantages of lactation, has aroused interest in expressing foreign proteins in various tissues of more prolific species such as rabbits and mice. It appears that the eggs and semen of transgenic animals might be good alternatives to mammary gland-based systems (Dyck *et al.*, 2003).

13.28. PHARMACEUTICAL AND MEDICAL APPLICATIONS OF PROTEOMICS

Advances in complex proteome technologies accelerate site-specific drug development. Promising areas of research include: delineation of altered protein expression, at the whole-cell or tissue levels, but also in subcellular structures; in protein complexes and in biological fluids; the development of novel biomarkers for diagnosis and early detection of disease; and the identification of new targets for therapeutics; and the potential for accelerating drug discovery through more effective strategies to evaluate therapeutic effectiveness and toxicity. Celis *et al.* (1984) have focused on establishing 2D proteomic databases useful for skin biology and in bladder cancer. They used noncultured cells such as keratinocytes (Celis *et al.*, 1992) to study the former and transitional and squamous cell carcinomas of the bladder (Celis *et al.*, 1999) for the later.

Proteomics holds particular promise in the following fields

• Identification of disease-related markers (biosensors, diagnostic kits)

• Identification of proteins as potential candidates in the development of vaccine targets

• Identification of disease-related targets

• Evaluation of process and bioavailability of drugs

• Evaluation of drug toxicity at tissue levels

• Validation of animal models

• Individualized drug design: pharmacoproteomics

At present, approximately 100 information categories (e.g., protein name, localization, regulation, expression, post-translational modifications) are available in database. It is possible to query the database searching by name, protein number, molecular weight, pI, organelle or cellular component, and to display its position on the 2-D image. This image can be compared to the master keratinocyte image. Nearly 100 polypeptides with known properties were stored as references. Again, the discovery of PCNA/cyclin, the first protein discovered by 2D gel technology, was carried out by Celis *et al*. It was found that PCNA/cyclin plays a significant role in DNA replication. New precision technology, based on protein structures and function makes it possible for clinicians to detect cancer earlier than ever and provide individualized treatment. Following the discovery of new proteins and gene maps, cancer researchers believed that proteomics is a revolutionary approach to detect cancer and other major illnesses (e.g., HIV) during their early phases and to tailor individualized therapy.

Proteomics has the potential to revolutionize diagnosis and disease management. Profiling serum protein patterns by means of surface-enhanced laser desorption/ionization time of flight (SELDI-TOFF) mass spectrometry is a novel approach to discover protein patterns that can be used to distinguish disease and disease-free states with high sensitivity and specificity. This method has shown great promise for early diagnosis of cancer (e.g., ovarian cancer). The study of Cellis *et al.* (1999) on bladder cancer was performed with the aim of unraveling the molecular mechanism of underlying tumor progression. For this purpose, approximately 700 tumors have been analyzed by utilizing 2D gel technologies. Several biomarkers have been identified, assuming that they may be useful for classifying superficial lesions and determining the individuals at risk. Moreover, Cellis *et al.* have been working on identifying protein markers that may be valuable for diagnosis and follow-up of bladder cancer patients. To achieve this goal, they have focused on the establishment of a comprehensive 2D gel database of urine proteins. In 2001, both Lawrie *et al.* and Moskaluk coupled LCM (laser capture microdissection) with 2D gel proteomics to recover proteins from laser captured microdissected tissue in a form that can be used in 2D gel analysis and mass spectrometry. This may provide valuable information for protein profiling and data basing of human tissues in healthy and disease states.

Proteomics have been used to develop biomarkers. This is achieved by comparative analysis of protein expression in healthy and diseased tissues to identify expressed proteins to be used as new markers, by analysis of secreted proteins in cell lines and primary cultures, and by direct serum protein profiling. MALDI seems to be a good technique for direct protein analysis in biological fluids (e.g., the identification of the small proteins-defensin 1, 2 and 3 as related to the anti-HIV-1 activity of CD8 antiviral factor). Infectious diseases, still a leading cause of death worldwide, can also be cured by the aid of proteomics. The most significant obstacle in treatment of infectious disease is the development of drug resistance. This calls the need for developing effective new therapies. At this point, joint application of proteomics and microbiology may be valuable. Neidhardt characterized protein expression patterns in *E. coli* under different growth conditions. The identification of the complete sequence of a number of microbial genomes was helpful for identifying proteins encoded in these genomes. The identification of new potential drug and vaccine targets against *Plasmodium falciparum*, which is the main cause of malaria, sets a good example for this kind of work. Proteomics can be used to enlighten the numerous significant aspects of microbial disease pathogenesis and treatment.

Toxicology is one of the most important applications of proteomics. 2D gel electrophoresis has been used for screening toxic agents and probing toxic mechanisms. Comparison of protein expression during a follow-up study may lead to identification of changes in biochemical pathways. After compiling a large number of proteomic libraries of the compounds with known toxicity, it may be possible to retrieve useful information to assess the toxicity of a novel compound before it enters clinical trials.

SUGGESTED READING

* Aina OH. *Biopolymers* 66, 184 (2002).
* Alon U. *PNAS USA*, 96, 6745 (1999).
* Andersen DC, Krummen L. *Curr Opin Biotechnol* 13, 117 (2002).
* Anderson GB. Embryonic stem cells in agriculture. In *Transgenic Animals in Agriculture* (Murray JD *et al.*), pp. 59-66, CABI, Wallingford (1999).
* Arap W, *et al. Science* 279, 377 (1998).
* Arap W, *et al. PNAS USA* 99, 1527 (2002).
* Archer R. *Nat Biotechnol* 17, 834 (1999).
* Balbas P. *Escherichia coll Mol. Biotechnol* 19, 251 (2001).
* Berg DT, *et al. PNAS USA* 100, 4423 (2003).
* Berggren K, *et al. Electrophoresis* 21, 2509 (2000).

- Blaber M. *Trends in Biotech* 22, 1 (2003).
- Blackstock WP, Weir MP. *Trends Biotech* 17, 121 (1999).
- Blind M, *et al.* *PNAS (USA)* 96, 3606 (1999).
- Boder ET, Wittrup KD. *Methods Enzymol* 328, 430 (2000).
- Bodor N, Buckwald P. *Med Res Rev* 20, 58 (2000).
- Bodovitz S. *Drug Discovery World,* 50 (2003).
- Bodovitz S, Joos T. *Trends in Biotech* 22, 4 (2003).
- Boerman OC, *et al.* *Semin. Nucl Med* 30, 195 (2000).
- Bradbury A, *et al.* *Trends in Biotech* 21,312 (2003a).
- Bradbury A, *et al.* *Trends in Biotech* 21, 275(2003).
- Branch AD. *Trends Biochem Sci* 23, 45 (1998).
- Braun P, LaBaer J. *Trends in Biotech* 21, 383 (2003).
- Braun P, *et al.* *PNAS (USA)* 99, 2654 (2002).
- Brinster RL. *Science* 296, 2174 (2002).
- Brinster RL, Nagano M. *Semin Cell Dev Biol* 9, 401 (1998).
- Caflisch A. *Trends in Biotech* 21, 423 (2003).
- Cagney G, Emili A. *Nat Biotechnol.* 20J, 1631 (2002).
- Cagney G, Emili A. *Nat Biotechnol* 20J, 1631, 70 (2002).
- Carter P. *Nat Rev Cancer* 1, 118 (2001).
- Celis JE, Bravo R, Larsen PM, Fey SJ. *Leukemia Res* 8, 143 (1984).
- Celis JE, Celis P, Ostegaard M, *et al.* *Cancer Res* 59, 3003 (1999).
- Celis JE, Rasmusen HH, Madsen P. *et al.* *Electrophoresis* 13, 893 (1992).
- Chang DC. *Guide to Electroporation and Electrofusion.* Academic Press, NewYork (1991).
- Cho MJ, Juliano R. *Trends in Biotech* 14, 153 (1996).
- Christendat D. *Nat Struct Bio* 7, 903 (2000).
- Colas P. *Curr Opin Chem Biol* 4, 54 (2000).
- Curnis F. *Nat Biotechnol* 18, 1185 (2000).
- Dahiyat BL, Mayo SL. *Science* 278, 82 (1997).
- Davies J, Riechmann L. *Biotechnol* 13, 475 (1995).
- Davies J, Riechmann L. *Immunotechnology* 2,169 (1996).
- Debouck C, Goodfellow PN. *Nat Genet* 21, 48 (1999).
- DeGrado WF, *et al.* *Science* 243, 622 (1989).
- Dennis MS, *et al.* *J Biol Chem* 277, 35035 (2002).
- Desjarlais JR, Lazar GA. *Trends in Biotech* 21, 725 (2003).
- Dove A. *Nat Bioteclmol* 20, 339 (2002).
- Dumoulin M, *et al.* *Protein Sci* 11, 500 (2002).

- Dunker AK, Obradovic Z. *Nat Biotechnol* 19, 805 (2001).
- Dyck MK, Lacroix D, Pothier F, Sirard M. *Trends in Biotech* 21, J394 (2003).
- Dym M. *PNAS (USA)* 91, 11287 (1994).
- Dyson HJ, Wright PE. *Curr Opin Struct Biol* 12, 54 (2002).
- Ellerby HM, *et al. Nat Med* 5, 1032 (1999).
- Eyestone WH. *Theriogenology* 51, 509 (1999).
- Famulok M, Verma S. *Trends in Biotech* 20, 462 (2002).
- Fawell S, *et al. PNAS (USA)* 9I, 664 (1994).
- Figeys D, Pinto D. *Electrophoresis* 22, 208 (2001).
- Frank R. *Comb Chem High Throughput Screen* 5, 429-440 (2002).
- Freeman T. *Med Res Rev* 20, 197 (2000).
- Frenkel D, Smit B, (eds). *Understanding Molecular Simulations.* Academic Press, San Diego (2002).
- Friedrich G, Soriano P. *Methods Enzymol* 225, 681 (1993).
- Gane PJ, Dean PM. *Curr Opin Struct Biol* 10, 401 (2000).
- Garrett MD, Workman P. *Eur J Cancer* 35, 2010 (1999).
- Gavin AC, *et al. Nature* 415, 141 (2002).
- Golub TR *et al. Science* 286, 531 (1999).
- Gomperts BD, Fernandez JM. *Trends Biochem Sci* 10, 414 (1985).
- Good PD, *et al. Gene Ther* 4, 45 (1997).
- Green M, Loewenstein PM. *Cell* 55, 1179 (1988).
- Griffin TJ, *et al. Mol Cell Proteomics* 1, 323 (2002).
- Haab BB, Dunhamn MJ, Brown PO. *Genome Biol* 2, (2001).
- Hallborn J, Carlsson R. *Biotechniques* 33, 30 (2002).
- Hammarstrom M, *et al. Protein Sci* 11, 313 (2002).
- Harrison SJ, *et al. Transgenic Res* 11, 143 (2002).
- Hartwell LH, *et al. Nature* 402, C47 (1999).
- Hasty J, McMillen D, Collins JJ. *Nature* 420, 224 (2002).
- Hellinga HW. *Nat Struct Biol* 5, 525 (1998).
- Henry S, *et al. J Pharm Sci* 87, 922 (1998).
- Hinds KD, Kim SW. *Adv Drug Deliv Rev* 54, 505 (2002).
- Ho Y, *et al. Nature* 415, 180 (2002).
- Holt LJ, Herring C, Jespers LS, Woolven BP, Tomlinson IM. *Trends in Biotech* 20, 484 (2003).
- Honaramooz A, *et al. Theriogenology* 59, 536 (2003).
- Hoogenboom HR. *Trends in Biotech* 15, 62 (1997).
- Hoogenboom HR, *et al. Nucleic Acids Res* 19, 4133 (1991).

- Hoogenboom HR, Winter G. *J Mol Biol* 227, 381 (1992).
- Houdebine LM. *Curr Opin Biotechnol* 13, 625 (2002).
- Houdebine LM. *Reprod Nutr Dev* 35, 609 (1995).
- Hust M, Dubel S. *Trends in Biotech* 22, 8 (2004).
- Ito T, *et al. PNAS (USA)* 98, 4569 (2001).
- Ivarie R. *Trends in Biotech* 21, 14 (2003).
- Jeong H, *et al. Nature* 411, 41 (2001).
- Kabouridis PS, *Trends in Biotech* 21, 498 (2003).
- Kamal A, Thao L, Sensintaffar J, *et al. Nature* 425, 407 (2003).
- Kanikkannan N. *BioDrugs* 16, 339 (2002).
- Karplus M, McCammon JA. *Nature Struct Biol* 9, 646 (2002).
- Kawasaki H, Taira K. *EMBO Rep* 3, 443 (2002).
- Kigawa T, *et al. FEBS Lett* 442, 15 (1999).
- King RW, *et al. Science* 277, 973 (1997).
- Kitano H. *Science* 295, 1662 (2002).
- Koehler MP, *et al. Bioorg Med Chem Lett* 12, 2883 (2002).
- Kohler G, Milstein C. *Nature* 256, 495 (1975).
- Kolanus W, Zeitlmann L. *Curr Top Microbiol Immunol* 231, 33 (1998).
- Konopka K, *et al. Gene* 255, 235 (2000).
- Kruglyak L, Nickerson DA. *Nat Genet* 27, 234 (2001).
- Kumar HD. *Genomics and Cloning-Technology and Applications.* Affil. East West Press, New Delhi (2004).
- Kuwabara T, *et al. Trends in Biotech* 18, 462 (2000).
- Lang D, *et al. Science* 289, 1546 (2000).
- Lavitrano M, *et al. PNAS (USA)* 99, 14230 (2002).
- Lavitrano M, *et al. Cell* 57, 717 (1989).
- Lee NS, *et al. Nat Biotechnol* 20, 500 (2002).
- Lein S, Lowman HB. *Trends in Biotech* 21, 556 (2003).
- Li M. *Nat Biotechnol* 18, 1251 (2000).
- Lockhart DJ, Winzeler EA. *Nature* 405, 827 (2000).
- Looger, L.L., Hellinga. H.W. *J. Mol. Biol.* 307: 429-445 (2001).
- Luhrs P, *et al. J Immunol* 169, 5217 (2002).
- MacBeath G, Schreiber SL. *Science* 289, 1760 (2000).
- Malakauskas SM, Mayo SL. *Nat Strut Biol* 5, 470 (1998).
- Mann DA, Frankel AD. *EMBO J* 10, 1733 (1991).
- Marshall SA, Mayo SL. *J Mol Biol* 305, 619 (2001).

- McDermott J, Samudrala R. *Trends in Biotech* 22, 60 (2004).
- Milo R, Shen-Orr S, Itzkovitz S, *et al. Science* 298J, 824 (2002).
- Mitchell HP. *Nat Biotechnol* 20, 225 (2002).
- Mitragotri S *et al. Science* 269, 850 (1995).
- Miyagishi M, Taira K. *Nat Biotechnol* 20, 497 (2002).
- Mukhopadhyay D. *J Mol Evol* 50, 214 (2000).
- Nam JM, Thaxton CS, Mirkin CA. *Science* 301, 1884 (2003).
- Navarro JD, *et al. Trends in Biotech* 21, 263 (2003).
- Neckers L, Lee Y. *Nature* 425, 357 (2003).
- Nizak C, *et al. Science* 300, 984 (2003).
- Oda Y, *et al. PNAS (USA)* 96, 6591 (1999).
- Page MJ, *et al. Drug Discov Today* 4, 55 (1999).
- Pandey A, Mann M. *Nature* 405, 837 (2000).
- Parekh RB, Rohlff C. *Curr Opin Biotechnol* 8, 718 (1997).
- Patterson SD, Aebersold R. *Nat Genet* 311, 323 (2003).
- Ponting CP, Russell RB. *J Mol Biol* 302, 104 (2000).
- Raghothama C, Pandey A. *Trends in Biotech* 21, 467 (2003).
- Rain JC. *et al. Nature* 409, 211 (2001).
- Rangel-Aldao R. *Nat Biotechnol* 21, 491 (2003).
- Ricci MS, *et al. Protein Sci* 12, 1030 (2003).
- Riechmann LJ. *Mol Biol* 256, 957 (1996).
- Rives AW, Galitski T. *PNAS (USA)* 100, 1128 (2003)
- Roos DS. *Science* 291, 1260 (2001).
- Rossi JJ. *Trends in Biotech* 13, 301 (1995).
- Sagermann M, *et al. PNAS (USA)* 100, 9191 (2003).
- Sahin U, *et al. Curr Opin Immunol* 93, 709 (1997).
- Sarkar CA, *et al. Nat Biotechnol* 20, 908 (2002).
- Sawasaki T, *et al. PNAS (USA)* 99, 14652 (2002).
- Sblattero D, Bradbury A. *Nat Biotechnol* 18, 75 (2000).
- Schweitzer B, *et al. PNAS (USA)* 97, 10113 (2002).
- Service RF. *Science* 294, 2080 (2001).
- Service RF. *Science* 301, 1171 (2003).
- Shockley TR, *et al. Ann NY Acad Sci* 618, 367 (1991).
- Sidhu SS. *Curr Opin Biotechnol* 11, 610 (2000).
- Skerra A. *J Mol Recognit* 13, 167 (2000).
- Smith GP. *Science* 2283, 1315 (1985).

- Steen H, Pandey A. *Trends in Biotech* 20, 861 (2002).
- Stemmer WP. *Nature* 370, 389 (1994).
- Stiles JG. *Diabetes Metab Res Rev* 18, S29 (2002).
- Sundaram R, *et al. Biopolymers* 66, 200 (2002).
- Swartz JR, *Curr Opin Biotechnol* 12, 195 (2001).
- Torchilin VP, *et al. PNAS (USA)* 100, 1972 (2003)
- Tuschl T. *Nat Biotechnol* 20, 446 (2002).
- Tuschl T. *Chembiochem.* 2, 239 (2001).
- Uetz P, *et al. Nature* 403, 623 (2000).
- Varmus H. *Science* 240, 1427 (1988).
- Verkhivker GM, *et al. PNAS (USA)* 100, 5148 (2003).
- Wadia JS, Dowdy SF. *Curr Opin Biotechnol* 13, 52 (2002).
- Waldo GS. *Curr Opin Chem Biol* 7, 33 (2003).
- Wall RJ, *et al. J Daily Sci* 80, 2213 (1997).
- Warashina M, *et al. PNAS (USA)* 98, 5572 (2001).
- Weng Z, DeLisi C. *Trends in Biotech* 20, 29 (2002).
- Weng Z, DeLisi C. *Immunol Rev* 163, 251 (1998).
- Wieland T. The history of peptide chemistry. In *Peptides: Synthesis. Structures and Applications* (Gutte, B., ed.), pp. 1-38, Academic Press, New York (1995).
- Wilkins MR, Williams KL, Appel RD, Hochstrasser DF. *Proteome Research, New Frontiers in Functional Genomics.* Springer, Heidelberg, Germany (1997).
- Williams C. *Curr Opin Biotechnol* II, 42 (2000).
- Wingren C, Ingvarsson J, Lindstedt M, Borrebaeck CAK. *Nat Biotechnol* 21, 223 (2003).
- Wold F. *Annu Rev Biochem* 50, 783 (1981).
- Worn A, Pluckthun A. *J Mol Biol* 305, 989 (2001).
- Wright PE, Dyson HJ. *J Mol Biol* 293, 321 (1999).
- Yee A, *et al. PNAS (USA)* 99, 1825 (2002).
- Yu EW, Koshland DEJ. *PNAS (USA)* 98, 9517 (2001).
- Zeng J. *Comb Chem High Throughput Screen* 3, 355 (2000).
- Zhang R, Regnier FE. *J Proreome Res* 1, 139 (2002).
- Zhu H, Snyder M. *Curr Opin Chem Biol* 5, 40 (2001).
- Zwaveling S. *et al. J Immunol 169,* 350 (2002).

14

DRUG DISCOVERY, DELIVERY, SCREENING TECHNOGLOBALISM AND DRUG DEVELOPMENT

14.1. INTRODUCTION

One approach to the search and discovery of new bioactive compounds is to ensure that organisms growing on selective isolation culture plates represent novel or previously uninvestigated centers of taxonomic variation (Goodfellow and O'Donnell, 1989). The choice of organisms for pharmacological screening programs particularly those with a low throughput, is really a matter of distinguishing among known organisms and recognizing new ones. It has now become fairly easy to detect rare and novel microorganisms due to the increasing availability of sound classifications based on the integrated use of genotypic and phenotypic data (Jeffries and Dodd, 2000). This approach, termed polyphasic taxonomy, signifies successive or simultaneous studies on groups of organisms by means of suitable taxonomic methods that yield good-quality genotypic and phenotypic data. Several powerful methods are available for the acquisition of taxonomic data (Bull *et al.*, 2000).

The recently completed Human Genome Project is expected to exert a strong impact on the identification of potential drug targets - targets that can affect the designing of specific screens for therapeutic drugs. Some of the potential therapeutic targets such as Alzheimer disease, angiogenesis and asthma are human genome specific, multifactorial, and involve complex signal cascades (Bull *et al.*, 2000). These will probably dominate technology development in the coming years. Initial success in the rational design for targets such as HIV-I protease (Jones, 1998) has led to suitable methods for rational design involving gene identification, metabolic pathway analysis (Karp *et al.*, 1999), or analysis of protein-protein interactions e.g., fluorescent-protein biosensors (Giuliano and Taylor, 1998). It seems certain that in the coming year molecular genetics, robotics, miniaturization, massively parallel preparation and detection systems as well as automatic data analysis will drive the search for drug discovery leads (Bull *et al.*, 2000). Whole genome sequencing means that while the gene is viewed as the drug lead, rational design is seen as the path to drug development. However, natural products undoubtedly happen to be the result of a long and parallel experiment in combinatorial gene shuffling, mutagenesis and screening for the generation of bioactive compounds. Nevertheless, genomics and modern technology can greatly aid the quest for novel natural products by enhancing our understanding and knowledge of biodiversity and of those factors that regulate, e.g., microbial growth and expression, so complementing the synthetic and semi synthetic routes to drug development (Gelbert and Gregg, 1997).

In the current era of 'technoglobalism', new analytical techniques and innovations are enabling greater efficiency and a significant enhancement in therapeutic benefit of newly discovered compounds. Research, development, production and assessment of clinical trial outcomes from the analytical techniques will boost efficiency and improvement in the pharmaceutical industry. New paradigms, so essential for discovery, manufacturing and valuation of various development option may be expected to emerge from an explosive increase in bioinformatics and available information and shape future policies and options in biomedicine and healthcare.

Progress in applied, drug discovery-related cancer research has occurred at a fairly slow pace. Despite the advent of genomics, proteomics, and several other modern technologies, the advances in real patient benefit in terms of quality of life and survival have been quite modest. But there are recent indications that novel drug modalities could offer unexpected therapeutic potential that translates into real patient benefit.

The demand for therapeutics is growing in several developing countries. Diabetes, infectious diseases, HIV / AIDS and oncology are some of the leading health concerns in India, where the patient population is much higher than in other parts of the world. New therapeutics are being developed for "neglected diseases" that are so prevalent in the developing world. Products like Hepatitis B vaccines and Recombinant Human Insulin can have significant impact on reducing healthcare costs for countries like India. Integration of natural product chemistry and structure-based drug design is a good alternative to combinatorial chemistry and high-throughput screening. The remarkable structural diversity displayed by the metabolites of various living organisms makes these molecules attractive starting points for the drug discovery process. These scaffolds provide ample opportunities for chemical modifications to enhance affinity towards a target and to affect their pharmacokinetic properties.

The changing pharmaceutical market presents new opportunities and challenges in discovering and selecting drug candidates and in their clinical trials. One factor that contributes to escalating costs in drug discovery is the high attrition rate but it may well be possible to reduce the high cost of R&D by considering factors that contribute to the failure of drug candidates in clinical trials. The changing pharmaceutical market also demands therapies for unmet clinical needs, which usually involve molecules that prove effective on invalidated/unprecedented disease targets, and may require prolonged clinical trials.

Immunogenicity poses a major challenge in protein therapeutics; the presence of aggregates and higher order structures is thought to cause immunogenicity. This issue may be addressed by developing stable protein formulations, alongside use of automation and high-throughput methods, which can speed up moving a drug candidate faster to the clinic in a cost-effective manner. A speedy movement of potential drug candidates from laboratory to market is desirable for both the company and the patient. The first step in this long route is to develop a robust manufacturing procedure that will deliver drug for testing in a Phase I clinical trial. To handle the increased number of molecules requiring development, Amgen Inc. (USA) has developed a Monoclonal Antibody Platform. By utilizing a "flexible generic purification scheme" many more drug candidates can be explored with limited resources.

The increasing demands for mammalian cell culture derived products e.g., antibodies require manufacturers not only to increase capacity but also to improve process productivity. This goal may be achieved by the development of highly productive cell lines, efficient fermentation processes and high yielding downstream processes.

For drug discovery efforts, a wealth of useful information is provided by ongoing work on genomics, proteomics, combinatorial synthesis, and rapid analytical methods but data alone are not enough. This is borne out by the fact that in recent years, the number of new drugs approved annually by the U.S. Food and Drug Administration has not increased significantly even after a large increase in R&D investment. Productivity, in terms of the number of new drugs per unit of R&D spending has been falling in recent years and may well force a complete restructuring of the pharmaceutical industry. Considerable concern has also been expressed over a growing dependence on billion-dollar blockbusters (Szuromi *et al.,* 2004). It is being asked whether the blockbuster syndrome itself has become an obstacle to progress. In this context, Walsh (2004) emphasized the importance of the modular protein machinery that makes polypeptide and non-ribosomal peptide antibiotics. Genetic engineering of the machinery involved could possibly give us novel antibiotics. Noble *et al.,* (2004) focused on the contribution of structural genomics to drug design for the protein kinase family; conceivably such single target approaches may prove effective against genetically complex cancers. MacCoss and Baillie (2004) showed how the synthesis of very effective analogs of lead compounds is now benefiting well from the increasingly accessible data on bioavailability and toxicity. Jorgensen (2004) discussed how computational methods address these concerns and facilitate the design and screening of compounds for binding to potential bimolecular targets. Allen and Cullis (2004) have dealt with how drug delivery systems may improve targeting and reduce toxicity, especially for anticancer and antifungal agents. It is emerging that the "pipeline" problem may not be caused by a lack of research effort or even funding; overcoming the obstacles in drug discovery may require continued efforts to provide valuable insights into disease pathways and greater diversity of candidate drug molecules (Szuromi *et al.,* 2004).

Ever since antibiotics were discovered in the 1940s they have saved millions of lives. But with growing antibiotic use, the organisms they were designed to kill have become more resistant. Paradoxically, while the need for new drugs is rising, the number of effective new antibiotics has been declining.

14.2. BIODIAGNOSTICS

Biopharmaceuticals and biodiagnostics are at present probably the most important of all the products from biotechnology. Several biopharmaceuticals and thousands of diagnostics for cardiovascular diseases, cancer, infectious diseases, trauma, brain disorders, genetic disorders, asymptomatic diseases of old age, and for physiological states such as pregnancy and prediction of ovulation have been commercialized. Diagnostics provide a quick return on investment and the development of biodiagnostics is quite suited to Indian industry (Sharma, 1995).

Biotechnology-derived diagnostics include immunodiagnostics (radioisotopic, non-radioisotopic, or radiopharmaceutical imaging), DNA probes (radioisotopic. non-radioisotopic, polymerase chain reaction), RNA probes, Tests for defective genes, and Biosensors. Several formats of immunoassays are commercially available. Some (e.g., radioimmunoassay. microtitre plate ELISA and haemagglutinin assays) can be used in the laboratory, whereas some others (e.g., dipstick dot ELISA, card ELISA, immunoconcentration test, immunochromatographic stick test and sol-particle immunoassay) can be used in the home.

There is a clear industrial trend toward the development of home tests, ultra sensitive tests, transducer-based immunosensors and multifunctional and random-access analyzers. Development of these immunoassays is a great advance. The technology comprises a miniaturized multianalyte system enabling simultaneous, ultra sensitive measurement of an unlimited number of analytes in a single drop of blood or other biological fluid. Multianalyte miniaturized systems can revolutionize medicine, particularly endocrinology, allergy testing, screening of transfusion blood for blood grouping, viral contamination and genetic testing (Sharma, 1995).

Gene manipulation usually depends on the hybridization of a nucleic acid probe to a target DNA or RNA sequence. These probes help in the detection of microorganisms in clinical specimens and also changes (deletions or rearrangements) in specific sequences in the test DNA and DNA fingerprinting. In clinical microbiology, hybridization could replace a whole variety of conventional test procedures such as cultivation of test samples on a variety of media in a variety of different ways followed by microscopy, animal cell culture and immunoassay. Table 14.1 compares the merits and demerits of immunoassay and gene probe assays.

Two options to perform hybridization reactions are: (I) immobilization of one of the two nucleic acid molecules taking part in the reaction to a solid support, or (2) the hybridization of both the nucleic acids in solution. In the latter option, as both the target and the probe nucleic acids are free to move, the alignment and binding occur quickly, so the hybridization is much faster than on solid supports.

Table 14.1: Comparison of immunoassays and gene probe assays

Immunologic assay	Gene probe
Suitable if antigen or antibody is present	Works when nucleic acid sequence is present
Organism has to be cultured	Culture is not needed
Identification of all sero-types may require several antibodies	One probe alone is sufficient
Specimen to be tested should be fresh	Is effective even on old or ancient specimens

In immobilized hybridization reaction (also called "sandwich" hybridization), the probe is attached to the bottom of an ELISA microtitre plate or a tube and the reaction is carried out as shown in figure 14.1. Non-radioactive labels such as incorporation of biotinylated nucleotides and the substrate into polynucleotides enzymatically or by direct conjugation of an enzyme to polyethyleneimine using p-benzoquinone and the coupling of resulting conjugate to DNA with glutaraldehyde, have further simplified the gene probe assays. After hybridization to the target DNA, the hybrids are detected enzymatically.

There is considerable potential for growth of the biodiagnostics market in India. Biodiagnostics are developed on the basis of a clear understanding of the disease at molecular level. This is a more rational and less random approach than the conventional ways of developing drugs. Some important requirements for development of biodiagnostics and their status in India are outlined below.

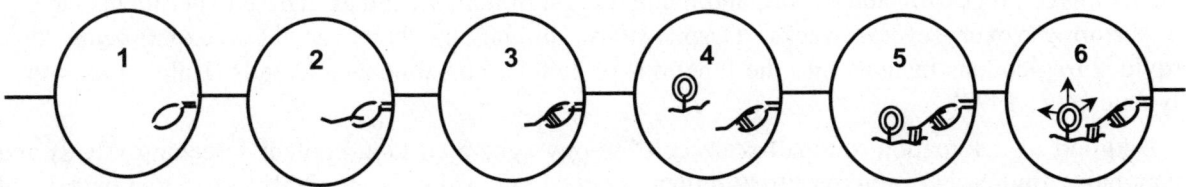

Fig. 14.1: The sandwich hybridization method as carried out in a microtitre plate. Numbers denote different states in the procedure. 1. Capture probe attached to well; 2. Addition of target DNA; 3. Target DNA hybridizes; 4. Addition of reporter (revealing) probe; 5. Revealing probe hybridizes; 6. Addition of reagents and detection of signal

Special reagents are required to develop biodiagnostics. A few examples are antigens (marker proteins), synthetic peptide antigens, polyclonal antibodies, monoclonal antibodies, antibody-enzyme conjugates, DNA probes, nucleic acid-enzyme conjugates, animal cells, tissues and microbial strains, foetal bovine serum, specialized culture media and thermostable enzymes. Most of these are imported. Microtitre plates, microtitre plate (strips), microtitre plate (breakable wells), solid support membranes, dipsticks, latex particles, chromatographic materials and dialysis membranes are also needed for developing biodiagnostics. Some of these are indigenously developed and have been commercialized, but high-quality materials for biodiagnostics have to be imported from advanced countries.

ELISA reader, ELISA plate washer, atomizer, multi-channel and single-channel micropipettes, micro and semi-micro-fluid dispensers, PCR-machine, ultrasonic cell disrupter, radioactivity counters, ultracentrifuge, microscopes, peptide and nucleic acid synthesizers and chromatographic equipment essential for the development of biodiagnostics are also imported even though some less sophisticated ones are being indigenously manufactured.

The biodiagnostics that have been approved for manufacture and marketing in India include HIV-1 and HIV-2 antibody ELISA, HBsAg ELISA, immunological color test for urinary hCG, latex agglutination inhibition test for hCG, monoclonal anti A and B blood grouping reagents, dipstick dot EIA for *S. typhi* antigens, rapid agglutination card test for syphilis, and foecal occult blood test for colorectal cancer (Sharma, 1995).

14.3. HIGH CONTENT SCREENING

Although recent advances in genomics and proteomics have profoundly stimulated investigations of DNA, RNA and proteins in living organisms, the complexity of interactions between these and other biomolecules, and between these and their physical and chemical environment, makes it very difficult to easily assign function and determine molecular mechanisms underlying life processes (Abraham *et al.*, 2004). In the living cell, biomolecules function in sub cellular organelles, which can reveal valuable functional information by examining the intracellular localization, transport and temporal and spatial control of the activity of these biomolecules (Giuliano and Taylor, 1998; Zhang *et al.*, 2002). Fluorescence light microscopy techniques, coupled with electronic imaging, are particularly useful tools for such studies in view of their compatibility with living cells; they allow molecule-specific measurements to be made with considerable sensitivity (Abraham *et al.*, 2004).

Cell biological investigations based on use of fluorescence microscopy have usually been practiced on a small scale to collect image data from a limited number of experimental samples, each not exceeding 10^3 cells per experiment. These small-scale systems are quite laborious and involve tedious image processing and export, and manipulation of numerical data. These experiments have to be performed over several weeks. Despite these limitations, however these experiments have provided tremendous insights into the functions of cellular constituents and cells (Hahn *et al.*, 1992; Plymale *et al.*, 1999).

Addition of automation to small-scale cell biology generated high content screening (HCS) and quantitative fluorescence microscopy (Giuliano *et al.*, 1997; Taylor *et al.*, 2001). HCS can be defined as the automation of high-content cell biological investigation of arrayed cells including all the various stages such as experimental design, sample preparation, image acquisition, archiving, processing and analysis, and cellular knowledge mining. HCS has proven useful as an early drug-discovery platform for defining the functions of genes, proteins and other biomolecules in normal and abnormal cellular functions. HCS is likely to have a strong impact on the implementation of huge-scale cell biology in biomedical research and biotechnology. Large-scale cell biology typically allows analysis of $> 10^6$ cells per experiment (unlike only about 10^3 as in small-scale biology). However, large-scale biology cannot replace creative small-scale biology. Once some new concept has emerged from small-scale biology, it should be subjected to suitable combinatorial experiments that involve variations of several parameters such as cell type, substrate chemistry, concentrations of agonists or antagonists, treatment durations, types of cellular variables measured per experiment, and number and frequency of time points. These experiments may also help in dissecting biochemical or metabolic pathways rapidly by pertinent measurements made in intact cells (Aridor and Hannan, 2000).

Large-scale cell biology augmented by HCS can potentially extend the utility of genomics. Genome-wide screens for analyzing the effect of suppression or amplification of protein expression have been used to (i) determine pathway components, and the temporal sequence of events in a given pathway, and (ii) validate molecular targets for therapeutic intervention (Schwartz, 1997; Ziauddin and Sabatini, 2001; Papetti and Herman, 2002).A variety of appropriate and integrated HCS tools required for successful implementation of large-scale cell biology are now available from Cellomics, Inc. (www.cellomics.com) to support automated experimentation and discovery, based on fixed end point and live-cell kinetic assays (Giuliano *et al.,* 2003).

Ultra modern hardware, software, and biological components have been used to build a large-scale HCS reader termed the Kinetic Scan (KSR) for live-cell kinetic analyses. The KSR offers a complete, automated solution for monitoring cellular processes in large arrays of individual living cells with high spatial and temporal resolution. It comprises advanced optics, automated scanning hardware. Liquid handling, environmental control, high-speed auto focus capability, image acquisition and analysis, and informatics tools to process the collected data (Abraham *et al.,* 2004; Giuliano *et al.,* 2003).

The tools of HCS have made it possible to perform automated high content cell biology on a large scale. They offer a reliable solution for addressing all the activities comprising cell-based experimentation and discovery. It is being anticipated that the present state of cell biology might be quite similar to that of the field of DNA sequencing in the pregenomic era before the advent of high-throughput automated DNA sequencers. Just as the advent of automated DNA sequencing, informatics and bioinformatics tools to handle vast amounts of genomic information greatly enlarged the scope of genomic investigation leading to rapid analysis of entire genomes, HCS and the integration of tools such as automated systems for high content cellular analysis and data management and knowledge mining, may very probably drive an analogous revolution in cell biology (Abraham *et al.,* 2004).

14.4. ORGANIC CHEMISTRY IN DRUG DISCOVERY

Organic chemistry has played a critical role in the pharmaceutical industry as a chief driver in the drug discovery process. Several new synthetic methods and technologies are now available to the chemist for understanding drug metabolism and chemical toxicology (MacCoss and Baillie, 2004). These new technologies and synthetic techniques are being used for rational drug design i.e. combinatorial chemistry, automated synthesis, and compound purification and identification. The advent of high-throughout screening (HTS) has allowed many targets to be screened.

Similarly, with the advent of much faster synthetic technologies, particularly nuclear magnetic resonance (NMR), lipid separations, and automated synthesis, the cycle time for synthetic manipulation of analogs has declined greatly. Compounds can be assayed both *in vitro* and *in vivo* at a much higher speed than was previously possible. Lipinski *et al.,* (1997) postulated the "rule of five" which turned out to be a good working hypothesis for predicting good drug like properties in new compounds. In the discovery setting, the rule of five predicts that poor absorption or permeation of drugs is more likely when a drug molecule possesses either (i) more than 5 hydrogen bond donors, (ii) 10 hydrogen bond acceptors, (iii) a molecular weight greater than 500kDa, or (iv) a calculated logP greater than 5. Careful attention has to be given to molecular weights, as well as to the physicochemical properties of lead molecules, such as lipophilicity (logP) and aqueous solubility (which influence oral bioavailability and the need for producing a parenteral formulation), together with animal pharmacokinetics, which may be cautiously extrapolated to predict corresponding behavior in humans (MacCoss and Baillie, 2004).

Studies on absorption, distribution, metabolism, and excretion (ADME) of lead compounds in animal species also provide valuable information on routes (such as renal, biliary, or metabolic) of clearance. This helps in the selection of compounds that show a balance between elimination pathways and thus would not be unduly dependent on a single organ for excretion.

As many potential drug candidates in early trials often fail because of clinical toxicity, the chemist needs to be well conversant with issues of toxicology. While the potential for genotoxicity can be assessed directly through a number of *in vitro* assays, this is not so for endo-organ toxicities (such as drug-induced liver damage) or immune-mediated toxicities (idiosyncratic reactions) (Uetrecht, 2003). However, some drug-related adverse events are mediated by a chemically reactive, electrophilic metabolite or metabolites, as opposed to the parent drug itself: this makes the generation of such electrophiles an undesirable feature of any drug candidate. Appropriate *in vitro* "trapping" experiments and assessments of covalent binding of lead drug candidates to protein both *in vitro* and *in vivo* enable the medicinal chemist working in drug metabolism to identify routes of metabolic activation and, through appropriate structural modification, to minimize this potential liability (Evans *et al.,* 2004; MacCoss and Baillie, 2004).

While the synthesis of many molecules laden with ADME, physical property, or toxicological shortcomings can sometime provide hits or leads, they usually do not shorten the time to the successful translation of such a hit into a drug candidate. According to MacCoss and Baillie, a "hit" is a non optimized structure obtained from some screening process on a target protein. It is usually a weak binder with a non-optimized pharmacokinetic profile. Likewise, a "lead" is a structure derived from an early "hit" and, although still not fully optimized, has some appropriate characteristics to be a precursor of a drug entity. Often a good lead shows some proof-of-concept activity in an *in vivo* pharmacological model, but has not been fully optimized for pharmacokinetic properties or undesirable off target activities.

14.5. IDENTIFICATION OF DRUG TARGET — THE INTERACTOME

Recently completed genome sequences have provided valuable pointers to potential drug targets. Even though sequencing of the human genome has been completed, exciting developments in the field of target identification are yet to materialize. Technological advances are enabling challenging biological questions to be addressed intelligently. One major challenge is to understand the highly complex physiology that underlies drug targets. What is needed is to identify interactions between drug targets (which are usually proteins such as receptors and enzymes) and also the proteins and other molecules that regulate them. We must first understand the complex and dynamic interaction of many proteins and different messengers and hormones determining the function of our cells and organs, and then choose potentially the most promising target for drug interaction that would give the most favorable ratio of wanted versus unwanted effects (Smith, 2004).

The modus operandi for the future drug-discovery program should be based on a tight integration of computer sciences and mathematics with experimental biology and chemistry. The data have to be assessed and interpreted by proper use of informatics systems. Genomics offers one approach to investigating physiology. The human, mouse, and rat genomes have already been sequenced.

Although much emphasis has been placed on proteomics for target identification, DNA microarray technology continues to be in the forefront as the technique of choice for identifying genes involved in susceptibility to disease. It is expected that target discovery and identification will soon benefit from the DNA microarrays of the complete human genome. Several companies are marketing this technology. For instance, in July 2003, NimbleGen (Madison, Wisconsin) marketed a chip containing 200,000 probes, with an average of five probes per gene. Since October 2003, the Human Genome U 133 plus 2.0 arrays has been marketed by Affymetrix (Santa Clara, California) with 1.3 million probes; it can analyze the expression of about 47,000 different transcripts. The most recent human whole-genome chip, launched in 2004 is from Agilent Technologies (Palo Alto, California). It is a double-density format chip with about 41.000 genes and, with the company's ImaGene image analysis software it is compatible with most commercial microarray scanners for 25 mm x 75 mm chips.

Microarrays are being widely used to study gene expression and to detect single-nucleotide polymorphisms. They may soon be used in assays to study the many forms that a protein target may take as a result of alternative splicing. There is also the clear possibility to apply microarrays not only in target identification but also genome-wide association studies of complex genetic diseases, e.g., to find genes that cause complex diseases in unrelated clinical populations. Finding genes causing a global disease makes a good drug target. The advent of microarrays has made individual genotyping feasible, and one can realistically compare the genomes of people with and without a disease at high-enough resolution to find potential drug targets (Smith, 2004).

Unfortunately the complete human-gene chips do have some limitations also. Firstly, in general, gene chips measure correlative rather than causative events. Second, because much cellular regulation occurs at the level of proteins, increased transcript production as measured by gene chips does not necessarily always correlate with production of protein; even if more protein is produced, it may require post-translation modification or relocation within a cell and so may not be active. Indeed, modifications of proteins introduce an additional complication that is not necessarily addressed by human-gene chips.

It is well known that complex interactions between proteins are crucial to their function. This means that determining the routes through which a potential drug target acts in the cell and its interactions with other proteins are extremely important. To tackle this problem, work is underway to map and study the 'interactome'-the detailed listing of which protein interacts with which other in an organism. In fact, the first such interactome has already been produced for *Drosophila melanogaster* (Smith, 2004). This work on *Drosophila* seems to point to a connection between proteins that are altered in human diseases and the 'druggable' classes of enzymes—enzymes that bind and are altered by small-molecule drugs.

14.6. CHEMOGENOMICS

Unlike the current drug-development route of target—drug—phenotype, researchers in the new field of chemogenomics start with a known drug that causes an interesting disease-relevant phenotype *in vitro* or *in vivo* and then identify the cellular target(s) for that drug. Chemogenomics has because a powerful tool in target identification because one can start with an active small molecule (Smith, 2004). Chemogenomics is in effect drug discovery in reverse. In this a drug compound with known effect is taken. The organism or the cell is exposed to this compound and the effect produced is studied so as to understand the mechanism of action as well as potential causes of side effects. It also helps in devising a more intelligent subsequent screening of compounds with better, more relevant assay readouts (Smith, 2004).

14.7. COMPUTATIONAL CHEMISTRY

The use of computers and computational methods in diverse aspects of drug discovery has been increasing in recent years. Specialists in the application of computational tools can deliver new drug candidates faster and at lower cost than those not familiar with such tools. Most drugs come through long routes starting with identification of a biomolecular target of potential therapeutic value. This potential candidate is subjected to detailed biological study, including animal studies. A multidisciplinary research team then sets out to find clinical candidates or drug like compounds that can be used in human clinical trials—compounds which selectively bind to the molecular target and interfere with its activity (Jorgensen, 2004). This is followed by screening of molecular libraries. Any resulting leads are optimized in a cycle that features design, synthesis and assaying of numerous analogs, and animal studies. In some cases it is possible to determine the crystal structure of complexes of some analogs with the biomolecular target. In these cases "structure-based drug design" (SBDD) and the efficient optimization of leads becomes possible (Maryanoff, 2004). SBDD has already led to the introduction of about 50 compounds into clinical trials and to several drug approvals. Here computation has a role in the structure refinement using simulated annealing, development of the underlying molecular mechanics (MM) force fields, structure display, and building and MM evaluation of analogs (Jorgensen, 2004).

Toward the end of the preclinical period of drug discovery, when several potential compounds have been identified, the focus shifts to concerns over differences in pharmacological issues relating to bioavailability, duration of action, and toxicity. Commonly, vigorous metabolic activity reduces bioavailability, so, for instance, reactive hydrogen can be replaced by a halogen to block a metabolic process. As solubility or cell permeability is central to bioavailability, attempts are made to improve it. Other concerns relate to the action of efflux pumps, active transport, potential drug-drug interactions, drug distribution in blood and tissue. Binding to plasma proteins, microbial resistance, and mutagenicity, nephrotoxicity, hepatotoxicity, and ventricular irregularity (Welling, 1997). The complex differences between animals and humans can be addressed through human clinical trials. There are the differences among humans, themselves. These individual differences lead to the future of pharmacogenomics (Licinio and Wong, 2002). Drug discovery being a complex process, a systematic use of a variety of modern computational tools facilitates understanding of this process. These tools usually include software developed by chemists for structure drawing, database entry-management-query, two-dimensional to three-dimensional structure conversion, molecular visualization, quantum chemistry, molecular mechanics, conformational searching, molecular dynamics, and biomolecular structure refinement, etc (Jorgensen, 2004).

14.8. VIROGENOMICS AND ANTIVIRAL DRUG DISCOVERY

The post-genomic revolution is all set to benefit in three ways: Firstly because viruses need the host to replicate they are vulnerable to inhibition of cellular pathways. Knowledge of complete genomic sequences of both virus and host can allow the study of this interaction on a global scale. Exploiting transcriptomics and proteomics while carrying out large-scale gene knockdown experiments can facilitate the identification of novel anti-viral targets. Second, such extensive parallel assay systems as DNA microarrays can greatly benefit viral diagnostics. Third, a meaningful interaction of genetics and genomics will make possible the analysis of viral strains and mutants on a huge scale. Besides the already well-known effects of viral infection on host cell transcriptional patterns, there is now a strong interest in applying functional genomics methods to the discovery of new targets and therapies for viral disease (DeFilippis *et al.,* 2003).

Genomics science may be considered to have been born in 1977, which described the first complete genome sequence of a bacteriophage. Over 1535 full viral genome sequences are known by now. Modern endeavors have made possible complete sequencing of the human genome as well as that of model organisms. Research in 'Virogenomics' is aimed at studying the interaction between the products of two genomes using post-genomic methods such as DNA microarrays. As viruses depend on a host organism for their multiplication this approach can enhance our understanding of virus-host interactions. Virogenomics research can potentially lead to new treatment for viral diseases because whole genome sequences (virus and host) represent the complete collection of possible antiviral targets. Till hitherto, antiviral drug discovery tended to focus on viral gene products but now a search for host cell targets has emerged as an attractive alternative.

Already, published studies have shown that a given virus induces or represses a given set of genes. What is needed is to find which of the many host cell gene products are essential for virus survival or for virally induced disease progression. It is these gene products that can be good targets for inhibiting virus infection, pathogenesis, or virus-induced tumor formation. Recent advances in gene knockdown technology can speed up the rate of identification of host cell pathways crucial to virus replication. Diagnostic virology is found to be strongly impacted by microarray technology because probes for thousands of viral species and strains can be matched against an unknown specimen.

Ramsay (1998) and Lockhart and Winzeler (2000) discussed the application of microarray technology in biomedicine. Microarrays are platforms made of glass, silicon, or nylon; these platforms contain oligo- or poly-nucleotides (targets) which are either identical or complementary to known genes. Analysis and search of biological samples is done by synthesis from sample mRNA of fluorescently labeled probes hybridized to target sequences. Gene expression can be estimated by measuring fluorescence emission with a suitable laser scanner. It is now possible to immobilize up to 20,000 different genes on a single array; this allows study of the transcriptional activity of entire eukaryotic genomes in parallel. It is possible to examine viral genes, host genes or any such combination on a single array. Microarray technology can also be used to immobilize specific probes for many different viral species, different viral strains, or complex DNA viruses (DeFilippis *et al.*, 2003).

Microarrays have proved useful for genotyping many small viruses (but not retroviruses, papillomaviruses and parvoviruses whose genomes are less than about 10 genes); for characterization of strain variability and identification of virus type(s) present in a clinical sample (An *et al.*, 2003). Microarrays have been designed using polynucleotides of conserved regions from a broad range of common viruses (Wang *et al.*, 2002). Random PCR amplification from infected samples can help in detecting infecting viruses by examining specific patterns of hybridization-it was this technique that confirmed that the agent of severe acute respiratory syndrome (SARS) is a member of the corona-virus family (DeFilippis, 2003). Diagnostic microarrays are destined to have valuable applications in biological warfare and bioterrorism. DNA microarrays can allow rapid diagnosis of individuals for exposure to different biothreats such as poxviruses, plague, anthrax and tularemia, and help in finding whether viral strains and types used in an attack have been genetically altered (DeFilippis *et al.*, 2003).

14.9. DNA MICROARRAY ANALYSIS OF VIRUS-INFECTED HOST CELLS

Viral mutant can lead to a change in the host cell transcriptional profile. The deletion of non-essential genes sometimes restores a 'normal' phenotype in tissue culture while the microarray fingerprint of such a mutant is still very different from the wild type if the deleted gene happens to be involved in manipulating host cell pathways that are not essential *in vitro* but have an important role *in vivo* (DeFilippis *et al.,* 2003). Use of DNA microarrays can therefore not only point to the function of nonessential viral genes but also prove helpful in classifying viral mutants generated by random approaches.

Besides metabolism, cellular pathways related to transcription and translation, signal transduction, host defense and cell cycle control are commonly altered either in response to, or as a result of viral infection. Transcriptional changes in virally infected cells can either be the result of anti-viral, or 'pro'-viral, or bystander host responses. One quite common anti-viral response is expression of interferon stimulated genes (ISGs) during infection by diverse, unrelated viruses. ISGs tend to block virus replication and to circumvent or impair this host response (Katze *et al.,* 2002). As the ability to prevent or inhibit this induction might conceivably contribute to virulence, it can be a potential target pathway for antiviral treatments. Antiviral therapy could be based on targeting viral proteins that interfere with the induction of ISGs, thereby releasing the innate immune response to combat viral infection (DeFilippis *et al.,* 2003).

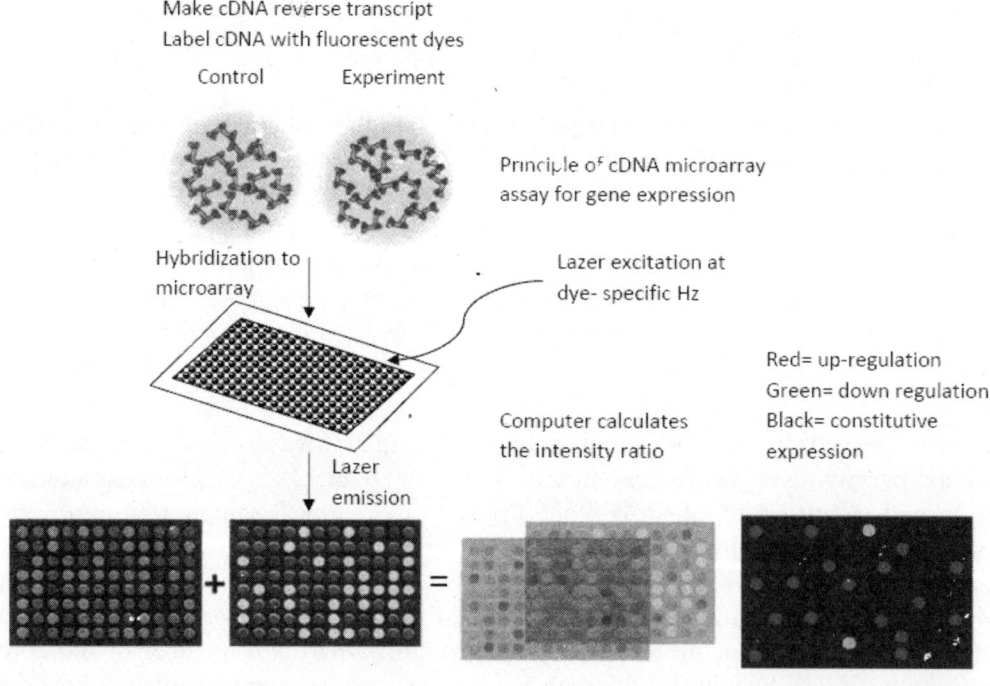

Fig.14.2: Principle of cDNA microarray assay of gene expression

Viruses often employ an anti-host strategy, which complicates transcriptome analysis; this strategy involves interference with cellular RNA metabolism. Global inhibition of transcription or RNA degradation can therefore be wrongly construed as gene repression in a comparative analysis (Geiss *et al.*, 2001). In such cases, microarray analysis is used to screen for host cell mRNAs that survive viral attack thus potentially representing novel antiviral host factors. Unlike those host pathways which represent an antiviral response, some others can be beneficial or even essential for viral replication. Inhibiting these 'pro'-viral factors can be an effective strategy for antiviral drug discovery (Schang, 2002). While global gene expression profiling can reveal host cell genes that promote viral growth, how to pick genes that might be important for viral replication is a daunting task.

Viral oncogenesis exemplifies virus modulation of host cell gene expression in which functional genomics can reveal novel targets and treatments. Since oncogenic transformation occurs through misregulation of gene expression, it is in the field of cancer research that transcriptomics and proteomics are likely to have the most immediate and direct benefiting for patients (Yeatman, 2003). Infected cells are transformed by viruses because viral oncogenes trigger cellular pathways that ultimately cross growth restrictions. The implication is that the study of viral transformation using functional genomics methods can unravel suitable targets relevant to the development of cancer in general.

14.10. GENE KNOCKDOWN APPROACHES

In principle at least, methods of functional genomics can identify new antiviral targets or targets for the treatment of diseases caused by viruses. However, pinpointing the changes that occur in host cells during virus infection is a daunting task. Till recently the availability of specific inhibitors warranted studying a particular host cell gene upregulated in a virally infected cell. But now we can make use of improved gene knockdown methods using antisense RNA or RNA interference (RNAi) (Heasman, 2002; McManus and Sharp, 2002). New antisense oligomers have the merit of high specificity and long life. The most recent method for analyzing gene inhibition studies is based on RNAi or siRNA; small (21-23 nucleotide) RNA duplexes interfere with the transcription program by degrading homologous mRNA (Hamilton and Baulcombe, 1999). RNA gene silencing mechanisms are quite common in plants, fungi, nematodes, *Drosophila* and mammalian cells, although the mechanism by which siRNA cleaves the target sequence is not clear.

Today, it is possible to use both new-generation antisense oligomers and siRNA to knockdown expression of genes found by DNA microarrays to be upregulated in virally infected organisms. Such a combination of microarray and knockdown methods is particularly attractive for viral systems because, instead of *de novo* induction, microarrays often indicate strong alterations in the level of a given transcript upon infection, thereby making it unnecessary to completely shut down expression of a target—it can suffice to reduce the level of induction back to the pre-infection state.

In some viral systems, siRNA targeted against viral or host cell genes inhibits viral replication (Coburn and Cullen, 2002; Bitko and Barik, 2001). Jiang and Milner (2002) reported that human papillomavirus and hepatitis C virus replication are modulated with siRNA (DeFilippis *et al.*, 2003). Brummelkamp *et al.* (2002) demonstrated the therapeutic potential of siRNA by retroviral delivery of siRNA that could suppress human pancreatic carcinoma, leading to loss of tumorigencity. The recent revolution in gene inhibition by antisense and siRNA can facilitate the validation of a large number of potential targets identified by DNA microarrays or other methods. Whole-genome screens with siRNA can enable a complete evaluation and validation of the role of host cell gene products for viral replication. It seems that the characterization of the functional host gene products essential for virus replication and disease is a problem that may be addressed effectively in the near future (DeFilippis *et al.,* 2003).

14.11. METAL-BASED PHARMACEUTICALS

Metal ions promote responses in living organisms that range from deficiency to toxicity. Metal ions contained within well-designed molecules already constitute a great boon for the medicinal pharmacopoeia. However, whether essential or not, the threshold for toxicity can be very low. One of the challenges of designing metal-based drugs is to balance the potential toxicity of an active formulation with the substantial positive impact of these increasingly common therapeutic and diagnostic aids.

Besides being essential nutrients, many metal ions are becoming increasingly prevalent components of diagnostic or therapeutic agents to treat many diseases and metabolic disorders (Orvig and Abrams, 1999; Farrell, 1999). The essential ions for humans include not only such expected known elements as zinc, copper, and manganese but also many that were previously thought of only as poisons, such as selenium and molybdenum (FNB, 2001). Included in the "possibly essential" list are such unexpected candidates as arsenic, nickel, silicon, and vanadium (NRC, 1989). Nutritional studies on various metals have shown that essentiality is no counter argument to toxicity, and vice versa. Therefore, it is important that appropriate intakes of metal-based therapeutics should be carefully defined (Thompson and Orvig. 2003). Indeed, the Swiss physician Paracelsus had stated in the 16th century "All substances are poisons: there is none which is not a poison". The right dose differentiates a poison and a remedy. For example, platinum, even though not an essential element is a crucial therapeutic adjuvant in cancer therapy, despite its well-known toxic potential.

Marginal deficiencies of essential minerals are involved in the pathogenesis of such chronic diseases as coronary heart disease, diabetes mellitus, nephropathy, and epilepsy. Also, overdose of a metal ion can lead to serious ill health. Pharmacologically beneficial intake ranges are usually somewhat higher than recognized windows of optimal intake for nutrients; this makes toxicity a bane for those designing metal-based pharmaceuticals. In fact, not only the right dose, but also the right metal-ligand combination, is critical. In a metal containing compound, the ligand is usually an organic compound that binds the metal ion(s) and modifies its properties. An important aspect of inorganic drug design relates to how the ligand affects bioavailability (bioavailability is the amount of a dose that is functionally usable by an organism).

14.12. THERAPEUTIC PRINCIPLES

The field of medicinal inorganic chemistry is generally considered to have numerous applications but no unifying principles. Recently, however, the following principles have emerged (i) dose makes the difference between boon or bane; (ii) the entire chemical entity, not just the metal ion, matters; (iii) a prerequisite for quantitative studies is the capacity for accurate measurement; and (iv) the bioavailability of a metal-containing compound determines its relative biochemical impact (Thompson and Orvig, 2003).

For chemotherapeutic applications the oxidation state of a metal is a critical factor as it is an indicator of its optimal dose and bioavailability. For example, Cr(VI) compounds are highly toxic, whereas Cr(III) compounds are much less so. Work is underway on vanadium compounds representative of three different physiologically compatible oxidation states of vanadium, V(V), V(IV), and V(III), as orally available insulin-enhancing therapeutics for diabetes (Thompson and Orvig, 2003). In diabetic animals, vanadium has normalized blood glucose and lipids; human clinical trials have also shown modest restoration of insulin sensitivity. V (IV) compounds are relatively more effective as glucose-lowering agents than their V(III) and V(V) analogs.

Many metalloenzymes are being examined for exploring the possibilities of developing synthetic mimics to revolutionize industrial catalysis, and this approach has its parallels in medicinal chemistry. It appears that the increasingly purposeful design of metal-based therapeutics leading to fairly well defined absorption, distribution, metabolism, and excretion of metal-based therapeutics can improve the boon-bane balance for metal ions in medicine in the coming years.

14.13. NEW PHARMACEUTICALS FROM MARINE ORGANISMS

The pressing need for the development of new pharmaceuticals is borne out even today by our inability to cure cancer, AIDS, Alzheimer's disease and arthritis (to mention but a few). Of all the natural sources for drugs, the marine environment happens to be the last great frontier. Marine ecosystems have been only recognized recently to contain sources of many novel new drugs. Chemists have been unraveling the structures of novel organic compounds produced by marine plants and animals, and surprisingly found a dramatically different environment for biosynthesis, one including new building blocks and incorporating unprecedented enzymatic reactions. This led to the recognition that marine sources have considerable potential to generate new drugs. The pharmaceutical industry now regards the oceans as a major frontier for medical research.

Many unique bioactive substances have been extracted from marine plants and invertebrate animals (Fenical, 1997). Most of the compounds initially discovered were not effective in treating diseases, but some could act as pharmacological probes as they have the potential to revolutionize our understanding of the underlying biochemistry of disease. Unique marine molecules such as manoalide and okadaic acid have been discovered. Manoalide was isolated in Hawaii from the sponge *Luffariella variabilis* and was the first substance ever observed to inhibit phospholipase A_2 selectively, an enzyme involved in many inflammatory diseases. Okadaic acid, a cyclic polyether first isolated from the sponge *Halichondria okadai,* is a highly selective inhibitor of the enzyme protein phosphatase, allowing it to be used to probe basic cellular phosphorylation processes. Besides these early discoveries, hundreds of bioactive metabolites have subsequently been discovered.

Many marine derived agents are at various stages of preclinical development. For cancer treatment, the information is readily available from the U.S. National Cancer Institute (NCI). Over one half of the NCI's natural products programs involve exploration of marine sources. At least six marine drugs are currently being clinically evaluated, for example, ecteinascidin 743, a novel alkaloid isolated from the mangrove ascidian *Ecteinascidia turbinata,* bryostatin-l, a macrolide antitumor agent isolated from the common fouling bryozoan *Bugula neritina,* dolastatin-l 0, a linear peptide found in the sea hare *Dolabella auricularia* and Halichondrin B, a complex anticancer agent first isolated from the sponge *Halichondria okadia.* Curacin A isolated from the marine cyanobacterium *Lyngbya majuscula* has promising effect on cancer cell division. Curacin A and a discodermolide from the deep water sponge *Discodermia dissobeta,* interact with the spindle protein tubulin in a similar fashion to Taxol, which is a clinically used drug. As Taxol has proven superior to older drugs in the treatment of certain forms of cancer, these new agents may hold similar promise.

Marine compounds also have the potential to treat diseases other than cancer. The pseudopterosins, a series of diterpenoid glycosides isolated from the Caribbean Sea whip *Pseudopterogorgia elisabethae,* shows impressive anti-inflammatory properties on the skin. The pseudopterosins modify the inflammatory response of human white blood cells, and control a major degradative component of the inflammation reaction. This property has prompted the development of a new additive, recently used by Estee Lauder in the 'Resilience' line of skin care products. A derivative of the natural product, methopterosin, is being tested for a wide range of inflammatory diseases including arthritis, psoriasis and asthma (Fenical, 1997).

The marine drug discovery effort has relied upon the enormous diversity of plants and animals found mainly in shallow waters throughout the tropical oceans. Here, species diversity is high and drug discovery can capitalize on the large number of species represented. However, these resources are limited and collectable marine organisms are likely to be almost completely explored within the next few decades. Where should scientists turn to ensure a continuing flow of new drugs'? Drugs can now be developed by diverse methods including computer-aided drug design and combinatorial synthesis. Drug discovery from nature, however, may survive, because of the huge diversity of microorganisms found in the oceans. The microorganisms found in the sea provide great opportunity to discover new drugs. The microbial adaptations to growing in the ocean are basically different from those in land based organisms (Attaway and Zaborsky, 1993). Nutrients are scarce in the sea, forcing many microorganisms to associate with the nutrient rich plants and animals found there. Microbial symbiosis is common and associational specificity high, and competition for resources at the microscopic level is intense. To cope with this situation microorganisms make a variety of chemical compounds for defense and competition. These compounds constitute the foundation for the development of marine microorganisms as a major drug resource. Many marine microbial compounds are chemically unique; the anti-inflammatory salinamides and the bromine containing antibiotic marinone exemplify the structural novelty observed in marine bacteria. Many marine fungi being unique to the ocean provide opportunities for the isolation of unique drugs.

14.14. NOVEL ANTI-PRION DRUGS

Prions, misfolded proteins that can propagate their altered conformational state, causes certain neurodegenerative diseases termed spongiform encephalopathies (Prusiner. 1998). The most surprising fact about prion proteins is that even on their own and without information from a nucleic acid they can act as powerful infectious agents (Prusiner, 1982, 1998). Till hitherto there was no treatment for prion diseases. But some anti-prion drugs are now been developed.

Transmissible spongiform encephalopathies are caused by an abnormal form of the membrane-bound PrP protein, a protein expressed at the surface of numerous cell types, including neurons (Saupe, 2003). Prusiner (1998) stated that during the course of the disease, an abnormal protease-resistant form of PrP (termed PrP^{sc} for scrapie) accumulates and converts the normal form (PrP^c) to PrP^{sc}. Wickner (1994) showed that a long-known bizarre genetic element of yeast is actually a prion protein, supporting the concept of a nucleic acid-free transmission of genetic information and defying the central dogma of molecular biology (Uptain and Lindquist, 2002).

But even though conceptually identical, there exist several differences between yeast and mammalian types of prion. Yeast prions neither kill cells nor cause 'disease' (Couzin, 2002). Prion-infected yeast strains can even grow better than wild type under certain growth conditions (True and Lindquist, 2000). Indeed, in yeast, prions might conceivably be adaptive. Further, unlike the membrane-bound PrP, fungal prions are cytosolic proteins. But PrP and the fungal prion proteins both can polymerize into amyloid aggregates, which may possibly represent either the replicative form of prions or terminal aggregation by-products.

Aguzzi *et al.* (2001) and White *et al.* (2003) have discussed immunological and pharmacological approaches to the development of prion disease therapies. Branched polyamines, cysteine protease inhibitors, tetrapyrrole compounds and tricyclic derivatives have been reported to promote PrP^{sc}

clearance in cell culture assays (Supattapone *et al.,* 2002) including the antimalarial drug quinacrine and the antipsychotic chlorpromazine. Also, various chemical treatments, e.g., mM concentrations of guanidine chloride (GuHCl) can cure yeast prions. Bach *et al.,* (2003) reported identification of new antiprion drugs, by screening a chemical library for molecules active against yeast prions, followed by a colorimetric assay to detect prion loss.

This screening technique led to be successful identification of six active molecules all being tricyclic derivatives. It appears that these compounds could have a broad, general effect on various prion proteins (Saupe, 2003). An interesting observation was that quinacrine and chlorpromazine, found to clear Prpsc in mammalian cell culture models, also cleared yeast prions. This point to the possibility that quinacrine and chlorpromazine could as well have been identified as anti-prion drugs using this yeast-based assay. Indeed, this assay may turn out to be a convenient screen for identifying novel anti-prion molecules.

According to Follette (2003), the drugs identified using the *in vitro* cell-culture assay, including quinacrine, do not prevent development of prion disease in live animals. Yet, being inexpensive, fast and simple, this yeast-based screening assay might prove potentially useful as an initial high-throughput screen used upstream of secondary screens using mammalian cell cultures, and ultimately, infected animals. Yeast prion propagation being strongly linked to amyloid aggregation, the screening developed by Bach *et al.,* could also facilitate the identification of molecules involved in other protein misfolding disorders with significant effects on human health, such as Parkinson's and Alzheimer's disease (Saupe, 2003). An added merit of yeast is that the eukaryotic cellular environment is much more relevant to the safety of protein-folding disorders in humans than a bacterial cell environment.

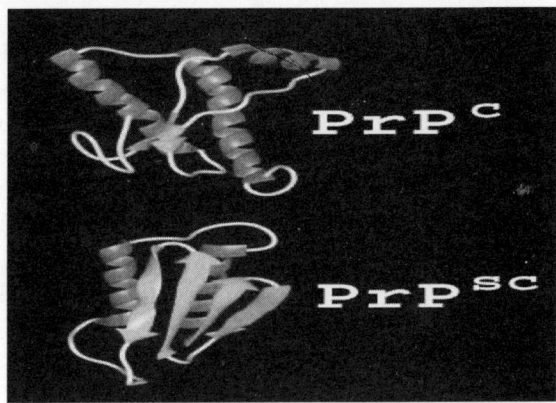

Fig. 14.3: Structure of prion

14.15. ION CHANNEL DRUG DISCOVERY

Being involved in regulating vital electrical functions in the body, ion channels can be good therapeutic drug targets for various disorders. In some cases, they are the direct cause of undesirable side effects. Ion channels are made of macromolecular protein complexes found within the cell membrane lipid bilayer. They make suitable targets for several drugs for treating such disorders as hypertension, arrhythmias, seizures, pain, stroke and diabetes. These channels comprise distinct protein subunits encoded by different genes (Catterall, 1995, 2000, 2000a; Jiang *et al.,* 2002; Bennett and Guthrie, 2003). Recent advances in our knowledge of ion channel structure function relationships have prompted vigorous search for ion channel targets in the worldwide drug discovery market (Ebneth, 2002).

Disease-causing mutations have been identified in ion channel genes. Mutations that lead to complete loss of function or even gain-of-function have been identified (Ackerman, 1998; Barchi, 1998; Hille, 2001). Some examples of disorders resulting in ion channel gene mutations include cardiac arrhythmias, migraine, muscle paralysis, and seizures (Hubner and Jentsch, 2002). Despite their crucial importance as targets, however, ion channels have till hitherto been neglected because of the paucity of methods to measure their activity directly by high-throughput screening (HTS). Several new technologies have been developed to address this lacuna (Owen and Silverthorne, 2002). Three classes of methods are available for evaluating ion channel pharmacology: (i) ligand binding or displacement; (ii) membrane potential measurements; and (iii) flux measurements. Usually ion channels are studied in Chinese hamster ovary cells, human embryonic kidney cells or *Xenopus* oocytes. The growing demand for improved ion channel screening technologies can be met only by generating novel ion channel cell lines (Bennett and Guthrie. 2003).

Because ion channels mediate the permeability of various ion concentrations on either side of the plasma membrane, changes in membrane potential reflect changes in ion channel conductance caused e.g., by drugs. This is the rationale for employing membrane potential as a measure of ion channel activity. Considerable progress has been recorded with systems that measure changes in membrane potential optically by using voltage-sensitive dyes. Cell lines have been produced with improved detection windows *via* mutations that change ion channel opening probability, which shift membrane potential to more favorable values. More conductances may be introduced to produce a membrane potential that shifts only when a few target channels are changed by the drug. It is also possible to employ fluorescent voltage-sensitive dyes to measure membrane-potential changes across the cellular membrane, either by electrical-potential-dependent redistribution of dye or by fluorescence resonance energy transfer (FRET) between a dye pair. FRET dye-pairs increase sensitivity and reduce background (Numann and Negulescu, 2001). The optical signal can be measured in a multi-well plate-reader and it changes in keeping with changes in membrane potential. Evaluation of concentration dependent effects on membrane potential helps in assessing drug-channel interactions.

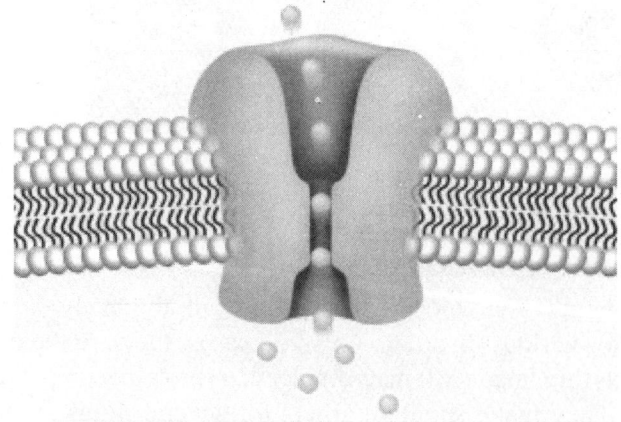

Fig. 14.4: Structure of ion channel

Another approach uses cell-based ion flux assays based on the detection of ion movement through the open channel. These assays require some means to activate the channel. Tracer ions detectable with spectroscopy can be incorporated, including radioactive or unnatural ions (e.g., Rb^+) or native ions (such as Ca^{2+}) may be used with fluorescent dyes. Detection involves radioactive decay of tracer ion, fluorescent plate-readers, spectroscopy or electronics (Bennett and Guthrie, 2003).

Ion-selective fluorescent probes that can estimate intracellular ionic concentrations are widely used in the pharmaceutical industry for screening with ion channels, primarily to detect calcium. Hamill *et al.*, (1981) developed a voltage-clamp technique that uses electronic negative-feedback circuits to control transcellular membrane potential and measures ionic flux (ion current) directly through open ion channels (Hille, 2001). Since the membrane potential does not change, the ionic current in a voltage-clamped cell is a direct index of the opening probability of the channels and yields valuable information on inhibitors and activators.

Membrane potential may also be altered at different rates to reveal channel state-dependent drug interactions. This can lead to drugs that act on demand in cells that cycle membrane potential at different rates (e.g., neuronal spike frequency or cardiac tachyarrhythmias). Some more recent technologies for ion channel screening rely on voltage clamp methods to measure channel behavior. Automating and industrializing the voltage-clamp method can be achieved by using cells that express the ion channel targets of interest (Papke and Porter Papke, 2002; Kiss *et al.*, 2003).

Trends in ion channel screening technologies have focused on increasing throughput and enhancing information content of assays through electrophysiological approaches. The ability to study ion channels by voltage clamp and their time-voltage and state-dependent drug interactions with enhanced throughput are now playing a crucial role in the development of novel, safe ion channel-targeted drugs (Bennett and Guthrie, 2003).

14.16. ANTIBODIES AS DRUGS

Antibodies are highly targeted proteins that constitute one of the more effective weapons of the immune system. If we could produce large amounts of specific antibodies against proteins involved in disease they should act like effective drugs. Unfortunately, however, the antibodies have until recently performed poorly in the clinic. Developments in genetic engineering, cancer biology, immunology and genomics have now allowed antibodies to express their therapeutic potential.

Table 14.2: Some monoclonal antibody therapies approved by the US food and drug administration

Product	Type	Condition	Company	Approved
Orthoclone OKT3	Mouse	Transplant rejection	Johnson & Johnson	1986
ReoPro	Chimeric	Cardiovascular disease	Eli Lilly	1994
Rituxan	Chimeric	Non-Hodgkin's lymphoma	Genentech	1997
Zenapax	Humanized	Respiratory syncytial virus	Medimmune	1998
Herceptin	Humanized	Metastatic breast cancer	Genentech	1998
Mylotarg	Humanized	Acute myelogenous toxin lined leukamia	American home Products	2000

Monoclonal antibodies are being mass-produced in the lab to recognize an individual molecular target. In USA, the Food and Drug Administration has approved about a dozen of them to treat cancer and transplant rejection and to combat autoimmune diseases such as rheumatoid arthritis (see Table 14.2). Hundreds of other monoclonal antibodies are in clinical trials worldwide.

Antibodies are Y-shaped proteins, consisting of two identical light and two identical heavy chains of polypeptides. The arms of the Y identify and bind to the antibody's specific molecular target, or antigen. When that happens, the portions of the heavy chains that extend into the stem of the Y alert and recruit the other components of the immune system to attack the structure to which the antibody is bound (Gura, 2002).

By fusing antibody-producing cells from immunized mice with antibody secreting mouse cells derived from a type of cancer called myeloma, Kohler and Milstein in 1975 generated hybrid cell lines that could be cloned and cultured indefinitely. When injected into mice, these immortalized cells grew into tumors producing large amounts of monoclonal antibodies. Today, it is possible to produce large quantities of monoclonals without any need to grow tumors in mice. While mouse antibodies worked well in rodent models of disease they however created problems when injected into human patients. The patient's immune systems quickly recognized the mouse antibodies as foreign proteins, and generated 'human anti mouse antibodies' that cleared the mouse proteins from the bloodstream sometime resulting in a fatal allergic response (Winter and Milstein, 1991).

But one mouse antibody passed through clinical trials. This monoclonal, termed Orthoclone OKT3 is used to help prevent the rejection of transplanted organs. It works by targeting a glycoprotein on the surface of T-cells that would otherwise recognize the organ as foreign. In effect, Orthoclone OKT3 shuts down one arm of the immune system-which helps to explain why it does not get cleared from the bloodstream quickly (Gura, 2002).

Scientists turned to genetic engineering of both mouse antibody-producing cells and hybridomas, mixing and matching DNA from mouse and human antibody genes with a view to make antibodies that would not be rejected by the human immune system. In one of these chimeras, genes encoding mouse antibody arms were simply grafted onto those for human antibody stems, producing antibodies that were roughly 30% mouse, 70% human.

These chimeric antibodies could communicate with the human immune system. But usually the chimaeras were attacked by the immune system. Later, the mouse component of chimeric antibodies was pruned down to only 5–10%. Three loops of amino acids within the variable region each antibody arms were known to act as the 'glue' to bind antibody to antigen. So everything but the genes for these loops was replaced with human sequences. The resulting 'humanized' mouse monoclonals seemed to evade the human immune system.

In 1994, Eli Lilly marketed the first chimeric antibody, ReoPro, which lessens the risk of blood clots in patients with cardiovascular disease by targeting a receptor protein on the surface of platelets. In 1997, Roche introduced the first humanized monoclonal antibody Zenapax that fights organ rejection by inhibiting a receptor on activated white blood cells, which would otherwise stimulate tissue rejection.

Now companies have moved onto solid tumors, which are harder to treat than lymphomas and leukaemia. Herceptin, marketed by Genentech, blocks a growth receptor on the surface of breast cancer cells. The effectiveness of monoclonals against cancer might be improved by attaching toxins or radionuclides to the antibodies. In 2002, IDEC Pharmaceuticals of San Diego received approval for Zevalin, a radioactive antibody for use against non-Hodgkin's lymphoma. Some researchers are contemplating the use of cocktails of monoclonal antibodies that will simultaneously target different molecules in multiple cell-signaling pathways. Another interesting approach is adopted by some companies, e.g., Abgenix to work with mice engineered to have immune systems that are human, as far as their production of antibodies is concerned. The rodents' ability to produce mouse antibodies was at first knocked out by deleting regions of the rodent's heavy and light-chain genes and then the equivalent human genes were added (Fishwild *et al.*, 1996). Now one only needs to inject the rodents with the antigen of choice and the animals start producing completely human compatible antibodies.

The chief problem with antibodies is their exorbitant cost. The proteins are usually generated by cell cultures in bioreactors; the purified antibodies can cost as much as US$ 1,000 per gram compared with $5 per gram for typical small molecules produced by chemical synthesis. Attempts are underway to improve the efficiency of antibody production in cell culture, but eventually they are likely to move to streamlined cell-free systems a step that would surely place antibodies in the clinical mainstream (Gura, 2002).

14.17. PROBIOTICS AS ALTERNATIVES TO ANTIBIOTICS

Two important classes of probiotics (lactic acid bacteria, LAB) present in several dairy products such as yogurt are lactobacilli and bifidobacteria. These bacteria are quite safe for use in humans (McFarland and Elmer, 1995; Teitelbaum and Walker, 2002; Ahmed, 2003). They potentially act through maintenance of mucosal intestinal resistance to infectious diseases; prevention of vaginitis; production of antimicrobial metabolites and nutraceuticals; immunomodulation; relief of constipation and prevention of antibiotic-associated diarrhea; metal detoxification; cholesterol and blood pressure reduction; regression of tumors and reduction in carcinogen and mutagen production (Kruger *et al.*, 2002; Brudnak. 2002; Ahmed. 2003). Most probiotics are readily available over the counter without prescription in supermarkets, grocery and health food stores. Unfortunately, the use of some probiotics is not always free of risk. Several cases of *Salmonella boulardii* septicemia have been reported and it is conceivable that probiotic use might detract from the currently prescribed high doses of antibiotics

Table 14.3: Safety assessment of probiotic lactic acid bacteria (LAB)

Properties	Safety factors to be evaluated
Intrinsic properties	Adhesion, antibiotic resistance; plasmids and their transfer
Metabolic Products	Concentrations, safety
Toxicity	Acute and subacute effects
Mucosal effects	Adhesion invasion; intestinal mucus degradation
Dose-response effects	Oral administration in volunteers
Clinical assessment	Side effects if any
Epidemiological studies	Critical surveillance of large populations following introduction of novel strains and products

LAB is Gram-positive, non-spore-forming, economically important bacteria found naturally in foods and the human intestine. They represent a genetically diverse group including some species of *Carnobacterium, Enterococcus, Lactobacillus, Lactococcus, Leuconostoc, Pediococcus, Streptococcus, Vagococcus and Weissella*. The genus *Lactobacillus* is quite heterogeneous, with >60 species of which about a third are strictly heterofermentative (Stiles and Holzapfel, 1997). Some 18 species of *lactobacilli* act as probiotics, and there may be about a dozen sp. of *Bifidobacterium*. Many LABS are safe for use in food; some species of *Streptococcus* and *Enterococcus* are pathogens. As attempts are being made to produce new probiotic strains by genetic modification, any possible safety concerns will need to be addressed. Adams (1999) proposed several tests for this purpose. In fact, some genetic systems (e.g., plasmid vectors, chromosome modification systems) have already been exploited to analyze and modify LAB, particularly *Lactococcus lactis* and others of industrial interest (Brondsted and Hammer, 1999; Renault, 2002; Dubnau and Lovett, 2002).

However, a few LABS have been modified by recombinant-DNA technology because of consumer resistance to their introduction in markets, especially in Europe. Starter strains can be produced by mutation and genetic modification. Single gene mutations have been introduced to produce lactococcal variants in lactose metabolism, citrate uptake and proteolytic activity. But the number of traits that can be modified by this method is limited. To avoid the problems associated with random mutagenesis, Mollet (1999) successfully used recombinant-DNA technology to improve the flavor and stability of buttermilk through metabolic engineering of *L. lactis*.

This genetically engineered strain is currently being used in a starter in the USA and in Denmark but has not found favour in the rest of Europe (Henriksen *et al.,* 1999; Gaskell *et al.,* 1999; Ahmed, 2002). Strains showing enhanced proteolytic properties have been produced by transfer of genes encoding certain peptidases of highly proteolytic strains of *L. helveticus* and *L. delbrueckii* into *L. lactis* using a food-grade cloning system (Wegmann, 1999; Joutsjoki *et al.,* 2002). Inter-LAB cloning can be used for introducing new functions. Genes may also be introduced from distant bacterial strains to produce GMOs.

14.18. NOVEL DRUGS THROUGH APOPTOSIS

Programmed cell death (apoptosis) plays an important role not only in development but also in some physiological processes. Apoptosis, accompanied by inflammation, is also a principal pathophysiological process that underlies several diseases. Apoptosis therefore provides many opportunities for the discovery and development of drugs (Alam, 2003). Certain drugs modulate apoptosis, being either pro-apoptotic or anti-apoptotic. Some important diseases that may be treated by apoptosis-modulating drugs are listed in Table 14.4. These diseases may also be classified by their requirement for either drugs that promote apoptosis (primarily anti-cancer drugs) or those that inhibit it. The anti-apoptotic opportunities may be acute versus chronic types of diseases.

The spectrum of apoptosis-inducing drugs and acute and chronic anti-apoptotic drugs points to the utility of apoptosis modulation as a therapy. Specific, targeted drugs that selectively induce apoptosis in some types of cancer are already available (Kaufman and Earnshaw, 2000; Evan and Vousden, 2001). However, Anti-apoptotic drugs for chronic diseases are not yet available. Several pro-apoptotic drugs for treating cancer are currently being developed. The anti-apoptotic drugs that are most advanced in the development are targeting such acute disease indications as stroke, myocardial infarction and sepsis, in which the role of apoptosis has been best defined and inhibitors of the apoptotic pathway have proven to be effective in various animal models.

The potential of novel targeted approaches for the treatment of cancers arises from selective induction of apoptosis in cancer cells in preference to normal cells (that is, the newer drugs will act as tumor-selective apoptosis-inducing agents). Indeed, two rather new drug development approaches for cancer treatment, which are most popular strategies in the whole of R&D, are angiogenesis inhibition and apoptosis induction.

Table 14.4 Examples of human diseases involving apoptosis

Neurodegenerative
Stroke, Traumatic brain injury and/or spinal cord injury, Alzheimer's, Parkinson's, Multiple sclerosis
Cardiovascular
Myocardial ischemia, Congestive heart failure
Others
Alopecia, Anemia, Burns, Cancer, Gastric ulcers, Infections, HIV, Transplant, Pancreatitis, Muscular dystrophy

Most apoptosis-inducing drugs being developed do not target the apoptosis machinery directly; rather they induce apoptosis indirectly by targeting cell proliferative or cell-survival signals (Kaufman and Earnshaw, 2000; Evan and Vousden, 2001). Some companies, however, have initiated discovery and development programs that target the apoptosis machinery directly to induce apoptosis in tumor cells. One of these approaches is an antisense oligonucleotide targeting the gene encoding an anti-apoptotic protein, BCL-2 (Banerjee, 2001). Another approach is directed towards another anti-apoptotic protein, X-linked inhibitor of apoptosis (XIAP); an antisense oligonucleotide targeting XIAP is currently in pre-clinical development (Hu *et al.,* 2003).

14.19. ACUTE APOPTOTIC DISEASE

The three acute medical conditions involved in many in-hospital deaths are ischemic stroke, myocardial infarctions and sepsis. Apoptosis seems to be active in the pathophysiology of each of these. Anti-apoptotic agents have shown pharmacological activity in animal models of these disorders. Anti-apoptotic drugs in pharmaceutical development are generally targeting these disorders (Alam, 2003; MacManus and Buchan, 2000; Love, 2003; James, 1998).

However, most of the companies which are interested in finding and developing anti-apoptosis treatments have not realized or appreciated this potential in the treatment of chronic diseases, probably because chronic anti-apoptotic therapy might adversely affect the normal physiological processes. Although the application of anti-apoptotic therapies for chronic disease is still in the remote future, a deeper understanding of the apoptotic pathways associated with principal chronic disorders could result in drugs that impact apoptosis in a disease-specific manner to slow the irreversible progression of the disease (Alam, 2003).

14.20. NANOCONTAINERS FOR DRUG DELIVERY

As unfavorable solubility, stability, and toxicity lower the therapeutic efficacy of many drugs. Suitable drug delivery systems can provide a concentration of drugs in an aqueous milieu above the intrinsic solubility limit of the free drug by increasing drug stability, and by targeting delivery to the required cells, thereby lowering the required dosage (Savic *et al.,* 2003; Saltzman, 2001). Block copolymer micelles, which are usually spherical, nanosized (10 to 100 nm), supramolecular assemblies of amphiphilic copolymers with a core-shell-type architecture have great potential for delivering hydrophobic drugs. The core of the micelles accommodates predominantly hydrophobic drugs. The shell is a brush like protective corona, which ensures the water dispensability of the micelles (Dumitriu, 2002).

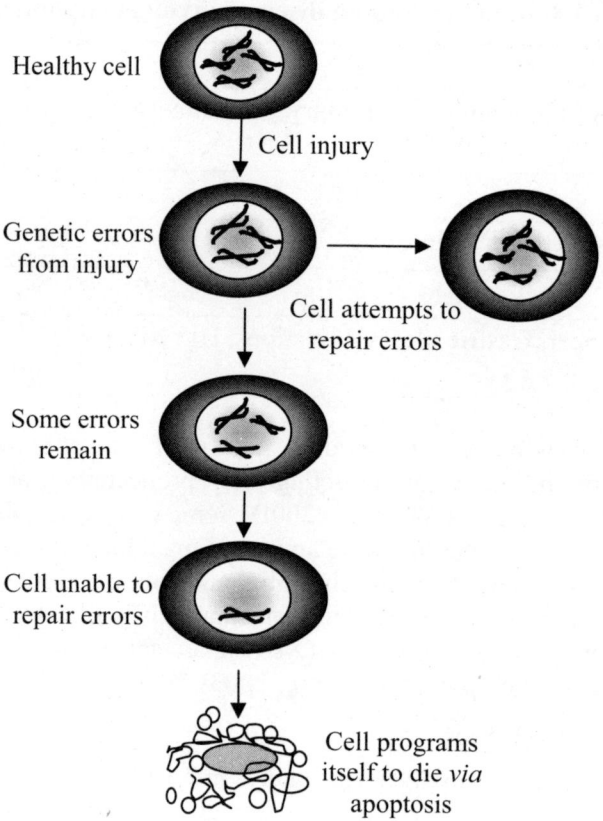

Healthy cell

Cell injury

Genetic errors
from injury

Cell attempts to
repair errors

Some errors
remain

Cell unable to
repair errors

Cell programs
itself to die *via*
apoptosis

Fig. 14.5: Events involved in apoptosis

Micelles formed by self-assembly of amphiphilic block copolymers (5–50 nm) in aqueous solutions are of great interest for drug delivery applications. The drugs can be physically entrapped in the core of block copolymer micelles and transported at concentrations that can exceed their intrinsic water- solubility. Moreover, the hydrophilic blocks can form hydrogen bonds with the aqueous surroundings and form a tight shell around the micellar core. As a result, the contents of the hydrophobic core are effectively protected against hydrolysis and recognition by the reticuloendothelial system and therefore preliminary elimination of the micelles from the bloodstream. A final feature that makes amphiphilic block copolymers attractive for drug delivery applications is the fact that their chemical composition, total molecular weight and block length ratio can be easily changed, which allows control of the size and morphology of the micelles. Functionalization of block copolymers with cross-linkable groups can increase the stability of the corresponding micelles and improve their temporal control. Substitution of block copolymer micelles with specific ligands is a very promising strategy to a broader range of sites of activity with a much higher selectivity (Fig. 14.7). The chief advantages of block copolymer micelles are their size, their high and controllable drug loading capacity, their biocompatibility, and the high diversity of drugs they can accommodate. But to effect targeted delivery at the sub cellular level of the hydrophobic (albeit often toxic agents) incorporated into the water-soluble, biocompatible, block copolymer micelles, a good understanding of the cellular distribution of micelles and micelle-incorporated agents is essential. To address these problem Savic *et al.*, used organelle-selective dyes in combination with confocal microscopy and a fluorescent-labeled polymer to gain good insight into the sub cellular distribution of block copolymer micelles. Their block copolymer micelles were made of poly (caprolactone)-β-poly (ethylene oxide) (PCL-β-PEO) block copolymer with tetramethylrhodamine-5-carbonyl azide (TMRCA) covalently attached to the PCL end of the polymer. Experiments using dyes as labels, conducted by Savic *et al.*, implicated several organelles as chief micelle targets, including mitochondria and the Golgi apparatus and pointed to the possibility of the delivery of certain inhibitors and activators of the cell signaling pathways. An understanding of their cellular distribution is essential to achieve selective delivery of drugs at the subcellular level. Triple labeling confocal microscopy in live cells has revealed the localization of micelles in several cytoplasmic organelles, including mitochondria, but not in the nucleus. Moreover, micelles change the cellular distribution of and increase the amount of the agent delivered to the cells. These micelles may thus be worth exploring for their potential to selectively deliver the drugs to the specified sub cellular targets.

14.21. PROTEIN KINASE INHIBITORS

Some serious diseases such as cancer and diabetes arise from perturbation of protein kinase-mediated cell signaling pathways. According to Manning *et al.*, (2002), the human genome codes for about 518 protein kinases that share a catalytic domain conserved in sequences and structures but which otherwise differ in the way their catalysis is regulated. There is an ATP-binding pocket between the two lobes of the kinase fold. This site, along with less conserved surrounding pockets, has attracted focus of inhibitor design based on differences in kinase structure and liability in order to achieve selectivity. Some drugs undergoing clinical trials target all stages of signal transduction: from the receptor tyrosine kinases that initiate intracellular signaling, through second-messenger generators and kinases involved in signaling cascades, to the kinases that regulate the cell cycle that governs cellular fate (Noble *et al.,* 2004).

Structures have not only inspired drug design but also illuminated the mechanism of inhibition. Structures have given insights into targeting of the inactive or active form of the kinase for in turn targeting of the global constellation of residues at the ATP site or less conserved additional pockets or single residues, and also in the targeting of noncatalytic domains (Noble *et al.,* 2004). Extensive structural studies have led to identification of the properties of the protein kinase ATP-binding sites that are exploited by the fairly potent and selective subset of promising inhibitors in clinical trials. The ATP-binding site presents several distinctive features from which the sites of different kinases that are potential drug targets have been categorized on the basis of shape and amino acid composition (Schiering *et al.,* 2003; Noble *et al.,* 2004).

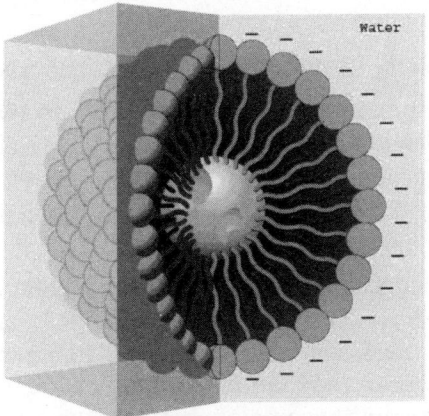

Fig.14.6: Micelles

Although structural results are definitely useful for antikinase drug development, the crucial consideration for successful therapy design is the choice of a suitable target. After characterization of the human genome (Manning *et al.,* 2002), genomic scale structure determination can be achieved and could contribute to both target selection and the careful design of inhibitor specificity. This in turn should help to mitigate the drug toxicity that so often leads to kinase inhibitor failure at the stage of clinical trials. It may also broaden the spectrum of diseases, particularly diseases of the poor people in which the pharmaceutical industry is not very interested. These diseases might be addressed by antikinase therapy. In the discovery of lead compounds, experimental and theoretical approaches are being developed to exploit structural information to cut short the long process (Noble *et al.,* 2004).

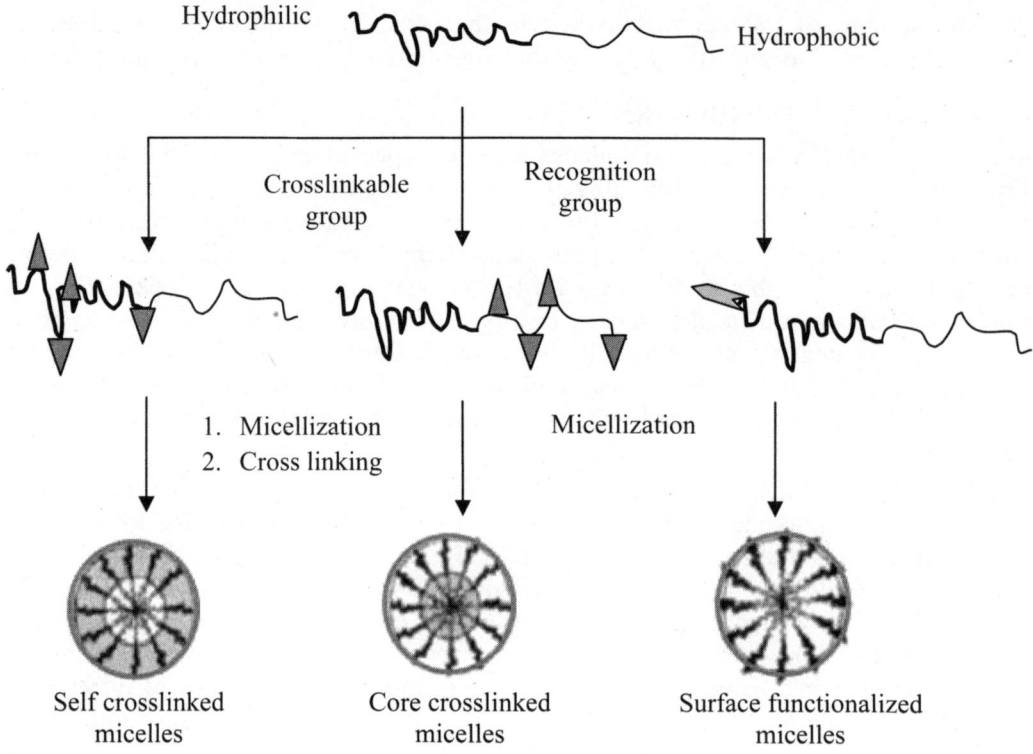

Fig. 14.7: Block copolymer micelles

14.22. POLYKETIDE AND NON RIBOSOMAL PEPTIDE ANTIBIOTICS

Polyketides (PKs) and nonribosomal peptides (NRPs) make up two families of natural products that can be biosynthesized by multimodular enzymes acting in assembly line arrays. The monomeric building blocks are organic acids and amino acids. Copolymerization *via* mixed modules of enzymatic machinery is used to assemble hybrid PK-NRP molecules of useful structural complexity and therapeutic activity (Walsh, 2004).

Our greatly increased knowledge about gene clusters that code for enzymes for the biosynthesis of many therapeutically useful PK, NRP, and hybrid PK-NRP natural products has facilitated the identification of many such clusters available in public databases. For example, the genome of the avermectin producer, *Streptomyces avermitilis* (Omura *et al.,* 2001) has revealed 24 additional polyketide synthase (PKS) or nonribosomal peptide synthase (NRPS) clusters for unidentified secondary metabolites, pointing to natural product biosynthetic capacity being tremendously underestimated by the products detected in fermentations.

PKs and NRPs made on multimodular enzymatic assembly lines often attain the conformations that establish biological activity by cyclization constraints introduced by tailoring enzymes. The dedicated tailoring enzymes are encoded by genes clustered with the assembly line genes for coordinated regulation. NRP heterocyclizations to thiazoles and oxazoles can occur on the elongating framework of acyl-S enzyme intermediates, whereas tandem cyclic PK polyether formation of furans and pyrans can be initiated by post-assembly line epoxidases. Macrocyclizations of NRP, PK, and hybrid NRP-PK scaffolds occur in assembly line chain termination steps. Post-assembly line cascades of enzymatic oxidations also create cross linked and cyclized architectures that generate the mature scaffolds of natural products (antibiotics). The modularity of the natural product assembly lines and permissivity of tailoring enzymes offer prospects for reprogramming to create novel antibiotics with optimized properties (Walsh, 2004).Diverse tools, genes, enzymes and variant monomers are now available for manipulations of natural products structures to explore the function of novel biological activities.

14.23. ENGINEERING OF YEASTS FOR PRODUCING DRUGS

Many drugs are based on proteins and Pharma Company's sometime attempt to formulate some proteins into medicines. One major obstacle in these efforts is that most proteins carry small groups of sugar molecules, some of which can trigger a dangerous immune reaction.

Most therapeutic proteins require the co-translational addition of glycans to specific asparagine residues of the protein to ensure proper folding and subsequent stability in the human serum. For therapeutic use in humans, glycoproteins require human-like N-glycosylation. Certain yeasts and filamentous fungi are suitable industrial fermentation organisms and can be readily grown to high cell density in culture. Moreover, glycoproteins from fungal systems contain nonhuman *N-glycans* of the high mannose type that are immunogenic in humans and so of limited therapeutic value (Hamilton *et al.,* 2003). However, fungi and mammals do share some early steps of protein N-glycosylation.

Although, mammalian cell cultures can tack on sugars correctly, they are more costly. The methylotrophic yeast *Pichia pastoris* is frequently used for the expression of heterologous proteins. It provides a cheaper means to produce sugared proteins correctly. Yeast cells make proteins with sugar attachments found commonly on human proteins. This process can manufacture existing protein therapeutics at lower cost and can also intensify search for new glycoprotein drugs, enabling researchers to easily attach different sugars to screen for the most effective combination (Service, 2004).

It is usually sugars that help proteins fold properly and stabilize when circulating in the blood. But different species attach different combinations of sugars in patterns that immune cells exploit to distinguish host proteins from invaders. Whereas yeast cells attach the sugar mannose, human cells add galactose and sialic acid, producing proteins in yeast appears to be fairly simple. In both yeast and humans, proteins are made in the endoplasmic reticulum, attached to complexes of mannose and other sugars, and later transported to the Golgi apparatus for further processing. In yeast, more mannose groups are then added. In humans, however, the enzyme mannosidase breaks off the mannose groups, while some other enzymes attach some other sugars. This prompted researchers to reason that if yeast cells could be engineered to express mannosidase, the cells wouldn't produce the mannose-rich sugar complexes that are so immunogenic to humans. Early attempts failed. It was then suspected that mannosidase in engineered yeast was not finding its way to the Golgi apparatus. So they inserted a more efficient mannosidase and engineered a yeast strain with glycoproteins containing very few mannose groups. Even then, the resulting proteins did not harbor the sugars commonly found in humans. But now, Hamilton *et al.,* have linked peptide cell targeting codes to certain enzymes that attach sugars found on human proteins and then added the genes for these hybrids to mannosidase-producing yeast. This combination has successfully produced large amounts of humanlike proteins. In fact, this engineered yeast not only turns out introduced proteins in human form but the cells also make the same modifications to all their own cellular proteins. But one limitation is that the humanized yeast proteins still fail to express the sugar sialic acid, whose presence enables proteins to evade clearance mechanisms in the body and circulate longer. If and when that machinery also can be added to yeast, the technique might be gainfully applied to produce cheaper protein therapeutics. The ability to generate human glycoproteins with homogenous N-glycan structures in a fungal host is a welcome step toward producing therapeutic glycoproteins.

14.24. SCALING-UP OF FERMENTATION PROCESSES

Proper optimization of fermentation processes increases the yield of the final product provided that the process complies with good manufacturing practices, the available equipment and the expected final scale of operation. Some genetically modified microorganisms overproduce recombinant proteins and most of the processes use only three such species, namely; *Escherichia coli, Saccharomyces cerevisiae,* and *Pichia pastoris.* Standard processes for each organism serve as a basis for the development of a tailored process. Thiry and Cingolani (2002) have devised an efficient approach to scaling up of fermentation processes for biopharmaceutical purposes, in a multidisciplinary environment.

Before starting the expensive optimization work, the stability of the strain should be established, at least for the number of generations necessary for cell banking and largest-scale fermentation, including the pre-cultures expression systems based on plasmids can be unstable, the stability differing for each plasmid and also depending on the host strain. High instabilities correlate with low copy number plasmids (Futcher and Cox, 1984). The size of the inserted DNA also affects the stability — the larger the plasmid the less stable it is. Culture conditions such as temperature, composition of the medium, and growth rate also affect the plasmid stability. Significant plasmid loss occurs over the post exponential growth phase and plasmid instability tends to enhance during gene expression. Antibiotics are sometimes used to stabilize plasmids.

The codon usage of the desired gene should be optimized to facilitate expression in the chosen microorganism (Thiry and Cingolani, 2002). As the fermentation protocol affects the impurity profile, it can strongly affect the efficacy of the downstream processing (DSP). The conditions of fermentation can determine whether the protein of interest will be in its soluble or insoluble form which also will affect the DSP and consequently the quality and yield of the purified product. Overproduction at high yield can cause depletion of certain essential factors needed for appropriate conformation of the protein.

Fermentation may be carried out in batch, fed-batch or continuous mode. Continuous culture is not very popular in the pharmaceutical industry in view of the higher probability of mutation and contamination. Batch processes are quite simple and robust but the only way to achieve high cell density is the more complex fed-batch mode that allows the metabolism of the strain to be controlled. The medium can be either completely defined or include some peptones. Complex media elicit better growth but are difficult to analyze; they also generate variations among different batches. Defined media give reproducible growth and the purity in the supernatant for secreted protein is better than with complex media (Lee, 1996).

The use of raw materials of animal origin should be avoided. When this is not possible, the raw materials must be produced in a country free from transmissible spongiform encephalopathies (TSEs).The pH optimization of the medium is essential for those proteins which can grow in a wide range of pH values. The choice of pH depends on the stability of the recombinant protein expressed. Working with *Pichia pastoris* at low pH avoids protease degradation. This yeast cannot grow at pH below 2.2 for fed-batch processes, exponential feeding allows the cells to be grown at a constant growth rate conducive to expression of recombinant proteins. Scaling up can affect such factors as the number of generations, the mutation probability, medium sterilization, the quality of temperature and pH regulations, agitation-aeration and pressure. The best way to scale-up a process is to first scale-down to the pilot scale the conditions of culture that will be used at the final scale of production and then to elevate the scale-the broth will become more and more heterogeneous in this way (Kwanmin, 1989; Enfors *et al.*, 2001; Thiry and Cingolani, 2002).

14.25. DRUG DELIVERY SYSTEMS

Some drug delivery systems (DDS) such as lipid or polymer-based nanoparticles have effectively improved the pharmacological and therapeutic properties of drugs administered parenterally, after some early problems encountered in the clinical applications of particulate DDS were overcome. Several DDS formulations of anticancer and antifungal drugs have now been approved for clinical use. There is also much interest in exploiting the advantages of DDS for *in vivo* delivery of new drugs derived from proteomics or genomics research and for their use in ligand-targeted therapeutics (Allen and Cullis, 2004).

DDS based on particulate carriers, composed primarily of lipids and/or polymers, and their associated therapeutics improves many of the pharmacological characteristics of conventional ("free") drugs. DDS can be designed either to change the pharmacokinetics (PK) and biodistribution (BD) of their associated drugs, or to serve as drug reservoirs (e.g., sustained release systems), or both. Table 14.5 shows some problems related to the free drugs that can be ameliorated by the use of DDS. The PK and BD tend to be a composite of the PK and BD of the free drug and the PK and BD of the carrier. However, the balance depends on the rate at which the drug is released from the carrier. Drug release rates have significant implications for the therapeutic effects of DDS. In polymer-drug conjugates or liposome systems, the drug is inactive (not bioavailable) while associated with the carrier, and failure to release the drug from the carrier at proper time usually results in a reduced therapeutic effect relative to the free drug. On the other hand, rapid release of the drug from the carrier can produce therapeutic effects similar to those seen upon administration of the free drug. The maximum tolerated dose (MTD) of the drug may either increase, decrease, or remain the same, depending on the properties of the drug itself, the effect of the DDS on the PK and BD of the drug, and the drug release rate (Allen and Cullis, 2004).

Allen and Cullis (2004) analyzed the issues related to the use of small-scale DDS (nanoparticles and microparticles with diameters not exceeding -200 nm) for parenteral (primarily intravenous) applications. These include liposomes and other lipid-based carriers such as micelles, lipid emulsions, lipid-drug complexes, polymer-drug conjugates, polymer microspheres, and certain ligand-targeted products such as immunoconjugates.Several DDS are available on the market (Table 14.6). Many of the currently approved DDS for parenteral administration are liposomal or lipid-based formulations or therapeutic molecules linked to polyethylene glycol (PEG). Important attributes of a good DDS include potency, stability, solubility, molecular weight, and charge. In general the fewer molecules that a DDS can carry, the more potent the drug is. If unduly high quantities of the carrier are used, problems of carrier toxicity, metabolism and elimination, or biodegradability can occur. Each liposome can entrap thousands of drug molecules, so drug potency is not a serious issue for this type of carrier. But, even the relatively high carrying capacity of liposomes can become problematic for very large therapeutic molecules such as proteins, particularly if small liposome diameters are chosen for reasons of biodistribution. Drug solubility can be critical in liposomal DDS.

According to Gabizon *et al.*, (2003), in general, when a drug is associated with a carrier, its clearance decreases (its half-life increases), the volume of distribution decreases and the area under the time-versus concentration curve increases. In the case of larger particulate carriers, e.g., liposomes, polymer-drug conjugates, and microspheres, the carrier size (typically 50-200 nm in diameter) confines it primarily to the blood compartment.

Some DDS have attracted criticism because of their pharmaceutical and commercial properties such as complexity, cost, storage stability, and intellectual property (IP) issues. IP issues are often difficult to resolve because control of the product requires an IP position not only on the drug, but also on the carrier technology. For liposomes and PEG-protein conjugates, these difficulties have been largely overcome, as indicated by the regulatory and commercial acceptance of these products. Two-year or longer stability has been achieved for these products in a wet or lyophilized form. No doubt the cost per treatment for DDS is often higher than the cost per treatment of the free drugs; but when we take into account the total cost, including the cost of treating drug-related side effects, the DDS become cost-competitive and comparable with free drugs (Smith *et al.*, 2002).

14.26. CELL-BASED THERAPIES

Living cells provide the starting material for a variety of new strategies for the treatment of diseases provided that some bureaucratic and technical obstacles are overcome. The best example of using living cells to treat disease is that of blood transfusion. Today, novel cell-based products have acquired potential as drug delivery vehicles, immunotherapies, and engineered tissues to regenerate damaged tissue. Cell-based therapies, however, encounter political hurdles. Controversies over cloning and human embryonic stem (ES) cells are delaying research. Still some experimental therapies are finding their way into the clinic.

A decade ago, most biotechnology companies were convinced that cell-based therapies were safe; thousands of patients received bone marrow transplants as part of their cancer treatments. These transplants allow cancer patients to survive potentially lethal doses of chemotherapy and radiation. The high doses of cytotoxic drugs and radiation destroy hematopoietic stem cells; the treated bone marrow cells thus give rise to all blood cell types, leaving patients prone to life-threatening infections and anemia (Dove, 2002). Hematopoietic stem cells should be salvaged from a patient's bone marrow before chemotherapy and radiation were administered; the rescued cells can then subsequently used to reconstitute his/her impaired immune system. Theoretically, this regimen was better than chemotherapy, which might leave the immune system intact but would not eradicate the cancer completely.

But companies investing in cell-based therapies have suffered huge losses. The combination of chemotherapy and cell transplantation, worked well for lymphomas and some cancers; nevertheless, clinical studies did not show any benefit for treating breast cancers, which affect the largest number of patients. In the face of such setbacks, surviving companies offering cell-based therapy have changed their research priorities. Some now hope to use cells as a delivery system for therapeutics, others are trying to make immune cells to act as cancer vaccines, and a few are attempting to coax cells to regenerate damaged tissues. Each company faces varying degrees of resistance from market forces, government regulators, and the human immune system (Dove, 2002).

The most straightforward application of cell-based therapies is probably the delivery of biological. Commonly a therapeutic protein is expressed in cultured cells, then purified and injected into the patient. Some companies wish to implant the cells directly. The merit of this approach is that protein-expressing cells usually deliver a steady, potentially more physiological, concentration of the protein (Bergers and Hanahan, 2001).

Table 14.5: Some non-ideal properties of drugs and their therapeutic implications

Problems	Implication	Effect of DDS
Low solubility	Hydrophobic drugs may precipitate in aqueous media. Toxicities are associated with the use of excipients such as camphor (the solubilizer for paclitaxal in Taxol).	By providing both hydrophilic and hydrophobic environments, lipid micelles or liposomes enhance drug solubility.
Rapid breakdown of the drug	Drug can lose activity following *in vivo* administration.	Protects the drug from premature degradation and functions as a sustained release system. Lower doses of drug are needed.
Unfavorable pharmacokinetics	Drug is cleared too rapidly, e.g., by the kidney, so requiring high dose or continuous infusion.	Substantially alters the PK of the drug and reduces clearance. Rapid renal clearance of small molecules is avoided.
Poor bio-distribution	Drugs widely distributed in the body affect normal tissues resulting in dose-limiting side effects (e.g., the cardiac toxicity of doxorubicin)	Particulate DDS lowers the volume of distribution reducing side effects in sensitive, non target tissues.
Non selectivity for target tissues	Distribution of the drug to normal tissue results in side effects that restrict the dose that can be administered. Low drug concentrations in target tissues give suboptimal therapeutic effects.	Increases drug concentration in diseased tissues such as tumors. Ligand mediated targeting of the DDS further improves drug specificity.

Some other possible benefits of cell-based drug delivery systems may be: the ability to get more drugs present, to get more of it directed to a specific site, or to just make it easier for the patient. In general, cell-based therapies are of two broad kinds but most companies concentrate on just one. Autologous therapies take a patient's own cells, modify or expand them *ex vivo,* and then inject them back into the same patient. The patient's immune system recognizes the therapeutic cells as "self" and does not reject them. Each treatment has to be custom made, and various logistical and regulatory obstacles need to be overcome. In the alternative, allografting approach, a company produces only one cell type for a given indication, and transplants those cells into all suitable patients. This bypasses the logistical problem of "individualized" cell therapy but allografts must cross the barrier of the human immune system, which efficiently identifies and eliminates "non-self" cells. Most companies which are developing cells as drug-delivery systems have chosen the allograft approach, but immunosuppressants are needed to prevent graft rejection, leaving patients susceptible to subsequent secondary infections.

Table 14.6: Some drug delivery systems (DDS) approved in various countries

Drug or therapeutic agent (trade name), manufacturer(s)	Indication
Liposomal amphotericin B (AmBisome), Gilead, Fujisawa	Fungal infections, leishmaniasis
PEG-adenosine deaminase (Adagen), Enzon	Severe combined immunodeficiency disease
Styrene maleic acid and neocarzinostatin copolymer in Ethiodol (SMANCS/Lipiodol, Zinostatin stimalamer), Yamanouchi	Hepatocellular carcinoma
Stealth (PEG-stabilized) liposomal doxorubicin (Doxil/Caelyx), ALZA, Schering Plough	Refractory ovarian or breast cancer
Liposomal cytosine arabinoside (DepoCyt), SkyePharma	Lymphomatous meningitis, neoplastic meningitis
Denileukin diftitox or interleukin 2-diptheria toxin fusion protein (ONTAK), Seragen	Cutaneous T-cell lymphoma
Liposomal verteporfin (Visudyne), QLT, Novartis	Wet macular degeneration plus laser treatment
PEG-interferon a-2b (PEG-lntron), Enzon, Schering-Plough	Hepatitis C
^{90}Y-ibritumomab tiuxetan or ^{90}Y anti-CD20 (Zevalin), IDEC	Relapsed or refractory non-Hodgkin's lymphoma

To overcome this problem, BioHybrid and other companies encapsulate the cells to protect them from the immune system. The capsule must be permeable enough to allow nutrients to enter and therapeutic proteins to escape, but they are required to be benign in absolute term to the immune system. Islet cells based transplants could potentially reduce the risk of the many serious sequellae of diabetes, such as the damage to peripheral blood vessels that can lead to gangrene and amputation.

14.27. LIVING MISSILES

Some cell types have properties that could be exploited to medical advantage. For example, Oxford BioMedica's cell therapy program harnesses the basic instincts of macrophages to accumulate in infected, inflamed, and hypoxic regions, which develop in cancers, arteriosclerosis, and inflamed joints. The company's MacroGen technology helps in extracting the patient's macrophages and transducing these with a gene, in this case one encoding the liver enzyme CYP2B6, which metabolizes a prodrug into an anti-tumor toxin.

The fact that skeletal muscle cells are relatively accessible, abundant and long-lived makes them highly suitable material for a drug-delivery system. Cell based therapy genetically modifies these cells to express therapeutic proteins, and then organizes the cells into 2 cm-long implants. The implants are inserted just below the skin for general protein release, or directly into the affected tissue for more local delivery (for example, of angiogenic factors) to the heart.

Layton Biosciences found that human neuronal stem cells preferentially migrate toward brain tumors. They intend to use such cells to deliver a cancer prodrug, which would then be metabolized by tumor cells into a cytotoxic agent. Neurotech uses immortalized retinal epithelial cells for treatment of degenerative diseases of the eye. The retinal cells are genetically modified to secrete therapeutic peptides or proteins, and are injected either directly or within a protective capsule (Dove. 2002).

No doubt, the immune system bars successful cell-based drug delivery, but it remains the chief instrument for generating effective cell-based immunotherapies. In general, cell-based immunotherapy employs dendritic cells, a subset of antigen presenting cells responsible for identifying non-self antigens, processing them, and initiating an immune reaction. Because dendritic cells recruit highly specific cytotoxic killer T-cells to perform their dirty work, researchers are working on T-cells directly. Companies working on allografts plan to establish a limited number of cell lines that can be differentiated into dendritic cells under laboratory conditions, trained to respond to tumor antigens, and implanted. Tom Okarma of Geron Company (Menlo Park) is a strong believer in the allograft approach; he describes his company's cultured ES cells as a self-renewing starting material to produce the therapeutic cell. However, although Geron has developed a uniform, cost - effective production technique, which produces the cell with the same efficiency as a monoclonal antibody, the chief disadvantage — as with all allografts is that the cells are recognized as foreign by the patient's immune system. Other companies are pursuing autologous cell therapies in which a patient's own hematopoietic stem cells are removed, trained to respond to tumor cells, and then reinjected. This solves the problem of immune rejection, but raises the formidable economic and regulatory challenges of producing a customized therapy for each patient. Maus *et al.*, (2002) have developed "artificial antigen-presenting cells". These cells express surface receptors that activate dendritic cells. Using this cell line, antigen-specific killer T-cells could be generated directly. This approach should prove useful in future cell-based cancer therapies.

14.28. REPAIR AND REPLACEMENT

By far the most exciting area of cell-based therapy has been regenerative medicine, which involves the use of cells to rebuild diseased or damaged tissues. Engineering complex organs *ex vivo* is still a long way off but approaches that involve injecting a small number of cells into damaged tissue may possibly treat some of the world's most devastating diseases.

As with drug delivery and immunotherapy, companies have to choose between autologous and allograft approaches in regenerative medicine. Proponents of allografts might dodge immune rejection by concentrating on immunologically isolated parts of the body, such as the brain, e.g., by focusing on two kinds of neuronal cells now: dopaminergic cells for Parkinson's disease and glial cells to replace damaged oligodendrocytes. Both cell types, which are derived from embryonic stem (ES) cells, are already undergoing trials in animal models. Geron has succeeded in coaxing its ES cells to differentiate into other cell types, such as hepatocytes. Although regenerating livers using cell transplants is a remote goal, in the near future liver cells should prove useful for toxicology studies of experimental medicine (Dove, 2002).In the short term, advocates of autologous transplantation seem to be pulling ahead in regenerative medicine race. Aastrom Biosciences for instance has started clinical trials using a cell mixture to replace bone lost in osteoporosis, and the company is about to start a trial using the same mixture for bone grafting to repair spinal fusions and leg fractures, using an automated cell-manufacturing system to grow sufficient quantities of the patient's own bone marrow.

Meanwhile, the immune system still presents a significant barrier to allografts, but perhaps not a lasting one. In fact stem cells themselves may provide the solution to their own rejection. Earlier studies of bone marrow transplants produced an interesting result: people who received bone marrow from a donor often became tolerant of the donor's antigens. However, when the same patient later received an organ donation from the same donor, the organ was often tolerated even without immunosuppressive drugs (Ciancio, 2001). In 2001, Kaufman *et al.*, coaxed human ES cells to form colonies of hematopoietic cells similar to those in bone marrow. This point to the possibility, that the same strategy could someday be applied to cell-based therapies.

Ultimately, both allografts and autologous cell transplants are likely to be modified and targeted in diverse ways to increase their potency. Conceivably, in a decade, we may not even have to take the dendritic cells out of the patient, handle them in the lab, and put them back; more sophisticated means to target them directly might well be developed by then. In that case, cell based therapies may behave much like stem cells themselves — able not only to sustain themselves, but also to produce progeny with quite different characteristics (Dove, 2002).

14.29. ENCAPSULATED CELLS FOR DISEASE TREATMENT

The new field of encapsulated cell technology (ECT) has developed rapidly in the past decade, with considerable improvement in the development and optimization of construct technologies for producing and characterizing new 3D devices. Advances in cell biology and genetics are providing novel cell lines that are well suited for immobilization applications in agriculture, the food industry and especially in health care (Orive *et al.,* 2002; Dove, 2002).

ECT implants consist of cells that have been genetically modified to produce a desired therapeutic factor that are encapsulated in a section of semi-permeable hollow fiber membrane. The diffusive characteristics of the hollow fiber membrane are designed to promote long-term cell survival by allowing influx of oxygen and nutrients while simultaneously preventing direct contact of the encapsulated cells with the cellular and molecular elements of the immune system. The cells continuously produce the therapeutic protein, which diffuses out of the implant at the target site. ECT therefore enables the controlled, continuous delivery of therapeutic factors directly to the retina, bypassing the blood-retina barrier. Long-term protein delivery (18 months) in the vitreous cavity of the eye has consistently been achieved when ECT devices containing human cells genetically engineered to secrete CNTF have been implanted in a highly disparate mammalian species (rabbits). In addition, the implants can be retrieved, providing an added level of safety as well as the ability to reverse or adjust therapy, if needed. Various aspects of ECT are summarized in Figure 14.8.

ECT based products can be tailored to address the three main clinical manifestations of retinal diseases: degeneration of photoreceptors and/or ganglion cells in the neural retina, vascular proliferation, and inflammation. A number of proteins have been discovered in the field of ophthalmology that possesses powerful neurotrophic, anti-angiogenic and anti-inflammatory properties. These proteins have the potential to significantly slow or halt disease processes in the eye. ECT represents a unique platform for the safe and effective delivery of various factors for the treatment of chronic ophthalmic diseases as follows:

• **neurotrophic factors** for the treatment of retinal degeneration in Retinitis Pigmentosa (RP), Geographic Atrophy (serious condition associated with the *Dry* form of Age-related Macular Degeneration), Glaucoma, Retinal Vein Occlusion and others.

• **anti-angiogenic factors** for the treatment of vascular proliferation in Diabetic Retinopathy and the Wet form of AMD, and for the treatment of abnormal vascular permeability for various forms of Macular Edema.

• **anti-inflammatory factors** for the treatment of Ocular Inflammations (Uveitis)

A variety of cell lines can be enclosed within semi permeable and biocompatible immobilization devices that facilitate the bi-directional diffusion of molecules. Nutrients, oxygen, waste products and biotherapeutic products freely diffuse across the membrane whereas high molecular weight antibodies, immunocytes and other immunologic moieties tend to be excluded. The characteristic immunobarrier of these devices has a doubly protective function-immunoisolating the transplanted tissue from the host's immune response, while also protecting it from biological risk. These properties make possible the transplantation of cells and tissues without immunosuppressive drugs and the delivery of therapeutic peptides either in a local or systemic manner, especially in conditions that require a long-term administration protocol (Wang *et al.,* 1997).

ECT is best applied in medicine for the controlled and continuous delivery of biological products to the host. Once transplanted, the biologics are produced and constantly secreted *de novo,* maintaining more physiological and effective concentration of the therapeutic proteins. Another merit of a cell-based approach within 'artificial extracellular matrices' is the targeting of the therapeutic strategy because it allows implanting microcapsules proximally to the therapeutic target, thereby getting more of the drug to the specific site of need and minimizing systemic blood-drug concentrations and the possible side effects. Alginate-encapsulated cells secreting endostatin (an anti-angiogenic endogenous peptide) have been used to treat experimental glioblastomas (Orive *et al.,* 2002).

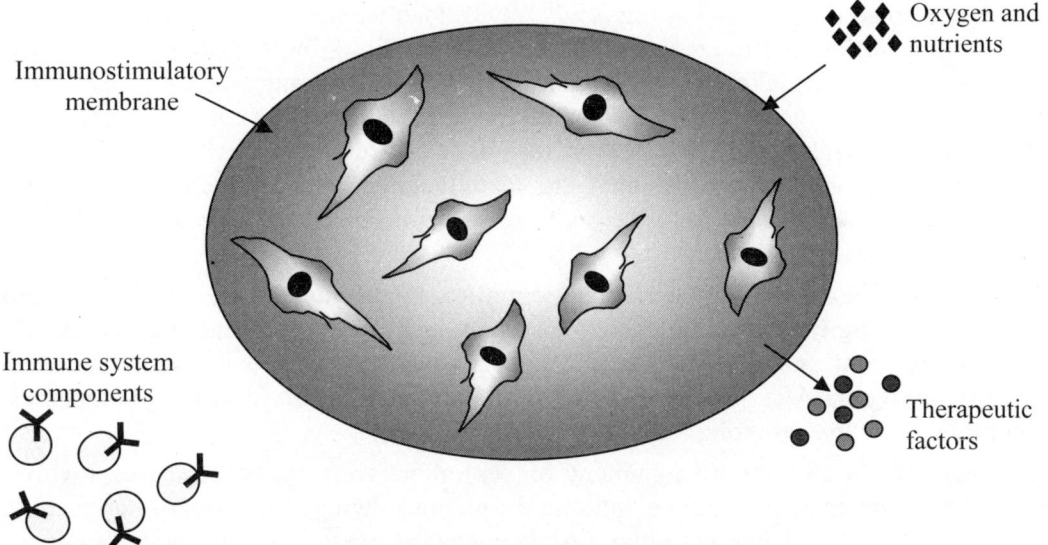

Fig.14.8: The salient features of ECT

Implanting immobilized cells adjacent to certain developing tumor cells may reduce tumor growth substantially while increasing intratumoral apoptosis. ECT has also been useful in patients of pancreatic cancer to evaluate the safety of local activation of low dose ifosfamide after treatment with encapsulated cells expressing a cytochrome P450 enzyme; in these patients, beads were delivered and controlled by supra-selective angiography to the intra-arterial placement. Median survival was doubled in the treatment group and the one-year survival rate was three times better. ECT also enhances biosafety because the polymer matrix and surrounding membrane prevent uncontrolled cell growth; in rare cases if problems do arise during treatment, the encapsulated drug containing cells can be removed easily. Another merit is that, compared with gene therapy approaches, encapsulated cells do not interfere with or modify the genome of the host. Organ failure or tissue loss, after disease or trauma, is a frequent and serious concern of health care system, especially in view of the acute shortage of donor organs.

ECT can be a valid strategy to overcome these limitations and, in due course, can generate enormous market opportunity for biotechnology companies. Indeed, the progress of ECT (Shapiro *et al.,* 2000) now benefits several areas, e.g., hemophilia, cancer, diabetes, neurodegenerative diseases, lysosomal storage diseases and renal failure (Table 14.8).

Several biotechnology industries have recently re-oriented their research fields, focusing either on pharmaceutical technology or on cell biology and genetics. The former aims at the design and improvement of polymeric materials to elaborate varied immobilization devices with adequate mechanical resistance, degradability, permeability, biocompatibility and immunocompatibility properties (Angelova and Hunkeler, 1999). The later deal with the suitable cell lines for therapy. The commonest strategy is that of allo- and xeno-grafting, in which transplantation is between individuals within the same species or across a species barrier, respectively. It is also possible to genetically modify a selected cell type by treatment with DNA so that the pattern of gene expression is changed, which makes it a cost-effective method of drug delivery.

One chief approach of companies engaged in ECT is to develop bioartificial pancreases for diabetes treatment (Read *et al.,* 2001; Wang *et al.,* 1997). Islet technology (St. Paul, MN, USA) uses highly purified alginate for islet microencapsulation. Large hollow-fibers (called sheets) with 2 to 3 million islets is the approach adopted by Islet Sheet Medical (San Francisco, CA, USA) to conceal immobilized cells from the host's immune system (Orive *et al.,* 2002). Another recently developed controlled molecular weight cutoff bioreactor for diabetes treatment has insulin-secreting cells enclosed within implantable biocapsules that are manufactured with a carefully designed silicon semipermeable membrane. Glucose from the body freely diffuses into the bioreactor and triggers the immobilized cells to produce insulin.

Dedicated research in cell biology and engineering has contributed much to the development of novel construct technologies, and to the evaluation of a range of new cells and improvements in cell sourcing and culture stabilization. Clinical trials have been made to evaluate the safety and efficacy of several bioartificial liver (BAL) devices. But the prime aim and objectives of ECT companies are to develop a complete new liver— a long term, lofty goal.

ECT is potentially useful in the treatment of central nervous system diseases involving the continuous deterioration of both cognitive and motor functions owing to the loss of nerve cells, either chronically as in Parkinson's, Huntington's and Alzheimer's diseases, or acutely as in trauma or stroke of the brain or spinal cord (Read *et al.,* 2001; AI-Hendy *et al.,* 1995). A new neurotrophic factor named Neublastin has been patented in Denmark; this is derived from a glial cell line. It increases the number of surviving tyrosine hydroxylase-immunoreactive neurons when added to cultures of fetal dopamine neurons. Neublastin is used for the treatment of the peripheral nervous system and multiple sclerosis. Some companies working on ECT are pursuing other research areas, such as skin replacement, venous ulcers and retinal disorders (Table 14.10).

One cause of concern associated with ECT is the clinical and public risk of xenotransplantation-possible jump of infectious agents, particularly the porcine endogenous retrovirus (PERV), from the recipient to others, and the danger of causing man-made pandemics (Pitkin and Mullon, 1999). It appears that human clinical trials of whole organ xenotransplants may be 'premature' (Butler, 1999) as they face serious scientific hurdles.

Table 14.7: Selected companies working on cell-based therapies (after Dove, 2002)

Company	Technology	Major Disease focus
Cell-based drug delivery		
BioHybrid Technologies (Shrewsbury, MA)	Encapsulation system for allografts	Encapsulated pancreatic islet cell allografts
Islet Sheet Medical (San Francisco, CA)	Encapsulated pancreatic islet cells	Retrievable bioartificial pancreas for diabetes
Neurotech (Evry, France)	Encapsulation system for allografts	Therapeutic protein delivery to eye and brain
Oxford BioMedica (Oxford, UK)	MacroGen (macrophages as gene delivery systems)	Pro-drug activating enzyme (CYP2B6) for treating cancers
Layton Biosciences (Sunnyvale. CA)	Human neuronal stem cells	CNS disorders (stroke. tumors, Parkinson's disease, Alzheimer's disease)
Cell Based Delivery (Providence, RI)	Implantable protein-expressing muscle tissue allografts	Therapeutic protein delivery for chronic diseases
Cell-based immunotherapy		
Aastrom Bioscience (Ann Arbor. Ml)	Autologous cell processing system, bone marrow and umbilical cord blood stem cells	Dendritic cell-based cancer vaccine. solid tissue and blood regeneration with stem cells
CellExSys (Seattle, WA) Geron (Menlo Park, CA)	*Ex vivo* production of cytotoxic T lymphocytes Human ES cells; dendritic cell vaccines	Cell-based treatments for hepatitis Band C, cancer Cell-based treatments for cancer, diabetes, osteoarthritis
Cell retrieval and expansion		
Gamida-Cell (Jerusalem, Israel)	Expanding stem cell populations *ex vivo*	Hematopoietic stem cells from umbilical cord blood for use in high-dose chemotherapy
Nexell Therapeutics (Irvine, CA)	Isolating hematopoietic stem cells	Stem cell therapy for chronic granulomatous disease and other hereditary blood disorders;cancer vaccines
TEl Biosciences (Boston, MA) Select Therapeutics (Woburn, MA)	Signaling molecules to induce stem cell differentiation 3-dimensional matrix for growing cells *ex vivo*	Tissue engineering using derived cell types Expansion of hematopoietic stem cells for bone marrow transplants, cytotoxic T cells to treat cancer

The 2002 US Pharmacopoeia and national formulary have approved the cell-based products as a new class of therapy product, suggesting some possible therapeutic indications (Anon., 2002) (Table 14.9). These new products may be combined with natural or synthetic biomaterials to form controlled drug delivery systems or tissue constructs (Orive *et al.*, 2002). It appears that in the coming years, a profound rationalization in the design, production and purification of polymeric biomaterials and devices will be required (Angelova and Hunkeler, 1999). One possibility may be to induce pre-vascularization at the site of cell transplantation, supplying enough nutrients and oxygen to the immobilized cells in the host, to be achieved by co-encapsulating angiogenic factors secreting cells or by designing biomaterials that release these factors in response to physiological cues (Lee *et al.*, 2000).

Table 14.8: Some reports on microencapsulated cell-based therapy

Disease	Mechanism of action
Cancer	Endostatin producing kidney cells encapsulated in sodium alginate
Haemophilia	Human factor IX secreting C2C 12 cells encapsulated in alginate PLL beads
Huntington' s	CNTF-producing BHK cells immobilized in hollow fibers
Parkinsons	GDNF-secreting BHK cells entrapped in hollow fibers
Dwarfism	Growth hormone secreting C2C12 cells encapsulated in alginate PLL beads
Renal failure	Alginate-PLL encapsulated *Escherichia coli* DH5 transfected with the urease gene
Diabetes	Encapsulated porcine islets

Abbreviation: Poly-L-lysine, PLL

14.30. PUBLIC DISEASE RESEARCH

Respiratory infections, malaria and tuberculosis happen to be the major causes of death and morbidity in Africa, Asia and South America. There are no effective, affordable and easy-to-use medicines to fight these infectious diseases. Market prospects rather than global health needs guide drug development, so the pipeline of new drugs for these neglected diseases is virtually empty. Less than 10 per cent of the world expenditure on health research and development (R&D) is devoted to the major health problems of 90 per cent of the population.

In the current transition towards a global knowledge economy, public sector policies are increasingly considering public research as an investment that should generate financial returns. Scientists are not only expected to publish their research and advance science, but also to promote and actively pursue the possible commercialization of research findings. This so-called valorization of research has become an important objective in the biotechnology and health sector where financial returns can be highly attractive. With valorization prospects being now included in the evaluation criteria for public research, research choices inevitably reflect market opportunities. Thus, the same market failure that deters the pharmaceutical industry from investing in neglected diseases also discourages public research.

New approaches to ensuring drug development for neglected diseases expect a significant contribution of public sector research. But the mere existence of scientific expertise does not suffice the purpose. Where the market fails, a global non-profit strategy for drug development needs to be developed and implemented within the public sector. In the expected valorization of public research, noncommercial pursuit of public health interests and social returns need to be emphasized over the economic goals.

14.31. PUBLIC-PRIVATE PARTNERSHIP IN DRUG DEVELOPMENT

Drug expenditure fairly accurately mirrors the global distribution of wealth. The annual world market for drugs is worth about US$ 310 billion, of which 90 per cent is spent in North America, Europe and Japan. Africa accounts for only one per cent of world drug sales. Pharmaceutical research and development (R&D) is both time and cost intensive, being mainly done by the private sector. Commercializing a new drug takes about twelve years and costs around US$ 250 million. Investment in R&D therefore depends on how attractive distinct markets may be. The pharmaceutical sector is motivated by profit to supply goods and services to the most lucrative markets. In a world of increasing wealth inequality, it is the poorest populations that are in most need of medicines for basic diseases. Thus there is a gap to be bridged between business practice and human need.

In 1998, global spending on health research by both the public and private sectors was about US$ 70 billion per year, but less than 10 per cent of this was devoted to diseases or conditions that account for 90 per cent of the global disease burden. Between 1975 and 1997, 1223 new pharmaceutical compounds were launched on the market, out of which only 11 were designed for tropical diseases (Lehmann, 2001). There is a glaring lack of market incentives to deal with neglected diseases such as malaria, tuberculosis and dengue fever. The financial and human resources channeled by the pharmaceutical sector into the diseases that most afflict the poor are miniscule in comparison to the enormous sums spent on finding cures for diseases that predominate in wealthy nations, such as heart disease and cancer.

14.32. PUBLIC-PRIVATE PARTNERSHIPS AND VENTURE PHILANTHROPY

Healthcare issues have become increasingly globalized. Every year, for instance, Human Immunodeficiency Virus/Acquired Immunodeficiency Syndrome (HIV/AIDS), malaria and tuberculosis kill about 5 million people in developing countries. This death toll has strong social, political and economic consequences not only for the countries concerned but also for the whole world—Industrialized countries are now realizing that with increasing international travel and exchange, every year about 120,000 people carry malaria, for instance, back to Europe.

Neither public nor private sectors alone have the means and incentive to produce medicines to counter tropical diseases. Attempts are therefore being made to bring together the pharmaceutical industry with its knowledge of product development and the public sector with its expertise in basic biology and field studies (Lehmann, 2001).

14.33. VIRTUAL PHARMACEUTICAL COMPANIES

Virtual pharmaceutical companies (VPCs) have sprung up to overcome market failures in pharmaceutical research. They combine entrepreneurial attitudes and social responsibility to make drugs available for developing countries. There are now several public-private cooperation ventures that adopt the approach of virtual pharmaceutical companies to neglected diseases (Box). VPCs have to contend with conflicting aims: on the one hand, they have to create incentives for private industry partners; on the other hand, they wish to make drugs available at reasonable prices. The conflicting aims have prompted VPCs to pursue a 'social venture capital' model for project funding. Whereas traditional venture capitalists seek equity in return for their investments, VPCs seek a commitment that drugs or vaccines will be provided to developing countries at a low price with a low profit margin. In exchange, private partners are permitted to use patents derived from the collaboration to produce products for profitable markets in industrialized countries.

VPCs deal with both drugs and vaccines, using appropriate approaches. The biology of vaccines is more complicated than that of drugs. The infectors of malaria and HIV are highly variable and their scientific knowledge is quite limited. Also no medical treatment can build up resistance. This means that the administration of a drug requires greater attention than vaccinations, which normally can be achieved by a single or two-time treatment. Further the motivations of individuals in the two cases are different. Drugs are demanded by sick people who are willing to spend to become healthy again; vaccines are preventive, so healthy people often feel no need to allocate resources simply because there is a risk of disease. Individuals sometime do not realize that they are at risk and, therefore, successful prevention by vaccination depends on political will and the capacity of public health services to carry out vaccination programs. Another difference relates to market incentives—the pharmaceutical industry finds it much more lucrative to develop treatments than one-time prevention. However, the vaccine market is highly concentrated and dominated by only four transnational companies: Glaxo Smith Kline (UK), Merck (USA), American Home Products (USA), and Aventis (France) (Lehmann, 2001). In industrialized countries several vaccines have been developed but they have reached the developing world very slowly. For example, a vaccine against Hepatitis B has been available since 1981, but it could only reach 40 per cent of infants worldwide and virtually none in the Sub-Saharan Africa.

Table 14.9: Indications of encapsulated cell therapy products

Indication	Product description
Pain	Cells secreting endorphins or catecholamines encapsulated in a hollow fibers
Diabetes	Encapsulated β-islet cells secreting insulin in response to glucose levels.
Wound healing/ Tissue repair	Sheet of allogeneic keratinocytes layered on a sheet of dermal fibroblasts
Defects in knee cartilage	Autologous chondrocytes
Cartilage-derived structures	Autologous or allergenic chondrocytes in biocompatible matrix
Bone repair	Mesenchymal stem cells in a biocompatible matrix
Neurodegenerative diseases	Allergenic or xenogeneic neuronal cells

14.34. THE INTERNATIONAL AIDS VACCINE INITIATIVE (IAVI)

Globally, about five million people become infected with HIV each year. Over 90 per cent of them live in developing countries. Since the HIV strains in these regions differ from those prevalent in industrialized countries, it is unattractive for the private sector to invest in developing a vaccine, and the public sector in industrialized countries has also neglected vaccine research. Instead, resources have mainly been concentrated on delaying the onset of AIDS after an HIV infection and the treatment of the symptoms. No reliable vaccine is yet available (IAVI, 2000). The International AIDS Vaccine Initiative (IAVI) was set up in 1996 to remedy this gap. IAVI intends to maximize the number of promising vaccine candidates in clinical trials. The initiative currently has six AIDS vaccine candidates under development. Projects include a partner in a developing country; this ensures that vaccine candidates match the relevant strains of HIV. IAVI funds both public research institutions and private companies. It follows a two-part approach to industrial involvement in the field of HIV vaccines:

Table 14.10: Selected companies working on ECT

Company*	Research area	Product description
Organogenesis (Canton, MA)	Skin replacement	*Apligraf:* A living, bi-layered skin substitute for venous and diabetic foot ulcers.
LifeCell (Branchburg, NJ)	Skin replacement	*Alloderm* : suitable for plastic surgery
Advanced Tissue Sciences (La Jolla, CA)	Skin replacement	*TransCyte* : a skin substitute
Cell Based Delivery (Providence, Rl)	Solid tumors and cardiovascular disease	*ImPACT system:* genetically modified cell-based delivery of peptides for the treatment of solid tumors, hormonal growth deficiency and cardiovascular and musculoskeletal diseases,
Neurotech S.A, (Evry, France)	Eye and brain	The delivery of drugs to the eye and brain
Novocell (Irvine, CA)	Diabetes	Immobilized pancreatic islet cells
Islet technology (St. Paul, MN)	Diabetes	Highly purified alginate for islet encapsulation
Islet Sheet Medical (San Francisco, CA)	Diabetes	Islet cells in an artificial polymer matrix
BioHybrid Technologies (Shrewsbury, MA)	Diabetes	Biocompatible gelatinous material for islet immobilization
Titan Pharmaceuticals, Inc. (San Francisco, CA)	Parkinson's disease	Spheramine: Dopamine secreting human retinal pigmented
Nsgene A/S (Copenhagen, Denmark)	Parkinson's disease	Epithelial cells on gelatin micro carriers.

* All except Neutotech and NsGene are located in the USA.

Push mechanisms: Direct and indirect investment into academic institutions and smaller biotechnology companies to stimulate early-stage vaccine R&D. Pull mechanisms: Creation of markets and profits for larger pharmaceutical companies to stimulate interest in large-scale testing, production and distribution in many countries. Except for a small contribution from Glaxo Smith Kline, no major vaccine producing company is yet collaborating with IAVI (IAVI, 2000).

14.35. THE GLOBAL TB ALLIANCE

With two million deaths a year, tuberculosis exerts a serious impact on developing countries. Tuberculosis is the major opportunistic infection of HIV disease in poor country settings. The *Global Alliance for TB Drug Development* (TB Alliance) was founded in 2000. It aims at commercializing a new anti-TB drug by 2010. This should provide better treatment than that possible with the drugs currently available because treatment will be shortened to two or three months and/or the frequency of drug administration will be reduced to once a day. Its efficacy against multi-drug resistant TB will be enhanced. It will provide more effective treatment against latent TB infection (Global TB Alliance, 2000).

In the field of agrobiotechnology the dissemination of proprietary technologies has occasionally been criticized as a top-down manoeuvre to legitimize the development of new techniques. For example, *Monsanto's* delivery of genetically modified potatoes and the so-called 'Golden Rice' by *Syngenta* were questioned as to their usefulness for the problems and people they supposedly address. By and large, pharmaceutical companies cannot be criticized on the same grounds. For one thing, they did not launch these partnerships themselves, but were relatively passively drawn into them. Furthermore, the scale and impact of diseases such as malaria, tuberculosis or HIV/AIDS make it hard to dismiss a contribution to alleviating these diseases as a public relations stunt by private companies (Lehmann, 2001).

14.36. DNA VACCINE TRIAL

Clinical trials of a two-component *Human Immunodeficiency Virus* (HIV) vaccine are now underway in Oxford (UK) and Nairobi (Kenya). Both components are based on HIV subtype A, the predominant strain in East Africa. This vaccine is the first one based on an HIV strain common in Africa to have entered even this first phase of clinical testing, which evaluates a vaccine's safety profile and yields some preliminary data on its ability to induce immune responses (Hanke, 2000).

Worldwide, there are some half a dozen different broad categories ~ vaccines undergoing early clinical testing, but only one (VaxGen's HIV envelope-based subunit vaccine) that has reached so-called Phase III trials which evaluate whether a vaccine does effectively prevent disease (Levings and Kahn, 2001).The new vaccine was developed through a Vaccine Development Partnership (VOP) between University of Oxford, the University of Nairobi and the IAVI, with vaccine production taking place at Cobra Pharmaceuticals in the UK and at Impfstoffwerk Dessau-Tornar GmbH (lOT) in Germany. The University of Nairobi's new HIV Vaccine Evaluation Unit, housed in the Department of Medical Microbiology, is carrying out clinical and laboratory work for the trial.

14.37. PRIME-BOOST STUDIES

Phase I testing of the first vaccine component - "naked" DNA containing selected HIV genes and individual epitopes (the portions of proteins that evoke immune responses) has revealed no adverse effects in the volunteers. Trials of the second vaccine component, which contains the same HIV genes inserted into harmless viral vector (the Vaccinia virus strain Modified Virus Ankara, MVA), began in Oxford in March 2001 (with eight volunteers). Later, the two components are planned to be tested in combination by vaccinating people first with HIV-DNA and then with the HIV-MVA vector. This strategy, known as a "prime-boost", has been found empirically to induce more potent immune responses in animals (rhesus macaques) than either component alone. The first prime-boost trial began in Oxford in August 2001.

Each of the components is designed to stimulate broad immune responses by T-lymphocytes, the arm of the immune system, which recognizes and destroys host cells infected by viruses, against multiple HIV epitopes. (In contrast, the B-Iymphocytes produce antibodies, which lead to the destruction of free virus in the blood). The epitopes have been identified in persons infected with subtype A HIV strains circulating in Kenya, but many of them are also found among other HIV subtypes (Levings and Kahn, 2001).The scientific rationale for a T-cell based AIDS vaccine arose out of studies with sex-workers in Africa. A small minority of these prostitutes remains seronegative despite continual exposure to HIV, and contains significant levels of HIV-specific T -cells in their bloodstream.

14.38. GLOBAL PUBLIC-PRIVATE PARTNERSHIPS FOR NEGLECTED DISEASES

Health problems of developing countries are no longer being financed solely through public funding. New partnerships are emerging between the public and private sectors. One of these new forms of health development and governance is Public Private Partnerships (PPPs).The research, development and delivery of drugs for neglected diseases is increasingly being undertaken by Public Private Partnerships but concerns have been raised about some of their key characteristics such as the inequality of the partners or their relationship with international organizations.

One central issue in analyzing these new institutional structures is how effective they are in addressing the health needs of the poor, and what their impact is on public and inter-governmental health work at field level. A growing number of PPPs now focus on medical R&D and the delivery of drugs and vaccines. However, the term partnership might be a misnomer (Walt and Lush, 2001). Areas of concern are the structural inequality between partners, and the burdens placed on the administrative and health care facilities of poor countries responsible for implementing the drug programs and health regimes developed by PPPs. The political and scientific arena is perhaps not as simple as the term 'public-private' suggests. PPPs are not just cooperation between the R&D facilities of public institutes and private companies. Private also includes private foundations whose philanthropic agendas are colored by the ideologies of their founders and trustees.

Global Public Private Partnerships (GPPPs) include novel governance mechanisms that are moving away from hierarchical, vertical, inter-governmental institutions (e.g., the World Health Organization) towards horizontal, participative, coordinating arrangements between private philanthropic organizations, companies, public research institutes and others. Walt and Lush (2001) described GPPPs as a specific form of governance, a mechanism of mobilizing political resources in situations where those resources are widely dispersed between private and public actors.

A burgeoning number of public-private entities have been established to address particular problems (Buse and Walt, 2000). Many are supply-driven, for example, by donations from the pharmaceutical industry, and for reasons, which range from a shift to greater corporate social responsibility or image building to market penetration. Other GPPPs are demand-driven, being largely initiated by the public sector, to overcome market failure in developing countries, for reasons which range from professional concern and public health ethos to fears of cross-border contamination of the population by infectious diseases. Industry participation in these entities has so far been relatively meager (Walt and Lush, 2001).

While the links between public and private sectors need to be encouraged, two issues should be kept in view to ensure that goodwill and enthusiasm is not dissipated. Firstly, too many GPPPs can lead to fragmentation and will not be sustainable. Secondly, the health sector needs to be strengthened and better organized so that health systems can effectively deliver new tools such as new vaccines and drugs. In order to build up health systems, painstaking and consultative processes are needed to ensure effective implementation in developing countries. Virtually, most drugs and vaccines have to be delivered through services, and this is where effort should be focused (Walt and Lush, 2001).

SUGGESTED READING

- Abraham VC, Taylor DL, Haskins K. *Trends in Biotech* 22, 15 (2004).
- Ackerman MJ. *Mayo Clin Proc* 73, 250 (1998).
- Adams MR. *J Biotechnol* 68, 171 (1999).
- Aguzzi A. *Nat Rev Neurosci* 2, 745 (2001).
- Ahmed FE. *Trends in Biotech* 20, 215 (2002).
- Ahmed FE. *Trends in Biotech* 21, 491 (2003).
- Alam JJ. *Trends in Biotech* 21, 479 (2003).
- Al-Hendy A, Hortelano G, Tannenbaum GS, *et al. Hum Gene Ther* 6, 165 (1995)
- Allen TM, Cullis R. *Science* 303, 1818 (2004).
- An HJ, Cho NH, Lee SY, *et al. Cancer* 97, 1672 (2003).
- Angelova N, Hunkeler D. *Trends in Biotech* 17, 409 (1999).
- Anon. U.S. *Pharmacopeia and National Formulary,* 10463, 2762 (2002).
- Aridor M, Hannan LA. *Traffic* 1, 836 (2000).
- Attaway D, Zaborsky O. (eds.). *Advances in Marine Biotechnology.* Vol. 1. *Pharmaceutical and Bioactive Natural Products.* Plenum Press, New York (1993).
- Bach S, Talarek N, Andrieu T, *et al., Nat Biotechnol* 21, 1075 (2003).
- Banerjee D. *Curr Opin Investig Drugs* 2, 574 (2001).
- Barchi RL. *Curr Opin Neurol* 11, 461 (1998).
- Bennett PB, Guthrie HRE. *Trends in Biotech* 21, 563 (2003).
- Bergers G, Hanahan D. *Nat Biotechnol* 19, 20 (2001).
- Bitko V, Barik S. *BMC Microbiol* 1, 34 (2001).
- Brondsted L, Hammer K. *Appl Environ Microbiol* 65, 752 (1999).
- Brudnak MA. Probiotics as an adjuvant to detoxification protocols. *M ed. Hypotheses,* 58, 382 (2002).
- Brummelkamp TR. *Cancer Cell 2*, 243 (2002).
- Bull AT, Ward AC, Goodfellow M. *Microbiol Mol Biol Rev* 64, 573 (2000).
- Buse K, Walt G. Global public-private partnerships: Part II - what are the healths issues for global governance? *Bulletin of the World Health Organization* 78, 699 (2000).
- Butler D. *Nature* 397, 281 (1999).
- Catterall WA. *Annu Rev Biochem* 64, 493 (1995).
- Catterall WA. *Neuron* 26, 13 (2000).
- Catterall WA. *Annu Rev Cell Del Biol* 16, 521 (2000).

- Celesia G. *Neurophysiol* 112, 2 (2000).
- Ciancio TD. *Transplantation* 71, 827 (2001).
- Coburn GA, Cullen BR. *J Virol* 76, 9225 (2002).
- Couzin J. *Science* 297, 758 (2002).
- DeFilippis. V., Raggo, C., Moses, A., Friih. K.. *Trends in Biotech.*, 21, 452-457 (2003).
- Dove A. *Nat Bioteclmol* 20, 777 (2002).
- Dubnau D, Lovett CM. Transformation and recombination. In *Bacillus subtilis and its Closest Relatives: from Gene to Cells* (Sonenehein, A.L. *et al.*, eds), ASM Press, pp. 453-471, Baltimore (2002).
- Dumitriu S. (Ed.). *Polymeric Biomaterials* Dekkar, New York (2002).
- Ebneth A. *Drug Discov Today* 7, 227 (2002).
- Enfors SO, Jahic M, Rozkov A, *et al.*, *J Biotechnol* 85, 175 (2001).
- Evan GJ, Vousden KH. *Nature* 411, 342 (2001).
- Evans DC, Watt AP, Nicoll-Griffith DA, Baillie TA. *Chem Res Toxicol* 17, 3 (2004).
- Farrell NP. (Ed.). *Uses of Inorganic Chemistry in Medicine.* Royal Society of Chemistry, Cambridge, UK, (1999).
- Fenical W. *Trends in Biotech* 15, 341 (1997).
- Fishwild DM, O'Donnell SL, Bengoechea T, *et al.*, *Nat Biotechnol* 14, 845 (1996).
- Follette P. *Science* 299, 191 (2003).
- Friedlander RM. *N Engl J Med* 348, 1365 (2003).
- Futcher AB, Cox BS. *J Biotechnol* 157, 283 (1984).
- Gabizon A, Shmeeda H, Barenholz Y. *Clin Pharmacokinet* 42, 419 (2003).
- Gaskell G, Bauer MW, Durant J, *et al.*, *Science* 285, 384 (1999).
- Geiss GK, An MC, Bumgarner RE, Hammersmark E, *et al.*, *J Virol* 75, 4321 (2001).
- Gelbert LM, Gregg RE. *Curr Opin Biotechnol* 8, 669 (1997).
- Giuliano KA, Haskins JR, Taylor DL, *et al.*, *Assay Drug Develop Technol* 1, 565 (2003).
- Giuliano KA, DeBiasio RL, Dunlay T, *et al.*, *J Biolmol Screen* 2, 249 (1997).
- Giuliano KA, Taylor DL. *Trends in Biotech* 16, 135 (1998).
- Goodfellow M, O'Donnell AG. Search and discovery of industrially significant actinomycetes, In Baumberg S, Hunter IS, Rhodes PM. (eds.). p. 343-383.*Microbial Products.* Cambridge University Press, Cambridge (1989).
- Gura T. *Nature* 417, 584 (2002).
- Hahn K, DeBiasio R, Taylor DL, *et al.*, *Nature* 359, 736 (1992).
- Hamill OP, Marty A, Neher E, *et al.*, *P flugers Arch* 391, 85 (1981).
- Hamilton AJ, Baulcombe DC. *Science* 286, 950 (1999).
- Hamilton SR, Bobrowicz P, Bobrowicz B, *et al.*, *Science* 301, 1244 (2003).

- Hanke T, McMichael AJ. *Nature Medicine* 6, 951 (2000).
- Heasman J. *Dev Biol* 243, 209 (2002).
- Henriksen CM, Nilsson D, Hansen S., *et al., Int Dairy J* 9, 17 (1999).
- Hille B. *Ion Channels of Excitable Membranes*. Simmer Associates, Sunderland (2001).
- Hu Y, Cherton-Horvat G, Dragowska V. *et al., Cancer Res* 9, 2826 (2003).
- Hubner CA, Jentsch TJ. *Mol Genet* 11, 2435 (2002).
- James TN. *Coron Artery Dis* 9, 291 (1998).
- Jeffries P, Dodd JC. Molecular ecology of mycorrhizal fungi, p. 73-103. In Priest FG, Goodfellow M. (ed.). *Applied Microbial Systematics*. Kluwer, Dordrecht (2000).
- Jiang M, Milner J. *Oncogene* 21, 6041 (2002).
- Jones PS. *Antiviral Chem Chemother* 9, 283 (1998).
- Jorgensen WL. *Science* 303, 1813 (2004).
- Joutsjoki V, Luoma S, Tamminen M. *et al., J Appl Microbiol* 92, 1159 (2002).
- Karp PC, Riley M, Paley SM, Pellegrin-Toole A, Krummenacker M. *Nucleic Acids Res* 27, 55 (1999).
- Katze MG, He Y, Gale MJ, *et al., Nat Rev Immunol* 2, 675 (2002).
- Kaufman DS, Hanson ET, Lewis RL, *et al., PNAS* (USA) 983, 10716 (2001).
- Kaufman SH, Earnshaw WC. *Exp Cell Res* 256, 42 (2000).
- Kiss L, Bennett PB, Uebele VN, *et al., Assay and Drug Dev Tech* 1, 127 (2003).
- Kohler G, Milstein C. *Nature* 256, 495 (1975).
- Krüger C, Hu Y, Pan Q. *et al., Nat Biotechnol* 20, 702 (2002).
- Kwanmin JJ, *Biopharm* 2, 30 (1989).
- Lee KY, Peters MC, Anderson KW. *et al., Nature* 408, 998 (2000).
- Lee SY. *Trends in Biotech* 14, 98 (1996).
- Lehmann V. *Biotechnology and Development Monitor* 46, 2 (2001).
- Levings B, Kahn R. *Biotechnology and Development Monitor* 46, 8 (2001).
- Licinio J, Wong ML. (Ed.). *Pharmacogenomics*: *The Search for Individualized Therapies*. Wiley-VCH, Weinheim (2002).
- Lipinski CA, Lombardo F, Dominy BW, Feeney PJ. *Adv Drug Delivery Rev* 23 (1997).
- Lockhart DJ, Winzeler EA. *Nature* 405, 827 (2000).
- Love S. *Neuropsycho-pharmacol Biol Psychiary* 27, 267 (2003).
- MacCoss M, Baillie TA. *Science* 303, 1810 (2004).
- MacManus JP, Buchan AM. *J Neurotrauma* 17, 899 (2000).
- Manning G, Whyte DE, Martinez R, Hunter T, Sudarsanam S. *Science* 298, 1912 (2002).
- Maryanoff BE. *J Med Chem* 47, 769 (2004).
- Maus MV, Thomas AK, Leonard DG. *et al., Nat Biotechnol* 20, 143 (2002).

- McFarland LV, Elmer GW. *Microecol Ther* 23, 46 (1995).
- McManus MT, Sharp PA. *Nat Rev Genet*, 3, 737 (2002).
- Mollet B. *Int Dairy J* 9, 11 (1999).
- Noble MEM, Endicott JA, Johnson LN. *Science* 1800 (2004).
- Numann R, Negulescu PA. *Trends Cardiovasc Med* 11, 54 (2001).
- Omura S, Ikeda H, Ishikawa J, *et al., PNAS* (USA) 98, 12215 (2001).
- Orive G, Hernandez RM, Gascon AR. *et al., Trends in Biotech* 20, 382 (2002).
- Orvig C, Abrams MJ. (Eds.). Special issue on Medicinal Inorganic Chemistry. *Chem. Rev.* 99: (No.9) (1999).
- Owen D, Silverthorne A. *Drug Discovery World,* 48 (2002).
- Plymale DR, Haskins JR, de la Iglesia FA. *et al., Nat Med* 5, 351 (1999).
- Papetti M, Herman IM. *Am J Physiol Cell Physiol* 282, C947 (2002).
- Papke RL, Porter Papke JK. *AxoBits* 36, 6 (2002).
- Petit-Zeman S. *Nat Biotechnol* 9, 201 (2001).
- Pirmohamed M, Park BK. *Toxicology* 192, 23 (2003).
- Pitkin Z, Mullon C. *Artf Organs* 23, 829 (1999).
- Prusiner SB. *Science* 216, 13, 414 (1982).
- Prusiner SB. *PNAS* (USA) 95, 13363 (1998).
- Ramsay G. *Nat Biotechnol,* 16, 40 (1998).
- Read TA, Farhadi M, Bjerkvig R, *et al., Cancer Res* 61, 6830 (2001).
- Renault P. *Biochimie* 84, 1073 (2002).
- Saltzman WM. *Drug Delivery: Engineering Principles for Drug Therapy.* Oxford Univ. Press, New York (2001).
- Sansom MS, Shrivastava IH, Bright JN, *et al., Biochim Biophys Acta* 1565, 294 (2002).
- Saupe SJ. *Trends in Biotech* 21, 516 (2003).
- Savic R, Luo L, Eisenberg A, Maysinger D. *Science* 300, 615 (2003).
- Schang LM. *J Antimicrob Chemother* 50, 779 (2002)
- Schiering N, Knapp S, Marconi M, *et al., PNAS* (USA) 100, 12654 (2003).
- Schwartz MA. *J Cell Biol* 139, 575 (1997).
- Service RF. *Science* 303, 798 (2004).
- Service RF. *Science* 294, 2080 (2001).
- Shapiro AM, Lakey JR, Ryan EA, *et al., N Engl J Med* 343, 230 (2000).
- Sharma NC, *Nat Acad Sci India* 65(B), II (Suppl.) pp. 229 (1995).
- Smith C. *Nature* 428, 225 (2004).
- Smith DH, Adams JR, Johnston SR, *et al., Ann Oncol* 133, 1590 (2002).
- Stiles ME, Holzapfel WH. *Int J Food Microbiol* 36, 1 (1997).

- Supattapone S, Nishina K, Rees JR. *Biochem Pharmacol* 63, 1383 (2002).
- Szuromi P, Vinson V, Marshall E. *Science* 303, 1795 (2004).
- Taylor DL, Woo ES, Giuliano KA. *Curr Opin Biotechnol* 12, 75 (2001).
- Teitelbaum JE, Walker WA. *Annu Rev Nutr* 22, 107 (2002).
- Terwogt JMM, Groenewegen G, Pluim D, *et al., Cancer Chemother Pharmacol* 49, 201 (2002).
- Thiry M, Cingolani D, *Trends in Biotech* 20, 103 (2002).
- Thompson KH, Orvig C. *Science* 300, 936 (2003).
- True HL, Lindquist SL. *Nature* 407, 477 (2000).
- Uetrecht J. *Drug Discov Today* 8, 832 (2003).
- Uptain SM, Lindquist S. *Annu Rev Microbiol* 56, 703 (2002).
- Waldmeier PC, *Biol Psychiatry* 27, 303 (2003).
- Walsh CT. *Science* 303, 1805 (2004).
- Walt G, Lush L. *Biotechnology and Development Monitor* 46, 9 (2001).
- Wang D, Coscoy L, Zylberberg M, *et al., PNA* (USA) 99, 15687 (2002).
- Wang T, Lacík I, Brissová M, *et al., Nat Biotechnol* 15, 358 (1997).
- Wegmann U. *Appl Environ Microbiol* 65, 4729 (1999).
- Welling PG. *Pharmacokinetics-Processes, Mathematics, and Applications. (*Ed. 2.) Amer. Chem. Soc., Washington, D.C. (1997).
- White AR, Enever P, Tayebi M. *Nature* 422, 80 (2003).
- Whittaker MM, Whittaker JW. *Protein Expr Purif* 20, 105 (2000).
- Wickner RB. *Science* 264, 566 (1994).
- Winter G, Milstein C. *Nature* 349, 293 (1991).
- Yeatman TJ. *Ann Surg Oncol* 10, 7 (2003).
- Zhang J, Campbell RE, Ting AY, *et al., Nat Rev Mol Cell Biol* 3, 906 (2002).
- Ziauddin J, Sabatini DM. *Nature* 411, 107 (2001).

IMMUNOLOGICAL TECHNIQUES AS ADVANCED BIOTECHNOLOGICAL TOOLS

15.6. ENZYME IMMUNOASSAY (EIA)

15.6.1. The enzyme-multiplied immunoassay technique (EMIT)

15.6.2. Enzyme-linked immunosorbent assay (ELISA)

15.7. FLOW INJECTION IMMUNOASSAY (FIIA)

15.8. ANTIBODY ABSORPTION TEST

15.9. IMMOBILIZATION TEST

15.10. POLYMERASE CHAIN REACTION (PCR)

15.11. DNA FINGERPRINTING

15.11.1. DNA microarray

15.11.2. Restriction fragment length polymorphism (RFLP)

15.12. MISCELLANEOUS DIAGNOSTIC TESTS

15.12.1. The patch test

15.12.2. Skin test

15.13. BIOSENSORS: IMMUNOSENSORS

15.1. INTRODUCTION

Immunodiagnostic tests used for the diagnosis have been used particularly in medical sciences extensively and also in many scientific disciplines for various identifications. The concept of immunoassay was first described in 1945 when Landsteiner suggested that antibodies could bind selectively to small molecules (haptens) while they may remain or made conjugate to a larger carrier molecule. Such tests constitute the basis of many analytical methods where antibodies are used as reagents, while the results of such tests help in diagnostic interpretation. The format of these tests has been equally varied; covering simple manual methods monitored by radioisotopes or enzymes; fully automated systems with integrated sophisticated detection; immunosensors; and 'dip-stick' tests even for home use as exemplified by the home pregnancy test. The wide repertoire of immunoassays available is undoubtedly a reflection of considerable success of assays in different disciplines. The historical development of immunoassays illustrates the multi-disciplinary contribution, beginning with the work of Krause on the reaction of soluble antigens and antiserum in the 1890s. In the early 1900s Bechold tried to discriminate between individual reactions of several antigens and antisera in complex mixtures by exploiting diffusion in gels.

Since the emergence of concept, immunoassays have witnessed phenomenal growth with a spectrum of range and scope of their applications. A vast array of different assay strategies has been developed to meet out the requirements with sensitivity, accuracy and convenience. The development of increasingly sensitive labels and detection equipments resulted in a drastic improvement in the sensitivity of immunoassay systems, allowing an ever-increasing range of analytes to be measured accurately. At the same time they are developed to be simple, inexpensive with the necessary reliability, accuracy and sensitivity which make immunoassay technology usable to much more diverse areas including home testing, near-patient monitoring and large screening programmes in developing countries. Recent developments in molecular biology techniques have further made the production of fusion antibody conjugates possible, which can incorporate the improvements in sensitivity and cost of reagents. However, dissatisfaction with various aspects of existing immunoassay technology necessitates the continued development of this already widely diverse subject.

The advantages of immunoassay technology include the following: low detection limits, wide range of analytes selectivity, high throughput of samples, reduced sample preparation cost and time, versatility for target analytes, cost effectiveness for large numbers of samples, adaptability to practical use. As is the case with every analytical method, immunoassay technology has limitations too, which include: interferences from sample matrices, cross reactivity to structural analogs of the target analyte, poor suitability for some multi-analyte applications, low availability of reagents, longer assay development time than some classical analytical methods, a large number of anticipated samples are required to justify the development of a new assay for a given analyte of interest.

The immunoassay is clearly not the best analytical method for all analytes in all situations. For example, gas–liquid chromatography (GLC) still remains the method of choice for the analysis of volatile compounds. Though, immunoassay technology is important for the analyst because it complements the classical methods, by providing a confirmatory means and method for many compounds and stands as the only reasonable analytical choice. Most immunoassays can be used to obtain quantitative results with similar or greater sensitivity, accuracy and precision than conventional analytical methods.

15.1.1. Principles of Immunoassays

Immunoassays are based on the reaction of an analyte or antigen (Ag) with a selective antibody (Ab) to give a product (Ag–Ab) that can be measured. The reactants are in a state of equilibrium that is characterized by the law of mass action. Several types of labels have been used in immunoassays, including radioactivity, enzymes, fluorescence, luminescence and phosphorescence. Each of these labels has advantages, but the most common label for clinical and environmental analysis is the use of enzymes as used with colorimetric substrates.

Enzyme immunoassays can be divided into two general categories: homogeneous and heterogeneous immunoassays. Heterogeneous immunoassays require the separation of bound and unbound reagents (antibody or antigen) during the assay. This separation is readily accomplished by washing the solid phase (such as test-tubes or microtiter plate wells) with a buffer system. Homogeneous immunoassays however do not require separation and washing steps, moreover the enzyme label must function within the sample matrix. As a result, assay interference caused by the matrix may be problematic for samples of environmental origins (i.e., soil, water, etc.). For samples of clinical origin (human or veterinary applications), high target analyte concentrations and relatively consistent matrices are often present. Thus for clinical or field applications, the homogeneous immunoassay format is popular, whereas the heterogeneous format predominates for environmental matrices.

15.2. ANTIGEN-ANTIBODY REACTIONS

The antigen-antibody reaction, a bimolecular association similar to an enzyme-substrate interaction is essentially an irreversible chemical alteration. The reaction involves various non-covalent interactions between the antigenic determinant or epitope of the antigen and the variable region of the antibody. The non-covalent interactions include:

(1) Hydrogen bonds

(2) Ionic bonds

(3) Hydrophobic interactions

(4) Van der Waals interactions

Antigenic determinant + $V_{H/L}$ of antibody $\rightarrow$ Antigen-Antibody reaction

The antibody can combine only with antigen which is identical or nearly identical with the inducing antigen; it does not combine with unrelated antigens, When the molecules of antibody and antigen are brought together in solution, they interact with each other forming a link between an antigen-antibody site in the immunoglobulin molecule, (part of the Fab fragment and other antigenic determinant parts). The molecules which are held together by non covalent intermolecules are effective only when the antigen-binding site and the antigenic determinant groups are able to make close contact. The closer the contact better could be fit and hence, stronger is the antigen-antibody bond. The strength of the sum total of non-covalent interactions between a single antigen binding site on an antibody and a single epitope determines the affinity of the antibody for that epitope. The affinity at one binding site therefore does not always reflect the true strength of the antibody-antigen interaction. When a complex antigen containing multiple, repeating antigenic determinants are mixed with antibodies containing multiple binding sites, the interaction of antibody with antigen at one site tends to increase the probability of reaction at a second site. The strength of such multiple interactions between a multivalent antibody and antigen is called avidity. Thus avidity of an antibody is a better measure than the affinity of its binding capacity within biological systems.

15.2.1. Precipitin Reactions

The interaction between an antibody and antigen molecule in soluble form, proceeds with the formation of a lattice that eventually develops into a visible precipitate. The formation of soluble antigen-antibody complex occurs within minutes while their visual recognition is very slow which often takes a day or two to reach completion. Formation of an antigen-antibody lattice depends on the valency of both the antibody and antigen. The prime requirement being the antigen must be either bivalent or polyvalent and must possess at least two copies of the same epitope or different epitopes with different antibodies present in polyclonal antisera. A precipitin reaction will not take place with monovalent Fab fragments or monovalent antigens.

15.2.1.1. Precipitin reactions in fluids

Precipitin reaction, a simple reaction that occurs between antibody and antigen molecules in soluble form can be explained as follows. A quantitative precipitin reaction can be performed by placing a known amount of antibody in a series of test tubes and by adding a measured amount of antigen to the tubes. The formed precipitate is separated and measured. A precipitin curve is obtained by plotting the amount of precipitate against the antigen concentrations. It can be well understood that maximum precipitate occurs when the ratio of antibody to antigen is optimum. This is projected as the equivalence zone. As a large multimolecular lattice is formed at the **equivalence zone** it precipitates out due to large size. The other two zones are the **antibody excess zone** and **antigen excess zone.** This test is rapid qualitative test for determining the presence of antibody or antigen. This is performed by adding antiserum to small tube and layering antigen on its top. If the antiserum contains antibodies specific for the test antigen, then the antibody and antigen diffuse towards each other and form a visible band of precipitate at the interface within few minutes. This, test is of importance in detecting and identifying antigens having applications in the typing of streptococci or pneumococci.

15.2.1.2. Precipitin reactions in gel (or) Immunodiffusion reactions

Precipitin reactions are not only performed in fluids but also they are conducted in agar matrix. The diffusion of antibody in antigen bearing agar or vice versa, results into the formation of a visible line of precipitate. This line appears at the region of equivalence and no visible precipitate forms/occurs in the region of antigen excess and/or antibody excess. These immunodiffusion reactions can be used in determining the relative concentration of antibodies or antigens or to determine the relative purity of an antigen preparation. Immunodiffusion technique can further be classified into two techniques which are used commonly.

1. Radial immunodiffusion or Mancini method

2. Double immunodiffusion or Ouchterlony method

15.2.1.2.1. Radial immunodiffusion or Mancini method

Radial immunodiffusion method is a simple quantitative assay wherein an antigen sample is placed in a well and allowed to diffuse into agar that contains a suitably diluted antiserum. A precipitin ring is formed at the zone of equivalence. The area of precipitin ring is proportional to the concentration of antigen. Comparing the area with a standard curve, the concentration of antigen can be determined. This technique is widely used to quantitatively measure serum IgM, IgG and 19A by incorporating suitable anti-isotype antibody into the agar. It has gained wide application in determining concentrations of serum complement components. However, the test limits to the concentrations of antigens above 10μg/ml. An **Oudin test** (Fig. 15.1) is a varied type of precipitation in gel that involves single diffusion. Antiserum, incorporated into agar, is placed in a narrow test tube. This is overlaid with an antigen solution which diffuses into the agar to yielding precipitation rings. It also called single radial diffusion test. A band of precipitation forms at the equivalence point.

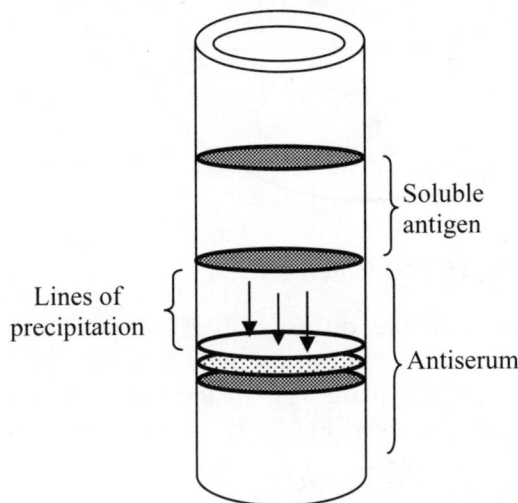

Soluble antigen

Lines of precipitation

Antiserum

Fig. 15.1: Oudin test

15.2.1.2.2. Double immunodiffusion or Ouchterlony method

Unlike Mancini method, in this method both antigen and antibody are placed in separate wells they diffuse radially towards each other thereby establishing a concentration gradient. This method plays as a tool in determining the relationship between antigens and the number of different antigen-antibody systems present. The patterns of precipitate lines that form when two different antigen preparations are placed in adjacent wells indicate whether or not they share the epitopes. This can be explained by an example wherein two antigens share identical epitopes, here, the antiserum forms a single precipitin line with each antigen that grows towards each other and fuses to form a patterned *identity*. However, when the antigens are unrelated, the antiserum forms independent precipitin lines that cross each other proving ***non-identity***. This crossing is possible as the unrelated antigen and antibody do not precipitate and hence free to diffuse apart. A third type of identity namely ***partial*** *identity* is seen when two antigens share the same epitopes but one or the other has a unique epitope. In this case, the antibodies to the common epitope form a line of identity, but antibodies to the unique epitope(s) diffuse past the precipitating line forming spur. A precipitin line is formed with the unique epitope(s) of the more complex antigen. This test is, however suffers some limitations of which the prime one being the time as it takes around 18-24 h in this case. This can however be overcome by using counter-current electrophoresis (Fig.15.2).

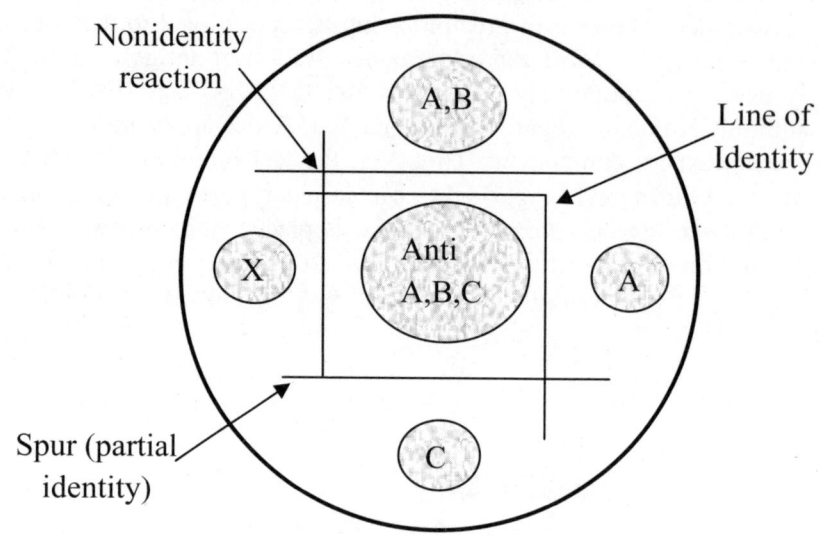

Fig.15.2: Ouchterlony test

The **Oakley-Fulthorpe test** is a double diffusion type of precipitation test performed by incorporating antibody into agar which is placed in the tube followed by a layer of plain agar. A solution of antigen is placed on top of the plain agar in the tube and precipitation occurs where antigen and antibody meet in the plain agar layer (Fig.15.3).

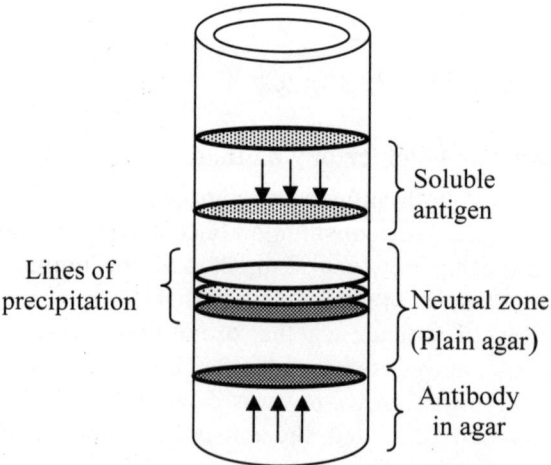

Fig.15.3: Oakley-Fulthorpe test

Hormone immunoassays

Multiple hormones, including thyroid-stimulating hormone, human growth hormone, insulin, glucagon's, and many others may be measured by an immunoassay using either radioactively labelled reagents or through enzyme colour reactions using the ELISA technique. Labelled and unlabelled hormones are allowed to compete for binding sites with an anti-hormone antibody. This is followed by the separation of bound from unbound hormone by using one of several techniques.

The solid-phase radioimmunoassay

The solid-phase radioimmunoassay requires the attachment of antigen (or antibody) to an insoluble support, which can be used to capture antibodies (or antigens) in a specimen to be assayed. Antibodies in a serum sample are exposed to an excess of antigen on an insoluble support and sufficient time is allowed for antigen–antibody interaction. This is followed by washing and the application of radiolabelled anti-Fc antibodies specific for the Fc regions of the captured antibodies. After washing, quantification of the bound antibody is determined from the amount of radioactivity adhering to the insoluble support. Various materials may be used as an appropriate insoluble support. These include Sepharose® beads or tissue culture plate wells. An unrelated protein must be used to coat the insoluble support prior to application of the specific antibody to saturate areas of the insoluble support where antigen is not located.

15.2.1.3. Immunoelectrophoresis

Immunoelectrophoresis is a qualitative technique that can detect antibody concentration of 3-20 µg/ml. When a large number of different antigens are present in a solution, it is difficult to separate the precipitin bands for each of the antigen-antibody reaction by simple diffusion method as discussed above. In such situations, where, multicomponent analysis is required, electrophoresis could be used effectively. Here, the antigen mixture is first electrophorized and separated by application of a charge. Then troughs are cut into the agar gel parallel to the direction of electric field and to this is added an antiserum. Following this, incubation is carried out in a humid chamber where the antigen and antibody diffuse towards each other leading to the formation of precipitin bands.

Immunoelectrophoresis is a technique widely used in detection of serum proteins. It is also helpful in determining whether a patient has an immunodeficiency or not. Other than simple electrophoresis are rocket electrophoresis and two-dimensional electrophoresis.

15.2.1.4. Rocket electrophoresis

One among the two immunoelectrophoresis which involve applications of only negatively charged antigen is subjected to electrophoresis in a gel containing antibody. The name of the technique so derived because of the shape or the precipitate formed due to antigen-antibody interaction which is in a rocket shape. The method is limited to negatively charged antigens only.

15.2.1.5. Two-dimensional immunoelectrophoresis

A modified version or the rocket electrophoresis is the two-dimensional immunoelectrophoresis. It is of quantitative method for the estimation of the antigen in a complex mixture. In this method, the antigen is separated into its components by electrophoresis. The gel is then laid over another agar gel containing antiserum, and electrophoresis is repeated at right angles to the previously conducted. This appears in the form of precipitin peaks.

15.2.1.6. Ammonium sulphate precipitation

The ammonium sulphate method is a means of measuring the primary antigen binding capacity of antisera and detects both precipitating and non-precipitating antibodies. It offers an advantage over equilibrium dialysis in that large non-dializable protein antigens may be used. This assay is based on the principle that certain proteins are soluble in 50% saturated ammonium sulphate, whereas antigen–antibody complexes are not. Thus, complexes may be separated from unbound antigen. Spontaneous precipitation will occur if a precipitating-type antibody is used, until a point of antigen excess is reached where complex aggregation no longer occurs and soluble complexes are formed. Upon the addition of an equal volume of saturated ammonium sulphate solution (SAS), these complexes become insoluble, leaving radiolabelled antigen in solution. SAS fractionation does not significantly alter the stoichiometry of the antibody–antigen reaction and inhibits the release or exchange of bound antigen. Thus, radioactivity of this "induced" precipitate is a measure of the antigen-binding capacity of the antisera as opposed to a measure of the amount of antigen or antibody spontaneously precipitated.

The **Lancefield precipitation test** is a ring precipitation test developed by Rebecca Lancefield to classify streptococci according to their group-specific polysaccharides. The polysaccharide antigen is derived by treatment of cultures of the microorganisms with HCl, formimide, or a *Streptomyces albus* enzyme. Antiserum is first placed into a serological tube, followed by layering the polysaccharide antigen over it. A positive reaction is indicated by precipitation at the interface.

15.2.2. Agglutination reactions

The agglutination reaction is similar in principle to the precipitation reaction. The interaction between antibody and a particulate antigen results in visible clumping called agglutination. In this reaction, the antigen is a part of the surface of some particulate material such as a red cell, bacterium or some inorganic particle which has been coated with antigen. Addition of antibody to a suspension of such particles combines with the surface, antigens and links them together to form clearly visible aggregates or agglutinates. However, a practical difficulty in this test is the occasional inhibition of agglutination in the first tube of an antiserum dilution series agglutination occurring only in those tubes which contain more dilute antiserum. The excess antibodies inhibit agglutination reactions this effect is known as *prozone effect,* which may be caused by several mechanism. Firstly, due to the stabilizing effects of high protein concentration on the particles. The protein coats the particle increases their net charge and so brings about increased electrostatic repulsion between individual particles thus opposing the efforts of the antibody molecule to link the particles and together. Secondly, when high concentrations of antibodies bind to the antigen but do not induce agglutination. Such antibodies are called incomplete antibodies. IgG often represents this class.

15.2.2.1. Hemagglutination

Agglutination reactions are routinely performed in typing ABO antigens. Here, the red blood cells (RBCs) are mixed on a slide with antisera to the A and B blood group antigens. If the antigen is present on the cells, they agglutinate, forming a visible clump on the slide (Fig. 15.4).

15.2.2.2. Bacterial agglutination

Any bacterial infection could result in to the elicitation of the production of the serum antibodies specific to the particular surface antigen of the respective bacterial cells. Using agglutination reactions, the presence of such antibodies can be detected. One of the classical applications of the agglutination test is the **Widal test** used for the demonstration of the antibodies to Salmonellae in serum specimens taken from suspected enteric fever cases. The test is performed by taking serum samples of infected patients and is serially diluted in a series of tubes to which the bacteria is added. The last tube showing the visible agglutination will reflect the sera antibody titer of the patient for the particular bacteria. The agglutination titer is defined as the reciprocal of the last serum dilution that elicits a positive agglutination reaction. For example, if the dilution 1/256 shows agglutination but the dilution 1/512 does not, then the agglutination titer of the patient's serum is 256. For some bacteria, high serum titer is obtained up to 1/50,000 and still shows agglutinations. Agglutination reactions also provide a way to type bacteria.

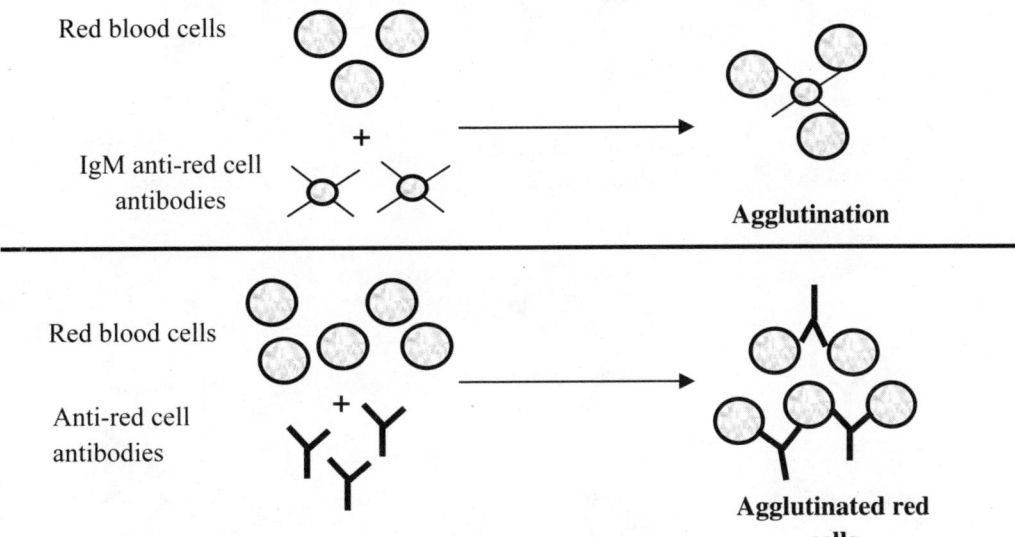

Fig. 15.4: Diagrammatic presentation of agglutination reaction

15.2.2.3. Passive agglutination

Agglutination reactions can be extended to soluble antigens by the technique of passive agglutination. The technique is very simple yet sensitive. Here, the soluble antigen is mixed with red blood cells that have been treated with tannic acid or chromium chloride, in order to promote the adsorption of the antigen to the surface of the cells. Serially diluted serum containing antibody is taken into micro titer plate well, to this is added the antigen coated red blood cells. Agglutination is assessed by the size of the characteristic spread pattern of agglutinated RBC at the bottom of the well. Passive agglutination is more sensitive than precipitin reactions which can detect antibody concentrations as low as 0.001μg/ml.

15.2.2.4. Agglutination inhibition

Agglutination inhibition is a modification of the agglutination assay and is highly sensitive method by which small quantities of antigen can be detected (0.001-0.01 μg/ml). It is a widely used diagnostic procedure. The presence of antibody in the patient's serum is thus detected by its ability to link with virus particles and prevent them from bringing about agglutination of the red cells.

Red cells and inert particles such as polystyrene particles can be coated with various antigens and these coated particles are then used in a variety of diagnostic tests (Fig.15.5). One such test is the test for pregnancy wherein latex coated particles with human chronic gonadotropin (HCG) and antibody to HCG are used. Addition of urine from a pregnant woman, which contains HCG, inhibits agglutination of the latex particles and thus confirms the pregnancy. Similarly, thyroid antibody test using thyroglobulin cells or latex particles can be used. Hormone-coated red cells or inert particles are used in many hormonal assay procedures which are based on the inhibition of the antibody-induced agglutination of the hormone 'coated particles by hormone added to the sample under test. Agglutination inhibition also has wide clinical application in identification if an individual is exposed to a specific type of virus that causes agglutination of red blood cells. Example, the myxoviruses causing influenza and mumps have the property of bringing about agglutination of red blood cells.

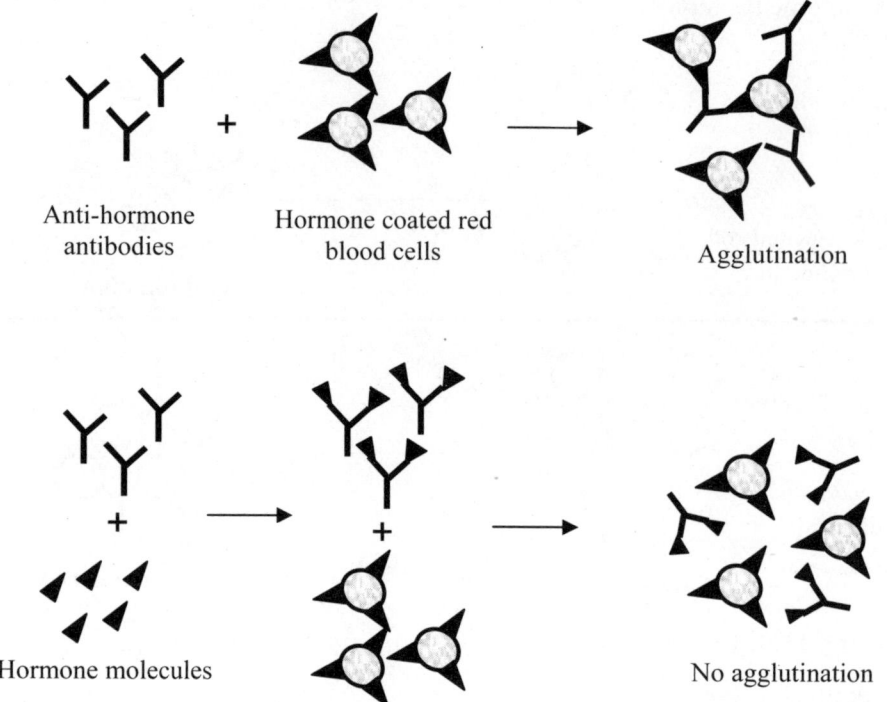

Fig. 15.5: Diagrammatic presentation of agglutination inhibition

The **Paul-Bunnell test** is an assay for heterophile antibodies in infectious mononucleosis patients. It is a hemagglutination test in which infectious mononucleosis patient serum induces sheep red blood cell agglutination. Absorption of the serum with guinea pig kidney tissue removes antibody to the Forssmann antigen but does not remove the sheep red blood cell agglutinin which can be absorbed with ox cells. This hemagglutinin is distinct from antibodies against the causative agent of infectious mononucleosis, i.e., the Epstein-Barr virus.

The **red cell-linked antigen antiglobulin test** is a passive hemagglutination test in which the red cells serve only as carriers for antigen coated on their surfaces. It can identify either agglutinating antibodies or non-agglutinating (incomplete) antibodies by the aggregation or clumping of antigen-bearing red cells. To perform the assay, the test serum is incubated with red cells treated with antigen, which are then washed and antibody against human globulin is added.

The **sheep red blood cell agglutination test** is an assay in which sheep erythrocytes are either agglutinated by antibody or are used as carrier particles for an antigen adsorbed on to their surface, in which case they are passively agglutinated by antibodies specific for the adsorbed antigen.

The ***Treponema pallidum* hemagglutination assay (TPHA)** is a test for antibodies specific for *T. pallidum* used formerly to diagnose syphilis. *T. pallidum* antigens were coated onto sheep red blood cells treated with tannic acid and formalin. Aggregation of the antigen-coated red cells signifies that antibody is present.

Rose-Waaler test: Sheep red blood cells are treated with a sub-agglutinating quantity of rabbit anti-sheep erythrocyte antibody. These particles may be used to identify rheumatoid factor in the serum of rheumatoid arthritis (RA) patients. Agglutination of the IgG-coated red cells constitutes a positive test and is based upon immunological cross reactivity between human and rabbit IgG molecules. It may be positive in collagen vascular diseases other than RA, but it has still proven beneficial in diagnosis.

The **antiglobulin consumption test** is an assay to test for the presence of an antibody in serum which is incubated with antigen-containing cells or antigen-containing particles. After washing, the cells or particles are treated with antiglobulin reagents and incubated further. If any antibody has complexed with the cells or particles, antiglobulin will be taken up. Antiglobulin depletion from the mixture is evaluated by assaying the free antiglobulin in the supernatant through combination with incomplete antibody-coated erythrocytes. No hemagglutination however reveals that the antiglobulin reagent has been consumed in the first step of the reaction and thus suggests that the original patient's serum contains the antibody under question or detection.

Tanned red cells are prepared by treating a suspension of erythrocytes with a 1:20,000 to 1:40,000 dilution of tannic acid that renders their surfaces capable of adsorbing soluble antigen. Thus, they have been widely used as passive carriers of soluble antigens in passive hemagglutination reactions. By adding toluene diisocyanate, the protein can become covalently bound to the red cell surface. However, this is not necessary for routine hemagglutination reactions. The **tanned red cell test** is a passive hemagglutination assay in which red blood cells are used only as carrier particles for soluble antigens. Agglutination of the cells by specific antibody signifies a positive reaction. To render erythrocytes capable of adsorbing soluble protein antigens to their surface, the cells are treated with a weak tannic acid solution. This promotes cell surface attachment of the soluble protein antigen.

The **latex fixation test** is a technique in which latex particles are used as passive carriers of soluble antigens adsorbed to their surfaces. Antibodies specific for the adsorbed antigen then cause agglutination of the coated latex particles. This has been widely used and constitutes the basis of an RA test in which pooled human IgG molecules are coated on the surface of latex particles which are then agglutinated by anti-immunoglobulin antibodies present in the sera of RA patients (Fig.15.6). **Latex particles** are inert particles of defined size that are used as carriers of either antigens or antibodies in latex agglutination immunoassays. An example is the RA test in which latex particles are coated with pooled human IgG that serves as antigen. These IgG-coated particles are agglutinated by rheumatoid factor (anti-immunoglobulin antibody) that may be detected in an RA patient's serum.

Mixed agglutination describes the aggregation (agglutination) produced when morphologically dissimilar cells that share a common antigen are reacted with antibody specific for this epitope. The technique is useful in demonstrating antigens on cells that by virtue of their size or irregular shape are not suitable for study by conventional agglutination tests. It is convenient to use an indicator, such as a red cell that possesses the antigen that is being sought. Thus, the demonstration of mixed agglutination in which the indicator cells are linked to the other cell type suspected of possessing the common antigen constitutes a positive test.

The **RPR (rapid plasma reagin) test** is an agglutination test used in screening of syphilis. Anti-lipoidal (non-treponemal) antibodies (reagins) develop in the host usually within 4 to 6 weeks after infection with *Treponema pallidum*. In the patients with primary syphilis, 93% develop a positive RPR.

Slide agglutination test refers to the aggregation of particulate antigen such as red blood cells, microorganisms, or latex particles coated with antigen within 30 sec following contact with specific antibody. The reactants are usually mixed by rocking the slide back and forth, and agglutination is observed both macroscopically and microscopically. The test has been widely used in the past for screening, but is unable to distinguish reactions produced by cross reacting antibodies which can be ruled out in a tube test that allows dilution of the antiserum.

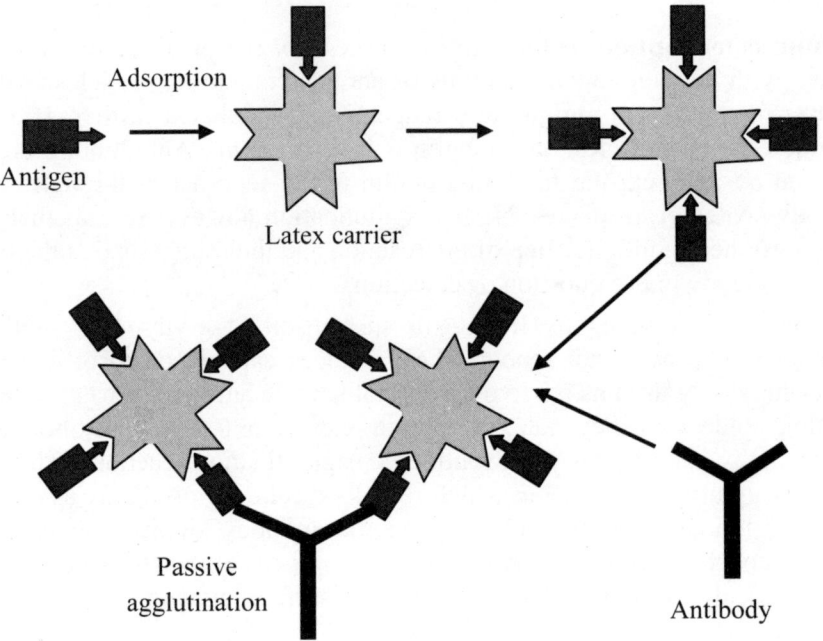

Fig. 15.6: Latex fixation test

The **tube agglutination test** is an agglutination assay that consists of serial dilutions of antiserum in serological tubes to which particulate antigen, such as microorganisms, is added.

The **Weil-Felix reaction** is a diagnostic agglutination test in which *Proteus* bacteria are agglutinated by the sera of patients with typhus. The reaction is based upon the cross reactivity of the carbohydrate antigen shared between *Rickettsiae* and selected *Proteus* strains. Various rickettsial diseases can be diagnosed on the basis of the reaction pattern of antibodies in the blood sera of rickettsial disease patients with O-agglutinable strains of *Proteus* OX19, OX2, and OX12.

The **Widal reaction** is a bacterial agglutination test employed to diagnose enteric infections caused by *Salmonella*. Doubling the dilutions of patient's serum which are subsequently combined with a suspension of microorganisms known to cause enteric fever such as *S. typhi*, *S. paratyphi* B, and *S. paratyphi* A and C. The microorganisms used in the test should be motile, smooth, and should present in the specific phase. To assay H agglutinins, formalin-treated suspensions are used, and to assay O agglutinin, alcohol-treated suspensions are employed. The Widal test is positive on the tenth day of the disease and may be false-positive if an individual previously received a TAB vaccine. Thus, it is important to repeat the test and observe a rising titre rather than to merely observe a single positive test. Widal originally described the test to diagnose *S. paratyphi* B infection.

The **passive agglutination test** is an assay conducted to recognize antibodies against soluble antigens that are attached to erythrocytes, latex, or other particles by either adsorption or chemical linkage. In the presence of antibodies specific for the antigen, aggregation of the passenger particles occurs. Examples of this technique include the RA latex agglutination test, the tanned red cell technique, the bentonite flocculation test, and the bis-diazotized benzidine test.

The **Takatsy method** is a technique that employs tiny spiral loops on the end of a handle that resembles those used for wire loops by bacteriologists. The loops are carefully engineered to retain a precise volume when immersed in a liquid. They are used to prepare doubling dilutions of a test liquid in microtitre wells of test plates. As the loops are passed from one well to the next, a spiral motion helps to discharge the contents into the well diluents and mix it. Several loops can be manipulated by one operator at the same time using a single plastic plate with multiple wells. This method has been applied in hemagglutination assays.

The **vaginal mucous agglutination test** is an assay for antibodies in bovine vaginal mucous from animals infected with *Campylobacter fetus*, *Trichomonas fetus*, and *Brucella abortus*. The mucous can be used in the same manner as serum for a slide or tube agglutination test employing the etiologic microorganisms as on antigen.

15.2.3. Complement fixation

The complement system which comprises of a group of serum proteins plays an important role in immune response. The complement system acts in a cascade fashion, i.e. the activation of one complement results in the activation of the next. The complement system collectively makes up much of the globulin fraction of serum. These proteins are as such in an inactive state. However, they are activated after the binding of antibodies to antigens and are specifically directed against the target molecules identified by the antibodies. Since the complement activation involves the binding of the components to antibody-antigen complexes and to each other with their consequent removal from serum, this event is called **complement fixation**.

Compartment activation takes place following two pathways: the classical and alternative pathways. When a complement binds to an antigen-antibody complex, it becomes "fixed" and "used-up". Complement fixation tests are very sensitive and are used to detect extremely small amounts of an antibody for a suspect microorganism. The sequence of complement fixation is well depicted in Figure 15.7. A known antigen is mixed with test serum lacking complement (Fig. 15.7a). The mixture is kept aside in order to form a complex if any. Now, complement is added to the mixture (Fig. 15.7b). If immune complexes are present, they will fix and the complement is consumed. This is followed by the addition of sensitized indicator cells, usually sheep red blood cells previously coated with complement fixing antibodies. Lysis of these indicator cells (Fig. 15.7c) results if an immune complex is not formed in the first step (Fig. 15.7a) of the test. Absence of lysis shows that specific antibodies are present in the test serum and the complement has been consumed by the immune complex.

Wassermann test used in the diagnosis of syphilis is an example of complement fixation test. Currently, it is used in the diagnosis of certain viral, fungal, rickettsial, chlamydial and protozan diseases. The **Wassermann reaction** is a complement fixation assay used extensively in the past to diagnose syphilis. Cardiolipin extracted from ox heart served as antigen which reacts with antibodies present in patients with syphilis. Biologic false-positive reactions using this test require the use of such confirmatory tests as the FTA-ABS test, the Reiter's complement fixation test, or the *Treponema pallidum* immobilization test. Both FTA and TPI tests involve the use of *T. pallidum* as antigen.

C1q binding assay for circulating immune complexes (CIC)

There are two categories of methods that assay circulating immune complexes: (1) The specific binding of CIC to complement components, such as C1q or the binding of complement activation fragments within the CIC to complement receptors, as in the Raji cell assay. (2) Precipitation of large and small CIC by polyethylene glycol. The C1q binding assay measures those CIC which are capable of binding C1q, a subcomponent of the C1 component of complement and capable of activating the classical complement pathway.

The **gonococcal complement fixation test** is an assay that uses as antigen an extract of *Neisseria gonorrhoea*. It is of little value in diagnosing early cases of gonorrhoea that appear before the generation of an antibody response, but may be used to identify late manifestations in untreated individuals.

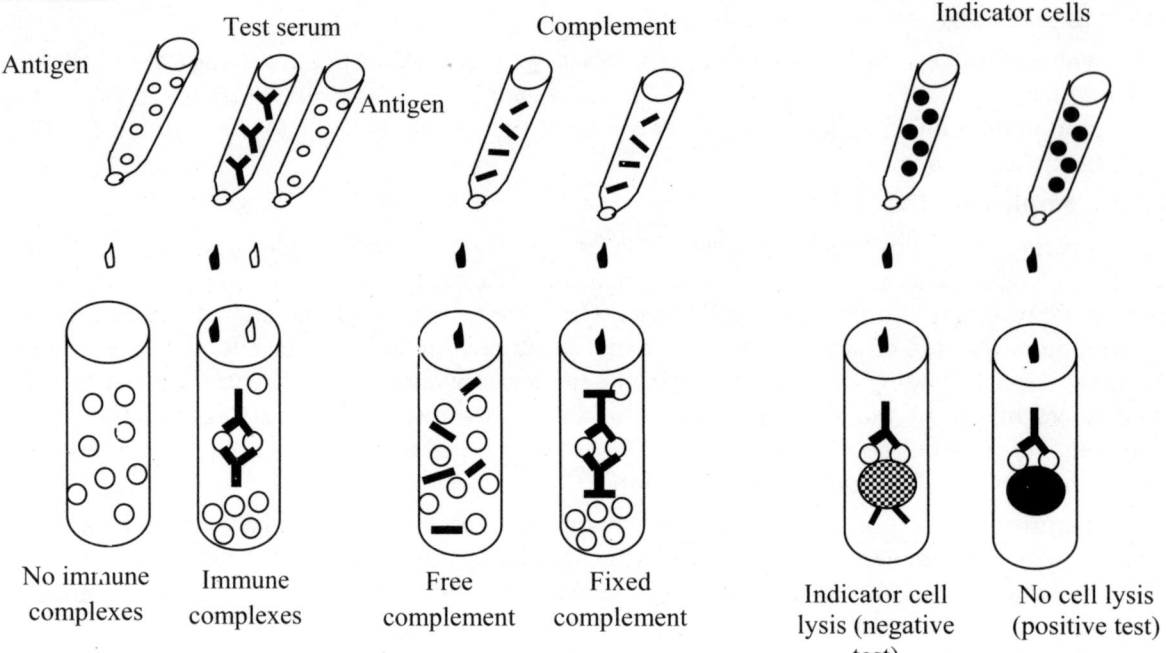

Fig. 15.7: Diagrammatic presentation of complement fixation test

A **complement fixation assay** is a serologic test based on the fixation of complement by antigen–antibody complexes. It has been applied to many antigen–antibody systems and was widely used earlier in the century as a serologic test for syphilis.

Reiter complement fixation test (historical) is a diagnostic test for syphilis that used an antigen derived from a protein extract of *Treponema pallidum* (the Reiter strain). This test identified antibodies formed against *Treponema* group antigens.

15.2.4. Neutralization reactions

15.2.4.1. Toxin neutralization

Neutralization reactions are antigen-antibody reactions that determine whether the activity of a toxin or virus has been neutralized by an antibody. Immunity to a disease like diphtheria depends on the production of specific antibodies that inactivate the toxins produced by the bacteria. This process is known as toxin neutralization. Once the toxin gets neutralized, the toxin-antibody complex is either unable to attach to receptor sites on host target cells or unable to enter the cell. Antiserum containing neutralizing antibody against a toxin is called antitoxin.

15.2.4.2. Viral neutralization

Fixation of classical pathway complement component C4b to the virus aids to the neutralization process. Antibodies such as IgG, IgM and IgA bind to some virus during their extracellular phase and inactivate them. This antibody-mediated viral inactivation is called **viral neutralization**.

Viral neutralization assays are used to detect viral infections. Serum containing viral antibodies can be introduced into tissue culture cells or embryonated egg cells. Viral neutralization occurs in the cases where antibodies against the virus are present and they prevent the virus from infecting the culture cells.

15.3. IMMUNOFLUORESCENCE

Fluorescent dye or fluorochrome can be used in the estimation of antibody or antigen binding to a cell. The antibody or antigen molecule can be tagged with a fluorescent dye and the light emitted by the dye at excitation wave length serves as a measure of the amount of antibody bound. The most commonly used dyes include fluorescein and rhodamine. Both the dyes can be conjugated to the Fc portion of the antibody molecule. Fluorescein absorbs blue light at 490 nm and emits an intense yellow-green fluorsecene at 517 nm, while rhodamine absorbs a yellow-green light at 515 nm and emits a deep red fluorescence at 546 nm.

Immunofluroscence has a wide variety of application. Antibody tagged with fluorescent dyes can be used in identifying a number of lymphocyte subpopulation. They are also helpful in identifying bacterial species, antigen-antibody complexes in autoimmune diseases, in detecting complement components in tissues, and to localize hormones and other cellular products stained *in situ*. Immunofluorescence can be carried out either by direct or indirect method. In the former method, the fluorochrome is directly bound to the specific antibody (primary antibody) while in the latter the primary antibody is unlabelled and is detected with an additional fluorochrome-labeled reagent. A third method also exists in which biotin-conjugated anti-isotype antibody acts as the second antibody and the fluorochrome-conjugated avidin, a protein that has high affinity binds to the biotin. The indirect method has an edge over the direct method. The first being that the primary antibody need not to be conjugated with the label. The second being the sensitivity of the method which is increased because of the multiple fluorochrome reagents that bind to each primary antibody. **Fluorescence** is the emission of light of one wavelength by a substance irradiated with light of a different wavelength.

Fluorescence microscopy employs a special microscope which uses ultraviolet light to illuminate a tissue or cell stained with a fluorochrome-labelled substance such as an antibody against an antigen of interest in the tissue. When returning from an excited state to a ground state, the tissue emits fluorescent light, which permits the observer to localize an antigen of interest in the tissue or cell. **Natural fluorescence** is **autofluorescence**. A **sandwich immunoassay** is a technique in which the analyte is bound to a solid phase and a labelled reagent subsequently bound immunochemically to the analyte. **Fluorescence quenching** is a method to ascertain association constants of antibody molecules interacting with ligands. Fluorescence quenching result from excitation energy transfer where, certain electronically excited residues in protein molecules, such as tryptophan and tyrosine, transfer energy to a second molecule which is bound to the protein. Maximum emission is a wavelength of approximately 345 nm. The attachment of the acceptor molecule need not be covalent. This transfer of energy occurs when the absorbance spectrum of the acceptor molecule overlaps with that of the emission spectrum of the donor and takes place via resonance interaction. There is no need for direct contact between the two molecules for energy transfer. If the acceptor molecule is non-fluorescent, diminution of energy occurs through non-radiation processes.

On the other hand, if the acceptor molecule is fluorescent, the transfer of radiation to it results in its own fluorescence (sensitized fluorescence). Fluorescence quenching techniques can provide very sensitive quantitative data on antibody–hapten interactions.

Fluorescent protein tracing employs fluorescent dyes are used in place of non-fluorescent dyes because they are detectable in a much lower concentration. Radioactive labelling is employed usually if the substance to be detected is present in minute amounts. Fluorescent labelling, however, provides simplicity to the technique and precise microscopic observation of fluorescence. Fluorescent microscopic preparations require several hours and permit localization at the cellular level, whereas autoradiogram requires a longer period and are localized at the tissue level. Either fluorescein (apple green fluorescence) or rhodamine (reddish-orange fluorescence) compounds may be used for tracing.

Immunofluorescence is a method used for the detection of antigen or antibody in cells or tissue sections using fluorescent labels, termed fluorochromes followed by fluorescent light microscopic examination. The most commonly used fluorochromes include fluorescein isothiocyanate, which imparts an apple-green fluorescence, and rhodamine B isothiocyanate, which imparts a reddish orange tint. This method, developed by Albert Coons in the 1940s, has a wide application in diagnostic medicine and research. In addition to antigens and antibodies, complement and other immune mediators may also be detected by this method. It is based on the principle that following adsorption of light by molecules, they dispose of their increased energy by various means, such as emission of light of longer wavelength. Fluorescence is the process whereby emission is of relatively short duration (10^{-6} to 10^{-9} sec) omitted on return of the excited molecules to the ground state. The active groups in protein that allow them to attach fluorochromes include free amino and carboxyl groups at the ends of each polypeptide chain, many free amino groups and lysine side chains, many free carboxyl groups in asparatic and glutamic acid residues, the guanidine group of arginine, the phenolic group of tyrosine, and the amino groups of histidine and tryptophan. Labelling antibody molecules with fluorochromes does not alter their antigen-binding specificity. Several immunofluorescence techniques are available. In the direct test, smears of the substance to be examined are fixed with the help of heat or methanol followed by flooding with a fluorochrome-antibody conjugate. This is followed by incubating in a moist chamber for 30−60 min at 37°C, after which the smear is washed first with buffered saline for 5–10 min and second in tap water for another 5−10 min. These washing procedures remove non conjugated globulin. After adding a small drop of buffered glycerol and the cover slip, the smear may be examined with the fluorescence light microscope. In the indirect test, which is more sensitive than the direct, a smear or tissue section is first flooded with unlabeled antibody specific for the antigen being sought. After washing, fluorescein-labelled anti-immunoglobulin of the species of the primary antibody is layered over the section. After appropriate incubation and washing, the section is cover slipped and examined as in the direct method. Other variations, such as complement staining, are also available. The indirect method is more sensitive than the direct method and considerably less expensive than one fluorochrome-labelled anti-immunoglobulin may be used with multiple primary antibodies specific for different antigens. The technique is widely used to diagnose and classify renal diseases, bullous skin diseases, and for the study of cells and tissues in connective tissue disorders such as SLE.

Membrane immunofluorescence refers to the reaction of a fluorochrome-labelled antibody with cell surface receptors of viable cells. This reaction of fluorescent antibody with surface antigens rather than internal antigens constitutes the basis for many immunologic assays such as labelling of lymphocytes with reagents for immune-phenotyping by flow cytometry, patching, and capping, and to detect changes in surface antigens through antigenic variation.

Nonspecific fluorescence is fluorescence emission that does not reflect antigen–antibody interaction and may confuse interpretation of immunofluorescence tests. Either free fluorochrome or fluorochrome tagging of proteins other than antibody such as serum albumin, α globulin, or β globulin may contribute to nonspecific fluorescence. Nonspecific staining is accounted for inappropriate controls.

The **double-layer fluorescent antibody technique** is an immunofluorescence method used to identify antigen in a tissue section or cell preparation on a slide by first covering and incubating it with antibody or serum containing antibody that is not labelled with a fluorochrome. After appropriate time allowed for interaction, the preparation is washed followed by a second application of fluorochrome-labelled antibody such as goat or rabbit antihuman immunoglobulin to the tissue or cell preparation and incubation. This technique has greater sensitivity than does the single-layer immunofluorescent method. Examples include the application of serum from a patient with Good pasture's syndrome to a normal kidney section acting as substrate followed by incubation and washing, and then covering with fluorochrome-labelled goat antihuman IgG to detect anti-glomerular basement membrane antibodies in the patient's serum. A similar procedure is used in detecting antibodies against intercellular substance antigens in the serum of patients with pemphigus vulgaris.

The **direct fluorescence antibody method-** It employs antibodies, either polyclonal or monoclonal, labelled with a fluorochrome such as fluorescein isothiocyanate, which yields an apple green colour under immunofluorescence microscopy, or rhodamine isothiocyanate, which yields a reddish-orange colour, to identify a specific antigen. This technique is routinely used in immunofluorescence evaluation of renal biopsy specimens as well as skin biopsy preparations to detect immune complexes comprised of the various immunoglobulin classes or complement components. **Direct immunofluorescence** refers to the use of fluorochrome-labelled antibody to identify antigens, especially those of tissues and cells. An example is the immunofluorescence evaluation of renal biopsy specimens.

Indirect immunofluorescence refers to as the interaction of unlabeled antibody with cells or tissues expressing antigen for which the antibody is specific, followed by treatment of this antigen–antibody complex with fluorochrome labelled anti-immunoglobulin that interacts with the first antibody, forming a so-called sandwich. The **indirect fluorescence antibody technique** is a method that identifies antibody or antigen using a fluorochrome-labelled antibody which combines with an intermediate antibody or antigen rather than directly with the antibody or antigen being sought. The indirect test has a greater sensitivity compared to those of the direct fluorescence antibody technique. It is often referred to as the sandwich or double-layer method.

A **fluorescence-activated cell sorter (FACS)** is an instrument that measures the size, granularity, and fluorescence of cells attributable to bound fluorescent antibodies, as individual single cell flows in a stream past photo detectors. Single-cell analysis by this method is termed as flow cytometry, and the machine used to make these measurements and/or sort cells is known as a flow cytometer or cell sorter.

Immunophenotyping uses monoclonal antibodies and flow cytometry to reveal cell surface or cytoplasmic antigens that yield information that may reflect clonality and cell lineage classification. This type of data is valuable clinically in aiding the diagnosis of leukaemia and lymphomas through the use of a battery of B cell, T cell, and myeloid markers. However, immunophenotyping results must be used only in conjunction with morphologic criteria when reaching a diagnosis of leukaemia or lymphoma.

Chemiluminescence is the conversion of chemical energy into light by an oxidation reaction. A high-energy peroxide intermediate, such as luminol, is produced by the reaction of a precursor substance exposed to peroxide and alkali.

The emission of light energy by a chemical reaction may occur during reduction of an unstable intermediate to a stable form. Chemiluminescence measures the oxidative formation of free radicals such as superoxide anion by polymorphonuclear neutrophils and mononuclear phagocytes. Light is released from these cells after they have taken up luminol (5-amino-2,3-dihydro-1,4-phthalazinedione). This is a mechanism that measures the respiratory burst in phagocytes. The oxidation of luminol increases intracellular luminescence. Chronic granulomatous disease may be diagnosed by this technique.

15.4. PROTEIN SEPARATION TECHNIQUES

Proteins may be purified using both electrophoresis and chromatography. Individual techniques are discussed separately. See affinity chromatography; isoelectric focussing; SDS-polyacrylamide gel electrophoresis (SDS-PAGE).

Southern blotting is a procedure used to identify DNA sequences. Following extraction of DNA from cells, it is digested with restriction endonucleases to cut DNA at precise sites into fragments. This is followed by separation of the DNA fragments according to size by electrophoresis in agarose gel, denaturation with sodium hydroxide, and transfer of the single-stranded DNA to a nitrocellulose membrane by blotting. This is followed by hybridization with a 35S- or 32P-radiolabeled probe of complementary DNA. Alternatively, a biotinylated probe may be used. Autoradiography or substrate digestion identifies the location of the DNA fragments that have hybridized with the complementary DNA probe. Specific sequences in cloned and in genomic DNA can be identified by Southern blotting. Whereas DNA analysis is referred to as Southern blot, RNA analysis is referred to as a Northern blot, and protein analysis is referred to as a Western blot. A North-western blot is one in which RNA-protein hybridizations are formed.

Western blotting method is similar to the Southern blotting method that is used for detecting DNA fragments and Northern blotting used for detecting mRNAs. The method can be used in identifying a specific protein in a complex mixture of proteins, or antibody to a given protein, by separating the protein electrophoretically on a polyacrylamide slab gel in the presence of sodium dodecyl sulfate (SDS) (Fig. 15.8). The protein bands are then transferred to a nitro-cellulose membrane by electrophoresis and individual protein bands are identified by flooding the nitro-cellulose membrane with radio labeled monoclonal or polyclonal antibody. The antigen- antibody complex that is formed can be visualized by autoradiography. In case of non availability of labeled specific antibody, antigen-antibody complex can be detected by adding a secondary anti-isotype antibody which is either radiolabelled or enzyme labeled. Western blotting method has been used in the identification of the envelope and core proteins of HIV and the antibodies of these components in the serum of HIV-infected individuals.

South-western blot is a method that combines Southern blotting that identifies DNA segments, with Western immunoblotting that characterizes proteins. A protein may be hybridized to a molecule of single-stranded DNA bound to the membrane. South-western blotting is helpful in delineating nuclear transcription-related proteins. The **Cleveland procedure** is a form of peptide map in which protease-digested protein products, with sodium dodecyl sulfate (SDS) present, are subjected to SDS-PAGE. This produces a characteristic peptide fragment pattern that is typical of the protein substrate and enzyme used. **Blot** refers to the transfer of DNA, RNA, or protein molecules from an electrophoretic gel to a nitrocellulose or nylon membrane by osmosis or vacuum, followed by immersing the membrane in a solution containing a complementary, i.e., mirror-image molecule corresponding to the one on the membrane. This is known as a hybridization blot.

Northern blotting is a method used to identify specific mRNA molecules. Following denaturation of RNA in a particular preparation with formaldehyde to cause the molecule to unfold and become linear, the material is separated by size through gel electrophoresis and blotted onto a natural cellulose or nylon membrane. This is then exposed to a solution of labelled DNA "probe" for hybridization. This step is followed by autoradiography. Northern blotting corresponds to a similar method used for DNA fragments which is known as Southern blotting.

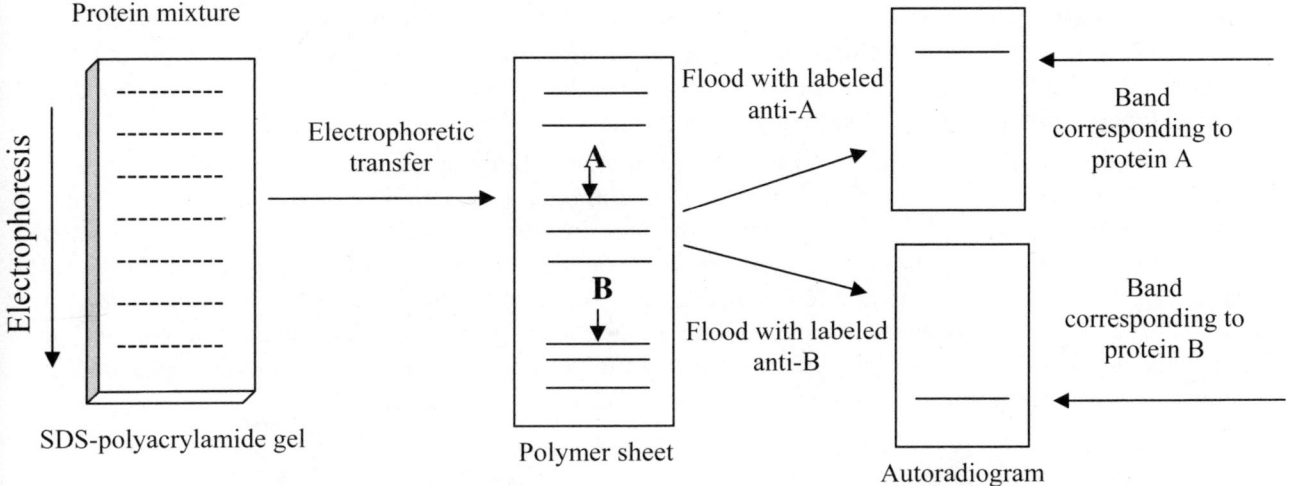

Fig. 15.8: Schematic presentation of Western blot method

***In-situ* hybridization** is a technique that is used to identify specific DNA or RNA segments in cells or tissues or in viral plaques or colonies of microorganisms. DNA in cells or tissue fixed on glass slides must be denatured with formamide before hybridization with a radio labelled or biotinylated DNA or RNA probe that is complementary to the tissue mRNA being sought. Proof that the probe have hybridized to its complementary strand in the tissue or cell under study must be by autoradiography or enzyme-labelled, probes depending on the technique being used. **Molecular hybridization probe** is a molecule of nucleic acid, which is labelled with a radionuclide or fluorochrome that can reveal the presence of complementary nucleic acid through molecular hybridization such as *in situ*. **FISH (fluorescence *in situ* hybridization)** is a method that determines ploidy by examining interphase (non-dividing) nuclei in cytogenetic and cytological samples.

In the **cell-mediated lympholysis (CML) test**, responder (effectors) lymphocytes are cytotoxic for donor (target) lymphocytes after the two are combined in culture. Target cells are labelled by incubation with 51Cr at 37°C for 60 min. Following combination of effectors and target cells in tissue culture, the release of 51Cr from target cells injured by cytotoxicity represents a measure of cell mediated lympholysis (CML). The CML assay gives uniform results. It is relatively simple to perform, and is rather easily controlled. The effecter cells can result from either *in-vivo* sensitization following organ grafting or can be induced *in vitro*. Variations in effecter to target cell ratios can be employed for quantification.

In the **mixed lymphocyte reaction (MLR),** lymphocytes from potential donor and recipient are combined in tissue specificities of the stimulator cells that are not present in the responder cells lead to blastogenesis of the responder lymphocytes. This leads to an increase in the synthesis of DNA and cell division. This process is followed by introduction of a measured amount of triturated thymidine, which is incorporated into the newly synthesized DNA.

The mixed-lymphocyte reaction usually measures a proliferative response and not an effecter-cell-killing response. The test is important in bone marrow and organ transplantation to evaluate the degree of histo-incompatibility between donor and recipient. Both $CD4^+$ and $CD8^+$ T lymphocytes proliferate and secrete cytokines in the MLR which is also called as mixed-lymphocyte culture.

15.5. RADIOIMMUNOASSAY (RIA)

The increasing use of immunological methods in the accurate estimation of polypeptide hormones has paved a way for the development of the estimation methods. One such method where the accuracy is up to the concentration of 0.0001 μg/ml is the radioimmunoassay (RIA). The method is now widely used in quantitative estimation of hormones, serum proteins, drugs and vitamins.

The principle of the assay method involves competitive binding of a radiolabelled antigen and unlabelled antigen to a high affinity antibody. Commonly used labeling material is the gamma-emitting isotope such as $^{125}1$. The method involves mixing of labeled antigen to antibody at a concentration that just saturates the antigen-binding sites of the antibody molecule. Now, on increasing the amount of unlabelled antigen the bound antigen (labeled) is displaced due to competitive binding between the labeled and unlabelled antigen. By increasing the amount of unlabeled antigen the free but labeled antigen in solution can be estimated and thus it is possible to determine the concentration of antigen, which combines antibody affinity sites.

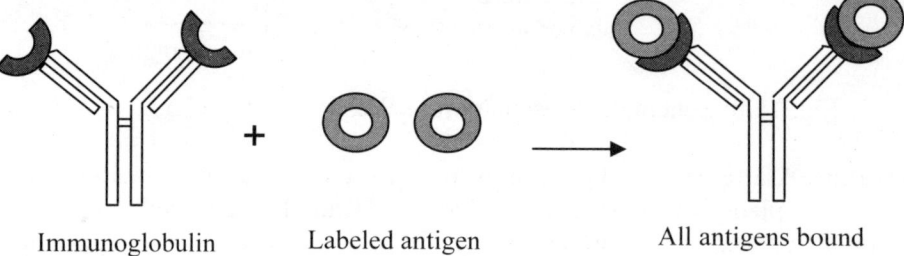

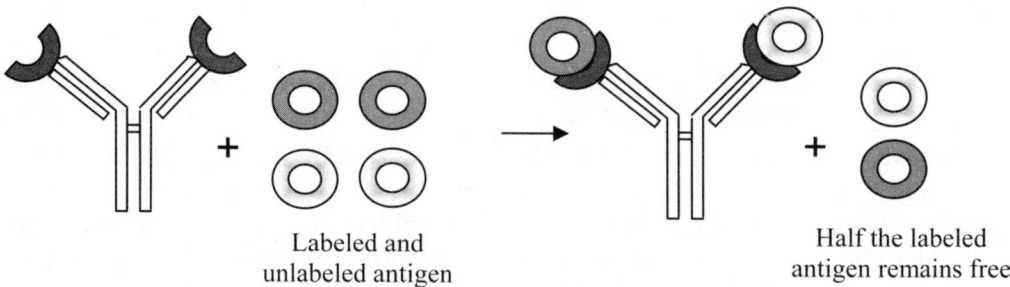

Fig. 15.9: Radioimmunoassay

15.5.1. The radioallergosorbent test (RAST)

RAST is a technique to detect specific IgE antibodies in a patient's serum. This solid-phase method involves binding of the allergen–antigen complex to an insoluble support such as dextran particles or Sepharose®. The serum from a patient is then passed over the allergen-support complex, which permits specific IgE antibodies in the serum to bind with the allergen. After washing off the nonreactive protein, radiolabelled antihuman IgE antibody is then placed in contact with the insoluble support where it reacts with the bound IgE antibody. Both the allergen and the anti-IgE antibody must be present in excess for the test to be accurate. The amount of radioactivity on the beads is proportional to the quantity of serum antibody that is allergen specific (Fig. 15.10).

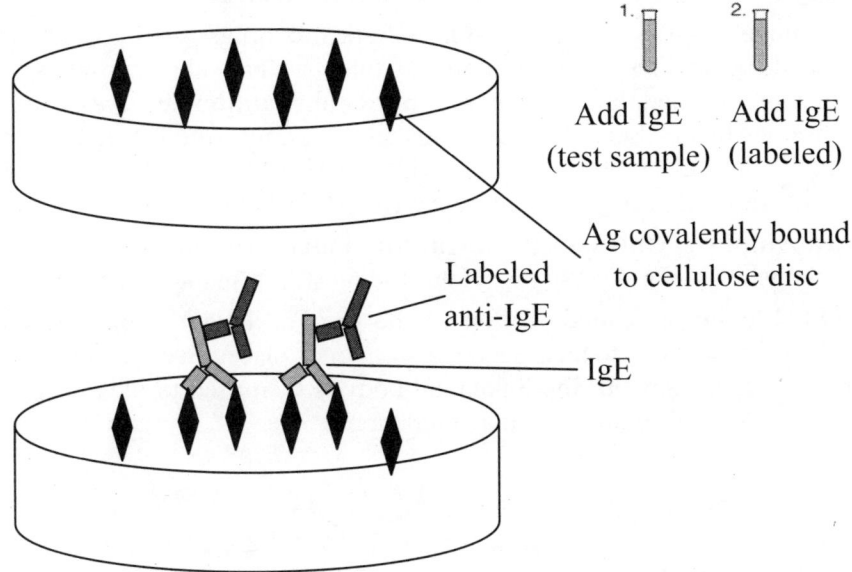

Fig. 15.10: Radioallergosorbent test (RAST)

15.5.2. The radioimmunosorbent test (RIST)

RIST is a solid-phase radioimmunoassay used to determine the serum IgE concentration. A standard quantity of radiolabelled IgE is added to the serum sample to be assayed. The mixture is then combined with Sephadex® or Dextran beads coated with antibody to human IgE. Following incubation and washing, the quantity of radiolabelled IgE bound to the beads is measured. The patient's IgE competes with the radiolabelled IgE or antibody attached to the beads. Therefore, the decrease in labelled IgE attached to the beads compared to a control in which labelled IgE combines with the beads without competition represents the patient's serum concentration of IgE. The radioallergosorbent test by comparison assays IgE levels reactive with a specific allergen.

15.5.3. The immuno-radiometric assay (IRMA)

IRMA is a quantitative method that assays certain plasma proteins based on a "sandwich" technique using radiolabelled antibody, rather than radiolabelled hormone competing with hormone from a patient in the radioimmunoassay (RIA) (Fig. 15.11). The **hook effect** is an artefact that may be seen in IRMA that occurs when a hormone being assayed is in very high concentration. The excess amount cannot be measured by the detector system since it attains and crosses a theoretical limit. The decreased counts with the labelled antibody at the elevated hormone concentration yield spuriously low results. Thus, IRMA is not an appropriate method to assay hormones present in relatively high concentrations, such as gastrin, prolactin, or HCG. The hook effect requires measurement of two separate concentrations to establish linearity.

15.6. ENZYME IMMUNOASSAY (EIA)

EIA is a technique employed to measure immunochemical reactions based on enzyme catalytic properties. The three widely used techniques include a heterogeneous EIA technique, ELISA, and two homogeneous techniques, enzyme-multiplied immunoassay technique (EMIT) and cloned enzyme donor immunoassay (CEDIA).

15.6.1. The enzyme-multiplied immunoassay technique (EMIT)

EMIT is an immunoassay used to monitor therapeutic drugs such as antitumor, antiepileptic, antiasthmatic, and metabolites of cocaine and of other agents subject to abuse. It is a one phase, competitive enzyme-labelled immunoassay. **Antihistone antibodies** are associated with several autoimmune diseases that include SLE, drug-induced lupus, juvenile RA, and RA. H-1 antibodies are the most common in SLE followed by anti-H2B, anti-H2A, anti-H3, and anti-H4, respectively. Antihistone antibodies are usually assayed by the ELISA technique.

Collagen disease/lupus erythematosus diagnostic panel refers to a battery of serum tests for the diagnosis of collagen vascular disease that yields the most information for the least cost.

The **ELISPOT assay** is a modification of the enzyme linked immunosorbent assay (ELISA) which involves the capture of products secreted from cells placed in contact with antigen or antibody fixed to a plastic surface. An enzyme-linked antibody is then used to identify the captured products by cleaving a colourless substrate to yield a colour spot.

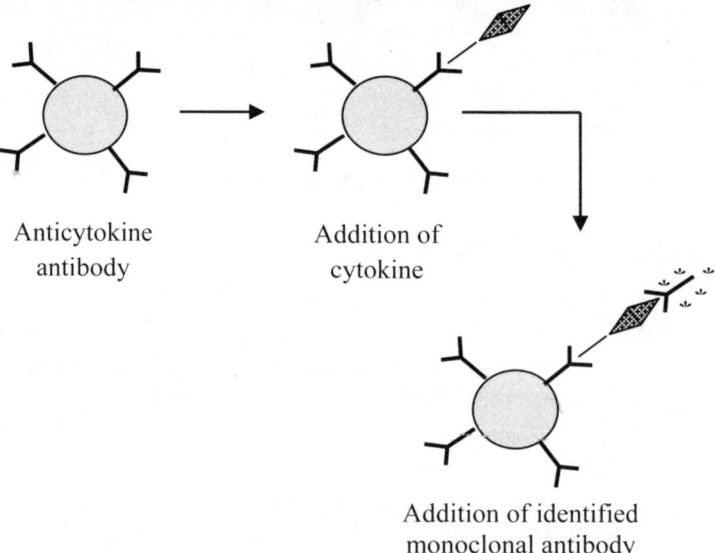

Anticytokine
antibody

Addition of
cytokine

Addition of identified
monoclonal antibody

Fig. 15.11: Immunoradiometric assay (IRMA)

15.6.2. Enzyme-linked immunosorbent assay (ELISA)

Enzyme-linked immunosorbent assay, commonly known as ELISA, is a. the latest method. In principle, the method is similar to that of the RIA which involves competitive binding. This method differs from the above that it does not involve in use of any radio-labeled material and the sensitivity of the method is equally good (0.0001-0.001 µg/ml). Above all, the method is sage and cheaper as compared to RIA. Here, the enzyme conjugated to an antibody reacts with a colorless substrate to generate a colored reaction product. The color is measured spectrophotometrically. A variety of enzymes such as horseradish peroxidase, alkaline phosphatase, p-nitorphenyl phosphatase have been used to link to the antibody or antigen molecule as may be the case. When mixed with a suitable substrate each of these enzymes generates a colored reaction product.

A number of different ELISA methods have been developed which can be used as per the requirement for either determining the antigen or the antibody. First, a standard curve is prepared using known concentrations of antibody or antigens from which the unknown concentration of the sample can be determined.

The various methods include **indirect ELISA** (Fig.15.12a) where the antigen is bound to the plastic plate; the antibody to be assayed constituted the second layer and the enzyme -linked to immunoglobulin as the top layer. The enzyme substrate is finally added and the color change is estimated spectrophotometrically. Next fall's the sandwich technique (Fig.15.12b) where the micro titer well is first coated with an antibody and the sample containing antigen is then added and allowed to react with the bound antibody. Now the well is washed and the second enzyme linked specific antibody is added and allowed to react. Subsequently, the substrate is added and the color produced is measured. Third comes the **competitive ELISA** (Fig.15.12c), which involves the principle similar to RIA. First, incubation of the antibody with the sample containing antigen is allowed. The antigen-antibody mixture is then added to an antigen coated micro titer well. As the antigen concentration increases, the amount of antibody available for binding of the antigen coated well decreases. If a substrate, i.e. enzyme-conjugated secondary antibody specific for the primary antibody is added, the amount of primary antibody bound in the well can be estimated quantitatively.

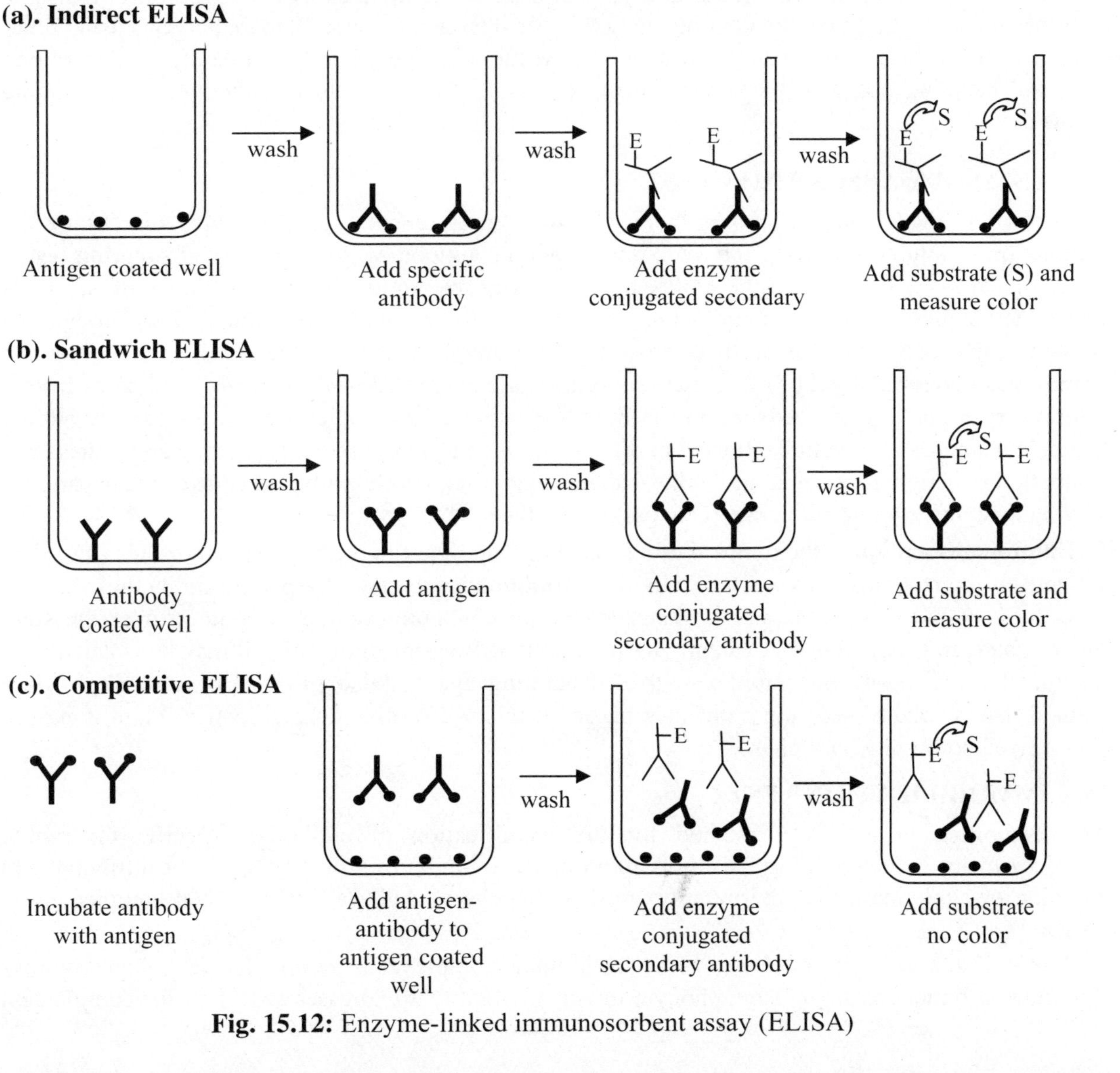

(a). Indirect ELISA

(b). Sandwich ELISA

(c). Competitive ELISA

Fig. 15.12: Enzyme-linked immunosorbent assay (ELISA)

15.7. FLOW INJECTION IMMUNOASSAY (FIIA)

In FIIA, antibodies are immobilized to form an affinity column and analyte is pumped over the column. The loading of the antibodies with analyte is followed by pumping over the column enzyme tracers that compete with the pesticide for the limited binding sites of the antibodies. Generally, the indirect format produces a result inversely proportional to the pesticide concentration. FIIA can be used with electrochemical, spectrophotometric, fluorimetric and chemiluminescence detection methods. Conventional UV visible spectrophotometry is also suitable for the FIIA detection of bioligand interactions.

FIIA has been used for the detection of diuron and atrazine in water. The method was developed as a cost-effective screen for determining compliance with the European drinking water directive. The column material was regenerated up to 1600 times over a 2.5 month period. FIIA is a powerful analytical tool for semi-continuous, high sample throughput applications and may serve as an alternative or complementary technique to solid-phase immunoassay by providing real-time monitoring data. In addition, the continuous flow system is easier to automate than assays using tubes or microplates. More rapid results and sensitive detections are possible by miniaturizing the column and fluid handling and with the development of sensors that can detect antibody–antigen binding events directly.

15.8. ANTIBODY ABSORPTION TEST

Absorption is the elimination of antibodies from a mixture by adding soluble antigens or the elimination of soluble antigens from a mixture by adding antibodies. An **antibody absorption test** is a serological assay based upon the ability of a cross-reactive antigen to diminish a serum sample's titre of antibodies against its homologous antigen, i.e., the antigen that stimulated its production. Cross reactive antibodies, as well as cross reactive antigens, may be detected in this way. An **immunoabsorbent** is a gel or other inert substances are also employed to absorb antibodies from a solution or to purify them. **Adsorption** is the elimination of antibodies from a mixture by adding particulate antigen or the elimination of particulate antigen from a mixture by adding antibodies. The incubation of serum-containing antibodies such as agglutinins with red blood cells or other particles may remove them through sticking to the particle surface.

Immunoabsorption is the removal of a selected group of antibodies by antigen or the removal of antigen by interaction with specific antibody. **Immunoadsorbents** are specific antibodies that are chemically bound to solid supports. When a mixture containing antigen is poured over the solid support, antigen is bound non-covalently to the immunoadsorbent from which it may be isolated after treating the sorbent–ligand complex with a denaturing agent. **Adsorption chromatography** is a method that is used to separate molecules based on their adsorptive characteristics. Fluid is passed over a fixed-solid stationary phase.

15.9. IMMOBILIZATION TEST

An immobilization test is a method for the identification of antibodies specific for motile microorganisms by determining the ability of antibody to inhibit motility. This may be attributable to adhesion or agglutination of the microorganisms' flagella or cell wall injury when complement is present.

The **Raji cell assay** is an *in vitro* assay for immune complexes in serum. The technique employs Raji cells, a lymphoblastoid B lymphocyte tumor cell line that expresses receptors for complement receptor 1, complement receptor 2, FCγ and C1q receptors. The cell line does not express surface immunoglobulins. Following combination of Raji cells with the serum sample, the immune complex is bound and quantified using radiolabelled F(ab′)2 fragments of antibodies against IgG.

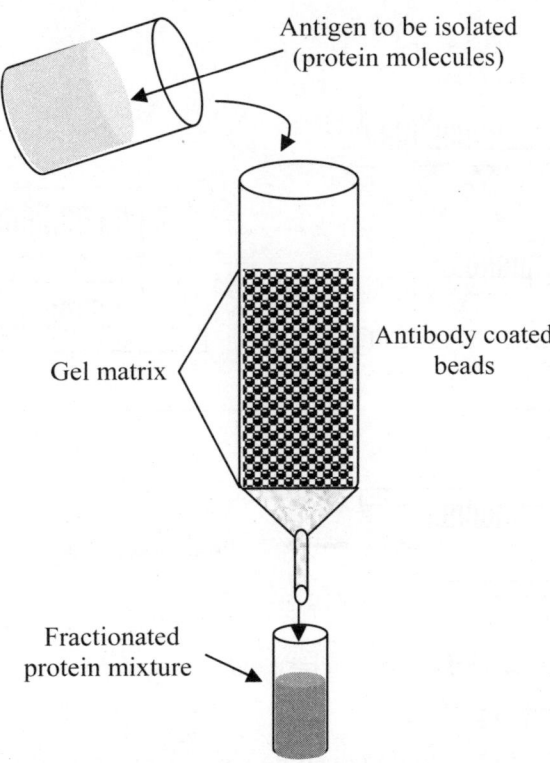

Fig. 15.13: Absorption chromatography is a method to separate molecules based on their absorptive characteristics

15.10. POLYMERASE CHAIN REACTION (PCR)

The polymerase chain reaction is a technique that is used to amplify a small DNA segment beginning with as little as 1 μg. The segment of double-stranded DNA is placed between two oligonucleotide primers through many cycles of amplification. Amplification takes place in a thermal cycler, with one step occurring at a high temperature in the presence of DNA polymerase that is able to withstand the high temperature. Within a few hours, the original DNA segment is transformed into millions of copies. PCR methodology has been used for multiple purposes, including detection of human immunodeficiency virus 1(HIV-1), the prenatal diagnosis of sickle cell anaemia and gene rearrangements in lymphoproliferative disorders, among numerous other applications. The technique is used principally to prepare enough DNA for analysis by available DNA methods and is used widely in DNA diagnostic work. PCR has 99.99% sensitivity. **PCR** is an abbreviation for polymerase chain reaction. **Reverse transcriptase polymerase chain reaction (RT-PCR)** is a technique employed to amplify RNA sequences. Reverse transcriptase is used to convert an RNA sequence into a cDNA sequence that is amplified by PCR using gene-specific primers. This technique is a variation of the polymerase chain reaction (PCR) employed to amplify a complementary cDNA of a gene of interest (Fig. 15.14).

Taq polymerase or *Thermus aquaticus* polymerase. A heat-resistant DNA polymerase, that greatly facilitates use of the polymerase chain reaction to amplify minute quantities of DNA from various sources into a sufficiently large quantity that can be analyzed.

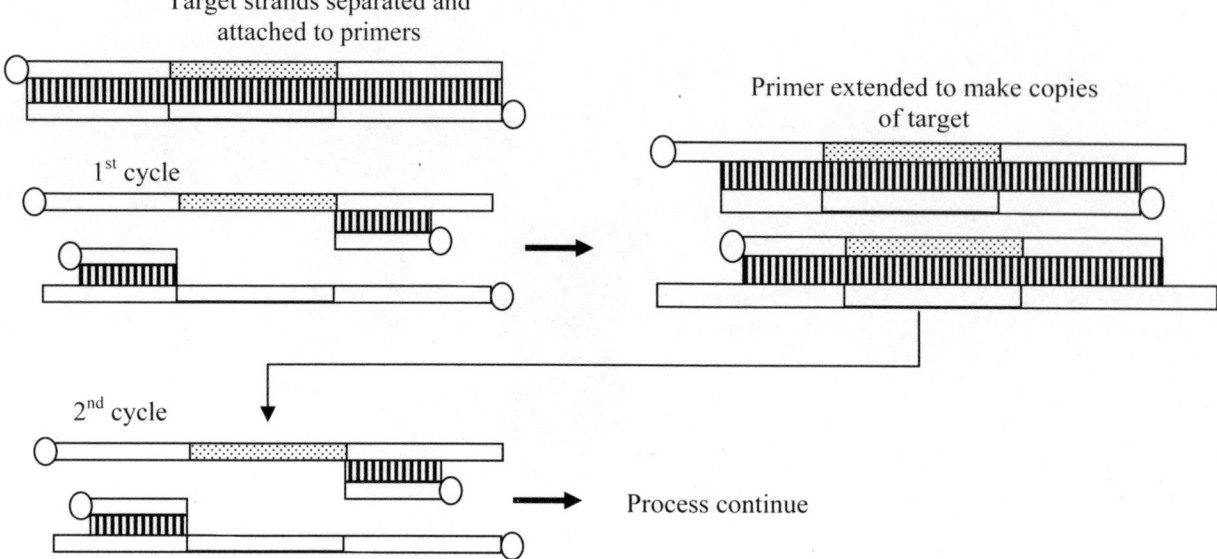

Fig. 15.14: Polymerase chain reaction (PCR)

15.11. DNA FINGERPRINTING

DNA fingerprinting is a method used to demonstrate short, tandem-repeated highly specific genomic sequences known as minisatellites. There is only a 1 in 30 billion probability that two persons would have the identical DNA fingerprint. It has greater specificity than restriction fragment length polymorphism (RFLP) analysis. Each individual has a different number of repeats. The insert-free wild-type M13 bacteriophage identifies the hypervariable minisatellites. The sequence of DNA that identifies the differences is confined to two clusters of 15-bp repeats in the protein III gene of the bacteriophage. The specificity of this probe, known as the Jeffries probe, renders it applicable to parentage testing, human genome mapping, and forensic science. RNA may also be split into fragments by an enzymatic digestion followed by electrophoresis. A characteristic pattern for that molecule is produced and aids in identifying it.

15.11.1. DNA microarray

This is a technique in which a different DNA is placed on a small section of a microchip. The microarray is then used to evaluate expression of RNA in normal or neoplastic cells.

Dot blot is a rapid hybridization method to partially quantify a specific RNA or DNA fragment found in a specimen without the need for a Northern or Southern blot. After serially diluting DNA, it is "spotted" on a nylon or nitrocellulose membrane and then denatured with NaOH. It is then exposed to a heat-denatured DNA fragment probe that is believed to be complementary to the nucleic acid fragment whose identity is being sought. The probe is labelled with 32P or 35S. When the two strands are complementary, hybridization takes place. This is detected by autoradiography of the radiolabelled probe.

Enzymatic, nonradioactive labels may also be employed. **Multilocus probes (MLPs)** (Fig. 15.15) are probes used to identify multiple related sequences distributed throughout each person's genome. Multilocus probes may reveal as many as 20 separate alleles. Because of this multiplicity of alleles, there is only a remote possibility that two unrelated persons would share the same pattern, i.e., about 1 in 30 billion. There is, however, a problem in deciphering the multibanded arrangement of minisatellite RFLPs, as it is difficult to ascertain which bands are allelic. Mutation rates of minisatellite HVRs remain to be demonstrated but are recognized occasionally.

15.11.2. Restriction fragment length polymorphism (RFLP)

RFLP refers to genome diversity in DNA from different subjects revealed by restriction map comparisons. It is based on differences in restriction fragment lengths which are determined by sites of restriction endonuclease cleavage of the DNA molecules. This is revealed by preparing Southern blots using appropriate molecular hybridization probes. Polymorphisms may be demonstrated in exons, introns, flanking sequences, or any DNA sequence. Variations in DNA sequence show Mendelian inheritance. Results are useful in linkage studies and can help to identify defective genes associated with inherited disease.

RFLP is a method that is used to identify local DNA sequence variations of humans or other animals that may be detected by the use of restriction endonucleases. These enzymes cut double stranded DNA at points where they recognize a very specific oligonucleotide sequence, resulting in DNA fragments of different lengths that are unique to each individual animal or person. The fragments of different sizes are separated by electrophoresis. The technique is useful for a variety of purposes, such as identifying genes associated with neurologic diseases (e.g., myotonic dystrophy) which are inherited as autosomal dominant genes or in documenting chimerism. The fragments may also be used as genetic markers to help identify the inheritance patterns of particular genes.

Single locus probes (SLPs) are probes that hybridize at only one specific locus. These probes identify a single locus of variable number of tandem repeats (VNTRs) and permit detection of a region of DNA repeats found in the genome only once and located at a unique site on a certain chromosome. Therefore, an individual can have only two alleles that SLPs will identify, as each cell of the body will have two copies of each chromosome, one from the mother and the other from the father. When the lengths of related alleles on homologous chromosomes are the same, there will be only a single band in the DNA typing pattern. Therefore, the use of an SLP may yield either a single or double-band result from each individual. Single locus markers such as the pYNH24 probe developed by White may detect loci that are highly polymorphic, exceeding 30 alleles and 95% heterozygosity. SLPs are used in resolving cases of disputed parentage.

A λ **cloning vector** is a genetically engineered λ phage that can accept foreign DNA and can be used as a vector in recombinant DNA studies. Phage DNA is cleaved with restriction endonucleases, and foreign DNA is inserted. Insertion vectors are those with a single site where phage DNA is cleaved and foreign DNA is inserted. Substitution or replacement vectors are those which possess two sites spanning a DNA segment that can be excised and replaced with foreign DNA.

Sequence-specific priming (SSP) is a method that employs a primer with a single mismatch in the 3′-end that cannot be employed efficiently to extend a DNA strand because the enzyme Taq polymerase, during the PCR reaction, and especially in the first PCR cycles which are very critical, does not manifest 3′ -5′ proofreading endonuclease activity that can remove the mismatched nucleotide.

If primer pairs are designed to have perfectly matched 3′-ends with only a single allele, or a single group of alleles and the PCR reaction is conducted under stringent conditions, a perfectly matched primer pair results in an amplification product, whereas a mismatch at the 3′-end primer pair will not provide any amplification product. A positive result, i.e., amplification, defines the specificity of the DNA sample. In this method, the PCR amplification step provides the basis for identifying polymorphism. The post amplification processing of the sample consists only of a simple agarose gel electrophoresis to detect the presence or absence of amplified product. DNA amplified fragments are visualized by ethidium bromide staining and exposure to UV light. A separate technique detects amplified product by colour fluorescence. The primer pairs are selected in such a manner that each allele should have a unique reactivity pattern with the panel of primer pairs employed. Appropriate controls must be maintained.

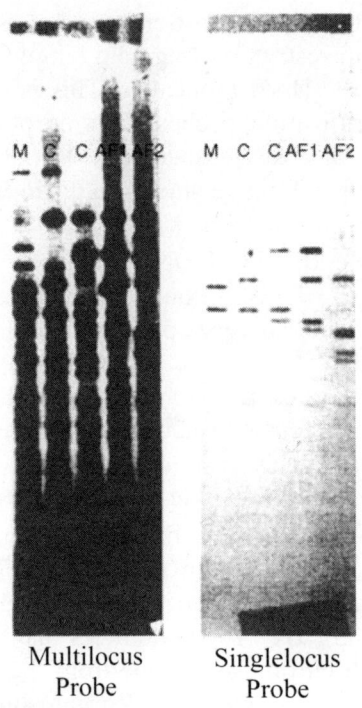

Multilocus   Singlelocus
Probe   Probe

Fig. 15.15: Multilocus probes (MLPs)

The **plaque-forming cell (PFC) assay** is a technique that is used for demonstrating and enumerating cells forming antibodies against a specific antigen. Mice are immunized with sheep red blood cells (SRBC). After a specified period of time, a suspension of splenic cells from the immunized mouse is mixed with antigen (SRBC) and spread on a suitable semisolid gel medium. After or during incubation at 37°C, complement is added. The erythrocytes that have anti-SRBC antibody on their surface will be lysed. Circular areas of haemolysis appear in the gel medium. If viewed under a microscope, a single antibody-forming cell can be identified in the centre of the lytic area. There are several modifications of this assay, as some antibodies other than IgM may fix complement less efficiently. In order to enhance the effects, an antiglobulin antibody called developing antiserum is added to the mixture. The latter technique is called indirect PFC assay. The **PFC (plaque-forming cell)** is an *in vitro* technique in which antibody-synthesizing cells derived from the spleen of an animal immunized with a specific antigen produce antibodies that lyse red blood cells coated with the corresponding antigen in the presence of complement in a gel medium. The reaction bears some resemblance to β hemolysis produced by streptococci on a blood agar plate. When examined microscopically, a single antibody-producing cell can be detected in the centre of the plaque-forming unit.

Jerne plaque assay is a technique to identify and enumerate cells synthesizing antibodies. Typically, spleen cells from a mouse immunized against sheep red blood cells are combined with melted agar or agarose in which sheep erythrocytes are suspended. After gentle mixing, the suspension is distributed into Petri plates where it gels. This is followed by incubation at 37°C, after which complement is added to the dish with the help of a pipette. Thus, the sheep erythrocytes (SRBC) surrounding cells secreting IgM antibody against SRBC are lysed by the added complement, producing a clear zone of haemolysis resembling the effect produced by β haemolytic streptococci on blood agar. IgG antibody against sheep erythrocytes can be identified by adding anti-IgG antibody to aid lysis by complement. Whereas modifications of this method have been used to identify cells producing antibodies against a variety of antigens or haptens conjugated to the sheep red cells, it can also be used to ascertain the immunoglobulin class being secreted. This method is also known as the **haemolytic plaque assay.**

The **reverse plaque method** is a method that identifies antibody-secreting cells regardless of their antibody specificity. The antibody-forming cells are suspended in agarose and incubated at 37°C in Petri plates with sheep red cells coated with protein A. Anti-Ig and complement are also present. Cells synthesizing and secreting immunoglobulin become encircled by Ig–anti-Ig complexes and then linked to the protein A expressed on the erythrocyte surfaces. This leads to hemolytic plaques (zones of lysis). Thus, any class of immunoglobulin can be identified by this technique ley appropriate choice of the antibody.

The **Cunningham plaque technique** is a modification of the haemolytic plaque assay in which an erythrocyte monolayer between a glass slide and cover slip is used without agar for the procedure.

Microlymphocytotoxicity is a widely used technique for HLA tissue typing. Lymphocytes are separated from heparinised blood samples by layering over Ficoll-Hypaque, centrifuging and removing lymphocytes from the interface, or with beads. After appropriate washing, these purified lymphocytes are counted and aliquots dispensed into microtitre plate wells containing predispensed quantities of antibody. When used for human histocompatibility (HLA) testing, antisera used in the wells are specific for the known HLA antigenic specificities. After incubation of the cells and antisera, rabbit complement is added and the plates are again incubated. The extent of cytotoxicity induced is then determined by incubating the cells with trypan blue, which enters the dead cells staining them blue but leaves live cells unstained. The plates are read by using an inverted phase contrast microscope. A scoring system from 0 to 8 (where 8 implies >80% of target cells killed) is employed to indicate cytotoxicity. Most of the sera used to date are multispecific, as they are obtained from multiparous females who have been sensitized during pregnancy by HLA antigens from their spouse. Monoclonal antibodies are being used with increasing frequency in tissue typing. This technique is useful to identify HLA-A, HLA-B, and HLA-C antigens. When purified, B cell preparations and specific antibodies against B cell antigens are employed; HLA-DR and HLA-DQ antigens can be identified.

In the **cell-mediated lympholysis (CML) test**, responder (effector) lymphocytes are cytotoxic for donor (target) lymphocytes from the two sources are combined in a culture. Target cells are labelled by incubation with 51Cr at 37°C for 60 min. Following combination of effector and target cells in tissue culture, the release of 51Cr from target cells injured due to cytotoxicity represents a measure of cell mediated lympholysis (CML). The CML assay gives uniform results; it is relatively simple to perform, and is rather easily controlled. The effector cells can result from either *in-vivo* sensitization following organ grafting or can be induced *in vitro*. Variations in effector to target cell ratios can be employed for quantification.

15.12. MISCELLANEOUS DIAGNOSTIC TESTS

15.12.1. The patch test

Patch test is an assay used to determine the cause of skin allergy, especially contact allergic (type IV) hypersensitivity. A small square of cotton, linen, or paper impregnated with the suspected allergen is applied to the skin for 24 to 48 h. The test is read by examining the site 1 to 2 d after applying the patch. The development of redness (erythema), edema, and formation of vesicles constitutes a positive test. The impregnation of tuberculin into a patch was used by Vollmer for a modified tuberculin test. There are multiple chemicals, toxins, and other allergens that may induce allergic contact dermatitis in exposed members of the population.

15.12.2. Skin test

Skin test is one of several assays in which a test substance is either injected into the skin or applied on to it to determine the host response. Skin tests have long been used to determine host hypersensitivity or immunity to a particular antigen or product of a microorganism. Examples include the tuberculin test, the Schick test, the Dick test, the patch test, the scratch test, etc.

The **Dick test** is a skin test used to signify the susceptibility to scarlet fever in subjects lacking protective antibody against the erythrogenic toxin of *Streptococcus pyogenes*. A minute quantity of diluted erythrogenic toxin is inoculated intradermally in the individual to be tested. An area of redness (erythema) occurs at the injection site 6 to 12 h following inoculation of the diluted toxin in individuals who do not have neutralizing antibodies specific for the erythrogenic toxin and therefore susceptible to scarlet fever. A heat-inactivated preparation of the same diluted toxin is also injected intradermally in the same individual as a control against nonspecific hypersensitivity to other products of the preparation.

The **tuberculin test** refers to the 24- to 48-h response to intradermal injection of tuberculin. If positive, it signifies delayed-type hypersensitivity (type IV) to the tuberculin and implies cell-mediated immunity to *Mycobacterium tuberculosis*. The intradermal inoculation of tuberculin or of purified protein derivative (PPD) leads to an area of erythema and in duration within 24 to 48 h in positive individuals. A positive reaction signifies the presence of cell-mediated immunity to *M. tuberculosis* as a consequence of past or current exposure to this microorganism.

The **prick test** is an assay for immediate (IgE-mediated) hypersensitivity in humans. The epidermal surface of the skin on which drops of diluted antigen (allergen) are placed, is pricked by a sterile needle. The **tine test** is a human tuberculin test that involves the intradermal inoculation of dried, old tuberculin using a four-pointed applicator that introduces the test substance 2 mm below the surface.

Histoplasmin is an extract from cultures of *Histoplasma capsulatum* that is injected intradermally, in the same manner as the tuberculin test, to evaluate whether an individual has cell-mediated immunity against this microorganism. The **histoplasmin test** is a skin test analogous to the tuberculin skin test, which determines whether or not an individual manifests delayed-type hypersensitivity (cell mediated) immunity to *Histoplasma capsulatum,* the causative agent of histoplasmosis in man. A positive skin test indicates an earlier or a current infection with *H. capsulatum.*

The **Schick test** is a test for susceptibility to diphtheria. Standardized diphtheria toxin is adjusted to contain 1/50 MLD in 0.1 ml, which is injected intracutaneously into the subject's forearm. Development of redness and in duration within 24 to 36 h after administration constitutes a positive test if it persists for 4 d or longer. The presence of 1/500 to 1/250 or more of a unit of antitoxin per millilitre of the patient's blood will result in a negative reaction because of neutralization of the injected toxin. Neither redness nor in duration appears if the test is negative. An individual with a negative test possesses sufficient antitoxin to protect against infection with *Corynebacterium diphtheriae,* whereas a positive test denotes susceptibility. A control is always carried out in the opposite forearm. For this test, toxin that has been diluted and heated to 70°C for 15 min is injected intracutaneously. Heating destroys the toxin's ability to induce local tissue injury; however, it does not affect the components of the diphtheria bacilli or of the medium that might evoke an allergic response in the individual. If the size and duration of the reaction at the injection site in the control approximates the reaction in the test arm, the result is negative. If the reaction is at least 50% larger and of longer duration on the test arm compared to the control, the individual is both allergic to the materials in the bacilli or in the medium and susceptible to the toxin. A positive Schick reaction suggests that diphtheria immunization is needed.

The **Casoni test** is a diagnostic skin test for hydatid disease in humans induced by *Echinococcus granulosus* infection. In sensitive individuals, a wheal and flareresponse develops within 30 min following intradermal inoculation of a tapeworm or hydatid cyst fluid extract. This is followed within 24 h by an area of indurations produced by this cell-mediated delayed-hypersensitivity reaction.

The **heaf test** is a type of tuberculin test in which an automatic multiple puncture device with six needles is used to administer the test material by intradermal inoculation. The multiple needles advance 2 to 3 mm into the skin.

The **Montenegro test** is a diagnostic assay for South American leishmaniasis induced by *Leishmania brasiliensis.* The intracutaneous injection of a polysaccharide antigen derived from the causative agent induces a delayed hypersensitivity response in the patient. They are not usually found in myositis, scleroderma, or Sjogren's syndrome.

Old tuberculin (OT) is a broth culture, heat-concentrated filtrates of medium in which Mycobacterium tuberculosis microorganisms were grown. It was developed by Robert Koch for use in tuberculin skin tests nearly a century ago.

Passive cutaneous anaphylaxis (PCA) is a skin test that involves the *in vivo* passive transfer of homocytotropic antibodies that mediates type I immediate hypersensitivity (e.g., IgE in man) from a sensitized to a previously non-sensitized individual by intradermally injecting the antibodies, which become anchored to mast cells through their Fc receptors. This is followed hours or even days later by intravenous injection of antigen mixed with a dye such as Evans Blue. Cross linking of the cell-fixed (e.g., IgE) antibody receptors by the injected antigen induces a type I immediate hypersensitivity reaction in which histamine and other pharmacological mediators of immediate hypersensitivity are released. Vascular permeability factors act on the vessels to permit plasma and dye to leak into the extra vascular space, forming a blue area that can be measured with callipers. In humans, this is called the Prausnitz-Küstner (PK) reaction.

15.13. BIOSENSORS: IMMUNOSENSORS

The biosensor technology enables rapid, sensitive measurements to be made using a simple procedure, with a device that is relatively easy to operate. Biosensors are compact, low-cost disposable devices which circumvent the need for frequent recalibration procedures. Only minimal sample preparation is needed and continuous measurements are usually obtainable using a biosensor in an on-line mode, such as in a fermentation broth or implanted within a subject (Cooper, 1992). A biosensor is a multicomponent system which incorporates a biological element which can recognize specifically the substance (analyte) to be measured. Enzymes and antibodies are often used to provide the biological sensing layer, and tissue slices, whole cells and multienzyme systems have been employed as the specific recognition system. A typical biosensor consists of a biologically sensitive layer combined with a base sensing device that produces an electrical signal when the biomolecule layer recognizes the substance to be measured.

The development of immunosensors is one of the most active research areas in immunodiagnostics. A large number of immunosensors, which combine the sensitivity and specificity of immunoassays with physical signal transduction, have been developed in recent years for pesticide analysis. A classical biosensor consists of three components, including a receptor (an antibody or binding protein), a transducer (e.g., an optical fibre or electrode) and signal processing electronics. The receptor is usually immobilized to the transducer surface, which enables it to detect interaction with analyte molecules. In contrast to immunoassays, immunosensors commonly rely on the reuse of the same receptor surface for many measurements. Direct signal generation potentially enables real-time monitoring of analytes, thus making immunosensors suitable tools for continuous environmental monitoring.

There are several classes and subclasses of immunosensors, each with advantages for environmental analysis. Piezoelectric sensors (including bulk acoustic and surface acoustic wave) use an external alternating electric field to directly measure the antibody–antigen interaction. Electrochemical sensors (including potentiometric, amperometric, capacitative and conductimetric) may offer inexpensive analytical alternatives for effluent monitoring. Optical sensors (including fibre-optic, evanescent wave biosensors and Mach–Zehnder interferometer sensors) measure the absorption or emission of a wavelength of light and base detection on fluorescence, absorbance, luminescence or total internal reflectance fluorescence. Surface plasmon resonance (SPR) is an optical electronic technique in which an evanescent electromagnetic field generated at the surface of a metal conductor is excited by light of a certain wavelength at a certain angle. An immunosensor has been developed for the detection of a trazine using SPR. Moreover, a grating coupler immunosensor was evaluated for the measurement of four s-triazine herbicides. One could detect terbutryn in the range 15–60nM using this biosensor. Because antibody based biosensors have no associated catalytic event to aid in transduction, they are far more complex than enzyme-based biosensors. In addition, they do not release their ligand quickly, leading to a slow response. Theoretically, biosensors are capable of continuous and reversible detection, but reversibility is difficult to achieve in practice because sensitive antibody–antigen interactions have high affinity constants. Because cost and time are critical factors in environmental monitoring, it is likely that the development of small-probe antibody-based biosensors yielding continuous readouts of an analyte at low concentration will not be rapid. However, research in the sensor field is certain to give improvements in many aspects of immunoassay technology, and antibody–hapten and receptor–ligand binding assays are being coupled to biological and physical transducers in many ingenious ways.

Antibodies can be generated in response to a wide range of antigens. However, the coupling of the antigen-antibody recognition event to a suitable transducer is often difficult. The lack of accompanying redox reaction or pH change on binding of antibody to antigen (or vice versa) has resulted in a predominance of enzyme-linked immunosensors in the literature. These sensors are based on the widely used enzyme-linked immunosorbent assay (ELISA) technique. When a layer of antibody is immobilized to, the electrode surface, the analyte antigen that can be assayed is inversely proportional to the amount of analyte present, and suitable choice of an enzyme label allows the antigen to be assayed electrochemically.

As protein surfaces are covered with charged residues, the binding of an antibody to its antigen obscures some of these residues leading to a change of surface charge, which could be measured. Biosensors find useful applications in immunology. A combination of immobilized antibody (or antigen) with an electronic device yields an immunosensor. In this system, the antigen acts as an analyte. The basic principle underlying immunoassays revolves round the interaction of the antigen or ligand (Ag) and its specific binding partner, the antibody (Ab), i.e.,

$$Ab + Ag = AbAg$$

The equilibrium constant (K) for this interaction fall in the range 10^5–10^{11} M. in the simplest immunoassays, the concentration of Ab is fixed. Thus, at equilibrium, the ratio of bound Ag to free Ag may be determined by adding a fixed amount of a tracer antigen.

The immunosensors are of two main types, namely, labeled and non-labelled (Table 15.1). Some frequently used labels include radioisotopes, enzymes, particles, fluorophores, and precipitins. Enzyme labels have, for instance, been incorporated into the immunosensor to work as effective chemical oxidase, alkaline phosphatase, glucoamylase, catalase, urease, glucose phosphate dehydrogenase, and malate dehydrogenase (Green, 1987). Labelling of immunosensors often enhances their sensitivity while retaining high selectivity. Examples of labeled immunosensors include enzyme immunosensing with an oxygen electrode and bioaffinity sensors with a preformed metastable ligand-receptor complex (Fig. 15.16). This latter type (bioaffinity) beiosensors are being used for determinating thyroxin, insulin, and biotin (Table 15.1).

Table 15.1: Properties of non-labelled and labeled immunosensors (after Aizawa, 1987)

Determinants	Biosensor type	Biosensor assembly	
		Receptor	Transducer
Albumin	I	Antialbumin	Ag/AgCl electrode
	EI	Antialbumin	O_2 electrode
IgG	EI	Anti-IgG (catalase label)	O_2 electrode
HCG	I	Anti-HCG	TiO_2 electrode
	EI	Anti-HCG (catalase label)	O_2 electrode
Alpha-Fetoprotein Antibody	EI	Anti-AFP (catalase label)	O_2 electrode
Syphilis	I	Cardiolipin	Ag/AgCl electrode
Blood group	I	Blood group substance	Ag/AgCl electrode

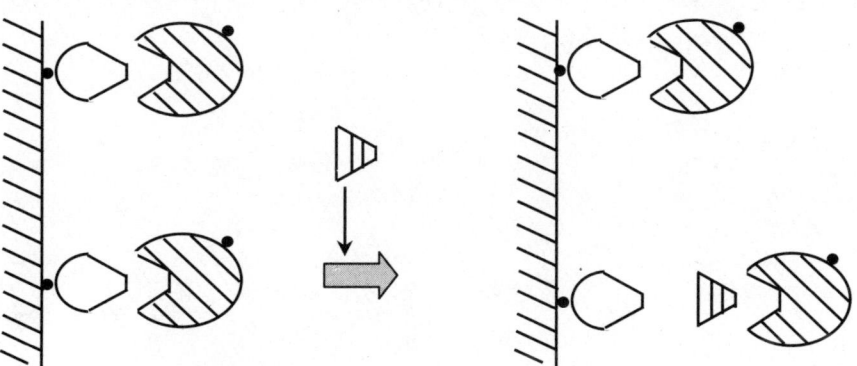

Fig. 15.16: Sketch of bioaffinity sensor

Non-labelled immunosensors include (1) potentiometric immunosensors with antigen- (or antibody-) coated membrane, and (2) potentiometric immunosensors with antibody-coated electrode. Some immunosensors developed for diagnosis of syphilis and for electrochemical typing, of blood are examples of category (1). Category (2) is exemplified by a TiO_2 electrode coated with covalently immobilized anti-human chorionic gonadotropin antibody.

SUGGESTED READING

- Arlson DP, Superko C, Mackey J, et al., *Focus* 12, 9 (1990).
- Caskey CT. *Science* 236, 1223 (1987).
- Debenham PG. *Trends Biotechnol* 10, 96 (1992).
- Hudson L, Hay FC. Practical Immunology, Blackwell Scientific Publications, Australia (1980).
- Roit IM, Brostoff J, Male DK. Immunology, 2 nd ed., C.V. Mosby, St. Louis (1989).
- Roitt I, Essential Immunology, Blackwell Scientific Publications, Australia (1986).
- Stites DP, Stobo JD, Wells JV. Basic and Clinical Immunology, 5 th edition, Lange Medical Publications (1984).
- Tizard IR. Immunology: An introduction, 2 nd ed., W.B. Saunders, Philadelphia (1988).
- Waldmann TA. *Sciences* 252, 1657 (1991).
- Weir DM. Handbook of Experimental Immunology, Blackwell Scientific Publications, Australia (1979).
- Weiss JB. *Clin Microbiol Rev* 8, 113 (1995).

16

DELIVERY APPROACHES FOR BIOTECHNOLOGICALS

16.1. INTRODUCTION

In the last three decades therapeutic peptides and proteins have risen to the prominence as potential drugs of the future. Biotechnology has played a key role in the development of peptide and protein drugs. Since its inception, the development and commercialization of protein based drugs have been the focus of the biotechnology industry. Management of illness through this class of pharmaceuticals has entered an era of rapid growth with their availability on a commercial scale. A new series of peptide and protein based pharmaceuticals have made their presence felt with the discovery of methods to clone and express the cDNA encoding heterologous proteins. The sequencing of the entire human genome has triggered an academic explosion with genomic informations. This will gave way to the discovery of new proteins with a better insight into the understanding of their function. The number of potential protein drug candidates will also emerge. The recent advances on large-scale fermentation and purification processes and analytical characterization have further widened the horizons. The proteins are now available in a much purer form in sufficient quantities and at a reasonable cost. The problem of immunogenicity and antigenicity has also been considerably reduced. Simultaneously, great efforts have been made in the understanding of the physiologic and pharmacologic behaviors of these biologic response modifiers and regulatory agents. Now they are known to carry out essentially all biological processes and reactions (e.g., as enzymes, ligands for signaling, antibodies, receptors and transcription factors). They have evolved to be highly specific and potent. Ailments that could be treated more effectively with this class of therapeutics include autoimmune diseases, cancer, mental disorders, hypertension and certain cardiovascular and metabolic diseases.

The peptide and protein drugs produced by recombinant DNA technology are the exact replicas of that obtained from natural sources. Despite the attractive features that proteins offer, a large majority of the therapeutics have some serious limitations. The chemical and structural complexities involved demand an effective delivery system in which the physicochemical and biologic properties, including molecular size, conformational stability, solubility, sensitivity to light, moisture and heat, biological half-life, immunogenicity, dose requirements, complex feedback control mechanisms, susceptibility to break down in both physical and biological environments, requirement for specialized mechanisms for transport across biological membranes are duly considered. Also, the use of proteins as drugs places distinct and different demands on these moieties. Endogenously, proteins are synthesized in small amounts as per biological needs, normally act in a transient fashion and are stabilized by the cellular and extracellular milieu. In contrast, the protein drugs are to be highly purified and concentrated and should have a shelf life of at least two years. Although many advances have been made towards their effective delivery, much work still remains before proteins become chemically viable and safe therapeutics.

In majority of the cases chronic therapy with these peptides and proteins is warranted. Generally they have an extremely short biological half-life. This trait precludes the parenteral delivery, as daily multiple injections would be required to maintain the therapeutic levels of drug, which has its inherent drawbacks. Oral administration is limited due to enzymatic degradation. Only after some viable novel delivery systems are developed to improve their systemic bioavailability, these peptide and protein drugs would be of therapeutic importance. Thus the challenges in biotechnology include not only cloning and synthesis of polypeptides but their effective nonparenteral delivery to the systemic circulation and to the site of their action as well. There is undoubtedly an urgent need to explore alternative non-parenteral routes of administration like buccal, nasal, pulmonary, ophthalmic, rectal, vaginal and transdermal. Alternatively, other approaches such as implants, self-regulatory delivery systems can equivocally be exploited. However, the transmucosal route mentioned in the preceding lines may impose additional biological barriers to this class of 'difficult' drugs in terms of tissue permeability, protease activity, etc.

Many peptides and proteins have been used as drugs since the commercial introduction in the 1920's and 30's of insulin, thyroid hormone and factor VIII. The initial report of the Human Genome Project was completed in 2000; 84% of protein bases were sequenced and almost 39,000 proteins were predicted. The number of peptide protein drugs is still limited (nearly 80 protein drugs have already been approved by the FDA, 80% of which are recombinant proteins). Recent developments in technology and science have provided the tool and opportunity to further expand the range of peptide- and protein-based drugs in an effort to combat poorly treated diseases and to increase patient quality of life. Such drugs, including synthetic vaccines, are also promising for protection against carcinogens and toxicants. While there has been rapid progress in molecular biology and production, progress in the formulation and development of peptide and protein drug delivery systems has only recently begun. This can be attributed primarily to lack of knowledge about the effects of route of administration and how physicochemical and chemical properties of peptides and proteins affectt the absorption and *in vivo* performance.

Most protein pharmaceuticals currently in use are generally delivered by parenteral routes such as *via* subcutaneous injections. The protein formulation used in these preparations is usually a solution or suspension, as with insulin. These formulations were developed initially to provide stability to the protein during storage; however there have been a number of efforts to produce a stable as well as controlled-release form of peptide and protein drugs. The development of conventional formulations to extend the dose interval may not be possible especially for insulin and some other protein drugs and hence repeated injections will possibly continue in future. New approaches are currently under investigations who seek upon possible solutions, such as using iontophoresis and other techniques, i.e. microneedles, which would facilitate acceptable patient compliance and also take into account life quality of the patients. Alternative routes of administration for peptide and protein pharmaceuticals, such as buccal , nasal, rectal, vaginal, and pulmonary have been under investigation and results of many of these efforts have been reported in the literature. The need to find a non-injectable/ non-invasive route of administration for peptides has shifted attention on oral administration. In considering the oral route of administration, there are several factors which will affect pharmacodynamics and pharmacokinetics of the drugs. As a result, the delivery of therapeutic peptides and proteins remains as a major priority for many researchers and pharmaceutical companies.

Many drug manufacturing companies are pursuing research programs in the oral delivery of peptides and proteins. This is a result of the advances in molecular biology, biotechnology and pharmaceutical technology, which together have made possible identification and commercial availability of many peptides and proteins with valuable therapeutic properties. Controlled delivery of peptide and protein drugs has some distinctive advantages:

- Conventional drug therapy requires periodic doses of therapeutic agents

-Controlled delivery and the formulation can provide maximum stability, activity and bioavailability,

- Some solubility problems can be seen in conventional formulations,

-Controlled delivery of peptide and protein drugs provides improved efficiency, reduced toxicity and improved patient convenience,

-Controlled drug delivery is delivery of drug at a rate or to a location determined by needs of the body or disease state over a specified or extended period of time during the therapy.

In view of the above, it is clear that there is a general requirement to understand and clarify the mechanisms of absorption for peptide and protein drugs as well as the properties of the drug and biological medium, such as solubility, dissolution rate, stability, molecular size and conformation, partition coefficient, charge, pH, binding and complexation, proteases, mucosal barrier, intestinal permeability, intestinal metabolism, route of administration, and hepatic metabolism.

Table 16.1: Some representative peptidal and proteinaceous drugs with their potential functions and/or biomedical applications

Peptide/Protein Drug(s)	Function(s) and/or Biomedical Applications
Cardiovascular-active	
Angiotensin II antagonist	Lowering blood pressure
Bradykinin	Improving peripheral circulation
Captopril	Heart failure management
Tissue plasminogen activator	Dissolution of blood clots
CNS-active	
Cholecystokinin	Suppressing appetite
β-endorphin	Relieving pain
Neuropeptide γ	Controlling feeding and drinking behavior
Nerve growth factor	Simulating nerve growth and repair
GI-active	
Gastrin antagonist	Reducing secretion of gastric acid
Pancreatic enzymes	Digestive supplement
Somatostatin	Reducing bleeding of gastric ulcers
Immunomodulating	
Bursin	Selective B-cell differentiating hormone
Cyclosporin	Inhibiting functions of T-lymphocyte
Enkephalins	Stimulating lymphocyte blastogenesis
Interferon	Enhancing activity of killer cells
Tumor necrosis factor	Controlling polymorphonuclear functions
Metabolism-modulating	
Human growth hormone	Treating hypopituitary dwarfism
Insulin	Treating diabetes mellitus
Luteinizing hormone	Inducing ovulation in women with hypothalamic amenorrhea
Vasopressin	Treating diabetes insipidus

16.2. PEPTIDE AND PROTEIN STRUCTURE

The proteins are relatively large molecules with complex architecture. The peptide chains in peptides and proteins are seldom linear and tend to adapt a variety of specific folded three-dimensional patterns and conformations. Conformation of the peptide chain is determined by the covalently bonded amino acid sequence, by disulfide bridges between cystein residues, and by total conformational energy (the sum of electrostatic energy, hydrogen-bonded energy, non-bonded energy and torsional energy). The properties that are affected by conformation include:

1. Physical properties such as solubility, and spectral properties, such as circular dichroism.
2. Chemical properties, since folding may stabilize reactive group by hydrogen bonding or may sterically shield them from reagents.
3. Biological properties, as the three-dimensional structures place catalytic groups into proper orientation for enzymatic activity or place backbone and side-chain groups into proper orientation for hormone-receptor interaction.
4. Stability to enzymatic cleavage since some of the amide groups susceptible to proteolysis is deterred due to sterical peptide chain orientation.

16.3. STABILITY PROFILE

One of the primary differences between the conventional drug entities and peptide/protein drugs is their poor stability profile. The degradation pathways of this class of drugs are due to chemical and physical instability. The high chemical and physical instability presents peculiar difficulties in the purification, separation, formulation, storage and delivery of these compounds. Physical instability involves transformations in the secondary, tertiary, or quaternary structures of the molecule. These changes are manifested as denaturation, aggregation precipitation and adsorption onto surfaces. Chemical instability involves alteration in the molecular structure producing a new chemical entity, by bond formation or cleavage. Changes brought about by physical and chemical instability almost always lead to partial or total loss of biological activity.

Table 16.2: Degradation pathways contributing to the instability of peptide(s) and protein drugs

Physical instability	Chemical instability
• Denaturation	• Deamidation
• Adsorption	• Oxidation and reduction
• Aggregation	• Proteolysis
• Precipitation	• Disulfide exchange
	• Racemization
	• β-elimination

16.4. BARRIERS TO PEPTIDE AND PROTEIN DELIVERY

The successful delivery of peptide and protein based pharmaceuticals is primarily determined by their ability to cross various barriers presented to it in the biological milieu. The various barriers encountered are presented:

Table 16.3: Barriers to peptide and protein drug delivery

- Enzymatic barrier
- Intestinal epithelial barrier
- Capillary endothelial barrier
- Blood brain barrier

16.5. CONTROLLED DELIVERY OF PEPTIDE AND PROTEIN DRUGS

16.5.1 Oral route

A primary objective of oral delivery systems is to protect protein and peptide drugs from acid and luminal proteases in the GIT. More recent efforts seem to focus on site-specific delivery systems. The site could be an organ, a cell subset or even an intracellular region with an objective of restricting the distribution of the peptide to the specific target site. This should allow for an increase in efficacy with a decrease in toxicity.

Various systems for achieving site-specific delivery of orally administered protein/peptide drugs have been discussed in recent years including coated systems based on pH changes and enzymatic activity of intestinal microflora, nanoparticles, liposomes, matrix devices and conjugate (degradable prodrug) formation. All of these have produced variable release profiles, often because the transit time through the colon can vary substantially from as low as 6 to as high as 30 h. Several of these approaches are somewhat complex and if they were to be translated into actual formulation of oral delivery systems, the products would be expensive and, therefore, unaffordable in most of the developing countries. In our laboratories, preliminary studies on microcapsules of chitosan-alginate modified with selected components such as HPMCAS, talc, microcrystalline cellulose, polymetacrylates and pectins were carried out. Protein release was determined at different pH covering the pH range of the gut. It was observed that microcapsules modified with talc and microcrystalline cellulose had higher protein retention in the core in all the pH tested. This shows that modification of the core of chitosan-alginate microcapsules could facilitate drug targeting to the colon. Rather than administering the protein itself, the DNA plasmid that codes for it is swallowed. This then captured in to the cells in the small intestine where it expresses the required protein drug using available materials in the cell. The protein is thereafter absorbed into the blood stream. The gene has a short half-life and hence must be administered regularly to be effective. The advantage is that it provides for safe, easily managed treatment unlike most gene-based therapies currently available. It is also hoped that this system will be relatively free from ectopic expressions usually experienced with gene therapies since the bulk of the administered genes remain within the intestine and is passed out with feaces along with sloughed cells of the intestinal epithelium.

Oral route is the most popular route of delivery from the patients' point of view. This route has mainly following advantages:

1. Convenient and acceptable.
2. Patient compliance is high.

However, successful oral therapy using peptide and protein drugs has been largely an eluded solution. The main barriers to their successful oral delivery are similar to that of traditional drug candidates, but these are more pronounced in the case of peptide/protein moieties. The options, however available to circumvent these barriers are much more limited specifically for peptides/proteins as all the issues leading to poor availability are to be addressed simultaneously. The main barriers to effective oral delivery of peptide/protein drugs are presented in Table 16.4.

Figure 16.1 Illustrates the various barriers to oral absorption. This is the reason why the oral bioavailability of peptide/protein drug is often less than 1%. With cyclosporin, thyrotropin-releasing hormone and leupeptins being the exceptions. Molecules that are absorbed via the lumen of the small intestine can either be taken up into the blood capillary or alternatively enter lymphatic lacteal located within the submucosal space. Molecules entering the blood are directed through the hepatic-portal system to the liver and are normally substantially metabolized before they reach the systemic circulation. This pre-systemic clearance often leads to insignificant correlation between membrane permeability, absorption and bioavailability.

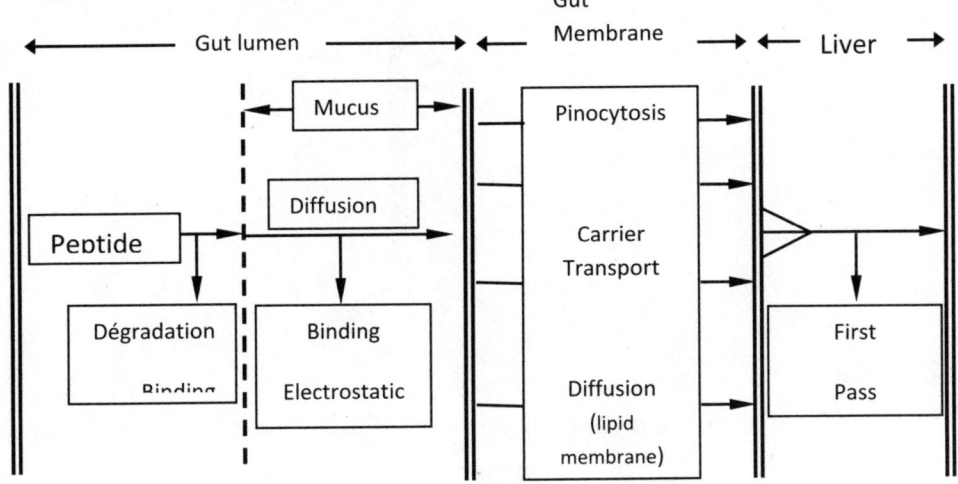

Fig. 16.1: Various barriers to oral absorption of peptides

Table 16.4: The main barriers to effective oral delivery

- Poor intrinsic permeability of peptides/proteins across biological membranes due to their large molecular size and hydrophilic nature;
- Susceptibility to enzymatic attack by intestinal proteases and peptidases and digestion into their constituent amino acids that lack the biological activity of the parent polypeptide;
- Rapid post-absorptive clearance;
- Physical instability i.e. tendencies to aggregate and/or non-specifically adsorbed on a variety of physical and biological surfaces.

However, in some cases there is an underlying physiological advantage in directing a peptide/protein to the liver prior to their entry into the systemic circulation. A classic example of such entity is insulin. On referring to its physiology we learn that endogenous insulin is released by the pancreas and first acts on the glucose reserves in respective organ before it acts peripherally. The liver removes half of the insulin presented to it through a single transhepatic circulation. Oral insulin delivery mimics the physiological pattern as it offers a mode to improve the portal levels of insulin and limits the peripheral hyperinsulinemia.into the tributaries of the hepatic portal vein leading to its direct delivery to the liver, the target organ, Uptake from the gut lumen into the lymphatic lacteal offers some advantages:

- Slow and sustained delivery (3-9 hours for onset of action) in contrast to that observed when molecules are delivered directly into blood capillaries (20-60 minutes for onset of action). The significant difference in blood profiles can be attributed to the fact that lymph moves at 1-2 ml/min while hepatic portal blood flows at a rate 1500 ml/min.
- Drugs can bypass liver, which is not the case with the molecules entering the blood capillaries. The relative proportion of drug taken up through these two different routes at a particular site within the gut is dependent on hydrophobic nature of the drug and formulation.

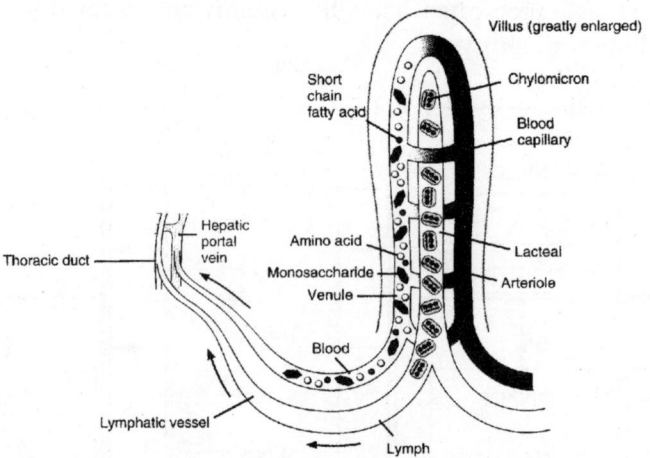

Fig. 16.2: Movement of absorbed moieties from the small intestine into the blood and lymph

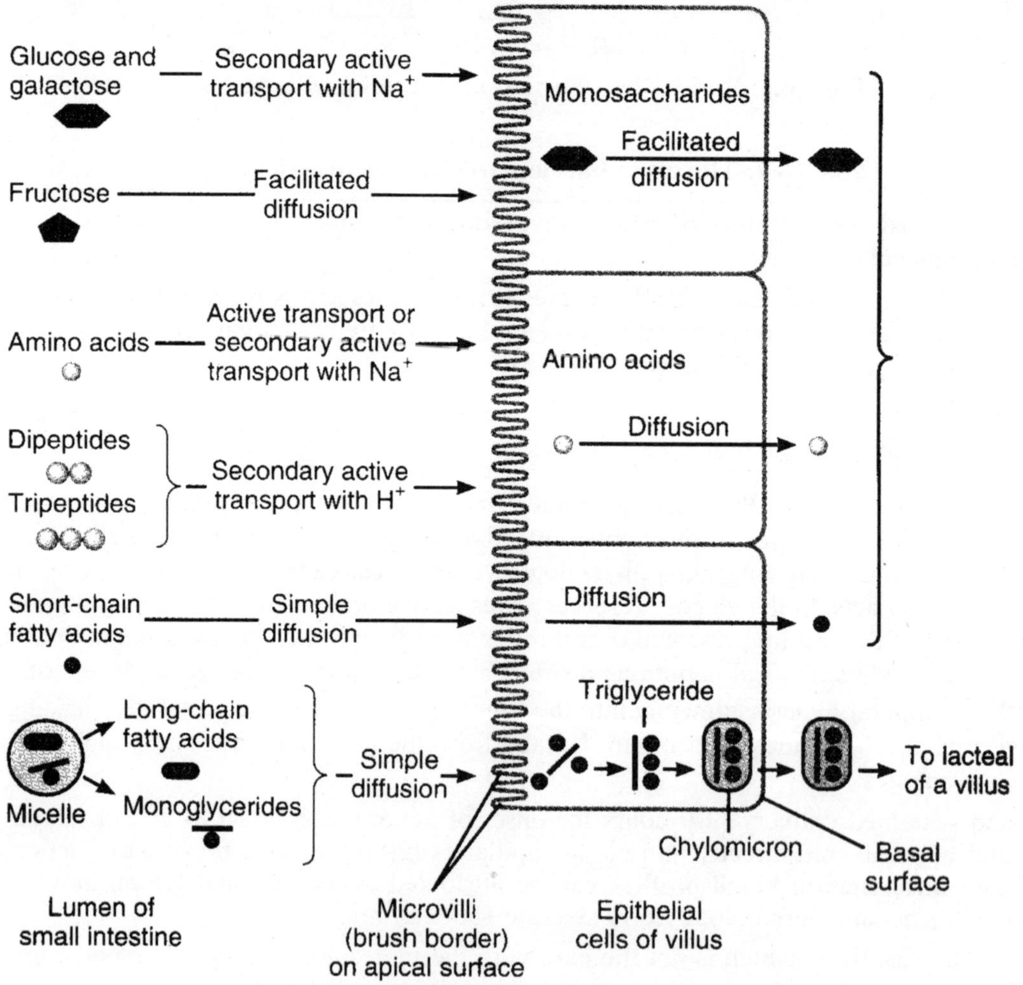

Fig. 16.3: Mechanistic diagram illustrating the movement of
moieties through epithelial cells of the villi

Finally, it has the potential to target moieties like cytokines and lymphokines to white blood cells present in the lymph system. In spite of extensive efforts, relatively little progress has been made to achieve the goal of safe, effective and commercially feasible oral formulations development for peptides/proteins. An absorption rate of some peptide/protein drugs is presented in Table 16.5.

The extent of bioavailability that is achieved with oral dosage forms is largely peptide/protein specific. For peptides having large therapeutic index and low manufacturing cost, a comparatively low bioavailability (e.g., 10%) may be acceptable. However, with peptides having a narrow therapeutic index and/or prohibitively high manufacturing costs, it may be desirable to have relatively high bioavailability (e.g., 30-50%). Various strategies have been evaluated and attempted to improve bioavailability of these bioactives.

Table 16.5: Gastrointestinal absorption of some peptides/proteins

% absorbed	Peptide/Protein	Molecular weight
< 2	Tetragastrin	483
	Pepstatinyl glycine	740
	1-Deamino-8-D-Arg vasopressin	1007
		1208
	Leuprolide	1250
	Empedopeptin	5700
	Insulin	40000
	Horse radish peroxidase	>50000
	Bovine serum albumin	
25-50	Alafosfain	196
	Dietary di- and tri- peptides	200-300
	Ampicillin	349
	Lysinopril	405
	Cyclosporin	1203
>50	Aminocephalosporins	350
	Enalapril	377
	Talampicillin	482

16.5.1.1. Approaches for enhancement of oral delivery of peptides and proteins

16.5.1.1.1. Modifications by chemical synthesis of prodrugs and analogues

Preparation of prodrugs and analogues of natural peptides/proteins is a rational approach towards achieving their improved delivery. This strategy of altering the peptide/protein structure by reversible (prodrug) or irreversible (analogue) chemical modification is aimed to transiently modify physicochemical properties of drugs, such as lipophilicity, charge, molecular size, solubility, configuration, isoelectric point, chemical stability, enzyme lability and affinity to carriers without compromising with the inherent pharmacological properties of parent drug. This modification assists in manipulation of the pharmacokinetic parameters, therapeutic value of the parent drug by facilitating membrane permeation and stability against degradation and thereby altering bioavailability.

Table 16.6: Approaches for oral delivery of peptide and protein drug(s)

Approach	Typical examples
Modifications by chemical synthesis of prodrugs and analogues	PEG derivatives, monosaccharide derivatives
Use of enzyme inhibitors	Bacitracin, chymostatin, aprotinin, soyabean trypsin inhibitor
Use of penetration enhancers	EDTA, sodium deoxycholate, saudium lauryl sulfate, oleic acid, zonula occludens toxin
Carrier systems	w/o/w emulsions, emulsomes, nano- and microparticles, bioadhesive systems

16.5.1.1.2. Use of enzyme inhibitors

Various enzyme inhibitors have been employed to achieve successful delivery of peptide and protein based drugs. The various enzymes that are involved in their degradation and their specific inhibitors are presented in Table 16.7.

Table 16.7: Enzymes and their specific inhibitors

Enzyme	Specific inhihitors
Acid protease (e.g., pepsin, rennin, cathepsin D, chymosin)	Diazoacetyl DL -norleucine methyl ester; 1,2-epoxy-3(Q-nitrophenoxy) propane; Pestatine
Aminopeptidases	Bestain, Bacitracin
Aminopeptidases B	Arphanamine
Ca^{2+} activated neutral protease	Protease inhibitor
Calpains I and II	Acetyl-leucyl-leucyl norleucinal
Chymotrypsin	Chymostatin; N-Tosyl-L-phenylalanine chloromethyl ketone
Endoprotease	α2-Macroglobulin
Glutathione-insulin transhydrogenase	Bacitracin
Metalloendoproteases	Phosphoramidon
Metalloprotease	Ethylenediamine tetra-acetic acid
Serine proteases (e.g., Elastase; Cathepsin; Trypsin; Thrombin; Kallikrein)	4-Amidinophenyl-methanesulfonyl fluoride Aprotinin 3 4- Dichloroisocoumarine Leupeptin Phenylmethanesulfonyl fluoride
Thiolproteases (e.g., Plasmin; Cathepsin B; Cathepsin L)	Cystain (N-[N(L-3-trans-carboxy-oxiran-2-carbonyl]-L-leucyl-1-[-agmatine] Leupeptin
Trypsin	Nα-Q-Tosyl-L-lysine chloromethyl ketone; Trypsin inhibitor

16.5.1.1.3. Use of penetration enhancers

The major pathways available for transport of peptide/protein drugs across a biomembrane are the transcellular and the paracellular routes. The transport across this pathway is dependent on the lipophilicity of the membrane and molecule, the molecular and the particulate size and surface associated charge. Penetration enhancers are compounds which, when added to a solute, increase its absorption across biological membranes. Peptide/protein drug moieties, due to their molecular size, often require penetration enhancers to achieve therapeutically significant levels of lumenal absorption.

The mechanisms involved in the improvement of intestinal permeation through transcellular route by absorption enhancers are:

- Interaction of absorption enhancers (e.g., mixed micelles, salicylic acid, acyl carnitine, middle chain fatty acids) with membrane lipid protein leads to membrane perturbation followed by an increase in the permeability. Saturated fatty acids with the same number of carbons show better results in comparison to the unsaturated fatty acids. This difference can be attributed to the presence of double bonds in the unsaturated fats that lead to the formation of fluid micelles. However, with saturated fats rigid micelles are formed having better disrupting properties than the fluid ones.

- Disorder of membrane status by decrease in membrane nonprotein thiol, e.g., diethyl maleate, salicylic acid.

The mechanisms involved in the improvement of intestinal membrane permeation by absorption enhancers through paracellular route include:

- Chelation between enhancer and Ca^{++}/Mg^{++} around tight junctions which force water through by osmosis, enhancing paracellular absorption of water-soluble drugs, e.g., EDTA/bile acids, middle chain fatty acids.

- Activation of junctional actomyosin contraction, e.g., glucose, amino acids, decanoyl carnitine, capric acid, mixed micelle.

16.5.1.1.4. Carrier systems

This strategy is particularly applicable in the case of poorly absorbed peptides/proteins, which are unstable in the g.i. lumen and their targeting to a specific tissue or organ is to be affected. The proper designing of the delivery system not only protects the drug from g.i. degrading components in the physical environment of the formulation prior to absorption, but also localizes the drug at or near the cellular membrane to maximize the driving force for passive permeation. Some of the delivery systems that have been explored include lipid vesicles, emulsions, emulsomes, particulate carriers and bioadhesive systems.

16.5.1.2. M cell targeted vaccine delivery

Oral vaccine delivery offers significant advantages over conventional parenteral routes. Most notably, oral delivery offers the potential for stimulating mucosal immune responses that protect against pathogen invasion at mucosal surfaces. In addition, oral vaccines are easy to administer, not requiring sterile needles or trained personnel, convenience and also the cost factors are of considerable significance in developing countries. Major factors currently hindering the development of oral vaccines include the need to present the vaccine antigen in such a form that it can both survive the hostile environment of the gastrointestinal tract and transported across the gastrointestinal epithelial barrier in sufficient quantities to stimulate protective immunity. Owing to their transcytotic capacity, M cells represent for an efficient potential portal for oral vaccine delivery.

M cells are epithelial cells specialized for sampling viruses and bacteria and perform a critical role in immune surveillance in mucosal tissues. The M cell apical surface is modified with less frequent microvilli and a thinner glycocalyx, and the basolateral membrane is invaginated to form an intraepithelial 'pocket' enclosing leukocytes. These alterations facilitate endocytosis and phagocytosis of microorganisms and transport across the epithelium. In certain tissues, M cell apical membranes exhibit distinct receptors which have been identified with monoclonal antibodies and lectins. Pathogenic bacteria and viruses can recognize the M cell surface and exploit its transcellular transport pathway to gain entry into host tissues. M cells sample and transport synthetic microspheres in a manner similar to microorganisms and thus play an essential role in the delivery of vaccines and drugs to mucosal lymphoid tissues. However, the efficiency of sampling of orally delivered microparticles by M cells is low. Strategies are being developed to target microparticles to M cell apical surfaces using M cell-selective probes in order to increase sampling efficiency and bioavailability of drugs and vaccines. Such targeting strategies are likely be critical in the development of more effective vaccines and drugs to be administered through mucosal routes. Specifically targeting vaccine delivery vehicles to the intestinal M cells may enhance the efficacy of oral vaccines. This may be achieved by coating delivery vehicles with ligands that selectively bind to M cell surfaces. Since M cells may be differentiated from enterocytes by cell surface carbohydrate expression, lectins represent one such group of ligands which may permit M cell targeting of orally administered vaccines.

16.5.1.3. Oral gene delivery

In vivo production of proteins through oral gene therapy has also been investigated. Rather than administering the protein itself, the DNA plasmid that codes for it is swallowed. This then attaches to the cells in the small intestine where it manufactures the required protein drug using available materials in the cell. The protein is thereafter absorbed into the blood stream. The gene has a short half-life and hence must be administered regularly to be effective. The advantage is that it provides for safe, easily managed treatment unlike most gene-based therapies currently available. It is also hoped that this system will be relatively free from ectopic expressions usually experienced with gene therapies since the bulk of the administered genes remain within the intestine and is passed out with feaces along with sloughed cells of the intestinal epithelium.

16.5.2. Nasal delivery

The nasal route has been chiefly employed for producing local action on the mucosa. But this route appears to hold immense promise for the delivery of peptides/proteins. The intranasal delivery of peptide was tried as early as 1920s with oxytocin and insulin. But it was only recently that it has received significant attention as a feasible route for peptide delivery. Anatomically the length of the nasal cavity is approximately 12 cm with a total volume of 15 ml. It is approximately 3 mm thick and covers about $150 cm^2$ areas. The nasal mucosa is highly vascularised. Drug absorption via nasal mucosa enters the systemic arterial circulation prior to traversing the liver. The nasal mucosa is relatively more permeable to peptides as compared to routes like oral and transdermal. The bioavailability of peptides through this route is reported to be of the order of 1 to 20%. This depends on the physical properties and molecular weight of the peptide but can be extremely variable.

Peptidal drug moieties like calcitonin, ACTH, insulin and interferon are reported to have appreciable absorption through nasal mucosa. Lypressin, a synthetic analogue of vasopressin has been introduced commercially as an intranasal dosage form following clinical trials. Encouraging results have also been obtained with GnRH, LHRH, buserelin, enkephalins and GHRF. The nasal route has been used to administer pituitary hormones, like vasopressin and oxytocin, for many years.

16.5.3. Transdermal delivery

Until recently, the utility of intact skin as a port for continuous transdermal delivery of drugs has been confined to topical medication and application. With an insight into the anatomy and physiology of the skin and percutaneous absorption it is now evident that through this route benefits equivalent to i.v. drug infusion (i.e., direct entry into the systemic circulation and control over drug levels) can be closely obtained while inherent hazards may effectively be excluded. Thus, this route not only exhibits improved patient compliance but also offers some advantages which prove it to be superior in regard to peptide/protein delivery.

Table 16.8: Approaches for transdermal delivery of peptide/protein based drugs

- Iontophoresis
- Phonophoresis
- Penetration enhancers
- Prodrugs

16.5.4. Pulmonary delivery

The respiratory tract offers an alternative site for systemic, however non-invasive delivery of peptides/proteins. Most of these drugs are readily absorbed through the lungs once they enter the deep lung tissues via transcytosis. Macromolecular drugs on administration through inhalation are reported to attain a bioavailability in the range of 20-95% as compared to s.c. injection.

The respiratory tract is mainly consisted of a naso-pharyngeal region, a tracheo-bronchial region and lungs. The local delivery of mucolytic and proteolytic agents, bronchodilators and sympathomimetic agents to the respiratory tract is accomplished via the airways as they provide larger surface area ($70m^2$) as compared to other mucosal sites including nasal, buccal, rectal and vaginal. In order to utilise the potential of pulmonary route for the systemic administration of peptides/proteins it seems necessary to understand the permeability characteristics of lungs, absorption mechanism in or through the lungs, lung metabolising capacity, factors controlling dose deposition and safety considerations. About 90% of the absorptive surface area of the lungs is represented by the alveoli. The latter is comprised of heterogenous population of epithelial cells. Out of these cells, a small group of cells known as type III cells exists as free alveolar macrophages. The epithelial cells remain in intimate contact with the vasculature. The distance between air and blood is much less than 1 μm. However, due to its involvement in free exchange of gases it becomes and functions as a major barrier to the large molecule, for example, horseradish peroxidase with a molecular weight of 40,000 deposited on airside and fails to reach the interstitium. The principal resistance is offered largely by alveolar epithelium where the cells are tightly intercalated. The pore openings in alveolar membrane are 6-10 $A^°$ and in pulmonary capillary membrane 40-50 $A^°$.

16.5.5. Rectal delivery

The rectum is a body cavity of the body through which absorption of drug(s) susceptible to gastric pH and environment is possible. Drugs can be easily inserted and localized in the rectum. The human rectum is about 15–20 cm in length and contains approx. 2-3 ml of inert mucus fluid when it is empty. The surface area of human rectum is 200–400 cm^2 in comparison to 2,000,000 cm^2 of the small intestine. Thus, it can be anticipated that the absorption through the rectum would be considerably less than the upper git. The rectal mucosa is devoid of any villi and therefore in resting state, it appears as non-motile.

Table 16.9: Advantages of rectal route are:

- It is highly vascularized.
- It avoids to a large extent the first pass or pre-systemic metabolism.
- It is suitable for drugs that can cause nausea/vomiting and irritate the gi mucosa on oral administration.
- In case of adverse reaction or drug overdose, the drug absorption can be interrupted.
- A large dose of drug can be administered.
- Drug can be targeted to the lymphatic system.

The large intestine is drained by three veins (de Boer). These veins do intermingle due to the presence of anastomoses. But still, the inferior and middle rectal veins drain into the inferior vena cava and thus bypass the portal system and as a consequence presystemic metabolism in the liver. The superior rectal vein drains into the portal vein. The large intestine is also drained by the lymphatics. It has been demonstrated that in the lower colon the drainage is mostly lymphatic. With an increase in the molecular weight of a compound, its lymphatic uptake is favored. Compounds with molecular weight greater than 2,000 preferably make an entry into the lymphatic fluid. Due to the bypass of the hepatic portal system, a considerable portion of the rectally absorbed drug enters ultimately the general circulation directly. However, it is established that the tight intercellular junctions of the columnar epithelium of the rectal mucosa limit the absorption and bioavailability of peptides/proteins.

The various factors affecting absorption from the rectum are:

- Amount of liquid present in the rectum.
- pH and buffer capacity of the rectal fluid
- Surface tension and viscosity of the rectal fluid
- Luminal pressure exerted by the rectal wall which enhances rectal absorption
- Solubility, partition coefficient, pKa of the drug
- Particle size and surface properties of the drug

16.5.6. Parenteral delivery

Parenteral mode of drug delivery has been the major route of choice for protein/peptide, owing to their poor absorption and metabolic instability when given by other alternative routes. For instance after intravenous administration the onset of action is fast and no absorption related issues are involved. Nevertheless, the fast clearance of drugs remains to be a major constraint. Potent nature of these moieties specifically demands their targeting to the specific receptors in order to improve their therapeutic index by optimising the access, amplitude and nature of interactions. This route precisely offers some unique possibilities for the targeting of drug moieties. If peptides are presented at high dosage levels, there stands the possibility of generation of immune responses and other undesirable deleterious side effects and interactions. Targeting thus protects both the drug and body from these contraindicative manifestations. Targeting assumes a focal objective since protein, owing to their large size, may be unable to leave the drug compartment to reach their active sites due to their inability to cross various membranes and barriers.

Moreover, for these drug moieties pulsed delivery is the preferred mode of delivery rather than the continuous delivery as it mimics the physiologic delivery pattern. This also avoids the down-regulation of receptors, which is major fallout of continuous administration. However, all these advantages are overruled by poor acceptance by the patients at large.

The drug delivery systems for parenteral delivery include those intended for intravenous, intramuscular, intraarteial, subcutaneous, intraperitoneal and intrathecal use. The drug carrier systems employed for defined and controlled delivery of drug through this route are particulates, as well as soluble carriers.

16.5.6.1. Hydrophilic polymer protectants

Another approach for modifying the pharmacodisposition of peptide/protein drug is the surface modifications by polymer chemistry approaches as they increase their apparent size and/or reduce their undesired interaction with blood and tissue components. Physicochemical interaction between a protein and the immune system components mediates immunosurveillance. Opsonization by fibrinogen, fibronectin or other blood components is followed by recognition and thereby removal of the formed immune complexes by the cells. Opsonised materials are entrapped into the cells after adherence to, and vesiculation of, phagocytosing cell membranes. If the adhesive forces between the therapeutic protein, blood macromolecules and cell-surface macromolecules are reduced, it is possible to minimize both opsonization and adherence *per se*. Surfacial modification by introducing a hydrated polymer at the surface generates a high potential energy barrier by creating a sterically stabilized surface. The presence of energetically unfavorable surface prevents the approach of macromolecules and thereby improves upon their tolerance within the vasculature. Some of the hydrophilic biopolymeric protectants are enlisted in Table 16.10.

As mentioned earlier the conjugation of protein with hydrophobic polymer elicits the following changes:

- **Stability:** An improvement in the chemical and physicochemical stability is significant. The resistance of peptide/protein against proteolysis and heat denaturation is also enhanced. Modification of the antigenic sites or sterical hindrance as offered by the polymer moiety block its interaction with the detrimental components.

- **Decrease in immunogenicity:** Reduction in the aggregation of therapeutic peptide/protein and/or masking of antigenic determinants brings about an overall reduction in the immunogenic profile.

- **Duration of action:** Since the uptake of conjugated proteins by the MPS is avoided, they can remain in the circulation for relatively a longer period of time. This may be helpful in developing a long-term circulating depot of protein therapeutics and even may improve the statistical probability for a competing process to occur (e.g., extravasation or interaction with an intravascular target cell).

16.5.7. Ocular delivery

Delivery of therapeutic proteins/ peptides has received a great attention over the last few years. However, limitations such as membrane permeability, large size, metabolism and solubility restrict their efficient delivery. A number of approaches have been used to overcome these limitations. Poor membrane permeability of hydrophilic peptides may be improved by structurally modifying the compound, thus increasing their membrane permeability. Ocular route is not a preferred route for systemic delivery of such large molecules.

However, for the treatment of local eye disorders these classes of molecules are carefully delivered in the form of nanomedicine. Immunoglobulin G has been effectively delivered to retina by transscleral route with insignificant systemic absorption. Many peptidal drugs such as vancomycin, ganciclovir and Vasoactive Peptide have been delivered to ocular sites with the help of nanocarriers such as PLGA nanoparticles and liposomes. Dipeptide ester prodrugs of ganciclovir based on valine (Val) and glycine (Gly) have been developed and found capable of improving ocular bioavailability and therapeutic activity of ganciclovir.

Table 16.10: Hydrophilic polymer protectants employed for therapeutic proteins

Protein	Projected use of conjugate
Albumin	
Asparaginase	Cancer
Dextran	
Carboxypeptidase G_2	Enzyme replacement therapy
β-Galactosidase	Enzyme replacement therapy
L-Asparaginase	Cancer (lower antigen reactivity and increased circulatory persistence)
Purine nucleosides	Inhibitors of adenosine deaminase
Urokinase	Fibrinolytic
N-(2-Hydroxypropyl)methacrylamide)	
Antibodies	Cancer seeking agents
Octylphenoxy Polyoxy Ethanols	
Interleukin 2	Cancer
Poly-D-Alanyl Peptides	
Asparaginase	Cancer
Polyethylene Glycols	
Adenosine deaminase	AD deficiency
Bilirubin oxidase	Bilirubinemia
Interleukin 2	Cancer
Islet-activating protein	Insulinogenic activity
L-Asparaginase	Malignant hematological disorders
Proteins	Radioprotection
Superoxide dismutase	Kidney transplantation, burns, reperfusion damage
Tissue plasminogen activator	Thrombolysis
Uricase	Altered antigenicity
Urokinase	Coagulant, fibrinolytic
Polyoxyethylene Sorbitans	
Interleukin 2	Cancer

Table 16.13 summarizes the work that has been carried out in the area of ocular delivery of proteins and peptides. The ocular route holds immense potential for peptides/proteins intended for pathological ophthalmologic conditions.

Table 16.11: Marketed preparation of proteins based on microspheres

Drug	Trade name	Company	Route	Application
Leuprolide acetate	Lupron Depot*	Takeda-Abott	3 months depot suspension	Prostate cancer
Recombinant human growth hormone	Nutropine Depot*	Genetech-Alkermes	Monthly S/C injection	Growth hormone deficiency
Goserelin acetate	Zoladex*	I.C.I.	S/C Implant	Prostate cancer
Octreotide acetate	Sandostatin LAR* depot	Novartis	Injectable S/C suspension	GH suppression, anticancer
Triptorelin	Decapepryl*	Debiopharm	Injectable Depot	LHRH agonist
Recombinant bovine somatropin	Posilac	Mansanto	Injectable depot oil based injection	To increase milk production in cattle

Table 16.12: Peptide/proteins employed for treatment of ophthalmic disorders

Peptide/protein	Therapeutic indication
Enkephalins, substance P	Anti-inflammatory
Aqueous humor dynamics	Atrial naturetic factor, LHRH, neurotensin, vasopressin
Cyclosporin, interferon	Generate immune response
Epidermal growth factor, fibronectin, insulin-like growth factor, mesodermal growth factor	Healing of wounds

The systemic delivery of peptide/protein drugs has been attempted through the ocular route. The concept behind ocular drug delivery to the systemic circulation exploits the stable dynamics of the lachrymal system that exports the drug to the nasal cavity from where considerable systemic absorption results. However, the localized bioavailability of the drugs remains poor through this route due to the existence of physiological barriers like tear dilution, lachrymal drainage and protein binding. Further the drug should have amphiphilic biphasic solubility profile to permeate the corneal membrane.

Peptide/protein administration through conjunctiva has been investigated as a potential alternative and convenient route of delivery. Attempts have been made through this route for administering insulin to control hyperglycemia and prevent retinopathy in diabetics. Significant absorption through conjunctival membranes with 500units/ml insulin solution has been reported. However, palpebral movements and tears swiftly wash away the insulin solution. Also the volume of the conjunctival sac in man is at the most 50 μl. This necessitates development of concentrated drug solutions so that the volume of administration can be reduced.

Viscosity of the insulin solution has been increased to control retention of drug solution. Sodium hyaluronic acid which is inherently present in the ocular vitreous fluid was employed at a concentration of 0.36% w/v to increase the viscosity almost 40-fold. Significant improvement in the insulin bioavailability and concomitant reduction in plasma glucose concentration was observed in diabetic dogs.

The feasibility of ocular peptide/protein delivery using eye drops as a delivery system is limited. The eye drops exhibit low bioavailability, low therapeutic efficacy and short duration of activity. To address these limitations eye inserts can be developed and employed.

Another device based on absorbable gelatin sponge has been successfully used to improve upon the above-mentioned limitations. It offers other benefits as well. The device is fabricated by punching a disc of gelatin. The drug solution is sorbed into the disc and the wet matrices are dried under vacuum. This device has been employed for insulin delivery and encouraging results were recorded. The key factors in prolonging the systemic absorption profile include the dissolution of the drug without causing any depot effect.

The benefits of this device are listed below:

- Relatively simple and cheap manufacturing procedure.
- On hydration the device becomes soft and pliable and hence comfortable.
- The treatment can be terminated simply by removal of the device from the eye.
- Gives rapid and prolonged blood glucose suppression up to 10 hours.
- Does not elicit any physical signs of eye irritation like lachrymation, redness, etc.
- On treatment with at least 5% acetic acid or 1% hydrochloric acid it does not require any absorption enhancer to promote systemic delivery of insulin.
- It regulates mass entry of the drug into the systemic circulation.

16.6. NANOCARRIERS FOR CONTROLLED DELIVERY OF PROTEINS AND PEPTIDES

The term "nanoparticle" is broadly applied in the description of almost every pharmaceutical carrier or imaging agent system, so further classification is needed for clarit. One group of nanocarriers includes single-chain polymer–drug conjugates, polymer colloids prepared by techniques such as emulsion polymerization, crosslinked nanogel matrices, dendrimers, and carbon nanotubes. For this group, the carrier is a single synthetic molecule with covalent bonds and a relatively large molar mass. Other types of nanocarriers, often termed nanoparticles, comprise self-assemblies of smaller molecules, which are aggregated through intermolecular forces. Liposomes and polyplexes are the most studied members of this class of particles, but this class of carriers also includes aggregates such as polymersomes and other assemblies of block copolymers, colloidosomal aggregates of latex particles, and protein or peptide assemblies. The dynamic nature of these types of systems depends upon the intermolecular forces in play and the biological conditions. Nanocarriers include also complexes based upon fullerenes, silica, colloidal gold, gold nanoshells, quantum dots, and superparamagnetic particles.

The use of a properly designed carrier for the sustained and targeted delivery of pharmaceuticals offers several advantages compared with classic administration: it can increase the amount of drug that reaches the targeted area, improve the transportation mechanism and protect the drug against inactivation, degradation and metabolization phenomena. The main characteristics that the carrier must show are:

- The ability to encapsulate the drug without deactivating it;
- The possibility for releasing the drug under proper conditions and according to proper
- kinetics;
- A high stability and long circulation time after administration;
- The capability to actively or passively deliver the drug to a target area.

Table 16.13: Studies reported related to ocular delivery of proteins and peptides

Drug	Type	Remarks
IgG protein	Protein (Transscleral delivery)	IgG protein delivered to the retina and choroid in an optimum concentration for the treatment of chorio-retinal disorders with negeligible systemic absorption
Vancomycin (peptide)	Peptide PLGA microparticles	PLGA microparticles loaded with peptide drug showed high and prolonged concentration of vancomycin &increased level of AUC (2 fold) as compared to aqueous solutions
Ganciclovir (GCV)	Peptide	Glycine-valine-GCV is the effective and lead candidate for the treatment of HCMV
Vasoactive intestinal peptide(VIP)	Peptide	Treatment of ocular inflammation by modulating the macrophages and t-cell activaton in the immune system
VIP	Peptide (liposomes)	For the treatment of endotoxin induced uveitis (EIU) as liposomal delivery increased its efficiency and bioavailability
Ganciclovir (GCV)	Peptide (Valine-Glycine-GCV produg)	Diester GCV prodrugs demonstrated excellent chemical stability, high aqueous solubility and markedly enhanced antiviral potency against the herpes viruses without any increase in cytotoxicity

Above all, the use of nanosized carriers offers a way to cross biological barriers that would otherwise forbid the drug to accede to the site of interest, as it often happens in the central nervous system or in the gastrointestinal tract. Nanocarriers have a high surface area to volume ratio, thus providing improved pharmacokinetics and biodistribution of drugs while minimizing toxicity, thanks to specific targeted transport. Moreover, they can improve the solubility of many drugs and prolong the shelf-life and *in vivo* stability of peptides, proteins and oligonucleotides. In particular, the use of biodegradable materials, which has already been reviewed, minimizes the risk for hypersensitivity reactions and ensures good tissue compatibility. Among the potential nanocarriers, colloidal systems such as liposomes and nanoparticles have aroused considerable interest and have been extensively reviewed.

Complex drug delivery systems are thus a potential alternative to the conventional formulations of proteins, in which the protein is usually either lyophilized, in suspension, or in an aqueous solution. The optimal release pattern may vary between proteins and between indications, and adaptable formulations are therefore required. Some proteins require sustained release, while others require controlled, immediate or pulsed release. Release can be obtained with different particulate drug delivery systems. Liposomes, solid-lipid nanoparticles, polymeric nanoparticles and virosomes are the most commonly used nanocarriers for protein delivery.

In many cases, targeted or untargeted liposomes and nanoparticles are rapidly cleared from the blood stream by the RES; although this event is usually considered a disadvantage, it can lead to the aim of activating macrophages if required by certain therapies. Since macrophages are mostly located in the spleen and liver, their ability to catch particles can be used to selectively deliver substances to these organs. Otherwise, specific chemical modification of the carrier can be performed in order to make the system able to avoid the RES. Surface modification of nanocarriers is commonly performed to give them suitable biological properties, to prolong their life in the blood stream, to limit the uptake by macrophages, and to make them able to target specific organs or tissues.

Nanoparticles, such as liposomes, polymeric micelles, lipoplexes and polyplexes have been extensively studied as targeted drug carrier systems over the past three decades. A wide variety of active agents can be incorporated into or complexed with these particles, varying from low molecular weight drug molecules to macromolecules such as proteins and nucleic acids. An important requirement to the systemic intravenous use of this targeted nanomedicine approach is the ability of the nanoparticles to circulate in the bloodstream for a prolonged period of time. To achieve this, PEG is often used as a coating material. It is generally assumed that PEG creates a so-called "steric stabilization" effect: the PEG molecules form a protective hydrophilic layer on the surface of the nanoparticle that opposes interaction with blood components. As a result, the PEG coating reduces uptake by macrophages of the mononuclear phagocyte system (MPS) and provides relatively long plasma residence times. Until now, PEG is still the most widely used material for achieving steric stabilization. Nevertheless, successful attempts have been made to design alternative polymers, for example polymers based on polyoxazoline, poly(vinyl alcohol), polyglycerol, poly(N-vinyl-2-pyrrolidinone), poly(*N*-(2-hydroxypropyl)methacrylamide) and poly(amino acid)s. For all these coating materials, prolonged circulation times of nanoparticles as compared to non-coated nanoparticles have been reported.

It is generally assumed that the macrophage-resistant property of sterically protected particles is due to suppression in surface opsonization (protein adsorption facilitating uptake) and protein adsorption. However, recent evidence shows that sterically stabilized particles are prone to opsonization, particularly by the opsonic components of the complement system. Moghimi and Szebeni evaluated these phenomena and discussed theories that reconcile complement activation and opsonization with prolonged circulation times. With respect to particle longevity, the physiological state of macrophages also plays a critical role. For example, stimulated or newly recruited macrophages can recognize and rapidly internalize sterically protected nanoparticles by opsonicindependent mechanisms.

Moreover, steric stabilization is not desirable for all steps in the drug targeting process. The prolonged circulation time is needed to enable extravasation at sites with increased vascular permeability such as tumors and inflamed sites (enhanced permeability and retention (EPR) effect). However, after localizing to the pathological site, nanoparticles should deliver their contents in an efficient manner to achieve a sufficient therapeutic response. The polymer coating may hinder drug release and target cell interaction and can therefore be an obstacle in the realization of the therapeutic response. Attempts have been made to enhance the therapeutic efficacy of sterically stabilized nanoparticles by means of shedding, *i.e.,* loss of the coating after arrival at the target site. This "unmasking" process may facilitate drug release and/or target cell interaction processes. The shedding concept provides a potential solution for several situations in which the polymer coating can have a negative effect on the delivery process.

Systemically administered nanomedicines should have diameters ranging from 10–200 nm: nanocarriers must be larger than 10 nm to avoid first-pass elimination through the kidneys and smaller than 200 nm to avoid sequestration by the spleen and liver. The size of the fenestrations in tumor vasculature also puts an upper limit on the size of nanocarriers that exploit the EPR effect to accumulate in tumors. Tumor vasculature fenestrations vary depending on a myriad of factors, but usually do not exceed several hundred nanometers. Nanocarrier size has been shown to influence circulation half-life and tissue accumulation. Size is not the only important property of drug nanocarriers. Surface properties can increase nanoparticle stability, prolong circulation in the blood and dramatically influence opsonization and uptake by the RES. The route of administration can also affect nanoparticle biodistribution and targeting. The preferred route of administration for nanocarriers is often by intravenous injection. Other routes of administration have generally proven less efficacious, usually because low drug reaches the target tissues. On the other hand, subcutaneous or intradermal injections may be preferable for lymphatic targeting whereas intraperitoneal injection may be more efficacious for brain targeting.

16.6.1. Liposomes

Liposomes are micro or nanometric vesicles composed of amphiphilic species, such as lipids or phospholipids, that spontaneously form one (unilamellar) or more (multilamellar) concentric bilayers separated by water compartments. Lipids expose their hydrophilic head outwards, while the hydrophobic tail is directed inwards in the bilayer. Depending on the number of bilayers, the particle size can range from about 20 nm to several micrometers.

Liposomes show very versatile properties in terms of size, surface charge and lipid composition, and their ability to incorporate almost any drug independent of its solubility in water makes these microreservoir systems useful for delivery purposes. There is a large variety of lipids employable for the preparation of liposomes, comprising for instance mixtures of stearic acid and Tween 80, mixtures of distearoyl phosphatidylcholine, distearoyl phosphatidylglycerol, and cholesterol, diplasmenylcholine, mixtures of distearoyl phosphatidylcholine, dimyristoyl phosphatidylglycerol, and cholesterol, mixtures of castor oil, phosphatidylcholine and polyethylene glycol coupled to distearoylphosphatidylethanolamine. The stability of protein-based drugs can be maintained using adequate incorporation processes such as reverse-phase evaporation, injection and freeze-thaw.

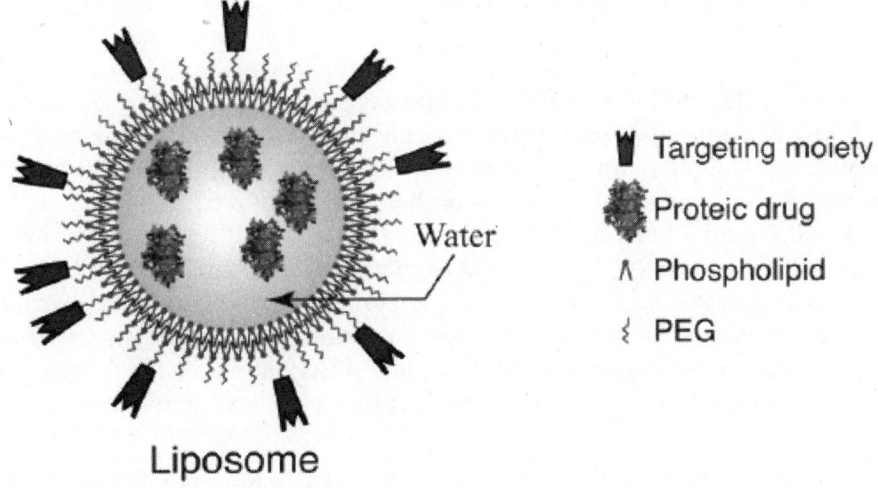

Fig. 16.4: Targeted delivery of proteins using liposome as carrier

Liposomes also proved to be safe *in vivo* and were even tested as possible candidates to improve the safety in prescribing drugs during pregnancy. Liposomes can be exploited for drug delivery *via* pulmonary route. This method exhibits numerous benefits as an alternative for repeated injection of drugs like insulin. Encapsulation of insulin into liposomal carriers for pulmonary delivery (dry powder inhalation) showed good hypoglycemic effect with low blood glucose level and long-lasting period and a relatively high pharmacological bioavailability.

Liposomes are suitable carriers for the delivery of pro-apoptotic membrane proteins into cancer cells to induce cell death. Voltage-dependent anionic channel (VDAC) and Bak are two mitochondrial outer membrane proteins involved in the activation of the intrinsic apoptotic pathway that have been successfully conjugated to liposomes and delivered into HCT116p53+/+ and HCT116p53−/− cells. It is well known that the use of liposomes as suitable carriers for drug delivery is prone to issues connected with the phagocytic activity of macrophages. The clearance of liposomes from the blood stream depends not only on mechanical filtration and membrane fusion events, but also on interactions with serum proteins and cellular receptors. Cellular receptors do not directly recognize the liposome as a foreign body, but they recognize specific serum proteins that bind the liposome surface (opsonins). Once the liposome has been internalized into a cell by endocytosis, several strategies can be used to achieve endosomal escape of liposome-encapsulated drugs. A recent technique consists of providing the cell with photosensitizer molecules, which primarily accumulate in endosomal membranes, and then exposing the system to light. Upon illumination, reactive singlet oxygen species form and damage the endosomal membrane, which becomes permeable to endocyted molecules (photochemical internalization). This method was successfully used to induce cytotoxicity in EGFreceptor positive human ovarian cancer cells, thanks to the plant toxin saporin encapsulated into targeted liposomes.

Liposomes can also undergo lipid exchange with high-density lipoproteins in blood, leading to liposome disintegration. The intrinsic instability of liposomes in the body environment causes fast release of the loaded drug. This means a peak in drug concentration a short time after administration (burst effect). Liposomes can be protected against the burst effect, e.g., by encapsulation in alginate shells crosslinked with Ba2+ ions. They can also be properly designed in order to minimize the macrophage uptake and prolong their circulation time after intravenous injection. The most exploited modification used to reach this goal is PEGylation. When the linear, non-toxic, flexible and hydrophilic PEG polymer that shows anti-opsonizing properties is grafted on the liposome surface, it forms a hydrophilic layer that shields the liposome surface charge. Its steric hindrance and hydrophilicity prevent opsonins from settling on the liposome surface, making it difficult for RES cells to recognize and interact with liposomes. For this reason, such liposomes are commonly named stealth liposomes, long-circulating liposomes or sterically stabilized liposomes. It has been reported that free PEG and bound PEG produce opposite effects: free PEG causes fusion of the particles, while bound PEG protects them PEG-functionalized lipids exhibit dose-independent pharmacokinetics in animals and humans, and the ability to cross biological barriers *in vivo*. These features allow PEGylated liposomes improved delivery and therapeutic efficacy of anti-cancer drugs. An important aspect to be considered in liposome PEGylation is the choice of the PEG-lipid conjugate alkyl chain, which can in some cases produce immunogenicity after repeated administration.

Woodle *et al* investigated the value of novel systemically long-circulating liposomes to prolong the duration of an antidiuretic hormone, arg8-vasopressin (VP), as a representative of low molecular weight peptides with rapid clearance. The cholesterol content was found to have a controlling effect on VP release in serum. Three types of liposomes were tested in VP-deficient Brattleboro rats. One contained phosphatidylserine (PS), which was rapidly cleared from the circulation. In the other two liposomes, PS was replaced by either phosphatidylglycerol or a novel phospholipid derivatized with polyethylene glycol (PE-PEG); both showing prolonged circulation. The duration of the prolonged bioactivity was not dose dependent, but the amplitude was. This is attributed to VP release from liposomes, which were distributed intact to another compartment without being taken up by the RES. The authors concluded that liposomes could be applied to prolong the biological activity of a therapeutic peptide by balancing liposome circulation time, release rate, and dose.

Kedar *et al* demonstrated that recombinant human interleukin-2 (IL-2) can be successfully encapsulated in unilamellar, long-circulating, sterically stabilized liposomes. They also compared the immunomodulatory and anti-tumor effects of IL-2, pegylated IL-2 (PEG-IL-2) and liposome encapsulated IL-2 (SSL-IL-2) in mice. They found that SSL-IL-2 was significantly more effective than IL-2 in increasing leukocyte number in the blood and spleen and triggering spleen lymphokineactivated killer cell activity. The survival of mice with advanced metastatic carcinoma (previously treated with cyclophosphamide chemotherapy) was two to six times greater following administration of SSL-IL-2 than IL-2. Moreover, successful treatment with SSL-IL-2 required lower cumulative doses and fewer administrations. PEG-IL-2 was a more potent immunostimulator than SSL-IL-2 in normal mice, and as effective as SSL-IL-2 in tumor-bearing mice. PEG-IL-2, however, caused marked toxicity, including severe thrombocytopenia.

PEGylation is also frequently used to prepare radiolabeled liposomes for imaging techniques. PEGylated liposomes labeled with 111In administered intravenously to rats affected by *Staphylococcus aureus* showed that their clearance from the blood stream is similar to that of control 111In-IgG. On the contrary, the uptake by the inflammatory site was twice that of the control, making the inflammation visible by scintigraphy one hour after injection.

However, PEGylation is not the only modification reaction that can be carried out on liposomes. To improve the efficacy of ligand binding to a liposome membrane, Yagi *et al.,* developed a novel lipid analog based on amino acids for liposome modification. This lipid consists of three peptide derivatives and two fatty acids, and it was used to prepare liposomes incorporating the HIV-TAT peptide (domain of human immunodeficiency virus TAT protein). This is a protein transduction domain commonly employed to investigate the delivery of macromolecules, nucleic acids and liposomes into cells. Liposomes containing the lipid analog bearing HIV-TAT peptide exhibited efficient cellular uptake.

Other peptides can be used to modify liposomes surface. Octaarginine oligopeptide (R8) bound on the surface of liposomes can enhance cell internalization by macropinocytosis. R8-modified liposomes can escape from macropinosomes into the cytosol, preserving the encapsulated drug from degradation.Green fluorescence protein was chosen as a model protein and efficiently delivered into mitochondria thanks to highly mitochondrion-fusogenic lipid formulation of the liposomes. Lipid modification can also alter the drug-loading efficacy by inducing changes in the membrane properties, such as micropolarity, microviscosity and free volume. Incorporation of cholesterol proved to reduce the partitioning of porphyrins, while methyl oleate and PEGylated lipids noticeably increased the value of the relevant binding constants. Another important feature deriving from lipid modification is the insertion of functional groups able to bind ligands to the surface of liposomes. Ligands can react with the functional groups either before or after the liposome formation.

16.6.2. Virosomes

The natural ability of viruses to enter and infect specific cell types can be exploited to deliver drugs into the cytosol. Indeed, the virus shell has the ability to bind to target cell receptors and to fuse with the membrane. Clearly, to use this kind of nanocarrier for drug delivery, the viral genetic information must be removed from the virus shell in order to avoid infection of the cell. The emptied viral shell (virosome) can be used to deliver molecules (e.g., DNA, RNA, antigens , vaccines) directly into cells, especially in gene therapy. Virosomes are often obtained from influenza virus by solubilization of the viral membrane followed by ultracentrifugation and reconstitution of the envelope by elimination of the detergent. Since virus derivatives often show high immunogenic properties, fusogenic viral envelope proteins or their synthetic analogs can be combined with liposomes to obtain fusogenic capacities while minimizing the immune response. The drug loading technique can also affect the delivery efficiency. Plasmid DNA can be delivered to target cells thanks to reconstituted influenza virosomes with good results *in vitro*, while *in vivo* the virosome-associated DNA is rapidly degraded by nuclease enzymes. The use of dicaproylphosphatidylcholine for solubilization of the viral membrane prevents its degradation by nucleases, thus making the DNA-virosome suitable for *in vivo* use.

16.6.3. Solid lipid nanoparticles

Solid lipid nanoparticles (SLNs) were first described in the nineties. They are made of solid lipids well tolerated by the body (e.g., glycerides composed of fatty acids, which are commonly used in emulsions for parenteral nutrition, cholesterol, glycerol behenate (Compritol® 888 ATO) glyceryl palmitostearate (Precirol® ATO 5), glyceryl monostearates (Imwitor® 900), tripalmitin and other triglycerides such as tristearin, trilaurin, hard fats such as Witepsol series, cetyl palmitate, lipid acids such as stearic acid, palmitic acid, thus minimizing the risk of acute and chronic toxicity. SLNs are solid at room temperature, thus allowing reduced mobility for incorporated drugs, which is a desirable feature for controlled drug release. Their diameter usually varies between 50 nm and 1 µm, and they can be stabilized using non-toxic surfactants, polymers or both. Large-scale production can be performed in a cost-effective and relatively simple way using hot or cold high-pressure homogenization (HPH) or microemulsion techniques. Other possible preparation methods, such as emulsification-solvent evaporation, solvent injection, solvent emulsification-diffusion and ultrasonication, require the use of organic solvents and do not allow for easy scale up.

Among particulate formulations, solid lipid nanoparticles have been successfully explored for drug delivery because they combine the benefits of liquid lipid-based colloidal systems (e.g., emulsions and liposomes) and solid systems. These products possess excellent tissue biocompatibility, biodegradability, composition flexibility and small size, making them suitable for a variety of applications. Furthermore, they have been found to enhance the drug bioavailability after oral or local administration. On the other hand, solid lipid particle manufacturing techniques are not easily adaptable to protein processing as they operate under high temperature, pressure, and shear stress, which are detrimental to protein stability. To overcome these issues, techniques based on supercritical fluids have been developed to process polymer and lipid materials and produce particulate pharmaceuticals. These techniques can be properly adapted to produce pharmaceutical grade protein delivery system formulations as they can avoid denaturation and degradation phenomena. Recently, Salmaso *et al.,* described a novel supercritical fluid gas microatomization process for the preparation of protein-loaded lipid particles. They demonstrated that the gas micro-atomization process was suitable for the fabrication of lipid nanoparticles loaded with insulin and recombinant human growth hormone (rh-GH), two proteins of relevant pharmaceutical interest with significantly different physicochemical properties.

When using hot or cold HPH, the lipid is heated to approximately 5–10 °C above its melting point, and then the drug is dissolved in the melt. For the hot homogenization technique, the drugcontaining molten lipid is placed into a hot aqueous surfactant solution and stirred to obtain a good dispersion. The pre-emulsion is homogenized using a piston-gap homogenizer and the hot O/W nanoemulsion is then cooled down to room temperature, so that the lipid can crystallize again forming solid lipid nanoparticles. Crystallization can also be initiated at lower temperatures or by lyophilization. Cold homogenization technique is employed in the case of highly temperature-sensitive drugs or hydrophilic drugs. Both hot and cold HPH exclude the use of organic solvents, which could deactivate the drug or produce undesired effects in the body. The HPH equipment can affect the particle characteristics.

To prepare SLNs by the microemulsion technique, a mixture of water, surfactant (e.g., phospholipids) and co-surfactant (e.g., short-chain fatty acids) is heated to the lipid melting temperature and added under gentle stirring to the lipid melt. The compounds must be mixed in the correct ratio to provide a clear stable system for microemulsion formation: nanodrop diameter should be less than 150 nm. The microemulsion is then dispersed in a cold aqueous medium (2–3 °C) under mild mechanical mixing; the precipitated spherical particles have diameters of 70-200 nm. Because of their lipid nature, SLNs are particularly well suited to load synthetic lipophilic drugs. Investigation of drug release kinetics and mechanism performed with etracaine, etomidate and prednisolone model drugs showed how this kind of carrier can be useful in the prolonged release of lipophilic drugs, while hydrophilic drugs would be partially lost during the hot homogenization process because of partitioning between the molten lipid and the water phase. SLNs prepared by hot HPH technique were loaded with tamoxifen, a nonsteroidal antiestrogen used in hormone-positive early breast cancer, and their antiproliferative activity was studied *in vitro* in the MCF-7 cell line. The resulted anti-tumor activity was comparable with that of the free drug, and the particle size was suitable for parenteral administration. *In vivo* studies proved that SLNs stabilized with tristearin enhance the half-life and mean residence time in plasma of the anticancer drug tamoxifen citrate.

The use of SLN for the delivery of peptides and proteins was recently reviewed by Almeida *et al.*, In one of the first studies concerning the incorporation of peptide-based species into lipid particles, SLNs were loaded with lysozyme, an enzyme capable of hydrolyzing 1,4-β- linkages in peptidoglycan and in chitodextrins; the protein maintained its activity during the process, thus proving that some proteins can endure the harsh procedures of formulation by HPH, making possible the use of SLN as antigen carriers for vaccine delivery. Encapsulation of the model decapeptide gonadorelin in solid lipid nanoparticles prepared was performed by solvent diffusion in an aqueous system. The rather slow *in vitro* gonadorelin release proved the suitability of SLNs as a prolonged release formulation for hydrophilic peptide drugs. SLNs were also evaluated as potential carriers for the delivery of recombinant yak interferon-α, which exhibits antiviral activity against vesicular stomatitis virus in Madin-Darby bovine kidney (MDBK) cells. SLNs with an average particle size of 124 nm were prepared by the double emulsion solvent evaporation (w/o/w) method. *In vitro* release study, antiviral activity measurements and cytotoxicity assays proved that interferonloaded SLN could be a useful formulation for controlled release in veterinary therapeutics.

Non-stealth SLNs usually accumulate in liver Kupffer cells after intravenous injection. In the case of liver diseases (hepatitis, hepatic neoplasms, visceral leishmaniasis), this feature can be exploited as a targeting strategy, but in other cases passive targeting should be avoided. Because of their physicochemical properties (particle size, surface charge, hydrophobicity), SLNs are mostly recognized by macrophages. Several modifications have been made to achieve long circulation times by avoiding RES uptake as discussed for stealth liposomes. SLNs surface can be modified by hydrophilic polymers or copolymers to make the particles stealth toward RES. PEG stearate modified SLNs showed reduced uptake by mouse macrophages after intraperitoneal injection, and the reduction was proportional to the PEG chain length.

SLNs are suitable nanocarriers for brain delivery. The brain takes up SLNs probably because of the surface adsorption of blood proteins such as apolipoproteins, which can favor the adherence to endothelial cells of the blood-brain barrier (BBB). This effect was studied for the trypanocidal drug diminazene formulated as a lipid-drug conjugate; the drug is hydrophilic and cannot cross the BBB, but the lipid-drug conjugate can cross the barrier thus reducing central nervous system infection of *Trypanosoma brucei* infected mice. A nanoparticulate system, consisting of lipid nanoparticles coated with chitosan (CS), was developed for the oral administration of peptide drugs. In particular, they investigated the nanoparticle ability to incorporate and deliver the model peptide salmon calcitonin (sCT). The results showed that a CS coating could be formed around the lipid nanoparticles by simple incubation in CS solution. In addition, sCT could be efficiently associated to the nanoparticles. Following an initial burst, the systems provided a continuous and slow release of the associated peptide. Constantinides *et al* developed self-emulsifying water-in-oil microemulsions incorporating medium-chain glycerides. Formulation of calcein (a water-soluble marker molecule), or SK&F 106760 (a water-soluble RGD peptide) resulted in significant bioavailability enhancement in rats relative to their aqueous formulations.

16.6.4. Polymeric nanoparticles

Polymeric nanoparticles are nanosized colloidal materials able to encapsulate, adsorb or covalently bind drugs. Since most polymer properties can be easily modified, nanoparticles constitute a versatile drug delivery system, which can be tailored to make the particles able to penetrate through biological barriers and to deliver drugs to cells or into intracellular compartments. Only a limited number of polymers can be used for the formulation of nanoparticles designed to deliver drugs *in vivo*. Indeed, a suitable polymer must be quickly eliminated from the body to allow repeated administrations while avoiding accumulation. The polymer itself and its degradation products must be non toxic and non immunogenic. Finally, the prepared nanoparticles should be endowed with suitable bulk properties to encapsulate the selected drug and tunable surface properties to modulate their *in vivo* fate.

There exist several protocols to manufacture polymer nanospheres, encapsulating a wide variety of therapeutic biomolecules. At the laboratory scale, the protocol may be as simple as the emulsification of a concentrated aqueous solution of protein or the freeze-dried solid, in solvent, followed by secondary emulsion in aqueous continuous phase: water-in-oil-in-water (w/o/w) or solid-in-oil-inwater (s/o/w) double emulsion–solvent evaporation. However, this apparent simplicity is misleading, since there remain almost intractable problems of protein unfolding and degradation, relevant with respect to fabrication, storage and release.

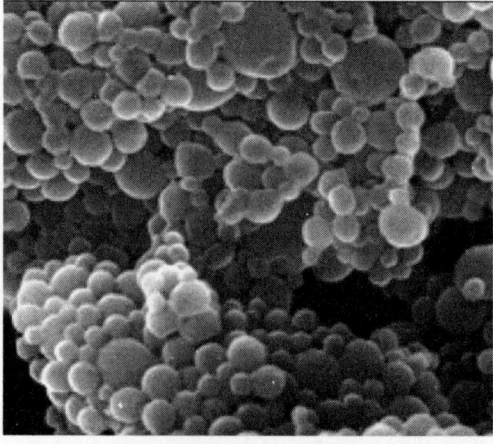

Fig. 16.5: SEM photograph of Polymeric nanoparticles

SUGGESTED READING

- Acartürk F, Degım Z, Degım T. Investigation of the absorption of insulin through vagina in rabbits, AAPS Annual Meeting and Exposition. 10-14, Toronto, Canada (2002).

- Adessi C, Sotto C. *Frontiers in Med Chem* 1, 513 (2004).

- Adessi C,Sotto C. *Curr. Med. Chem* 9, 963 (2002).

- Amidon G. *Pharm News* 2, 32 (1995).

- Arhewoh IM, Okhamafe AO. *JMBR* 3, 7 (2004).

- Banga AK. Structure and analysis of therapeutic peptides and proteins. In Therapeutic Peptides and Proteins: Formulation, Processing and Delivery Systems. Technomic Publishing Co. Inc., Pennsylvania, (1995).

- Barichello JM, Morishita M, Takayama K, *et al.*, *Int J Pharm* 184, 189 (1999).

- Berkland C, Kipper MJ, Narasimhan B, Kim K, Pack D. *J Cont Rel* 94, 129 (2004).

- Bittner B, Morlock M, Koll H, *et al.*, *Eur J Pharm Biopharm* 45, 295 (1998).

- Blanco-Prieto MJ, Campanero MA, Besseghir K, *et al.*, *J Cont Rel* 96, 437 (2004).

- Bodde HE, Brink IV, Koerten HK, *et al.*, *J Cont Rel* 1, 227 (1991).

- Borkx RD, Bisland SK, Gariepy J. *J Controlled Release* 78, 115 (2001).

- Bourke SL, Kohn J. *Adv Drug Del Rev* 55, 447 (2003).

- Carino GP, Jacob JS, Mathiowitz E. *J Cont Rel* 65, 261 (2000).

- Çelebi N, Alemdaroglu-Isbasar C, Degim Z, Erdogan D, Nacar A, Özogul C. The effects of EGF containing liposome formulations on burn wound healing: a histological study, Proceedings, European Conference on Drug Delivery and Pharmaceutical Technology. May 10-12, Sevilla, Spain (2004).

- Celebi N, Cilek A, Ocak F, Krisnada A. Preparation and characterization of microemulsion using lecithin as surfactants for oral administration of insulin, Pharmacy and Pharmaceutical Sciences World Congress. 61st International Congress of FIP,1-6 Sept 2001; Singapore, Abstracts, p.72.

- Celebi N, Erden N, Gönül B, *et al.*, *J Pharm Pharmacol* 46, 386 (1994).

- Celebi N, Türkyilmaz A, Gönül B, Alkan-Onyuksel H. In: Hincal A, Kas HS, Eds., Physical characterization and stability of a microemulsion for potential oral administration of a peptide, Biomedical Science and Technology, Recent Developments in the Pharmaceutical Sciences. Plenium Press, New York, 65 (1998).

- Celebi N, Türkyilmaz A, Gönül B, *et al.*, *J Cont Rel* 83, 197 (2002).

- Chia HH, Yang YY, Chung TS. *J Control Rel* 75, 11 (2001).

- Cilek A, Celebi N, Ocak F, Tay A. Oral absorption of recombinant insulin from microemulsion in rats, EUFEPS World Conference on Drug Absorption and Drug Delivery Benefiting from New Biology and Informatics. Copenhagen, Denmark, June 18-20, 2001; Proceedings. Abstracts, p. 81-82.

- Cilek A. Development of insulin containing microemulsion formulations and *in vivo* evaluations, Master Degree thesis, Gazi University, Faculty of Pharmacy, Department of Pharmaceutical Technology. Ankara, 2001.

- Cleland JL. Protein delivery from biodegradable microspheres, In: Sanders LM, Hendren RW. Eds., Protein Delivery: Physical Systems. Plenium Press, New York, 1, (1997).

- Cournarie F, Savelli MP, Bretez VRF, *et al.*, *Eur J Pharm Biopharm* 58, 477 (2004).

- Davis SS, Hardy JG, Fara JW. *Gut* 27, 886 (1986).

- Davis SS, Illum L, Tomlinson E. Delivery systems for peptide drugs. NATO ASI Series A. Life Sciences. Plenum Press, New York. 125 (1986).

- Degim IT, Ilbasmis S, Dundaroz R, *et al.*, *Pediatr Nephrol* 18, 1032 (2003).

- Degim T, Pugh WJ, Hadgraft J. *Int J Pharm* 167, 229 (1998).

- Degim Z, Çelebı N, Sayan H, *et al.*, *Amino Acids* 22, 187 (2002).

- Degim Z, Degim T, Acartürk F, Erdogan D, Özogul C, Köksal M. Rectal administration of insulin-chitosan formulations: an experimental study in rabbits, Proceedings, 30th Annual Meeting & Exposition of the Controlled Release Society. Scotland, United Kingdom (2003).

- Denton JB, Konishi Y, Scheraga HA. *Biochemistry* 21, 5155 (1982).

- Dogru ST, Calıs S, Oner F. *J Clin Pharm Ther* 25, 435 (2000).

- Doscherholmen A, Macmalion J, Ripley D. *J Lab clin Med* 78, 839 (1971).

- Eldridge JH, Hammond CJ, Meulbroek A, *et al.*, *J Controlled release* 11, 205 (1990).

- Fanning AS, Jameson BJ, Jesaitis LA. *J Biol Chem* 273, 29745 (1998).

- Fattal E, Couvreur P, Pecquet S. *Ann Pharm Fr* 60, 44 (2002).

- Fishbein I, Chorny M, Rabinovich L, *et al.*, *J Cont Rel* 65, 221 (2000).

- Gaidamakova EK, Backer MV, Backer JM. *J Controlled Release* 74, 314 (2001).

- Genta I, Perugini P, Pavanetto F, *et al.*, *J Cont Rel* 77, 287 (2001).

- Gesellchen PD, Santerre RF. Synthesis of peptides and proteins by chemical and biotechnological means, In: Lee VHL Ed., Peptide and Protein Drug Delivery. Marcel and Dekker Inc., New York, 57 (1991).

- Gonnela PA, Siminoski K, Ri A. *J Clin Invest* 50, 22 (1987).

- Gonzalez Barcena D, Kastin AJ, Miller MC. *Lancet* 2, 1126 (1975).

- Hans ML, Lowman AM. *Curr Opp Sol State and Mat Sci* 6, 319 (2002).

- Herr G, Wahl D, Kussweyyer W. *Ann Chir Gynaecol* 82, 99 (1993).

- Hıncal AA, Calıs S, Microsphere preparation by solvent evaporation method, In: Wise DL. Ed., Handbook of Pharmaceutical Controlled Release Technology. Marcel Dekker Inc., New York, 329 (2000).

- Humphrey MJ, Ringrose PS. *Drug Met Rev* 17, 283 (1986).

- Illum L, Fisher AN, Jabbal-Gill I. *Int J Pharm* 222, 109 (2001).

- Isbasar C, Degim Z, Çelebi N. Development and *in vitro* evaluation of chitosan gel and liposome formulation of EGF, Proceedings, 30th Annual Meeting & Exposition of the Controlled Release Society, Scotland. July 19-23, United Kingdom (2003).

- Janes KA, Fresneau MP, Marazuela A. *J Controlled Release* 73, 255 (2001).

- Jang HS, Kim HJ. Kim JM, Lee *et al.*, *Mol Ther* 9, 464 (2004).

- Johnson OL, Cleland JL, Lee HJ, *et al.*, *Nat Med* 2, 795 (1996).

- Kalia YN, Naik A, Garrison J, *et al.*, *Adv Drug Del Rev* 56, 619 (2004).

- Kamath KR, Park K. *Adv Drug Del Rev* 11, 984 (1993).

- Kari B. *Diabetes* 35, 217 (1986).

- Katakam M, Ravis WR, Banga AK. *J Cont Rel* 49, 21 (1997).

- Keljo DJ, Hamilton JR. *Am J Physiol* 244, G637 (1983).

- Khoo SM, Edwards GA, Porter CJH *et al.*, *J Pharm Sci* 90, 1599 (2001).

- Kim YJ, Choi S, Koh JJ, *et al.*, *Pharm Res* 18, 548 (2001).

- Kimura T *Pharm Int* 5, 75 (1984).

- Kimura T,Saishin I. 1818 – 1824. In: Encyclopedia of controlled drug delivery, Edith Marthiowitz. (Edn) John Wiley and Sons Inc. New York. 2, 739 , (1999).

- Kompella UB, Lee VHL. *Adv Drug Del Rev* 46, 211 (2001).

- kompella UB, Lee VHL. *Adv Drug Del Rev* 46, 211 (2001).

- Kompella UB,Lee VHL. *Adv Drug Del Rev* 46, 211 (2001).

- Kopeck J, Kopekova P, Minko T. *J Controlled Release* 74, 147 (2001).

- Krishnaiah YSR, Veer RV, Dinesh KB. *J Controlled Release* 77, 87 (2001).

- Lakshmi S, Katti DS, Laurencin CT. *Adv Drug Del Rev* 55, 467 (2003).

- Langkjaer J, Brange J, Grodsky GM, *et al.*, *J Cont Rel* 51, 47 (1998).

- Lavasanifar A, Samuel J, Kwon GS. *Adv Drug Del Rev* 54, 169 (2002).

- Leach JB, Schmidt CE. *Biomaterials* 26, 125 (2005).

- Lee VHL. Changing needs in drug delivery in the era of peptide and protein drugs, In: Lee HHL Ed., Peptide Protein Delivery. Macel and Dekker Inc., New York, 1 (1990).

- Leferve ME, Joel DD (1977). et al, *advanced drug delivery reviews* 47, 21 (2001).

- Lemoine D, Preat V. *J Cont Rel* 54, 15 (1998).

- Leoni L, Desai TA. *Adv Drug Del Rev* 56, 211 (2004).

- Liu X, Sun O, Wang H, Zhang L, Wang JY. *Biomaterials* 26, 109 (2005).

- Machay M. *Biotech Gen Eng Rev* 8, 251 (1990).

- Mackay M, Phillips J, Hastewell J. *Adv Drug Del Rev* 28, 253 (1997).

- Mackay M, Phillips J, Hastewell J. *Adv Drug Del Rev* 28, 253 (1997).

- Margreiter R. *Lancet* 359, 741 (2002).

- Matsuzawa A, Morishita M, Takayama K *et al.*, *Biol Pharm Bull* 18, 1718 (1995).

- Mehta RC, Jeyanthi R, Calıs S, *et al.*, *J Cont Rel* 29, 375 (1994).

- Mi FL, Shyu SS, Lin YM, Wu YB, Peng CK, Tsai HY. *Biomaterials* 24, 5023 (2003).

- Mitra S, Gaur U, Ghosh PC, Maitra A. *J Controlled Release* 74, 317 (2001).

- Mitragotri S, Kost J. *Adv Drug Del Rev* 56, 589 (2004).

- Morishita M, Matsuzawa A, Takayama K, *et al.*, *Int J Pharm* 172, 189 (1998).

- Muranishi S, Takada K, Hoshikawa H, Murakami M. Enhanced absorption and lymphatic transport of macromolecules via the rectal route. In Delivery system for Peptide drugs. Davis SS *et al* (Eds). Plenum Press. New York 177 (1987).

- Muranishi S, Yamamoto A. Mechnism of absorption enhancement through the gastrointestinal epithelium. In: Drug absorption enhancement. Taylor and Francis (Eds) 67 (1994).

- Okhamafe AO, Amsden B, Chu W, *et al.*, *J Microencapsulation* 13, 497 (1996).

- Okhamafe AO, Goosen MFA. Control of membrane permeability in Microcapsules. In; Fundamentals of animal cell encapsulation and immobilization. Goosen Mattheus (Edn) CRC Press, Inc. USA (1993).

- Okhamafe AO, Goosen MFA. Modulation of membrane permeability. In; Cell encapsulation technology and therapeutics. Goosen Mattheus (Edn) Birkhäuser Boston, USA. 53 (1999).

- Onuki Y, Morishita M, Takayama K, *et al.*, *Int J Pharm* 198, 147 (2000).

- Onuki Y, Morishita M, Takayama K. *J Cont Rel* 97, 91 (2004).

- Pastorino F, Stuart D, Ponzoni M. etal., *J Controlled Release* 14, 69 (2001).

- Pillai O, Nair V, Panchagnula R. *Int J Pharm* 269, 109 (2004).

- Pliquett UF, Gusbeth CA. *J Bioelectrochem* 51, 41 (2000).

- Pontiroli AE. *J Cont Rel* 13, 247 (1990).

- Prausnitz MR. *Adv Drug Del Rev* 56, 581 (2004).

- Pulapura S, Li C, Kohn J. *Biomaterials* 11, 666 (1990).

- Rathi RC, Zentner GM. US Patent 6.004.573, (1999).

- Ribeiroa CC, Barriasa CC, Barbosaa MA. *Biomaterials* 25, 4363 (2004).

- Sali A, Shakhnovic E, Karplus M. *J Mol Biol* 235, 1614 (1994).

- Santiago N, Milstein S, Rivera T, Garcia E, Zaidi T, Hong H, *et al.*, *Pharm Res* 10, 1243 (1993).

- Schachter DM, Kohn J. *J Cont Rel* 78, 143 (2002).

- Schatzlein AG, Rutherford C, Corrihons F, *et al.*, *J Controlled Release* 74, 357 (2001).

- Schwendeman SP. *Crit Rev Ther Drug Carrier Syst* 19, 73 (2002).

- Senel S, Kremer MJ, Kas S, *et al.*, *Biomaterials* 21, 2067 (2000).

- Shinji S, Suzuki N, Kikuchi H, Hiwatori K. *Int J Pharm* 149, 93 (1997).

- Silbart LK, Karen DF. *Science* 243, 1462 (1989).

- Sinha VR, Bansal K, Kaushik R, *et al.*, *Int J Pharm* 278, 1 (2004).

- Sinha VR, Singla AK, Wadhawan S, *et al.*, *Int J Pharm* 274, 1 (2004).

- Sinha VR, Trehan A. *J Cont Rel* 90, 261 (2003).

- Smith PL. *J Cont Rel* 46, 99 (1997).

- Stevenson BR, Keon BH. *Annu Rev Cell Dev Biol* 14, 89 (1998).

- Stubbe B, Martis B, Moonter GV. *J Controlled Release* 75, 103 (2001).

- Suzuki A, Morishita M, Kajita M, *et al.*, *J Pharm Sci* 87, 1196 (1998).

- Takenaga M, Yamaguchi Y, Kitagawa A, *et al.*, *J Cont Rel* 79, 81 (2002).

- Tobio M. *Colloids Surf B* 18, 315 (2000).

- Tollefsen S, Tjelle TE, Schneider J, *et al.*, *Vaccine* 20, 3370 (2002).

- Veronese FM, Marsilio F, Caliceti P, *et al.*, *J Cont Rel* 52, 227 (1998).

- Veuillez F, Kalia YN, Jacques Y, Deshusses J, Buri P. *Eur J Pharm Biopharm* 51, 93 (2001).
- Wathm N. *Gen Eng News* 14, 1 (1994).
- Watnasirichaikul S, Rades T, Tucker IG, *et al.*, *Int J Pharm* 235, 237 (2002).
- Weert M, Hennink WE, Jiskoot W. *Pharm Res* 17, 1159 (2000).
- Wenzel JGW, Balaji KSS, Koushik K, *et al.*, *J Cont Rel* 85, 51 (2002).
- Wheatley MA, Chang M, Park E, Langer R. *J Appl Pol Sci* 43, 2123 (1991).
- Wilson PJ, Basit AW. *Int J Pharmaceutics* 300, 89 (2005).
- Wright JC, Leonard ST, Stevenson CL. *et al.*, *J Cont Rel* 75, 1 (2001).
- Wua TJ, Huanga HH, Lana CW. *Biomaterials* 25, 651 (2004).
- Wyatt TL, Whaley KJ, Cone RA, *et al.*, *J Cont Rel* 50, 93 (1998).
- Yano H, Hirayama F, Kamada M. *J Controlled Release* 79, 103 (2002).
- Yeh MK. *J Microencapsul* 7, 743 (2000).
- Yeo Y, Basaran OA, Park K. *J Cont Rel* 93, 161 (2003).
- Yetkin G, Celebi N, Agabeyoglu I, Gökcora N. *STP Pharma Sciences* 9, 249 (1999).
- Yetkin G, Celebi N, Ozer C, *et al.*, *Int J Pharm* 277, 163 (2004).
- Yetkin G, Celebi N, Ozogul C, *et al.*, *STP Pharma Sciences* 11, 187 (2001).
- Yewey GL, Duysen EG, Cox SM, Dunn RL. In: Sanders LM, Hendren RW Eds., Delivery of proteins from a controlled release injectable implant. Protein Delivery: Physical Systems. Plenium Press, New York 93 (1997).
- Yokohama S, Yamashita K, Toguchi H. *J Pharm Dyn* 7, 101 (1984).
- Young L, Jernigan RL, Covell DG. *Protein Science* 3, 717 (1994).
- Zentner GM, Rathi R, Shih C, *et al.*, *J Cont Rel* 72, 203 (2002).
- Zhang X, Wu D, Chu CC. *Biomaterials* 25, 4719 (2004).
- Zhou S, Deng X, He S, *et al.*, *J Pharm Pharmacol* 54, 1287 (2002).

INDEX

Reader's Note

Reader's Note